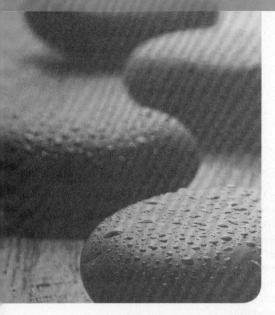

Essentials of Psychiatric Nursing

Mary Ann Boyd, PhD, DNS, RN, PMHCNS-BC

Professor Emerita
Southern Illinois University Edwardsville
Edwardsville, Illinois

Clinical Faculty
St. Louis University
St. Louis, Missouri

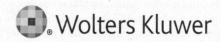
. Wolters Kluwer

Philadelphia • Baltimore • New York • London
Buenos Aires • Hong Kong • Sydney • Tokyo

Publisher: Julie Stegman
Acquisitions Editor: Natasha McIntyre
Marketing Manager: Todd McQueston
Product Development Editor: Meredith Brittain
Editorial Assistant: Dan Reilly
Production Project Manager: Cynthia Rudy
Design Coordinator: Terry Mallon
Illustration Coordinator: Jennifer Clements
Manufacturing Coordinator: Karin Duffield
Prepress Vendor: Aptara, Inc.

9 8 7 6 5 4 3 2 1

Printed in China

Library of Congress Cataloging-in-Publication Data

Boyd, M. (Mary Ann), author.
 Essentials of psychiatric nursing : contemporary practice/Mary Ann Boyd.
    p. ; cm.
 Includes bibliographical references and index.
  ISBN 978-1-4963-3214-1 (paperback)
 I. Title.
 [DNLM: 1. Mental Disorders–nursing.   2. Psychiatric Nursing–methods.
WY 160]
 RC440
 616.89'0231–dc23

                                                    2015035020

LWW.com

To Jason, Andrea, and Lisa with love and pride.

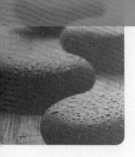

Contributors

CONTRIBUTORS TO *ESSENTIALS OF PSYCHIATRIC NURSING*

Beverly Baliko, PhD, RN
Associate Professor
College of Nursing
University of South Carolina
Columbia, South Carolina
Chapter 30: Mental Health Care for Survivors of Violence

Andrea C. Bostrom, PhD, PMHCNS-BC
Professor
Kirkhof College of Nursing
Grand Valley State University
Grand Rapids, Michigan
Chapter 21: Schizophrenia and Related Disorders

Mary R. Boyd, PhD, RN
Associate Professor
College of Nursing
University of South Carolina
Columbia, South Carolina
Chapter 30: Mental Health Care for Survivors of Violence

Stephanie Burgess, PhD, APRN, FNP-BC
Associate Dean for Nursing Practice & Clinical
  Professor
College of Nursing
University of South Carolina
Columbia, South Carolina
Chapter 30: Mental Health Care for Survivors of Violence

Sheri Compton-McBride, MS, RN
Director of Clinical Acquisitions and Instructor
School of Nursing
Southern Illinois University Edwardsville
Edwardsville, Illinois
Chapter 26: Sleep–Wake Disorders

Judith M. Erickson, PhD, PMHCNS-BC
Dean
Harriet Rothkopf Heilbrunn School of Nursing
Long Island University
Long Island, New York
Chapter 16: Anxiety and Panic Disorders

Cheryl Forchuk, RN, PhD
Associate Director of Nursing Research
University of Western Ontario
Lawson Health Research Institute
Arthur Labatt Family School of Nursing and
  Department of Psychiatry
London, Ontario
Chapter 8: The Nurse-Patient Relationship

Kimberlee Hansen, RN, MS, NP
Nurse Practitioner
Jefferson Barracks Division
VA St. Louis Health Care System
St. Louis, Missouri
Chapter 22: Personality and Impulse-Control Disorders

Emily J. Hauenstein, PhD, LCP, MSN, RN
Unidel Katherine L. Esterly Chair in Health Sciences and
  Senior Associate Dean of Nursing & Healthcare
College of Health Sciences
University of Delaware
Newark, Delaware
Chapter 15: Suicide Prevention

Victoria Soltis-Jarrett, PhD, PMHCNS-BC,
  PMHNP-BC
Associate Clinical Professor and Coordinator of the
  PMHNP Program
University of North Carolina at Chapel Hill
Chapel Hill, North Carolina
Chapter 23: Somatic Symptom and Dissociative Disorders

Sandra P. Thomas, PhD, RN, FAAN
Professor and Chair, PhD Program in Nursing
University of Tennessee
Knoxville, Tennessee
Chapter 13: Management of Anger, Aggression, and
    Violence

Barbara Jones Warren, PhD, RN, CNS-BC, PMH,
    FAAN
Professor, Clinical Nursing
Specialty Director, Psychiatric and Mental Health
    Nursing
National Institutes of Health/American Nurses
    Association Ethnic/Racial Minority Fellow
The Ohio State College of Nursing
Columbus, Ohio
Chapter 19: Depression

Jane H. White, PhD, PMH-CNS, BC
Vera E. Bender Professor of Nursing and Associate
    Dean for Research and Graduate Programs
School of Nursing
Adelphi University
Garden City, New York
Chapter 24: Eating Disorders

CONTRIBUTORS TO *PSYCHIATRIC NURSING: CONTEMPORARY PRACTICE, 5TH EDITION ENHANCED UPDATE*

Beverly Baliko, PhD, RN
Associate Professor
College of Nursing
University of South Carolina
Columbia, South Carolina
Chapter 40: Caring for Survivors of Violence

Ann R. Bland, PhD, PMHCNS/NP-BC
Admissions Nurse
Holly Hill Hospital
Raleigh, North Carolina
Chapter 27: Borderline Personality Disorder

Andrea C. Bostrom, PhD, PMHCNS-BC
Professor
Kirkhof College of Nursing
Grand Valley State University
Grand Rapids, Michigan
Chapter 22: Schizophrenia

Mary R. Boyd, PhD, RN
Associate Professor
College of Nursing
University of South Carolina
Columbia, South Carolina
Chapter 40: Caring for Survivors of Violence

Stephanie Burgess, PhD, APRN, FNP-BC
Associate Dean for Nursing Practice & Clinical
    Professor
College of Nursing
University of South Carolina
Columbia, South Carolina
Chapter 40: Caring for Survivors of Violence

Jeanne A. Clement, EdD, PMHCNS-BC, FAAN
Associate Professor Emeritus
College of Nursing
The Ohio State University
Columbus, Ohio
Chapter 12: Cognitive Interventions in Psychiatric
    Nursing

Sheri Compton-McBride, MS, RN
Director of Clinical Acquisitions and Instructor
School of Nursing
Southern Illinois University Edwardsville
Edwardsville, Illinois
Chapter 32: Sleep–Wake Disorders

Catherine Gray Deering, PhD, APRN, BC
Professor
Clayton State University
Morrow, Georgia
Chapter 15: Mental Health Promotion for Children and
    Adolescents
Chapter 34: Mental Health Assessment of Children and
    Adolescents

Peggy El-Mallakh, PhD, RN
Assistant Professor
College of Nursing
University of Kentucky
Lexington, Kentucky
Chapter 5: Mental Health Care in the Community

Judith M. Erickson, PhD, PMHCNS-BC
Dean
Harriet Rothkopf Heilbrunn School of Nursing
Long Island University
Long Island, New York
Chapter 26: Anxiety, Obsessive-Compulsive, Trauma,
    and Stressor-Related Disorders

Cheryl Forchuk, RN, PhD
Associate Director of Nursing Research
University of Western Ontario
Lawson Health Research Institute
Arthur Labatt Family School of Nursing and
    Department of Psychiatry
London, Ontario
Chapter 9: Communication and the Therapeutic
    Relationship

Vanya Hamrin, RN, MSN, APRN, BC
Associate Professor
School of Nursing
Vanderbilt University
Nashville, Tennessee
Chapter 34: Mental Health Assessment of Children and
    Adolescents

Kimberlee Hansen, RN, MS, NP
Nurse Practitioner
Jefferson Barracks Division
VA St. Louis Health Care System
St. Louis, Missouri
Chapter 28: Antisocial Personality and Other
    Personality and Impulse-Control Disorders

Emily J. Hauenstein, PhD, LCP, MSN, RN
Unidel Katherine L. Esterly Chair in Health Sciences
    and
Senior Associate Dean of Nursing & Healthcare
College of Health Sciences
University of Delaware
Newark, Delaware
Chapter 21: Suicide Prevention

Peggy Healy, MSN, RN-BC, PMHN
Program Manager, Mental Health Clinic
VA St. Louis Health Care System
St. Louis, Missouri
Chapter 36: Mental Health Assessment of Older Adults

Gail L. Kongable, RN, MSN, FNP
Nurse Practitioner, Family Medicine of Albemarle
University of Virginia
Charlottesville, Virginia
Chapter 42: Caring for Medically Compromised
    Persons

**Ruth Beckmann Murray, EdD, MSN, RN, N-NAP,
    FAAN**
Professor Emerita
Doisy College of Health Sciences, School of Nursing
St. Louis University
St. Louis, Missouri
Chapter 38: Caring for Persons Who Are Homeless and
    Mentally Ill

Nan Roberts, MSN, PMHCNS-BC
Advanced Practice Nurse
St. Charles, Missouri
Chapter 23: Schizoaffective, Delusional, and Other
    Psychotic Disorders

**Victoria Soltis-Jarrett, PhD, PMHCNS-BC,
    PMHNP-BC**
Associate Clinical Professor and Coordinator of the
    PMHNP Program
University of North Carolina at Chapel Hill
Chapel Hill, North Carolina
Chapter 29: Somatic Symptom and Related Disorders

Georgia L. Stevens, PhD, APRN, PMHCNS-BC
Director
P.A.L. Associates
Partners in Aging and Long-Term Caregiving
Washington, D.C.
Chapter 17: Mental Health Promotion for Older Adults

Roberta Stock, MSN, PMHCNS-BC
Advanced Practice Nurse
Community Treatment, Inc.
Jefferson County Missouri Community Mental Health
    Centers
Crystal City, Missouri
Chapter 23: Schizoaffective, Delusional, and Other
    Psychotic Disorders

Sandra P. Thomas, PhD, RN, FAAN
Professor and Chair, PhD Program in Nursing
University of Tennessee
Knoxville, Tennessee
Chapter 19: Management of Anger, Aggression, and
    Violence

**Barbara Jones Warren, PhD, RN, CNS-BC, PMH,
    FAAN**
Professor, Clinical Nursing
Specialty Director, Psychiatric and Mental Health
    Nursing
National Institutes of Health/American Nurses
    Association Ethnic/Racial Minority Fellow
The Ohio State College of Nursing
Columbus, Ohio
Chapter 24: Depression

Jane H. White, PhD, PMH-CNS, BC
Vera E. Bender Professor of Nursing and Associate
    Dean for Research and Graduate Programs
School of Nursing
Adelphi University
Garden City, New York
Chapter 30: Eating Disorders

Deborah McNeil Whitehouse, DSN, APRN, BC
Dean
College of Health Sciences
Eastern Kentucky University
Richmond, Kentucky
Chapter 27: Borderline Personality Disorder

Rhonda K. Wilson, MS
Quality Manager
Chester Mental Health Center
Chester, Illinois
Chapter 41: Caring for Persons With Mental Illness
and Criminal Behavior

Richard Yakimo, PhD, PMHCNS-BC, N-NAP
Assistant Professor
University of Missouri—St. Louis
College of Nursing
St. Louis, Missouri
Chapter 16: Mental Health Promotion for Young and
    Middle-Aged Adults
Chapter 38: Caring for Persons Who Are Homeless and
    Mentally Ill

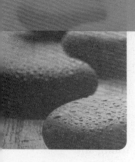

Reviewers

Kim Siarkowski Amer, PhD, RN
Associate Professor
School of Nursing
DePaul University
Chicago, Illinois

Catherine Batscha, DNP, PMHNP-BC,
  PMHCNS-BC
Assistant Professor
University of Louisville
Louisville, Kentucky

Lorraine Buchanan, MSN, RN
Clinical Assistant Professor
School of Nursing
University of Kansas
Kansas City, Kansas

Sheila J. Capp, PhD, RN
Professor of Nursing
Blessing-Rieman College of Nursing
Quincy, Illinois

Ellen Condron, MSN, BSN
Associate Professor of Nursing
Fairmont State University
Coordinator, Nursing of Children
Fairmont, West Virginia

Kim Cooper, MSN, RN
Dean, School of Nursing
Ivy Tech Community College
Terre Haute, Indiana

Flor A. Culpa-Bondal, PhD, RN, CNS/PMH-BC
Associate Professor
School of Nursing
College of Health Sciences
Georgia College and State University
Milledgeville, Georgia

Susanne Duelm, RN, BA
Faculty II
Baptist Health System
School of Health Professions
San Antonio, Texas

Judy Glaser, DNP, RN, PMHCNS-BC, PMHNP-BC
Assistant Professor
PMHNP Program Track Coordinator
Georgia Regents University
College of Nursing, Athens
Athens, Georgia

Betsy D. Gulledge, PhD, RN, CNE, NEA-BC
Associate Dean of Nursing/Assistant Professor
Jacksonville State University
Jacksonville, Alabama

Cynthia A. Hoppe, DNS, RN
Professor of Nursing
Delgado Community College
Charity School of Nursing
New Orleans, Louisiana

Alton McLendon, MSN, BSN, RN
Interim Chair of Nursing
Georgia Perimeter College
Clarkston, Georgia

Elizabeth Mcquinn, MSN, PMHCNS-BC
Psychiatric Clinical Nurse Specialist
Noblesville, Indiana

Cheryl L. Miller, EdD, MSN, RN
Professor of Nursing
Chattanooga State Community College
Chattanooga, Tennessee

Cynthia K. Neff, MSN, RN
Professor
Allegany College of Maryland
Cumberland, Maryland

Shelley Rayborn, MSN, PHN, RN
Evening/Weekend Program Coordinator
Associate Degree Nursing Program
St. Catherine University
Minneapolis, Minnesota

Donna F. Rye, MSN, RN
Assistant Professor
Cox College
Springfield, Missouri

Janene Luther Szpak, DNP, PMHNP-BC
Associate Professor
Robert Morris University
School of Nursing and Health Sciences
Moon Township, Pennsylvania

Laureen M. Tavolaro-Ryley, MSN, RN, CNS
Independence Foundation Chair in Nursing
Community College of Philadelphia
Philadelphia, Pennsylvania

Arlene Trolman, EdD, MEd, MS, BS, RN
Associate Professor
Adelphi University
College of Nursing and Public Health
Garden City, New York

Laura Pruitt Walker, DHEd, MSN, RN, COI
Assistant Professor
Jacksonville State University College of Nursing
Jacksonville, Alabama

K. Russell Walker, MSN, RN
Assistant Professor of Nursing
MacMurray College
Jacksonville, Illinois

Alexandra Winter, EdD, MSN, RN
Nursing Faculty
Metropolitan Community College
Omaha, Nebraska

Amy Yeates, DNP, MS, BSN
Visiting Instructor
Illinois Wesleyan University
Bloomington, Illinois

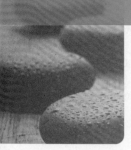

Preface

Mental health care is no longer segregated to long-term care facilities or acute psychiatric facilities. Psychiatric-mental health nursing knowledge and skills are integral to nursing practice. Mental health care is integrated into mainstream health care and is delivered in all settings. Today the practicing nurse is required to have an extensive understanding of mental health disorders and the impact of the illness and treatment on the quality of life of the individual and family. Recovery from mental illness is a journey involving a partnership between health care professionals and the person with a mental health disorder. This individual not only needs support and treatment to recover from a serious disorder but also help in eradicating the stigma associated with a mental illness.

Essentials of Psychiatric Nursing provides students with the evidence-based knowledge to develop recovery-oriented nursing interventions with the person with mental illness. Nursing curricula emphasize different aspects of the underlying body of knowledge. Some nursing programs teach psychiatric nursing content in the beginning of the curriculum with an emphasis on basic communication skills and an overview of mental health disorders. Other programs emphasize mental health more than mental disorders. And many programs focus on the nursing care of persons with mental disorders. *Essentials of Psychiatric Nursing* was developed to meet the needs of programs that primarily emphasize communication skills, mental health promotion, and current, evidence-based, recovery-oriented nursing care of persons with common mental health disorders.

The text presents complex concepts in easy-to-understand language with multiple examples and explanations. The text is filled with meaningful information and is applicable to all areas of nursing practice.

Pedagogical features in the book, including NCLEX Notes, Critical Thinking Questions, Fame & Fortune highlights, and summaries of entertainment videos, as well as Nursing Care Plans available online at http://thepoint .lww.com/BoydEssentials, offer opportunities for students to challenge the stigma associated with mental disorders. Case studies are central to the mental disorders discussions and provide students with the opportunity to link real-life experiences to theoretical concepts.

Our goal is to prepare nursing leaders who challenge the status quo, partner with their patients in the delivery of care, and use the latest evidence in their nursing practice.

Text Organization

Unit I, Essentials of Mental Health Care, discusses mental health and mental disorders as they relate to the concept of wellness. In Chapter 1, students will learn about the concepts of stigma and recovery. Chapter 2 discusses cultural and spiritual issues, and Chapter 3 covers patient rights and legal issues. Unit II, Psychiatric-Mental Health Nursing Frameworks, provides a foundation for beginning practice with an explanation of ethics, standards, and nursing in Chapter 4; the theoretical foundation in Chapter 5; and the biologic foundations in Chapter 6.

Unit III, Knowledge and Skills of Psychiatric-Mental Health Nursing, contains two communication chapters: Chapter 7, which focuses on therapeutic communication, and Chapter 8, which discusses the nurse-patient relationship. In addition, in this unit students will learn about psychiatric-mental health nursing assessment with a brief overview of typical nursing interventions in Chapter 9, pharmacology and other biologic interventions in Chapter 10, and group interventions in Chapter 11.

The chapters in Unit IV, Prevention of Mental Disorders, are not specific to persons with mental disorders. Content in this unit is applicable to all nursing practice settings. This unit presents a model of stress that is supported by strong evidence and that can be applied to all areas of nursing. Chapter 13 explains how to understand and manage angry and aggressive patients. Content in the other chapters in this unit, including crisis intervention (Chapter 14) and suicide prevention (Chapter 15), are also applicable to care of persons with or without mental disorders.

The bulk of the content related to mental disorders is found in Unit V, Care and Recovery for Persons with Mental Health Disorders, which consists of 12 chapters

(Chapters 16 through 27). Each chapter defines a mental disorder(s) according to the *Diagnostic and Statistical Manual of Mental Disorders*, Fifth Edition *DSM-5*, and identifies key nursing assessment and intervention strategies to promote recovery of persons with mental illness. Case studies are threaded throughout each chapter to demonstrate, in easy-to-understand language, the concepts being discussed. Students have the opportunity to access videos that demonstrate nurses interacting with persons with the disorder.

Unit VI, Care of Special Populations, consists of three chapters discussing mental health needs of special populations. Chapter 28 focuses on the mental disorders of children, and Chapter 29 is about the neurocognitive disorders of older adults. Chapter 30 comprehensively covers care of persons who are victims of violence.

Pedagogical Features

Essentials of Psychiatric Nursing incorporates a multitude of pedagogical features to focus and direct student learning:

- **Expanded Table of Contents** allows readers to find and refer to concepts from one location.
- **Learning Objectives, Key Terms,** and **Key Concepts** in the chapter openers cue readers on what will be encountered and what is important to understand in each chapter.
- **Summary of Key Points** lists at the end of each chapter provide quick access to important chapter content to facilitate study and review.
- **Critical Thinking Challenges** ask questions that require students to think critically about chapter content and apply psychiatric nursing concepts to nursing practice.
- **Movies** list current examples of movies that depict various mental health disorders and that are widely available on DVD for rent or purchase. Viewing points are provided to serve as a basis for discussion in class and among students.

Special Features

- **NCLEX Notes** help students focus on important application areas to prepare for the NCLEX.
- **Case Studies** are threaded throughout the Unit V disorder chapters. Each chapter begins with a case study that is highlighted throughout the chapter. This case study is used as the prototype in the Nursing Care Plan (at http://thepoint.lww.com/Boyd Essentials) and the Therapeutic Interaction. A link to this same case study on thePoint, is provided for students to view via video the symptoms and the nursing care for a patient with a specific disorder.

- **Emergency Care Alerts** highlight important situations in psychiatric nursing care that the nurse should recognize as emergencies.
- **Fame and Fortune** features highlight famous people who have made important contributions to society despite dealing with mental health problems. In many instances, the public remained unaware of these disorders. The feature emphasizes that mental disorders can happen to anyone and that people with mental health problems can be productive members of society.
- **Diagrams, illustrations, and photos** colorfully illustrate the interrelationship of the biologic, psychological, and social domains of mental health and illness.
- **Nursing Management of Selected Disorders** sections provide an in-depth study of the more commonly occurring major psychiatric disorders.
- **Nursing Care Plans,** based on case scenarios and available at http://thepoint.lww.com/BoydEssentials, present clinical examples of patients with a particular diagnosis and demonstrate plans of care that follow patients through various diagnostic stages and care delivery settings.
- **Research for Best Practice** boxes highlight today's focus on evidence-based practice for *best practice*, presenting findings and implications of studies that are applicable to psychiatric nursing practice.
- **Therapeutic Dialogue** boxes compare and contrast therapeutic and nontherapeutic conversations to encourage students by example to develop effective communication skills.
- **Psychoeducation Checklists** identify content areas for patient and family education related to specific disorders and their treatment. These checklists support critical thinking by encouraging students to develop patient-specific teaching plans based on chapter content.
- **Clinical Vignette** boxes present reality-based clinical portraits of patients who exhibit the symptoms described in the text. Questions are posed to help students express their thoughts and identify solutions to issues presented in the vignettes.
- **Drug Profile** boxes present a thorough picture of commonly prescribed medications for patients with mental health problems. Examples include lorazepam (Ativan), an anxiolytic, and mirtazapine (Remeron), an antidepressant. The profiles complement the text discussions of biologic processes known to be associated with various mental health disorders.
- **Key Diagnostic Characteristics** summaries describe diagnostic criteria, target symptoms, and associated findings for select disorders, described in the *DSM-5* by the American Psychiatric Association.

- **Patient education**, **family**, and **emergency icons** highlight content related to these topics to help link concepts to practice.

Teaching/Learning Package

To facilitate mastery of this text's content, a comprehensive teaching and learning package has been developed to assist faculty and students.

- Lippincott CoursePoint: **Lippincott CoursePoint is a comprehensive, digital, integrated course solution for nursing education.** Lippincott CoursePoint is designed for the way students learn, providing content in context, exactly where and when students need it. Lippincott CoursePoint is an integrated learning solution featuring:
  - Leading content in context: Content provided in the context of the student learning path engages students and encourages interaction and learning on a deeper level.
    - The interactive ebook features content updates based on the latest evidence-based practices and provides students with anytime, anywhere access on multiple devices.
    - Multimedia resources, including videos, animations, and interactive tutorials, walk students through knowledge application and address multiple learning styles.
    - Full online access to *Stedman's Medical Dictionary for Health Professions and Nursing* ensures students work with the best medical dictionary available.
  - Powerful tools to maximize class performance: Course-specific tools, such as adaptive learning powered by *prepU*, provide a personalized learning experience for every student.
  - Real-time data to measure students' progress: Student performance data provided in an intuitive display lets instructors quickly spot which students are having difficulty or which concepts the class as a whole is struggling to grasp.
- prepU: **Adaptive Learning | Powered by prepU is an adaptive learning system that helps every student learn more, while giving instructors the data they need to monitor each student's progress, strengths, and weaknesses.** This tool is such a value to students because they learn and retain course material in an adaptive learning environment catered to their individual needs. It helps students focus their study time much more effectively, as they are focused on practicing what they don't know, instead of spending time on the concepts they already understand. And instructors are able to better evaluate student comprehension and differentiate instruction, and can identify common misunderstandings in realtime and correct them.

Instructor Resources

Tools to assist you with teaching your course are available upon adoption of this text at http://thepoint.lww.com/BoydEssentials.

- The **Test Generator** lets you put together exclusive new tests from a bank containing hundreds of questions to help you in assessing your students' understanding of the material. Test questions correspond to chapter learning objectives.
- A sample **Syllabus** provides guidance for structuring your course.
- **Learning Management System cartridges.**
- An **ebook** allows access to the book's full text and images online.
- **Strategies for Effective Teaching** offer creative approaches.
- **Access to All Student Resources** is also provided.
- An extensive collection of materials is provided for each book chapter:
  - **Pre-Lecture Quizzes** (and answers) are quick, knowledge-based assessments that allow you to check students' reading.
  - **PowerPoint Presentations** provide an easy way for you to integrate the textbook with your students' classroom experience, either via slide shows or handouts. Multiple-choice and true/false questions are integrated into the presentations to promote class participation and allow you to use i-clicker technology.
  - **Guided Lecture Notes** walk you through the chapters, objective by objective, and provide you with corresponding PowerPoint slide numbers.
  - **Discussion Topics** (and suggested answers) can be used as conversation starters or in online discussion boards.
  - **Assignments** (and suggested answers) include group, written, clinical, and Web assignments.
  - **Case Studies** with related questions (and suggested answers) give students an opportunity to apply their knowledge to a client case similar to one they might encounter in practice.
  - An **Image Bank** lets you use the photographs and illustrations from this textbook in your PowerPoint slides or as you see fit in your course.

Student Resources

An exciting set of free resources is available to help students review and apply important concepts. Students can access these resources at http://thepoint.lww.com/BoydEssentials using the codes printed in the front of their textbooks.

- **NCLEX-Style Review Questions** for each chapter help students review important concepts and practice for the NCLEX.
- **Watch & Learn Videos:**
  - **Online video series**, *Lippincott Theory to Practice Video Series: Psychiatric–Mental Health Nursing*, includes videos of true-to-life patients displaying mental health disorders, allowing students to gain experience and a deeper understanding of mental health patients. The video series allows viewing of complete patient interviews and also gives the opportunity to view snippets of those interviews, for closer analysis or classroom discussion. The innovative videos explore topics such as Depression, Eating Disorders, and Addiction.
  - A **Watch & Learn Video Clip** on cognitive functions is included from *Lippincott Video Guide to Psychiatric–Mental Health Nursing Assessment*.
- **Practice & Learn Activities:**
  - Most of these activities relate to the *Lippincott Theory to Practice Video Series: Psychiatric–Mental Health Nursing videos* mentioned above. Each activity presents a recap of the case followed by suggested background readings, related learning objectives, insights into the patient's thinking, and discussion questions.
  - Other case studies, from *Lippincott Interactive Case Studies in Psychiatric–Mental Health Nursing*, relate to therapeutic communication, antidepressants, and dementia.

- **MOVIE viewing GUIDES** highlight films depicting individuals with mental health disorders and provide students the opportunity to approach nursing care related to mental health and illness in a novel way.
- **Clinical Simulations** on schizophrenia, depression, and the acutely manic phase walk students through case studies and put them in real-life situations.
- **Journal Articles** provided for each chapter offer access to current research available in Wolters Kluwer journals.
- In addition, as indicated in the table of contents and in the appropriate places in the book, the following are found on the book's companion website at http://thepoint.lww.com/BoydEssentials: **Chapter 27** (Sexual Disorders: Nursing Care of Persons with Sexual Dysfunction), **Chapter 30** (Mental Health Care for Survivors of Violence), **Appendix A** (Brief Psychiatric Rating Scale), **Appendix B** (Abnormal Involuntary Movement Scale (AIMS)), **Appendix C** (Simplified Diagnosis for Tardive Dyskinesia (SD-TD), and the **glossary**.
- Plus a **Spanish-English audio glossary, Lippincott Nursing Drug Handbook App, Nursing Professional Roles and Responsibilities, Heart and Breath Sounds, and Learning Objectives** from the textbook.

Mary Ann Boyd, PhD, DNS, RN, PMHCNS-BC

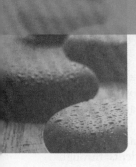

Acknowledgments

This text is a result of many long hours of diligent work by the contributors, editors, and assistants. Psychiatric nurses are constantly writing about and discussing new strategies for caring for persons with mental disorders. Consumers of mental health services provide directions for nursing care and validate the importance of nursing interventions. I wish to acknowledge and thank these individuals.

Natasha McIntyre, Matt Hauber, Meredith Brittain, Christine Abshire, Cindy Rudy, and Loftin Montgomery of Wolters Kluwer, as well as Karan Singh Rana of Aptara, were extraordinary partners in this project during the development of this text. I want to especially acknowledge their attention to detail and commitment to the completion of this edition. They provided direction, support, and valuable input throughout this project.

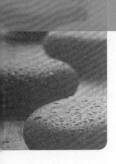

Contents

Chapter 27 is available at http://thepoint.lww.com/BoydEssentials and in the CoursePoint ebook.

Chapter 30 is available at http://thepoint.lww.com/BoydEssentials
and in the CoursePoint ebook.

Appendices A, B, C, and the Glossary are available at http://
thepoint.lww.com/BoydEssentials and in the CoursePoint ebook.

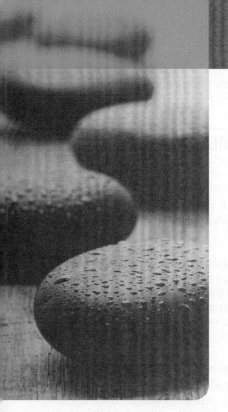

1

Mental Health and Mental Disorders

Fighting Stigma and Promoting Recovery

Mary Ann Boyd

KEY CONCEPTS

- mental health
- mental disorders
- stigma
- recovery
- wellness

LEARNING OBJECTIVES

After studying this chapter, you will be able to:

1. Relate the concept of mental health to wellness.

2. Identify the rationale for promoting wellness for people with mental health challenges.

3. Differentiate the concepts of mental health and mental illness.

4. Discuss the significance of epidemiological evidence in studying the occurrence of mental disorders.

5. Describe the consequences of the stigma of mental illness on individuals and families.

6. Identify recovery components and their role in the treatment of mental illness.

KEY TERMS

- cultural syndrome • DSM-5 • epidemiology • incidence • label avoidance • mental disorder • mental health • point prevalence • prevalence • public stigma • rate • self-stigma • social change • syndrome

To understand health and illness in any practice area, nurses need a basic understanding of mental health and its relationship with wellness. This chapter discusses concepts of mental health and wellness, the diagnosis of mental disorders, how the stigma of mental illness can be a barrier to treatment, and the importance of focusing on recovery from mental illness.

MENTAL HEALTH AND WELLNESS

Mental health is conceptualized by the World Health Organization (WHO) as a state of well-being in which the individual realizes his or her own abilities, can cope with life's normal stresses, can work productively and fruitfully and can make a contribution to society.

A person cannot be healthy without being "mentally" healthy, but it is possible to be mentally healthy and have a mental or physical disorder (World Health Organization [WHO], 2013a). Mental health is essential to personal well-being, interpersonal relationships, and contributing to the community.

> **KEYCONCEPT**   **Mental health** is the emotional and psychological well-being of an individual who has the capacity to interact with others, deal with ordinary stress, and perceive one's surroundings realistically (adapted from American Nurses Association, American Psychiatric Nurses Association, International Society of Psychiatric–Mental Health Nurses, 2014).

Related to the concept of mental health, wellness is defined as a "purposeful process of individual growth, integration of experience, and meaningful connection with others, reflecting personally valued goals and strengths and resulting in being well and living values" (McMahon & Fleury, 2012). Wellness involves having a purpose in life, being actively involved in satisfying work and play, having joyful relationships, having a healthy body and living environment, and being happy (U.S. Department of Health and Human Services, Substance Abuse & Mental Health Services Administration [U.S. DHHS, SAMHSA], 2010) (see Fig. 1.1). Mental health problems significantly impact the process of wellness: Many people with mental health problems die decades earlier than the general public from preventable diseases (Schuffman, Druss, & Parks, 2009; Whiteford et al., 2013). Poverty, unemployment, underemployment, trauma, and lack of education, common in people who have mental health issues, often prevent the achievement of wellness (U.S. DHHS, SAMHSA, 2010).

OVERVIEW OF MENTAL HEALTH DISORDERS

Mental disorders can disrupt mental health and result in one of the most common causes of disability. In this text, the terms "mental disorder" and "mental illness" will be used interchangeably.

> **KEYCONCEPT**   **Mental disorders** are clinically significant disturbances in cognition, emotion regulation, or behavior that reflect a dysfunction in the psychological, biological, or developmental processes underlying mental dysfunction. They are usually associated with distress or impaired functioning (American Psychiatric Association [APA], 2013).

A mental illness or mental disorder is a **syndrome,** a set of symptoms that cluster together that may have multiple causes and may represent several different disease states that have not yet been defined. Unlike many medical diseases, mental disorders are defined by clusters of behaviors, thoughts, and feelings, not underlying biologic pathology. Laboratory tests are not generally used in diagnosing mental disorders.

The landmark study *Global Burden of Disease 2010* found an alarming impact of mental and behavioral disorders on health and productivity in the world. Depression is one of the leading disease burdens in middle- and high-income countries such as the United States. By 2030, depression is projected to be the leading burden worldwide (WHO, 2013b). In the United States, 1 in 4 adults, or 57.7 million people, has a diagnosable mental disorder in any given year (National Institute of Mental Health, 2013).

Evidence for this very high occurrence of mental disorders is established through epidemiological research. **Epidemiology,** the study of patterns of disease distribution and determinants of health within populations, contributes to the overall understanding of the mental health status of population groups, or aggregates, and associated factors. Epidemiological studies examine associations among possible factors related to an area of investigation, but they do not determine causes of illnesses. The Centers for Disease Control and Prevention (CDC) tracks and reports mental health epidemiological data. Throughout this book, epidemiological data are included in discussions of mental health problems and mental disorders. See Box 1.1 for an explanation of terms.

Diagnosis of Mental Health Conditions

Mental disorders are organized and diagnosed according to the criteria published in the *Diagnostic and Statistical*

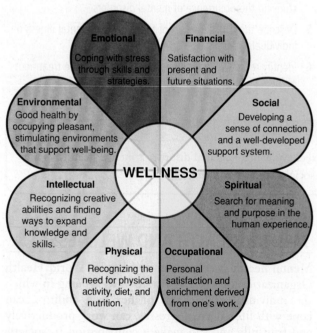

FIGURE 1.1 Eight dimensions of wellness. Adapted from Swarbrick, M. (2006). A wellness approach. *Psychiatric Rehabilitation Journal, 29*(4), 311–314. (U.S. DHHS, SAMHSA, 2010)

Disability Assessment Schedule 2.0 is an instrument that can be used for measuring the amount of impairment that the individual experiences.

Some disorders are influenced by cultural factors (see Chapter 2), and others are considered cultural syndromes that represent a specific pattern of symptoms that occur within a specific cultural group or community (APA, 2013). There is little research that reliably describes cultural syndromes, but there are two conditions, *ataque de nervios* and *susto*, that are frequently reported in small number of persons (Razzouk, Nogueira, & Mari Jde, 2011) (Box 1.2).

Stigma

Stigma, one of major treatment barriers facing individuals with mental health problems and their families, was highlighted in the President's New Freedom Commission on Mental Health *Report* in 2003. People with mental health symptoms have been stoned to death, hanged, and publicly humiliated. Stigma leads to community misunderstanding, prejudice, and discrimination.

> **KEYCONCEPT** **Stigma** can be defined as a mark of shame, disgrace, or disapproval that results in an individual being shunned or rejected by others. Public stigma, self-stigma, and label avoidance are three types of stigma people with mental illnesses experience.

Public Stigma

Public stigma occurs after individuals are publicly "marked" as being mentally ill. When individuals with mental illness act or say things that are odd or unusual or tell others that they have a mental illness, they are at risk of being publicly identified as having a mental illness and are subject to prejudice and discrimination. Common stereotypes include being dangerous, unpredictable,

Manual of Mental Disorders–5 (*DSM-5;* APA, 2013). The current *DSM-5* system contains subtypes and other specifiers that further classify disorders. Although the *DSM-5* specifies criteria for diagnosing mental disorders, there are no absolute boundaries separating one disorder from another, and disorders often have different manifestations at different points in time.

In a mental disorder, alterations in behaviors, thoughts, and feelings are unexpected and are outside normal, culturally defined limits. If a behavior is considered normal within a specific culture, it is not viewed as a psychiatric symptom. For example, members of some religious groups "speak in tongues." To an observer, it appears that the individuals are having hallucinations (see Chapter 21), but this behavior is normal for this group within a particular setting.

The amount of disability or impairment in functioning is an important consideration when assessing a person with a mental disorder. A person's ability to understand, communicate, and get along with others is important in the recovery process. If symptoms impair an individual's ability to independently perform self-care and daily activities, recovery will be more difficult. The WHO and incapable of functioning independently. People with mental illness are sometimes treated as if they are responsible for their disabilities and are inaccurately accused of being weak or immoral (Corrigan, Morris, Michaels, Rafacz, & Rüsch, 2012). Stigmatization robs individuals of work, independent living, and meaningful relationships (see Fame & Fortune, p. 4).

The media often perpetuates negative stereotypes of persons with mental health issues. Films are especially important in influencing the public perception of mental illness because the media tend to be especially effective in shaping opinion in situations in which strong opinions are not already held. Although some films present sympathetic portrayals of people with mental illness and professionals who work in the field of mental health (e.g., *Beautiful Mind, Benny and Joon, The Soloist*), many more do not. People with mental illness are portrayed most often as aggressive, dangerous, and unpredictable. Films such as *Friday the 13th* (1980) and *Nightmare on Elm Street* (1984) perpetuate the myth that all people who leave psychiatric hospitals are violent and dangerous. Movies such as *The Exorcist* (1973) suggest to the public that mental illness is the equivalent of possession by the devil. These films in part account for the continuing stigma of mental illness.

When people with mental illnesses or emotional problems are stigmatized by society, they are often ostracized by the society in which they live. The stigma associated

---

FAME & FORTUNE

Thomas Eagleton, LL.B (1929–2007)

U.S. Senator from Missouri (1968–1987)

PUBLIC PERSONA

Thomas Eagleton was born in St. Louis, Missouri. He graduated from Amherst College in 1950 and Harvard Law School in 1953. He was elected circuit attorney of St. Louis and Attorney General of Missouri in 1960. He was elected to the U.S. Senate in 1968 and served in the Senate for 19 years. He was instrumental in the Senate's passage of the Clean Air and Water Acts and sponsored the Eagleton Amendment, which halted the bombing in Cambodia and effectively ended American involvement in the Vietnam War. He was active in matters dealing with foreign relations, intelligence, defense, education, health care, and the environment. He served in public office for more than 30 years, wrote three books, and held the title of Professor of Public Affairs at Washington University in St. Louis. The U.S. Courthouse in downtown St. Louis was named for him.

PERSONAL REALITIES

Thomas Eagleton was nominated to run for vice president at the 1972 Democratic Party convention with George McGovern as the presidential candidate. After the convention, Mr. Eagleton's hospitalization and treatment for depression was revealed. He was replaced on the Democratic presidential ticket within a few weeks.

Source: *The Biographical directory of the United States Congress, 1774–present.* Retrieved March 8, 2007, from http://bioguide.congress.gov/scripts/biodisplay.pl?index=E000004.

FAME & FORTUNE

Barret Robbins (1973–)

NFL Center

PUBLIC PERSONA

Barret Robbins was a shining football star when he played at Texas Christian University and was a member of the Phi Kappa Sigma fraternity. He was drafted by the Oakland Raiders in the second round of the 1995 draft. He became one of NFL's best centers and was elected to the Pro Bowl in 2002.

PERSONAL REALITIES

Barret Robbins was first diagnosed with bipolar disorder after his disappearance 2 days before Super Bowl XXXVII when he was hospitalized after a mania-driven drinking binge. He had been hospitalized for depression during college. Since the time he lost his career, he has been on a very rocky road to recovery. He has been arrested, shot, and separated from his family. He was recently released from a period of jail following an assault on a police detective release from a treatment facility ("Miami Beach Det. Reveals Details About Run-In With Ex-NFL Star," http://miami.cbslocal.com/2012/09/24/miami-beach-det-reveals-details-about-run-in-with-ex-nfl-star/). He is hopeful that he will be able to stay on his medication and away from substances to regain his life.

---

with all forms of mental illness is strong but generally increases the more an individual's behavior differs from the cultural norm.

Mental health treatment and providers are also objects of stigma. In films, psychiatric hospitals are often portrayed as dangerous and unwelcoming places, such as in *The Snake Pit* (1948), *One Flew Over the Cuckoo's Nest* (1975), *Instinct* (1999), *Twelve Monkeys* (1995), *Sling Blade* (1996), *Girl, Interrupted* (1999), *Don Juan Demarco* (1994), *A Beautiful Mind* (2001), and *Analyze That* (2002). Nurses are dressed in white in contrast to the dark, gloomy surroundings, and patients have little to do other than to walk the halls of the institution, acting odd. Psychiatrists, psychologists, and other health professionals who work with people with mental illnesses are often portrayed as "arrogant and ineffectual," "cold-hearted and authoritarian," "passive and apathetic," or "shrewd and manipulative" (Wedding, Boyd, & Niemiec, 2009).

One of the best ways to counteract the negative effects of stigma is to have contact with the stigmatized group (Corrigan et al., 2012). Another way is to use nonstigmatizing language. Just as a person with diabetes mellitus should not be referred to as a "diabetic" but rather as a "person with diabetes," a person with a mental disorder should never be referred to as a "schizophrenic" or "bipolar" but rather as a "person with schizophrenia" or a "person with bipolar disorder." Using words such as "psycho," "nuts," "funny farm," and "maniac" reinforces negative images of mental illness. Jokes that depict people with mental illness as stupid, dangerous, or incompetent perpetuate negative myths.

Self-Stigma

Self-stigma occurs when negative stereotypes are internalized by people with mental illness. Patients are aware of the public's negative view of mental illness and agree with the public's perceptions. They begin to believe that they are unpredictable, cannot become productive members of society, or have caused their illness. As a result of the application of the negative stereotype to self, they have low self-esteem (Corrigan et al., 2012).

Label Avoidance

Label avoidance, avoiding treatment or care in order not to be labeled as being mentally ill, is another type of stigma, and one of the reasons, that so few people with mental health problems actually receive help (Ciftci, Jones, & Corrigan, 2013). By avoiding treatment, they avoid the stigma of mental illness. For example, negative views of mental illness by several of the Asian cultures influence the willingness of its members to seek treatment. They may ignore their symptoms or refuse to seek treatment because of the stigma associated with being mentally ill (Ciftci et al., 2013; Lee et al., 2009).

RECOVERY FROM MENTAL ILLNESS

Recovery is the single most important goal for individuals with mental disorders (U.S. DHHS, SAMHSA, 2009). The following definition of recovery was released following a lengthy consensus process that began in 2010 and involved government agency officials, experts, consumers, family members, advocates, researchers, managed care representatives, and others.

> **KEYCONCEPT** **Recovery** from mental disorders and/or substance use disorders is a process of change through which individuals improve their health and wellness, live a self-directed life, and strive to reach their full potential (U.S. DHHS, SAMHSA, 2012).

Recovery-oriented treatment is based on the belief that mental illnesses and emotional disturbances are treatable and that recovery is an expectation. There are four dimensions that support recovery, including *health*

BOX 1.3

Research for Best Practice: Nurse and Patient Recovery Skills

Aston, V. & Coffey, M. (2011). Recovery: What mental health nurses and service users say about the concept of recovery. Journal of Psychiatric and Mental Health Nursing, 19(3), 257–263.

THE QUESTION: How do nurses and consumers view recovery-oriented care?

METHODS: Data were collected from a group of consumers and another group of nurses. Open-ended questions guided the discussions, which took place at a local drop-in center and day hospital. Data were recorded and underwent a rigorous process of analysis

FINDINGS: Four recovery-oriented practice themes emerged that impact both consumers and nurses. The first theme was the meaning of recovery. Both groups were uncertain of the in-depth meaning of recovery. The second theme was semantics, that is, the use of language to describe recovery and its process. Both groups found the word "recovery" difficult to associate with mental health but could not come up with a better term. The nurses were also unclear about their role within recovery. The third theme was therapeutics—specifically relationships between nurses and patients. Both the nurses and patients described difficulty in developing a collaborative relationship with each other because they were accustomed to the typical dependent nurse–patient relationship. The last theme related to the concept of a journey. Recovery is usually described as a journey, but not everyone will go through the journey. However, those who go through the journey describe it as a long and winding road.

IMPLICATIONS FOR NURSING: Traditional views are not easily changed. Being involved in decision making helps the patient transition from a dependent-driven relationship to a collaborative recovery-oriented one. Lack of information and training along with working in rigid task-oriented systems create frustration and lack of role clarity for both the nurse and the consumer.

(managing disease and living in a physically and emotionally healthy way), *home* (a safe and stable place to live), *purpose* (meaningful daily activities and independence, resources, and income), and *community* (relationships and social networks). Consumers and families have real and meaningful choices about treatment options and providers. In recovery-oriented care, the person with a mental health problem develops a partnership with a clinician to manage the illness, strengthen coping abilities, and build resilience for life's challenges (Box 1.3).

Mental health recovery benefits not only the individual and family but also society by ultimately reducing the global burden of mental health problems. Recovery is guided by 10 fundamental principles; see Box 1.4.

Individuals with mental illnesses can regain mental health with the support of families, mental health providers, and society. The contributions of these individuals strengthen communities and support the overall health of a nation.

BOX 1.4

Guiding Principles of Recovery

Recovery emerges from hope: The belief that recovery is real provides the essential and motivating message of a better future—that people can and do overcome the internal and external challenges, barriers, and obstacles that confront them.

Recovery is person-driven: Self-determination and self-direction are the foundations for recovery, as individuals define their own life goals and design their unique path(s).

Recovery occurs via many pathways: Individuals are unique with distinct needs, strengths, preferences, goals, culture, and backgrounds including trauma experiences that affect and determine their pathway(s) to recovery. Abstinence is the safest approach for those with substance use disorders.

Recovery is holistic: Recovery encompasses an individual's whole life, including mind, body, spirit, and community. The array of services and supports available should be integrated and coordinated.

Recovery is supported by peers and allies: Mutual support and mutual aid groups, including the sharing of experiential knowledge and skills, as well as social learning, play an invaluable role in recovery.

Recovery is supported through relationship and social networks: An important factor in the recovery process is the presence and involvement of people who believe in the person's ability to recover; who offer hope, support, and encouragement; and who also suggest strategies and resources for change.

Recovery is culturally-based and influenced: Culture and cultural background in all of its diverse representations including values, traditions, and beliefs are key in determining a person's journey and unique pathway to recovery.

Recovery is supported by addressing trauma: Services and supports should be trauma-informed to foster safety (physical and emotional) and trust, as well as to promote choice, empowerment, and collaboration.

Recovery involves individual, family, and community strengths and responsibility: Individuals, families, and communities have strengths and resources that serve as a foundation for recovery.

Recovery is based on respect: Community, systems, and societal acceptance and appreciation for people affected by mental health and substance use problems—including protecting their rights and eliminating discrimination—are crucial in achieving recovery.

(U.S. DHHS, SAMHSA, 2012)

SUMMARY OF KEY POINTS

■ Mental health is the emotional and psychological well-being of an individual. To be mentally healthy means that one can interact with others, deal with daily stress, and perceive the world realistically. Mental disorders are health conditions characterized by alterations in thinking, mood, or behavior and are associated with distress or impaired functioning.

■ Epidemiology is important in understanding the distribution of mental illness and determinants of health within a given population. The rate of occurrence refers to the proportion of the population that has the disorder. Incidence is the rate of new cases within a specified time. Prevalence is the rate of occurrence of all cases at a particular point in time.

■ Stigma toward mental illness can be viewed in three ways. Public stigma marks a person as having a mental illness. When a person with a mental illness shares the public's negative view of mental illness, self-stigma occurs. If a person with a mental illness does not seek treatment because of fear of being labeled "mentally ill," label avoidance occurs.

■ The *DSM-5* organizes psychiatric diagnoses according to behaviors and symptom patterns.

■ Cultural syndromes are specific disorders found within a particular locality or culture. There is little research on the syndromes, but *ataque de nervios* and *susto* are well documented.

■ Mental health recovery is the single most important goal for the mental health delivery system. Recovery is viewed a process of changes through which individuals improve their health and wellness, live a self-directed life, and strive to reach their full potential.

CRITICAL THINKING CHALLENGES

1. A person who is seeking help for a mental disorder asks why the individual's physical health is important to the nurse.

2. Compare the meaning of the epidemiological terms *prevalence*, *incidence*, and *rate*. Access the CDC's website (www.cdc.gov), and identify major mental health problems in the United States.

3. Examine the description of people with mental illness in the media, including television programs, news, and newspapers. Are negative connotations evident?

4. Examine how family and friends describe people with mental illness. Do you think their description of mental illness is based on fact or myth? Explain.

5. Explain the three forms of stigma and give examples.

6. Discuss the negative impact of labeling someone with a psychiatric diagnosis.

7. Using the components of mental health recovery as a framework, compare the goals for a person with schizophrenia with those with a medical disease such as diabetes.

Beautiful Dreamers: **1992, Canada.**
This film is based on a true story about poet Walt Whitman's visit to an asylum in London, Ontario, Canada. Whitman, played by Rip Torn, is shocked by what he sees and persuades the hospital director to offer humane treatment. Eventually, the patients wind up playing the townspeople in a game of cricket.
Viewing Points: Observe the stigma that is associated with having a mental illness.

REFERENCES

American Psychiatric Association. (2013). *Diagnostic and statistical manual of mental disorders* (5th ed). Arlington, VA: Author.

American Nurses Association, American Psychiatric Nurses Association, & International Society of Psychiatric–Mental Health Nurses. (2014). *Psychiatric–mental health nursing: Scope and standards of practice.* 2nd edition. Silver Spring, MD: American Nurses Association.

Ciftci, A., Jones, N., & Corrigan, P. W. (2013). Mental health stigma in the Muslim community. *Journal of Muslim Mental Health, 7*(1), 17–31.

Corrigan, P. W, Morris, S. B., Michaels, P. J., Rafacz, J. D., & Rüsch, N. (2012). Challenging the public stigma of mental illness: A meta-analysis of outcome studies, *Psychiatric Services, 63*(10), 963–973. doi:10.1176/appi.ps.005292011

Lee, S., Juon, H. S., Martinez, G., Hsu, C. E., Robinson, E. S., Bawa, J., et al. (2009). Model minority at risk: Expressed needs of mental health by Asian American young adults. *Journal of Community Health, 34*(2), 144–152.

McMahon, S., & Fleury, J. (2012). Wellness in older adults: A concept analysis. *Nursing Forum, 47*(1), 39–51.

National Institute of Mental Health. (2013). *The numbers counts: Mental disorders in American.* Retrieved June 18, 2014, from http://www.nimh.nih.gov/health/publications/the-numbers-count-mental-disorders-in-america/index.shtml

President's New Freedom Commission Mental Health. (2003). *Achieving the promise: Transforming mental health care in America—Final report* (DHHS Publication No. SMA-03–3832). Retrieved June 30, 2009, from http://www.mentalhealthcommission.gov/report/FinalReport/toc.html

Razzouk, D, Nogueira, B, & Mari Jde, J. (2011). The contribution of Latin American and Caribbean countries on culture bound syndromes studies for the ICD-10 revision: Key findings from a working in progress. *Revista Brasileira de Psiquiatria, 33*(suppl. 1), S5–20.

Schuffman, D., Druss, B. G., & Parks, J. J. (2009). State mental health policy: Mending Missouri's safety net—Transforming systems of care by integrating primary and behavioral health care. *Psychiatric Services, 60*(5), 585–588.

U.S. DHHS, SAMHSA. (2009). Transforming mental health care in America: Federal action agenda—First steps. Retrieved June 18, 2014, from http://www.samhsa.gov/federalactionagenda/NFC_FMHAA.aspx

U.S. DHHS, SAMHSA. (2010). The eight dimensions of wellness (Publication No. SMA12-4568). Retrieved from http://store.samhsa.gov/product/SAMHSA-s-Wellness-Initiative-Eight-Dimensions-of-Wellness/SMA12-4568

U.S. DHHS, SAMHSA. (2012). SAMHSA's working definition of recovery updated. Retrieved June 18, 2014, from http://blog.samhsa.gov/2012/03/23/defintion-of-recovery-updated/#.U4MD_kAQOuY.

Wedding, D., Boyd, M. A., & Niemiec, R. (2009). *Movies and mental illness* (3rd ed). Göttingen, Germany: Hogrefe & Huber.

Whiteford, H. A. Degenhardt, L., Rehm, J., Baxter, A. J., Ferrari, A. J., Erskine, H. E., et al. (2013). Global burden of disease attributable to mental and substance use disorders: Findings from the Global burden of Disease Study 2010. *Lancet. 382*(9904), 1575–1586.

WHO. (2013a). *Comprehensive mental health action plan 2013–2020. Sixty-six World Health Assembly, Agenda Item 13.3.* Geneva, Switzerland: Author.

WHO. (2013b). *Depression. A hidden burden.* Geneva, Switzerland: Author. Retrieved June 18, 2014, from http://www.who.int/mental_health/management/depression/flyer_depression_2012.pdf?ua=1

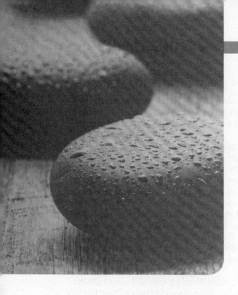

2
Cultural and Spiritual Issues Related to Mental Health Care

Mary Ann Boyd

KEY CONCEPTS

- culture
- cultural competence
- spirituality

LEARNING OBJECTIVES

After studying this chapter, you will be able to:

1. Discuss the ways that cultural competence is demonstrated in psychiatric-mental health nursing.

2. Describe the beliefs about mental health and illness in different cultural and social groups.

3. Differentiate concepts of religion and spirituality.

4. Discuss the role of spirituality and religiousness in persons with mental illness.

5. Discuss the beliefs of major religions and their role in shaping views on mental illnesses.

KEY TERMS

- acculturation • cultural explanations • cultural identity • cultural idiom of distress • linguistic competence
- religiousness

All cultural groups have sets of values, beliefs, and patterns of accepted behavior, and it is often difficult for those of one culture to understand those of another. This is especially true regarding mental illness—whereas some cultures view it as a condition for which the ill person must be punished and ostracized from society, other cultures are more tolerant and believe that family and community members are key to the care and treatment of mentally ill people. Nurses' and patients' religious backgrounds and cultural heritages may be different, so it is important for nurses to understand clearly the thinking and perspectives of other cultures and groups.

This chapter examines cultural and social mores of various cultural and religious groups. Understanding cultural and religious beliefs and the significance of spirituality is especially important when caring for people with mental health problems. These beliefs and practices can define and shape the experience of being

mentally ill and influence the willingness to seek care. Treating mental disorders is intertwined with people's attitudes about themselves, their beliefs, values, and ways.

> **KEYCONCEPT** **Culture** is not only a way of life for people who identify or associate with one another on the basis of some common purpose, need, or similarity of background but also the totality of learned, socially transmitted beliefs, values, and behaviors that emerge from its members' interpersonal transactions.

Cultures are dynamic and continually changing. When immigrants arrive in the United States with their own cultures, they begin to adapt to their new environment. **Acculturation** is the term used to describe the socialization process by which minority groups learn and adopt selective aspects of the dominant culture. Their culture changes as a result of the influences of the new environment. Eventually, a new minority culture evolves that is different than the native culture and also different from the dominante culure, which in turn is transformed by the new residents.

Everyone has a **cultural identity**, or set of cultural beliefs with which one looks for standards of behavior. Because culture is broadly defined, many people consider themselves to have multiple cultural identities. The dominant culture for much of the U.S. history, has been based on the beliefs, norms, and values of white Americans of Judeo-Christian origin. Even though the United States is rapidly changing, most health care professionals are primarily products of an education system of white American culture. All persons and organizations function within a culture.

CULTURAL AND LINGUISTIC COMPETENCE

Psychiatric–mental health nurses have an obligation to be culturally and linguistically competent to provide quality care. There are several definitions of cultural and linguistic competence, but there is a general consensus that cultural and linguistic competence involves an adjustment or recognition of one's own culture in order to understand the culture of another person. **Linguistic competence**, the capacity to communicate effectively and convey information that is easily understood by diverse audiences, is an important part of cultural competence (Goode & Jones, 2009). A nurse who is culturally competent understands and appreciates cultural differences in health care practices and similarities within, among, and between groups.

> KEYCONCEPT **Cultural competence** is a set of academic and interpersonal skills that are respectful of and responsive to the health beliefs, health care practices, and cultural and linguistic needs of diverse patients to bring about positive health care outcomes (U.S. Department of Health and Human Services [U.S. DHHS], 2013).

Cultural competence is demonstrated in several ways. Valuing patients' culture beliefs and recognizing the need to bridge language barriers are essential behaviors. There are linguistic variations within cultural groups as well as cultural variations within a language group. Speaking the same language does not guarantee shared meaning and understanding. Communication may be adversely affected when patients are unable to fully express themselves in English. Understanding the impact of literacy levels is integral to providing culturally competent care. Demonstrating an understanding that literacy levels contribute to the interpretation of personal, psychological experiences is critical (U.S. DHHS, 2013).

CULTURAL AND SOCIAL FACTORS AND BELIEFS ABOUT MENTAL ILLNESS

Cultural beliefs and practices influence how patients communicate and manifest their symptoms, cope with their illnesses, and receive family and community support. The *DMS-5* differentiates **cultural idiom of distress**, a commonly used term or phrase that describes the suffering within a cultural group from **cultural explanations**, perceived causes for symptoms (APA, 2013). For example, the term, *nervios*, is an idiom used by Hispanics in the Western Hemisphere that explains a wide range of somatic and emotional symptoms such as headache, irritability, nervousness, insomnia, and difficulty concentrating. The term *susto*, (extreme fright causing the soul to leave the body) is believed to be the cause of a group of varied symptoms including appetite disturbance, sleep problems, low self-worth among people in Central and South America.

Social factors also contribute to the development of mental disorders. Ethnic and racial minorities in the United States live in a social environment of inequality that increases their exposure to racism, discrimination, violence, and poverty, which contribute to the experience of their illnesses (U.S. DHHS, 2013). Racially and ethnically diverse groups are less likely to receive mental health services and more likely to receive poorer quality care. Poverty is found in all cultural groups and is present in other groups, such as older adults, people with physical disabilities, individuals with psychiatric impairments, and single-parent families. In the United States, one third of people living below the poverty line are single mothers and their children; 27.2% of African Americans live below the poverty level, as do 25.6% of Hispanic Americans and 9.7% of white Americans (DeNavas-Walt, Proctor, & Smith, 2013). Currently in the United States, the poverty guidelines for a family of four is a yearly income of $23,850 or less in the 48 mainland states; $29,820 or less in Alaska; and $27,430 or less in Hawaii (U.S. Census, 2014).

Families living in poverty are under tremendous financial and emotional stress, which may trigger or exacerbate mental problems. Along with the daily stressors of trying to provide food and shelter for themselves and their families, their lack of time, energy, and money prevents them from attending to their psychological needs. Often, these families become trapped in a downward economic spiral as tension and stress mount. The inability to gain employment and the lack of financial independence only add to the feelings of powerlessness and low self-esteem. Being self-supporting gives one a feeling of control over life and bolsters self-esteem. Dependence on others or the government causes frustration, anger, apathy, and feelings of depression and meaninglessness. Alcoholism, depression, and child and partner abuse may become a means of coping with such hopelessness and despair. The homeless population is the group most at risk for being unable to escape this spiral of poverty.

Hispanic Americans

The number of Hispanic Americans living in the United States has been gradually increasing, and this group is now the largest minority in the United States. From 2000 to 2008, there was a 75% increase in population, from 35.3 to 53 million, representing 17% of the U.S. population. Countries of origin include Mexico (65%), Central and South American (16%), Puerto Rico (8%), and Cuba (4%). Hispanic populations are largest in urban areas, such as New York, Chicago, Los Angeles, San Francisco, and Miami–Fort Lauderdale (U.S. Census Bureau, 2013).

Studies indicate that Hispanic Americans tend to use all other resources before seeking help from mental health professionals. Reasons for this are unclear, but barriers for treatment include beliefs that mental health facilities do not accommodate their cultural needs (e.g., language, beliefs, values), cost of care, and concerns regarding immigration status (Lee, Laiewski, & Choi, 2014; Kalthman, de Mendoza, Gonzales, & Serrano, 2013) (Box 2.1).

African Americans

In 2012, the estimated population of African Americans was 44.5 million, or 12.8% of the United States population (U.S. Census Bureau, 2013). Although African Americans share many beliefs, attitudes, values, and behaviors, there are also many subcultural and individual differences based on social class, country of origin, occupation, religion, educational level, and geographic location. Many African Americans have extensive family

---

BOX 2.1

Cultural Competence and Mental Health

- Learn about the patient's country of origin before assessment.
- Conduct a thorough social and cultural assessment.
- Demonstrate genuine interest in and respect for the individual.
- Educate patients about mental health issues, including available treatments, benefits of obtaining services, and contributions and abilities of individuals with a mental illness.
- Do not assume that all individuals of a racial or ethnic group are the same.
- Being quiet and lack of eye contact may be culturally appropriate and may indicate shyness, not depression or another mental illness.
- Tailor interventions to the individual; one intervention does not work for everyone.

Adapted from Acosta, H. (2009). *Hispanic mental health: Do and don'ts when working with Hispanics in mental health.* Retrieved on July 16, 2009, from http://www.culturallycompetentmentalhealthnj.org.

BOX 2.2

Research for Best Practice: African American Men and Women's Attitudes, Stigma and Coping

Ward, E. C., Wiltshire, J. C., Detry, M. A., & Brown, R. L. (2013). African American men and women's attitude toward mental illness, perceptions of stigma, and preferred coping behaviors. Nursing Research, 62(3), 185–194.

THE QUESTION: What are the attitudes toward mental illness, perceived stigma, and preferred coping behaviors related to seeking treatment of mental illness in African American women?

METHODS: An exploratory, cross-sectional survey design was used. Community-dwelling African Americans (n = 272) age 25 to 85 years rated their beliefs, coping preferences, and perceived stigma associated with seeking treatment for mental illness.

FINDINGS: The findings suggested that these participants understood some of the causes of mental illness, identified many of the symptoms of mental illness, and believed that treatment controlled the mental illness. Their attitudes suggested that they were not very open to acknowledging psychological problems and were concerned about the stigma associated with mental illnesses. While somewhat open to mental health services, they preferred religious coping, especially in the older and middle-aged participants.

IMPLICATIONS FOR NURSING: The nurse should consider the impact of stigma on the willingness to seek treatment for mental illness. There is a need for psychoeducation interventions designed to increase openness to psychological problems and reduce stigma.

---

networks in which members can be relied on for moral support, help with child rearing, provide financial aid, and help in crises. In many African American families, older members are treated with great respect. But African Americans with mental illness suffer from the stresses of double stigma—not only from their own cultural group but also from longtime racial discrimination. To make matters worse, racial discrimination may come from within the health community itself (Box 2.2).

Several studies show that diagnoses and treatment for African Americans often are racially biased (Eack, Bahorik, Newhill, Neighbors, & Davis, 2012). African Americans are disproportionately diagnosed as having schizophrenia when compared to other groups. Evidence suggests that the overdiagnosis in research studies may be related to whether the interviewer perceived that the patient was honest in reporting symptoms. A trusting, open, and collaborative therapeutic relationship during the diagnostic process is essential in order to conduct a meaningful assessment (Eack et al., 2012).

Asian Americans, Polynesians, and Pacific Islanders

In 2012, more than 18.9 million (4.4% of the U.S. population) Asian Americans, Polynesians, and Pacific

Islanders lived in the United States, and this group represents one of the fastest growing minority populations in the United States. This large multicultural group includes Chinese, Filipino, Japanese, Asian Indian, Korean, Vietnamese, Laotian, Cambodian, Hawaiian, Samoan, and Guamanian people. Most Chinese, Japanese, Korean, Asian Indian, and Filipino immigrants have migrated to urban areas; the Vietnamese have settled throughout the United States (U.S. Census Bureau, 2013).

Generally, Asian cultures have a tradition of denying or disguising the existence of mental illnesses. In many of these cultures, it is an embarrassment to have a family member treated for mental illness, which may explain the extremely low utilization of mental health services. Only 17% of those experiencing problems seek care (Lee et al., 2009).

Asian Americans may experience a culture-bound syndrome, such as neurasthenia, which is characterized by fatigue, weakness, poor concentration, memory loss, irritability, aches and pains, and sleep disturbances. Associated with the Korean culture, *hwa-byung*, "suppressed anger syndrome," is characterized by subjective and expressed anger, sensations of heat, and feelings of hate (Lee et al., 2012). Research regarding specific mental health problems in Asian cultures is sparse, but various data suggest that rates of suicide within Native Hawaiian adolescents are higher than those of other adolescents in the United States (Suicide Prevention Resource Center, 2013).

Native Americans

In 2012, the estimated population of Native Americans was more than 6.3 million people, over 1% of the U.S. population (U.S. Census Bureau, 2013). Native American cultures emphasize respect and reverence for the earth and nature, from which come survival and comprehension of life and one's relationships with a separate, higher spiritual being and with other human beings. Shamans, or medicine men, are central to most cultures. They are healers believed to possess psychic abilities. Healing treatments rely on herbal medicines and healing ceremonies and feasts. Self-understanding derives from observing nature; relationships with others emphasize interdependence and sharing.

Traditional views about mental illnesses vary among the tribes. In some, mental illness is viewed as a supernatural possession, as being out of balance with nature. In certain Native American groups, people with mental illnesses are stigmatized. However, the degree of stigmatization is not the same for all disorders. In tribal groups that make little distinction between physical and mental illnesses, there is little stigma. In other groups, a particular event, such as suicide, is stigmatized. Different ill-

nesses may be encountered in different Native American cultures and gene pools.

Women of Minority Groups

Women within minority groups may experience more conflicting feelings and psychological stressors than do men in trying to adjust to both their defined role in the minority culture and a different role in the larger predominant society. Compared to men, more Asian American women suffer from depression, yet are less likely than white women to seek out mental health care (Appel, Huang, Ai, & Lin, 2011).

Rural Cultures

Most mental health services are located in urban areas because most people live near cities. Those living in rural areas have limited access to health care which leads to fewer people being diagnosed with a mental health problem. Even though rural residents are less likely than urban residents to have mental health diagnoses or receive mental health care, the suicide rate is higher in the rural areas with firearms most commonly used (Searles, Valley, Hedegaard, & Betz, 2013). Rural areas are also diverse in both geography and culture. For example, access to mental health for those in the deep South is different from access for those with the same problems in the Northwest. Treatment approaches may be accepted in one part of the country but not in another. Suicide rates are higher in rural areas when compared to urban areas.

SPIRITUALITY, RELIGION, AND MENTAL ILLNESS

Both spirituality and religion are factors that may influence beliefs about mental illness and impact treatment and recovery.

> **KEYCONCEPT**   **Spirituality** develops over time and is a dynamic, conscious process characterized by two movements of transcendence (going beyond the limits of ordinary experiences): either deep within the self or beyond the self. Self-transcendence involves self-reflection and living according to one's values in establishing meaning to events and a purpose to life. Transcendence beyond self is characterized by a feeling of connection and mutuality to a higher power (Vachon, Fillon, & Achille, 2009).

Related but different than spirituality, **religiousness** is the participation in a community of people who gather around common ways of worshiping. Spirituality can be expressed through adhering to a particular religion. Religious beliefs often define an individual's relationship

TABLE 2.1 MAJOR WORLD RELIGIONS AND BELIEF FORMS		
Source of Power or Force (Deity)	**Historical Sacred Texts or Beliefs**	**Key Beliefs or Ethical Life Philosophy**
Buddhism		
Buddha Individual responsibility and logical or intuitive thinking Buddhist subjects include: • *Lamaism* (Tibet), in which Buddhism is blended with spirit worship • *Mantrayana* (Himalayan area, Mongolia, Japan), in which intimate relationship with a guru and recitations of secret mantras are emphasized; belief in sexual symbolism and demons • *Ch'an* (China) *Zen* (Japan), in which self-reliance and awareness through intuitive understanding are stressed. • *Satori* (enlightenment) may come from "sudden insight" or through self-discipline, meditation, and instruction	Tripitaka (scripture) Middle Path (way of life) The Four Noble Truths Eightfold Path (guides for life) The Texts of Taoism (include the Tao Te Ching of Lao Tzu and The Writings of Chuang Tzu) Sutras (Buddhist commentaries) Sangha (Buddhist Community)	Buddhism attempts to deal with problems of human existence such as suffering and death. Life is misery, unhappiness, and suffering with no ultimate reality in the world or behind it. The cause of all human suffering and misery is desire. The "middle path" of life avoids the personal extremes of self-denial and self-indulgence. Visions can be gained through personal meditation and contemplation; good deeds and compassion also facilitate the process toward nirvana, the ultimate mode of existence. The end of suffering is the extinction of desire and emotion and ultimately the unreal self. Present behavior is a result of past deed.
Christianity		
God, a unity in tripersonality; Father, Son, and Holy Ghost	Bible Teachings of Jesus through the apostles and the church fathers	God's love for all creatures is a basic belief. Salvation is gained by those who have faith and show humility toward God. Brotherly love is emphasized in acts of charity, kindness, and forgiveness.
Confucianism		
No doctrine of a god or gods or life after death Individual responsibility and logical and intuitive thinking	Five Classics (Confucian thought) Analects (conversations and sayings of Confucius)	A philosophy or a system of ethics for living rather than a religion that teaches how people should act toward one another. People are born "good." Moral character is stressed through sincerity in personal and public behavior. Respect is shown for parents and figures of authority. Improvement is gained through self-responsibility, introspection, and compassion for others.
Hinduism		
Brahma (the Infinite Being and Creator that pervades all reality) Other gods: Vishnu (preserver), Shiva (destroyer), Krishna (love)	Vedas (doctrine and commentaries)	All people are assigned to castes (permanent hereditary orders, each having different privileges in society; each was created from different parts of Brahma): 1. *Brahmans:* includes priests and intellectuals 2. *Kshatriyas:* includes rulers and soldiers 3. *Vaisya:* includes farmers, skilled workers, and merchants 4. *Sudras:* includes those who serve the other three castes (servants, laborers, peasants) 5. *Untouchables:* the outcasts; those not included in the other castes
Islam		
Allah (the only God) Has two major sects: • *Sunni* (orthodox): traditional and simple practices are followed; human will is determined by outside forces • *Shiite*, practices are rapturous and trancelike; human beings have free will	Koran (the words of God delivered to Mohammed by the angel Gabriel) Hadith (commentaries by Mohammed) Five Pillars of Islam (religious conduct) Islam was built on Christianity and Judaism	God is just and merciful; humans are limited and sinful. God rewards the good and punishes the sinful. Mohammed, through the Koran, guides people and teaches them truth. Peace is gained through submission to Allah. The sinless go to Paradise, and the evil go to Hell. A "good" Muslim obeys the Five Pillars of Islam.

TABLE 2.1	MAJOR WORLD RELIGIONS AND BELIEF FORMS (*CONTINUED*)	
Source of Power or Force (Deity)	Historical Sacred Texts or Beliefs	Key Beliefs or Ethical Life Philosophy
Judaism		
God	Hebrew Bible (Old Testament) Torah (first five books of Hebrew Bible) Talmud (commentaries on the Torah)	Jews have a special relationship with God: obeying God's law through ethical behavior and ritual obedience earns the mercy and justice of God. God is worshiped through love, not out of fear.
Shintoism		
Gods of nature, ancestor worship, national heroes	Tradition and custom (the way of the gods) Beliefs were influenced by Confucianism and Buddhism	Reverence for ancestors and a traditional Japanese way of life are emphasized. Loyalty to places and locations where one lives or works and purity and balance in physical and mental life are major motivators of personal conduct.
Taoism		
All the forces in nature	Tao-te-Ching ("The Way and the Power")	Quiet and happy harmony with nature is the key belief. Peace and contentment are found in the personal behaviors of optimism, passivity, humility, and internal calmness. Humility is an especially valued virtue. Conformity to the rhythm of nature and the universe leads to a simple, natural, and ideal life.
Tribal Beliefs		
Animism: Souls or spirits embodied in all beings and everything in nature (trees, rivers, mountains) *Polytheism:* Many gods, in the basic powers of nature (sun, moon, earth, water)	Passed on through ceremonies, rituals, myths, and legends Oral history, rather than written literature, is the common medium	All living things are related. Respect for powers of nature and pleasing the spirits are fundamental beliefs to meet the basic and practical needs for food, fertility, health, and interpersonal relationships and individual development. Harmonious living is comprehension and respect of natural forces.

Summary of Other Belief Forms

- *Agnosticism:* the belief that whether there is a God and a spiritual world or any ultimate reality is unknown and probably unknowable
- *Atheism:* the belief that no God exists because "God" is defined in any current existing culture of society
- *Maoism:* the faith that is centered in the leadership of the Communist Party and all the people; the major belief goal is to move away from individual personal desires and ambitions toward viewing and serving all people as a whole
- *Scientism:* the belief that values and guidance for living come from scientific knowledge, principles, and practices; systematic study and analysis of life, rather than superstition, lead to true understanding and practice of life.

Adapted from Axelson, J. A., & McGrath, P. (1998, 1993, 1985). *Counseling and development in a multicultural society.* Pacific Grove, CA: Brooks/Cole Publishing Company, a division of International Thomson Publishing Inc. Used with permission of the publisher.

within a family and community. Many different religions are practiced throughout the world. Judeo-Christian thinking tends to dominate Western societies. Other religions, such as Islam, Hinduism, and Buddhism, dominate Eastern and Middle Eastern cultures (Table 2.1). Because religious beliefs often influence approaches to mental health, it is important to understand the basis of various religions that appear to be growing in the United States. Both religion and spirituality can provide support and strength in dealing with mental illnesses and emotional problems.

People with mental illness benefit from spiritual assessment and interventions (see Chapter 9). Perception of well-being and health in persons with severe mental illness has been positively associated with spirituality and religiousness. To carry out spiritual interventions, the nurse enters a therapeutic relationship with the patient and uses the self as a therapeutic tool (Box 2.3). Examples of spiritual interventions include meditation; guided imagery; and, when appropriate, prayer to connect with inner sources of solace and hope.

BOX 2.3

Research for Best Practice: Coping Strategies of Family Members

Eaton, P. M., Davis, B. L., Hammond, P. V., Condon, E. H., & Zina, T. M. (2011). Coping strategies of family members of hospitalized psychiatric patients. Nursing Research and Practice. doi:10.1155./2011/392705

THE QUESTION: What are the coping strategies of family members of hospitalized patients with psychiatric disorders?

METHODS: A descriptive, correlational, mixed method research approach was guided by the Neuman Systems Model as forty-five family members of hospitalized patients with psychiatric disorders were asked to complete the Family Crisis Oriented Personal Evaluation Scale and semi-structured interviews.

FINDINGS: Family members used more emotion-coping strategies rather than problem-solving strategies. The coping strategies used included communicating with immediate family, acceptance of their situation, passive appraisal, avoidance, and spirituality.

IMPLICATIONS FOR NURSING: Families are impacted by psychiatric hospitalizations of members and need nursing support in order to have the energy to provide care and support to their family member. Spirituality is one of the coping strategies that can be supported.

SUMMARY OF KEY POINTS

- The term *culture* is defined as a way of life that manifests the learned beliefs, values, and accepted behaviors that are transmitted socially within a specific group.

- Everyone has a cultural identity, which helps define expected behavior.

- Cultural and linguistic competence is based on a set of skills that allows individuals to increase their understanding and appreciation of cultural differences and similarities within, among, and between groups. Cultural competence is demonstrated by valuing the culture beliefs, bridging any language gap, and considering the patient's literacy level when planning and implementing care.

- Mental illnesses are stigmatized in many cultural groups. A variety of cultural and religious beliefs underlie the stigmatization.

- Access to mental health treatment is particularly limited for those living in rural areas or those who live in poverty.

- Spirituality can be a source of strength and support for both the patient with mental illness and the nurse providing the care.

- Religious beliefs are closely intertwined with beliefs about health and mental illness.

CRITICAL THINKING CHALLENGES

1. Assess your cultural competence with groups that have the following heritage: African, Asian, Hispanic, and Native American.
2. Compare beliefs about mental illnesses within African and Asian American groups.
3. Compare the access to mental health services in your state or county in rural areas versus urban areas.
4. Discuss the differences between spirituality and religiousness. Is it possible that someone can be spiritual and not religious?
5. Identify the religious groups that are associated with the following sacred texts: Bible, Koran, Vedas, Texts of Taoism, Talmud.

House of Sand and Fog: **(2003).**
Colonel Massoud Amir Behrani, an Iranian immigrant played by Ben Kingsley, has spent most of his savings trying to enhance his daughter's chances of a good marriage. The rest of his funds were spent at an auction on a repossessed house owned by Kathy Nicoli (Jennifer Connelly), an emotionally unstable, depressed young woman who failed to pay property taxes. The struggle for the house ensues with tragic results.

Viewing Points: Identify the cultural differences between the Behrani and Nicoli families. Are any cultural stereotypes depicted in the film? Discuss the role of prejudice and discrimination in the outcome of the movie. How did Kathy's mental illness and relationship with the police officer influence the negotiation for the house?

REFERENCES

American Psychiatric Association. (2013). *Diagnostic and statistical manual of mental disorders, DSM-5* (5th ed). Arlington, VA: American Psychiatric Association.

Appel, H.B., Huang, B., Ai, A. L., & Lin, C. J. (2011). Physical, behavioral, and mental health issues in Asian American women: Results from the national Latino Asian American study. *Journal of Women's Health (2002), 20*(11), 1703–1711.

DeNavas-Walt, C., Proctor, B. D., & Smith, J. C. (2013). *Income, Poverty, and Health Insurance Coverage in the United States: 2012. U.S. Census Bureau Current population reports* (pp. 60–245). Washington, DC: U.S. Government Printing Office.

Eack, S. M., Bahorik, A. L., Newhill, C. E., Neighbors, H. W., & Davis, L. E. (2012). Interviewer-perceived honesty as a mediator of racial disparities in the diagnosis of schizophrenia. *Psychiatric services (Washington, D.C.), 63*(9), 875–880.

Eaton, P. M., Davis, B. L., Hammond, P. V., Condon, E. H., & McGee, Z. T. (2011). Coping strategies of family members of hospitalized psychiatric patients. *Nursing Research and Practice.* doi:10.1155/2011/392705

Goode, T. D., & Jones, W. (2009). Linguistic Competence. National Center for Cultural Competence, Georgetown University Center for Child and Human Development. Washington, DC. http://nccc.georgetown.edu/documents/Definition%2520of%2520Linguistic%2520Competence.pdf

Kaltman, S., de Mendoza, A. H., Gonzales, F. A., & Serrano, A. (2013). Preferences for trauma-related mental health services among Latina immigrants from Central America, South America, and Mexico.

Psychological Trauma: Theory, Research, Practice, and Policy. doi:10.1037/a0031539

Lee, J., Min, S. K., Kim, K. H., Kim, B., Cho, S. J., Lee, S. H., et al. (2012). Differences in temperament and character dimensions of personality between patients with Hwa-byung, an anger syndrome, and patients with major depressive disorder. *Journal of Affective Disorders, 138*(1–2), 110–116.

Lee, S. L., Juon, H. S., Martinez, G, Hsu, C. E., Robinson, E. S., Bawa J, et al. (2009). Model minority at risk: Expressed needs of mental health by Asian American young adults. *Journal of Community Health, 34*(2), 144–152.

Lee, S., Laiewski, L., & Choi, S. (2014). Racial-ethnic variation in U.S. mental health service use among Latino and Asian non-U.S. citizens. *Psychiatric Services, 65*(1), 68–74.

Searles, V. B., Valley, M. A., Hedegaard, H., Betz, M. E. (2013). Suicides in urban and rural counties in the United States, 2006-2008. *Crisis: The Journal of Crisis Intervention and Suicide Prevention,* 1–9. doi:10,1027/0227-5910/a000224

Suicide Prevention Resource Center. (2013). *Suicide among racial/ethnic populations in the U.S. Asians, Pacific Islander, and Native Hawaiians. Fact sheet.* Suicide Prevention Action Network USA. Retrieved December 4, 2010, from http://www.spanusa.org

U.S. Census Bureau. (2014). U.S. Census Bureau. Statistical Abstract of the United States: 2012 (131st ed) Washington, DC, 2011. http://www.census.gov.

U.S. Census Bureau. (2014). State and County Quick Facts. Data derived from Population Estimates, American Community Survey, Census of Population and Housing, State and County Housing Unit Estimates, County Business Patterns, Nonemployer Statistics, Economic Census, Survey of Business Owners, Building Permits. http://quickfacts.census.gov/qfd/states/00000.html

U.S. Department of Health and Human Services. (2013). Cultural competency. Office of Minority Health. http://minorityhealth.hhs.gov/templates/browse.aspx?lvl=2&lvlID=11

U.S. Department of Health and Human Services. (2010). The delayed update of the HHS poverty guidelines for the remainder of 2010. *Federal Register, 75*(148), 45628.

Vachon, M., Fillion, L., & Achille, M. (2009). A conceptual analysis of spirituality at the end of life. *Journal of Palliative Medicine, 12*(1), 53–59.

Ward, E. C., Wiltshire, J. C., Detry, M. A., & Brown, R. L. (2013). African American men and women's attitude toward mental illness, perceptions of stigma, and preferred coping behaviors. *Nursing Research, 62*(3), 185–194.

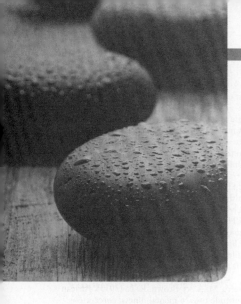

3
Patient Rights and Legal Issues

Mary Ann Boyd

KEY CONCEPT

- self-determinism

LEARNING OBJECTIVES

After studying this chapter, you will be able to:

1. Define *self-determinism* and its implications in mental health care.

2. Discuss the legal protection of the rights of people with mental disorders.

3. Discuss the legal determination of competency.

4. Delineate the differences between voluntary and involuntary treatment.

5. Discuss the difference between privacy and confidentiality.

6. Discuss HIPAA and mandates to inform and their implications in psychiatric–mental health care.

7. Describe the mentally ill populations in forensic settings.

8. Discuss the stigma of mental illness and criminality.

9. Describe legal outcomes for persons with mental illness in forensic systems.

10. Identify the importance of accurate, quality documentation in electronic and non-electronic patient records.

KEY TERMS

- accreditation • advance care directives • assault • breach of confidentiality • competence • confidentiality • external advocacy system • forensic • incompetent • informed consent • internal rights protection system • involuntary commitment • least restrictive environment • living will • medical battery • negligence • power of attorney • privacy • voluntary admission • voluntary commitment

Because individuals with mental disorders are often vulnerable to mistreatment and abuse, their legal rights and the ethical health care practices of mental health providers are ongoing concerns for psychiatric–mental health nurses. For example, can a person be forced into a hospital if his or her behavior is bizarre but harmless? What human rights can be denied to a person who has a mental disorder and under what circumstances? These questions are not easily answered. This chapter summarizes some of the key patient rights and legal issues that underlie psychiatric–mental health nursing practice across the continuum of care.

SELF-DETERMINISM: A FUNDAMENTAL RIGHT AND NEED

At the foundation of many questions related to the rights of mental health patients is the issue of self-determinism and preservation of this right.

> **KEYCONCEPT** **Self-determinism** promotes growth and well-being toward human potential through having basic psychological needs met including autonomy (initiation and control of one's actions), competence (perceived effectiveness in social interactions), and relatedness (connections and belongingness with others) (Deci & Ryan, 2012).

A self-determined individual is internally motivated to make choices based on personal goals, not to please others or to be rewarded. That is, a person engages in activities that are interesting, challenging, pleasing, exciting, or fun, requiring no rewards other than the positive feelings that accompany them because of inner goals, needs, drives or preferences. Personal autonomy and avoidance of dependence on others are key values of self-determinism, which is integral to the recovery process (see Chapter 1).

In mental health care, self-determinism is the right to choose one's own health-related behaviors, which at times differ from those recommended by health professionals. A patient's right to refuse treatment, to choose the second or third best health care recommendation rather than the first, and to seek a second opinion are all self-deterministic acts. In mental health care, adhering to treatment regimens may be at odds with the self-deterministic views of an individual. Supporting a person's ability to choose treatment becomes complex because of related issues of competency, informed consent, voluntary and involuntary commitment, and public safety; these issues are discussed later in this chapter.

PROTECTION OF PATIENT RIGHTS

Because people with psychiatric problems are vulnerable to mistreatment and abuse, laws have been passed that guarantee them legal protection. These laws offer protection of self-determinism, protection against discrimination in employment, and protection against mistreatment in health care settings.

Self-Determination Act

The *Patient Self-Determination Act* (PSDA) was implemented on December 1, 1991, as a part of the Omnibus Budget Reconciliation Act of 1990 and requires hospitals, health maintenance organizations, skilled nursing facilities, home health agencies, and hospices receiving Medicare and Medicaid reimbursement to inform patients at the time of admission of their right to be a central part of any and all health care decisions made about them or for them. Patients have the following rights:

- Be provided with information regarding advance care documents.
- Be asked at admission or enrollment whether they have an advance care document and that this fact be recorded in the medical record.
- Be provided with information on their rights to complete advance care documents and refuse medical care (Omnibus Budget Reconciliation Act, 1990).

The Act also requires health care institutions receiving Medicare and Medicaid reimbursement to educate health care personnel and the local community about advance care planning.

Advance Care Directives in Mental Health

At different times during the course of an illness, people with mental disorders may be unable to make sound decisions regarding their treatment and care. Fortunately, advance care directives legally protect them from their periodic poor decision-making abilities. A competent individual can make a decision about a treatment—a decision that can be honored even if the person is no longer able to make decisions. (See later discussion for how competency is determined.)

Advance care directives are written instructions for health care when individuals are incapacitated. Living wills and appointment directives, often referred to as power of attorney or health proxies, are recognized under state laws and their courts. A **living will** states what treatment should be omitted or refused in the event that a person is unable to make those decisions. A durable **power of attorney** for health care appoints a proxy, usually a relative or trusted friend, to make health care decisions on an individual's behalf if that person is incapacitated.

An advance directive does not need to be written, reviewed, or signed by an attorney. It must be witnessed by two people and notarized and applies only if the individual is unable to make his or her own decisions as a result of being incapacitated or if, in the opinion of two physicians, the person is otherwise unable to make decisions for him- or herself.

Psychiatric advance directives (PADs) are relatively new legal instruments and allow patients, while competent, to document their choices of treatment and care. This declaration must be made in advance and signed by the patient and two witnesses. Through the use of a PAD, individuals are empowered to direct their treatment such as choice of medication and hospitalization. Although a physician can override this declaration during times when the patient's decision-making capacity is clearly distorted because of mental illness, the patient must be informed first and the order made by the court. During periods of competency, the PAD can be revoked.

[handwritten margin note: Must be competent to change]

Bill of Rights for Mental Health Patients

Rights of people with mental disorders receive additional protection beyond that afforded to patients in other health care areas (Box 3.1). The *Mental Health Systems Act* [42 U.S.C. 9501 et seq.] of 1980 requires that each state review and revise, if necessary, its laws to ensure that mental health patients receive these human rights protections and services that they require.

BOX 3.1

Bill of Rights for Persons Receiving Mental Health Services

- The right to treatment and services under conditions that support the person's personal liberty and restrict such liberty only as necessary to comply with treatment needs, laws, and judicial orders.
- The right to an individualized, written, treatment or service plan (to be developed promptly after admission), treatment based on the plan, periodic review and reassessment of needs and appropriate revisions of the plan, including a description of services that may be needed after discharge.
- The right to ongoing participation in the planning of services to be provided and in the development and periodic revision of the treatment plan, and the right to be provided with a reasonable explanation of all aspects of one's own condition and treatment.
- The right to refuse treatment, except during an emergency situation, or as permitted under law in the case of a person committed by a court for treatment.
- The right not to participate in experimentation in the absence of the patient's informed, voluntary, written consent, the right to appropriate protections associated with such participation, the right to an opportunity to revoke such consent.
- The right to freedom from restraints or seclusion, other than during an emergency situation.

- The right to a humane treatment environment that affords reasonable protection from harm and appropriate privacy.
- The right to confidentiality of records.
- The right to access, upon request, one's own mental health care records.
- The right (in residential or inpatient care) to converse with others privately and to have access to the telephone and mails unless denial of access is documented as necessary for treatment.
- The right to be informed promptly, in appropriate language and terms, of the rights described in this section.
- The right to assert grievances with respect to infringement of the Bill of Rights, including the right to have such grievances considered in a fair, timely, and impartial procedure.
- The right of access to protection, service, and a qualified advocate in order to understand, exercise, and protect one's rights.
- The right to exercise the rights described in this section without reprisal, including reprisal in the form of denial of any appropriate, available treatment.
- The right to referral as appropriate to other providers of mental health services upon discharge.

From Title V of the Mental Health Systems Act [42 U.S.C. 9501 et seq.]. Retrieved from http://www4.law.cornell.edu/uscode/42/10841.html.

Americans with Disabilities Act and Job Discrimination

The *Americans With Disabilities Act* of 1990 (ADA) ensures that people with disabilities, such as severe mental disorders,

FAME & FORTUNE

Elizabeth Parsons Ware Packard (1816–1895)

Author and Social Reformer

PUBLIC PERSONA

Elizabeth Packard, social reformer in the latter half of the 19th century, lived in Chicago and later in Springfield, Illinois. She supported herself and her six children through her writings and books that exposed the abuse of patients committed to insane asylums of the day. After her children were grown, Elizabeth Packard lobbied legislators in the Illinois state capital on behalf of her reforms.

PERSONAL REALITIES

In 1864, Elizabeth Packard was committed to the Illinois State Hospital for the Insane based solely on her husband's assertion that her religious views were different from his. In reality, she was not sufficiently subordinate to her husband. Illinois law at the time permitted any married man to consign his wife to the asylum with no requirement other than consent of the asylum superintendent. Elizabeth Packard was incarcerated in the hospital for 3 years, during which time she rejected any treatment offered.

Source: Lightner, D. L. (1999). *Asylum, prison, and poorhouse: The writings and reform work of Dorothea Dix in Illinois.* Carbondale and Edwardsville, IL: Southern Illinois University Press.

have legal protection against discrimination in the workplace, housing, public programs, transportation, and telecommunications. An employer is free to select the most qualified applicant available, but if the most qualified person has a mental disorder, this law mandates that reasonable accommodations need to be made for that individual. Accommodations are any adjustments to a job or work environment, such as restructuring a job, modifying work schedules, and acquiring or modifying equipment (U.S. Equal Employment Opportunity Commission, 2013).

Internal Rights Protection Systems

Mental health care systems have **internal rights protection systems,** or mechanisms to combat any violation of their patients' rights. *Public Law 99-319, the Protection and Advocacy for Mentally Ill Individuals Act of 1986*, requires each state mental health provider to establish and operate a system that protects and advocates for the rights of individuals with mental illnesses and investigates any incidents of abuse and neglect.

External Advocacy Systems

Health organizations such as the American Hospital Association, American Healthcare Association, and the American Public Health Association serve as advocates for the rights and treatment of mental health patients and are a part of an **external advocacy system.** They are financially and administratively independent from the mental health agencies. These groups advocate through negotiation and recommendations but have no legal authority. They can resort to litigation that leads to lawsuits and consent decrees (legal mandates that are monitored by the U.S. Department of Justice) or, in some instances, a denial of accreditation to the health care institution by their certifying body.

Accreditation of Mental Health Care Delivery Systems

Patient rights are also assured of protection by an agency's **accreditation**, the recognition or approval of an institution according to the accrediting body's criteria. Accrediting bodies such as The Joint Commission require patient rights standards. The Centers for Medicare and Medicaid Services (CMS) sets patient rights standards for institutions seeking Medicare and Medicaid funding. Community mental health centers are not accredited by either the Joint Commission or CMS but by another agency, the Commission on Accreditation of Rehabilitation Facilities.

TREATMENT AND PATIENT RIGHTS

In caring for patients receiving mental health services or treatment, it is important for nurses to understand several issues related to the patient's rights to determine choices about his or her own treatment. These issues are related to competency, informed consent, least restrictive environment, and voluntary and involuntary treatment.

Competency

One of the most important concepts underlying the legal rights of individuals is competency to consent to or to refuse treatment. Although competency is a legal determination, it is not clearly defined across the states. It is generally agreed that **competence**, or the degree

to which the patient can understand and appreciate the information given during the consent process, refers to a patient's cognitive ability to process information at a specific time. A patient may be competent to make a treatment decision at one time and not be competent at another time. Competence is also decision specific, so that a patient may be competent to decide on a simple treatment with a relatively clear consequence but may not be competent to decide about a treatment with a complex set of outcomes. A competent patient can refuse any aspect of the treatment plan.

Competency is different from rationality, which is a characteristic of a patient's decision, not of the patient's ability to make a decision. An irrational decision is one that involves hurting oneself pointlessly, such as stopping recommended treatment even though symptoms return. A person who is competent may make what appears to be an irrational decision, and it cannot be overruled by health care providers; however, if a person is judged **incompetent** (i.e., unable to understand and appreciate the information given during the consent process), it is possible to force treatment on the individual. Strong arguments are, however, made against forced treatment under these circumstances. Forced treatment denigrates individuals, and according to self-determinism theory and recovery concepts, individuals are not as likely to experience treatment success if it is externally imposed.

How is it determined that a patient is competent? Mental health legal experts generally agree that four areas should be directly assessed (Applebaum, 2007). Table 3.1 outlines these assessment areas. A patient who is competent to give informed consent should be able to achieve the following:

- Communicate choices.
- Understand relevant information.
- Appreciate the situation and its consequences.
- Use a logical thought process to compare the risks and benefits of treatment options.

TABLE 3.1	DETERMINATION OF COMPETENCY	
Assessment Area	Definition	Patient Attributes
Communicate choices	Ability to express choices	Patient should be able to repeat what he or she has heard
Understand relevant information	Capacity to comprehend the meaning of the information given about treatment	Patient should be able to paraphrase understanding of treatment
Appreciate the situation and its consequence	Capacity to grasp what the information means specifically to the patient	Patient should be able to discuss the disorder, the need for treatment, the likely outcomes, and the reason the treatment is being suggested
Use a logical thought process to compare the risks and benefits of treatment options	Capacity to reach a logical conclusion consistent with the starting premise	Patient should be able to discuss logical reasons for the choice of treatment

Adapted from Applebaum, P. (2007). Assessment of patients' competence to consent to treatment. *New England Journal of Medicine*, 357(18), 1834–1840.

Informed Consent

Individuals seeking mental health care must provide **informed consent**, a legal procedure to ensure that the patient knows the benefits and costs of treatment. To provide informed consent for care, the patient must be given adequate information upon which to base decisions and actively participate in the decision-making process. Informed consent is not an option but is mandated by state laws. In most states, the law mandates that a mental health provider must inform a patient in such a way that an average reasonable person would be able to make an educated decision about the interventions.

Informed consent is complicated in mental health treatment. A patient must be competent to give consent, but the individual's decision-making ability often is compromised by the mental illness. This dilemma might be illustrated by a situation in which a person who is informed of medication side effects refuses treatment, not because of the potential negative impact of the medication but because he or she denies the illness outright. The health care provider knows that when the person begins taking the medication, the symptoms of the illness will subside, and the decision-making ability will return.

Most institutions have policies that outline the nursing responsibilities within the informed consent process. The nurse has a key role in the process of informed consent, from structuring the written informed consent document to educating the patient about a particular procedure. The nurse makes sure that consent has been obtained before any treatment is given. Informed consent is especially important in research projects involving experimental drugs or therapies.

Least Restrictive Environment

The right to refuse treatment is related to a larger concept—the right to be treated in the **least restrictive environment**, which means that an individual cannot be restricted to an institution when he or she can be successfully treated in the community. In 1975, the courts ruled that a person committed to psychiatric treatment had a right to be treated in the least restrictive environment (Dixon *v.* Weinberger, 1975). Medication cannot be given unnecessarily. An individual cannot be restrained or locked in a room unless all other "less restrictive" interventions are tried first.

Voluntary and Involuntary Treatment

Accessing the mental health delivery system is similar to seeking any other type of health care. Whether in a public or private system, the treatment setting is usually outpatient. Treatment strategies (e.g., medication, psychotherapy) are recommended and agreed on by both the provider and the individual. Arrangements for treatment and follow up are then made. The patient leaves the outpatient setting and is responsible for following the plan.

Inpatient treatment is generally reserved for patients who are acutely ill or have a forensic commitment. If hospitalization is required, the person enters the treatment facility, participates in the treatment planning process, and follows through with the treatment. The individual maintains all civil rights and is free to leave at any time even if it is against medical advice. In most settings, this type of admission is called a **voluntary admission**. If an individual is admitted to a public facility, the state statute may refer to the process as **voluntary commitment** rather than admission; however, in both instances, full legal rights are retained.

Involuntary commitment is the confined hospitalization of a person without the person's consent but with a court order. There are also legal provisions for people to be involuntarily committed to outpatient mental health facilities through state civil laws. Because involuntary commitment is a prerogative of the state agency, each state and the District of Columbia have separate commitment statutes; however, three common elements are found in most of these statutes. The individual must be (1) mentally disordered, (2) dangerous to self or others, or (3) unable to provide for basic needs (i.e., "gravely disabled").

Patients who are involuntarily committed have the right to receive treatment, but they also may have the right to refuse it. Arguments over the rights of civilly committed patients to refuse treatment first surfaced in 1975 when a federal district court judge issued a temporary restraining order prohibiting the use of psychotropic medication against the patient's will at a state hospital in Boston. Today, laws about commitment and refusal of medication vary from state to state. Many states recognize the rights of involuntarily committed patients to refuse medication (National Mental Health Information Center, 2007). The state trend is to grant patients the right to refuse treatment whether they are competent or incompetent.

Commitment procedures vary considerably among the states. Most have provisions for an emergency short-term hospitalization of 48 to 92 hours authorized by a certified mental health provider without court approval. At the end of that period, the individual either agrees to voluntary treatment or extended commitment procedures are begun. The judge must order the commitment, and the individual is afforded several legal rights, including notice of the proceedings, a full hearing (jury trial if requested) in which the government must prove the grounds for commitment, and the right to legal counsel at state expense.

NCLEXNOTE   Which patient is most likely a candidate for involuntary commitment? A patient who refuses to take medication or one who is singing in the street in the middle of the night disturbing the neighbors?

Answer: The patient who is singing in the night disturbing the neighbors. Rationale: Patients have a right to refuse medication in many states and provinces. Refusing medication does not pose an immediate danger to self or others. The patient who is singing in the street is more likely to be judged as a danger to self or to others.

PRIVACY AND CONFIDENTIALITY

In addition to issues related to self-determinism, privacy and confidentiality are rights that need to be protected for mental health patients. **Privacy** refers to that part of an individual's personal life that is not governed by society's laws and government intrusion. Protecting an individual from intrusion is a responsibility of health care providers. **Confidentiality** can be defined as an ethical duty of nondisclosure. Providers who receive confidential information must protect that information from being accessed by others and resist disclosing it. Confidentiality involves two people: the individual who discloses and the person with whom the information is shared. If confidentiality is broken, a person's privacy is also violated; however, a person's privacy can be violated but confidentiality maintained. For example, if a nurse observes an adult patient reading pornography alone in his or her room, the patient's privacy has been violated. If the patient asks the nurse not to tell anyone and the request is honored, confidentiality is maintained.

A **breach of confidentiality** is the release of patient information without the patient's consent in the absence of legal compulsion or authorization to release information (Wettstein, 1994). For example, discussing a patient's problem with one of his or her relatives without the patient's consent is a breach of confidentiality. Even sharing patient information with another professional who is not involved in the patient's care is a breach of confidentiality because the individual has not given permission for the information to be shared. Maintaining confidentiality is not as easy as it first appears. For example, family members are legally excluded from receiving any information about an adult member without consent even if that member is receiving care from the family. Ideally, a patient gives consent for information to be shared with the family or has psychiatric advance care directive.

HIPAA and Protection of Health Information

The Health Insurance Portability and Accountability Act of 1996 (HIPAA) provides legal protection in several areas of health care, including privacy and confidentiality. This act protects working Americans from losing existing health care coverage when changing jobs and increases opportunities for purchasing health care. It regulates the use and release of patient information, especially electronic transfer of health information. Effective April 2003, HIPAA regulations require patient authorization for the release of information with the exception of that required for treatment, payment, and health care administrative operations. The release of information related to psychotherapy requires patient permission. The underlying intent is to prevent the release of information to agencies not related to health care, such as employers, without the patient's consent. When information is released, the patient must agree to the exact information that is being disclosed, the purpose of disclosure, the recipient of the information, and an expiration date for the disclosure of information (U.S. Department of Health and Human Services, 2002).

The American Recovery and Reinvestment Act of 2009 includes several provisions affecting the management of health information. For the most part, this law focuses on maintaining privacy of electronic transfer and storage of health information and communication. In the clinical area, one way of maintaining privacy is by restricting access to records by staff members unless there is a specific reason such as caring for a patient.

Mandates to Inform

At certain times, health care professionals are legally obligated to breach confidentiality. When there is a judgment that the patient has harmed any person or is about to injure someone, professionals are mandated by law to report it to authorities. The legal "duty to warn" was a result of the 1976 decision of *Tarasoff v. Regents of the University of California*. In this case, a 26-year-old graduate student told university psychologists about his obsession with another student, Tatiana Tarasoff, whom he subsequently killed. Tatiana Tarasoff's parents initiated a separate civil action and brought suit against the therapist, the university, and the campus police, claiming that Tatiana's death was a result of negligence on the part of the defendants.

The plaintiffs claimed that the therapists should have warned Ms. Tarasoff that the graduate student presented a danger to her and that he should have been confined to a hospital. Both claims were originally dismissed in the lower courts, but in 1974, the California Supreme Court reversed the lower courts' decisions and said that Ms. Tarasoff should have been warned. The high court said that psychotherapists have a duty to warn the foreseeable victims of their patients' violent actions. Because of the outcry from professional mental health organizations, the court agreed to review the case, and in 1976, the original decision was revised by the ruling that psychotherapists have a duty to exercise reasonable care in protecting the foreseeable victims of their patients' violent actions. The results of this case have had far-reaching consequences and have influenced many decisions in the United States. Although many lawsuits have been based on the Tarasoff case, most have failed. Usually, if there are clear threats of violence toward others, the therapist is mandated to warn potential victims.

> **NCLEXNOTE**   What guides the intervention for a patient who tells the nurse that he (she) wants to hurt a family member: mandate to inform or HIPAA?
> Answer: Mandate to inform. Rationale: Because others are at risk for injury, the Tarasoff decision will prevail.

CRIMINAL JUDICIAL PROCESSES

In mental health, the term **forensic** pertains to legal proceedings and mandated treatment of persons with a mental illness. Individuals with mental illnesses are at higher risk for arrest than the general population (Fisher et al., 2011) and are more likely to have encounters with the criminal justice system and be convicted of a crime than those without a mental illness (Bradley-Engen, Cuddeback, Gayman, Morrissey, & Mancuso, 2010). Despite the large number of people with mental illnesses that commit crimes, the majority of the encounters with the justice system occur when individuals with mental illness are victims of crime (Ascher-Svanum, Nyhuis, Faries, Ball, & Kinon, 2010).

As the number of state hospitals was dramatically reduced beginning in the 1960s, the number of persons with mental illness incarcerated in jails and prisons increased. A large number of persons with mental illness are confined to U.S. prisons and jails. More than half of all prison and jail inmates have (or have had) a mental health problem (Thompson, 2011). It is estimated that approximately 705,600 state prison inmates, 78,800 federal prisoners, and 479,900 inmates in local jails have mental health problems (Thompson, 2011).

Individuals with mental illnesses are treated in a variety of forensic settings, including county jails, correctional facilities, psychiatric hospitals, and the community. Inpatient services in most state hospitals now focus on those individuals who commit crimes or who are charged with an offense. The number of admissions to state psychiatric hospitals is increasing for the first time since the 1970s because of an increase of forensic patients (Manderscheid, Atay, & Crider, 2009).

Stigma of Criminality

These patients suffer the combined effects of the stigma of mental illness and criminality. Although stigma is an issue for all persons with a mental illness, it is magnified for those who have committed a crime. There is often

reluctance on the part of mental health professionals to treat these patients, especially if murder and childhood sexual abuse are involved. Even if the worry is unfounded, clinicians express safety concerns for themselves and other patients and may refuse to care for these patients.

When nonforensic patients receive the maximum benefit from hospitalization, they are normally discharged into the community. For forensic patients, the community often wants a more stringent discharge threshold and unrealistically expects the hospital to guarantee compliance with community rules and structure. Treatment and the criminal justice systems are often in conflict with each other.

Fitness to Stand Trial

Once a mental illness is diagnosed in a person who has committed a crime, the individual's **fitness to stand trial** is determined. Fitness means that a person is able to consult with a lawyer with a reasonable degree of rational understanding of the facts of the alleged crime and of the legal proceedings as spelled out in the court case of *Dusky vs. U.S.* of 1960 (Beran & Tommey, 1979, p. 12). A person is found **unfit to stand trial (UST)** if, because of mental or physical condition, he or she is unable to understand the nature and purpose of the proceedings or to assist in the defense (West, 2010).

In most states, when an individual with a mental illness is found UST, hospitalization in a forensic mental health facility follows. The goal of this hospitalization is to help the person become "fit" to stand trial, not to treat the mental illness. Sometimes the patient's mental illness has to be treated to attain fitness. Simply stated, to be fit to stand trial, the person must be able to communicate with counsel and assist in the defense; be able to appreciate his or her presence in relation to time, place, and things; be able to understand that he or she is in a court of justice charged with a criminal offense; show an understanding of the charges and their consequences, as well as court procedures and the roles of the judge, jury, prosecutor, and defense attorney; and have sufficient memory to relate the circumstances surrounding the alleged criminal offense.

An individual cannot be "unfit" forever. If fitness cannot be attained usually within 1 year, a hearing is held, during which the facts of the alleged crime are presented to a judge who rules on the case. If the charges are dismissed, the judge could order a civil commitment. If there is sufficient evidence to convict, the individual could be sent back to the hospital for further treatment to attain fitness. The maximum length of this additional treatment is based on the severity of the charge. For those accused of sexual-related offenses (because of mental disorder), states usually have special statutes for hospitalization and discharge (e.g., registration and community notification).

Not Guilty But Mentally Ill

Once fitness to stand trial is established, the trial or hearing can proceed. One possible outcome is **not guilty by reason of insanity (NGRI)**. The accused is judged to not know right from wrong or to be unable to control his or her actions at the time of the crime. The rationale underlying this ruling is one of fairness. It is unfair to hold a person responsible if that individual does not know that the action is wrong or does not have control over his or her behavior.

Nearly all individuals found NGRI are also subject to involuntary commitment in a "secure" setting. The patient cannot leave hospital grounds without court approval. A person sentenced NGRI is given a date that is equal to the time or sentence to be served if he or she had been guilty of the crime.

Guilty but Mentally Ill

Different from NGRI, in which "not guilty" individuals are committed to the mental health system, **guilty but mentally ill (GBMI)** is a criminal conviction, and the person is sent to the correctional system. Mental illness is considered a factor in the crime but not to the extent that the individual is incapable of knowing right from wrong or controlling their actions. The sentence for the GBMI is the same type of determinate sentence any inmate receives. Before release, every effort is made to ensure that patients will receive proper follow-up care in the community and close monitoring by parole staff. Both NGRI and GBMI persons are treated for their mental disorders, but one is treated in jail and the other in a hospital. The conditions of release are different. Whereas individuals with a GBMI are subject to the correctional system's parole decisions, those with an NGRI are discharged from the hospital through the courts upon recommendations of the forensic mental health professionals.

Probation

Probation is a sentence of conditional or revocable release under the supervision of a probation officer for a specified time. For individuals with a mental illness who have committed minor offenses, probation is sometimes used instead of jail as long as care in a treatment facility can be arranged. If treatment and rehabilitation are successful, criminal charges may be dropped and a prison record avoided. Probation is also used when a criminal has served time and continued monitoring is needed after being released from the correctional facility.

Misconceptions Regarding Insanity Pleas

There are many misconceptions about the insanity plea. One is that the insanity defense provides a loophole through which criminals can escape punishment for illegal acts. In reality, the insanity defense is extremely difficult to use even in the cases of severely ill individuals. As a result, despite popular belief, the insanity defense is used in fewer than 1% of criminal cases

Countless newspaper articles, talk shows, and news commentaries concerning the insanity defense have bombarded the public. Some of the cases have been highly publicized. One such case was that of John Hinckley, who attempted to assassinate President Ronald Reagan in 1981 and who was found NGRI. On psychiatric examination, Hinckley was found to be living in a "fantasy world with magical and grandiose expectations of impressing and winning over" his love, actress Jodie Foster (Goldstein, 1995, p. 309). Hinckley attempted to commit a historic deed that would make him famous and unite him with the love object of his delusions. His acquittal stimulated public cries for reform of the insanity defense. Within 2.5 years of John Hinckley's acquittal, 34 states changed their insanity defense statutes to limit its use or to prevent the premature release of dangerous people.

ACCOUNTABILITY FOR NURSES AND OTHER MENTAL HEALTH CARE PROFESSIONALS

Nurses and other health care professionals are accountable for the care they provide in mental health as well as any other practice area.

Legal Liability in Psychiatric Nursing Practice

Malpractice is based on a set of torts (a civil wrong not based on contract committed by one person that causes injury to another). An **assault** is the threat of unlawful force to inflict bodily injury upon another. An assault must be imminent and cause reasonable apprehension in the individual. Battery is the intentional and unpermitted contact with another. **Medical battery**, intentional and unauthorized harmful or offensive contact, occurs when a patient is treated without informed consent. For example, a clinician who fails to obtain consent before performing a procedure is subject to being accused of medical battery. Also, failure to respect a patient's advance directives is considered medical battery. False imprisonment is the detention or imprisonment contrary to provision of the law. Facilities that do not discharge voluntarily committed patients upon request can be subject to this type of litigation.

Negligence is a breach of duty of reasonable care for a patient for whom a nurse is responsible that results in personal injuries. A clinician who does get consent but does not disclose the nature of the procedure and the risks involved is subject to a negligence claim. Five elements are required to prove negligence: duty (accepting assignment to care for patient), breach of duty (failure to practice according to acceptable standards of care), cause in fact (the injury would not have happened if the standards had been followed), cause in proximity (harm actually occurred within the scope of foreseeable consequence), and damages (physical or emotional injury caused by breach of standard of care). Simple mistakes are not negligent acts.

Lawsuits in Psychiatric Mental Health Care

Few lawsuits are filed against mental health clinicians and facilities compared with other health care areas. If psychiatric nurses are included in lawsuits, they are usually included in the lawsuit filed against agency. Common areas of litigation surround the nursing care of patients who are suicidal or violent. Maintaining and documenting an appropriate standard of care (see Chapter 6) can protect nurses from complicated legal proceedings. The following can help prevent negative outcomes of malpractice litigations:

- Evaluate risks, especially when privileges broaden or care is transferred.
- Document decisional processes and reasons for choices among alternatives.
- Involve family in important decisions.
- Make decisions within team model and document this shared responsibility.
- Adhere to agency's policy and procedures.
- Seek consultation and record input.

Nursing Documentation

Careful documentation is important both to help ensure protection of patient rights and for nurse accountability. Documentation can be handwritten or electronic. It is very common in psychiatric facilities that all disciplines record one progress note. Nursing documentation is based on nursing standards (see Chapter 6) and the policies of the particular facility. Many documentation styles are problem focused. That is, documentation is structured to address specific problems that are identified on the nursing care plan or interdisciplinary treatment plan. No matter the setting or structure of the documentation, nurses are responsible for documenting the following:

- Observations of the patient's subjective and objective physical, psychological, and social responses to mental disorders and emotional problems
- Interventions implemented and the patient's response
- Observations of therapeutic and side effects of medications
- Evaluation of outcomes of interventions

Particular attention should be paid to the reason the patient is admitted for care. If the person's initial problem was suicide or homicidal ideation, the patient should routinely be assessed for suicidal and homicidal thoughts even if the treatment plan does not specifically identify suicide and homicide as potential problems. Careful documentation is always needed for patients who are suicidal, homicidal, aggressive, or restrained in any way. Medications prescribed on an as-needed (PRN) basis also require a separate entry, including reason for administration, dosage, route, and response to the medication.

A patient record is the primary documentation of a patient's problems, verifies the behavior of the patient at the point of care, and describes the care provided. The patient record is considered a legal document. Courts consider acts not recorded as acts not done. Patients also have legal access to their records. For handwritten documentation, the entries should always be written in pen with no erasures. If an entry is corrected, it should be initialed by the person making the correction. All entries should be clear, well written, and void of jargon. Judgmental statements, such as "patient is manipulating staff" have no place in patients' records. Only meaningful, accurate, objective descriptions of behavior should be used. General, stereotypic statements, such as "had a good night" or "no complaints" are meaningless and should be avoided.

With the universal use of electronic records, meaningful documentation is sometimes more difficult. Many institutions require health care workers to enter observations, assessment data, and interventions into a template that requires a "click" in a box on the monitor screen. Additional narrative entries are usually required to provide quality, individualized care. Nurses are held to the same standards of practice and documentation when entering electronic data as when entering data a non-electronic record.

SUMMARY OF KEY POINTS

- The right of self-determination entitles all patients to refuse treatment, to obtain other opinions, and to choose other forms of treatment. It is one of the basic patients' rights established by Title II, Public Law 99-139, outlining the Universal Bill of Rights for Mental Health Patients.

- Laws and systems are established to protect the rights of people with mental health issues. Some of these include the Self-Determination Act, advance directives, a patient Bill of Rights, the Americans with Disabilities Act, internal rights protection systems, external advocacy systems, and accreditation of mental health care delivery systems.

■ The internal rights protection system and the external advocates combat violations of human rights.

■ Informed consent is another protective right that helps patients decide what can be done to their bodies and minds. It must be obtained from a competent individual before any treatment is begun to ensure that the information is not only received but understood.

■ A competent person can refuse any treatment. Incompetence is determined by the court when the patient cannot understand the information.

■ The right to the least restrictive environment entitles patients to be treated in the least restrictive setting and by the least restrictive interventions and protects patients from unnecessary confinement and medication.

■ Involuntary commitment procedures are specified at the state level. Patients who are involuntarily committed have the right to refuse treatment and medication.

■ Patient privacy is protected through HIPAA regulations related to the transfer and storage of information. A breach in confidentiality is legally mandated when there is a threat of violence toward others.

■ There are special legal terms and considerations for individuals who have mental disorders and commit crimes. Those determined to be *unfit to stand trial* are mentally incompetent and unable to understand the proceedings against them or assist in their own defense. These patients are committed to a mental health facility for treatment until they achieve fitness. Those determined to be *not guilty by reason of insanity* are those who demonstrate that they had no understanding of their actions and no control over them when they committed the crime. These patients are committed to a mental health facility for treatment and then discharged after treatment.

■ *Guilty but mentally ill* applies to those who demonstrate that they knew the wrongfulness of their actions and had the ability to act otherwise. These patients enter the correctional system and receive treatment for their disorder but are returned after treatment to serve their sentences. For mentally disordered sex offenders, states usually have special statutes for hospitalization and discharge. Prisoners who develop mental illness while in prison are transferred to a mental hospital, treated, and returned to prison to complete their sentences.

■ The goal for the person in a forensic setting is to coordinate mental health services and to provide a wide range of services that will help him or her successfully live within his or her community.

■ Nursing documentation is guided by practice standards and policies of the agency. Nurses are responsible for individualized documentation in both electronic and non-electronic health records.

CRITICAL THINKING CHALLENGES

1. Consider the relationship of self-determinism to competence by differentiating patients who are competent to give consent and those who are incompetent. Discuss the steps in determining whether a patient is competent to provide informed consent for a treatment.

2. Define competency to consent to or refuse treatment and relate the definition to the Self-Determination Act.

3. A patient is involuntarily admitted to a psychiatric unit and refuses all medication. After being unable to persuade the patient to take prescribed medication, the nurse documents the patient's refusal and notifies the prescriber. Should the nurse attempt to give the medication without patient consent? Support your answer.

4. A person who is homeless with a mental illness refuses any treatment. Although he is clearly psychotic and would benefit from treatment, he is not a danger to himself or others and seems to be able to provide for his basic needs. His family is desperate for him to be treated. What are the ethical issues underlying this situation?

5. Discuss the purposes of living wills and health proxies. Discuss their use in psychiatric–mental health care.

6. Identify the legal and ethical issues underlying the Tarasoff case and mandates to inform.

7. Compare the authority and responsibilities of the internal rights protection system with those of the external advocacy system.

8. Describe the differences between UST, NGRI, and GBMI. What are the criteria to be met by patients who are UST before they are determined to be fit to stand trial?

 Nuts: 1987. Starring Barbra Streisand, Richard Dreyfuss, Maureen Stapleton, Eli Wallach, and Robert Webber. A strong-willed, high-priced prostitute is accused of manslaughter. Her family and attorney want her to plead guilty by reason of insanity. The movie revolves around the family's attempt to have her declared incompetent to stand trial, which would commit her to a mental health center before she can go to trial. She insists on proving her sanity, and to discover the truth, her lawyer must battle his prejudice and her inexplicable belligerence.

Viewing Points: Watch how the family members attempt to use the competency hearings for maintaining family secrets.

REFERENCES

Applebaum, P. (2007). Assessment of patients' competence to consent to treatment. *New England Journal of Medicine, 357*(18), 1834–1840.

Ascher-Svanum, H., Nyhuis, A. W., Faries, D. E., Ball, D. E., & Kinon, B. J. (2010). Involvement in the U.S. criminal justice system and cost implications for persons treated for schizophrenia. *BMC Psychiatry, 10,* 11.

Beran, N. J., & Tommey, B. G. (1979). Mentally ill offenders and the criminal justice system. In Issues in forensic services (p. 1–23). New York: Proeger Publishers, Proeger Special Studios.

Bradley-Engen, M. S., Cuddeback, G. S., Gayman, M. D., Morrissey, J. P., & Mancuso, D. (2010). Trends in state prison admission of offenders with serious mental illness. *Psychiatric Services, 61*(12), 1263–1265.

Deci, E. L., & Ryan, R. M. (2012). Self-determination theory in health care and its relations to motivational interviewing: A few comments. *The International Journal of Behavioral Nutrition and Physical Activity, 9,* 24. http://www.ijbnapa.org/content/9/1/24

Dixon *v.* Weinberger, 405 F. Supp. 974 (D. D. C. 1975).

Fisher, W. H., Simon, L., Roy-Bujnowski, K., Grudzinskas, A., Wolff, N., Crockett, E., & Banks, S. (2011). Risk of arrest among public mental health services recipients and the general public. *Psychiatric Services, 62*(1), 67–72.

Goldstein, R. (1995). Paranoids in the legal system: The litigious paranoid and the paranoid criminal. *Psychiatric Clinics of North America, 18*(2), 303–315.

Manderscheid, R. W., Atay, J. E., & Crider, R. A. (2009). Changing trends in state psychiatric hospital use from 2002 to 2005. *Psychiatric Services, 60*(1), 29–34.

National Mental Health Information Center. (2007). *Know your rights.* Center for Mental Health Service. Substance Abuse and Mental Health Services Administration. Retrieved March 8, 2007, from http://mentalhealth.Samhoa.gov

Omnibus Budget Reconciliation Act of 1990. Public Law No. 101–158, Paragraph 4206, 4751.

Tarasoff v. Regents of the University of California, 551P. 2d 334 (Cal. 1976).

Thompson, M. (2011). Gender, race, and mental illness in the criminal justice system. *Corrections & mental health: An update of the National Institute of Corrections.* National Institute of Corrections. Retrieved from http://community.nicic.gov/blogs/mentalhealth/archive/2011/03/02/gender-race-and-mental-illness-in-the-criminal-justice-system.aspx.

U.S. Department of Health and Human Services. (2002). Standards for privacy of individually identifiable health information; final rule. *Federal Register, 65,* 53182–53273.

U.S. Equal Employment Opportunity Commission, Office of the Americans with Disabilities Act. (2013). *The Americans with Disabilities Act: Questions and answers.* Washington, DC: U.S. Government Printing Office. Retrieved from www.eeoc.gov.

West, T. (Ed.). (2010). West Illinois criminal law and procedure, 2010 edition (pp. 640–641). Chicago, IL: Thompson Reuters.

Wettstein, R. (1994). Confidentiality. In J. Oldham & M. Riba (Eds.), *Review of psychiatry* (Vol. *13,* pp. 343–364). Washington, DC: American Psychiatric Press.

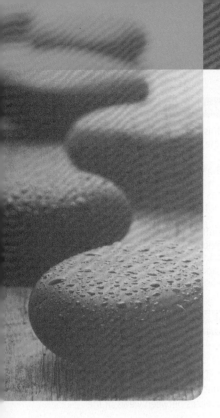

UNIT II
PSYCHIATRIC-MENTAL HEALTH NURSING FRAMEWORKS

4
Ethics, Standards, and Nursing Frameworks

Mary Ann Boyd

KEY CONCEPTS

- autonomy
- beneficence

- biopsychosocial framework
- standardized nursing language

LEARNING OBJECTIVES

After studying this chapter, you will be able to:

1. Identify ethical frameworks used in psychiatric nursing practice.

2. Delineate the scope and standards of psychiatric–mental health nursing practice.

3. Discuss the impact of psychiatric–mental health nursing professional organizations on practice.

4. Integrate the biopsychosocial framework within the wellness and recovery models.

5. Discuss the basic tools of psychiatric nursing.

6. Discuss selected challenges of psychiatric–mental health nursing.

KEY TERMS

- advanced practice psychiatric–mental health registered nurse • clinical reasoning • fidelity • justice • nonmaleficence • nursing process • paternalism • psychiatric–mental health registered nurse • reflection • scope and standards of practice • veracity

This chapter opens with a discussion of the ethical concepts psychiatric nurses use on a daily basis. Integral to the understanding of the day-to-day practice of psychiatric–mental health nursing, the scope and standards of practice are then highlighted. This chapter integrates the biopsychosocial framework into the recovery and wellness models. The discussion of the challenges of psychiatric

nursing sets the stage for the rest of the text through an overview of the dynamic nature of this specialty.

ETHICS OF PSYCHIATRIC NURSING

Psychiatric–mental health nursing actions are guided by the *Guide to the Code of Ethics for Nurses* (Box 4.1)

BOX 4.1

Code of Ethics for Nurses

1. The nurse practices with compassion and respect for the inherent dignity, worth, and unique attributes of every person.
2. The nurse's primary commitment is to the patient, whether an individual, family, group, community, or population.
3. The nurse promotes, advocates for, and strives to protects the rights, health, and safety of the patients.
4. The nurse has authority, accountability, and responsibility for nursing practice; makes decisions, and takes action consistent with the obligation to promote health and to provide optimal care.
5. The nurse owes the same duties to self as to others, including the responsibility to promote health and safety, preserve wholeness of character and integrity maintain competence, and continue personal and professional growth.
6. The nurse participates in establishing, maintaining, and improving through individual and collective effort, establishes, maintains, and improves the ethical environment of the work setting and conditions of employment that are conducive to safe, quality health care.
7. The nurse in all roles and settings, advances the profession through research and scholarly inquiry, professional standards development, and the generation of both nursing and health policy.
8. The nurse collaborates with other health professionals and the public to protect human rights, promote health diplomacy, and reduce health disparities.
9. The profession of nursing, collectively through its professional organizations, must articulate nursing values, maintain the integrity of the profession, and integrate principles of social justice into nursing and health policy.

BOX 4.2

Basic Questions for Ethical Decision Making

- What do I know about this patient situation?
- What do I know about the patient's values and moral preferences?
- What assumptions as I making that need more data to clarify?
- What are my own feelings (and values) about the situation, and how might they be influencing how I view and respond to this situation?
- Are my own values in conflict with those of the patient?
- What else do I need to know about this case, and where can I obtain this information?
- What can I never know about this case?
- Given my primary obligation to the patient, what should I do to be ethical?

Davis, A. (2008). Provision two. In M. Fowler (Ed.). *Guide to the code of ethics for nursing: Interpretation and application* (p. 18). Washington, DC: Nursebooks.org.

NCLEXNOTE   Be prepared to think in terms of patient scenarios that depict the principles of beneficence versus autonomy and identify differences between views of the patient and nurse.

(ANA, 2015). The *Code* serves to inform both nurses and society of the profession's ethical expectations and requirements and provides a framework within which nurses can make ethical decisions. Psychiatric nurses face ethical problematic situations daily. To determine the best ethical action, the nurse can reflect on a series of questions, outlined in Box 4.2.

Autonomy and beneficence are fundamental ethical concepts.

KEYCONCEPTS   According to the principle of **autonomy**, each person has the fundamental right of self-determination. According to the principle of **beneficence**, the health care provider uses knowledge of science and incorporates the art of caring to develop an environment in which individuals achieve their maximal health care potential.

These principles can conflict when the patient is being guided by the principle of autonomy and the nurse by the principle of beneficence. For example, a patient wants to stop taking medication (autonomy), and the nurse urges the patient to continue (beneficence).

Other ethical principles that guide mental health care include justice, nonmaleficence, paternalism, veracity, and fidelity. **Justice** is the duty to treat all fairly, distributing the risks and benefits equally. Justice becomes an issue in mental health when a segment of a population does not have access to health care. Basic goods should be distributed, so that the least advantaged members of society are benefited. **Nonmaleficence** is the duty to cause no harm, both individual and for all. **Paternalism** is the belief that knowledge and education authorize professionals to make decisions for the good of the patient. Mandatory use of seat belts and motorcycle helmets is an example of paternalism. This principle can be in direct conflict with the mental health recovery belief of self-determinism (see Chapter 3). **Veracity** is the duty to tell the truth. This is easier said than done. Patients may ask questions when the truth is unknown. For example, if I take my medication, will the voices go away? **Fidelity** is faithfulness to obligations and duties. It is keeping promises. Fidelity is important in establishing trusting relationships.

NCLEXNOTE   Tracking ethical decisions that the psychiatric nurse encounters in the inpatient versus outpatient setting may be a topic for examination.

SCOPE AND STANDARDS OF PRACTICE

The practice of psychiatric nursing is regulated by law but guided by **scope and standards of practice**.

The legal authority to practice nursing is granted by the states and provinces, but scope and standards of practice are defined by the profession of nursing. The ANA and the psychiatric nursing organizations (discussed later in this chapter) collaborate in defining the boundaries of psychiatric-mental health nursing and informing society about the parameters of practice. The standards are authoritative statements that describe the responsibilities for which the practitioners are accountable.

Scope of Psychiatric–Mental Health Nursing Areas of Concern

The areas of concern for the psychiatric–mental health nurse include a wide range of actual and potential mental health problems or psychiatric disorders, such as emotional stress or crisis, self-concept changes, developmental issues, physical symptoms that occur with psychological changes, and symptom management of patients with mental disorders. To understand the problem and select an appropriate intervention, integration of knowledge from the biologic, psychological, and social domains is necessary.

Standards of Practice

Six standards of practice are organized according to the nursing process and include: assessment, diagnosis, outcome identification, planning, implementation, and evaluation (Box 4.3). The **nursing process** serves as the foundation for clinical decision making and provides a framework for nursing practice.

Each of these six standards includes competencies for which **Psychiatric-Mental Health Registered Nurse (PMH-RN)** and **Advanced Practice Psychiatric-Mental Health Registered Nurses (PMH-APRN)** are accountable. The fifth standard, implementation, has several subcategories that define standards for specific interventions. These standards of practice define the parameters of psychiatric-mental health nursing practice. It is important that nurses are prepared to practice according to these standards. Nurses ultimately are held accountable by society for practicing according to their standards.

BOX 4.3
Standards of Practice

STANDARD 1. ASSESSMENT
The PMH registered nurse collects and synthesizes comprehensive health data that are pertinent to the healthcare consumer's health and/or situation.

STANDARD 2. DIAGNOSIS
The PMH registered nurse analyzes the assessment data to determine diagnoses, problems, and areas of focus for care and treatment, including level of risk.

STANDARD 3. OUTCOMES IDENTIFICATION
The PMH registered nurse identifies expected outcomes and the healthcare consumer's goals for a plan individualized to the healthcare consumer or to the situation.

STANDARD 4. PLANNING
The PMH registered nurse develops a plan that prescribes strategies and alternatives to assist the healthcare consumer in attainment of expected outcomes.

STANDARD 5. IMPLEMENTATION
The PMH registered nurse implements the specified plan.

Standard 5A Coordination of Care
The PMH registered nurse coordinates care delivery.

Standard 5B Health Teaching and Health Promotion
The PMH registered nurse employs strategies to promote health and a safe environment.

Standard 5C Consultation
The PMH advanced practice registered nurse provides consultation to influence the identified plan, enhance the abilities of other clinicians to provide services for healthcare consumers, and effect change.

Standard 5D Prescriptive Authority and Treatment
The PMH advanced practice registered nurse uses prescriptive authority, procedures, referrals, treatments, and therapies in accordance with state and federal laws and regulations.

Standard 5E Pharmacological, Biological, and Integrative Therapies
The PMH advanced practice registered nurse incorporates knowledge of pharmacological, biological, and complementary interventions with applied clinical skills to restore the healthcare consumer's health and prevent further disability.

Standard 5F Milieu Therapy
The PMH advanced practice registered nurse provides, structures, and maintains a safe, therapeutic, recovery-oriented environment in collaboration with healthcare consumers, families, and other healthcare clinicians.

Standard 5G Therapeutic Relationship and Counseling
The PMH registered nurse uses the therapeutic relationship and counseling interventions to assist healthcare consumers in their individual recovery journeys by improving and regaining their previous coping abilities, fostering mental health, and preventing mental disorder and disability.

Standard 5H Psychotherapy
The PMH advanced practice registered nurse conducts individual, couples, group, and family psychotherapy using evidence-based psychotherapeutic frameworks and the nurse-client therapeutic relationship.

STANDARD 6. EVALUATION
The PMH registered nurse evaluates progress toward attainment of expected outcomes.

Standards of Professional Performance

Ten standards of professional performance for psychiatric-mental health nurses follow the six standards of practice. These standards define and inform society about the professional role of psychiatric-mental health nurses and include ethics, education, evidence-based practice and research, quality of practice, communication, leadership, collaboration, professional practice evaluation, resource utilization, and environmental health. Each standard of performance includes expected competencies (ANA et al., 2014) (Table 4.1).

Levels of Practice

There are two levels of psychiatric-mental health nursing practice. The first level is the PMH-RN with educational preparation within a bachelor's degree, associate's degree, or a diploma program. The next level is the PMH-APRN with educational preparation within a master's degree or doctoral degree program. At the PMH-APRN level, two sub-categories exist including the mental health clinical specialist (PMHCNS) and psychiatric-mental health nurse practitioner (PMHMP) (Box 4.4).

Psychiatric–Mental Health Nursing Practice

According to *the Psychiatric–Mental Health Nursing: Scope and Standards of Practice*, the **psychiatric–mental health nurse** is a registered nurse who demonstrates specialized competence and knowledge, skills, and abilities in caring for persons with mental health issues and problems and psychiatric disorders. Competency is obtained through both education and experience. The preferred educational preparation is at the baccalaureate level with

---

BOX 4.4

Clinical Activities of Psychiatric–Mental Health Nurses

PSYCHIATRIC–MENTAL HEALTH REGISTERED NURSE
Health promotion and health maintenance
Intake screening, evaluation, and triage
Case management
Provision of therapeutic and safe environments
Milieu therapy
Promotion of self-care activities
Administration of psychobiologic treatment and monitoring responses
Complementary interventions
Crisis intervention and stabilization
Psychiatric rehabilitation

ADVANCED PRACTICE REGISTERED NURSE
Psychopharmacological interventions
Psychotherapy
Community interventions
Case management
Program development and management
Clinical supervision
Consultation and liaison

---

credentialing by the American Nurses Credentialing Center (ANCC) or a recognized certification organization. (ANA et al., 2014).

Nursing practice at this level is "characterized by the use of the nursing process to treat people with actual or potential mental health problems, psychiatric disorders and co-occurring psychiatric and substance use disorders (ANA 2014, pg. 25). By using the nursing process, the PMH-RN promotes and fosters health and safety, assesses dysfunction and areas of strength, and assists individuals in achieving personal recovery goals. The nurse performs a wide range of interventions, including

TABLE 4.1	STANDARDS OF PROFESSIONAL PERFORMANCE	
Standard	**Area of Performance**	**Description**
Standard 7	Ethics	Integrates ethical provisions in all areas of practice.
Standard 8	Education	Attains knowledge and competency that reflect current nursing practice.
Standard 9	Evidence-Based Practice & Research	Integrates evidence and research findings into practice.
Standard 10	Quality of Practice	Systematically enhances the quality and effectiveness of nursing practice.
Standard 11	Communication	Communicates effectively in a variety of formats in all areas of practice.
Standard 12	Leadership	Provides leadership in the professional practice setting and the profession.
Standard 13	Collaboration	Collaborates with the healthcare consumer, family, interprofessional health team, and others in the conduct of nursing practice.
Standard 14	Professional Practice Evaluation	Evaluates one's own practice in relation to the professional practice standards and guidelines, relevant statutes, rules, and regulations.
Standard 15	Resource Utilization	Considers factors related to safety, effectiveness, cost, and impact on practice in the planning and delivery of nursing services.
Standard 16	Environmental Health	Practices in an environmentally safe and healthy manner.

From American Nurses Association, American Psychiatric Nurses Association & International Society of Psychiatric–Mental Health Nurses (2014). *Psychiatric–Mental Health Nursing: Scope and Standards of Practice*, 2nd Edition. Silver Spring, MD: Nursesbooks.org.

health promotion and health maintenance strategies, intake screening and evaluation and triage, case management, milieu therapy, promotion of self-care activities, psychobiologic inter-ventions, complementary interventions, health teaching, counseling, crisis care, and psychiatric rehabilitation. An overview of psychiatric nursing interventions is presented in Unit 3.

Advanced Practice

The PMH-APRN is also a licensed registered nurse but is educationally prepared at the master's level and is nationally certified as a clinical nurse specialist or a psychiatric nurse practitioner by the ANCC. The DNP (doctorate in nursing practice) requires advanced education in systems function, analysis, health policy, and advocacy may be at the PMH-RN level (RN administrators or educators) or at the APRN level (ANA et al., 2014). Researchers are prepared at the highest education level preparation with a doctorate in nursing science (DNS, DNSc) or a doctor of philosophy (PhD) degree.

Psychiatric–Mental Health Nursing Organizations

Whereas the establishment and reinforcement of standards go a long way toward legitimizing psychiatric–mental health nursing, professional organizations provide leadership in shaping mental health care. They do so by providing a strong voice for meaningful legislation that promotes quality patient care and advocates for maximal use of nursing skills.

The ANA is one such organization. Although its focus is on addressing the emergent needs of nursing in general, the ANA supports psychiatric–mental health nursing practice through liaison activities, such as advocating for psychiatric–mental health nursing at the national and state levels and working closely with psychiatric–mental health nursing organizations.

The APNA and the ISPN are two organizations for psychiatric nurses that focus on mental health care. The APNA is the largest psychiatric–mental health nursing organization, with the primary mission of advancing psychiatric–mental health nursing practice; improving mental health care for culturally diverse individuals, families, groups, and communities; and shaping health policy for the delivery of mental health services. The ISPN consists of four specialist divisions: the Association of Child and Adolescent Psychiatric Nurses, International Society of Psychiatric Consultation Liaison Nurses, Society for Education and Research in Psychiatric–Mental Health Nursing, and Adult and Geropsychiatric-Mental Health Nurses. The purpose of ISPN is to unite and strengthen the presence and the voice of psychiatric–mental health nurses and to promote quality care for individuals and

families with mental health problems. The International Nurses Society on Addictions (INTNSA) is committed to the prevention, intervention, treatment, and management of addictive disorders. These organizations have annual meetings at which new research is presented. Student memberships are available.

THE BIOPSYCHOSOCIAL FRAMEWORK

The holistic, biopsychosocial model (Fig. 4.1) is well recognized as an organizing framework for understanding the interactive domains of an individual's mental health and matching appropriate interventions with patient's needs. This model is easily integrated with the recovery and wellness models and guides recovery-oriented care. The biopsychosocial framework is useful in standardized nursing languages such as NANDA International/Nursing Interventions Classification (NIC)/Nursing Outcomes Classification (NOC), Clinical Care Classification, and the Omaha system (Martin, 2005; Saba, 2012; Schwirian, 2013).

> **KEYCONCEPT**   The **biopsychosocial framework** consists of three separate but interdependent domains: biologic, psychological, and social. Each domain has an independent knowledge and treatment focus but interacts and is mutually interdependent with the other domains.

Biologic Domain

The *biologic* domain consists of the biologic theories related to mental disorders and problems as well as *all* of the biologic activity related to other health problems. Biologic theories and concepts also relate to functional

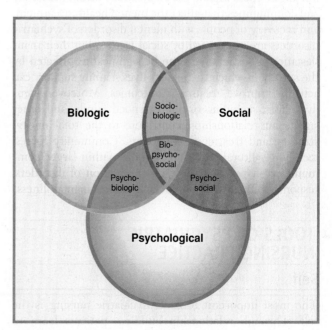

FIGURE 4.1 The biopsychosocial model.

health patterns such as exercise, sleep, and adequate nutrition to mental health conditions. In addition, the neurobiologic theories also serve as a basis for understanding and administering pharmacologic agents (see Chapters 6 and 10).

Psychological Domain

The *psychological* domain contains the theoretical basis of the psychological processes—thoughts, feelings, and behavior (intrapersonal dynamics) that influence one's emotion, cognition, and behavior. The psychological and nursing sciences generate theories and research that are critical in understanding patients' symptoms and responses to mental disorders. Although there are neurobiologic changes in mental disorders, symptoms are psychological. For example, even though manic behavior is caused by dysfunction in the brain, there are no laboratory tests to confirm a diagnosis, only a pattern of behavior.

Many psychiatric nursing interventions are behavioral, such as cognitive approaches, behavior therapy, and patient education. Therapeutic communication techniques require nurses to develop awareness of their own, as well as their patients', internal feelings and behavior. For mental health nurses, understanding their own and their patients' intrapersonal dynamics and motivation is critical in developing a therapeutic relationship (see Chapter 7).

Social Domain

The *social* domain includes theories that account for the influence of social forces encompassing the patient, family, and community within cultural settings. Social and nursing sciences explain the connections within the family and communities that affect the mental health, treatment, and recovery of people with mental disorders. Psychiatric disorders are not caused by social factors, but their manifestations and treatment can be significantly affected by the society in which the patient lives. Family support can actually improve treatment outcomes. Moreover, family factors, including origin, extended family, and other significant relationships, contribute to the total understanding and treatment of patients. Community forces, including cultural and ethnic groups within larger communities, shape the patient's manifestation of disorders, response to treatment, and overall view of mental illness.

TOOLS OF PSYCHIATRIC NURSING PRACTICE

Self

The most important tool of psychiatric nursing is the self. Through relationship building, patients learn to trust the nurse, who then guides, teaches, and advocates

for quality care and treatment. Throughout this book, the patient–nurse relationship is emphasized.

Clinical Reasoning and Reflection

Sound **clinical reasoning** depends on the critical thinking skills and reflection. During critical thinking activities, such as problem solving and decision making, nurses analyze evaluate, explain, infer, and interpret biopsychosocial data. Some critical thinking activities, such as nursing assessments, take time, but many decisions are moment-to-moment, such as deciding whether a patient can leave a unit or whether a patient should receive a medication.

Reflection involves continual self-evaluation through observing, monitoring, and judging nursing behaviors with the goal of providing ideal interventions. Reflection skills are used in all aspects of psychiatric nursing practice, from enhancing of self awareness and examining nurse–patient interactions to evaluation of the system of care.

Interdisciplinary Care

The psychiatric–mental health nurse can expect to collaborate with other professionals and the patient in all settings. In the hospital, a patient may see a psychiatrist or psychiatric nurse practitioner who treats the symptoms and prescribes the medication; a case manager who coordinates care; a psychiatric social worker for individual psychotherapy; a psychiatric nurse for management of responses related to the mental disorder, administration of medication, and monitoring side effects; and an occupational therapist for transition into the workplace. In the community clinic, a patient may meet weekly with a therapist, monthly with a mental health provider who prescribes medication, and twice a week with a group leader in a day treatment program. All of these professionals bring a specialized skill to the patient's care.

Plan of Care

Just like patients in medical–surgical settings, patients receiving psychiatric mental health services have written plans of care. The patient and family (if appropriate) should be a participant in the development of the plan. If only nursing care is being provided, such as in-home care, a recovery-oriented nursing care plan may be used. If other disciplines are providing services to the same patient, which often occurs in a hospital, an interdisciplinary recovery plan may be used with or instead of a traditional nursing care plan. When an interdisciplinary plan is used, components of the nursing care plan should always be easily identified. The nurse provides the care that is judged to be within the scope of practice of the psychiatric–mental health nurse. Thus, the traditional nursing care plan may or may not be used, depending on institutional policies.

Whether a nursing care plan or an interdisciplinary recovery plan is used, these plans are important because they are individualized to a patient's needs. They are sometimes approved by third-party payers who reimburse the cost of the service. In this text, the emphasis is on developing nursing care plans because they serve as a basis of practice and can be included in a multidisciplinary or interdisciplinary individual treatment plan.

CHALLENGES OF PSYCHIATRIC NURSING

The challenges of psychiatric nursing are increasing. New knowledge is being generated, technology is shaping health care into new dimensions, and nursing practice is becoming more specialized and autonomous. This section discusses a few of the challenges.

Knowledge Development, Dissemination, and Application

Knowledge is rapidly expanding in the psychiatric–mental health field. Genetic research has opened a new area of investigation into the etiology of several disorders such as schizophrenia, bipolar disorders, dementia, and autism. Psychoneuroimmunology is investigating the role of the immune system in the development of mental disorders. The presence of comorbid medical disorders gains increasing importance in the treatment of mental disorders. For example, hypertension, hypothyroidism, hyperthyroidism, and diabetes mellitus all affect the treatment of psychiatric disorders. The challenge for psychiatric nurses today is to stay abreast of the advances in total health care in order to provide safe, competent care to individuals with mental disorders.

Additional challenges for psychiatric nurses include updating their knowledge, so that significant results of studies can be applied to the care of patients. Accessing new information through journals, electronic databases, and continuing education programs takes time and vigilance but provides a sound basis for application of new knowledge.

Overcoming Stigma

Nurses can play an important role in dispelling myths of mental illnesses. Stigma often prevents individuals from seeking help for mental health problems (see Chapter 1). Reducing stigma is every nurse's responsibility, whether or not the nurse practices psychiatric nursing. To reduce the burden of mental illness and improve access to care,

nurses can educate all of their patients about the etiology, symptoms, and treatment of mental illnesses.

Integration of Mental Health Care and Medical Care

There was a time when psychiatric nursing care was viewed as being separate from medical nursing. This is no longer true. Even though the focus is on mental health issues, the psychiatric nurse practices from a holistic perspective and considers the medical needs of the patient and their impact on the individual's mental health. The practice of psychiatric nursing is even more challenging as mental health promotion approaches include wellness concepts and approaches.

Health Care Delivery System Challenges

Additional continuing challenges for psychiatric nurses include providing nursing care within integrated community-based services where culturally competent, high-quality nursing care is needed to meet the emerging mental health care needs of patients. In caring for patients who require support from the social welfare system in the form of housing, job opportunities, welfare, and transportation, nurses need to be knowledgable about these systems. Moreover, in some settings, the nurse may be the only one who has a background in medical disorders, such as human immunodeficiency virus, acquired immunodeficiency syndrome, and other somatic health problems. Assertive community treatment reduces inpatient service use, promotes continuity of outpatient care, and increases the stability of people with serious mental illnesses. The nurse is involved in moving the currently fragmented health care system toward one focusing on consumer needs.

Impact of Technology and Electronic Health Records

Technologic advances have an unprecedented impact on the delivery of psychiatric nursing care and present new challenges. With the use of electronic health records, protection of patient confidentiality is more difficult in some ways. Patient records, once stored in remote areas and rarely viewed, are now readily available and easily accessed. Nurses need to be vigilant in maintaining privacy and confidentiality.

Electronic documentation enables nursing terminologies to be standardized and readily available to the nurse. The advantage of a standardized nursing language is improved patient care through better communication among nurses and other disciplines, increased visibility of nursing interventions, enhanced data collection, useful

TABLE 4.2	EXAMPLES OF THE RELATIONSHIP OF THE BIOPSYCHOSOCIAL MODEL TO STRUCTURED NURSING LANGUAGES		
	Interventions		
Nursing Language	*Biologic*	*Psychological*	*Social*
NANDA International, NIC, and NOC *Diagnosis:* Insomnia	Encourage use of sleep medications that do not contain REM sleep suppressors.	Assist to eliminate bedtime stressors.	Regulate environmental stimuli.
Clinical Care Classification (CCC) *Diagnosis:* Sleep Pattern Disturbance	Care related to improving pattern of sleep.	Teach sleep pattern control.	Manage sleep pattern control.
Omaha System *Diagnosis:* Insomnia	Take medication therapy as prescribed.	Establish routine. Use guided imagery.	Use community resources.

Saba, V. K. (2007). *Clinical care classification (CCC) system. A guide to nursing documentation.* New York: Springer Publishing Company.

Smith, K. J. & Craft-Rosenberg, M. (2010). Using NANDA, NIC, NOC in an undergraduate nursing practicum. *Nurse Educator*, 35(4), 162–166.

Martin, K. S. (2005). *The Omaha system: A key to practice, documentation, and information management* (2nd ed). St. Louis: Elsevier Saunders.

outcome evaluations, and greater adherence to standards of care (Schwirian, 2013).

> **KEYCONCEPT** A **standardized nursing language** is readily understood by all nurses to describe care. It provides a common means of communication.

There are several terminology sets being evaluated for use in electronic records (Schwirian, 2013). Table 4.2 provides an example of how some of these standardized languages relate to the biopsychosocial framework. These terminologies vary in their scope of practice and their applicability to psychiatric nursing practice. For example, NANDA International/NIC/NOC is more inclusive of mental health phenomena than the Perioperative Nursing Data Set (PNDS). To be useful in psychiatric nursing, standardized languages must specifically address re-sponses to mental disorders and emotional problems.

Telemedicine is a reality and takes many forms, from communicating with remote sites to completing educational programs. It is important that patients have the opportunity to use technology to learn about their disorders and treatment. Because many of the disorders can affect cognitive functioning, it is also important that software programs be developed that can be used by these individuals to facilitate cognitive functioning.

SUMMARY OF KEY POINTS

■ Standards for ethical behaviors for professional nurses are set by national professional organizations such as the ANA.

■ There are several ethical principles to consider when providing psychiatric nursing care, including autonomy, beneficence, justice, nonmaleficence, paternalism, veracity, and fidelity.

■ *Psychiatric-Mental Health Nursing: Scope and Standards of Practice, published in 2014,* establishes the areas of concern, standards of practice according to the nursing process, and standards of professional performance and differentiates between the functions of the basic and advanced practice nurse.

■ Several professional nursing organizations provide leadership in shaping mental health care, including the ANA, the APNA, ISPN, and INTNSA.

■ The biopsychosocial framework focuses on the three separate but interdependent dimensions of biologic, psychological, and social factors in the assessment and treatment of mental disorders. This comprehensive and holistic approach to mental disorders is the foundation for effective psychiatric–mental health nursing practice is integrated into recovery and wellness models.

■ Nursing care plans and interdisciplinary treatment plans are written plans of care that are developed for each patient. Clinical reasoning skills are needed for developing and revising these tools.

■ The psychiatric–mental health nurse interacts with other disciplines and many times acts as a coordinator in the delivery of care. There is always a plan of care for a patient, but it may be a nursing care plan or an individualized treatment plan that includes other disciplines.

■ New challenges facing psychiatric nurses are emerging. Interpretation of research findings will assume new importance in the care of individuals with psychiatric disorders. The roles of nurses are expanding as nursing care becomes an established part of the community-based health care delivery system.

CRITICAL THINKING CHALLENGES

1. A 19-year-old patient with schizophrenia announces that he and a 47-year-old patient with bipolar disorder will be married the following week. They ask the nurse to witness the wedding. Discuss which ethical principles may be in conflict.

2. Compare the ethical concepts of *autonomy* and *beneficence*. Focus on the difference between legal consequences and ethical dilemmas.

3. Compare the variety of patients for whom psychiatric–mental health nurses care. Factors to be considered are age, health problems, and social aspects.

4. Visit the ANA's website for a description of the psychiatric–mental health nurse's certification credentials. Compare the basic level functions of a psychiatric nurse with those of the advanced practice psychiatric nurse.

5. Explain the biopsychosocial framework and apply it to the following three clinical examples:

   a. A first-time father is extremely depressed after the birth of his child, who is perfectly healthy.

   b. A child is unable to sleep at night because of terrifying nightmares.

   c. An older woman is resentful of moving into a senior citizens residence even though the decision was hers.

6. Discuss the purposes of the following organizations in promoting quality mental health care and supporting nursing practice. Visit the organizations' websites for more information.

   a. American Nurses Association
   b. American Psychiatric Nurses Association
   c. International Society of Psychiatric–Mental Health Nurses
   d. International Nurses Society on Addictions

REFERENCES

American Nurses Association, American Psychiatric Nurses Association & International Society of Psychiatric–Mental Health Nurses (2014). *Psychiatric–Mental Health Nursing: Scope and Standards of Practice*, 2nd. Edition. Silver Spring, MD: Nursesbooks.org.

Davis, A. (2008). Provision two. In M. Fowler (Ed.): *Guide to the code of ethics for nurses: Interpretation and Application* (p. 18). Washington, DC: Nursebooks.org.

Martin, K. S. (2005). *The Omaha system: A key to practice, documentation, and information management* (2nd ed.). St. Louis: Elsevier Saunders.

Saba, V. K. (2012). Clinical care classification system. *Sabacare.* http://www.sabacare.com/About/?PHPSESSID=b9e97459af41b2c80d-194d7434aa7800

Schwirian, P. M. (2013). Informatics and the future of nursing: Harnessing the power of standardized nursing terminology. *Bulletin of the Association for Information Science and Technology, 39*(5), 20–24.

Smith, K. J. & Craft-Rosenberg, M. (2010). Using NANDA, NIC, NOC in an undergraduate nursing practicum. *Nurse Educator, 35*(4), 162–66.

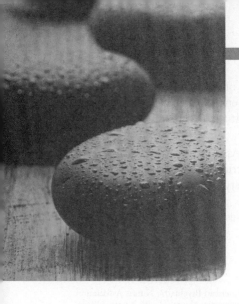

5
Theoretical Basis of Psychiatric Nursing

Mary Ann Boyd

KEY CONCEPTS

- anxiety
- empathic linkage

LEARNING OBJECTIVES

After studying this chapter, you will be able to:

1. Discuss psychosocial theories that support psychiatric nursing practice.

2. Identify the underlying theories that contribute to the understanding of human beings and behavior.

3. Compare the key elements of each theory that provides a basis for psychiatric–mental health nursing practice.

4. Identify common nursing theoretic models used in psychiatric–mental health nursing.

KEY TERMS

- behaviorism • classical conditioning • cognitions • cognitive theory • connections • countertransference • defense mechanisms • disconnections • empathy • family dynamics • formal support systems • informal support systems • interpersonal relations • libido • modeling • object relations • operant behavior • psychoanalysis • self-efficacy • self-system • social distance • transaction • transference • unconditional positive regard

This chapter presents an overview of selected psychodynamic, cognitive-behavioral, developmental, social, and nursing theories that serve as the knowledge base for psychiatric–mental health nursing practice. Many of these theories are covered in more depth in other chapters. Biologic theories are discussed in Chapters 6 and 10.

PSYCHODYNAMIC THEORIES

Psychodynamic theories explain the development of mental or emotional processes and their effects on behavior and relationships. Many of the psychodynamic concepts and models that are important in psychiatric nursing began with the Austrian physician Sigmund Freud (1856–1939). Since his time, Freud's theories have been enhanced by interpersonal and humanist models. These theories proved to be especially important in the

development of therapeutic relationships, techniques, and interventions (Table 5.1).

Psychoanalytic Theory

In Freud's psychoanalytic model, the human mind is conceptualized in terms of conscious mental processes (an awareness of events, thoughts, and feelings with the ability to recall them) and unconscious mental processes (thoughts and feelings that are outside awareness and are not remembered).

Study of the Unconscious

Freud believed that the unconscious part of the human mind is only rarely recognized by the conscious, as in remembered dreams (see Movies at the end of this

TABLE 5.1	PSYCHODYNAMIC MODELS		
Theorist	**Overview**	**Major Concepts**	**Applicability**
Psychoanalytic Models			
Sigmund Freud (1856–1939)	Founder of psychoanalysis Believed that the unconscious could be accessed through dreams and free association Developed a personality theory and theory of infantile sexuality	Id, ego, superego Consciousness Unconscious mental processes Libido Object relations Anxiety and defense mechanisms Free associations, transference, and countertransference	Individual therapy approach used for enhancement of personal maturity and personal growth
Anna Freud (1895–1982)	Application of ego psychology to psychoanalytic treatment and child analysis with emphasis on the adaptive function of defense mechanisms	Refinement of concepts of anxiety, defense mechanisms	Individual therapy, childhood psychoanalysis
Neo-Freudian Models			
Alfred Adler (1870–1937)	First defected from Freud Founded the school of individual psychology	Inferiority	Added to the understanding of human motivation
Carl Gustav Jung (1875–1961)	After separating from Freud, founded the school of psychoanalytic psychology Developed new therapeutic approaches	Redefined libido Introversion Extroversion Persona	Personalities are often assessed on the introversion and extroversion dimensions
Otto Rank (1884–1939)	Introduced idea of primary trauma of birth Active technique of therapy, including more nurturing than Freud Emphasized feeling aspect of analytic process	Birth trauma Will	Recognized the importance of feelings within psychoanalysis
Erich Fromm (1900–1980)	Emphasized the relationship of the individual to society	Society and individual are not separate	Individual desires are formed by society
Melanie Klein (1882–1960)	Devised play therapy techniques Believed that complex unconscious fantasies existed in children younger than 6 months of age Principal source of anxiety arose from the threat to existence posed by the death instinct	Pioneer in object relations Identification	Developed different ways of applying psychoanalysis to children; influenced present-day English and American schools of child psychiatry
Karen Horney (1885–1952)	Opposed Freud's theory of castration complex in women and his emphasis on the oedipal complex Argued that neurosis was influenced by the society in which one lived	Situational neurosis Character	Beginning of feminist analysis of psychoanalytic thought
Interpersonal Relations			
Harry Stack Sullivan (1892–1949)	Impulses and striving need to be understood in terms of interpersonal situations	Participant observer Parataxic distortion Consensual validation	Provided the framework for the introduction of the interpersonal theories in nursing
Humanist Theories			
Abraham Maslow (1908–1970)	Concerned himself with healthy rather than sick people Approached individuals from a holistic-dynamic viewpoint	Needs Motivation	Used as a model to understand how people are motivated and needs that should be met
Frederick S. Perls (1893–1970)	Awareness of emotion, physical state, and repressed needs would enhance the ability to deal with emotional problems	Reality Here-and-now	Used as a therapeutic approach to resolve current life problems that are influenced by old, unsolved emotional problems
Carl Rogers (1902–1987)	Based theory on the view of human potential for goodness Used the term *client* rather than *patient* Stressed the relationship between therapist and client	Empathy Positive regard	Individual therapy approach that involves never giving advice and always clarifying client's feelings

chapter). The term *preconscious* is used to describe unconscious material that is capable of entering consciousness.

Personality and Its Development

Freud's personality structure consists of three parts: the id, ego, and superego (Freud, 1927). The *id* is formed by unconscious desires, primitive instincts, and unstructured drives, including sexual and aggressive tendencies that arise from the body. The *ego* consists of the sum of certain mental mechanisms, such as perception, memory, and motor control, as well as specific defense mechanisms (discussed below). The ego controls movement, perception, and contact with reality. The capacity to form mutually satisfying relationships is a fundamental function of the ego, which is not present at birth but is formed throughout the child's development. The *superego* is that part of the personality structure associated with ethics, standards, and self-criticism. A child's identification with important and esteemed people in early life, particularly parents, helps form the superego.

Object Relations and Identification

Freud introduced the concept of **object relations**, the psychological attachment to another person or object. He believed that the choice of a sexual partner in adulthood and the nature of that relationship depended on the quality of the child's object relationships during the early formative years.

The child's first love object is the mother, who is the source of nourishment and the provider of pleasure. Gradually, as the child separates from the mother, the nature of this initial attachment influences future relationships. The development of the child's capacity for relationships with others progresses from a state of narcissism to social relationships, first within the family and then within the larger community. Although the concept of object relations is fairly abstract, it can be understood in terms of a child who imitates her mother and then becomes like her mother in adulthood. This child incorporates her mother as a love object, identifies with her, and grows up to become like her. This process is especially important in understanding an abused child who, under certain circumstances, becomes an adult abuser.

Anxiety and Defense Mechanisms

For Freud, anxiety is the reaction to danger and is experienced as a specific state of physical unpleasantness. **Defense mechanisms** are coping styles that protect a person from unwanted anxiety. Although they are defined differently than in Freud's day, defense mechanisms still play an explanatory role in contemporary psychiatric–mental health practice. Defense mechanisms are discussed in the chapter on Communication and the Therapeutic Relationship (Chapter 9).

Sexuality

The energy or psychic drive associated with the sexual instinct, or **libido**, literally translated from Latin to mean "pleasure" or "lust," resides in the id. When sexual desire is controlled and not expressed, tension results and is transformed into anxiety (Freud, 1905). Freud believed that adult sexuality is an end product of a complex process of development that begins in early childhood and involves a variety of body functions or areas (oral, anal, and genital zones) that correspond to stages of relationships, especially with parents.

Psychoanalysis

Freud developed **psychoanalysis**, a therapeutic process of accessing the unconscious conflicts that originate in childhood and then resolving the issues with a mature adult mind. As a system of psychotherapy, psychoanalysis attempts to reconstruct the personality by examining free associations (spontaneous, uncensored verbalizations of whatever comes to mind) and the interpretation of dreams. Therapeutic relationships had their beginnings within the psychoanalytic framework.

Transference and Countertransference

Transference is the displacement of thoughts, feelings, and behaviors originally associated with significant others from childhood onto a person in a current therapeutic relationship (Moore & Fine, 1990). For example, a woman's feelings toward her parents as a child may be directed toward the therapist. If a woman were unconsciously angry with her parents, she may feel unexplainable anger and hostility toward her therapist. In psychoanalysis, the therapist uses transference as a therapeutic tool to help the patient understand emotional problems and their origin.

Countertransference, on the other hand, is defined as the direction of all of the therapist's feelings and attitudes toward the patient. Countertransference becomes a problem when these feelings and perceptions are based on other interpersonal experiences. For example, a patient may remind a nurse of a beloved grandmother. Instead of therapeutically interacting with the patient from an objective perspective, the nurse feels an unexplained attachment to her and treats the patient as if she were the nurse's grandmother. The nurse misses important assessment and intervention data.

Neo-Freudian Models

Many of Freud's followers ultimately broke away, establishing their own forms of psychoanalysis. Freud did not receive criticism well. The rejection of some of his basic tenets often cost his friendship as well. Various psychoanalytic schools have adopted other names because their doctrines deviated from Freudian theory.

Adler's Foundation for Individual Psychology

Alfred Adler (1870–1937), a Viennese psychiatrist and founder of the school of individual psychology, was a student of Freud's who believed that the motivating force in human life is an intolerable sense of inferiority. Some people try to avoid these feelings by developing an unreasonable desire for power and dominance. This compensatory mechanism can get out of hand, and these individuals become self-centered and neurotic, overcompensate, and retreat from the real world and its problems.

Today, Adler's theories and principles are adapted and applied to both psychotherapy and education. Adlerian theory is based on principles of mutual respect, choice, responsibility, consequences, and belonging.

Jung's Analytical Psychology

One of Freud's earliest students, Carl Gustav Jung (1875–1961), a Swiss psychoanalyst, created a model called analytical psychology. Jung believed in the existence of two basically different types of personalities: extroverted and introverted. Whereas extroverted people tend to be generally interested in other people and objects of the external world, introverted people are more interested in themselves and their internal environment. According to Jung, both extroverted and introverted tendencies exist in everyone, but the libido usually channels itself mainly in one direction or the other. He also developed the concept of *persona*—what a person appears to be to others in contrast to who he or she really is (Jung, 1966).

Horney's Feminine Psychology

Karen Horney (1885–1952), a German American psychiatrist, challenged many of Freud's basic concepts and introduced principles of feminine psychology. Recognizing a male bias in psychoanalysis, Horney was the first to challenge the traditional psychoanalytic belief that women felt disadvantaged because of their genital organs. Freud believed that women felt inferior to men because their bodies were less completely equipped, a theory he described as "penis envy." Horney rejected this concept, as well as the oedipal complex, arguing that there are significant cultural reasons why women may strive to obtain qualities or privileges that are defined by a society as being masculine. For example, in Horney's time, most women did not have access to a university education, the right to vote, or economic independence. She argued that women truly were at a disadvantage because of the paternalistic culture in which they lived (Horney, 1939).

Other Neo-Freudian Theories

Otto Rank: Birth Trauma

Otto Rank (1884–1939), an Austrian psychologist and psychotherapist, was also one of Freud's students. He attributed all neurotic disturbances to the primary trauma of birth. For Rank, human development is a progression from complete dependence on the mother and family to physical independence coupled with intellectual dependence on society and finally to complete intellectual and psychological emancipation. A person's will guides and organizes the integration of self.

Erich Fromm: Societal Needs

Erich Fromm (1900–1980), an American psychoanalyst, focused on the relationship of society and the individual. He argued that individual and societal needs are not separate and opposing forces; their relationship is determined by the historic background of the culture. Fromm also believed that the needs and desires of individuals are largely formed by their society. For Fromm, the fundamental purpose of psychoanalysis and psychology is to bring harmony and understanding between the individual and society (Fromm-Reichmann, 1950).

Melanie Klein: Play Therapy

Melanie Klein (1882–1960), an Austrian psychoanalyst, devised play therapy techniques to demonstrate how a child's interaction with toys reveals earlier infantile fantasies and anxieties. She believed that complex, unconscious fantasies exist in children younger than 6 months of age. She is generally acknowledged as a pioneer in presenting an object relations viewpoint to the psychodynamic field, introducing the idea of early identification, a defense mechanism by which one patterns oneself after another person, such as a parent (Klein, 1963).

Harry Stack Sullivan: Interpersonal Forces

Interpersonal theories stress the importance of human relationships; instincts and drives are less important. Harry Stack Sullivan (1892–1949), an American psychiatrist, viewed **interpersonal relations** as a basis of human development and behavior. He believed that the health or sickness of one's personality is determined by the characteristic patterns in which one deals with other people. For example, one man is passive aggressive to everyone who contradicts him. This maladaptive behavior began when he was unable to express his disagreement to his parents. Health depends managing the constantly changing physical, social, and interpersonal environment as well as past and current life experiences (Sullivan, 1953).

Humanistic Theories

Humanistic theories are based on the belief that all human beings have the potential for goodness. Humanist therapists focus on patients' ability to learn about and accept themselves. They do not investigate repressed memories. Through therapy, patients explore personal capabilities in order to develop self-worth. They learn to experience the world in a different way.

Rogers' Client-Centered Therapy

Carl Rogers (1902–1987), an American psychologist, introduced client-centered therapy. **Empathy**, the capacity to assume the internal reference of the client in order to perceive the world in the same way as the client, is used in the therapeutic process (Rogers, 1980). The counselor is genuine but nondirect and also uses **unconditional positive regard**, a nonjudgmental caring for the client. In this therapy, the counselor's attitude and nonverbal communication are crucial. The therapist's emotional investment (i.e., true caring) in the client is essential in the therapeutic process (Rogers, 1980).

Gestalt Therapy

Another humanistic approach is Gestalt therapy, developed by Frederick S. (Fritz) Perls (1893–1970), a German-born former psychoanalyst who immigrated to the United States. Perls believed the root of human anxiety is frustration with inability to express natural biologic and psychological desires in modern civilization. The repression of these basic desires causes anxiety. In Gestalt therapy, these unmet needs are brought into awareness through individual and group exercises (Perls, 1969).

Abraham Maslow's Hierarchy of Needs

Abraham Maslow's (1921–1970) hierarchy of needs is fixture in social science and nursing (Maslow, 1970) (Figure 5.1). In nursing, Maslow's model is used to prioritize care. Basic needs (food, shelter) should be met before higher level needs (self-esteem) can be met.

Applicability of Psychodynamic Theories to Psychiatric–Mental Health Nursing

Several psychodynamic concepts are important in the practice of psychiatric–mental health nursing, such as

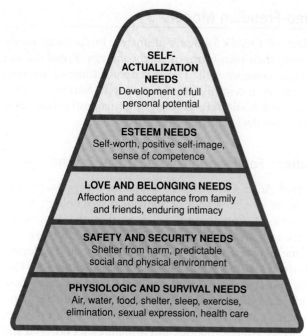

FIGURE 5.1   Maslow's hierarchy of needs.

interpersonal relationships, defense mechanisms, transference, countertransference, and internal objects. In particular, a therapeutic interpersonal relationship is a core of psychiatric–mental health nursing intervention (see Chapter 10 for nursing interventions). Even though there is general consensus that most of these theories are useful, the nurse should continue to critically analyze them for utility and relevance. For example, Maslow's theory may be useful when a person with mental illness is homeless and wants food and shelter. But, another person in a similar situation may reject food and shelter because self-esteem is associated with being free to reject the confines of an institution. In this case, self-esteem need is more important than food or shelter.

Recently, there is renewed interest in psychodynamic treatment for depression. Psychodynamic therapists have a strong emphasis on affect and emotional expression, examination of topics that the patient avoids, recurring patterns of behaviors, feelings, experiences, and relationship, the past and its influence on the present, interpersonal relationships, and exploration of wishes, dreams, and fantasies (Luyten & Blatt, 2012).

COGNITIVE-BEHAVIORAL THEORIES
Behavioral Theories

Behavioral theories attempt to explain how people learn and act. Behavioral theories never attempt to explain the cause of mental disorders; instead, they focus on normal human behavior. Research results are then applied to the clinical situation. Two areas of behavioral theories

TABLE 5.2	BEHAVIORAL THEORISTS		
Theorist	Overview	Major Concepts	Applicability
Stimulus–Response			
Edwin R. Guthrie (1886–1959)	Continued with understanding conditioning as being important in learning	Recurrence of responses tends to follow a specific stimulus	Important in analyzing habitual behavior
Ivan P. Pavlov (1849–1936)	Classical conditioning	Unconditioned stimuli Unconditioned response Conditioned stimuli	Important in understanding learning of automatic responses such as habitual behaviors
John B. Watson (1878–1958)	Introduced behaviorism Believed that learning was classical conditioning called *reflexes* Rejected distinction between mind and body	Principle of frequency Principle of recency	Focuses on the relationship between the mind and body
Reinforcement Theories			
B. F. Skinner (1904–1990)	Developed an understanding of the importance of reinforcement and differentiated types and schedules	Operant behavior Respondent behavior Continuous reinforcement Intermittent reinforcement	Important in behavior modification
Edward L. Thorndike (1874–1949)	Believed in the importance of effects that followed behavior	Reinforcement	Important in behavior modification programs

relevant to psychiatric–nursing practice are stimulus–response theories and reinforcement theories (Table 5.2).

Early Stimulus–Response Theories

Pavlovian Theory

One of the earliest behavioral theorists was Ivan P. Pavlov (1849–1936), who noticed that stomach secretions of dogs were stimulated by triggers other than food reaching the stomach. He found that the sight and smell of food triggered stomach secretions, and he became interested in this anticipatory secretion. Through his experiments, he was able to stimulate secretions with a variety of other laboratory nonphysiologic stimuli. Thus, a clear connection was made between thought processes and physiologic responses.

In Pavlov's model, there is an unconditioned stimulus (not dependent on previous training) that elicits an unconditioned (i.e., specific) response. In his experiments, meat is the unconditioned stimulus, and salivation is the unconditioned response. Pavlov taught the dog to associate a bell (conditioned stimulus) with the meat (unconditioned stimulus) by repeatedly ringing the bell before presenting the meat. Eventually, the dog salivated when he heard the bell. This phenomenon is called **classical conditioning** (or pavlovian conditioning) (Pavlov, 1927/1960).

John B. Watson and the Behaviorist Revolution

At about the same time Pavlov was working in Russia, **behaviorism**, a learning theory that only focuses on objectively observable behaviors and discounts any independent activities of the mind, was introduced in the United States by John B. Watson (1878–1958). He rejected the distinction between body and mind and emphasized the study of objective behavior (Watson & Rayner, 1920). He developed two principles: frequency and recency. The *principle of frequency* states that the more often a response is made to a stimulus, the more likely the response to that stimulus will be repeated. The *principle of recency* states that the closer in time a response is to a particular stimulus, the more likely the response will be repeated.

Reinforcement Theories

Edward L. Thorndike

A pioneer in experimental animal psychology, Edwin L. Thorndike (1874–1949) studied the problem-solving behavior of cats to determine whether animals solved problems by reasoning or instinct. He found that neither choice was completely correct; animals gradually learn the correct response by "stamping in" the stimulus–response connection. The major difference between Thorndike and behaviorists such as Watson was that Thorndike believed that reinforcement of positive behavior was important in learning. He was the first reinforcement theorist, and his view of learning became the dominant view in American learning theory (Thorndike, 1916).

B. F. Skinner

One of the most influential behaviorists, B. F. Skinner (1904–1990), studied **operant behavior** or conditioning.

In this type of learning, the focus is on the consequence of the behavioral response, not a specific stimulus. If a behavior is reinforced or rewarded with success, praise, money, and so on, the behavior will probably be repeated. For example, if a child climbs on a chair, reaches the faucet, and is able to get a drink of water successfully, it is more likely that the child will repeat the behavior (Skinner, 1935). If a behavior does not have a positive outcome, it is less likely that the behavior will be repeated. Nurses use this knowledge to create behavior management plans to reinforce healthy, positive behaviors.

Cognitive Theories

The initial behavioral studies focused on human actions without much attention to the internal thinking process. When complex behaviors could not be accounted for by strictly behavioral explanations, thought processes became new subjects for study. **Cognitive theory**, an outgrowth of different theoretic perspectives, including the behavioral and the psychodynamic, attempted to link internal thought processes with human behavior (Table 5.3).

Albert Bandura's Social Cognitive Theory

Learning by watching others is the basis of Albert Bandura's (b. 1925) social cognitive theory. He developed his ideas after being concerned about television violence contributing to aggression in children. He showed learning occurs by internalizing behaviors of others through a process of **modeling** called pervasive imitation, or one person trying to be like another. The model does not have to be a real person but could be a character in history or generalized to an ideal person (Bandura, 1977, 1986).

An important concept of Bandura's is **self-efficacy**, a person's sense of his or her ability to deal effectively with the environment (Bandura, 1993). Efficacy beliefs influence how people feel, think, motivate themselves, and behave. The stronger the self-efficacy, the higher the goals people set for themselves and the firmer their commitment to them (McIntosh, 2003; Shin, Yun, Pender, & Jang, 2005).

One of Bandura's recent contributions is showing that intentions and self-motivation play roles in determining behavior, significantly expanding the reinforcement model. He believes that the human mind is not only reactive to a stimulus but is also creative, proactive, and reflective (Bandura, 2001).

Aaron Beck: Thinking and Feeling

American psychiatrist Aaron T. Beck (b. 1921) of the University of Pennsylvania devoted his career to understanding the relationship between cognition and mental health. For Beck, **cognitions** are verbal or pictorial events in the stream of consciousness. He realized the importance of cognitions when treating people with depression. He found that depression improved when patients began viewing themselves and situations in a positive light.

He believes that people with depression have faulty information-processing systems that lead to biased cognitions. These faulty beliefs cause errors in judgment that become habitual errors in thinking. These individuals incorrectly interpret life situations, judge themselves too harshly, and jump to inaccurate negative conclusions. A person may truly believe that he or she has no friends, and therefore no one cares. On examination, the evidence for the beliefs is based on the fact that there has been no contact with anyone because of moving from one city to another. Thus, a distorted belief is the basis of the cognition. Beck and his colleagues continue to develop cognitive therapy, a successful approach for the treatment of depression (Beck, 2005). Recent research supports the variability of beliefs between different generations within the same culture indicating the importance of understanding underlying beliefs (Box 5.1).

Applicability of Cognitive-Behavioral Theories to Psychiatric–Mental Health Nursing

Basing interventions on behavioral theories is widespread in psychiatric nursing. For example, patient education interventions are usually derived from the behavioral

TABLE 5.3	COGNITIVE THEORISTS		
Theorist	Overview	Major Concepts	Applicability
Aaron Beck (b. 1921)	Conceptualized distorted cognitions as a basis for depression	Cognitions Beliefs	Important in cognitive therapy
Kurt Lewin (1890–1947)	Developed field theory, a system for understanding learning, motivation, personality, and social behavior	Life space Positive valences	Important in understanding motivation for changing behavior
Edward Chace Tolman (1886–1959)	Introduced the concept of cognitions: believed that human beings act on beliefs and attitudes and strive toward goals	Negative valences Cognition	Important in identifying person's beliefs

BOX 5.1

Research for Best Practice: Differences in Beliefs in First- and Second-Generation Mothers

Mamisachvili, L., Ardiles, P., Mancewicz, G., Thompson, S., Rabin, K., & Ross, L. E. (2013). Culture and postpartum mood problems: Similarities and differences in the experiences of first- and second-generation Canadian women. Journal of Transcultural Nursing, 24(2), 162–170.

THE QUESTION: Are there similarities and differences in experiences of postpartum mood problems (PPMP) between first- and second-generation Canadian women?

METHODS: In this exploratory qualitative study, the researchers interviewed nine first-generation and eight second-generation women to explore potential role of cultural values, beliefs, and immigration experiences in postpartum mood problems.

FINDINGS: While both generations experienced conflicts with their parents or in-laws regarding child rearing and the negative effects of PPMP stigma, the second-generation women were surprised that they needed support and experienced a loss of self. In these women, their PPMP is also related to not meeting their own and societal expectations of maternal roll fulfillment.

IMPLICATION FOR NURSING: There is variation in the beliefs associated with the state of depression. Understanding underlying belief systems is critical for providing the appropriate interventions.

theories. Teaching patients new coping skills for their symptoms of mental illnesses is another example. Changing an entrenched habit involves helping patients identify what motivates them and how these new lifestyle habits can become permanent. In psychiatric units, behavioral interventions include the privilege systems and token economies. Behavioral approaches are discussed throughout this text.

DEVELOPMENTAL THEORIES

Developmental theories explain normal human growth and development over time. Many developmental theories

are presented in terms of stages based on the assumption that normal development proceeds longitudinally from the beginning to the ending stage.

Erik Erikson: Psychosocial Development

Freud and Sullivan both published treatises on stages of human development, but Erik Erikson (1902–1994) outlined the psychosocial developmental model that is most often used in nursing. Erikson's model is an expansion of Freud's psychosexual development theory. Whereas Freud's model emphasizes intrapsychic experiences, Erikson's recognizes the role of the psychosocial environment. For example, parental divorce disrupts the family interaction pattern, and the financial and housing environment impact the development of the children.

Each of Erikson's eight stages are organized by age and developmental conflicts: basic trust versus mistrust, autonomy versus shame and doubt, initiative versus guilt, industry versus inferiority, identity versus role diffusion, intimacy versus isolation, generativity versus stagnation, and ego integrity versus despair. Successful resolution of a conflict or crisis leads to essential strength and virtues (Table 5.4). For example, a positive outcome of the trust versus mistrust crisis is the development of a basic sense of trust. If the crisis is unsuccessfully resolved, the infant moves into the next stage without a sense of trust. According to this model, a child who is mistrustful will have difficulty completing the next crisis successfully and, instead of developing a sense of autonomy, will more likely be full of shame and doubt (Erikson, 1963).

Identity and Adolescence

One of Erikson's major contributions is the recognition of the turbulence of adolescence and identity formation. When adolescence begins, childhood ways are given up,

TABLE 5.4	ERIKSON'S EIGHT AGES OF MAN	
Approximate Chronologic Age	**Developmental Conflict***	**Long-Term Outcome of Successful Resolution**
Infant	Basic trust vs. mistrust	Drive and hope
Toddler	Autonomy vs. shame and doubt	Self-control and willpower
Preschool-aged child	Initiative vs. guilt	Direction and purpose
School-aged child	Industry vs. inferiority	Method and competence
Adolescence	Identity vs. role diffusion	Devotion and fidelity
Young adult	Intimacy vs. isolation	Affiliation and love
Adulthood	Generativity vs. stagnation	Production and care
Maturity	Ego integrity vs. despair	Renunciation and wisdom

*Successful outcome is evidenced by the development of the characteristic listed first.

Adapted from Erikson, E. (1963). *Childhood and society* (pp. 273–274). New York: Norton.

and bodily changes occur. An identity is formed. Trying to reconcile a personal view of self with society's perception can be overwhelming and lead to role confusion and alienation (Erikson, 1968).

Research Evidence for Erikson's Models

Evidence is mixed that every person follows the eight stages of development as outlined by Erikson. In an early study, male college students who measured low on identity also scored low on intimacy ratings (Orlofsky, Marcia, & Lesser, 1973). These results lend support to the idea that identity precedes intimacy. In another study, intimacy was found to begin developing early in adolescence before the development of identity (Ochse & Plug, 1986). Studying fathers with young children, Christiansen and Palkovitz (1998) found that *generativity* (defined as the need or drive to produce, create, or effect a change) was associated with a paternal identity, psychosocial identity, and psychosocial intimacy. In addition, fathers who had a religious identification also had higher generativity scores than did others.

A longitudinal study of 86 men beginning at age 21 years with reassessment 32 years later at age 53 years supports Erikson's psychosocial eight-stage model (Westermeyer, 2004). In this study, 48 men (56%) achieved generativity at follow-up. Successful young adults as predicted by Erikson's model at midlife lived within a warm family environment; had an absence of troubled parental discipline; experienced a mentor relationship; and, most importantly, had favorable peer group relationships.

Erikson's model may apply differently to men and women. In one study, generativity is associated with well-being in both men and women, but in men, generativity is related to the urge for self-protection, self-assertion, self-expansion, and mastery. In women, the antecedents may be the desire for contact, connection, and union (Ackerman, Zuroff, & Moskowitz, 2000).

Studies show that generativity is significantly associated with successful marriage, work achievements, close friendships, altruistic behaviors, and overall mental health. Generativity is also associated with optimism and forgiveness in dealing with grandparenting problems within the family (Ehlman & Ligon, 2012; Pratt, Norris, Cressman, Lawford, & Hebblethwaite, 2008).

Jean Piaget: Learning in Children

One of the most influential people in child psychology is Jean Piaget (1896–1980), who contributed more than 40 books and 100 articles on child psychology alone. Piaget's theory views intelligence as an adaptation to the environment. He proposes that cognitive growth is like embryologic growth: an organized structure becomes more and more differentiated over time. Piaget's system explains how knowledge develops and changes (Table 5.5).

Each stage of cognitive development represents a particular structure with major characteristics. Piaget's theory was developed through observation of his own children and therefore never received formal testing.

The major strength of his model is its recognition of the central role of cognition in development and the discovery of surprising features of young children's thinking. For example, children in middle childhood become capable of considering more than one aspect of an object or situation at a time. Their thinking becomes more complex. They can understand that the area of a rectangle is determined by the length *and* width. For psychiatric–mental health nurses, Piaget's model provides a framework to recognize different levels of thinking in the assessment and intervention processes. For example, the assessment of concrete thinking is typical of some people with schizophrenia who are unable to perform abstract thinking.

Carol Gilligan: Gender Differentiation in Moral Development

Carol Gilligan (b. 1936) argues that most development models are male centered and therefore inappropriate for girls and women. She challenges Erik Erikson (psychosocial development) and Kohlberg's (moral) theories as being biased against women because they are based on primarily privileged, white men and boys. For Gilligan, attachment within relationships is the important factor for successful development. After comparing male and female personality development, she highlights differences (Gilligan, 2004). In developing identity, boys separate from their mothers, and girls attach. Girls probably learn to value relationships and become interdependent at an earlier age. They learn to value the ideal of care, begin to respond to human need, and want to take care of the world by sustaining attachments so no one is left alone. Her model of moral development, *Ethic of Care*, is divided into three stages beginning with *preconventional* or selfishness (what is best for me) to *conventional* or responsibility to others (self-sacrifice is goodness) to *postconventional* or do not hurt others or self (she is a person too) (Gilligan, 2011).

Gilligan's conclusion that female development depends on relationships has implications for everyone who provides care to women. Traditional models that advocate separation as the primary goal of human development immediately place women at a disadvantage. By negating the value and importance of attachments within relationships, the natural development of women is impaired. If Erikson's model is applied to women, their failure to separate then becomes defined as a developmental failure (Gilligan, 1982).

TABLE 5.5	PIAGET'S PERIODS OF INTELLECTUAL DEVELOPMENT		
Age (years)	Period	Cognitive Developmental Characteristics	Description
Birth to 2	Sensorimotor	Divided into six stages, characterized by (1) inborn motor and sensory reflexes, (2) primary circular reaction and first habit, (3) secondary circular reaction, (4) use of familiar means to obtain ends, (5) tertiary circular reaction and discovery through active experimentation, and (6) insight and object permanence	The infant understands the world in terms of overt, physical action on that world. The infant moves from simple reflexes through several steps to an organized set of schemes. Significant concepts are developed, including space, time, and causality. Above all, during this period, the child develops the scheme of the permanent object.
2–7	Preoperational	Deferred imitation; symbolic play, graphic imagery (drawing); mental imagery; and language Egocentrism, rigidity of thought, semilogical reasoning, and limited social cognition	Child no longer only makes perceptual and motor adjustment to objects and events. Child can now use symbols (mental images, words, gestures) to represent these objects and events; uses these symbols in an increasingly organized and logical fashion.
7–11	Concrete operations	Conservation of quantity, weight, volume, length, and time based on reversibility by inversion or reciprocity; operations: class inclusion and seriation	Conservation is the understanding of what values remain the same. For example, if liquid is poured from a short, wide glass into a tall, narrow one, the preoperational child thinks that the quantity has changed. For the concrete operation child, the amount stays the same.
11 through the end of adolescence	Formal operations	Combination system whereby variables are isolated and all possible combinations are examined; hypothetical-deductive thinking	Mental operations are applied to objects and events. The child classifies, orders, and reverses them. Hypotheses can be generated from these concrete operations.

Jean Baker Miller: A Sense of Connection

Jean Baker Miller (1927–2006) conceptualized female development within the context of experiences and relationships. Consistent with the thinking of Carol Gilligan, the Miller relational model views the central organizing feature of women's development as a sense of connection to others. The goal of development is to increase a woman's ability to build and enlarge mutually enhancing relationships (Miller, 1994). **Connections** (mutually responsive and enhancing relationships) lead to mutual engagement (attention), empathy, and empowerment. In relationships in which everyone interacts beneficially, mutual psychological development can occur. **Disconnections** (lack of mutually responsive and enhancing relationships) occur when a child or adult expresses a feeling or explains an experience and does not receive any response from others. The most serious types of disconnection arise from the lack of response that occurs after abuse or attacks. The theory is currently evolving and serves as a model for psychotherapy and nursing practice on psychiatric units (Riggs & Bright, 1997; Walker & Rosen, 2004).

Applicability of Developmental Theories to Psychiatric–Mental Health Nursing

Developmental theories are used in understanding childhood and adolescent experiences and their manifestations as adult problems. When working with children, nurses can use developmental models to help gauge development and mood. However, because most of the models are based on the assumptions of the linear progression of stages and have not been adequately tested, applicability has limitations. Most do not account for gender differences and diversity in lifestyles and cultures.

SOCIAL THEORIES

Numerous social theories underlie psychiatric–mental health nursing practice. Chapter 3 presents some of the sociocultural issues and discusses various social groups. This section represents a sampling of important social theories that a nurse uses. This discussion is not exhaustive and should be viewed by the student as including a few of the important social theoretic perspectives.

Family Dynamics

Family dynamics are the patterned interpersonal and social interactions that occur within the family structure over the life of a family. Family dynamics models are based on systems theory in which the change of one part affects the total functioning of the system. The family is viewed organizationally as an open system in which one member's actions influence the functioning of the total system. Family theories that are important in psychiatric–mental health nursing are based on systems models but have rarely been tested for wide-range validity. Specific family theories are discussed in depth in Chapter 14: Family Assessment and Interventions.

Family theories are especially useful to nurses who are assessing family dynamics and planning interventions. Family systems models are used to help nurses form collaborative relationships with patients and families dealing with health problems. Generalist psychiatric–mental health nurses will not be engaged in family therapy. However, they will be caring for individuals and families. Understanding family dynamics is important in every nurse's practice. Many family interventions are consistent with these theories (see Chapter 14). Many of the symptoms of mental disorders, such as hallucinations or delusions, have implications for the total family and affect interactions.

Formal and Informal Social Support

Assisting patients in the recovery process means helping patients identify supportive family and community systems. **Formal support systems** are large organizations, such as hospitals and nursing homes that provide care to individuals. **Informal support systems** are family, friends, and neighbors. Individuals with strong informal support networks actually live longer than those without this type of support. Adolescents who are survivors of sexual assault are more likely to seek support from informal support systems than formal supports (Fehler-Cabral & Campbell, 2013). In addition, classic studies showed that those without informal support have significantly higher mortality rates when the causes of death are accidents (e.g., smoking in bed) or suicides (Litwak, 1985).

An important concept is **social distance**, the degree to which the values of the formal organization and primary group members differ. In the United States, the most closely located, accessible, and available family member is expected to provide the care to a family member. Spouses are the first choice, then children, other family members, friends, and finally formal support. On the other, care-related stress can result in the informal caregiver changing the balance by placing a family member in an institution (Friedemann, Newman, Buckwalter, & Montgomery, 2014).

Formal and informal support systems are balanced when they are at a midpoint of social distance, that is, close enough to communicate but not so close to destroy each other—neither enmeshment nor isolation (Litwak, Messeri, & Silverstein, 1990; Messeri, Silverstein, & Litwak, 1993). Conflicts arise when the relationship becomes unbalanced. For example, if the primary group and the formal care system begin performing similar caregiving services, there may be disagreements. Balance is reestablished when the formal system increases the social distance by developing relationships and providing support to the caregiver and reducing contact with the patient. Thus, a balance is maintained between the two systems. In another instance, when a patient relies only on the health care provider for care and support (e.g., calls the nurse every day, visits the physician weekly, refuses any help from family), balance can be reestablished by linking the patient to an informal support system for help with some of the caregiving tasks.

By applying frameworks of formal and informal support systems to their patients, psychiatric nurses can understand the complex social forces that patient's with mental disorders and their caregivers experience (McPherson, Kayes, Moloczij, & Cummins, 2013) (Box 5.2). Nurses can help adjust the social distance between the formal and informal systems by identifying communication barriers and helping the two groups work together. For example, a patient misses an appointment because of a lack of transportation. The case manager helps the patient communicate the problem to the system to obtain another appointment. Informal caregivers are valued by the case manager, who recognizes the important services performed by family and friends. Thus, linkages between mental health providers (formal support) and the consumer network (informal support) are reinforced.

BOX 5.2

Research for Best Practice: Formal and Informal Services

McPherson, K. M., Kayes, N. K., Moloczij, N., & Cummins. C. (2013). Improving the interface between informal carers and formal health and social services: A qualitative study. International Journal of Nursing Studies, 51(3), 418–429. doi:10.1016/j.inurstu.2013.07.006

THE QUESTION: Is there a connection between informal and formal care givers? How can positive connections or interface be developed and maintained between them?

METHODS: Qualitative interviewing of formal and informal care givers (n = 70) using focus groups and individual interviews.

FINDINGS: Four themes emerged including (1) quality of care for the patient, (2) knowledge exchange (valuing each other's perspectives), (3) need for flexibility services, and (4) reducing the caregiver burden.

IMPLICATIONS FOR NURSING: Positive interface of formal and informal caregiver can ensure quality care for individuals.

Role Theories

A role is a person's social position and function within an environment. Anthropologic theories explain members' roles that relate to a specific society. For example, the universal roles of healer may be assumed by a nurse in one culture and a spiritual leader in another. Societal expectations, social status, and rights are attached to these roles. Psychological theories, which are concerned about roles from a different perspective, focus on the relationship of an individual's role: the self. The responsibilities of a parent are often in conflict with the personal needs for time alone. All of the neo-Freudian and humanist models that have been discussed focus on reciprocal social relationships or interactions that determine how the mind develops.

Role theories emphasize the importance of social interaction in either the individual's choice of a particular role or society's recognition of it. Psychiatric–mental health nursing uses role concepts in understanding group interaction and the role of the patient in the family and community (see Chapters 12 and 13). In addition, milieu therapy approaches discussed in later chapters are based on the patient's assumption of a role within the psychiatric environment.

Sociocultural Perspectives

Margaret Mead: Culture and Gender

American anthropologist Margaret Mead (1901–1978) is widely known for her studies of primitive societies and her contributions to social anthropology. She conducted studies in New Guinea, Samoa, and Bali and devoted much of her studies to the patterns of child rearing in various cultures. She was particularly interested in the cultural influences determining male and female behavior (Mead, 1970). Influenced by Carl Jung and Erik Erikson, she had a vision of unity and diversity of the psychosocial development of a single human species (Sullivan, 2004). Although her research is often criticized as not having scientific rigor and being filled with misinterpretations, it is accepted as a classic in the field of anthropology (Sullivan, 2004). She established the importance of culture in determining human behavior.

Madeleine Leininger: Transcultural Health Care

Concern about the impact of culture on the treatment of children with psychiatric and emotional problems led Madeleine Leininger (1924–2012) to develop a new field, transcultural nursing, directed toward holistic, congruent, and beneficent care. Leininger developed the *Theory of Culture Care Diversity and Universality*, which explains diverse and universal dimensions of human caring (Figure 5.2).

Nursing care in one culture is different from another because definitions of health, illness, and care are culturally defined (Leininger & McFarland, 2006). The goal of Leininger's theory is to discover culturally based care (Leininger, 2007).

Applicability of Social Theories to Psychiatric–Mental Health Nursing

The use of social and sociocultural theories is especially important for psychiatric–mental health nurses. In any individual or family assessment, the sociocultural aspect is integral to mental health. It would be impossible to complete an adequate assessment without considering the role of the individual within the family and society. Interventions are based on the understanding and significance of family and cultural norms. It would be impossible to interact with the family in a meaningful way without an understanding of the family's cultural values. In the inpatient setting, the nurse is responsible for designing the social environment of the unit as well as ensuring that the patient is safe from harm. To accomplish this complex task, an understanding of the unit as a small social community helps the nurse use the environment in patient treatment (see Chapter 10). In addition, many group interventions are based on sociocultural theories (see Chapter 13).

NURSING THEORIES

Nursing theories are useful to psychiatric–mental health nursing in conceptualizing the individual, family, or community and in planning nursing interventions (see Chapter 10). The use of a specific theory depends on the patient situation. For example, in people with schizophrenia who have problems related to maintaining self-care, Dorothea Orem's theory of self-care is useful. By contrast, Hildegarde Peplau's theories are appropriate when a nurse is developing a relationship with a patient. Because of the wide range of possible problems requiring different approaches, familiarity with several nursing theories is essential.

Interpersonal Relations Models

Hildegarde Peplau: The Power of Empathy

Hildegarde Peplau (1909–1999) introduced the first systematic theoretic framework for psychiatric nursing and focused on the nurse–patient relationship in her book *Inter-personal Relations in Nursing* in 1952 (Peplau, 1952). She led psychiatric–mental health nursing out of the confinement of custodial care into a theory-driven professional practice. One of her major contributions was the introduction of the nurse–patient relationship (see Chapter 9).

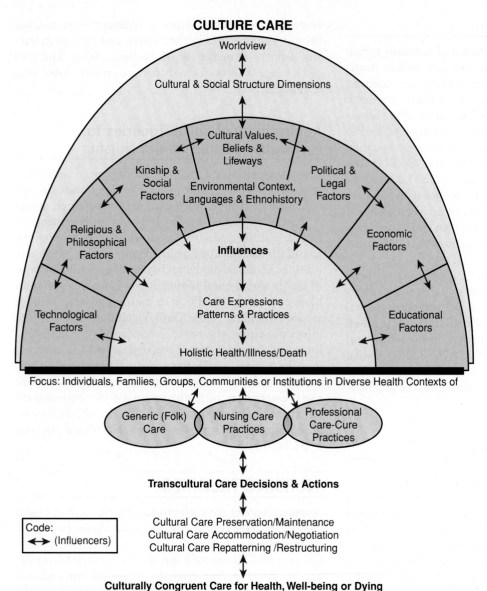

CULTURE CARE

Worldview

Cultural & Social Structure Dimensions

Cultural Values, Beliefs & Lifeways

Kinship & Social Factors

Environmental Context, Languages & Ethnohistory

Political & Legal Factors

Religious & Philosophical Factors

Influences

Economic Factors

Technological Factors

Care Expressions Patterns & Practices

Educational Factors

Holistic Health/Illness/Death

Focus: Individuals, Families, Groups, Communities or Institutions in Diverse Health Contexts of

Generic (Folk) Care

Nursing Care Practices

Professional Care-Cure Practices

Transcultural Care Decisions & Actions

Code:
⟷ (Influencers)

Cultural Care Preservation/Maintenance
Cultural Care Accommodation/Negotiation
Cultural Care Repatterning /Restructuring

Culturally Congruent Care for Health, Well-being or Dying

FIGURE 5.2 Leininger's Sunrise Model to depict theory of cultural care diversity and universality. Reprinted with permission from the estate of Dr. Madeleine Leininger.

Peplau believed in the importance of the environment, defined as external factors considered essential to human development (Peplau, 1992): cultural forces, presence of adults, secure economic status of the family, and a healthy prenatal environment. Peplau emphasized the importance of empathic linkage.

> **KEYCONCEPT** **Empathic linkage** is the ability to feel in oneself the feelings experience by another person.

The interpersonal transmission of anxiety or panic is the most common empathic linkage. According to Peplau, other feelings, such as anger, disgust, and envy, can also be communicated nonverbally by way of empathic transmission to others. Although the process is not yet understood, she explains that empathic communication occurs. She believes that if nurses pay attention to what they feel during a relationship with a patient, they can gain invaluable observations of feelings a patient is experiencing and has not yet noticed or talked about.

Anxiety is a key concept for Peplau, who contends that professional practice is unsafe if this concept is not understood.

> **KEYCONCEPT** **Anxiety**, according to Peplau, is an energy that arises when expectations that are present are not met.

If anxiety is not recognized, it continues to rise and escalates toward panic. There are various levels of anxiety, each having its observable behavioral cues (Box 5.3). These cues are sometimes called *defensive*, but Peplau argues that they are often "relief behaviors." For example, some people may relieve their anxiety by yelling and swearing; others seek relief by withdrawing. In both instances, anxiety was generated by an unmet security need.

> **BOX 5.3**
> ## Levels of Anxiety
>
> **Mild:** awareness heightens
> **Moderate:** awareness narrows
> **Severe:** focused narrow awareness
> **Panic:** unable to function

NCLEXNOTE Peplau's model of anxiety continues to be an important concept in psychiatric nursing. Severe anxiety interferes with learning. Mild anxiety is useful for learning.

The **self-system** is another important concept in Peplau's model. Drawing from Sullivan, Peplau defined the self as an "anti-anxiety system" and a product of socialization. The self proceeds through personal development that is always open to revision but tends toward stability. For example, in parent–child relationships, patterns of approval, disapproval, and indifference are used by children to define themselves. If the verbal and nonverbal messages have been derogatory, children incorporate these messages and also view themselves negatively.

The concept of need is important to Peplau's model. Needs are primarily of biologic origin but need to be met within a sociocultural environment. When a biologic need is present, it gives rise to tension that is reduced and relieved by behaviors meeting that need. According to Peplau, nurses should recognize and support the patients' patterns and style of meeting their health care needs.

Ida Jean Orlando

In 1954, Ida Jean Orlando (1926–2007) studied the factors that enhanced or impeded the integration of mental health principles in the basic nursing curriculum. From this study, she published *The Dynamic Nurse–Patient Relationship* to offer nursing students a theory of effective nursing practice. She studied nursing care of patients on medical–surgical units, not people with psychiatric problems in mental hospitals. Orlando identified three areas of nursing concern: the nurse–patient relationship, the nurse's professional role, and the identity and development of knowledge that is distinctly nursing (Orlando, 1961). A nursing situation involves the behavior of the patient, the reaction of the nurse, and anything that does not relieve the distress of the patient. Patient distress is related to the inability of the individual to meet or communicate his or her own needs (Orlando, 1961, 1972).

Orlando helped nurses focus on the whole patient rather than on the disease or institutional demands. Her ideas continue to be useful today, and current research supports her model (Olson & Hanchett, 1997). A small nursing study investigated whether Orlando's nursing

theory–based practice had a measurable impact on patients' immediate distress when compared with nonspecified nursing interventions Orlando's approach consisted of the nurse validating the patient's distress before taking any action to reduce it. Patients being cared for by the Orlando group experienced significantly less stress than those receiving traditional nursing care (Potter & Bockenhauer, 2000).

Existential and Humanistic Theoretical Perspectives

Rosemarie Rizzo Parse

The *Humanbecoming Theory* views humans as indivisible, unpredictable, ever-changing coauthors and experts about their lives (Parse, 1998, 2007). Three major themes underlie this theory: meaning (personal meaning to the situation), rhythmicity (the paradoxical patterning of the human-universe mutual processes—the ups and downs of life), and transcendence (power and originating of transforming) (Parse, 1996, 1998, 2008). The postulates involved in living a human life are *illuminating* (unbound knowing extended to infinity), *paradox* (intricate rhythm expressed as a pattern preference), *freedom* (liberation), and *mystery* (unexplainable) (Parse, 2007).

As one of the more abstract nursing theories, *humanbecoming* can used in understanding patients' life experiences and connecting psychologically with a patient. This theory has been widely studied in nursing and adds qualitative dimension to understanding the patient's human experience. For example, one of the studies addressed the positive effects of feeling strong within a community (Doucet, 2012).

Jean Watson

The theory of transpersonal caring was initiated by Jean Watson (b. 1940). Watson believes that caring is the foundation of nursing and recommends that specific theories of caring be developed in relation to specific human conditions and health and illness experiences (Watson, 2005). Her conceptualizations transcend conventional views of illness and focus on the meaning of health and quality of life (Watson, 2007). There are three foundational concepts of her theory:

* Transpersonal Caring–Healing Relations: a relational process related to philosophic, moral, and spiritual foundation
* 10 Caritas Process: the original 10 Carative Factors have evolved into the 10 Caritas Processes (Box 5.4)
* Caritas Field: a field of consciousness created when the nurse focuses on love and caring as his or her way of being and consciously manifests a healing presence with others.

BOX 5.4

Nursing: Human Science and Human Care Assumptions, and Factors in Care

ASSUMPTIONS

1. Caring can be effectively demonstrated and practiced only interpersonally.
2. Caring consists of factors that result in the satisfaction of certain human needs.
3. Effective caring promotes health and individual or family growth.
4. Caring responses accept a person not only as he or she is now but also as what he or she may become.
5. A caring environment offers the development of potential while allowing the person to choose the best action for him- or herself at a given point in time.
6. Caring is more "healthogenic" than is curing. It integrates biophysical knowledge with knowledge of human behavior to generate or promote health and provide ministrations to those who are ill. A science of caring is complementary to the science of curing.
7. The practice of caring is central to nursing.

10 CARITAS PROCESSES™

1. Embrace altruistic values and practice loving kindness with self and others.
2. Instill faith, hope, and honor in others.
3. Be sensitive to self and others by nurturing individual beliefs and practices.
4. Develop helping–trusting–caring relationships.
5. Promote and accept positive and negative feelings as you authentically listen to another's story.
6. Use creative scientific problem-solving methods for caring decision making.
7. Share teaching and learning that addresses the individual needs and comprehension styles.
8. Create a healing environment for the physical and spiritual self that respects human dignity.
9. Assist with basic physical, emotional, and spiritual human needs.
10. Be open to mystery and allow miracles to enter.

From Watson Caring Science Institute, International Caritas Consortium. (2010). *Dr. Jean Watson's Human Caring Theory: Ten caritas processes.* http://www.watsoncaringscience.org/about-us/caring-science-definitions-processes-theory/

Watson's theory is especially applicable to the care of those who seek help for mental illness. This model emphasizes the importance of sensitivity to self and others; the development of helping and trusting relations; the promotion of interpersonal teaching and learning; and provision for a supportive, protective, and corrective mental, physical, sociocultural, and spiritual environment. A transpersonal caring intervention guide offers protocols to assist nurses in using caring intentionally and effectively in practice (Gallagher-Lepak & Kubsch, 2009). Watson's model is a model in the acute health care settings to guide the establishment of genuine therapeutic relationships (Hogan, 2013).

Systems Models

Imogene M. King

The theory of goal attainment developed by Imogene King (1923–2007) is based on a systems model that includes three interacting systems: personal, interpersonal, and social. In this model, human beings interact with the environment, and the individual's perceptions influence reactions and interactions (Figure 5.3). Nursing involves caring for the human being, with the goal of health defined as adjusting to the stressors in both internal and external environments (King, 2007). She defines nursing as a "process of human interactions between nurse and patient whereby each perceives the other and the situation; and through communication, they set goals, explore means, and agree on means to achieve goals" (King, 1981, p. 144). This model focuses on the process that occurs between a nurse and a patient. The process is initiated to help the patient cope with a health problem that compromises his or her ability to maintain social roles, functions, and activities of daily living (King, 1992).

In this model, the person is goal oriented and purposeful, reacting to stressors, and is viewed as an open system interacting with the environment. The variables in nursing situations are as follows:

- Geographic place of the transacting system, such as the hospital
- Perceptions of the nurse and patient
- Communications of the nurse and patient
- Expectations of the nurse and patient
- Mutual goals of the nurse and patient

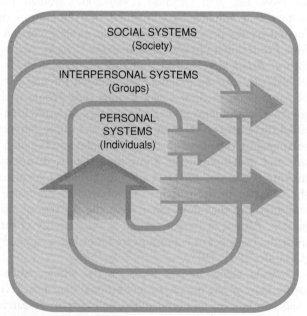

FIGURE 5.3 Imogene King's conceptual framework for nursing: dynamic interacting systems.

- The nurse and patient as a system of interdependent roles in a nursing situation (King, 1981, p. 88)

The quality of nurse–patient interactions may have positive or negative influences on the promotion of health in any nursing situation. It is within this interpersonal system of nurse and patient that the healing process is performed. Interaction is depicted in which the outcome is a **transaction**, defined as the transfer of value between two or more people. This behavior is unique, based on experience, and is goal directed.

King's work reflects her understanding of the systematic process of theory development. Her model continues to be developed and applied in national and international settings, including psychiatric–mental health care (Shanta & Connolly, 2013).

Betty Neuman

Betty Neuman (b. 1924) uses a systems approach as a model of nursing care. Neuman wants to extend care beyond an illness model, incorporating concepts of problem finding and prevention and the newer behavioral science concepts and environmental approaches to wellness. Neuman developed her framework in the late 1960s as chairwoman of the University of California at Los Angeles graduate nursing program. The key components of the model are a client system (physiological, psychological, sociocultural, developmental, spiritual) interacting with the environment. The wholistic model can be applied to prevention and treatment.

Neuman was one of the first psychiatric nurses to include the concept of stressors in understanding nursing care. The Neuman systems model is applied to a practice and educational setting, including community health, family therapy, renal nursing, perinatal nursing, and mental health nursing of older adults (Neuman & Fawcett, 2011; Beckman, Boxley-Harges, & Kaskel, 2012). This model has been applied to the practice and educational setting including international programs (Merks, Verberk, de Kuiper, & Lowry, 2012).

Dorothea Orem

Self-care is the focus of the general theory of nursing initiated by Dorothea Orem (1914–2007) in the early 1960s. The Self-Care Deficit Nursing Theory consists of three separate parts: a theory of self-care, theory of self-care deficit, and theory of nursing systems (Biggs, 2008; Orem & Taylor, 2011; Orem, 2001). The theory of self-care defines the term as activities performed independently by an individual to promote and maintain personal well-being throughout life. The central focus of Orem's theory is the self-care deficit theory, which describes how people can be helped by nursing. Nurses can help meet self-care

> ### BOX 5.5
> ### Research for Best Practice: Keys to Successful Self-Management of Medications
>
> *Swanlund, S. L., Scherck, K. A., Metcalfe, S. A., & Jesek-Hale, S. R. (2008). Keys to successful self-management of medications.* Nursing Science Quarterly, 21(3), 238–246.
>
> **QUESTION:** How do community-dwelling older adults manage their medications?
>
> **METHODS:** Guided by Orem's Self-Care Deficit Nursing Theory, 19 older adults were interviewed about their medication self-management practices.
>
> **FINDINGS:** Three themes emerged: successful self-management of medications, living orderly, and aging well. The clear message of this study is that self-management of medication is successful when habits are established and the use of medications is integrated into the person's lifestyle.
>
> **IMPLICATIONS FOR NURSING:** Many persons with mental disorders must take medications to control symptoms. Adherence to a medication regime is problematic, and there are high noncompliance rates. The results of this study suggest the strategies should be designed to reinforce the importance of routines and building medication use into the person's normal daily lifestyle.

requisites through five approaches: acting or doing for, guiding, teaching, supporting, and providing an environment to promote the patient's ability to meet current or future demands. The nursing systems theory refers to a series of actions a nurse takes to meet the patient's self-care requisites. This system varies from the patient being totally dependent on the nurse for care to needing only some education and support.

Orem's model is used in psychiatric–mental health nursing because of its emphasis on promoting independence of the individual and on self-care activities (Burdette, 2012; Seed & Torkelson, 2012). Although many psychiatric disorders have an underlying problem, such as motivation, these problems are generally manifested as difficulties conducting ordinary self-care activities (e.g., personal hygiene) or developing independent thinking skills. See Box 5.5 for an example.

Other Nursing Theories

Other nursing models are applied in psychiatric settings. Martha Rogers' model of unitary human beings and Calista Roy's adaptation model have been the basis of many psychiatric nursing approaches.

SUMMARY OF KEY POINTS

- The traditional psychodynamic framework helped form the basis of early nursing interpersonal interventions, including the development of therapeutic relationships and the use of such concepts as transference, countertransference, empathy, and object relations.

- The behavioral theories are often used in strategies that help patients change behavior and thinking.

- Sociocultural theories remain important in understanding and interacting with patients as members of families and cultures.

- Nursing theories form the conceptual basis for nursing practice and are useful in a variety of psychiatric–mental health settings.

CRITICAL THINKING CHALLENGES

1. Discuss the similarities and differences among Freud's ideas and those of the neo-Freudians, including Jung, Adler, Horney, and Sullivan.

2. Compare and contrast the basic ideas of psychodynamic and behavioral theories.

3. Compare and differentiate classic conditioning from operant conditioning.

4. Define the following terms and discuss their applicability to psychiatric–mental health nursing: classical conditioning, operant conditioning, positive reinforcement, and negative reinforcement.

5. List the major developmental theorists and their main ideas.

6. Discuss the cognitive therapy approaches to mental disorders and how they can be used in psychiatric–mental health nursing practice.

7. Define formal and informal support systems. How does the concept of social distance relate to these two systems?

8. Compare and contrast the basic ideas of the nursing theorists.

MOVIES

Freud: 1962. This film depicts Sigmund Freud as a young physician, focusing on his early psychiatric theories and treatments. His struggles for acceptance of his ideas among the Viennese medical community are depicted. This fascinating film is well done and gives an interesting overview of the impact of psychoanalysis.

Viewing Points: Watch for the impact on political thinking during the gradual acceptance of Freud's ideas. Discuss the "dream sequence" and its impact on the development of psychoanalysis as a therapeutic technique.

An Angel at My Table: 1989, New Zealand. This three-part television miniseries tells the story of Janet Frame, New Zealand's premiere novelist and poet. Based on her autobiography, the film portrays Frame as a shy, awkward child who experiences a family tragedy that alienates her socially. She studies in England to be a teacher, but her shyness and social ineptness cause extreme anxiety. Seeking mental health care, she receives a misdiagnosis of schizophrenia and spends 8 years in a mental institution. She barely escapes a lobotomy when she is notified of a literary award. She then begins to develop friendships and a new life.

Viewing Points: Observe Janet Frame's childhood development. Does she "fit" any of the models that are discussed in this chapter? Consider her life in light of Gilligan and Miller's theories that it is important for women to have a sense of connection.

REFERENCES

Ackerman, S., Zuroff, D. C., & Moskowitz, D. S. (2000). Generativity in midlife and young adults: Links to agency, communion, and subjective well-being. *International Journal of Aging and Human Development, 5*(1), 17–41.

Bandura, A. (1977). *Social learning theory.* Englewood Cliffs, NJ: Prentice-Hall.

Bandura, A. (1986). *Social Foundations of thought and action: A social-cognitive theory.* Englewood Cliffs, NJ: Prentice Hall.

Bandura, A. (1993). Perceived self-efficacy in cognitive development and function. American Educational Research Association Annual Meeting. *Educational Psychologist, 28*(2), 117–148.

Bandura, A. (2001). Social cognitive theory: An agentic perspective. *Annual Review of Psychology, 52,* 1–26.

Beck, A. T. (2005). The current state of cognitive therapy: A 40-year retrospective. *Archives of General Psychiatry, 62*(9), 953–959.

Beckman, S.J., Boxley-Harges, S.L., & Kaskel, B.L. (2012). Experience informs: Spanning three decades with the Neuman Systems Model. *Nursing Science Quarterly, 25*(4), 341–346.

Biggs, A. (2008). Orem's Self-Care Deficit Nursing Theory: Update on the state of the art and science. *Nursing Science Quarterly, 21*(3), 200–206.

Burdette, L. (2012). Relationship between self-care agency, self-care practices and obesity among rural midlife women. *Self-Care, Dependent-Care & Nursing, 19*(1), 5–14.

Christiansen, S. L., & Palkovitz, R. (1998). Exploring Erikson's psychosocial theory and development: Generativity and its relationship to paternal identity, intimacy, and involvement in childcare. *The Journal of Men's Studies, 7*(1), 133–156.

Doucet, T.J. (2012). Feeling strong: A Parse research method study. *Nursing Science Quarterly, 25*(1), 62–71.

Ehlman, K., & Ligon, M. (2012). The application of a generativity model for the older adults. *International Journal of Aging and Human Development, 74*(4), 331–344.

Erikson, E. (1963). *Childhood and society* (2nd ed). New York: Norton.

Erikson, E. (1968). *Identity: Youth and crisis.* New York: Norton.

Fehler-Cabral, F., & Campbell, R. (2013). Adolescent sexual assault disclosure: The impact of peers, families, and schools. *American Journal of Community Psychology, 52*(1–2), 73–83.

Freud, S. (1905). Three essays on the theory of sexuality. In J. Strachey, A. Freud, A. Strachey, & A. Tyson (Eds.). (1953). *The standard edition of the complete psychological works of Sigmund Freud* (pp. 135–248). London: Hogarth Press.

Freud, S. (1927). The ego and the id. In E. Jones (Ed.): (1957). *The international psychoanalytical library* (No. 12). London: Hogarth Press.

Friedemann, M., Newman, F. L., Buckwalter, K. C., & Montgomery R. J. (2014). Resource need and use of multiethnic caregivers of elders in their homes. *Journal of Advanced Nursing, 70*(3), 662–673.

Fromm-Rieichmann, F. (1950). *Principles of intensive psychotherapy.* Chicago: University of Chicago Press.

Gallagher-Lepak, S., & Kubsch, S. (2009). Transpersonal caring: A nursing practice guideline. *Holistic Nursing Practice, 23*(3), 171–182.

Gilligan, C. (1982). *In a different voice.* Cambridge, MA: Harvard University Press.

Gilligan, C. (2004). Recovering psyche: Reflections on life-history and history. *Annual of Psychoanalysis, 32*, 131–147.

Gilligan, C. (2011). *Joining the resistance*. Malden, MA: Polity Press.

Hogan, B. K. (2013). Caring as a scripted discourse versus caring as an expression of an authentic relationship between self and other. *Issues in Mental Health Nursing, 34*(5), 375–379.

Horney, K. (1939). *New ways in psychoanalysis*. New York: Norton.

Jung, C. (1966). On the psychology of the unconscious. The personal and the collective unconscious. In Jung, C (Ed.), *Collected works of C. G. Jung* (2nd ed, Vol. 7, pp. 64–79). Princeton, NJ: Princeton University Press.

King, I. (1981). *A theory for nursing: Systems, concepts, process*. New York: Wiley.

King, I. (1992). King's theory of goal attainment. *Nursing Science Quarterly, 5*(1), 19–26.

King, I. (2007). King's conceptual system, theory of goal attainment, and transaction process in the 21st century. *Nursing Science Quarterly, 20*(2), 109–116.

Klein, M. (1963). *Our adult world and other essays*. London: Heinemann Medical Books.

Leininger, M. (2007). Theoretical questions and concerns: Response from the Theory of Culture Care Diversity and Universality perspective. *Nursing Science Quarterly, 20*, 9–13.

Leininger, M., & McFarland, M. (2006). *Cultural care diversity and universality theory. A theory of nursing* (2nd ed). Seaburg, MA: Jones & Bartlett Publishers.

Litwak, E. (1985). Complementary roles for formal and informal support groups: A study of nursing homes and mortality rates. *Journal of Applied Behavioral Science, 21*(4), 407–425.

Litwak, E., Messeri, P., & Silverstein, M. (1990). The role of formal and informal groups in providing help to older people. *Marriage and Family Review, 15*(1–2), 171–193.

Luyten, P., & Blatt, S. J. (2012). Psychodynamic treatment of depression. *Psychiatric Clinics of North America, 35*(1), 111–129.

Maslow, A. (1970). *Motivation and personality* (rev. ed). New York: Harper & Brothers.

McIntosh, D. (2003). *Testing an intervention to increase self-efficacy of staff in managing clients perceived as violent*. University of Cincinnati, PhD dissertation. Retrieved March 7, 2007, from http://etd,iohiolink.edu/view.cgi?acc_num=ucin1069786693

McPherson, K. M., Kayes, N. K., Moloczij, N., & Cummins C. (2013). Improving the interface between informal carers and formal health and social services: A qualitative study. *International Journal of Nursing Studies, 51*(3), 418–429. doi:10.1016/j.ijnurstu.2013.07.006

Mead, M. (1970). *Culture and commitment: A study of the generation gap*. Garden City, NY: Natural History Press/Doubleday & Co.

Merks, A., Verberk, F., de Kuiper, M., Lowry, L. W. (2012). Neuman systems model in holland: An update. *Nursing Science Quarterly, 25*(4), 364–368.

Messeri, P., Silverstein, M., & Litwak, E. (1993). Choosing optimal support groups: A review and reformulation. *Journal of Health and Social Behavior, 34*(6), 122–137.

Miller, J. (1994). Women's psychological development. Connections, disconnections, and violations. In M. Berger (Ed.): *Women beyond Freud: New concepts of feminine psychology* (pp. 79–97). New York: Brunner Mazel.

Moore, B., & Fine, B. (Eds.). (1990). *Psychoanalytic terms and concepts*. New Haven, CT: The American Psychoanalytic Association and Yale University Press.

Neuman, B., & Fawcett, J. (Eds). (2011). *The Neuman systems model* (5th ed). Upper Saddle River, NJ: Prentice Hall.

Ochse, R., & Plug, C. (1986). Cross-cultural investigation of the validity of Erikson's theory of personality development. *Journal of Personality and Social Psychology, 50*(6), 1240–1252.

Olson, J., & Hanchett, E. (1997). Nurse-expressed empathy, patient outcomes, and the development of a middle-range theory. *Image: The Journal of Nursing Scholarship, 29*(1), 71–76.

Orem, D. (2001). *Nursing concepts of practice* (6th ed). St. Louis: Mosby.

Orem, D. E., & Taylor, S. G. (2011). Reflections on nursing practice science: The nature, the structure, and the foundation of nursing sciences. *Nursing Science Quarterly, 24*(1), 35–41.

Orlando, I. J. (1961). *The dynamic nurse–patient relationship*. New York: G. P. Putnam's Sons.

Orlando, I. J. (1972). *The discipline and teaching of nursing process*. New York: G. P. Putnam's Sons.

Orlofsky, J., Marcia, J., & Lesser, I. (1973). Ego identity status and the intimacy versus isolation crisis of young adulthood. *Journal of Personality and Social Psychology, 27*(2), 211–219.

Parse, R. R. (1996). Reality: A seamless symphony of becoming. *Nursing Science Quarterly, 9*, 181–184.

Parse, R. R. (1998). *The human becoming school of thoughts: A perspective for nurses and other health professionals*. London: Sage.

Parse, R. R. (2007). The human becoming school of thought in 2050. *Nursing Science Quarterly, 20*, 308–311.

Parse, R. R. (2008). The humanbecoming leading-following model. *Nursing Science Quarterly, 21*, 369–375.

Pavlov, I. P. (1927/1960). *Conditioned reflexes*. New York: Dover Publications.

Peplau, H. (1952). *Interpersonal relations in nursing*. New York: G. Putnam & Sons.

Peplau, H. (1992). Interpersonal relations: A theoretical framework for application in nursing practice. *Nursing Science Quarterly, 5*(1), 13–18.

Perls, F. (1969). *In and out of the garbage pail*. Lafayette, CA: Real People Press.

Potter, M. L., & Bockenhauer, B. J. (2000). Implementing Orlando's nursing theory. *Journal of Psychosocial Nursing and Mental Health Services, 38*(13), 14–21.

Pratt, M. W., Norris, J. E., Cressman, K., Lawford, H., & Hebblethwaite, S. (2008). Parents' stories of grandparenting concerns in the three-generational family: Generativity, optimism, and forgiveness. *Journal of Personality, 76*(3), 581–604.

Riggs, S. R., & Bright, M. S. (1997). Dissociative identity disorder: A feminist approach to inpatient treatment using Jean Baker Miller's relational model. *Archives of Psychiatric Nursing, 11*(4), 218–224.

Rogers, C. (1980). *A way of being*. Boston: Houghton Mifflin.

Seed, M. S., & Torkelson, D. J. (2012). Beginning the recovery journey in acute psychiatric care: Using concepts from Orem's self-care deficit nursing theory. *Issues in Mental Health Nursing, 33*(6), 394–398.

Shanta, L. L., & Connolly, M. (2013). Using King's interacting systems theory to link emotional intelligence and nursing practice. *Journal of Professional Nursing, 29*(3), 174–180.

Shin, Y., Yun, S., Pender, N. J., & Jang, H. (2005). Test of the health promotion model as a causal model of commitment to a plan for exercise among Korean adults with chronic disease. *Research in Nursing & Health, 28*(2), 117–125.

Skinner, B. F. (1935). The generic nature of the concepts of stimulus and response. *Journal of General Psychology, 12*, 40–65.

Sullivan, G. (2004). A four-fold humanity: Margaret Mead and psychological types. *Journal of the History of the Behavioral Sciences, 40*(2), 183–206.

Sullivan, H. (1953). *The interpersonal theory of psychiatry*. New York: Norton.

Thorndike, E. L. (1906). *The principles of teaching, based on psychology*. New York: A.G. Seiler.

Walker, M., & Rosen, W. B. (2004). *How connections heal: Stories from relational-cultural therapy*. New York: Guilford Press.

Watson, J. (2005). *Caring science as sacred science*. Philadelphia: F. A. Davis.

Watson, J. (2007). Theoretical questions and concerns: Response from a Caring Science Framework. *Nursing Science Quarterly, 20*, 13–15.

Watson, J. B., & Rayner, R. (1920). Conditioned emotional reactions. *Journal of Experimental Psychology, 3*, 1–14.

Westermeyer, J. F. (2004). Predictors and characteristics of Erikson's life cycle model among men: A 32-year longitudinal study. *International Journal of Aging & Human Development, 58*(1), 29–48.

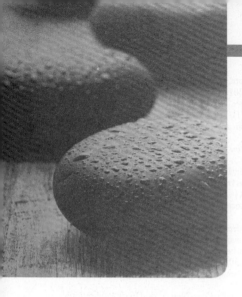

6

Biologic Foundations of Psychiatric Nursing

Mary Ann Boyd

KEY CONCEPTS

- neuroplasticity
- neurotransmitters

LEARNING OBJECTIVES

After studying this chapter, you will be able to:

1. Describe the association between biologic functioning and symptoms of psychiatric disorders.

2. Locate brain structures primarily involved in psychiatric disorders and describe the primary functions of these structures.

3. Describe basic mechanisms of neuronal transmission.

4. Identify the location and function of neurotransmitters significant to hypotheses regarding major mental disorders.

5. Discuss the role of genetics in the development of psychiatric disorders.

6. Discuss the basic utilization of new knowledge gained from fields of study, including psychoneuroimmunology and chronobiology.

KEY TERMS

- acetylcholine • amino acids • autonomic nervous system • basal ganglia • biogenic amines • biologic markers • brain stem • cerebellum • chronobiology • circadian cycle • cortex • dopamine • extrapyramidal motor system • frontal, parietal, temporal, and occipital lobes • functional imaging • GABA • genetic susceptibility • glutamate • hippocampus • histamine • limbic system • locus ceruleus • neurocircuitry • neurohormones • neurons • neuromodulators • neuropeptides • norepinephrine • phenotype • pineal body • population genetics • proband • psychoneuroimmunology • receptor • serotonin • structural imaging • synaptic cleft • working memory • zeitgebers

All behavior recognized as human results from actions that originate in the brain and its amazing interconnection of neural networks. Modern research has increased understanding of how the complex circuitry of the brain interacts with the external environment, memories, and experiences. Through the spinal column and peripheral nerves, along with other systems, such as the endocrine and immune systems, the brain constantly receives and processes information. As the brain shifts and sorts through the amazing amount of information it processes every hour, it decides on actions and initiates behaviors, allowing each person to act in entirely unique and very human ways.

Mental disorders cannot be traced to specific physiological problems but rather are complex syndromes consisting of biopsychosocial symptoms that more or less cluster together. Therefore, it is important for the nurse to understand basic nervous system functioning, as well as some of the research that is exploring the biologic basis of mental disorders.

This chapter reviews the basic information necessary for understanding neuroscience as it relates to the role of the psychiatric–mental health nurse. It reviews basic central nervous system (CNS) structures and functions, the peripheral nervous system (PNS), general functions of the major neurotransmitters and receptors, basic principles of neurotransmission, genetic models, circadian rhythms, and biologic tests. The chapter assumes that the reader has a basic knowledge of human biology, anatomy, and pathophysiology. It is not intended as a full presentation of neuroanatomy and physiology but rather as an overview of the structures and functions most critical to understanding the role of the psychiatric–mental health nurse. Psychiatric–mental health nurses must be able to make the connection between (1) patients' psychiatric symptoms, (2) the probable alterations in brain functioning linked to those symptoms, and (3) the rationale for treatment and care practices.

NEUROANATOMY OF THE CENTRAL NERVOUS SYSTEM

Although this section discusses functioning areas of the brain separately, each area is intricately connected with the others, and each functions interactively. The CNS contains the brain, brain stem, and spinal cord, and the PNS consists of the neurons that connect the CNS to the muscles, organs, and other systems in the periphery of the body. Whatever affects the CNS may also affect the PNS and vice versa.

Cerebrum

The largest region of the human brain, the cerebrum fills the entire upper portion of the cranium. The **cortex**, or outermost surface of the cerebrum, makes up about 80% of the human brain. The cortex is four to six cellular layers thick, and each layer is composed of cell bodies mixed with capillary blood vessels. This mixture makes the cortex gray brown (thus the term *gray matter*). The cortex consists of numerous bumps and grooves in a fully developed adult brain, as shown in Figure 6.1. This "wrinkling" allows for a large amount of surface area to be confined in the limited space of the skull. The increased surface area allows for more potential connections among cells within the cortex. The grooves are called *fissures* if they extend deep into the brain and *sulci* if they are shallower. The bumps or convolutions are called *gyri*. Together, they provide many of the landmarks for the subdivisions of the cortex. The longest and deepest groove, the longitudinal fissure, separates the cerebrum into left and right hemispheres. Although these two divisions are nearly symmetric, there is some variation in the location and size of the sulci and gyri in each hemisphere. Substantial variation in these convolutions is found in the cortex of different individuals.

Left and Right Hemispheres

The cerebrum can be roughly divided into two halves, or hemispheres. The left hemisphere is dominant in about 95% of people, but about 5% of individuals have mixed dominance. Each hemisphere controls functioning mainly on the opposite side of the body. Aside from controlling activities on the left side of the body, the right hemisphere

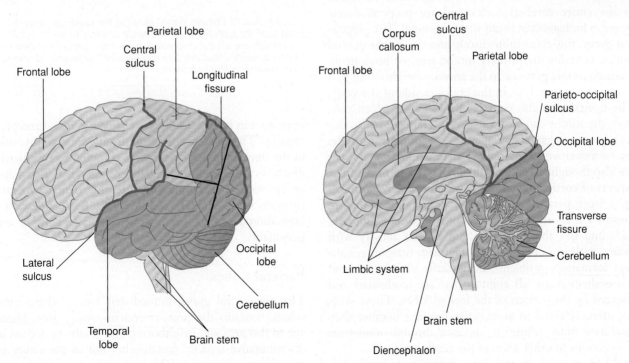

FIGURE 6.1   Lateral and medial surfaces of the brain. *Left,* The left lateral surface of the brain. *Right,* The medial surface of the right half of a sagittally hemisected brain.

also provides input into receptive nonverbal communication, spatial orientation and recognition, intonation of speech and aspects of music, facial recognition and facial expression of emotion, and nonverbal learning and memory. In general, the left hemisphere is more involved with verbal language function, including areas for both receptive and expressive speech control, and provides strong contributions to temporal order and sequencing, numeric symbols, and verbal learning and memory.

The two hemispheres are connected by the corpus callosum, a bundle of neuronal tissue that allows information to be exchanged quickly between the right and left hemispheres. An intact corpus callosum is required for the hemispheres to function in a smooth and coordinated manner.

Lobes of the Brain

The lateral surface of each hemisphere is further divided into four lobes: the **frontal, parietal, temporal, and occipital lobes** (see Figure 6.1). The lobes work in coordinated ways, but each is responsible for specific functions. An understanding of these unique functions is helpful in understanding how damage to these areas produces the symptoms of mental illness and how medications that affect the functioning of these lobes can produce certain effects.

Frontal Lobes

The right and left frontal lobes make up about one fourth of the entire cerebral cortex and are proportionately larger in humans than in any other mammal. The precentral gyrus, the gyrus immediately anterior to the central sulcus, contains the primary motor area, or homunculi. Damage to this gyrus or to the anterior neighboring gyri causes spastic paralysis in the opposite side of the body. The frontal lobe also contains Broca's area, which controls the motor function of speech. Damage to Broca's area produces expressive aphasia, or difficulty with the motor movements required for speech. The frontal lobes are also thought to contain the highest or most complex aspects of cortical functioning, which collectively makes up a large part of what we call personality. **Working memory** is an important aspect of frontal lobe function, including the ability to plan and initiate activity with future goals in mind. Insight, judgment, reasoning, concept formation, problem-solving skills, abstraction, and self-evaluation are all abilities that are modulated and affected by the actions of the frontal lobes. These skills are often referred to as *executive functions* because they modulate more primitive impulses through numerous connections to other areas of the cerebrum.

When normal frontal lobe functioning is altered, executive functioning is decreased, and modulation of

BOX 6.1
Frontal Lobe Syndrome

In the 1860s, Phineas Gage became a famous example of frontal lobe dysfunction. Mr. Gage was a New England railroad worker who had a thick iron-tamping rod propelled through his frontal lobes by an explosion. He survived, but suffered significant changes in his personality. Mr. Gage, who had previously been a capable and calm supervisor, began to show impatience, labile mood, disrespect for others, and frequent use of profanity after his injury (Harlow, 1868). Similar conditions are often called *frontal lobe syndrome*. Symptoms vary widely from individual to individual. In general, after damage to the dorsolateral (upper and outer) areas of the frontal lobes, the symptoms include a lack of drive and spontaneity. With damage to the most anterior aspects of the frontal lobes, the symptoms tend to involve more changes in mood and affect, such as impulsive and inappropriate behavior.

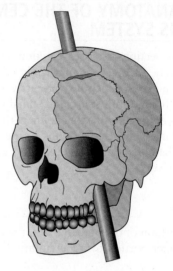

The skull of Phineas Gage, showing the route the tamping rod took through his skull. The angle of entry of the rod shot it behind the left eye and through the front part of the brain, sparing regions that are directly concerned with vital functions like breathing and heartbeat.

impulses can be lost, leading to changes in mood and personality. The importance of the frontal lobe and its role in the development of symptoms common to psychiatric disorders are emphasized in later chapters that discuss disorders such as schizophrenia, attention deficit hyperactivity disorder (ADHD), and dementia. Box 6.1 describes how altered frontal lobe function can affect mood and personality.

Parietal Lobes

The postcentral gyrus, immediately behind the central sulcus, contains the primary somatosensory area. Damage to this area and neighboring gyri results in deficits in discriminative sensory function but not in the ability to perceive sensory input. The posterior areas of the parietal lobe appear to coordinate visual and somatosensory information. Damage to this area produces complex sensory deficits, including neglect of contralateral sensory stimuli and spatial relationships. The parietal lobes contribute to the ability to recognize objects by touch, calculate, write, recognize fingers of the opposite hands, draw, and organize spatial directions (e.g., how to travel to familiar places).

Temporal Lobes

The temporal lobes contain the primary auditory and olfactory areas. Wernicke's area, located at the posterior aspect of the superior temporal gyrus, is primarily responsible for receptive speech. The temporal lobes also integrate sensory and visual information involved in control of written and verbal language skills as well as visual recognition. The hippocampus, an important structure discussed later, lies in the internal aspects of each temporal lobe and contributes to memory. Other internal structures of this lobe are involved in the modulation of mood and emotion.

Occipital Lobes

The primary visual area is located in the most posterior aspect of the occipital lobes. Damage to this area results in a condition called *cortical blindness*. In other words, the retina and optic nerve remain intact, but the individual cannot see. The occipital lobes are involved in many aspects of visual integration of information, including color vision, object and facial recognition, and the ability to perceive objects in motion.

Association Cortex

Although not a lobe, the association cortex is an important area that allows the lobes to work in an integrated manner. Areas of one lobe of the cortex often share functions with an area of the adjacent lobe. When these neighboring nerve fibers are related to the same sensory modality, they are often referred to as *association areas*. For example, an area in the inferior parietal, posterior temporal, and anterior occipital lobes integrates visual, somatosensory, and auditory information to provide the abilities required for basic academic skills. These areas, along with numerous connections beneath the cortex, are part of the mechanisms that allow the human brain to work as an integrated whole.

Subcortical Structures

Beneath the cortex are layers of tissue composed of the axons of cell bodies. The axonal tissue forms pathways that are surrounded by glia, a fatty or lipid substance, which has a white appearance and give these layers of neuron axons their name—white matter. Structures inside the hemispheres, beneath the cortex, are considered subcortical. Many of these structures, essential in the regulation of emotions and behaviors, play important roles in our understanding of mental disorders. Figure 6.2 provides a

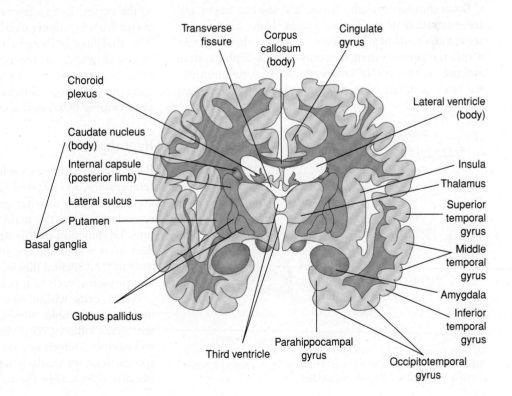

FIGURE 6.2 Coronal section of the brain, illustrating the corpus callosum, basal ganglia, and lateral ventricles.

coronal section view of the gray matter, white matter, and important subcortical structures.

The **basal ganglia** are subcortical gray matter areas in both the right and the left hemisphere that contain many cell bodies or nuclei. The primary subdivisions of the basal ganglia are the putamen, globus pallidus, and caudate. The basal ganglia are involved with motor functions and association in both the learning and the programming of behavior or activities that are repetitive and, done over time, become automatic. The basal ganglia have many connections with the cerebral cortex, thalamus, midbrain structures, and spinal cord. Damage to portions of these nuclei may produce changes in posture or muscle tone. In addition, damage may produce abnormal movements, such as twitches or tremors. The basal ganglia can be adversely affected by some of the medications used to treat psychiatric disorders, leading to side effects and other motor-related problems.

Limbic System

The **limbic system** is essential to understanding the many hypotheses related to psychiatric disorders and emotional behavior in general. The limbic system is called a "system" because it comprises several small structures that work in a highly organized way. These structures include the hippocampus, thalamus, hypothalamus, amygdala, and limbic midbrain nuclei. See Figure 6.3 for identification and location of the structures within the limbic system and their relationships to other common CNS structures.

Basic emotions, needs, drives, and instinct begin and are modulated in the limbic system. Hate, love, anger, aggression, and caring are basic emotions that originate within the limbic system. Not only does the limbic system function as the seat of emotions, but because emotions are often generated based on our personal experiences,

the limbic system also is involved with aspects of memory. Hypothesized changes in the limbic system play a significant role in many theories of major mental disorders, including schizophrenia, depression, and anxiety disorders (discussed in later chapters).

Hippocampus

The **hippocampus** is involved in storing information, especially the emotions attached to a memory. Our emotional responses to memories and our associations with other related memories are functions of how information is stored within the hippocampus. Although memory storage is not limited to one area of the brain, destruction of the left hippocampus impairs verbal memory, and damage to the right hippocampus results in difficulty with recognition and recall of complex visual and auditory patterns. Deterioration of the nerves of the hippocampus and other related temporal lobe structures found in Alzheimer's disease produces the disorder's hallmark symptoms of memory dysfunction.

Thalamus

Sometimes called the "relay-switching center of the brain," the thalamus functions as a regulatory structure to relay all sensory information, except smell, sent to the CNS from the PNS. From the thalamus, the sensory information is relayed mostly to the cerebral cortex. The thalamus relays and regulates by filtering incoming information and determining what to pass on or not pass on to the cortex. In this fashion, the thalamus prevents the cortex from becoming overloaded with sensory stimulus. The thalamus is thought to play a part in controlling electrical activity in the cortex. Because of its primary relay function, damage to a very small area of the thalamus may produce deficits in many cortical functions, thus, causing behavioral abnormalities.

Hypothalamus

Basic human activities, such as sleep–rest patterns, body temperature, and physical drives such as hunger and sex, are regulated by another part of the limbic system that rests deep within the brain and is called the hypothalamus. Dysfunction of this structure, whether from disorders or as a consequence of the adverse effect of drugs used to treat mental illness, produces common psychiatric symptoms, such as appetite and sleep problems.

Nerve cells within the hypothalamus secrete hormones, for example, antidiuretic hormone, which when sent to the kidneys, accelerates the reabsorption of water; and oxytocin, which acts on smooth muscles to promote contractions, particularly within the walls of the uterus. Because cells within the nervous system produce these

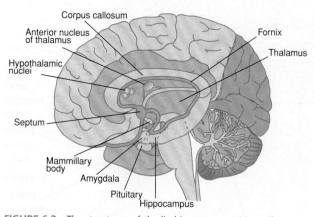

FIGURE 6.3 The structures of the limbic system are integrally involved in memory and emotional behavior. Theories link changes in the limbic system to many major mental disorders, including schizophrenia, depression, and anxiety disorders.

hormones, they are often referred to as **neurohormones** (hormones that are produced by cells within the nervous system) and form a communication mechanism through the bloodstream to control organs that are not directly connected to nervous system structures.

The pituitary gland, often called the *master gland*, is directly connected by thousands of neurons that attach it to the ventral aspects of the hypothalamus. Together with the pituitary gland, the hypothalamus functions as one of the primary regulators of many aspects of the endocrine system. Its functions are involved in control of visceral activities, such as body temperature, arterial blood pressure, hunger, thirst, fluid balance, gastric motility, and gastric secretions. Deregulation of the hypothalamus can be manifested in symptoms of certain psychiatric disorders. For example, in schizophrenia, patients often wear heavy coats during the hot summer months and do not appear hot. Before the role of the hypothalamus in schizophrenia was understood, psychological reasons were used to explain such symptoms. Now it is increasingly clear that such a symptom relates to deregulation of the hypothalamus's normal role in temperature regulation and is a biologically based symptom (Kreuzer et al., 2012).

Amygdala

The amygdala is directly connected to more primitive centers of the brain involving the sense of smell. It has numerous connections to the hypothalamus and lies adjacent to the hippocampus. The amygdala provides an emotional component to memory and is involved in modulating aggression and sexuality. Impulsive acts of aggression and violence have been linked to dysregulation of the amygdala, and erratic firing of the nerve cells in the amygdala is a focus of investigation in bipolar mood disorders (see Chapter 20).

Limbic Midbrain Nuclei

The limbic midbrain nuclei are a collection of neurons (including the ventral tegmental area and the locus ceruleus) that appear to play a role in the biologic basis of addiction. Sometimes referred to as the pleasure center or reward center of the brain, the limbic midbrain nuclei function to chemically reinforce certain behaviors, ensuring their repetition. Emotions such as feeling satisfied with good food, the pleasure of nurturing young, and the enjoyment of sexual activity originate in the limbic midbrain nuclei. The reinforcement of activities such as nutrition, procreation, and nurturing young are all primitive aspects of ensuring the survival of a species. When functioning in abnormal ways, the limbic midbrain nuclei can begin to reinforce unhealthy or risky behaviors, such as drug abuse. Exploration of this area of the brain is in its infancy but offers potential insight into addictions and their treatment.

Other Central Nervous System Structures

The **extrapyramidal motor system** is a bundle of nerve fibers connecting the thalamus to the basal ganglia and cerebral cortex. Muscle tone, common reflexes, and automatic voluntary motor functioning (e.g., walking) are controlled by this nerve track. Dysfunction of this motor track can produce hypertonicity in muscle groups. In Parkinson's disease, the cells that compose the extrapyramidal motor system are severely affected, producing many involuntary motor movements. A number of medications, which are discussed in Chapter 10, also affect this system.

The **pineal body** is located above and medial to the thalamus. Because the pineal gland easily calcifies, it can be visualized by neuroimaging and often is a medial landmark. Its functions remain somewhat of a mystery despite long knowledge of its existence. It contains secretory cells that emit the neurohormone melatonin and other substances. These hormones are thought to have a number of regulatory functions within the endocrine system. Information received from light–dark sources controls release of melatonin, which has been associated with sleep and emotional disorders. In addition, a modulation of immune function has been postulated for melatonin from the pineal gland.

The **locus ceruleus** is a tiny cluster of neurons that fan out and innervate almost every part of the brain, including most of the cortex, the thalamus and hypothalamus, the cerebellum, and the spinal cord. Just one neuron from the ceruleus can connect to more than 250,000 other neurons. Despite its small size, the wide-ranging neuronal connections allow this tiny structure to influence the regulation of attention, time perception, sleep–rest cycles, arousal, learning, pain, and mood. It also plays a role in information processing of new, unexpected, and novel experiences. Some think its function or dysfunction may explain why individuals become addicted to substances and seek out risky behaviors despite awareness of negative consequences.

The **brain stem**, which is located beneath the thalamus and composed of the midbrain, pons, and medulla, has important life-sustaining functions. Nuclei of numerous neural pathways to the cerebrum are located in the brain stem. They are significantly involved in mediating symptoms of emotional dysfunction. These nuclei are also the primary source of several neurochemicals, such as serotonin, that are commonly associated with psychiatric disorders.

The **cerebellum** is in the posterior aspect of the skull beneath the cerebral hemispheres. This large structure controls movements and postural adjustments. To regulate postural balance and positioning, the cerebellum

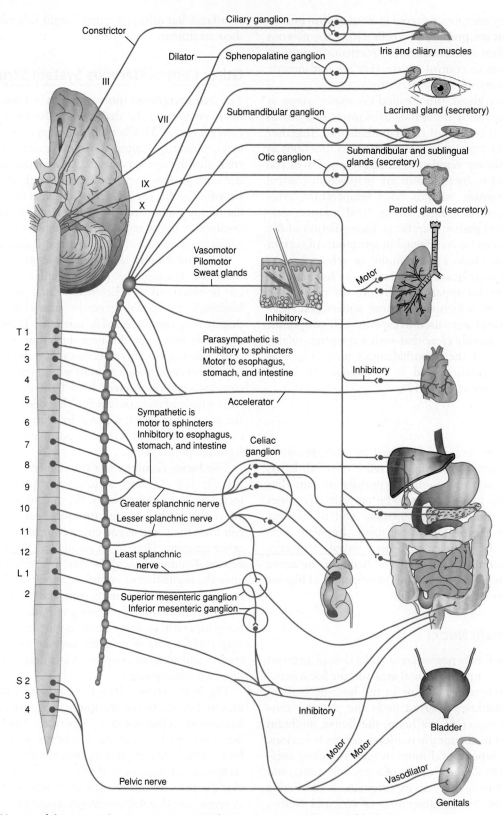

FIGURE 6.4 Diagram of the autonomic nervous system. Note that many organs are innervated by both sympathetic and parasympathetic nerves. (Adapted with permission from Chaffee, E. E., & Lytle, I. M. [1980]. *Basic physiology and anatomy*. Philadelphia: J. B. Lippincott.)

receives information from all parts of the body, including the muscles, joints, skin, and visceral organs, as well as from many parts of the CNS.

Autonomic Nervous System

Closely associated with the spinal cord but not lying entirely within its column is the **autonomic nervous system**, a subdivision of the PNS. It was originally given this name for being independent of conscious thought, that is, automatic. However, it does not necessarily function as autonomously as the name indicates. This system contains efferent (nerves moving away from the CNS), or motor system neurons, which affect target tissues such as cardiac muscle, smooth muscle, and the glands. It also contains afferent nerves, which are sensory and conduct information from these organs back to the CNS.

The autonomic nervous system is further divided into the sympathetic and parasympathetic nervous systems. These systems, although peripheral, are included here because they are involved in the emergency, or "fight-or-flight," response as well as the peripheral actions of many medications (see Chapter 10). Figure 6.4 illustrates the innervations of various target organs by the autonomic nervous system. Table 6.1 identifies the actions of the sympathetic and parasympathetic nervous systems on various target organs.

NEUROPHYSIOLOGY OF THE CENTRAL NERVOUS SYSTEM

At their most basic level, the human brain and connecting nervous system are composed of billions of cells. Most are connective and supportive glial cells with ancillary functions in the nervous system.

> **KEYCONCEPT** **Neuroplasticity** is a continuous process of modulation of neuronal structure and function in response to the changing environment.

The changes in neural environment can come from internal sources, such as a change in electrolytes, or from

TABLE 6.1	PERIPHERAL ORGAN RESPONSE IN THE AUTONOMIC NERVOUS SYSTEM	
Effector Organ	Sympathetic Response (Mostly Norepinephrine)	Parasympathetic Response (Acetylcholine)
Eye		
• Iris sphincter muscle	Dilation	Constriction
• Ciliary muscle	Relaxation	Accommodation for near vision
Heart		
• Sinoatrial node	Increased rate	Decrease is rare
• Atria	Increased contractility	Decrease in contractility
• Atrioventricular node	Increased contractility	Decrease in conduction velocity
Blood vessels	Constriction	Dilation
Lungs		
• Bronchial muscles	Relaxation	Bronchoconstriction
• Bronchial glands		Secretion
Gastrointestinal Tract		
• Motility and tone	Relaxation	Increased
• Sphincters	Contraction	Relaxation
• Secretion		Stimulation
Urinary Bladder		
• Detrusor muscle	Relaxation	Contraction
• Trigone and sphincter	Contraction	Relaxation
Uterus	Contraction (pregnant) Relaxation (nonpregnant)	Variable
Skin		
• Pilomotor muscles	Contraction	No effect
• Sweat glands	Increased secretion	No effect
Glands		
• Salivary, lachrymal		Increased secretion
• Sweat		Increased secretion

external sources, such as a virus or toxin. Because of neuroplasticity, nerve signals may be rerouted, cells may learn new functions, the sensitivity or number of cells may increase or decrease, and some nerve tissue may undergo limited regeneration. Brains are most plastic during infancy and young childhood, when large adaptive learning tasks should normally occur. With age, brains become less plastic, which explains why it is easier to learn a second language at the age of 5 years than 55 years. Neuroplasticity contributes to understanding how function may be restored over time after brain damage occurs, or how an individual may react over time to continuous pharmacotherapy regimens.

Neurons and Nerve Impulses

In the human body, approximately 10 billion nerve cells, or **neurons**, function to receive, organize, and transmit information (Figure 6.5). Each neuron has a cell body, or soma, which holds the nucleus containing most of the cell's genetic information. The soma also includes other organelles, such as ribosomes and endoplasmic reticu-

lum, which carry out protein synthesis; the Golgi apparatus, which contains enzymes to modify the proteins for specific functions; vesicles, which transport and store proteins; and lysosomes, which are responsible for degradation of these proteins. Located throughout the neurons, mitochondria, containing enzymes and often called the "powerhouse" are the sites of many energy-producing chemical reactions. These cell structures provide the basis for secreting numerous chemicals by which neurons communicate.

It is not just the vast number of neurons that accounts for the complexities of the brain but also the enormous number of neurochemical interconnections and interactions among neurons. A single motor neuron in the spinal cord may receive signals from more than 10,000 sources of interconnections with other nerves. Although most neurons have only one axon, which varies in length and conducts impulses away from the soma, each has numerous dendrites, receiving signals from other neurons. Because axons may branch as they terminate, they also have multiple contacts with other neurons.

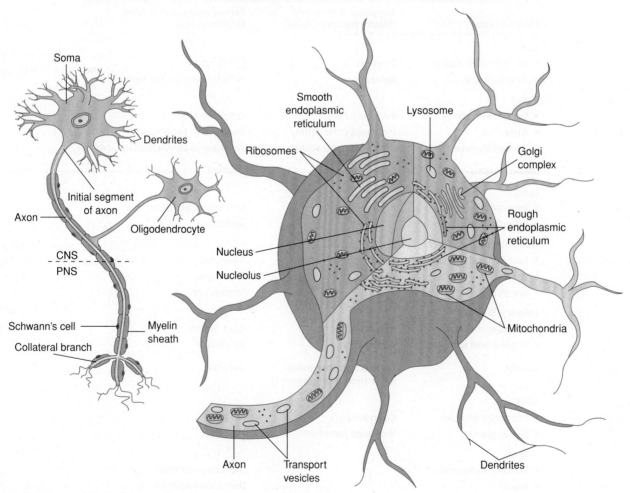

FIGURE 6.5 Cell body and organelles of neuron.

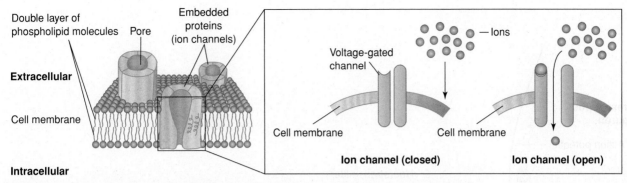

FIGURE 6.6 Initiation of a nerve impulse. The initiation of an action potential, or nerve impulse, involves the opening and closing of the voltage-gated channels on the cell membrane and the passage of ions into the cell. The resulting electrical activity sends communication impulses from the dendrites or axon into the body.

Nerve signals are prompted to fire by a variety of chemical or physical stimuli. This firing produces an electrical impulse. The cell's membrane is a double layer of phospholipid molecules with embedded proteins. Some of these proteins provide water-filled channels through which inorganic ions may pass (Figure 6.6). Each of the common ions—sodium, potassium, calcium, and chloride—has its own specific molecular channel. Many of these channels are voltage gated and thus open or close in response to changes in the electrical potential across the membrane. At rest, the cell membrane is polarized with a positive charge on the outside and about a 270-millivolt charge on the inside, owing to the resting distribution of sodium and potassium ions. As potassium passively diffuses across the membrane, the sodium pump uses energy to move sodium from the inside of the cell against a concentration gradient to maintain this distribution. An action potential, or *nerve impulse*, is generated as the membrane is depolarized and a threshold value is reached, which triggers the opening of the voltage-gated sodium channels, allowing sodium to surge into the cell. The inside of the cell briefly becomes positively charged and the outside negatively charged. Once initiated, the action potential becomes self-propagating, opening nearby sodium channels. This electrical communication moves into the soma from the dendrites or down the axon by this mechanism.

Synaptic Transmission

For one neuron to communicate with another, the electrical process described must change to a chemical communication. The **synaptic cleft**, a junction between one nerve and another, is the space where the electrical intracellular signal becomes a chemical extracellular signal. Various substances are recognized as the chemical messengers among neurons.

As the electrical action potential reaches the ends of the axons, called *terminals*, calcium ion channels are opened, allowing an influx of Ca^{++} ions into the neuron. This increase in calcium stimulates the release of neurotransmitters into the synapse. Rapid signaling among neurons requires a ready supply of neurotransmitter. These neurotransmitters are stored in small vesicles grouped near the cell membrane at the end of the axon. When stimulated, the vesicles containing the neurotransmitter fuse with the cell membrane, and the neurotransmitter is released into the synapse (Figure 6.7). The neurotransmitter then crosses the synaptic cleft to a receptor site on the postsynaptic neuron and stimulates adjacent neurons. This is the process of neuronal communication.

When the neurotransmitter has completed its interaction with the postsynaptic receptor and stimulated that cell, its work is done, and it needs to be removed. It can be removed by natural diffusion away from the area of high neurotransmitter concentration at the receptors by being broken down by enzymes in the synaptic cleft or through reuptake through highly specific mechanisms into the presynaptic terminal. The primary steps in synaptic transmission are summarized in Figure 6.7.

Neurotransmitters

As described in the overview above, neurotransmitters are key in the process of synaptic transmission. Neurotransmitters are small molecules that directly and indirectly control the opening or closing of ion channels. **Neuromodulators** are chemical messengers that make the target cell membrane or postsynaptic membrane more or less susceptible to the effects of the primary neurotransmitter.

> **KEYCONCEPT** **Neurotransmitters** are small molecules that directly and indirectly control the opening or closing of ion channels.

Excitatory neurotransmitters reduce the membrane potential and enhance the transmission of the signal between neurons. *Inhibitory neurotransmitters* have the opposite effect and slow down nerve impulses. Although some are synthesized from dietary precursors, such as

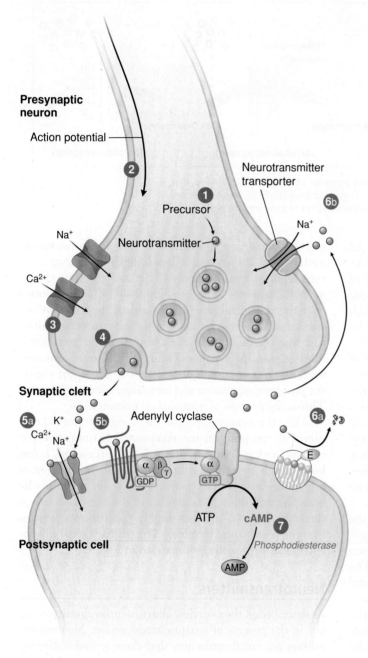

Presynaptic neuron

Action potential

Neurotransmitter transporter

Precursor

Neurotransmitter

Na^+

Ca^{2+}

Na^+

Synaptic cleft

K^+

Ca^{2+}

Na^+

Adenylyl cyclase

α β γ GDP

α GTP

E

ATP

cAMP

Postsynaptic cell

Phosphodiesterase

AMP

FIGURE 6.7 Steps in synaptic transmission. Synaptic transmission can be divided into a series of steps that couple electrical depolarization of the presynaptic neuron to chemical signaling between the presynaptic and postsynaptic cells. 1. Neuron synthesizes neurotransmitter from precursors and stores the transmitter in vesicles. 2. An action potential traveling down the neuron depolarizes the presynaptic nerve terminal. 3. Membrane depolarization activates voltage-dependent Ca^{2+} channels, allowing Ca^{2+} entry into the presynaptic nerve terminal. 4. The increased cytosolic Ca^{2+} enables vesicle fusion with the plasma membrane of the presynaptic neuron, with subsequent release of neurotransmitter into the synaptic cleft. 5. Neurotransmitter diffuses across the synaptic cleft and binds to one of two types of postsynaptic receptors. 5a. Neurotransmitter binding to ionotropic receptors causes channel opening and changes the permeability of the postsynaptic membrane to ions. This may also result in a change in the postsynaptic membrane potential. 5b. Neurotransmitter binding to metabotropic receptors on the postsynaptic cell activates intracellular signaling cascades; the example shows G protein activation leading to the formation of cAMP by adenylyl cyclase. In turn, such a signaling cascade can activate other ion-selective channels (not shown). 6. Signal termination is accomplished by removal of transmitter from the synaptic cleft. 6a. Transmitter can be degraded by enzymes (E) in the synaptic cleft. 6b. Alternatively, transmitter can be recycled into the presynaptic cell by reuptake transporters. 7. Signal termination can also be accomplished by enzymes (such as phosphodiesterase) that degrade postsynaptic intracellular signaling molecules (such as cAMP). (Reprinted with permission from Golan, D. E., Tashjian, A. H., Armstrong, E. J., and Armstrong, A. W. [2011]. *Principles of Pharmacology*, 3rd edition. Philadelphia: Wolters Kluwer.)

tyrosine or tryptophan, most synthesis occurs in the terminals or the neuron itself. Neurotransmitters are commonly classified as the following: cholinergic, biogenic amine (monoamines or bioamines), amino acid, and neuropeptides. Table 6.2 summarizes some of the key neurotransmitters and their proposed functions.

Acetylcholine

Acetylcholine (ACh) is the primary cholinergic neurotransmitter. Found in the greatest concentration in the

PNS, ACh provides the basic synaptic communication for the parasympathetic neurons and part of the sympathetic neurons, which send information to the CNS.

ACh is an excitatory neurotransmitter that is found throughout the cerebral cortex and limbic system. It arises primarily from cell bodies in the basal forebrain constellation, which provides innervations to the cerebral cortex, amygdala, hippocampus, and thalamus as well as from the dorsolateral tegmentum of the pons that projects to the basal ganglia, thalamus, hypothalamus, medullary reticular formation, and deep cerebellar

TABLE 6.2	CLASSIC AND PUTATIVE NEUROTRANSMITTERS: THEIR DISTRIBUTION AND PROPOSED FUNCTIONS		
Neurotransmitter	Cell Bodies	Projections	Proposed Function
Acetylcholine			
Dietary precursor: choline	Basal forebrain Pons Other areas	Diffuse throughout the cortex, hippocampus PNS	Important role in learning and memory Some role in wakefulness and basic attention Peripherally activates muscles and is the major neurochemical in the autonomic system
Monoamines			
Dopamine (dietary precursor: tyrosine)	Substantia nigra Ventral tegmental area Arcuate nucleus Retina olfactory bulb	Striatum (basal ganglia) Limbic system and cerebral cortex Pituitary	Involved in involuntary motor movements Some role in mood states, pleasure components in reward systems, and complex behavior (e.g., judgment, reasoning, insight)
Norepinephrine (dietary precursor: tyrosine)	Locus ceruleus Lateral tegmental area and others throughout the pons and medulla	Very widespread throughout the cortex, thalamus, cerebellum, brain stem, and spinal cord Basal forebrain, thalamus, hypothalamus, brain stem, and spinal cord	Proposed role in learning and memory, attributing value in reward systems, fluctuates in sleep and wakefulness Major component of the sympathetic nervous system responses, including "fight or flight"
Serotonin (dietary precursor: tryptophan)	Raphe nuclei Others in the pons and medulla	Very widespread throughout the cortex, thalamus, cerebellum, brain stem, and spinal cord	Proposed role in the control of appetite, sleep, mood states, hallucinations, pain perception, and vomiting
Histamine (precursor: histidine)	Hypothalamus	Cerebral cortex Limbic system Hypothalamus Found in all mast cells	Control of gastric secretions, smooth muscle control, cardiac stimulation, stimulation of sensory nerve endings, and alertness
Amino Acids			
GABA	Derived from glutamate without localized cell bodies	Found in cells and projections throughout the CNS, especially in intrinsic feedback loops and interneurons of the cerebrum Also in the extrapyramidal motor system and cerebellum	Fast inhibitory response postsynaptically, inhibits the excitability of the neurons and therefore contributes to seizure, agitation, and anxiety control
Glycine	Primarily the spinal cord and brain stem	Limited projection, but especially in the auditory system and olfactory bulb Also found in the spinal cord, medulla, midbrain, cerebellum, and cortex	Inhibitory Decreases the excitability of spinal motor neurons but not cortical
Glutamate	Diffuse	Diffuse, but especially in the sensory organs	Excitatory Responsible for the bulk of information flow
Neuropeptides			
Endogenous opioids (i.e., endorphins, enkephalins)	A large family of neuropeptides that has three distinct subgroups, all of which are manufactured widely throughout the CNS	Widely distributed within and outside of the CNS	Suppress pain, modulate mood and stress Likely involvement in reward systems and addiction Also may regulate pituitary hormone release Implicated in the pathophysiology of diseases of the basal ganglia
Melatonin (one of its precursors: serotonin)	Pineal body	Widely distributed within and outside of the CNS	Secreted in dark and suppressed in light, helps regulate the sleep–wake cycle as well as other biologic rhythms
Substance P	Widespread, significant in the raphe system and spinal cord	Spinal cord, cortex, brain stem, and especially sensory neurons associated with pain perception	Involved in pain transmission, movement, and mood regulation
Cholecystokinin	Predominates in the ventral tegmental area of the midbrain	Frontal cortex, where it is often colocalized with dopamine Widely distributed within and outside of the CNS	Primary intestinal hormone involved in satiety; also has some involvement in the control of anxiety and panic

CNS, central nervous system; GABA, gamma-aminobutyric acid; PNS, peripheral nervous system.

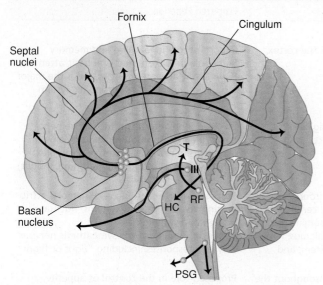

FIGURE 6.8 Cholinergic pathways. HC, hippocampal formation; PSG, parasympathetic ganglion cell; RF, reticular formation; T, thalamus. (Adapted with permission from Nolte, J., & Angevine, J. [1995]. *The human brain: In photographs and diagrams.* St. Louis: Mosby.)

nuclei (Siegel & Sapru, 2010) (Figure 6.8). These connections suggest that ACh is involved in higher intellectual functioning and memory. Individuals who have Alzheimer's disease or Down syndrome often exhibit patterns of cholinergic neuron loss in regions innervated by these pathways (e.g., the hippocampus), which may contribute to their memory difficulties and other cognitive deficits. Some cholinergic neurons are afferent to these areas bringing information from the limbic system, highlighting the role that ACh plays in communicating one's emotional state to the cerebral cortex.

Biogenic Amines

The **biogenic amines** (bioamines) consist of small molecules manufactured in the neuron that contain an amine group, thus the name. The catecholamines (amine attached to a catechol group) include dopamine, norepinephrine, and epinephrine, which are all synthesized from the amino acid tyrosine. Another monoamine, serotonin, is synthesized from tryptophan. Melatonin is derived from serotonin. All of these neurotransmitters are critical in many of the mental disorders.

Dopamine

Dopamine is an excitatory neurotransmitter found in distinct regions of the CNS and is involved in cognition, motor, and neuroendocrine functions. Dopamine is the neurotransmitter that stimulates the body's natural "feel good' reward pathways, producing pleasant euphoric sensation under certain conditions. It is involved in the regulation of action, emotion, motivation, and attention.

Dopamine levels are decreased in Parkinson's disease, and abnormally high activity of dopamine has been associated with schizophrenia (discussed in more detail in Chapter 22). Abnormalities of dopamine activity within the reward system pathways are suspected to be a critical aspect of the development of drug and other addictions. The dopamine pathways are distinct neuronal areas within the CNS in which the neurotransmitter dopamine predominates. Three major dopaminergic pathways have been identified.

The *mesocortical* and *mesolimbic pathways* originate in the ventral tegmental area and project into the medial aspects of the cortex (mesocortical) and the limbic system inside the temporal lobes, including the hippocampus and amygdala (mesolimbic). Sometimes they are considered to be one pathway and at other times two separate pathways. The mesocortical pathway has major effects on cognition, including such functions as judgment, reasoning, insight, social conscience, motivation, the ability to generalize learning, and reward systems in the human brain. It contributes to some of the highest seats of cortical functioning. The mesolimbic pathway also strongly influences emotions and has projections that affect memory and auditory reception. Abnormalities in these pathways have been associated with schizophrenia.

Another major dopaminergic pathway begins in the substantia nigra and projects into the basal ganglia, parts of which are known as the *striatum*. Therefore, this pathway is called the *nigrostriatal pathway*. This influences the extrapyramidal motor system, which serves the voluntary motor system and allows involuntary motor movements. Destruction of dopaminergic neurons in this pathway has been associated with Parkinson's disease.

The final dopamine pathway originates from projections of the mesolimbic pathway and continues into the hypothalamus, which then projects into the pituitary gland. Therefore, this pathway, called the *tuberoinfundibular pathway*, has an impact on endocrine function and other functions, such as metabolism, hunger, thirst, sexual function, circadian rhythms, digestion, and temperature control. Figure 6.9 illustrates the dopaminergic pathways.

Norepinephrine

Norepinephrine is an excitatory neurochemical that plays a major role in generating and maintaining mood states. Decreased norepinephrine has been associated with depression, and excessive norepinephrine has been associated with manic symptoms (Blier & El Mansari, 2013). Because norepinephrine is so heavily concentrated in the terminal sites of sympathetic nerves, it can be released quickly to ready the individual for a fight-or-flight response to threats in the environment. For this reason, norepinephrine is thought to play a role in the physical symptoms of anxiety.

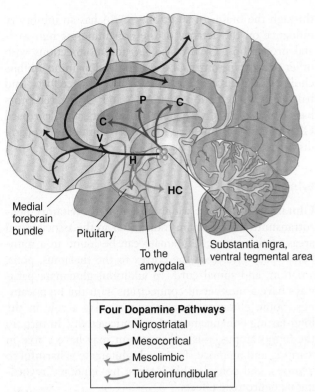

Four Dopamine Pathways
- Nigrostriatal
- Mesocortical
- Mesolimbic
- Tuberoinfundibular

FIGURE 6.9   Dopaminergic pathways. C, caudate nucleus; H, hypothalamus; HC, hippocampal formation; P, putamen; S, striatum; V, ventral striatum. (Adapted with permission from Nolte, J., & Angevine, J. [1995]. *The human brain: In photographs and diagrams.* St. Louis: Mosby.)

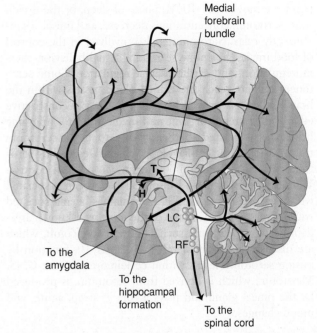

FIGURE 6.10   Noradrenergic pathways. H, hypothalamus; LC, locus ceruleus; RF, reticular formation; T, thalamus. (Adapted with permission from Nolte, J., & Angevine, J. [1995]. *The human brain: In photographs and diagrams.* St. Louis: Mosby.)

Nerve tracts and pathways containing predominantly norepinephrine are called *noradrenergic* and are less clearly delineated than the dopamine pathways. In the CNS, noradrenergic neurons originate in the locus ceruleus, where more than half of the noradrenergic cell bodies are located. Because the locus ceruleus is one of the major timekeepers of the human body, norepinephrine is involved in sleep and wakefulness. From the locus ceruleus, noradrenergic pathways ascend into the neocortex, spread diffusely (Figure 6.10), and enhance the ability of neurons to respond to whatever input they may be receiving. In addition, norepinephrine appears to be involved in the process of reinforcement, which facilitates learning. Noradrenergic pathways innervate the hypothalamus and thus are involved to some degree in endocrine function. Anxiety disorders and depression are examples of psychiatric illnesses in which dysfunction of the noradrenergic neurons may be involved. (Refer to Table 6.1 for the effects of ACh on various organs in the parasympathetic system.)

Serotonin

Serotonin (also called 5-hydroxytryptamine or 5-HT) is primarily an excitatory neurotransmitter that is diffusely distributed within the cerebral cortex, limbic system, and basal ganglia of the CNS. Serotonergic neurons also project into the hypothalamus and cerebellum. Figure 6.11 illustrates serotonergic pathways. Serotonin plays a role in emotions, cognition, sensory perceptions, and essential biologic functions, such as sleep and appetite. During the

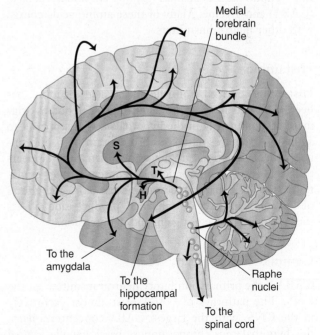

FIGURE 6.11   Serotonergic pathways. H, hypothalamus; S, septal nuclei; T, thalamus. (Adapted with permission from Nolte, J., & Angevine, J. [1995]. *The human brain: In photographs and diagrams.* St. Louis: Mosby.)

rapid eye movement (REM) phase of sleep, or the dream state, serotonin concentrations decrease, and muscles subsequently relax. Serotonin is also involved in the control of food intake, hormone secretion, sexual behavior, thermoregulation, and cardiovascular regulation. Some serotonergic fibers reach the cranial blood vessels within the brain and the *pia mater* where they have a vasoconstrictive effect. The potency of some new medications for migraine headaches is related to their ability to block serotonin transmission in the cranial blood vessels. Descending serotonergic pathways are important in central pain control. Whereas depression and insomnia have been associated with decreased levels of 5-HT, mania has been associated with increased 5-HT. Some of the most well-known antidepressant medications, such as Prozac and Zoloft, which are discussed in more depth in Chapter 10, function by raising serotonin levels within certain areas of the CNS. Melatonin, which is derived from serotonin, is produced by the pineal gland and plays a role in sleep, aging, and mood changes.

Amino Acids

Amino acids, the building blocks of proteins, have many roles in intraneuronal metabolism. In addition, amino acids can function as neurotransmitters in as many as 60% to 70% of the synaptic sites in the brain. Amino acids are the most prevalent neurotransmitters. Virtually all of the neurons in the CNS are activated by excitatory amino acids, such as glutamate, and inhibited by inhibitory amino acids, such as gamma-aminobutyric acid (GABA) and glycine. Many of these amino acids coexist with other neurotransmitters.

Histamine

Histamine, derived from the amino acid histidine, has been identified as a neurotransmitter. Its cell bodies originate predominantly in the hypothalamus and project to all major structures in the cerebrum, brain stem, and spinal cord. Its functions are not well known, but it appears to have a role in autonomic and neuroendocrine regulation. Many psychiatric medications can block the effects of histamine postsynaptically and produce side effects such as sedation, weight gain, and hypotension.

Gamma-Aminobutyric Acid

GABA is the primary inhibitory neurotransmitter for the CNS. The pathways of GABA exist almost exclusively in the CNS, with the largest GABA concentrations in the hypothalamus, hippocampus, basal ganglia, spinal cord, and cerebellum. GABA functions in an inhibitory role in control of spinal reflexes and cerebellar reflexes. It has a major role in the control of neuronal excitability through the brain. In addition, GABA has an inhibitory influence on the activity of the dopaminergic nigrostriatal projections. GABA also has interconnections with other neurotransmitters. For example, dopamine inhibits cholinergic neurons, and GABA provides feedback and balance. Dysregulation of GABA and GABA receptors has been associated with anxiety disorders, and decreased GABA activity is involved in the development of seizure disorders.

Glutamate

Glutamate, the most widely distributed excitatory neurotransmitter, is the main transmitter in the associational areas of the cortex. Glutamate can be found in a number of pathways from the cortex to the thalamus, pons, striatum, and spinal cord. In addition, glutamate pathways have a number of connections with the hippocampus. Some glutamate receptors may play a role in the long-lasting enhancement of synaptic activity. In turn, in the hippocampus, this enhancement may have a role in learning and memory. Too much glutamate is harmful to neurons, and considerable interest has emerged regarding its neurotoxic effects.

Conditions that produce an excess of endogenous glutamate can cause neurotoxicity by overexcitation of neuronal tissue. This process, called excitotoxicity, increases the sensitivity of glutamate receptors, produces overactivation of the receptors, and is increasingly being understood as a critical piece of the cascade of events involved in physical symptoms of alcohol withdrawal in dependent individuals. Excitotoxicity is also believed to be part of the pathology of conditions such as ischemia, hypoxia, hypoglycemia, and hepatic failure. Damage to the CNS from chronic malfunctioning of the glutamate system may be involved in the psychiatric symptoms seen in neurodegenerative diseases such as Huntington's, Parkinson's, and Alzheimer's diseases; vascular dementia; amyotrophic lateral sclerosis; and acquired immune deficiency syndrome (AIDS)–related dementia. Degeneration of glutamate neurons is implicated in the development of schizophrenia.

Neuropeptides

Neuropeptides, short chains of amino acids, exist in the CNS and have a number of important roles as neurotransmitters, neuromodulators, or neurohormones. Neuropeptides were first thought to be pituitary hormones, such as adrenocorticotropin, oxytocin, and vasopressin, or hypothalamic-releasing hormones (e.g., corticotropin-releasing hormone and thyrotropin-releasing hormone [TRH]). However, when an endogenous morphine-like substance was discovered in the 1970s, the term *endorphin*, or endogenous morphine, was introduced. Although the amino acids and monoamine neurotransmitters can be produced directly from dietary precursors in any part of the neuron, neuropeptides are, almost without exception, synthesized from messenger RNA in the cell body. Currently, two types of neuropeptides have been identified. Opioid neuropeptides, such as endorphins, enkephalins, and dynorphins, function in endocrine functioning and pain suppression. The nonopioid neuropeptides, such as substance P and somatostatin, play roles in pain transmission and endocrine functioning, respectively.

There are considerable variations in the distribution of individual neuropeptides, but some areas are especially rich in cell bodies containing neuropeptides. These areas include the amygdala, striatum, hypothalamus, raphe nuclei, brain stem, and spinal cord. Many of the interneurons of the cerebral cortex contain neuropeptides, but there are considerably fewer in the thalamus and almost none in the cerebellum.

Receptors

Embedded in the postsynaptic membrane are a number of proteins that act as receptors for the released neurotransmitters. Each neurotransmitter has a specific **receptor**, or protein, for which it and only it will fit.

Lock and Key

The "lock-and-key" analogy has often been used to describe the fit of a given neurotransmitter to its receptor site. The target cell, when stimulated by the neurotransmitter, will then respond by evoking its own action potential and either producing some action common to that cell or acting as a relay to keep the messages moving throughout the CNS. This pattern of the electrical signal from one neuron, converted to chemical signal at the synaptic cleft, picked up by an adjacent neuron, again converted to an electrical action potential, and then to a chemical signal, occurs billions of times a day in billions of different neurons. This electrical–chemical communication process allows the structures of the brain to function together in a coordinated and organized manner.

Receptor Sensitivity

Both presynaptic and postsynaptic receptors have the capacity to change, developing either a greater-than-usual response to the neurotransmitter, known as supersensitivity, or a less-than-usual response, called subsensitivity. These changes represent the concept of neuroplasticity of brain tissue discussed earlier in the chapter. The change in sensitivity of the receptor is most commonly caused by the effect of a drug on a receptor site or by disease that affects the normal functioning of a receptor site. Drugs can affect the sensitivity of the receptor by altering the strength of attraction or affinity of a receptor for the neurotransmitter, by changing the efficiency with which the receptor activity translates the message inside the receiving cell, or by decreasing over time the number of receptors.

These mechanisms may account for the long-term, sometimes severely adverse, effects of psychopharmacologic drugs, the loss of effectiveness of a given medication, or the loss of effectiveness of a medication after repeated use in treating recurring episodes of a psychiatric disorder. Disease may cause a change in the normal number or function of receptors, thereby altering their sensitivity. For example, depression is associated with a reduction in the normal number of certain receptors, leading to an abnormality in their sensitivity to neurotransmitters such as serotonin and norepinephrine (Bewernick & Schlaepfer, 2013). A decreased response to continued stimulation of these receptors is usually referred to as *desensitization* or *refractoriness*. This suspected subsensitivity is referred to as *downregulation* of the receptors.

Receptor Subtypes

The nervous system uses many different neurochemicals for communication, and each specific chemical messenger requires a specific receptor on which the chemical can act. More than 100 different chemical messengers have been identified, with new ones being uncovered. In addition to the sheer number of receptors needed to accommodate these chemicals, the neurotransmitters may produce different effects at different synaptic sites.

Each major neurotransmitter has several different subtypes of receptors, allowing the neurotransmitter to have different effects in different areas of the brain. The receptors usually have the same name as the neurotransmitter, but the classification of the subtypes varies. For example, dopamine receptors are named D1, D2, D3, and so on. Serotonin receptors are grouped in families such at 5HT 1a, 5HT 1b, and so on. The receptors for Ach have completely different names: muscarinic and nicotinic. Two specific subtype receptors have been identified for GABA: A and B.

Neurocircuitry

Brain structures such as the prefrontal cortex, striatum, hippocampus, and amygdala are linked through complex neural functional networks (Haber & Rauch, 2010; Sequira, Martin, & Vawter, 2012). Recent research indicates that a dysfunctional **neurocircuitry** underlies most psychiatric disorders (Figure 6.12). Various neurocircuits are the focus of study of different illness. For example, the cingulo-frontal-parietal network is associated with attention-deficit disorder, and the amygdalo-cortical circuitry is the focus in psychosis and schizophrenia.

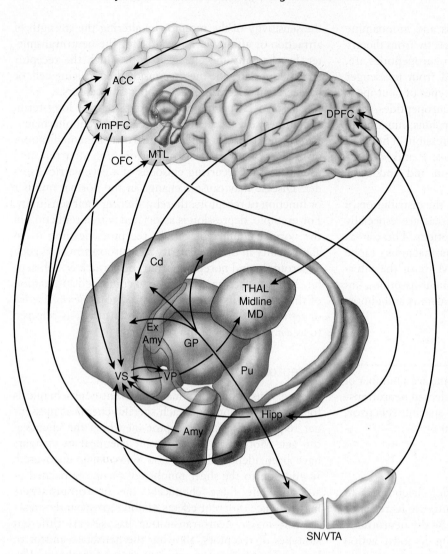

FIGURE 6.12 Key structures and pathways involved in neuropsychiatric disorders. *Arrows* illustrate projections. ACC, anterior cingulate cortex; Amy, amygdala; Cd, caudate nucleus; DPFC, dorsal prefrontal cortex; GP, globus pallidus; Ex Amy, extended amygdala; Hipp, hippocampus; MD, medial dorsal nucleus of the thalamus; MTL, medial temporal lobe; OFC, orbital frontal cortex; Pu, Putamen; SN, substantia nigra; Thal, thalamus; vmPFC, ventral medial prefrontal cortex; VP, ventral pallidum; VS, ventral striatum; VTA, ventral tegmental area. (Redrawn with permission from Haber, S. N., & Rauch, S. L. [2010]. Neurocircuitry: A window into the networks underlying neuropsychiatric disease. *Neuropsychopharmacology Reviews*, 35[1], 1–3.)

STUDIES OF THE BIOLOGIC BASIS OF MENTAL DISORDERS

As described earlier, mental disorders are complex syndromes consisting of clusters of biopsychosocial symptoms. These syndromes are not specific physiological disorders, and research efforts are focused on piecing the puzzle together. One important area of study is genetics; it is well established that genetic factors play an important role in the development of mental disorders. In addition, as the complexity of the nervous system and its interrelationship with other body systems and the environment has become more fully understood, new fields of study have emerged. One field worth noting is **psychoneuroimmunology** (PNI). Although it has long been observed that individuals under stress have compromised immune systems and are more likely to acquire common diseases, only recently have changes in the immune system been noted as widespread in some psychiatric illnesses. Another field, chronobiology, has provided new informa-

tion suggesting that dysfunction of biologic rhythms may not only result from a psychiatric illness but also contribute to its development.

Genetics

The sequence of the human genome is the beginning of our understanding of complex genetic connections that leads to a **phenotype** or observable characteristics or expressions of a specific trait. The genome provides researchers with a road map of the exact sequence of the three billion nucleotide bases that make up human organisms. Many thought that after the human genome was mapped, it would be easy to determine the genes responsible for mental disorders. Unfortunately, it is not that simple. Knowing the location of the gene and its sequence are just pieces of the complex puzzle. The location of the genes does not tell us which genes are responsible for a mental illness or how mutations occur.

King George III (1739–1830)

Bipolar Illness Misdiagnosed

PUBLIC PERSONA

Crowned King of England at age 22 years, George III headed the most influential colonial power in the world at that time. England thrived in the peacetime after the Seven Years' War with France but simultaneously taxed its American colonies so heavily and resolutely that the colonies rebelled. Could the American Revolution be blamed on King George III's state of mind?

PERSONAL REALITIES

At age 50 years, the king first experienced abdominal pain and constipation followed by weak limbs, fever, tachycardia, hoarseness, and dark red urine. Later, he experienced confusion, racing thoughts, visual problems, restlessness, delirium, convulsions, and stupor. His strange behavior included ripping off his wig and running about naked. Although he recovered and did not have a relapse for 13 years, he was considered to be mad. Relapses after the first relapse became more frequent, and the king was eventually dethroned by the Prince of Wales.

Was George's madness in reality a genetically transmitted blood disease that caused thought disturbances, delirium, and stupor? The genetic disease porphyria is caused by defects in the body's ability to make haem. The diseases are generally inherited in an autosomal dominant fashion. The retrospective diagnosis was not made until 1966 (Macalpine & Hunter, 1966). Before that, it was believed that he had bipolar disorder.

Other members of the royal family who had this hereditary disease were Queen Anne of Great Britain; Frederic the Great of Germany; George IV of Great Britain (son of George III); and George IV's daughter, Princess Charlotte, who died during childbirth from complications of the disease.

Source: Macalpine, I. & Hunter, R. (1966). The "insanity" of King George 3d: A classic case of porphyria. *British Medical Journal, 1*(5479), 65–71.

Population Genetics

Inheritance of mental disorders is studied by using epidemiologic methods that identifies risks and patterns of illness or traits from generation to generation. Beginning with a **proband**, a person who has the disorder or trait, **population genetics** relies on the following principle epidemiologic methods:

- **Family studies** analyze the occurrence of a disorder in first-degree relatives (biologic parents, siblings, and children), second-degree relatives (grandparents, uncles, aunts, nieces, nephews, and grandchildren), and so on.
- **Twin studies** analyze the presence or absence of the disorder in pairs of twins. The concordance rate is the measure of similarity of occurrence in individuals with a similar genetic makeup.
- **Adoption studies** compare the risk for the illness developing in offspring raised in different environ-

ments. The strongest inferences may be drawn from studies that involve children separated from their parents at birth.

Mental disorders and their symptoms are not an expression of a single gene. The transmission pattern does not follow classic Mendelian genetics in which the dominant allele (variant) on only one chromosome or recessive alleles on both chromosomes are responsible for manifestation of a disorder. Monozygotic (identical) twins do not manifest the same mental disorder with 100% concordance rate, but they have a higher rate of a disorder than dizygotic (fraternal) twins, who share roughly the same proportion of genes that ordinary siblings do (50%). Internal and external environmental events influence the development of a disorder with a genetic contribution. This interaction between the environment and a genetic predisposition underlies several mental disorders such as schizophrenia, autism, and ADHD.

Molecular Genetics

A gene comprises short segments of DNA and is packed with the instructions for making proteins that have a specific function. When genes are absent or malfunction, protein production is altered, and bodily functions are disrupted. In this fashion, genes play a role in cancer, heart disease, diabetes, and many psychiatric disorders. Although no conclusive evidence exists for a complete genetic cause of most psychiatric disorders, significant evidence suggests that strong genetic contributions exist for most (Sullivan, Daly, & O'Donovan, 2012).

Intracellular genes direct protein production responsible for genetic expression. Individual nerve cells outside of the cell respond to these changes, modifying proteins to adapt to the new environment. This dynamic nature of gene function highlights the manner in which the body and the environment interact and in how environmental factors influence gene expression.

The study of molecular genetics in psychiatric disorders is in its infancy. It is likely that psychiatric disorders are polygenic. This means that psychiatric disorders develop when genes interact with each other and with environmental factors such as stress, infections, poor nutrition, catastrophic loss, complications during pregnancy, and exposure to toxins. Thus, genetic makeup conveys vulnerability, or a risk for the illness, but the right set of environmental factors must be present for the disorder to develop in an at-risk individual (Sequeira, Martin, & Vawter, 2012).

Genetic Susceptibility

The concept of **genetic susceptibility** suggests that an individual may be at increased risk for a psychiatric disorder. Specific risk factors for psychiatric disorders are just beginning to be understood, and environmental influences are examples of risk factors. In the absence of one specific gene for the major psychiatric disorders, risk factor assessment is a logical alternative for predicting who is more likely to experience psychiatric disorders or certain conditions, such as aggression or suicidality (Wasserman, Terenius, Wasserman, & Sokolowski, 2010).

When considering information regarding risks for genetic transmission of psychiatric disorders, there are several key points to remember:

- Psychiatric disorders have been described and labeled quite differently across generations, and errors in diagnosis may occur.
- Similar psychiatric symptoms may have considerably different causes, just as symptoms such as chest pain may occur in relation to many different causes.
- Genes that are present may not always cause the appearance of the trait.
- Several genes work together in an individual to produce a given trait or disorder.
- A biologic cause is not necessarily solely genetic in origin. Environmental influences alter the body's functioning and often mediate or worsen genetic risk factors.

Psychoneuroimmunology

PNI examines the relationships among the immune system, nervous system, and endocrine system and our behaviors, thoughts, and feelings. The immune system is composed of the thymus, spleen, lymph nodes, lymphatic vessels, tonsils, adenoids, and bone marrow, which manufactures all the cells that eventually develop into T cells, B cells, phagocytes, macrophages, and natural killer (NK) cells (Figure 6.13). Many contemporary stress research studies are examining the role of the NK cells in the early recognition of foreign bodies. Lower NK cell function is related to increased disease susceptibility. NK cell function is affected by stress-induced physiologic arousal in humans. NK cell activity has been shown to vary in response to many emotional, cognitive, and physiologic stressors, including anxiety, depression, perceived lack of personal control, bereavement, pain, and surgery (Pace & Heim, 2011).

Overactivity of the immune system can occur in autoimmune diseases such as systemic lupus erythematosus (SLE), allergies, and anaphylaxis. Evidence suggests that the nervous system regulates many aspects of immune function. Specific immune system dysfunctions may result from damage to the hypothalamus, hippocampus, or pituitary and may produce symptoms of psychiatric disorders. Figure 6.14 illustrates the interaction between

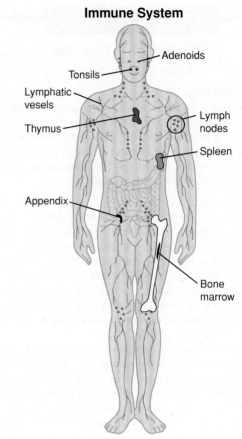

Immune System

FIGURE 6.13 The immune system.

stress and the immune system. This figure also demonstrates the true biopsychosocial nature of the complex interrelationship of the nervous system, the endocrine system, the immune system, and environmental or emotional stress.

Immune dysregulation may also be involved in the development of psychiatric disorders. This can occur by allowing neurotoxins to affect the brain, damaging neuroendocrine tissue, or damaging tissues in the brain at locations such as the receptor sites. Some antidepressants have been thought to have antiviral effects. Symptoms of diseases such as depression may occur after an occurrence of serious infection, and prenatal exposure to infectious organisms has been associated with the development of schizophrenia. Stress and conditioning have specific effects on the suppression of immune function (Pace & Heim, 2011).

Normal functioning of the endocrine system is often disturbed in people with psychiatric disorders. For example, thyroid functioning is often low in those with bipolar disorder, and people with schizophrenia have a higher incidence of diabetes (see Unit VI). The hypothalamus sends and receives information through the pituitary, which then communicates with structures in the peripheral aspects of the body. Figure 6.15 presents an example

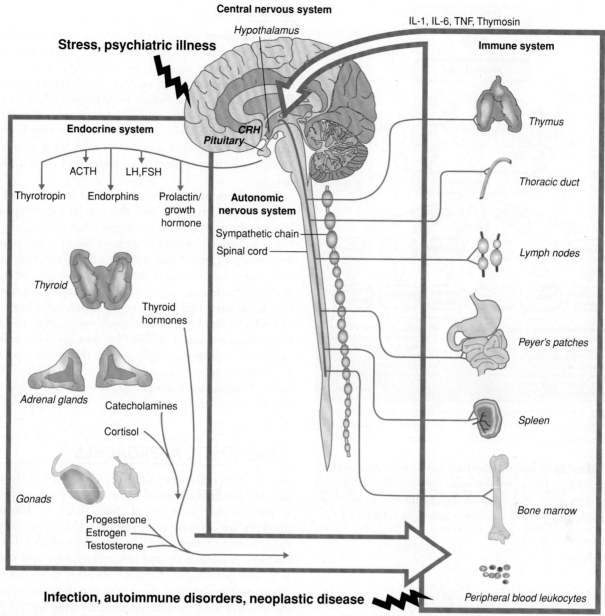

FIGURE 6.14 Examples of the interaction between stress or psychiatric illness and the immune system through the endocrine system. ACTH, adrenocorticotropic hormone; CRH, corticotropin-releasing hormone; FSH, follicle-stimulating hormone; IL, interleukin; LH, luteinizing hormone; TNF, tumor necrosis factor.

of the communication of the anterior pituitary with a number of organs and structures.

Axes, the structures within which the neurohormones are providing messages, are the most often studied aspect of the neuroendocrine system. These axes always involve a feedback mechanism. For example, the hypothalamus–pituitary–thyroid axis regulates the release of thyroid hormone by the thyroid gland using TRH hormone from the hypothalamus to the pituitary and thyroid-stimulating hormone (TSH) from the pituitary to the thyroid. Figure 6.16 illustrates the

hypothalamic–pituitary–thyroid axis. The hypothalamic–pituitary–gonadal axis regulates estrogen and testosterone secretion through luteinizing hormone and follicle-stimulating hormone. Interest in the endocrine system is heightened by various endocrine disorders that produce psychiatric symptoms. Addison's disease (hypoadrenalism) produces depression, apathy, fatigue, and occasionally psychosis. Hypothyroidism produces depression and some anxiety. Administration of steroids can cause depression, hypomania, irritability, and in some cases, psychosis. Some psychiatric

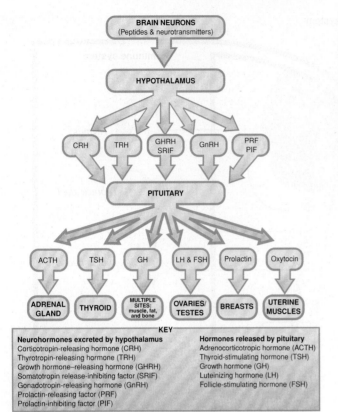

FIGURE 6.15 Hypothalamic and pituitary communication system. The neurohormonal communication system between the hypothalamus and the pituitary exerts effects on many organs and systems.

disorders have been associated with endocrine system dysfunction. For example, some individuals with mood disorders show evidence of dysregulation in adrenal, thyroid, and growth hormone axes (see Chapter 19).

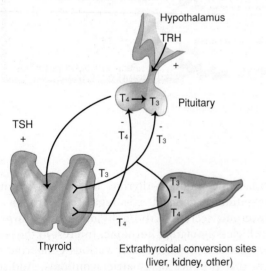

FIGURE 6.16 Hypothalamic–pituitary–thyroid axis. This figure shows the regulation of thyroid-stimulating hormone (TSH or thyrotropin) secretion by the anterior pituitary. Also depicted are the positive effects of thyrotropin-releasing hormone (TRH) from the hypothalamus and negative effects of circulating triiodothyronine (T_3) and T_3 from intrapituitary conversion of thyroxine (T_4).

Chronobiology

Chronobiology involves the study and measure of time structures or biologic rhythms. Some rhythms have a **circadian cycle**, or 24-hour cycle, but others, such as the menstrual cycle, operate in different periods. Rhythms exist in the human body to control endocrine secretions, sleep–wake, body temperature, neurotransmitter synthesis, and more. These cycles may become deregulated and may begin earlier than usual, known as a phase advance, or later than usual, known as a phase delay.

Zeitgebers are specific events that function as time givers or synchronizers and that set biologic rhythms. Light is the most common example of an external zeitgeber. The suprachiasmatic nucleus of the hypothalamus is an example of an internal zeitgeber. Some theorists think that psychiatric disorders may result from one or more biologic rhythm dysfunctions. For example, depression may be, in part, a phase advance disorder, including early morning awakening and decreased time of onset of REM sleep. Seasonal affective disorder may be the result of shortened exposure to light during the winter months. Exposure to specific artificial light often relieves symptoms of fatigue, overeating, hypersomnia, and depression (see Chapters 10, 19, and 26).

DIAGNOSTIC APPROACHES

Although no commonly used laboratory tests exist that directly confirm a mental disorder, they are still used as part of the diagnosis of these illnesses. **Biologic markers** are diagnostic test findings that occur only in the presence of the psychiatric disorder and include such findings as laboratory and other diagnostic test results and neuropathologic changes noticeable in assessment. These markers increase diagnostic certainty and reliability and may have predictive value, allowing for the possibility of preventive interventions to forestall or avoid the onset of illness. In addition, biologic markers could assist in developing evidence-based care practices. If markers are used reliably, it is much easier to identify the most effective treatments and to determine the expected prognoses for given conditions. The psychiatric–mental health nurse should be aware of the most current information on biologic markers so that information, limitations, and results can be discussed knowledgeably with the patient.

Laboratory Tests

For many years, laboratory tests have attempted to measure levels of neurotransmitters and other CNS substances in the bloodstream. Many of the metabolites of neurotransmitters can be found in the urine and cerebrospinal fluid (CSF) as well. However, these measures have had only limited utility in elucidating what is happening in the brain. Levels of neurotransmitters and metabolites in the bloodstream or urine do not necessarily equate with levels in the CNS. In addition, availability of the neurotransmitter or metabolite does not predict the availability of the neurotransmitter in the synapse, where it must act, or directly relate to the receptor sensitivity. Nonetheless, numerous research studies have focused on changes in neurotransmitters and metabolites in blood, urine, and CSF. These studies have provided clues but remain without conclusive predictive value and therefore are not routinely used.

Another laboratory approach to the study of some of the psychiatric disorders is the challenge test. A challenge test has been most often used in the study of panic disorders. These tests are usually conducted by intravenously administering a chemical known to produce a specific set of psychiatric symptoms. For example, lactate or caffeine may be used to induce the symptoms of panic in a person who has panic disorder. The biologic response of the individual is then monitored.

Beyond their role in helping to diagnose mental disorders, laboratory tests are also an active part of the normal care and assessment of patients with psychiatric disorders. Many physical conditions mimic the symptoms of mental illness, and many of the medications used to treat psychiatric illness can produce health problems. For these reasons, the routine care of patients with psychiatric disorders includes the use of laboratory tests such as complete blood counts, thyroid studies, electrolytes, hepatic enzymes, and other evaluative tests. Psychiatric–mental health nurses need to be familiar with these procedures and assist patients in understanding the use and implications of such tests.

Neurophysiologic Procedures

Several neurophysiological procedures are used in mental health for diagnostic purposes.

Electroencephalography

Electroencephalography (EEG) is a tried and true method for investigating what is happening inside the living brain. Developed in the 1920s, EEG measures electrical activity in the uppermost nerve layers of the cortex. Usually, 16 electrodes are placed on the patient's scalp. The EEG machine, equipped with graph paper and recording pens, is turned on, and the pens then trace the electrical impulses generated over each electrode. Until the use of computed tomography (CT) in the 1970s, the EEG was the only method for identifying brain abnormalities. It remains the simplest and most noninvasive method for

identifying some disorders. It is increasingly being used to identify individual neuronal differences.

An EEG may be used in psychiatry to differentiate possible causes of the patient's symptoms. For example, some types of seizure disorders, such as temporal lobe epilepsy, head injuries, or tumors, may present with predominantly psychiatric symptoms. In addition, metabolic dysfunction, delirium, dementia, altered levels of consciousness, hallucinations, and dissociative states may require EEG evaluation.

Spikes and wave-pattern changes are indications of brain abnormalities. Spikes may be the focal point from which a seizure occurs. However, abnormal activity often is not discovered on a routine EEG while the individual is awake. For this reason, additional methods are sometimes used. Nasopharyngeal leads may be used to get physically closer to the limbic regions. The patient may be exposed to a flashing strobe light while the examiner looks for activity that is not in phase with the flashing light or the patient may be asked to hyperventilate for 3 minutes to induce abnormal activity if it exists. Sleep deprivation may also be used. This involves keeping the patient awake throughout the night before the EEG evaluation. The patient may then be drowsy and fall asleep during the procedure. Abnormalities are more likely to occur when the patient is asleep. Sleep may also be induced using medication; however, many medications change the wave patterns on an EEG. For example, the benzodiazepine class of drugs increases the rapid and fast beta activity. Many other prescribed and illicit drugs, such as lithium, which increases theta activity, can cause EEG alterations.

In addition to reassuring, preparing, and educating the patient for the examination, the nurse should carefully assess the history of substance use and report this information to the examiner. If a sleep-deprivation EEG is to be done, caffeine or other stimulants that might assist the patient in staying awake should be withheld because they may change the EEG patterns.

Polysomnography

Polysomnography is a special procedure that involves recording the EEG throughout a night of sleep. This test is usually conducted in a sleep laboratory. Other tests are usually performed at the same time, including electrocardiography and electromyography. Blood oxygenation, body movement, body temperature, and other data may be collected as well, especially in research settings. This procedure is usually conducted for evaluating sleep disorders, such as sleep apnea, enuresis, or somnambulism. However, sleep pattern changes are frequently researched in mental disorders as well.

Researchers have found that normal sleep divisions and stages are affected by many factors, including drugs, alcohol, general medical conditions, and psychiatric disorders. For example, REM latency, the length of time it takes an individual to enter the first REM episode, is shortened in depression. Reduced delta sleep is also observed. These findings have been replicated so frequently that some researchers consider them biologic markers for depression.

Structural and Functional Imaging

Neuroimaging of the brain involves **structural imaging**, which visualizes the structure of brain and allows diagnosis of gross intracranial disease and injury, and **functional imaging**, which visualizes processing of information. One of the most well-known examples of structural imaging is magnetic resonance imaging (MRI), which produces two- or three-dimensional images of brain structures without the use of X-rays or radioactive tracers. An MRI creates a magnetic field around the patient's head through which radio waves are sent. A functional MRI (fMRI) that creates functional images relies on the properties of oxygenated and deoxygenated hemoglobin to see images of changes in blood flow. The advantage of fMRI is that it is possible to see how the brain works when different stimuli are presented and problems that exist, such as a stroke. The fMRI has replaced most use of positron emission tomography (PET), which measures blood flow and oxygen and glucose metabolism. The emissions from the injected radioactive tracers are rapidly decayed and limit the monitoring of PET to short tasks.

Neuroimaging has limited clinical use in mental health, with the exception of the diagnosis of some of the dementias, particularly Alzheimer's (Frisoni, Fox, Jack, Scheltens, & Thompson, 2010). Neuroimaging has promising potential for unlocking the pathophysiology of several mental disorders. With the introduction of the fMRI, it is now possible to study the circuitry and pinpoint genetic-based predisposing factors. An MRI technique, diffusion tensor imaging, allows for viewing macroscopic changes that occur at the axon level (Radanovic et al., 2013).

Other Neurophysiologic Methods

Evoked potentials (EPs), also called event-related potentials, use the same basic principles as an EEG. They measure changes in electrical activity of the brain in specific regions as a response to a given stimulus. Electrodes placed on the scalp measure a large waveform that stands out after the administration of repetitive stimuli, such as a click or flash of light. There are several different types of EPs to be measured, depending on the sensory area affected by the stimulus, the cognitive task required, or the region monitored, any of which can change the length of time until the wave occurrence. EPs are used extensively in psychiatric research. In clinical practice,

EPs are used primarily in the assessment of demyelinating disorders, such as multiple sclerosis.

However, brain electrical activity mapping studies, which involve a 20-electrode EEG that generates computerized maps of the brain's electrical activity, have found a slowing of electrical activity in the frontal lobes of individuals who have schizophrenia.

SUMMARY OF KEY POINTS

- Neuroscientists now view behavior and cognitive function as a result of complex interactions within the CNS and its plasticity, or its ability to adapt and change in both structure and function.

- Each hemisphere of the brain is divided into four lobes: the frontal lobe, which controls motor speech function, personality, and working memory—often called the executive functions that govern one's ability to plan and initiate action; the parietal lobe, which controls the sensory functions; the temporal lobe, which contains the primary auditory and olfactory areas; and the occipital lobe, which controls visual integration of information.

- The structures of the limbic system are integrally involved in memory and emotional behavior. Dysfunction of the limbic system has been linked with major mental disorders, including schizophrenia, depression, and anxiety disorders.

- Neurons communicate with each other through synaptic transmission. Neurotransmitters excite or inhibit a response at the receptor sites and have been linked to certain mental disorders. These neurotransmitters include Ach, dopamine, norepinephrine, serotonin, GABA, and glutamate.

- Although no one gene has been found to produce any psychiatric disorder, significant evidence indicates there most psychiatric disorders have a genetic predisposition or susceptibility. For individuals who have such genetic susceptibility, the identification of risk factors is crucial in helping to plan interventions to prevent development of that disorder or to prevent certain behavior patterns, such as aggression or suicide.

- PNI examines the relationship among the immune system; the nervous system; the endocrine system; and thoughts, emotions, and behavior.

- Chronobiology focuses on the study and measure of time structures or biologic rhythms occurring in the body and associates dysregulation of these cycles as contributing factors to the development of psychiatric disorders.

■ Biologic markers are physical indicators of disturbances within the CNS that differentiate one disease process from another, such as biochemical changes or neuropathologic changes. These biologic markers can be measured by several methods of testing, including challenge tests, EEG, polysomnography, EPs, CT scanning, MRI, PET, and single-photon emission computed tomography; the psychiatric nurse must be familiar with all of these methods.

CRITICAL THINKING CHALLENGES

1. A woman who has experienced a "ministroke" continues to regain lost cognitive function months after the stroke. Her husband takes this as evidence that she never had a stroke. How would you approach patient teaching and counseling for this couple to help them understand this occurrence if the stroke did damage to her brain?

2. Your patient has "impaired executive functioning." Consider what would be a reasonable follow-up schedule for this patient for counseling sessions. Would it be reasonable to schedule visits at 1:00 PM weekly? Is the patient able to keep to this schedule? Why or why not? What would be the best schedule?

3. Mr. S. is unable to sleep after watching an upsetting documentary. Identify the neurotransmitter activity that may be interfering with sleep. (Hint: Fight or flight.)

4. Describe what behavioral symptoms or problems may be present in a patient with dysfunction of the following brain area:
   a. Basal ganglia
   b. Hippocampus
   c. Limbic system
   d. Thalamus
   e. Hypothalamus
   f. Frontal lobe

5. Compare and contrast the functions of the sympathetic and parasympathetic nervous systems.

6. Discuss the steps in synaptic transmission, beginning with the action potential and ending with how the neurotransmitter no longer communicates its message to the receiving neuron.

7. Examine how a receptor's usual response to a neurotransmitter might change.

8. Compare the roles of dopamine and Ach in the CNS.

9. Explain how dopamine, norepinephrine, and serotonin all contribute to endocrine system regulation. Suggest some other transmitters that may affect endocrine function.

10. Discuss how the fields of psychoneuroimmunology and chronobiology overlap.

11. Compare the methods used to find biologic markers of psychiatric disorders reviewed in this chapter. Consider the potential risks and benefits to the patient.

REFERENCES

Bewernick, B. H., & Schlaepfer, T. E. (2013). Chronic depression as a model disease for cerebral aging. (Review). *Dialogues in Neuroscience, 15*(1), 77–85.

Blier, P., & El Mansari, M. (2013). Serotonin and beyond: Therapeutics for major depression. *Philosophical Transactions of the Royal Society of London. Series B, Biological Sciences, 368*(1615), 20120536. doi:10.1098/rstb.2012.0536

Frisoni, G. B., Fox, N. C., Jack, C. R., Scheltens, P., & Thompson, P. M. (2010). The clinical use of structural MRI in Alzheimer Disease. *Nature Reviews Neurology, 6*(2), 67–77.

Haber, S. N., & Rauch, S. L. (2010). Neurocircuitry: A window into the networks underlying neuropsychiatric disease. *Neuropsychopharmacology Reviews, 35*(1), 1–3.

Harlow, J. M. (1868). Recovery after severe injury to the head. *Publication of the Massachusetts Medical Society, 2,* 327.

Kreuzer, P., Landgrebe, M., Wittmann, M., Schecklmann, M., Poeppl, T. B., Hajak, G., et al. (2012). Hypothermia associated with antipsychotic drug use: A clinical case series and review of current literature. *Journal of Clinical Pharmacology, 52*(7), 1090–1097.

Macalpine, I., & Hunter, R. (1966). The "insanity" of King George 3d: A classic case of porphyria. *British Medical Journal, 1*(5479), 65–71.

Nolte, J., & Angevine, J. (1995). *The human brain: In photographs and diagrams.* St. Louis: Mosby.

Pace, T. W., & Heim, C. M. (2011). A short review on the psychoneuroimmunology of posttraumatic stress disorder: From risk factors to medical comorbidities. (Review). *Brain, Behavior, and Immunity, 25*(1), 6–13.

Radanovic, M., Pereira, F. R., Stella, F., Aprahamian, I., Ferreira, L. K., Forlenza, O. V., et al. (2013). White matter abnormalities associated with Alzheimer's disease and mild cognitive impairment: A critical review of MRI studies. (Review). *Expert Review of Neurotherapeutics, 13*(5), 483–493.

Sequeira, P. A., Martin, M. V., & Vawter, M. P. (2012). The first decade and beyond of transcriptional profiling in schizophrenia. (Review). *Neurobiology of Disease, 45*(1), 23–26.

Siegel, A., & Sapru, H. N. (2010). *Essential neuroscience* (2nd ed.) Philadelphia: Lippincott Williams & Wilkins.

Sullivan, P. F., Daly, M. F., & O'Donovan, M. (2012). Genetic architectures of psychiatric disorders: The emerging picture and its implications. (Review). *Nature Reviews Genetics. 13*(8), 537–551.

Wasserman, D., Terenius, L., Wasserman, J., & Sokolowski, M. (2010). The 2009 Nobel conference on the role of genetics in promoting suicide prevention and the mental health of the population. *Molecular Psychiatry, 15*(1), 12–17.

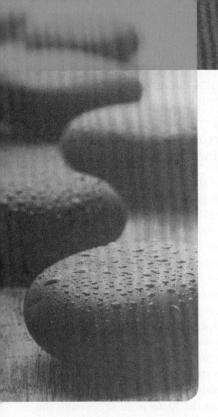

UNIT III

KNOWLEDGE AND SKILLS OF PSYCHIATRIC-MENTAL HEALTH NURSING

7

Therapeutic Communication

Mary Ann Boyd

KEY CONCEPTS

- self-awareness
- therapeutic communication

LEARNING OBJECTIVES

After studying this chapter, you will be able to:

1. Identify the importance of self-awareness in nursing practice.

2. Develop a repertoire of verbal and nonverbal communication skills.

3. Develop a process for selecting effective communication techniques.

4. Explain the physical, emotional, and social boundaries of a therapeutic interaction.

5. Discuss the significance of defense mechanisms.

KEY TERMS

- active listening • boundaries • communication blocks • content themes • defense mechanisms • introspective
- nonverbal communication • passive listening • process recording • self-disclosure • symbolism • verbal communication

Therapeutic communication is a basic skill of all nurses. When caring for a person with emotional problems or a mental disorder, therapeutic communication is critical in helping an individual participate in health seeking behaviors. The purposes of this chapter are to (1) help the nurse develop self-awareness and (2) develop therapeutic communication skills.

SELF-AWARENESS

Self-awareness is the process of understanding one's own beliefs, thoughts, motivations, biases, and limita-

tions and recognizing how they affect others. Without self-awareness, nurses will find it impossible to establish and maintain therapeutic relationships with patients. "Know thyself" is a basic tenet of psychiatric–mental health nursing (Box 7.1).

A well-developed sense of self-awareness can only come after nurses carry out self-examination. This process can provoke anxiety and is rarely comfortable, either when done alone or with help from others. Self-examination involves reflecting on the personal meaning of the current nursing situation. This reflection can relate to similar past situations and issues related to one's own

BOX 7.1

"Know Thyself"

- What physical problems or illnesses have you experienced?
- What significant traumatic life events (e.g., divorce, death of significant person, abuse, disaster) have you experienced?
- What prejudiced or embarrassing beliefs and attitudes about groups different from yours can you identify from your family, significant others, and yourself?
- Which sociocultural factors in your background could contribute to being rejected by members of other cultures?
- How would the above experiences affect your ability to care for patients?

personal values. Self-examination without the benefit of another's perspective can lead to a biased view of self. Conducting self-examinations with a trusted individual who can give objective but realistic feedback is best. The development of self-awareness requires a willingness to be **introspective** and to examine personal beliefs, attitudes, and motivations.

> **KEYCONCEPT** **Self-awareness** is the process of understanding one's own beliefs, thoughts, motivations, biases, and limitations, and recognizing how they affect others.

Know Thyself

Each nurse brings personal characteristics to a nurse-patient interaction. The patient's communication is immediately influenced by the nurse's physical characteristics: age, gender, body weight, height, ethnic or racial background, and any other observed physical characteristics. Additionally, the nurse's response to a patient can be influenced by unobservable personal physical characteristics, such as a an existing chronic illness. The nurse's psychological state also influences how he or she analyzes patient information and selects treatment interventions. An emotional state or behavior can inadvertently influence the therapeutic relationship. For example, a nurse who has just learned that her child is using illegal drugs and who has a patient with a history of drug use may inadvertently project a judgmental attitude toward her patient, which would interfere with therapeutic communication. The nurse needs to examine underlying emotions, motivations, and beliefs and determine how these factors shape behavior.

The nurse's social biases can be particularly problematic for the nurse–patient interaction. Although the nurse may not verbalize these values to patients, some are readily evident in the nurse's behavior and appearance. A patient may perceive biases in the nurse as a result of how the nurse acts or appears at work. Other sociocultural values may not be immediately obvious to the patient; for example, the nurse's religious or spiritual beliefs or feelings about death, divorce, abortion, or homosexuality.

These beliefs and thoughts can influence how the nurse interacts with a patient who is dealing with such issues.

Understanding Personal Feelings and Beliefs and Changing Behavior

Nurses must understand their own personal feelings and beliefs and try to avoid projecting them onto patients. The development of self-awareness will enhance the nurse's objectivity and foster a nonjudgmental attitude, which is so important for building and maintaining trust throughout the nurse–patient interaction. Soliciting feedback from colleagues and supervisors about how personal beliefs or thoughts are being projected onto others is a useful self-assessment technique. One of the reasons that ongoing clinical supervision is so important is that the supervisor really knows the nurse and can continually support positive interactions, observe for inappropriate communication, and question assumptions that the nurse may hold. Clinical supervision is different from administrative supervision in that the focus is on supporting the growth of the nurse and does not generally involve an administrative or reporting relationship.

After a nurse has identified and analyzed his or her personal beliefs and attitudes, behaviors that were driven by prejudicial ideas may change. The change process requires introspective analysis that may result in viewing the world differently. Through self-awareness and conscious effort, the nurse can change learned behaviors to engage effectively in therapeutic communication with patients. Nevertheless, sometimes a nurse realizes that some attitudes are too ingrained to support an effective interaction with a patient with different beliefs. In such cases, the nurse should refer the patient to someone with whom the patient is more likely to develop a successful therapeutic relationship.

COMMUNICATION TYPES AND TECHNIQUES

Effective communication skills, including verbal and nonverbal techniques, are the building blocks for all successful relationships (Box 7.2). **Verbal communication**, which is principally achieved by spoken words, includes the underlying emotion, context, and connotation of what is actually said. **Nonverbal communication** includes gestures, expressions, and body language. Both the patient and the nurse use verbal and nonverbal communication. To respond therapeutically, the nurse assesses and interprets all forms of patient communication.

> **NCLEXNOTE** In analyzing patient–nurse communication, nonverbal behaviors and gestures are communicated first. If a patient's verbal and nonverbal communications are contradictory, priority should be given to the nonverbal behavior and gestures.

BOX 7.2
Principles of Therapeutic Communication

- The patient should be the primary focus of the interaction.
- A professional attitude sets the tone of the therapeutic relationship.
- Use self-disclosure cautiously and only when the disclosure has a therapeutic purpose.
- Avoid social relationships with patients.
- Maintain patient confidentiality.
- Assess the patient's intellectual competence to determine the level of understanding.
- Implement interventions from a theoretic base.
- Maintain a nonjudgmental attitude. Avoid making judgments about the patient's behavior.
- Avoid giving advice. By the time the patient sees the nurse, he or she has had plenty of advice.
- Guide the patient to reinterpret his or her experiences rationally.
- Track the patient's verbal interaction through the use of clarifying statements.
- Avoid changing the subject unless the content change is in the patient's best interest.

KEYCONCEPT Therapeutic communication is the ongoing process of interaction through which meaning emerges.

Therapeutic and social interactions are very different. In a therapeutic communication, the nurse focuses on the patient and patient-related issues even when engaging in social activities with that patient. For example, a nurse may take a patient shopping and out for lunch. Even though the nurse is engaged in a social activity, the trip should have a definite purpose, and conversation should focus only on the patient. The nurse must not attempt to meet his or her own social or other needs during the activity.

Verbal Communication

The process of verbal communication involves a sender, a message, and a receiver. The patient is often the sender, and the nurse is often the receiver, but communication is always two-way (Figure 7.1). The patient formulates an idea, encodes that message (puts ideas into words), and then transmits the message with emotion. The patient's words and their underlying emotional tone and connotation communicate the individual's needs and emotional problems. The nurse receives the message, decodes it (interprets the message, including its feelings, connotation, and context), and then responds to the patient.

On the surface, this interaction is deceptively simple; unseen complexities lie beneath. Is the message the nurse receives consistent with the patient's original idea? Did the nurse interpret the message as the patient intended? Is the verbal message consistent with the nonverbal flourishes that accompany it? Validation is essential to ensure that the nurse has received the information accurately.

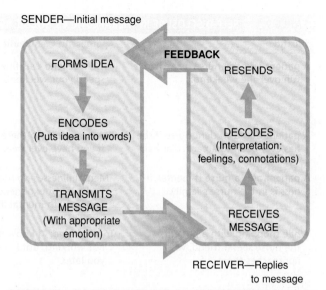

FIGURE 7.1   The communication process. (Adapted from Boyd, M. [1995]. Communication with patients, families, healthcare providers, and diverse cultures. In Strader, M. K., & Decker, P. J. [Eds.]. *Role transition to patient care management* [p. 431]. Norwalk, CT: Appleton & Lange.)

Limiting Self-Disclosure

One of the most important principles of therapeutic communication is to focus the interaction on the patient's concerns. **Self-disclosure**, telling the patient personal information, generally is not a good idea. The conversation should focus on the patient, not the nurse. If a patient asks the nurse personal questions, the nurse should elicit the underlying reason for the request. The nurse can then determine how much personal information to disclose, if any. In revealing personal information, the nurse should be purposeful and have identified therapeutic outcomes. For example, a male patient who was struggling with the implications of marriage and fidelity asked a male nurse if he had ever had an extramarital affair. The nurse interpreted the patient's statement as seeking role-modeling behavior for an adult man and judged self-disclosure in this instance to be therapeutic. He honestly responded that he did not engage in affairs and redirected the discussion back to the patient's concerns.

Nurses sometimes may feel uncomfortable avoiding patients' questions for fear of seeming rude. As a result, they might sometimes disclose too much personal information because they are trying to be "nice." However, being nice is not necessarily therapeutic. As appropriate, redirecting the patient, giving a neutral or vague answer, or saying, "Let's talk about you," may be all that is necessary to limit self-disclosure. In some instances, nurses may need to tell the patient directly that the nurse will not share personal information (Table 7.1).

TABLE 7.1	SELF-DISCLOSURE IN THERAPEUTIC VS. SOCIAL RELATIONSHIPS	
Situation	Appropriate Therapeutic Response	Inappropriate Social Response with Rationale
A patient asks the nurse if she had fun over the weekend.	"The weekend was fine. How did you spend your weekend?"	"It was great. My boyfriend and I went to dinner and a movie." (This self-disclosure has no therapeutic purpose. The response focuses the conversation on the nurse, not the patient.)
A patient asks a student nurse if she has ever been to a particular bar.	"Many people go there. I'm wondering if you have ever been there?"	"Oh yes—all the time. It's a lot of fun." (Sharing information about outside activities is inappropriate.)
A patient asks a nurse if mental illness is in the nurse's family.	"Mental illnesses do run in families. I've had a lot of experience caring for people with mental illnesses."	"My sister is being treated for depression." (This self-disclosure has no purpose, and the nurse is missing the meaning of the question.)
While shopping with a patient, the nurse sees a friend, who approaches them.	To her friend: "I know it looks like I'm not working, but I really am. I'll see you later."	"Hi, Bob. This is Jane Doe, a patient." (Introducing the patient to the friend is very inappropriate and violates patient confidentiality.)

Using Verbal Communication Techniques

Psychiatric nurses use many verbal techniques in establishing relationships and helping patients focus on their problems. Asking a question, restating, and reflecting are examples of such techniques. These techniques may at first seem artificial, but with practice, they can be useful. Table 7.2 lists some techniques along with examples.

Silence and Listening

One of the most difficult but often most effective communication techniques is the use of silence during verbal interactions. By maintaining silence, the nurse allows the patient to gather thoughts and to proceed at his or her own pace. It is important that the nurse not interrupt silences because of his or her own anxiety or concern of "not doing anything" if sitting quietly with a patient.

Listening is another valuable tool. Silence and listening differ in that silence consists of deliberate pauses to encourage the patient to reflect and eventually respond. Listening is an ongoing activity by which the nurse attends to the patient's verbal and nonverbal communication. The art of listening is developed through careful attention to the content and meaning of the patient's speech. There are two types of listening: passive and active. **Passive listening** involves sitting quietly and letting the patient talk. A passive listener allows the patient to ramble and does not focus or guide the thought process. This form of listening does not foster a therapeutic relationship. Body language during passive listening usually communicates boredom, indifference, or hostility (Figure 7.2).

Through **active listening**, the nurse focuses on what the patient is saying interprets the interaction, and responds to the message objectively. While listening, the nurse concentrates only on what the patient says and the underlying meaning. The nurse's verbal and nonverbal behaviors indicate active listening. The nurse usually responds indirectly using techniques such as open-ended statements, reflection (see Table 7.2), and questions that

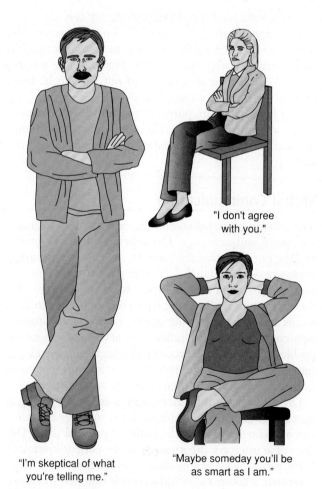

"I don't agree with you."

"I'm skeptical of what you're telling me."

"Maybe someday you'll be as smart as I am."

FIGURE 7.2 Negative body language.

TABLE 7.2	VERBAL COMMUNICATION TECHNIQUES		
Technique	Definition	Example	Use
Acceptance	Encouraging and receiving information in a nonjudgmental and interested manner	*Patient:* I have done something terrible. *Nurse:* I would like to hear about it. It's OK to discuss it with me.	Used in establishing trust and developing empathy
Confrontation	Presenting the patient with a different reality of the situation	*Patient:* My best friend never calls me. She hates me. *Nurse:* I was in the room yesterday when she called.	Used cautiously to immediately redefine the patient's reality. However, it can alienate the patient if used inappropriately. A nonjudgmental attitude is critical for confrontation to be effective.
Doubt	Expressing or voicing doubt when a patient relates a situation.	*Patient:* My best friend hates me. She never calls me. *Nurse:* From what you have told me, that does not sound like her. When did she call you last?	Used carefully and only when the nurse feels confident about the details. It is used when the nurse wants to guide the patient toward other explanations.
Interpretation	Putting into words what the patient is implying or feeling	*Patient:* I could not sleep because someone would come in my room and rape me. *Nurse:* It sounds like you were scared last night.	Used in helping the patient identify underlying thoughts or feelings
Observation	Stating to the patient what the nurse is observing	*Nurse:* You are trembling and perspiring. When did this start?	Used when a patient's behaviors (verbal or nonverbal) are obvious and unusual for that patient
Open-ended statements	Introducing an idea and letting the patient respond	*Nurse:* Trust means… *Patient:* That someone will keep you safe.	Used when helping patient explore feelings or gain insight
Reflection	Redirecting the idea back to the patient for classification of important emotional overtones, feelings, and experiences; it gives patients permission to have feelings they may not realize they have	*Patient:* Should I go home for the weekend? *Nurse:* Should you go home for the weekend?	Used when patient is asking for the nurse's approval or judgment; use of reflection helps nurse maintain a nonjudgmental approach
Restatement	Repeating the main idea expressed; lets patient know what was heard	*Patient:* I hate this place. I don't belong here. *Nurse:* You don't want to be here.	Used when trying to clarify what the patient has said
Silence	Remaining quiet but nonverbally expressing interest during an interaction	*Patient:* I am angry! *Nurse:* (Silence) *Patient:* My wife had an affair.	Used when patient needs to express ideas but may not know quite how to do it; with silence, the patient can focus on putting thoughts together
Validation	Clarifying the nurse's understanding of the situation	*Nurse:* Let me see if I understand.	Used when nurse is trying to understand a situation the patient is trying to describe

elicit additional responses from the patient. In active listening, the nurse should avoid changing the subject and instead follow the patient's lead. At times, however, it is necessary to respond directly to help a patient focus on a specific topic or to clarify his or her thoughts or beliefs about that topic.

NCLEXNOTE Self-disclosure can be used in very specific situations, but self-disclosure is not the first intervention to consider. In prioritizing interventions, active listening is one of the first to use.

Validation

Another important technique is *validation*, which means explicitly checking one's own thoughts or feelings with another person. To do so, the nurse must own his or her own thoughts or feelings by using "I" statements (Orlando, 1961). The validation generally refers to observation, thoughts, or feelings and seeks explicit feedback. For example, a nurse who sees a patient pacing the hallway before a planned family visit may conclude that the patient is anxious. Validation may occur with a statement

TABLE 7.3   TECHNIQUES THAT INHIBIT COMMUNICATION

Technique	Definition	Example	Problem
Advice	Telling a patient what to do	*Patient:* I can't sleep. It is too noisy. *Nurse:* Turn off the light and shut your door.	The nurse solves the patient's problem, which may not be the appropriate solution and encourages dependency on the nurse.
Agreement	Agreeing with a particular viewpoint of a patient	*Patient:* Abortions are sinful. *Nurse:* I agree.	The patient is denied the opportunity to change his or her view now that the nurse agrees.
Challenges	Disputing the patient's beliefs with arguments, logical thinking, or direct order	*Patient:* I'm a cowboy. *Nurse:* If you are a cowboy, what are you doing in the hospital?	The nurse belittles the patient and decreases the patient's self-esteem. The patient will avoid relating to the nurse who challenges.
Reassurance	Telling a patient that everything will be OK	*Patient:* Everyone thinks I'm bad. *Nurse:* You are a good person.	The nurse makes a statement that may not be true. The patient is blocked from exploring his or her feelings.
Disapproval	Judging the patient's situation and behavior	*Patient:* I'm so sorry. I did not mean to kill my mother. *Nurse:* You should be. How could anyone kill their mother?	The nurse belittles the patient. The patient will avoid the nurse.

such as, "I notice you pacing the hallway. I wonder if you are feeling anxious about the family visit?" The patient may agree, "Yes. I keep worrying about what is going to happen!" or disagree, "No. I have been trying to get into the bathroom for the last 30 minutes, but my roommate is still in there!"

Avoiding Blocks to Communication

Some verbal techniques block interactions and inhibit therapeutic communication (Table 7.3). One of the biggest blocks to communication is giving advice, particularly when others have already given the same advice. Giving advice is different from supporting a patient through decision making. The therapeutic dialogue presented in Box 7.3 differentiates between advice (telling the patient what to do or how to act) from therapeutic communication, through which the nurse and patient explore alternative ways of viewing the patient's world. The patient can then reach his or her own conclusions about the best approaches to use.

Nonverbal Communication

Gestures, facial expressions, and body language actually communicate more than verbal messages. Under the best circumstances, body language mirrors or enhances what is verbally communicated. However, if verbal and nonverbal messages conflict, the listener will believe the nonverbal message. For example, if a patient says that he feels fine but has a sad facial expression and is slumped in a chair away from others, the message of sadness and depression, rather than the patient's words, will be accepted. The same is true of a nurse's behavior. For example, if a nurse

tells a patient, "I am happy to see you," but the nurse's facial expression communicates indifference, the patient will receive the message that the nurse is bored.

People with psychiatric problems often have difficulty verbally expressing themselves and interpreting the emotions of others. Because of this, nurses need to continually assess the nonverbal communication needs of patients. Eye contact (or lack thereof), posture, movement (shifting in chair, pacing), facial expressions, and gestures are nonverbal behaviors that communicate thoughts and feelings. For example, a patient who is pacing and restless may be upset or having a reaction to medication. A clenched fist usually indicates that a person feels angry or hostile.

Nonverbal behavior varies from culture to culture. The nurse must, therefore, be careful to understand his or her own cultural context as well as that of the patient. For example, in some cultures, it is considered disrespectful to look a person straight in the eye. In other cultures, not looking a person in the eye may be interpreted as "hiding something" or as having low self-esteem. Whether one points with the finger, nose, or eyes and how much hand gesturing to use are other examples of nonverbal communication that may vary considerably among cultures. The nurse needs to be aware of cultural differences in communication in the context of each relationship and may need to consult with a cultural interpreter or use other learning opportunities to ensure that his or her communication is culturally congruent.

Nurses should use positive body language, such as sitting at the same eye level as the patient with a relaxed posture that projects interest and attention. Leaning slightly forward helps engage the patient. Generally, the nurse should not cross his or her arms or legs during therapeutic communication because such postures erect

BOX 7.3 • THERAPEUTIC DIALOGUE • **Giving Advice versus Recommendations**

Ms. J has just received a diagnosis of phobic disorder and has been given a prescription for fluoxetine (Prozac). She was referred to the home health agency because she does not want to take her medication. She is fearful of becoming suicidal. Two approaches are given below.

INEFFECTIVE COMMUNICATION (ADVICE)

Nurse: Ms. J, the doctor has ordered the medication because it will help with your anxiety.

Ms. J: Yes, but I don't want to take the medication. I'm afraid it will make me suicidal. Some psychiatric medication does that. I haven't had any attacks for 2 weeks, and it seems too risky since I'm doing better. I'm scared of the side effects.

Nurse: This medication has rarely had that side effect. You should try it and see if you have any suicidal thoughts.

Ms. J: [Remains silent for a while, crosses her legs, and looks away from the nurse and down at her feet] … okay.

(The nurse leaves, and Ms. J decides not take the medication. Within 1 week, Ms. J is taken to the emergency room with a panic attack.)

EFFECTIVE COMMUNICATION

Nurse: Ms. J, how have you been doing?

Ms. J: So far, so good. I haven't had any attacks for 2 weeks.

Nurse: I understand that the doctor gave you a prescription for medication that may help with the panic attacks.

Ms. J: Yes, but I don't want to take it. I'm afraid of becoming suicidal. Some of this psychiatric medication does that. I don't really want to take a needless risk since I've been feeling better.

Nurse: Those worries are understandable. Have you ever had feelings of hurting yourself?

Ms. J: Not yet.

Nurse: If you took the medication and had thoughts like that, what would you do?

Ms. J: I don't know, that's why I'm scared.

Nurse: I think I see your dilemma. This medication may help your panic attacks, but if the medication produces suicidal thoughts then it might compromise your progress and that's a pretty serious risk. Is that correct?

Ms. J: Yeah, that's it.

Nurse: What are the circumstances under which you would feel more comfortable trying the medication?

Ms. J: If I knew that I would not have suicidal thoughts. If I could be assured of that.

Nurse: I can't guarantee that, but perhaps we could create an environment in which you would feel safe. I could call you every few days to see if you are having any of these thoughts and, if so, I could help you deal with them and make sure you see the doctor to review the medication.

Ms. J: Oh, that helps. If you do that, then I think that I will be alright.

(Ms. J successfully takes the medication.)

CRITICAL THINKING CHALLENGE

- Contrast the communication in the first scenario with that in the second.
- What therapeutic communication techniques did the second nurse use that may have contributed to a better outcome?
- Are there any cues in the first scenario that indicate that the patient will not follow the nurse's advice? Explain.

barriers to interaction. Uncrossed arms and legs project openness and a willingness to engage in conversation (Figure 7.3). Any verbal response should be consistent with nonverbal messages.

Selection of Communication Techniques

In successful therapeutic communication, the nurse chooses the best words to say and uses nonverbal behav-iors that are consistent with these words. If a patient is angry and upset, should the nurse invite the patient to sit down and discuss the problem, walk quietly with the patient, or simply observe the patient from a distance and not initiate conversation? Choosing the best response begins with assessing and interpreting the meaning of the patient's communication—both verbal and nonverbal.

Nurses should not necessarily take verbal messages literally, especially when a patient is upset or angry. For

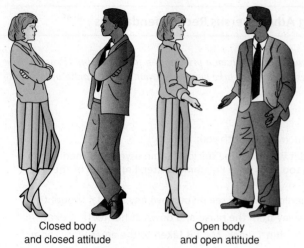

Closed body
and closed attitude

Open body
and open attitude

FIGURE 7.3 Open and closed body language.

example, one nurse walked into the room of a newly admitted patient who accused, "You locked me up and threw away the key." The nurse could have responded defensively that she had nothing to do with the patient being admitted; however, that response could have ended in an argument, and communication would have been blocked. Fortunately, the nurse recognized that the patient was communicating frustration at being in a locked psychiatric unit and did not take the accusation personally.

The next step is identifying the desired patient outcome. To do so, the nurse should engage the patient with eye contact and quietly try to interpret the patient's feelings. In this example, the desired outcome was for the patient to clarify the hospitalization experience. The nurse responded, "It must be frustrating to feel locked up." The nurse focused on the patient's feelings rather than the accusations, which reflected an understanding of the patient's feelings. The patient knew that the nurse accepted these feelings, which led to further discussion. It may seem impossible to plan reactions for each situation, but with practice, the nurse will begin to respond automatically in a therapeutic way.

Boundaries and Body Space Zones

Boundaries are the defining limits of individuals, objects, or relationships. Boundaries mark territory, distinguishing what is "mine" from "not mine." Human beings have many different types of boundaries. Material boundaries, such as fences around property, artificially imposed state lines, and bodies of water, define territory as well as provide security and order. Personal boundaries include physical, psychological, and social dimensions. Physical boundaries are those established in terms of physical closeness to others—who we allow to touch us or how close we want others to stand near us.

Psychological boundaries are established in terms of emotional distance from others—how much of our innermost feelings and thoughts we want to share. Social boundaries, such as norms, customs, and roles, help us establish our closeness and place within the family, culture, and community. Boundaries are not fixed but dynamic. When boundaries are involuntarily transgressed, the individual feels threatened and responds to the perceived threat. The nurse must elicit permission before implementing interventions that invade the patient's personal space.

Personal Boundaries

Every individual is surrounded by four different body zones that provide varying degrees of protection against unwanted physical closeness during interactions. These were identified by Hall (1990) as the intimate zone (e.g., for whispering and embracing), the personal zone (e.g., for close friends), the social zone (e.g., for acquaintances), and the public zone (usually for interacting with strangers) (Figure 7.4). The actual sizes of the different zones vary according to culture. Some cultures define the intimate zone narrowly and the personal zones widely. Thus, friends in these cultures stand and sit close while interacting. People of other cultures define the intimate zone widely and are uncomfortable when others stand close to them.

The variability of intimate and personal zones has implications for nursing. For a patient to be comfortable with a nurse, the nurse needs to protect the intimate zone of that individual. The patient usually will allow the nurse to enter the personal zone but will express discomfort if the nurse breaches the intimate zone. For the nurse, the difficulty lies in differentiating the personal zone from the intimate zone for each patient.

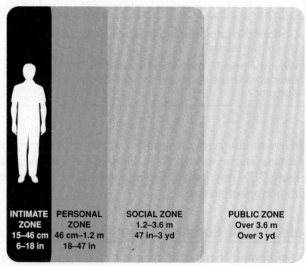

INTIMATE ZONE	PERSONAL ZONE	SOCIAL ZONE	PUBLIC ZONE
15–46 cm 6–18 in	46 cm–1.2 m 18–47 in	1.2–3.6 m 47 in–3 yd	Over 3.6 m Over 3 yd

FIGURE 7.4 Body space zones.

The nurse's awareness of his or her own need for intimate and personal space is another prerequisite for therapeutic interaction with the patient. It is important that a nurse feels comfortable while interacting with patients. Establishing a comfort zone may well entail fine-tuning the size of body zones. Recognizing this will help the nurse understand occasional inexplicable reactions to the proximity of patients.

Professional Boundaries and Ethics

For nurses, professional boundaries are also essential to consider in the context of the nurse–patient interaction. Patients are often at a very vulnerable point in their life, and nurses need to be aware of professional boundaries to avoid exploitation of the patient. For example, in a friendship, there is a two-way sharing of personal information and feelings, but in nurse–patient relationship interactions, the focus is on the patient's needs, and the nurse generally does not share personal information or attempt to meet his or her own needs through the relationship.

Defense Mechanisms

When communicating with patients, it is also important for the nurse to be aware of the defense mechanisms patients may use. The concept of "defense mechanisms" is an old one, originating in Freud's theory of psychoanalysis. While defense mechanisms might seem to indicate the existence of problematic mental state, this is not true. Healthy individuals in many different contexts use defense mechanisms. **Defense mechanisms,** (also known as coping styles), are psychological mechanisms that help an individual respond to and cope with difficult situations, emotional conflicts and external stressors. Some defense mechanisms (e.g., projection, splitting, acting out) are mostly maladaptive. Others (e.g., suppression, denial) may be either maladaptive or adaptive depending on the context in which they occur. The use of defense mechanisms becomes maladaptive when its persistent use interferes with the person's ability to function and quality of life (see Table 7.4).

For example, responding to a difficult life event altruistically is very often a healthy way to recover. On the other hand, defense mechanisms such as acting out, autistic fantasies, projection, and splitting are rarely adaptive. A defense mechanism such as repression can be a natural way to react to a traumatic experience, specifically when used in appropriate moderation. However, the unchecked repression of difficult thoughts or feelings can keep someone from coming to terms with their experiences. In developing a successful therapeutic relationship, and in establishing open communication, such knowledge of defense mechanisms will prove itself invaluable.

As nurses develop therapeutic communication skills, they will begin recognizing their patients, defense mechanisms. With experience, the nurse will evaluate the purpose of a defense mechanism and then determine whether or not it should be discussed with the patient. For example, if a patient is using humor to alleviate an emotionally intense situation, that may be very appropriate. On the other hand, if someone continually rationalizes antisocial behavior, the use of the defense mechanism should be discussed.

> **NCLEXNOTE** When studying defense mechanisms, differentiate similar defense mechanisms. For example, displacement, devaluation, and projection are similar, but not the same. Identify these mechanisms in your process recordings.

COMMUNICATION CONSIDERATIONS FOR PATIENTS WITH MENTAL HEALTH CHALLENGES

For patients with specific, known mental health problems or illnesses, the nurse must consider how these issues may impact the interactions.

Considering Specific Mental Health Issues

An individual's mental health challenges should be considered when selecting communication strategies. For example, patients may frequently be experiencing increased levels of anxiety. The nurse who understands that focal attention decreases as anxiety increases will use shorter and simpler statements or questions when the patient exhibits higher levels of anxiety.

Patients who are experiencing depression may have difficulty articulating their feelings or their thinking and responses may be slowed. The nurse will frequently use silence and empathic techniques throughout this interaction. The person who is depressed may also use communication styles such as overgeneralizing ("This always happens to me…everything always turns out for the worse…."). The nurse can assist the patient to be more specific (e.g., asking about a specific time or a specific exception).

When patients are experiencing schizophrenia, they may have hallmark symptoms such as hallucinations or delusions. If a person is having auditory hallucinations (hearing sounds that no one else does), the nurse's voice may be one of several the patient is hearing. Clear, short sentences may assist in getting the patient's attention on the nurse's voice. A person experiencing delusions may use pronouns vaguely ("they" did it) or other forms of vague or unclear communication. Clarifying and assisting the patient to be more specific may assist the patient's thinking as well as communication.

TABLE 7.4	SPECIFIC DEFENSE MECHANISMS AND COPING STYLES

The following defense mechanisms and coping styles are commonly used when the individual deals with emotional conflict or stressors (either internal or external).

Defense Mechanism	Definition	Example
Acting out	Using actions rather than reflections or feelings during periods of emotional conflict	A teenager gets mad at his parents and begins staying out late at night.
Affiliation	Turning to others for help or support (sharing problems with others without implying that someone else is responsible for them)	An individual has a fight with her spouse and turns to her best friend for emotional support.
Altruism	Dedicating life to meeting the needs of others (receives gratification either vicariously or from the response of others)	After being rejected by her boyfriend, a young girl joins the Peace Corps.
Anticipation	Experiencing emotional reactions in advance or anticipating consequences of possible future events and considering realistic, alternative responses or solutions	A parent cries for 3 weeks before her last child leaves for college. On the day of the separation, the parent spends the day with friends.
Autistic fantasy	Excessive daydreaming as a substitute for human relationships, more effective action, or problem solving	A young man sits in his room all day and dreams about being a rock star instead of attending a baseball game with a friend.
Denial	Refusing to acknowledge some painful aspect of external reality or subjective experience that would be apparent to others (*psychotic denial* used when there is gross impairment in reality testing)	A teenager's best friend moves away, but the adolescent says he does not feel sad.
Devaluation	Attributing exaggerated negative qualities to self or others	A boy has been rejected by his long-time girlfriend. He tells his friends that he realizes that she is stupid and ugly.
Displacement	Transferring a feeling about, or a response to, one object onto another (usually less threatening), substitute object	A child is mad at her mother for leaving for the day but says she is really mad at the sitter for serving her food she does not like.
Dissociation	Experiencing a breakdown in the usually integrated functions of consciousness, memory, perception of self or the environment, or sensory and motor behavior	An adult relates severe sexual abuse experienced as a child but does it without feeling. She says that the experience was as if she were outside her body watching the abuse.
Help-rejecting complaining	Complaining or making repetitious requests for help that disguise covert feelings of hostility or reproach toward others, which are then expressed by rejecting the suggestions, advice, or help that others offer (complaints or requests may involve physical or psychological symptoms or life problems)	A college student asks a teacher for help after receiving a bad grade on a test. Every suggestion the teacher has is rejected by the student.
Humor	Emphasizing the amusing or ironic aspects of the conflict or stressor	A person makes a joke right after experiencing an embarrassing situation.
Idealization	Attributing exaggerated positive qualities to others	An adult falls in love and fails to see the negative qualities in the other person.
Intellectualization	Excessive use of abstract thinking or the making of generalizations to control or minimize disturbing feelings	After rejection in a romantic relationship, the rejected explains the relationship dynamics to a friend.
Isolation of affect	Separation of ideas from the feelings originally associated with them	The individual loses touch with the feelings associated with a rape while remaining aware of the details.
Omnipotence	Feeling or acting as if one possesses special powers or abilities and is superior to others	An individual tells a friend about personal expertise in the stock market and the ability to predict the best stocks.
Passive aggression	Indirectly and unassertively expressing aggression toward others. There is a facade of overt compliance masking covert resistance, resentment, or hostility.	One employee doesn't like another, so he secretly steals her milk from the office refrigerator. She is unaware of his hostile feelings.
Projection	Falsely attributing to another one's own unacceptable feelings, impulses, or thoughts	A child is very angry at a parent but accuses the parent of being angry.

TABLE 7.4	SPECIFIC DEFENSE MECHANISMS AND COPING STYLES *(Continued)*	
Defense Mechanism	**Definition**	**Example**
Projective identification	Falsely attributing to another one's own unacceptable feelings, impulses, or thoughts. Unlike simple projection, the individual does not fully disavow what is projected. Instead, the individual remains aware of his or her own affect or impulses but misattributes them as justifiable reactions to the other person. Frequently, the individual induces the very feelings in others that were first mistakenly believed to be there, making it difficult to clarify who did what to whom first.	A child is mad at a parent, who in turn becomes angry at the child but may be unsure of why. The child then feels justified at being angry with the parent.
Rationalization	Concealing the true motivations for one's own thoughts, actions, or feelings through the elaboration of reassuring or self-serving but incorrect explanations	A man is rejected by his girlfriend but explains to his friends that her leaving was best because she was beneath him socially and would not be liked by his family.
Reaction formation	Substituting behavior, thoughts, or feelings that are diametrically opposed to one's own unacceptable thoughts or feelings (this usually occurs in conjunction with their repression)	A wife finds out about her husband's extramarital affairs and tells her friends that she thinks his affairs are perfectly appropriate. She truly does not feel, on a conscious level, any anger or hurt.
Repression	Expelling disturbing wishes, thoughts, or experiences from conscious awareness (the feeling component may remain conscious, detached from its associated ideas)	A woman does not remember the experience of being raped in the basement but does feel anxious when going into that house.
Self-assertion	Expressing feelings and thoughts directly in a way that is not coercive or manipulative	An individual reaffirms that going to a ball game is not what she wants to do.
Self-observation	Reflecting feelings, thoughts, motivation, and behavior and responding to them appropriately	An individual notices an irritation at his friend's late arrival and decides to tell the friend of the irritation.
Splitting	Compartmentalizing opposite affect states and failing to integrate the positive and negative qualities of the self or others into cohesive images	Self and object images tend to alternate between polar opposites: exclusively loving, powerful, worthy, nurturing, and kind or exclusively bad, hateful, angry, destructive, rejecting, or worthless. One friend is wonderful and another former friend, who was at one time viewed as being perfect, is now believed to be an evil person.
Sublimation	Channeling potentially maladaptive feelings or impulses into socially acceptable behavior	An adolescent boy is very angry with his parents. On the football field, he tackles someone very forcefully.
Suppression	Intentionally avoiding thinking about disturbing problems, wishes, feelings, or experiences	A student is anxiously awaiting test results but goes to a movie to stop thinking about it.
Undoing	Words or behavior designed to negate or to make amends symbolically for unacceptable thoughts, feelings, or actions	A man has sexual fantasies about his wife's sister. He takes his wife away for a romantic weekend.

As you read through the chapters on various mental challenges, consider how the signs and symptoms of each illness could have an impact on communication and the evolving therapeutic relationship.

Analyzing Interactions

Many patients with psychiatric disorders have difficulty communicating. For example, perceptual, cognitive, and information-processing deficits, which are typical of people with schizophrenia, can interfere with the patient's ability to express ideas, understand concepts, and accurately perceive the environment. Because communication is complex, mental health clinicians monitor their interactions with patients using various methods, including audio recording; video recording; and **process recording**, which entails writing a verbatim transcript of the interaction. A video or audio recording of an interaction provides the most accurate monitoring but is cumbersome to use. Process recording, one of the easiest methods to use, is adequate in most situations. Nurses should use it when first learning therapeutic communication and

TABLE 7.5	PROCESS RECORDING

Setting: The living room of Mr. S's home. Mr. S is 23 years old and was hospitalized for 2 weeks. His diagnosis is a bipolar mood disorder, and he is recovering from a depressive episode. His parents are in the room but cannot hear the conversation. Mr. S is sitting on the couch, and the nurse is sitting on a chair. This is the nurse's first visit after Mr. S's discharge from the hospital.

Patient	Nurse	Interpretation/Analysis
	How are you doing, Mr. S? (smiles and offers hand to shake)	*Plan:* Initially develop a sense of trust and initiate a therapeutic relationship.
I'm fine. It's good to be home (looking at floor, takes nurse's hand to briefly shake). I really don't like the hospital. (shakes his head while still looking at floor).	You didn't like the hospital?	Interpretation: Validating assumption that Mr. S does not want to return to hospital. Nonverbal communication may indicate sadness or low self-esteem. This needs further exploration.
No. The nurses lock you up (maintains eye contact with nurse, frowning, arms crossed). Are you a nurse?		Patient validates assumption regarding hospital, but nonverbal behavior indicates there may be further concerns.
	I'm a nurse. I'm wondering if you think that I will lock you up (maintains eye contact and open posture)?	Interpretation: Mr. S may be wondering what my role is and whether I will put him back in the hospital. This assumption needs to be validated, and my role needs clarification.
You could tell my mom to put me back in the hospital (maintains eye contact with nurse).	Any treatment that I recommend will be thoroughly discussed with you first. I am here to help you stay out of the hospital. I will not discuss anything with your mother unless you give me permission to do so (nurse maintains eye contact and open posture).	Use interpretation to clarify Mr. S's thinking. Mr. S is wondering about my relationship with his mother. Explain my role and confidentiality.
(Patient maintains eye contact and uncrosses arms.)		Patient's nonverbal communication appears to indicate he is more comfortable with this clarification.

during times when communication becomes a problem. In a process recording, the nurse records, from memory, the verbatim interaction immediately after the communication (Table 7.5).

The nurse then analyzes the content of the interaction in terms of the words and their meaning for both the patient and the nurse. The analysis is especially important because the ability to communicate verbally is often compromised in people with mental disorders. Because words may not have the same meaning for the patient as they do for the nurse, clarification of meaning becomes especially important. The analysis can identify symbolic meanings, themes, and blocks in communication.

Symbolism

Symbolism, the use of a word or phrase to represent an object, event, or feeling, is used universally. For example, automobiles are named for wild animals that represent speed, prowess, and beauty. In people with mental disorders, the use of words to symbolize events, objects, or feelings is often idiosyncratic, and they cannot explain their choices. For example, a person who is feeling scared and anxious may tell the nurse that bombs and guns are

exploding. It is up to the nurse to make the connection between the bombs and guns and the patient's feelings and then validate this with the patient. Because of the patient's cognitive limitations, the individual may express feelings only symbolically. Another example is found in Table 7.6.

Some patients, for example, some with developmental disabilities or organic brain difficulties, may have difficulty with abstract thinking and symbolism. Conversations may be interpreted literally. For example, in response to the question: "What brings you to the hospital?" a patient might reply, "The ambulance." In these situations, the nurse must be cautious to avoid using symbols or metaphors. Concrete language, that is, language reflecting what can be observed through the senses, will be more easily understood.

Content Themes

Verbal behavior is also interpreted by analyzing **content themes**. Patients often express concerns or feelings repeatedly in several different ways. After a few sessions, a common theme emerges. Themes may emerge symbolically, as in the case with the patient who constantly talks about the "guns and bombs." Alternatively, a theme may

TABLE 7.6   USE OF SYMBOLISM

Setting: Mr. A has been diagnosed with schizophrenia and expresses himself through the use of television characters. A nurse observed another patient shoving him against the wall. As the nurse approached the two patients, the other patient ran, leaving Mr. A noticeably shaking. The nurse checked to see if Mr. A was all right.

Patient	Nurse	Interpretation/Analysis
	Mr. A, are you OK? (approaches patient)	
Robin Hood saved the day. (trembling, arms crossed)		Mr. A could not say, "Thank you for helping me." Instead, he could only describe a fictional character's response.
	You feel that you are saved?	The nurse focused on what Mr. A must be feeling if he felt that he had been rescued.
It's a glorious day in Sherwood Forest! (trembling decreases; smiles at nurse)		He seems to be happy now.
	Mr. A, are you hurting anywhere? (eyes scan over patient, using concerned tone of voice)	The nurse wanted to check whether the patient had been hurt when pushed against the wall.
The angel of mercy put out the fire. (continues to smile and extends hand to shake hands with nurse)		The patient is apparently not hurting now.

simply be identified as a recurrent thread of a story that a patient retells at each session. For example, one patient often discussed his early abandonment by his family. This led the nurse to hypothesize that he had an underlying fear of rejection. The nurse was then able to test whether there was an underlying fear and to develop strategies to help the patient explore the fear (Box 7.4). It is important to involve patients in analyzing themes so they may learn this skill. Within the therapeutic relationship, the person who does the work is the one who develops the competencies, so the nurse must be careful to share this opportunity with the patient (Peplau, 1952, 1992).

Communication Blocks

Communication blocks are identified by topic changes that either the nurse or the patient makes. Topics are changed for various reasons. A patient may change the topic from one that does not interest him to one that he finds more meaningful. However, an individual usually changes the topic because he or she is uncomfortable with a particular subject. When a topic change is identified, the nurse or patient hypothesizes the reason for it. If the nurse changes the topic, he or she needs to determine why. The nurse may find that he or she is uncomfortable with the topic or may not be listening to the patient. Novice mental health nurses who are uncomfortable with silences or trying to elicit specific information from the patient often change topics.

The nurse must also record and interpret the patient's nonverbal behavior in light of the verbal behavior. Is the patient saying one thing verbally and another nonverbally? The nurse must consider the patient's cultural background. Is the behavior consistent with cultural norms? For example, if a patient denies any problems but is affectionate and physically demonstrative (which is antithetical to her naturally stoic cultural beliefs and behaviors), the nonverbal behavior is inconsistent with what is normal behavior for that person. Further exploration is needed to determine the meaning of the culturally atypical behavior.

KEYCONCEPT   The **nurse–patient relationship** is a dynamic process that changes with time. It can be viewed in steps or phases with characteristic behaviors for both the patient and the nurse.

BOX 7.4

Themes and Interactions

Session 1: Patient discusses the death of his mother at a young age.
Session 2: Patient explains that his sister is now married and never visits him.
Session 3: Patient says that his best friend in the hospital was discharged and he really misses her.
Session 4: Patient cries about a lost kitten.
Interpretation: Theme of loss is pervasive in several sessions.

SUMMARY OF KEY POINTS

- To deal therapeutically with the emotions, feelings, and problems of patients, nurses must understand their own cultural values and beliefs and interpersonal strengths and limitations.

CRITICAL THINKING CHALLENGES

1. Describe how you would do a suicide assessment on a distraught patient who comes to the physician's office expressing concerns about her ability to cope with her current situation. Describe how you would approach this patient if you determined she was suicidal. How might this assessment look different depending on the phase of the therapeutic relationship?

2. Describe how you would communicate with a patient who is concerned that the diagnosis of bipolar disorder will negatively affect his or her social and work relationships.

3. Your depressed patient does not seem inclined to talk about the depression. Describe the measures you would take to initiate a therapeutic relationship with him or her.

Analyze That: 2002. In this comedy sequel to *Analyze This* (1999), Billy Crystal plays psychiatrist Dr. Ben Sobel. The patient is Paul Vitti (Robert De Niro), a mobster who has been sent to prison. Vitti is either having a psychotic break or is faking one, and his former psychiatrist is called back to assess the situation. Vitti is sent to Sobel's home for treatment. Both the psychiatrist and patient have unresolved feelings related to the deaths of their fathers.

Viewing Points: The issue of therapeutic boundaries is a source of comedy in this film. What normal therapeutic boundaries are being violated? Whose needs are being met throughout the film? What would be appropriate if a patient evoked personal unresolved issues for the therapist?

REFERENCES

Barwick, M. A., Bennett, L. M., Johnson, S. N., McGowan, J., & Moore, J. E. (2012). Training health and mental health professionals in motivational interviewing: A systematic review. *Children and Youth Services Review, 34*(9), 1786–1795. doi:10.1016/j.childyouth.2012.05.012

Boyd, M. (1995). Communication with patients, families, healthcare providers, and diverse cultures. In M. Strader & P. Decker (Eds.). *Role transition to patient care management* (pp. 431). Norwalk, CT: Appleton & Lange.

Orlando, I. (1961). *Orlando's dynamic nurse-patient relationship: Function, process and principles.* New York: G.P. Putman's Sons.

Peplau, H. E. (1952, 1992). *Interpersonal relations in nursing.* New York: J. P. Putnam's Sons.

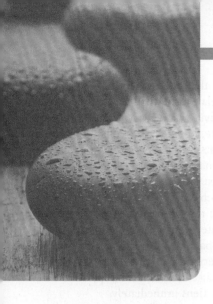

8
The Nurse-Patient Relationship

Cheryl Forchuk

KEY CONCEPT

- nurse–patient relationship

LEARNING OBJECTIVES

After studying this chapter, you will be able to:

1. Explain how the nurse can establish a therapeutic relationship with patients by using rapport and empathy.

2. Explain what occurs in each of the three phases of the nurse–patient relationship: orientation, working, and resolution.

3. Describe what characterizes a nontherapeutic or deteriorating nurse–patient relationship.

KEY TERMS

- countertransference • deteriorating relationship • empathy • empathic linkages • nontherapeutic relationship
- orientation phase • rapport • resolution • transference • working phase

The nurse–patient relationship is an important tool used to reach recovery goals. The purposes of this chapter are to (1) examine the specific stages or steps involved in establishing a therapeutic nurse-patient relationship, (2) explore the specific factors that make a nurse–patient relationship successful and therapeutic, and (3) differentiate therapeutic from nontherapeutic relationships.

EFFECTIVE COMMUNICATION NEEDS IN RELATIONSHIPS

When the nurse is establishing a nurse-patient relationship, the quality of communication is critical. This section describes the importance of rapport, empathy, recognition of empathic linkages, and the role of professional boundaries in nurse–patient interactions.

Rapport

Rapport, interpersonal harmony characterized by understanding and respect, is important in developing a trusting, therapeutic relationship. Nurses establish rapport through interpersonal warmth, a nonjudgmental attitude, and a demonstration of understanding. A skilled nurse will establish rapport that will alleviate the patient's anxiety in discussing personal problems.

People with psychiatric problems often feel alone and isolated. Establishing rapport helps lessen feelings of being alone. When rapport develops, a patient feels comfortable with the nurse and finds self-disclosure easier. The nurse also feels comfortable and recognizes that an interpersonal bond or alliance is developing. All of these factors—comfort, sense of sharing, and decreased anxiety—are important in establishing and building the nurse–patient relationship.

Empathy 👂

The use of empathy in a therapeutic relationship is central to psychiatric–mental health nursing. Empathy is sometimes confused with sympathy, which is the expression of compassion and kindness. **Empathy** is the ability to experience, in the present, a situation as another did at some time in the past. It is the ability to put oneself in another person's circumstances and to imagine what it would be like to share their feelings. The nurse does not actually have to have had the experience but has to be able to imagine the feelings associated with it. For empathy to develop, there must be a giving of self to the other individual and a reciprocal desire to know each other personally. The process involves the nurse receiving information from the patient with open, nonjudgmental acceptance and communicating this understanding of the experience and feelings so the patient feels understood.

Recognition of Empathic Linkages

While empathy is essential, it is important for the nurse to be aware of **empathic linkages**, the direct communication of feelings (Peplau, 1952). This commonly occurs with anxiety. For example, a nurse may be speaking with a patient who is highly anxious, and the nurse may notice his or her own speech becoming more rapid in tandem with the patient's. The nurse may also become aware of subjective feelings of anxiety. It may be difficult for the nurse to determine if the anxiety was communicated interpersonally or if the nurse is personally reacting to some of the content of what the patient is communicating. However, being aware of one's own feelings and analyzing them is crucial to determining the source of the feeling and addressing associated problems.

Professional Boundaries in a Nurse-Patient Relationship 👂

The importance of professional boundaries was discussed in Chapter 7. Maintaining professional boundaries may be more difficult in an ongoing therapeutic relationship. The patient may seek a friendship or sexual relationship with the nurse but this would be inconsistent with the professional role and is usually considered unethical.

Indicators that the relationship may be moving outside the professional boundaries are gift giving on either party's part, spending more time than usual with a particular patient, strenuously defending or explaining the patient's behavior in team meetings, the nurse feeling that he or she is the only one who truly understands the patient, keeping secrets, or frequently thinking about the patient outside of the work situation (Forchuk et al., 2006). State or provincial regulatory bodies will have either guidelines or firm rules regarding any legal or professional restrictions

about the amount of time that must pass prior to engaging in a romantic or sexual relationship with a former patient. Guidelines are comparatively vague about when a friendship would be appropriate, but such relationships are not appropriate when the nurse is actively providing care to the patient. Exceptions may be when a relationship preceded the nursing context and another nurse is unavailable to provide care, such as in a rural area. Similarly, relationships to meet the nurse's needs that are acquired through the nursing context, such as a relationship with a family member of the patient, also breach professional boundaries. When concerns arise related to therapeutic boundaries, the nurse must seek clinical supervision or transfer the care of the patient immediately.

THE NURSE–PATIENT RELATIONSHIP

The nurse–patient relationship is a dynamic process that changes with time. It can be viewed in steps or phases with characteristic behaviors for both patient and nurse. This text uses an adaptation of Hildegarde Peplau's model, which she introduced in her seminal work, *Interpersonal Relations in Nursing* (1952, 1992). Emerging evidence suggests that a well-developed nurse–patient relationship positively affects patient care.

Phases 👂

The nurse–patient relationship is conceptualized in three overlapping phases that evolve with time: orientation phase, working phase, and resolution phase. The **orientation phase** is the phase during which the nurse and patient get to know each other. During this phase, which can last from a few minutes to several months, the patient develops a sense of trust in the nurse. The second is the **working phase**, in which the patient uses the relationship to examine specific problems and learn new ways of approaching them. The final stage, **resolution phase**, is the termination stage of the relationship and lasts from the time the problems are actually resolved to the close of the relationship. The relationship does not evolve as a simple linear relationship. Instead, the relationship may be predominantly in one phase, but reflections of all phases can be seen in each interaction (Table 8.1).

> **KEYCONCEPT** The **nurse–patient relationship** is a dynamic process that changes with time. It can be viewed in steps or phases with characteristic behaviors for both the patient and the nurse.

Orientation Phase

The orientation phase begins when the nurse and patient meet and ends when the patient begins to identify problems to be examined. During the orientation phase, the

TABLE 8.1	PHASES OF THE NURSE–PATIENT RELATIONSHIP		
	Orientation	**Working**	**Resolution**
Patient	Seeks assistance Identifies needs Commits to a therapeutic relationship During the later part, begins to test relationship	Discusses problems and underlying needs Uses emotional safety of relationship to examine personal issues Tests new ways of solving problems Feels comfortable with nurse May use transference	May express ambivalence about the relationship and its termination Uses personal style to say "good-bye"
Nurse	Actively listens Establishes boundaries of the relationship Clarifies expectations Identifies countertransference issues Uses empathy Establishes rapport	Supports development of healthy problem solving Encourages patient to prepare for the future	Avoids returning to patient's initial problems Encourages independence Promotes positive family interactions

nurse discusses the patient's expectations, explains the purpose of the relationship and its boundaries, and facilitates the development of the relationship. It is natural for the nurse to be nervous during the first few sessions. The goal of the orientation phase is to develop trust and security within the nurse–patient relationship. During this initial phase, the nurse listens intently to the patient's history and perception of problems and begins to understand the patient and identify themes. The use of empathy facilitates the development of a positive therapeutic relationship.

First Meeting

During the first meeting, outlining both nursing and patient responsibilities is important. The nurse is responsible for providing guidance throughout the therapeutic relationship, protecting confidential information, and maintaining professional boundaries. The patient is responsible for attending agreed-upon sessions, interacting during the sessions, and participating in the nurse–patient relationship. The nurse should also explain clearly to the patient meeting times, handling of missed sessions, and the estimated length of the relationship. Issues related to recording information and how the nurse will work within the interdisciplinary team should also be made explicit.

Usually, both the nurse and the patient feel anxious at the first meeting. The nurse should recognize the anxieties and attempt to alleviate them before the meeting. The patient's behavior during this first meeting may indicate to the nurse some of the patient's problems in interpersonal relationships. For example, a patient may talk nonstop for 15 minutes or may brag of sexual conquests. What the patient chooses to tell or not to tell is significant. What a patient first does or says may not accurately indicate his or her true feelings or the situation. In the beginning, patients may deny problems or employ various forms of defense mechanisms or prevent the nurse from getting to know them. The patient is usually nervous and insecure during the first few sessions and may exhibit behavior reflective of these emotions, such as rambling. Typically, by the third session, the patient can focus on a topic.

Confidentiality in Treatment

Ideally, nurses include people who are important to the patient in planning and implementing care. The nurse and patient should discuss the issue of confidentiality in the first session. The nurse should be clear about any information that is to be shared with anyone else. The nurse shares significant assessment data and patient progress with a supervisor, team members, and a physician. Most patients expect the nurse to communicate with other mental health professionals and are comfortable with this arrangement. Restrictions regarding what can be shared and with whom are also covered by state or provincial mental health acts and health information acts.

Testing the Relationship

This first part of the orientation phase, called the "honeymoon phase," is usually pleasant. However, the therapeutic team typically hits rough spots before completing this phase. The patient begins to test the relationship to become convinced that the nurse will really accept him or her. Typical "testing behaviors" include forgetting a scheduled session or being late. Patients may also express anger at something a nurse says or accuse the nurse of breaking confidentiality. Another common pattern is for the patient to first introduce a relatively superficial issue as if it is the major problem. The nurse must recognize that these behaviors are designed to test the relationship and establish its parameters, not to express rejection or dissatisfaction with the nurse. The student nurse often feels personally rejected during the patient's testing and may even become angry with the patient. If the nurse simply accepts the behavior and continues to be available and consistent to the patient, these behaviors usually subside. Testing needs to be understood as a normal way that human beings develop trust.

Working Phase

When the patient begins identifying problems to work on, the working phase of the relationship has started. Problem identification can yield a wide range of issues, such as managing symptoms of a mental disorder, coping with chronic pain, examining issues related to sexual abuse, or dealing with problematic interpersonal relationships. Through the relationship, the patient begins to explore the identified problems and develop strategies to resolve them. By the time the working phase is reached, the patient has developed enough trust that he or she can examine the identified problems within the security of the therapeutic relationship. In the working phase, the nurse can use various verbal and nonverbal techniques to help the patient examine problems and to support the patient through the healing process.

Transference (unconscious assignment to others of the feelings and attitudes that the patient originally associated with important figures) and **countertransference** (the provider's emotional reaction to the patient based on personal unconscious needs and conflicts) become important issues in the working phase. For example, a patient could be hostile to a nurse because of underlying resentment of authority figures; the nurse, in turn, could respond defensively because of earlier experiences of anger. The patient uses transference to examine problems. During this phase, the patient is psychologically vulnerable and emotionally dependent on the nurse. The nurse needs to recognize countertransference and prevent it from eroding professional boundaries.

Many times, nurses are eager to implement rehabilitation plans. However, this cannot be done until the patient trusts the nurse and identifies what issues he or she wishes to work on in the context of the relationship.

Resolution Phase

The final stage of the nurse–patient relationship is resolution, which begins when the actual problems are resolved and ends with the termination of the relationship. During this phase, the patient is redirected toward a life without this specific therapeutic relationship. The patient connects with community resources, solidifies a newly found understanding, and practices new behaviors. The patient takes responsibility for follow-up appointments and interacts with significant others in new ways. New problems are not addressed during this phase except

in terms of what was learned during the working stage. The nurse assists the client in strengthening relationships, making referrals, and recognizing and understanding signs of future relapse.

Termination begins on the first day of the relationship when the nurse explains that this relationship is time limited and was established to resolve the patient's problems and help him or her handle them. Because a therapeutic relationship is dependent, the nurse must constantly evaluate the patient's level of dependence and continually support the patient's move toward independence. Termination is usually stressful for the patient, who must sever ties with the nurse who has shared thoughts and feelings and given guidance and support over many sessions.

Depending on previous experiences with terminating relationships, some patients may not handle their emotions well during termination. Some may not show up for the last session at all to avoid their feelings of sadness and separation. Many patients display anger about the relationship's ending. Patients may express anger toward the nurse or displace it onto others. For example, a patient may shout obscenities at another patient after being told that his therapeutic relationship with the nurse would end in a few weeks. One of the best ways to handle the anger is to help the patient acknowledge it, to explain that anger is a normal emotion when a relationship is ending, and to reassure the patient that it is acceptable to feel angry. The nurse should also reassure the patient that anger subsides after the relationship is over.

Another typical termination behavior is raising old problems that have already been resolved. The nurse may feel frustrated if patients in the termination phase present resolved problems as if they were new. The nurse may feel that the sessions were unsuccessful. In reality, patients are attempting to prolong the relationship and avoid its ending. Nurses should avoid addressing these problems. Instead, they should reassure patients that they already covered those issues and learned methods to control them. They should explain that the patient may be feeling anxious about the relationship's ending and redirect the patient to newly found skills and abilities in forming new relationships, including support groups and social groups. The final meeting should focus on the future (Box 8.1). The nurse can reassure the patient that the nurse will remember him or her, but the nurse should not agree to see the patient outside the relationship.

Nontherapeutic Relationships

Although it is hoped that all nurse–patient relationships will go through the phases of the relationship described earlier, this is not always the case. In a **nontherapeutic relationship**, the nurse and patient both feel very frustrated and keep varying their approach with each other in an attempt to establish a meaningful relationship. This

BOX 8.1 • THERAPEUTIC DIALOGUE • The Last Meeting

INEFFECTIVE APPROACH

Ms. J: Why did the other nurses bring you flowers and cards today?

Nurse: Well, that's because today is my last day, I'm transfering to the new hospital, across town.

Ms. J: Oh, um. I was just thinking, I need to talk to you about something important.

Nurse: What is it?

Ms. J: I have been worrying about my medication again.

Nurse: Oh, have you had any side effects?

Ms. J: No, but I might.

Nurse: I think you should tell the new nurse.

Ms. J: She is too new. She won't understand and you helped me last time. I feel so worried about your leaving. Is there any way you can stay? You said that you would check in, remember?

Nurse: Well, I could check on you tomorrow?

Ms. J: Oh, would you? I would really appreciate it if you would give me your new telephone number that way I can tell you if anything happens.

Nurse: I don't know what the number will be, but you might be able to find it online.

EFFECTIVE APPROACH

Ms. J: Why did the other nurses bring you flowers and cards today?

Nurse: Oh, hello Ms. J. Do you remember? Today is my last day.

Ms. J: Oh, yes. Well, I need to talk to you about something important.

Nurse: We talked about that. Anything "important" needs to be shared with the new nurse.

Ms. J: But I want to tell you. You really made me feel better last time.

Nurse: Thank you, but remember that you improved a lot because you know what to do in order to continue progressing. Saying good-bye can be very hard.

Ms. J: I'll miss you.

Nurse: Your feelings are very normal when relationships are ending. I will remember you in a very special way.

Ms. J: Can I please have your telephone number in case I need to talk to you?

Nurse: No, I can't give that to you. It is important that we say good-bye today. And, remember, you can always talk to the new nurse about your concerns.

Ms. J: Okay, I know. Good-bye. Good luck.

Nurse: Good-bye.

CRITICAL THINKING CHALLENGE

- What were some of the mistakes the nurse in the first scenario made?

- In the second scenario, how does therapeutic communication in the termination phase differ from effective communication in the working phase?

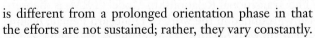

is different from a prolonged orientation phase in that the efforts are not sustained; rather, they vary constantly.

The nurse may try longer meetings, shorter meetings, being more or less directive, and varying the therapeutic stance from warm and friendly to aloof. Patients in this phase may try to talk about the past but then change to discussions of the "here and now." They will try talking about their family and in the next meeting talk about their work goals. Both *grapple and struggle* to come to a common ground, and both become increasingly frustrated with each other.

Eventually, the frustration becomes so great that the pair gives up on each other and moves to a phase of *mutual withdrawal*. The nurse may schedule seeing this patient at the end of the shift and "run out of time" so the meeting never happens. The patient will leave the unit or otherwise be unavailable during scheduled meeting times. If a meeting does occur, the nurse will try to keep it short, thinking, "What's the point—we just cover the same old ground anyway." The patient will attempt to keep it superficial and stay on safe topics ("You can always ask about your medications—nurses love to health teach, you know").

A **deteriorating relationship** is also nontherapeutic and has been shown to have predictable phases (Coatsworth-Puspoky, Forchuk, & Ward-Griffin, 2006). This relationship starts in the *withholding* phase during which the nurse is perceived as "withholding" nursing support. The nurse fails to recognize that the patient is a person with an illness or health needs. The patient feels uncomfortable, anxious, frustrated, and guilty about being ill and does not develop a sense of trust. A barrier exists between the patient and nurse.

The middle phase of a deteriorating relationship consists of two subphases: *avoiding* and *ignoring*. The patient begins to avoid the nurse and perceives that the nurse is avoiding him or her. The patient abides by the rules and because he or she does not want to cause problems. The nurse is perceived as rude and condescending. The nurse ignores and avoids the patient's requests for help; in turn, the patient becomes more anxious, frustrated, and fearful. Patients experiencing this phase report feelings of wanting to give up, being rejected, not being cared for, and not being listened to.

The end phase is named *struggling with and making sense of*. In the final phase of a nontherapeutic, deteriorating relationship, the patient struggles with and tries to understand the unsatisfactory relationship. The patient feels hopeless and frustrated as a result of the lack of support received by the nurse. In a deteriorating relationship, the patient and nurse begin as strangers and end as enemies.

Obviously, no therapeutic progress can be made in a nontherapeutic or deteriorating relationship. The nurse may be hesitant to ask for a therapeutic transfer, assuming that a relationship would similarly fail with another nurse. However, each relationship is unique, and difficulties in one relationship do not predict difficulties in the next. Clinical supervision early on may assist the development of the relationship, but often a therapeutic transfer to another nurse is required.

EXAMPLES OF STRATEGIES RELATED TO THERAPEUTIC RELATIONSHIPS

Motivational Interviewing

Motivational interviewing (MI) is a clinical method intended to engage a patient's own decision-making ability. By focusing and reinforcing the client's own arguments for change, MI can be used to achieve positive outcomes. This is an inherently collaborative process; through directed counseling, and focused discussions between the care provider and the patient. As a result, MI is inherently exploratory and adaptive.

There is a lot of evidence to suggest that MI produces positive health outcomes; however, evidence also suggests that external factors can influence the success of long-term outcomes. These external factors are often interpersonal and social (Berg, Ross, & Tikkanen, 2011). Because much of the success of MI depends on the quality of interaction between the care provider and the patient, good communication practices are essential for effective implementation of MI. Many of these problems are the result of the assumption that high-risk behaviors are entirely or mostly under the control of the individual (Berg et al., 2011). Careful attention to the effects of this assumption can make clear where MI may or may not be an ideal treatment option.

Because the success of MI is, in part, dependent on contingent factors, care providers require frequent instruction and feedback. Strong communication in the context of therapeutic relationships as discussed in this chapter, especially self-awareness, empathetic linkages, active listening, and the avoidance of unhelpful varieties of defense mechanisms, require on-going training and will affect therapeutic outcomes. While challenging to successfully implement, MI has produced positive health outcomes in many different settings (Barnett, Sussman, Smith, Rohrbach, & Spruijt-Metz, 2012; Barwick, Bennett, Johnson, McGowan, & Moore, 2012; Chen, Creedy, Lin, & Wollin, 2012; Cronk, Russell, Knowles, Matteson, Peace, & Ponferrada, 2012; Day, 2013). Every particular use of MI is likely to vary according to patient needs; Miller and Moyers (2006) have identified eight features of MI that should appear in every application of this technique:

1. "openness to collaboration with clients' own expertise,
2. proficiency in client centered counseling, including accurate empathy,
3. recognition of key aspects of client speech that guides the practice of MI,
4. eliciting and strengthening client change talk,
5. rolling with resistance,
6. negotiating change plans,
7. consolidating client commitment, and
8. switching flexibly between MI and other intervention styles." (pg. 3)

Transitional Relationship Model (TRM)/ Transitional Discharge Model (TDM)

The Transitional Relationship Model (TRM) is theoretically grounded in the work of Hildegard Peplau; healing occurs in relationships. Therapeutic relationships can be formed with either professionals or peer supporters. The TRM was first developed to ease the transition from hospital to community, but its use has now been expanded in a variety of transitional care processes. There are two essential components of the TRM:

1. the therapeutic relationship should be extended until a new relationship with another care provider is established (continuing relationships formed in the hospital

BOX 8.2

Research for Best Practice: Transitional Relationship Model

Forchuk, C., Martin, M. L., Jensen, E., Ouseley, S., Sealy, P., Beal, G., et al. (2013), Integrating an evidence-based intervention into clinical practice: 'Transitional relationship model'. Journal of Psychiatric and Mental Health Nursing, 20(7), 584–594. doi:10.1111/j.1365–2850.2012.01956.x

THE QUESTION: The Transitional Relationship Model (TRM) facilitates an effective discharge from the hospital to the community. Given this, what is the most effective way of implementing this model? What might facilitate the successful implementation of the TRM? What are the barriers to successful implementation?

METHODS: This study implemented the TRM in three waves, across six wards using a delayed implementation control group design to study how the addition of new information changed the implementation of the TRM. Following the experiences of the wards in which the TRM was initially implemented, recommendations for successful implementation of the model were developed for the subsequent waves of wards. Recommendations were developed using a combination of qualitative methods: monthly summaries, progress reports, meeting minutes, and focus groups.

FINDINGS: The results of this study can be divided into two categories: facilitators and barriers. The successful implementation of the TRM was aided by the use of educational modules (for both staff and peer training), on-site champions, and supportive documentation systems. Barriers included: feeling swamped or overwhelmed, "death by process," preexisting conflicts within teams, and changes in champions.

IMPLICATIONS FOR NURSING: The positive health outcomes associated with the TRM require careful preparation and constant attention to education, communication, and the effectiveness of the support given to caregivers.

until new therapeutic relationships in the community are formed) and,

2. trained peer support (often through a consumer survivor group) from a psychiatric survivor who has now successfully transitioned to the community.

In addition to producing positive therapeutic outcomes, the TRM also reduces time spent in hospital and readmissions (Reynolds, Lauder, Sharkey, Macivier, Veitch, & Cameron, 2004). See Box 8.2.

Technology and the Therapeutic Relationship

As technology develops and becomes increasingly accessible, traditional face-to-face communication can be replaced with technological interactions. Below are some of the most common forms of this communication:

Phone and video conferencing: this method is becoming increasingly popular, especially in remote areas where the land or the isolation of the clinic constitutes barriers to the development of a therapeutic relationship. However,

three important criteria must be conceded prior to the use of this technology:

- Nonverbal communication is more difficult to detect and access
- The patient must have reliable access to the technology
- An appropriate method of documentation much still be used

Internet communication: Above all else, any communication over the internet must be secure to maintain confidentiality. Hospital firewalls can be useful in establishing such connections (Forchuk et al., 2012). One must always be aware of a hospital's or research site's policies and best practices regarding communication online. Some commonly used platforms for online communication, such as Facebook, cannot meet the standards discussed above and so ought not to be used in communication with patients. However, the internet is an invaluable resource for educational and research purposes.

SUMMARY OF KEY POINTS

- The nurse–patient relationship is built on therapeutic communication, including verbal and nonverbal interactions between the nurse and the patient.

- Two of the most important communication concepts are empathy and rapport.

- In the nurse–patient relationship, as in all types of relationships, certain physical, emotional, and social boundaries and limitations need to be observed.

- The therapeutic nurse–patient relationship consists of three major and overlapping stages or phases: the orientation phase, in which the patient and nurse meet and establish the parameters of the relationship; the working phase, in which the patient identifies and explores problems; and the resolution phase, in which the patient learns to manage the problems and the relationship is terminated.

- The nontherapeutic relationship consists of three major and overlapping phases: the orientation phase, the grappling and struggling phase, and the phase of mutual withdrawal. A deteriorating relationship begins with a withholding phase, continues through the phases of avoiding and ignoring, and finally ends unsatisfactorily with a phase named "struggling with and making sense of."

CRITICAL THINKING CHALLENGES

1. A patient who has followed all of the nurse's recommendations is very late for his appointment and announces

that he is no longer going to take his medication. The nurse is quite surprised because she thought that he had adhering to treatment recommendations. What phase of the therapeutic relationship are they entering? Explain. Discuss three different patient behaviors that could during the resolution phase of the nurse-patient relationship. Discuss an ideal "working phase" of a nurse patient relationship.

2. Think of a time that you worked with a patient you did not like. What was behind the dislike? How did you handle the therapeutic relationship? What could you do differently?

Good Will Hunting: 1997. Robin Williams plays therapist Dr. Sean Maguire. His patient, Will Hunting (Matt Damon), is a janitor at MIT who is also a troubled genius. Through a strong relationship, Will begins to realize his potential. This film deals with intense blocks to communication, as well as issues around justice system use and class.
Viewing Points: Watch closely how the relationship develops between the characters played by Williams and Damon. How does the relationship change as the characters move through different stages of their relationship? Do you think that the level of self-disclosure depicted is therapeutic?

In Treatment: 2008. This television show is about a Washington-based psychotherapist, Paul Weston (Gabriel Byrne). The series runs throughout the week. From Monday to Thursday, Dr. Weston meets with patients and on Friday, he visits his own therapist. (Being analyzed yourself is an expectation for psychoanalysts.)
Viewing Points: What aspects of therapeutic relationships can you identify in Dr. Weston's session? Look for ways in which transference and countertransference are portrayed. How is self-awareness developed for Dr. Weston?

Silver Linings Playbook: 2012. This film portrays one man's struggle to return to society after he is released from a psychiatric inpatient hospital. Patrick (Bradley Cooper), who is trying to reconnect with his ex-wife and manage bipolar disorder, meets Tiffany (Jennifer Lawrence), who is struggling with depression following the death of her husband. Throughout the film, issues relating to stigma, establishing a therapeutic relationship, and how individuals suffering from mental illness may mutually support each other are dealt with.

Viewing Points: As part of Patrick's release, he is mandated to continue meeting with a therapist. Think of this in relation to the TDM model discussed above. How is it similar and how is it different? Others often stigmatize Patrick and Tiffany. Can you identify where this happens and how such treatment might be avoided? Reflect on the fact that many other characters seem to have undiagnosed mental illnesses (such as OCD and anxiety). How do the characters help and hurt each other as they deal with the challenges of mental illness?

REFERENCES

Barnett, E., Sussman, S., Smith, C., Rohrbach, L. A., & Spruijt-Metz, D. (2012). Motivational interviewing for adolescent substance use: A review of the literature. *Addictive Behaviors, 37*(12), 1325–1334. doi:10.1016/j.addbeh.2012.07.001

Barwick, M. A., Bennett, L. M., Johnson, S. N., McGowan, J., & Moore, J. E. (2012). Training health and mental health professionals in motivational interviewing: A systematic review. *Children and Youth Services Review, 34*(9), 1786–1795. doi:10.1016/j.childyouth.2012.05.012

Berg, R. C., Ross, M. W., & Tikkanen, R. (2011). The effectiveness of MI4MSM: How useful is motivational interviewing as an HIV risk prevention program for men who have sex with men? A systematic review. *AIDS Education and Prevention, 23*(6), 533–549. doi:10.1521/aeap.2011.23.6.533

Chen, S. M., Creedy, D., Lin, H. S., & Wollin, J. (2012). Effects of motivational interviewing intervention on self-management, psychological and glycemic outcomes in type 2 diabetes: A randomized controlled trial. *International Journal of Nursing Studies, 49*(6), 637–644. doi:10.1016/j.ijnurstu.2011.11.011

Coatsworth-Puspoky, R., Forchuk, C., & Ward-Griffin, C. (2006). "Nurse–client processes in mental health: Recipient's perspectives." *Journal of Psychiatric and Mental Health Nursing, 13*(3), 347–355.

Cronk, N. J., Russell, C. L., Knowles, N., Matteson, M., Peace, L., & Ponferrada, L. (2012). Acceptability of motivational interviewing among hemodialysis clinic staff: A pilot study. *Nephrology Nursing Journal, 39*(5), 385–391.

Day, P. (2013). Using motivational interviewing with young people: A case study. *British Journal of School Nursing, 8*(2), 97–99.

Forchuk, C., Carmichael, C., Golea, G., Johnston, N., Martin, M. L., Patterson, P., et al. (2006). *Nursing best practice guideline: Establishing therapeutic relationships (revision).* Toronto, Canada: Registered Nurses Association of Ontario.

Forchuk, C., Martin, M. L. Jensen, E., Ouseley, S., Sealy, P., Beal, G. et al. (2012). Integrating the transitional relationship model into clinical practice. *Archives of Psychiatric Nursing, 26*(5), 374–381.

Forchuk, C., Martin, M. L., Jensen, E., Ouseley, S., Sealy, P., Beal, G., et al. (2013). Integrating an evidence-based intervention into clinical practice: 'Transitional relationship model'. *Journal of Psychiatric and Mental Health Nursing, 20*(7), 584–594. doi:10.1111/j.1365-2850.2012.01956.x

Miller, W. R., & Moyers, T. B. (2006). Eight Stages in Learning Motivational Interviewing. *Journal of Teaching in the Addictions, 5*(1), 3–17. doi:10.1300/J188v05n01_02

Peplau, H. E. (1952, 1992). *Interpersonal relations in nursing.* New York: J. P. Putnam's Sons.

Reynolds, W., Lauder, W., Sharkey, S., Macivier, S., Veitch, T., & Cameron, D. (2004). The effects of transitional discharge model for psychiatric patients. *Journal of Psychiatric and Mental Health Nursing, 11*, 82–88.

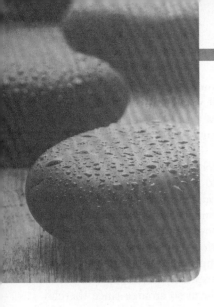

9
The Psychiatric-Mental Health Nursing Process

Mary Ann Boyd

KEY CONCEPTS

- assessment
- mental status examination
- nursing diagnosis
- outcomes
- nursing interventions

LEARNING OBJECTIVES

After studying this chapter, you will be able to:

1. Define the nursing process in psychiatric-mental health nursing.

2. Conduct a psychiatric-mental health nursing assessment.

3. Develop nursing diagnoses following a psychiatric-mental health nursing assessment.

4. Develop patient outcomes from a nursing diagnosis.

5. Apply psychiatric-mental health nursing interventions for persons with mental health problems and mental disorders.

6. Explain how patient outcomes are evaluated in psychiatric-mental health nursing.

KEY TERMS

- affect • behavior modification • behavior therapy • bibliotherapy • body image • chemical restraint • cognition • conflict resolution • containment • cognitive interventions • counseling • cultural brokering • de-escalation • distraction • dysphoric • euphoric • euthymic • guided imagery • home visits • insight • judgment • labile • milieu therapy • mood • open communication • patient observation • personal identity • psychoeducation • reminiscence • restraint • risk factors • seclusion • self-care • self-concept • self-esteem • simple relaxation techniques • spiritual support • structured interaction • token economy • validation

The nursing process is the model of care used in psychiatric-mental health nursing. In this text, the nursing process is organized around the areas of assessment, diagnosis and outcome development, intervention, and evaluation. Within this framework, this chapter delineates general areas of practice and is an introduction to some, but not all, of the commonly used interventions. Application of the nursing process to patients with specific psychiatric disorders and emotional problems are discussed in other chapters.

PSYCHIATRIC–MENTAL HEALTH NURSING ASSESSMENT

Assessment is the collection and interpretation of biopsychosocial information to determine health, functional status, and human responses to mental health problems. These responses are expressed through biologic, psychological, and social manifestations.

Assessment is not an isolated activity. Rather, it is a systematic and ongoing process that occurs throughout the nurse's care of the patient. The Psychiatric-Mental Health Nursing Assessment (Box 9.1) is a basic guide to collecting assessment data. Assessment information is entered into the patient's written or computerized record, which may be presented in several different formats, including forms, checklists, narratives, and problem-oriented notes.

> **KEYCONCEPT** **Assessment** is the deliberate and systematic collection and interpretation of biopsychosocial information or data to determine current and past health, functional status, and mental health problems, both actual and potential.

Assessment begins with the first contact with the patient and is based on the establishment of rapport with the patient (see Chapter 8). Legal consent must be given by the patient, and the nurse must follow the Health Insurance Portability and Accountability Act of 1996 (HIPAA) guidelines (see Chapter 3). The patient must develop a sense of trust before he or she will be comfortable revealing intimate life details. It is of paramount importance that the nurse has a healthy knowledge of him- or herself as well (Box 9.2). The nurse's own biases and values, which may be different from those of the patient, can influence the nurse's interpretation of assessment data. A careful self-assessment helps the nurse interpret the data objectively.

Patient Interviews

An assessment interview usually involves direct questions to obtain facts, clarify perceptions, validate observations, interpret the meanings of groups of facts, or compare information. The specific questions may take different forms. The nurse must clearly state the purpose of the interview and, if necessary, modify the interview process, so that both the patient and nurse agree on its purpose. The nurse may choose to use open- or closed-ended questions. Open-ended questions are most helpful when beginning the interview because they allow the nurse to observe how the patient responds verbally and nonverbally. They also convey caring and interest in the person's well-being, which helps to establish rapport. Nurses should use closed-ended questions when they need specific information. For example, "How old are you?" asks for specific information about the patient's age. These types of questions limit the individual's response but often serve as good follow-up questions for clarification of thoughts or feelings expressed.

Questions such as "How did you come to this clinic today?" allow patients to describe their experience in their own way. Some patients may answer this question concretely by saying, "I took a taxi" or "I came by car." Others may address this question by responding, "My family thought I should come, so they brought me"

or "Well, I got up this morning...I took a shower, got dressed...and then, well you know, it's difficult sometimes to decide." Each of these answers helps the nurse assess the patient's thinking process as well as evaluate the content of the response.

Clarification is extremely important during the assessment process. Words do not have the same meaning to all people. Education, language, culture, history, and experience may influence the meaning of words. Sometimes simple and direct questioning provides clarification. In other situations, the nurse may clarify by providing a specific example for a more global thought the patient is trying to express. For example, a patient may say, "Things have been so strange since the children left." The nurse may respond with, "Sometimes, parents feel sad and empty when their children leave home. They don't know what to do with their time." Frequently summarizing what has been said allows the patient the opportunity to correct the nurse's interpretation. For example, verbalizing a sequence of events that the patient has reported may help to identify omissions or inconsistencies. Restating information or reflecting feelings that the patient has described also allows opportunity for clarification. It is essential that nurses understand exactly what patients are attempting to communicate before beginning to intervene. Box 9.3 provides a summary of other behaviors that enhance the effectiveness of an assessment interview.

Many psychiatric symptoms are beyond a patient's awareness. Family members, friends, and other health care professionals are important sources of information. Before seeking information from others, the nurse must obtain permission from the patient. The nurse needs to provide the patient with a clear explanation of why the information is needed and how it will be used.

Assessment of the Biologic Domain

Many psychiatric disorders produce physical symptoms, such as the lack of appetite and weight loss associated with depression. A person's physical condition may also affect mental health, producing a recurrence or increase in symptoms. Many physical disorders may present first with symptoms considered to be psychiatric. For example, hypothyroidism often presents with feelings of lethargy, decreased concentration, and depressed mood. For these reasons, biologic information about the patient is always considered.

Current and Past Health Status

Beginning with a history of the patient's general medical condition, the nurse should consider the following:

- Availability of, frequency of, and most recent medical evaluation, including test results

BOX 9.1

Psychiatric-Mental Health Nursing Assessment

I. **Major reason for seeking help** _____

II. **Initial information**
   Name _____
   Age _____ Marital status _____ Gender _____ Ethnic identification _____

III. **Present and past health status** _____

	Normal	Treated	Untreated
Physical functions: System review	☐	☐	☐
Elimination	☐	☐	☐
Activity/exercise	☐	☐	☐
Sleep	☐	☐	☐
Appetite and nutrition	☐	☐	☐
Hydration	☐	☐	☐
Sexuality	☐	☐	☐
Self-care	☐	☐	☐
Existing physical illnesses	☐	☐	☐
Medications (prescription and over-the-counter)	Dosage	Side effects	Frequency
Significant laboratory tests	Values	Normal range	

IV. **Mental health problems**
   Major concerns regarding mental health problem _____
   Major loss/change in past year: No _____ Yes _____
   Fear of violence: No _____ Yes _____
   Strategies for managing problems/disorder _____

V. **Mental status examination**
   General observations (appearance, psychomotor activity, attitude) _____
   Orientation (time, place, person) _____
   Mood, affect, emotions _____
   Speech (verbal ability, speed, use of words correctly) _____
   Thought processes (tangential, logic, repetition, rhyming of words, loose connections, disorganized) _____
   Cognition and intellectual performance _____
   Attention and concentration _____
   Abstract reasoning and comprehension _____
   Memory (recall, short-term, recent, and remote) _____
   Judgment and insight _____

VI. **Significant behaviors (psychomotor, agitation, aggression, withdrawn)** _____

VII. **Self-concept (body image, self-esteem, personal identity)** _____

VIII. **Stress and coping patterns** _____

IX. **Risk assessment** _____
   Suicide: High _____ Low _____ Assault/homicide: High _____ Low _____
   Suicide thoughts or ideation: No _____ Yes _____
   Current thoughts of harming self _____
   Plan _____
   Means _____
   Means available _____
   Assault/homicide thoughts: No _____ Yes _____
   What do you do when angry with a stranger? _____
   What do you do when angry with family or partner? _____
   Have you ever hit or pushed anyone? No _____ Yes _____
   Have you ever been arrested for assault? No _____ Yes _____
   Current thoughts of harming others _____

X. **Functional status**
   Changes in functioning (work, school, home) _____

XI. **Social systems**
   Cultural assessment
      Cultural group _____
      Cultural group's view of health and mental illness _____
      What cultural rules do you try to live by? _____
      Important cultural foods _____
   Family assessment
      Family members _____
      Members important to patient _____
      Decision makers, family roles, supportive members _____
   Community resources _____

XII. **Spiritual assessment**

XIII. **Economic status**

XIV. **Legal status**

XV. **Quality of life**

Summary of significant data that can be used in formulating a nursing diagnosis
SIGNATURE/TITLE _____ Date _____

BOX 9.2

Self-Concept Awareness

Self-awareness is important in any interaction. To understand a patient's self-concept, the nurse must be aware of his or her own self-concept. By answering these questions, nurses can evaluate self-concept components and increase their self-understanding. The more comfortable the nurse is with him- or herself, the more effective the nurse can be in each and every patient interaction.

BODY IMAGE
- How do I feel about my body?
- How important is my physical appearance?
- How does my body measure up to my ideal body? (How would I like to appear?)
- What is positive about my body?
- What would I like to change about my body?
- How does my body image affect my self-esteem?

SELF-ESTEEM
- When do I feel confident and good about myself?
- When do I feel unimportant?
- What do I do when I feel good about myself? (Call friends, socialize?)
- What do I do when I have negative feelings about myself? (Withdraw, dress poorly?)
- When do I make negative statements?
- Am I able to correct my negative self-statements?

PERSONAL IDENTITY
- How do I describe myself?
- What three adjectives describe who I am?
- Do I identify with a particular cultural group, family role, or place of residence?
- What would I like to have on my tombstone?

BOX 9.3

Assessment Interview Behaviors

The following behaviors carried out by the nurse will enhance the effectiveness of the assessment interview:

- *Exhibiting empathy*—to show empathy to the patient, the nurse uses phrases such as, "That must have been upsetting for you" or "I can understand your hurt feelings."
- *Giving recognition*—the nurse gives recognition by listening actively: verbally encouraging the patient to continue, and nonverbally presenting an open, interested demeanor.
- *Demonstrating acceptance*—note that acceptance does not mean agreement or nonagreement with the patient but is a neutral stance that allows the patient to continue.
- *Restating*—the nurse tries to clarify what the patient is trying to say by restating it.
- *Reflecting*—the nurse presents the patient's last statement as a question. This gives the patient a chance to expand on the information.
- *Focusing*—the nurse attempts to bring the conversation back to the questions at hand when the patient goes off on a tangent.
- *Using open-ended questions*—general questions give the patient a chance to speak freely.
- *Presenting reality*—the nurse presents reality when the patient makes unrealistic or exaggerated statements.
- *Making observations*—the nurse says aloud what patient behaviors are observed to give the patient a chance to speak to those behaviors. For example, the nurse may say, "I notice you are twisting your fingers; are you nervous about something?"

- Past hospitalizations and surgical procedures
- Vision and hearing impairments
- Cardiac problems, including cerebrovascular accidents (strokes), myocardial infarctions (heart attacks), and childhood illnesses
- Respiratory problems, particularly those that result in a lack of oxygen to the brain
- Neurologic problems, particularly head injuries, seizure disorders, or any losses of consciousness
- Endocrine disorders, particularly unstable diabetes or thyroid or adrenal dysfunction
- Immune disorders, particularly human immunodeficiency virus (HIV) and autoimmune disorders
- Use, exposure, abuse, or dependence on substances, including alcohol, tobacco, prescription drugs, illicit drugs, and herbal preparations.

Physical Examination

Body Systems Review

After the nurse obtains historical information, he or she should examine physiologic systems to evaluate the patient's current physical condition. The psychiatric nurse should pay special attention to various systems that treatment may affect. For example, if a patient is being treated with antihypertensive medication, the dosage may need to be adjusted if an antipsychotic medication is prescribed. If a patient is overweight or has diabetes, some psychiatric medications can affect these conditions. Patients with compromised immune function (HIV, cancer) may experience mood alterations.

Neurologic Status

Particular attention is paid to recent head trauma; episodes of hypertension; and changes in personality, speech, or the ability to handle activities of daily living (ADLs). Cranial nerve dysfunction, reflexes, muscle strength, and balance are included in a thorough assessment. The nurse routinely assesses and documents movement disorders through the use of such tools as the Abnormal Involuntary Movement Scales (see Chapter 21).

Laboratory Results

The nurse reviews and documents any available laboratory data, especially any abnormalities. Hepatic, renal, or urinary abnormalities are particularly important to document because these systems metabolize or excrete many psychiatric medications. In addition, the nurse notes abnormal white blood cell and electrolyte levels. Laboratory data are especially important, particularly if the nurse is the only person in the mental health team who has a "medical" background (Table 9.1).

Physical Functions

Elimination

The nurse should inquire about and document the patient's daily urinary and bowel habits. Various medications can affect bladder and bowel functioning, so a baseline must be noted. For example, diarrhea and frequency of urination can occur with the use of lithium carbonate. Anticholinergic effects of antipsychotic medication can cause constipation and urinary hesitancy or retention.

Activity and Exercise

The patient's daily methods and levels of activity and exercise must be queried and documented. Activities are important interventions, and baseline information is needed to determine what the patient already enjoys or dislikes and whether he or she is getting sufficient exercise or adequate recreation. A patient may have altered activity or exercise in response to medication or therapies. In addition, many psychiatric medications cause weight gain, and nurses need to develop interventions that assist the patient to increase activities to counteract the weight gain.

Sleep

Changes in sleep patterns often reflect changes in a patient's emotions and are symptoms of disorders. If the patient responds positively to a question about changes in sleep patterns, it is important to clarify just what those changes are. For example, "difficulty falling asleep" means different things to different people. For a person who usually falls right to sleep, it could mean that it takes 10 extra minutes to fall asleep. For a person who normally takes 35 minutes to fall asleep, it could mean that it takes 90 minutes to do so.

Appetite and Nutrition

Changes in appetite and nutritional intake are assessed and documented because they can indicate changes in moods or relapse. For example, a patient who is depressed may not notice hunger or even that he or she does not have the energy to prepare food. Others may handle stressful emotions through eating more

than usual. This information also provides valuable clues to possible eating disorders and problems with body image.

Obesity is one of the major health problems of many Americans, but it is particularly problematic for persons with psychiatric disorders. Many of the medications are associated with weight gain. A baseline body mass index (BMI) should be determined as treatment is initiated.

Hydration

Gaining perspective on how much fluid patients normally drink and how much they are drinking now provides important data. Some medications can cause retention of fluids, and others can cause diuresis; thus, the patient's current fluid status must be understood.

Sexuality

Questioning a patient on issues involving sexuality requires comfort with one's own sexuality. Changes in sexual activity as well as comfort with sexual orientation are important to assess. Issues involving sexual orientation that are unsettled in a patient or between a patient and family member may cause anxiety, shame, or discomfort. It is necessary to explore how comfortable the patient is with his or her sexuality and sexual functioning. These questions should be asked in a matter-of-fact but gentle and nonjudgmental manner. Initiating the topic of sexuality may begin with a question such as "Are you sexually active?" Birth control medications may also alter mood.

Self-Care

Self-care is the ability to perform ADLs successfully. Often, a patient's ability to care for him- or herself or carry out ADLs, such as washing and dressing, are indicative of his or her psychological state. For example, a depressed patient may not have the energy change into clean clothes. This information may also help the nurse to determine actual or potential obstacles to a patient's compliance with a treatment plan.

Pharmacologic Assessment

The review of systems serves as a baseline from which the nurse may judge whether the initiation of a medication exacerbates symptoms or causes new ones to develop. It is important to determine which medications the patient takes now or has taken in the past. These include over-the-counter, herbal or nonprescription medications as well as prescribed medications. This assessment is important for reasons other than serving as a baseline. It helps

TABLE 9.1	SELECTED HEMATOLOGIC MEASURES AND THEIR RELEVANCE TO PSYCHIATRIC DISORDERS	
Test	Possible Results	Possible Cause or Meaning
Complete Blood Count (CBC)		
Leukocyte (white blood cell [WBC]) count	Leukopenia—decrease in leukocytes (white blood cells) Agranulocytosis—decrease in number of granulocytic leukocytes Leukocytosis—increase in leukocyte count above normal limits	May be produced by: antipsychotics, carbamazepine Lithium causes a benign mild to moderate increase (11,000–17,000/mcL). Neuroleptic malignant syndrome (NMS) can be associated with increases of 15,000 to 30,000/mm^3 in about 40% of cases.
WBC differential	"Shift to the left"—from segmented neutrophils to band forms	Shift often suggests a bacterial infection but has been reported in about 40% of cases of NMS.
Red blood cell (RBC) count	Polycythemia—increased RBCs	Primary form—true polycythemia caused by several disease states Secondary form—compensation for decreased oxygenation, such as in chronic pulmonary disease Blood is more viscous, and the patient should not become dehydrated.
	Decreased RBCs	Decrease may be related to some types of anemia, which requires further evaluation.
Hematocrit (Hct)	Elevations	Elevation may be caused by dehydration.
	Decreased Hct	Anemia may be associated with a wide range of mental status changes, including asthenia, depression, and psychosis. 20% of women of childbearing age in the United States have iron-deficiency anemia.
Hemoglobin (Hb)	Decreased	Another indicator of anemia; further evaluation of source requires review of erythrocyte indices.
Erythrocyte indices, such as red cell distribution width (RDW)	Elevated RDW	Finding suggests a combined anemia as in that from chronic alcoholism, resulting from both vitamin B$_{12}$ and folate acid deficiencies and iron deficiency Oral contraceptives also decrease vitamin B$_{12}$.
Other Hematologic Measures		
Vitamin B$_{12}$	Deficiency	Neuropsychiatric symptoms, such as psychosis, paranoia, fatigue, agitation, marked personality change, dementia, and delirium, may develop.
Folate	Deficiency	The use of alcohol, phenytoin, oral contraceptives, and estrogens may be responsible.
Platelet count	Thrombocytopenia—decreased platelet count	Some psychiatric medications, such as carbamazepine, phenothiazines, or clozapine, or other nonpsychiatric medications, may cause thrombocytopenia. Several medical conditions are other causes.
Serum Electrolytes		
Sodium	Hyponatremia—low serum sodium	Significant mental status changes may ensue. Condition is associated with Addison's disease, the syndrome of inappropriate secretion of antidiuretic hormone (SIADH), and polydipsia (water intoxication) as well as carbamazepine use.
Potassium	Hypokalemia—low serum potassium	Produces weakness, fatigue, electrocardiogram (ECG) changes; paralytic ileus and muscle paresis may develop. Common in individuals with bulimic behavior or psychogenic vomiting and use or abuse of diuretics; laxative abuse may contribute; can be life threatening.
Chloride	Elevation	Chloride tends to increase to compensate for lower bicarbonate.
	Decrease	Binging–purging behavior and repeated vomiting may be causes.
Bicarbonate	Elevation	Causes may be binging and purging in eating disorders, excessive use of laxatives, or psychogenic vomiting.
	Decrease	Decrease may develop in some patients with hyperventilation syndrome and panic disorder.

TABLE 9.1	SELECTED HEMATOLOGIC MEASURES AND THEIR RELEVANCE TO PSYCHIATRIC DISORDERS *(Continued)*	
Test	**Possible Results**	**Possible Cause or Meaning**
Renal Function Tests		
Blood urea nitrogen (BUN)	Elevation	Increase is associated with mental status changes, lethargy, and delirium. Cause may be dehydration. Potential toxicity of medications cleared via the kidney, such as lithium and amantadine, may increase.
Serum creatinine	Elevation	Level usually does not become elevated until about 50% of nephrons in the kidney are damaged.
Serum Enzymes		
Amylase	Elevation	Level appears to increase after binging and purging behavior in eating disorders and declines when these behaviors stop.
Alanine aminotransferase (ALT)—formerly serum glutamic pyruvic transaminase (SGPT)	ALT > AST	Disparity is common in acute forms of viral and drug-induced hepatic dysfunction.
	Elevation	Mild elevations are common with use of sodium valproate.
Aspartate aminotransferase (AST)—formerly serum glutamic oxaloacetic transaminase (SGOT)	AST > ALT	Severe elevations in chronic forms of liver disease and post-myocardial infarction may develop.
Creatine phospho-kinase (CPK)	Elevations of the isoenzyme related to muscle tissue	Muscle tissue injury is the cause. Level is elevated in neuroleptic malignant syndrome (NMS). Level is also elevated by repeated intramuscular injections (e.g., antipsychotics).
Thyroid Function		
Serum triiodothyronine (T_3)	Decrease	Hypothyroidism and nonthyroid illness cause decrease. Individuals with depression may convert less T_4 to T_3 peripherally but not out of the normal range. Medications such as lithium and sodium valproate may suppress thyroid function, but clinical significance is unknown.
	Elevations	Hyperthyroidism, T_3, toxicosis, may produce mood changes, anxiety, and symptoms of mania
Serum thyroxine (T_4)	Elevations	Hyperthyroidism is a cause.
Thyroid stimulating hormone (TSH or thyrotropin)	Elevations	Hypothyroidism—symptoms may appear very much like depression except for additional physical signs of cold intolerance, dry skin, hair loss, bradycardia, and so on. Lithium—may also cause elevations.
	Decrease	Considered nondiagnostic—may be hyperthyroidism, pituitary hypothyroidism, or even euthyroid status.

target possible drug interactions, determines whether the patient has already used medications that are being considered, and identifies whether medications may be causing psychiatric symptoms.

Assessment of the Psychological Domain

The psychological domain is the traditional focus of the psychiatric-mental health nursing assessment. By definition,

psychiatric disorders and emotional problems are manifested through psychological symptoms related to mental status, moods, thoughts, behaviors, and interpersonal relationships. This domain includes psychological growth and development. Assessing this domain is important in developing a comprehensive picture of the patient.

Responses to Mental Health Problems

Individual concerns regarding a mental health problem or its consequences are included in the mental health assessment. A mental disorder, like any other illness, affects patients and families in many different ways. It is safe to say that a mental illness changes a person's life, and the nurse should identify what the changes are and their meaning to the patient and family members. Many patients experience specific fears, such as losing their job, family, or safety. Included in this part of the assessment is identifying current strategies or behaviors the patient uses in dealing with the consequences of disorder. A simple question such as "How do you deal with your voices when you are with other people?" may initiate a discussion about responses to the mental disorder or emotional problem.

Mental Status Examination

The mental status examination establishes a baseline, provides a snapshot of where the patient is at a particular moment, and creates a written record. Areas of assessment include general observations, orientation, mood and affect, speech, thought processes, and cognition. Box 9.4 provides a narrative note of the results from a patient's mental status examination.

> **KEYCONCEPT** The **mental status examination** is an organized systematic approach to assessment of an individual's current psychiatric condition.

General Observations

At the beginning of the interview, the nurse should record his or her initial impressions of the patient. These general observations include the patient's appearance, affect, psychomotor activity, and overall behavior. How is the patient dressed? Is the dress appropriate for weather and setting? What is the patient's affect (emotional expression)? What behaviors is the patient displaying? For example, the same nurse assessed two male patients with depression. At the beginning of the mental status examination, the differences between these two men were very clear. The nurse described the

---

BOX 9.4

Narrative Mental Status Examination Note

The patient is a 65-year-old widowed man who is slightly disheveled. He is cooperative with the interviewer and judged to be an adequate historian. His mood and affect are depressed and anxious. He becomes tearful throughout the interview when speaking about his wife. His flow of thought is hesitant but coherent when he is speaking about his wife. He is oriented to time, place, and person. He shows good recent and remote memory. He is able to recall several items given him by the interviewer. The patient shows poor insight and judgment regarding his sadness since the loss of his wife. He repeatedly says, "Mary wouldn't want me to be sad. She would want me to continue with my life."

---

first patient as "a large, well-dressed man who is agitated and appears angry, shifts in his seat, and does not maintain eye contact. He interrupts often in the initial explanation of mental status." The nurse described the other patient as a "small, unshaven, disheveled man with a strong body odor who appears withdrawn. He shuffles as he walks, speaks very softly, appears sad, and avoids direct eye contact."

Orientation

The nurse can determine the patient's orientation by asking the date, time, and current location of the interview setting. If a patient knows the year but not the exact date, the interviewer can ask the season. A person's orientation tells the nurse the extent of confusion. If a patient does not know the year or the place of the interview, he or she is exhibiting considerable confusion.

Mood and Affect

Mood refers to the prominent, sustained, overall emotions that the person expresses and exhibits. Mood may be sustained for days or weeks, or it may fluctuate during the course of a day. For example, some patients with depression have a diurnal variation in their mood. They experience their lowest mood in the morning, but as the day progresses, their depressed mood lifts and they feel somewhat better in the evening. Terms used to describe mood include **euthymic** (normal), **euphoric** (elated), **labile** (changeable), and **dysphoric** (depressed, disquieted, restless).

Affect refers to the person's capacity to vary outward emotional expression. Affect fluctuates with thought content and can be observed in facial expressions, vocal fluctuations, and gestures. During the assessment, the patient may exhibit anger, frustration, irritation, apathy, and helplessness while his or her overall mood remains unchanged.

Affect can be described in terms of range, intensity, appropriateness, and stability. Range can be full or restricted. An individual who expresses several different emotions consistent with the stated feelings and content being expressed is described as having a *full range* of affect that is congruent with the situation. An individual who expresses few emotions has a restricted affect. For example, a patient could be describing the recent tragic death of a loved one in a monotone with little expression. In determining whether this response is normal, the nurse compares the patient's emotional response with the cultural norm for that particular response. *Intensity* can be increased, flat, or blunted. The nurse determines whether the emotional response is *appropriate* for the situation. For example, an inappropriate response is shown by a patient who has an extreme reaction to the death of the victims of the September 11 tragedy as if the victims were personal friends. Another patient said that his life stopped when the World Trade Center towers came down. He could not eat or sleep for weeks afterward. *Stability* can be mobile (normal) or labile. If a patient reports feeling happy one minute and reduced to tears the next, the person probably has an unstable mood. During the interview, the nurse should look for rapid mood changes that indicate lability of mood. A patient who exhibits intense, frequently shifting emotional extremes has a labile affect.

Speech

Speech provides clues about thoughts, emotional patterns, and cognitive organization. Speech may be pressured, fast, slow, or fragmented. Speech patterns reflect the patient's thought patterns, which can be logical or illogical. To check the patient's comprehension, the nurse can show a patient an object (e.g., pen, watch) and ask the person to name them. During conversation, the nurse assesses the fluency and quality of the patient's speech. The nurse listens for repetition or rhyming of words.

Thought Processes

The nurse assesses the patient for rapid change of ideas; inability or taking a long time to get to the point; loose or no connections among ideas or words; rhyming or repetition of words, questions, or phrases; or use of unheard of words. Any of these observations indicates abnormal thought patterns. The content of what the patient says is also important. What thought is the patient expressing? The nurse listens for unusual and unlikely stories, fears or behaviors; for example, "The FBI is tracking me" or "I am afraid to leave my house."

Cognition and Intellectual Performance

To assess the patient's **cognition**, that is, the ability to think and know, the nurse uses memory, calculation, and reasoning tests to identify specific areas of impairment. The cognitive areas include (1) attention and concentration, (2) abstract reasoning and comprehension, (3) memory, and (4) insight and judgment.

Attention and Concentration

To test attention and concentration, the nurse asks the patient, without pencil or paper, to start with 100 and subtract 7 until reaching 65 or to start with 20 and subtract 3. The nurse must decide which is most appropriate for the patient considering education and understanding. Subtracting 3 from 20 is the easier of the two tasks. Asking a patient to spell "world" backward is also useful in determining attention and concentration.

Abstract Reasoning and Comprehension

To test abstract reasoning and comprehension, the nurse gives the patient a proverb to interpret. Examples include "People in glass houses shouldn't throw stones," "A rolling stone gathers no moss," and "A penny saved is a penny earned."

Recall, Short-Term, Recent, and Remote Memory

There are four spheres of memory to check: recall, or immediate, memory; short-term memory; recent memory; and long-term, or remote, memory. To check immediate and short-term memory, the nurse gives the patient three unrelated words to remember and asks him or her to recite them right after telling them and at 5-minute and 15-minute intervals during the interview. To test recent memory, the nurse may question about a holiday or world event within the past few months. The nurse tests long-term or remote memory by asking about events years ago. If they are personal events and the answers seem incorrect, the nurse may check them with a family member.

Insight and Judgment

Insight and judgment are related concepts that involve the ability to examine thoughts, conceptualize facts, solve problems, think abstractly, and possess self-awareness. **Insight** is a person's awareness of his or her own thoughts and feelings and ability to compare them with the thoughts and feelings of others. It involves an awareness of how others view one's behavior and its meaning. For example, many patients do not believe that they have mental illness. They may have delusions and hallucinations or be hospitalized for bizarre and sometimes dangerous behavior, but they are completely unaware that their behavior is unusual or abnormal. During an interview, a patient may adamantly proclaim that nothing is wrong or that he or she does not have a mental illness. Even if a problem is recognized, the patient may lack insight regarding issues related to care.

Judgment is the ability to reach a logical decision about a situation and to choose a course of action after examining and analyzing various possibilities. Throughout the interview, the nurse evaluates the patient's ability to make logical decisions. For example, some patients may continually choose partners who are abusive. The nurse could logically conclude that these patients have poor judgment in selecting partners. Another way to examine a patient's judgment is to give a simple scenario and ask the person to identify the best response. An example of such a scenario is asking, "What would you do if you found a bag of money outside a bank on a busy street?" If the patient responds, "Run with it," his or her judgment is questionable.

Behavior

Throughout the assessment, the nurse observes any behavior that may have significance in understanding the patient's response or symptoms of the mental disorder or emotional problem. For example, a depressed patient may be tearful throughout the session, whereas an anxious patient may twist or pull his or her hair, shift in the chair, or be unable to maintain eye contact. The nurse may find that whenever a particular topic is addressed, the patient's behavior changes. The nurse needs to relate patterned behaviors to significant events by connecting behaviors with the assessment data. For example, a patient may change jobs frequently, causing family distress and financial problems. Exploration of the events leading up to job changes may elicit important information regarding the patient's ability to solve problems.

Self-Concept

Self-concept, which develops over a lifetime, represents the total beliefs about three interrelated dimensions of the self: body image, self-esteem, and personal identity. The importance of each of these dimensions varies among individuals. For some, beliefs about themselves are strongly tied to body image; for others, personal identity is most important. Still others develop personal identity from what others have told them over the years. The nurse carrying out an assessment must keep in mind that self-concept and its components are dynamic and variable. For example, a woman may have a consistent self-concept until her first pregnancy. At that time, the many physiologic changes of pregnancy may cause her body image to change. She may be comfortable and enjoy the "glow of pregnancy," or she may feel like a "bloated cow." Suddenly, her body image is the most important part of her self-concept, and how she handles it can increase or decrease her self-esteem or sense of personal identity. Thus, all of the components are tied together, and each one affects the others.

Self-concept is assessed through eliciting patients' thoughts about themselves, their ability to navigate in the world, and their nonverbal behaviors. A disheveled sloppy physical appearance outside cultural norms is an indication of poor self-concept. Negative self-statements, such as, "I could never do that," "I have no control over my life," and "I'm so stupid" reveal poor views of self. The nurse's own self-concept can shape the nurse's view of the patient. For example, a nurse who is self-confident and feels inwardly scornful of a patient who lacks such confidence may intimidate the patient through unconscious, judgmental behaviors or inconsiderate comments.

A useful approach to measuring self-concept is asking the patient to draw a self-portrait. For many patients, drawing is much easier than writing and serves as an excellent technique for monitoring changes. Interpretation of self-concept from drawings focuses on size, color, level of detail, pressure, line quality, symmetry, and placement. Low self-esteem is expressed by small size, lack of color variation, and sparse details in the drawing. Powerlessness and feelings of inadequacy are expressed through a lack of a head, a mouth, arms, feet, or in the drawing. A lack of symmetry (placement of figure parts or entire drawings off center) represents feelings of insecurity and inadequacy. As self-esteem builds, size increases, color tends to become more varied and brighter, and more detail appears. Figure 9.1 shows a self-portrait of a patient at the beginning of treatment for depression and another drawn 3 months later.

Body Image

Body image represents a person's beliefs and attitudes about his or her body and includes such dimensions as size (large or small) and attractiveness (pretty or ugly). People who are satisfied with their body have a more positive body image than those who are not satisfied. Generally, women attach more importance to their body

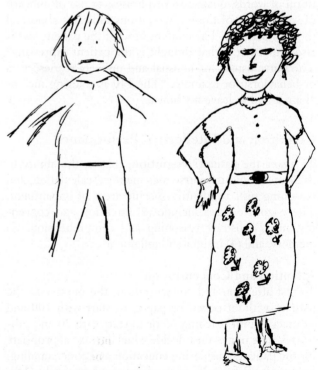

FIGURE 9.1 *Left:* Self-portrait of a 52-year-old woman at first group session following discharge from hospital for treatment of depression. *Right:* Self-portrait after 3 months of weekly group interventions.

image than do men and may even define themselves in terms of their body.

Patients express body image beliefs through statements about their bodies. Statements such as "I feel so ugly," "I'm so fat," and "No one will want to have sex with me" express negative body images. Nonverbal behaviors indicating problems with body image include avoiding looking at or touching a body part; hiding the body in oversized clothing; or bandaging a particularly sensitive area, such as a mole on the face. Cultural differences must be considered when evaluating behavior related to body image. For example, the expectation of some cultures is that women and girls will keep their bodies completely covered and wear loose-fitting garments.

> **NCLEXNOTE** Be prepared to assess reactions to a body image change (e.g., loss of vision, paralysis, colostomy, amputation).

Self-Esteem

Self-esteem is the person's attitude about the self. Self-esteem differs from body image because it concerns satisfaction with one's overall self. People who feel good about themselves are more likely to have the confidence to try new health behaviors. They are also less likely to be depressed. Negative self-esteem statements include "I'm a worthless person" and "I never do anything right."

Personal Identity

Personal identity is knowing "who I am." Every life experience and interaction contributes to knowing oneself better. Personal identity allows people to establish boundaries and understand personal strengths and limitations. In some psychiatric disorders, individuals cannot separate themselves from others, which shows that their personal identity is not strongly developed. A problem with personal identity is difficult to assess. Statements such as, "I'm just like my mother, and she was always in trouble," "I become whatever my current boyfriend wants me to be," and "I can't make a decision unless I check it out first" are all statements that require further exploration into the person's view of self.

Stress and Coping Patterns

Everyone has stress (see Chapter 12). Sometimes the experience of stress contributes to the development of mental disorders. Identification of major stresses in a patient's life helps the nurse understand the person and support the use of successful coping behaviors in the future. The nurse should explore how the patient deals with stress and identify successful coping mechanisms in order to encourage their use.

> **NCLEXNOTE** Every assessment should focus on stress and coping patterns. Identifying how a patient copes with stress can be used as a basis of care in all nursing situations. Include content from Chapter 12 when studying these concepts.

Risk Assessment

Risk factors are characteristics, conditions, situations, or events that increase the patient's vulnerability to threats to safety or well-being. Throughout this text, the sections concerning risk factors focus on the following:

- Risks to the patient's safety
- Risks for developing psychiatric disorders
- Risks for increasing, or exacerbating, symptoms and impairment in an individual who already has a psychiatric disorder.

Consideration of risk factors involving patient safety should be included in each assessment. Examples of these risks include the risk for suicide and violence toward others or the risk for events, such as falling, seizures, allergic reactions, or elopement (unauthorized absence from health care facility). Nurses assess factors on a priority basis. For example, threats of violence or suicide take priority.

Suicidal Ideation

During the assessment, the nurse needs to listen closely to whether the patient describes or mentions thinking about self-harm. If the patient does not openly express ideas of self-harm, it is necessary to ask in a straight-forward and gentle manner, "Have you ever thought about injuring or killing yourself?" If the patient answers, "Yes, I am thinking about it right now," the nurse knows not to leave the patient unobserved and to institute suicide precautions as indicated by the facility protocols. General questions to ask to ascertain suicidal ideation follow:

- Have you ever tried to harm or kill yourself?
- Do you have thoughts of suicide at this time? If yes, do you have a plan? If yes, can you tell me the details of the plan?
- Do you have the means to carry out this plan? (If the plan requires a weapon, does the patient have it available?)
- Have you made preparations for your death (e.g., writing a note to loved ones, putting finances in order, giving away possessions)?
- Has a significant episode in your life caused you to think this way (e.g., recent loss of spouse or job)?

If any of these responses are "yes," the nurse should explore the issue in detail, notify the supervisor, and clearly document the patient responses and nursing follow-up. The nurse is expected follow the agency policies.

Assaultive or Homicidal Ideation 🔲

When assessing a patient, the nurse also needs to listen carefully to any delusions or hallucinations that the patient shares. If the patient gives any indication that he or she must or is being told to harm someone, the nurse must first think of self-safety and institute assaultive precautions as indicated by the facility protocols. General questions to ascertain assaultive or homicidal ideation follow:

- Do you intend to harm someone? If yes, who?
- Do you have a plan? If yes, what are the details of the plan?
- Do you have the means to carry out the plan? (If the plan requires a weapon, is it readily available?)

Assessment of the Social Domain

The assessment continues with examination of the patient's social domain. The nurse inquires about inter-actions with others in the family and community (work, church, or other organizations); the patient's parents and their marital relationship; the patient's place in birth order; names and ages of any siblings; and relationships with spouse, siblings, and children. The nurse also assesses work and education history and community activities. The nurse observes how the patient relates to any family or friends who may be in attendance. This component of the assessment helps the nurse anticipate how the patient may get along with other patients in an inpatient setting. It also allows the nurse to plan for any anticipated difficulties.

Functional Status

An important aspect of the assessment is determining the functioning of the patient (i.e., is an adult working and living independently? is a student attending classes?). How the patient copes with strangers and those with whom he or she does not get along is also important information.

Social Systems

A significant component of the patient's life involves the social systems in which he or she may be enmeshed. The social systems to examine include the family, the culture to which the patient belongs, and the community in which he or she lives.

Family Assessment

How the patient fits in with and relates to his or her family is important to know. General questions to ask include the following:

- Who do you consider family?
- How important to you is your family?

- How does your family make decisions?
- What are the roles in your family, and who fills them?
- Where do you fit in your family?
- With whom in your family do you get along best?
- With whom in your family do you have the most conflict?
- Who in your family is supportive of you?

Cultural Assessment

Culture can profoundly affect a person's world view (see Chapter 2). Culture helps a person frame beliefs about life, death, health and illness, and roles and relationships. During cultural assessment, the nurse must consider factors that influence the manifestations of the current mental disorder. For example, a patient mentions "speaking in tongues." The nurse may identify this experience as a hallucination when, in fact, the patient was having a religious experience common within some branches of Christianity. In this instance, knowing and understanding such religious practices will prevent a misinterpretation of the symptoms.

The nurse can elicit important cultural information by asking the following questions:

- To what cultural group do you belong?
- Were you raised in an ethnic community?
- How do you define health?
- How do you define illness?
- How do you define good and evil?
- What do you do to get better when you are physically ill? Mentally ill?
- Whom do you see for help when you are physically ill? Mentally ill?
- By what cultural rules or taboos do you try to live?
- Do you eat special foods?

Community Support and Resources

Many patients are connected to community resources, and the nurse needs to assess what they are and the patterns of usage. For example, a patient who is homeless may know of a church where he or she can sleep but may go there only on cold nights. Or a patient may go to the community center daily for lunch to be with other people.

Spiritual Assessment

Among the many definitions of spirituality is one offered by Burkhardt and Nagai-Jacobson (1997). Spirituality is

> the unifying force of a person; the essence of being that shapes, gives meaning to, and is aware of one's self-becoming. Spirituality permeates all of life and is manifested in one's being, knowing, and doing.

It is expressed and experienced uniquely by each individual through and within connection to God, Life Force, the Absolute, the environment, nature, other people, and the self (Burkhardt & Nagai-Jacobson, 1997, p. 42).

Nurses must be clear about their own spirituality to be sure it does not interfere with assessment of the patient's spirituality. General questions to ask include the following:

- What gives your life meaning?
- What is the purpose of your life?
- What do you do to bring joy into your life?
- What life goals have you set for yourself?
- Do you think that stress in any way has caused your illness?
- Can you forgive others?
- Can you forgive yourself?
- Is your faith helpful to you in stressful situations?
- Is worship important to you?
- Do you participate in any religious activities?
- Do any religious beliefs control your life?
- Do you believe in God or a higher power?
- Do you pray?
- Do you meditate?
- Do you feel connected with the world?

NCLEXNOTE Identify emotional problems that are related to religion or spiritual beliefs such as conflicts between recommended treatments and beliefs.

Occupational Status

The nurse should document the occupation the patient is now in as well as a history of jobs. If the patient has changed jobs frequently, the nurse should ask about the reasons. Perhaps the patient has faced such problems as an inability to focus on the job at hand or to get along with others. If so, such issues require further exploration.

Economic Status

Finances are very private for many people; thus, the nurse must ask questions about economic status carefully. What the nurse needs to ascertain is not specific dollar amounts but whether the patient feels stressed by finances and has enough for basic needs.

Legal Status

Because of laws governing mentally ill people, ascertaining the patient's correct age, marital status, and any legal guardianship is important. The nurse may need to check the patient's medical records for this information.

Quality of Life

The patient's perspective on quality of life means how the patient rates his or her life. Does a patient feel his life is poor because he cannot purchase everything he wants? Does another patient feel blessed because the sun is shining today? Listening carefully to the patient's discussion of his or her life and how he or she measures the quality of that life provides important information about self-concept, coping skills, desires, and dreams.

NURSING DIAGNOSIS

After completing an assessment of the patient, the nurse generates nursing diagnoses based on the assessment data. With experience, the nurse can easily cluster the assessment data to support one nursing diagnosis over another. Nursing diagnoses are universally used in nursing practice and education. In this text, primarily NANDA diagnoses are used. See Box 9.5 for more information. For each disorder, data are presented to support related nursing diagnoses.

KEYCONCEPT A **nursing diagnosis** is a clinical judgment about an identified problem or need that requires nursing interventions and nursing management. It is based on data generated from a nursing assessment (Carpenito-Moyet, 2014).

DEVELOPING PATIENT OUTCOMES

Mutually agreed-upon goals flow from the nursing diagnoses and provide guidance in determining appropriate interventions. Initial outcomes are determined and then are monitored and evaluated throughout the care process. Measuring outcomes not only demonstrates clinical effectiveness but also helps to promote rational clinical decision making and is reflective of the nursing interventions.

KEYCONCEPT **Outcomes** are the changes—favorable or unfavorable—in a patient's health status that can be attributed to nursing care at a given point in time (Moorhead, Johnson, Maas, & Swanson, 2008). An outcome is concise, stated in few words and in neutral terms. Outcomes describe a patient's state, behavior, or perception. Outcomes are variable and can be measured (Table 9.2, p. 116).

Outcomes focus on the individual recipient of care (patient or family caregivers) and include patient statements, behaviors, or perceptions that are sensitive to or influenced by nursing interventions (Moorhead et al., 2008). Nurses are accountable for documenting patient outcomes; nursing interventions; and any changes in diagnosis, care plan, or both. Outcomes can be expressed in terms of the patient's actual responses (no longer reports hearing voices) or the status of a nursing diagnosis at a point in time after implementation of nursing interventions, such as Caregiver Role Strain resolved.

BOX 9.5

NANDA International Nursing Diagnoses (2015–2017)

HEALTH PROMOTION
Deficient Diversional Activity
Sedentary Lifestyle
Frail Elderly Syndrome
Risk for Frail Elderly Syndrome
Deficient Community Health
Risk-Prone Health Behavior
Ineffective Health Maintenance
Ineffective Self-Health Management
Readiness for Enhanced Health Management
Ineffective Family Health Management
Noncompliance
Ineffective Protection

NUTRITION
Insufficient Breast Milk
Ineffective Breastfeeding
Interrupted Breastfeeding
Readiness for Enhanced Breastfeeding
Ineffective Infant Feeding Pattern
Imbalanced Nutrition: Less Than Body Requirements
Imbalanced Nutrition: More Than Body Requirements
Readiness for Enhanced Nutrition
Obesity
Overweight
Risk for Overweight
Risk for Imbalanced Nutrition: More Than Body Requirements
Impaired Swallowing
Risk for Unstable Blood Glucose Level
Neonatal Jaundice
Risk for Neonatal Jaundice
Risk for Impaired Liver Function
Risk for Electrolyte Imbalance
Readiness for Enhanced Fluid Balance
Deficient Fluid Volume
Excess Fluid Volume
Risk for Deficient Fluid Volume
Risk for Imbalanced Fluid Volume

ELIMINATION AND EXCHANGE
Impaired Urinary Elimination
Readiness for Enhanced Urinary Elimination
Functional Urinary Incontinence
Overflow Urinary Incontinence
Reflex Urinary Incontinence
Stress Urinary Incontinence
Urge Urinary Incontinence
Risk for Urge Urinary Incontinence
Urinary Retention
Constipation
Risk for Constipation
Chronic Functional Constipation
Risk for Chronic Functional Constipation
Perceived Constipation
Diarrhea
Dysfunctional Gastrointestinal Motility
Risk for Dysfunctional Gastrointestinal Motility
Bowel Incontinence
Impaired Gas Exchange

ACTIVITY/REST
Insomnia
Sleep Deprivation
Readiness for Enhanced Sleep
Disturbed Sleep Pattern
Risk for Disuse Syndrome
Impaired Bed Mobility

Impaired Physical Mobility
Impaired Wheelchair Mobility
Impaired Sitting
Impaired Standing
Impaired Transfer Ability
Impaired Walking
Fatigue
Wandering
Activity Intolerance
Risk for Activity Intolerance
Ineffective Breathing Pattern
Decreased Cardiac Output
Risk for Decreased Cardiac Output
Risk for Impaired Cardiovascular Function
Risk for Ineffective Gastrointestinal Perfusion
Risk for Ineffective Renal Perfusion
Impaired Spontaneous Ventilation
Ineffective Peripheral Tissue Perfusion
Risk for Decreased Cardiac Tissue Perfusion
Risk for Ineffective Cerebral Tissue Perfusion
Risk for Ineffective Peripheral Tissue Perfusion
Dysfunctional Ventilatory Weaning Response
Impaired Home Maintenance
Readiness for Enhanced Self-Care
Bathing Self-Care Deficit
Dressing Self-Care Deficit
Feeding Self-Care Deficit
Toileting Self-Care Deficit
Self-Neglect

PERCEPTION/COGNITION
Unilateral Neglect
Acute Confusion
Chronic Confusion
Risk for Acute Confusion
Labile Emotional Control
Ineffective Impulse Control
Deficient Knowledge
Readiness for Enhanced Knowledge
Impaired Memory
Readiness for Enhanced Communication
Impaired Verbal Communication

SELF-PERCEPTION
Readiness for Enhanced Hope
Hopelessness
Risk for Compromised Human Dignity
Disturbed Personal Identity
Risk for Disturbed Personal Identity
Readiness for Enhanced Self-Concept
Chronic Low Self-Esteem
Situational Low Self-Esteem
Risk for Chronic Low Self-Esteem
Risk for Situational Low Self-Esteem
Disturbed Body Image

ROLE RELATIONSHIPS
Caregiver Role Strain
Risk for Caregiver Role Strain
Impaired Parenting
Readiness for Enhanced Parenting
Risk for Impaired Parenting
Risk for Impaired Attachment
Dysfunctional Family Processes
Interrupted Family Processes
Readiness for Enhanced Family Processes
Ineffective Relationship
Readiness for Enhanced Relationship

BOX 9.5

NANDA International Nursing Diagnoses (2015–2017) *(Continued)*

Risk for Ineffective Relationship
Parental Role Conflict
Ineffective Role Performance
Impaired Social Interaction

SEXUALITY
Sexual Dysfunction
Ineffective Sexuality Pattern
Ineffective Childbearing Process
Readiness for Enhanced Childbearing Process
Risk for Ineffective Childbearing Process
Risk for Disturbed Maternal–Fetal Dyad

COPING/STRESS TOLERANCE
Post-Trauma Syndrome
Risk for Post-Trauma Syndrome
Rape Trauma Syndrome
Relocation Stress Syndrome
Risk for Relocation Stress Syndrome
Ineffective Activity Planning
Risk for Ineffective Activity Planning
Anxiety
Defensive Coping
Ineffective Coping
Readiness for Enhanced Coping
Ineffective Community Coping
Readiness for Enhanced Community Coping
Compromised Family Coping
Disabled Family Coping
Readiness for Enhanced Family Coping
Death Anxiety
Ineffective Denial
Fear
Grieving
Complicated Grieving
Risk for Complicated Grieving
Impaired Mood Regulation
Readiness for Enhanced Power
Powerlessness
Risk for Powerlessness
Impaired Resilience
Readiness for Enhanced Resilience
Risk for Impaired Resilience
Chronic Sorrow
Stress Overload
Decreased Intracranial Adaptive Capacity
Autonomic Dysreflexia
Risk for Autonomic Dysreflexia
Disorganized Infant Behavior
Readiness for Enhanced Organized Infant Behavior
Risk for Disorganized Infant Behavior

LIFE PRINCIPLES
Readiness for Enhanced Hope
Decisional Conflict
Readiness for Enhanced Decision-making
Impaired Emancipated Decision-making
Readiness for Enhanced Emancipated Decision-making
Risk for Impaired Emancipated Decision-making
Moral Distress
Impaired Religiosity
Readiness for Enhanced Religiosity
Risk for Impaired Religiosity
Spiritual Distress
Risk for Spiritual Distress

SAFETY/PROTECTION
Risk for Infection
Ineffective Airway Clearance
Risk for Aspiration
Risk for Bleeding
Risk for Dry Eye
Risk for Falls
Risk for Injury
Risk for Corneal Injury
Risk for Perioperative Positioning Injury
Risk for Thermal Injury
Risk for Urinary Tract Injury
Impaired Dentition
Impaired Oral Mucous Membrane
Risk for Impaired Oral Mucous Membrane
Risk for Peripheral Neurovascular Dysfunction
Risk for Pressure Ulcer
Risk for Shock
Impaired Skin Integrity
Risk for Impaired Skin Integrity
Risk for Sudden Infant Death Syndrome
Risk for Suffocation
Delayed Surgical Recovery
Risk for Delayed Surgical Recovery
Impaired Tissue Integrity
Risk for Impaired Tissue Integrity
Risk for Trauma
Risk for Vascular Trauma
Risk for Other Directed Violence
Risk for Self-Directed Violence
Self-Mutilation
Risk for Self-Mutilation
Risk for Suicide
Contamination
Risk for Contamination
Risk for Poisoning
Risk for Adverse Reaction to Iodinated Contrast Media
Latex Allergy Response
Risk for Allergy Response
Risk for Latex Allergy Response
Risk for Imbalanced Body Temperature
Hyperthermia
Hypothermia
Risk for Hypothermia
Risk for Perioperative Hypothermia
Ineffective Thermoregulation

COMFORT
Impaired Comfort
Readiness for Enhanced Comfort
Nausea
Acute Pain
Chronic Pain
Labor Pain
Chronic Pain Syndrome
Impaired Comfort
Readiness for Enhanced Comfort
Risk for Loneliness
Social Isolation

GROWTH/DEVELOPMENT
Risk for Disproportionate Growth
Risk for Delayed Development

TABLE 9.2	EXAMPLE OF OUTCOMES	
Diagnosis	Outcome	Intervention
Impaired social interaction (isolates self from others)	Social involvement Indicators: 1. Interact with other patients. 2. Attend group meetings.	Using a contract format, explain role and responsibility of patients

This documentation is important for further research, cost, and continuity and quality of care studies.

NURSING INTERVENTIONS

Interventions can be either nurse-initiated treatment, which is an autonomous action in response to a nursing diagnosis, or physician-initiated treatment with an order written in the patient's record.

> KEYCONCEPT **Nursing interventions** are nursing actions or treatment, selected based on clinical judgment, that are designed to achieve patient, family, or community outcomes. Interventions can be direct or indirect.

There are several nursing interventions systems, including the Nursing Interventions Classification (NIC), the Clinical Care Classification system, and the Omaha nursing model. All of these systems are recognized by the American Nurses Association (ANA) (Bulechek, Butcher, Dochterman, & Wagner, 2013; Martin, 2005; Saba, 2012). See Chapter 4. In this text, the *Psychiatric-Mental Health Nursing: Scope and Standards of Practice* guides the use of interventions (ANA, APNA, & ISPN, 2014). Some are adapted from classification systems and others from the psychiatric-mental health nursing literature.

Interventions for the Biologic Domain

Biologic interventions focus on physical functioning and are directed toward the patient's self-care, activities and exercise, sleep, nutrition, relaxation, hydration, and thermoregulation as well as pain management and medication management.

Promotion of Self-Care Activities

Many patients with psychiatric–mental health problems can manage ADLs or self-care activities such as bathing, dressing appropriately, selecting adequate nutrition, and sleeping regularly. Others cannot manage such self-care activities, either because of their symptoms or as a result of the side effects of medications.

In the inpatient setting, the psychiatric-mental health nurse structures the patient's activities, so that basic self-care activities are completed. During acute phases of psychiatric disorders, the inability to attend to basic self-care tasks, such as getting dressed, is very common. Thus, the ability to complete personal hygiene activities (e.g., dental care, grooming) is monitored, and patients are assisted in completing such activities. In a psychiatric facility, patients are encouraged and expected to develop independence in completing these basic self-care activities. In the community, monitoring these basic self-care activities is always a part of the nursing visit or clinic appointment.

Activity and Exercise Interventions

In some psychiatric disorders (e.g., schizophrenia), people become sedentary and appear to lack the motivation to complete ADLs. This lack of motivation is part of the disorder and requires nursing intervention. In addition, side effects of medication often include sedation and lethargy. Encouraging regular activity and exercise can improve general well-being and physical health. In some instances, exercise behavior becomes an abnormal focus of attention, as may be observed in some patients with anorexia nervosa.

When assuming the responsibility of direct care provider, the nurse can help patients identify realistic activities and exercise goals. As leader or manager of a psychiatric unit, the nurse can influence ward routine. Alternatively, the nurse can delegate activity and exercise interventions to nurses' aides. Some institutions have other professionals (e.g., recreational therapists) available for the implementation of exercise programs. As a case manager, the nurse should consider the activity needs of individuals when coordinating care.

Sleep Interventions

Many psychiatric disorders and medications are associated with sleep disturbances. Sleep is also disrupted in patients with dementia; such patients may have difficulty falling asleep or may frequently awaken during the night. In Alzheimer's Disease, individuals may reverse their sleeping patterns by napping during the day and staying awake at night.

Nonpharmacologic interventions are always used first because of the side-effect risks associated with the use of sedatives and hypnotics (see Chapter 10). Sleep interventions to communicate to patients include the following:

- Go to bed only when tired or sleepy.
- Establish a consistent bedtime routine.
- Avoid stimulating foods, beverages, or medications.
- Avoid naps in the late afternoon or evening.
- Eat lightly before retiring and limit fluid intake.
- Use your bed only for sleep or intimacy.
- Avoid emotional stimulation before bedtime.

- Use behavioral and relaxation techniques.
- Limit distractions.

Nutrition Interventions

Psychiatric disorders and medication side effects can affect eating behaviors. For varying reasons, some patients eat too little, but others eat too much. For instance, homeless patients with mental illnesses have difficulty maintaining adequate nutrition because of their deprived lifestyle. Substance abuse also interferes with maintaining adequate nutrition, either through stimulation or suppression of appetite or neglecting nutrition because of drug-seeking behavior. Thus, nutrition interventions should be specific and relevant to the individual's circumstances and mental health. In addition, recommended daily nutritional allowances are important in the promotion of physical and mental health, and nurses should consider them when planning care.

Some psychiatric symptoms involve changes in perceptions of food, appetite, and eating habits. If a patient believes that food is poisonous, he or she may eat sparingly or not at all. Interventions are then necessary to address the suspiciousness as well as to encourage adequate intake of recommended daily allowances. Allowing patients to examine foods, participate in preparations, and test the safety of the meal by eating slowly or after

everyone else may be necessary. For patients who are paranoid, it is sometimes helpful to serve prepackaged foods.

Relaxation Interventions

Relaxation promotes comfort, reduces anxiety, alleviates stress, eases pain, and prevents aggression. It can diminish the effects of hallucinations and delusions. The many different relaxation techniques used as mental health interventions range from simple deep breathing to biofeedback to hypnosis. Although some techniques, such as biofeedback, require additional training and, in some instances, certification, nurses can easily apply simple relaxation, distraction, and imagery techniques.

Simple relaxation techniques encourage and elicit relaxation to decrease undesirable signs and symptoms. **Distraction** is the purposeful focusing of attention away from undesirable sensations, and **guided imagery** is the purposeful use of imagination to achieve relaxation or direct attention away from undesirable sensations (Box 9.6). These interventions are helpful for people experiencing anxiety; guided imagery is especially useful in stress management.

Relaxation techniques that involve physical touch (e.g., back rubs) usually are not used for people with mental disorders. Touching and massaging usually are not appropriate, especially for those who have a history of

---

BOX 9.6

Relaxation Techniques: Descriptions and Implementation

SIMPLE RELAXATION TECHNIQUES
- Create a quiet, nondisrupting environment with dim lights and a comfortable temperature.
- Instruct the patient to assume a relaxed position, wearing loose and comfortable clothing.
- Instruct the patient to relax and to let the sensations happen.
- Use a low tone of voice with a slow, rhythmic pace of words.
- Instruct the patient to take an initial slow, deep breath (abdominal breathing) while thinking about pleasant events.
- Use soothing music (without words) to enhance relaxation.
- Reinforce the use of relaxation by praising efforts and helping the patient to schedule time regularly for it.
- Evaluate and document the patient's response to relaxation.

DISTRACTION
- Distraction techniques include music, counting, television, reading, play, and exercise. Help the patient choose a technique that will work for him or her.
- Advise the patient to practice the distraction technique before he or she will need to use it.
- Have the patient develop a specific plan for how and when he or she will use distraction.
- Evaluate and document the patient's response to distraction.

GUIDED IMAGERY
- Help the patient choose a particular guided imagery technique (alone or with others).

- Discuss an image the patient has experienced as pleasurable and relaxing, such as lying on a beach, watching snow fall, floating on a raft, or watching the sun set.
- Individualize the images chosen, considering religious or spiritual beliefs, artistic interests, or other individual preferences.
- Make suggestions to induce relaxation (e.g., peaceful images, pleasant sensations, or rhythmic breathing).
- Use modulated voice when guiding the imagery experience.
- Have the patient travel mentally to the scene, and assist in describing the setting in detail.
- Use permissive directions and suggestions when leading the imagery, such as "perhaps," "if you wish," or "you might like."
- Have the patient slowly experience the scene. How does it look? smell? sound? feel? taste?
- Use words or phrases that convey pleasurable images, such as floating, melting, and releasing.
- Develop cleansing or clearing portion of imagery (e.g., all pain appears as red dust and washes downstream in a creek as you enter).
- Assist the patient in developing a method of ending the imagery technique, such as counting slowly while breathing deeply.
- Encourage expression of thoughts and feelings regarding the experience.
- Prepare the patient for unexpected (but often therapeutic) experiences, such as crying.
- Evaluate and document the patient's response.

Adapted from Bulechek et al. (2013).

physical or sexual abuse. Such patients may find touching too stimulating or misinterpret it as being sexual or aggressive.

Hydration Interventions

Assessing fluid status and monitoring fluid intake and output are often important interventions. Overhydration or underhydration can be a symptom of a disorder. For example, some patients with psychotic disorders experience chronic fluid imbalance. Many psychiatric medications affect fluid and electrolyte balance (see Chapter 10). For example, when taking lithium carbonate, patients must have adequate fluid intake and pay special attention to testing serum sodium levels. Interventions that help patients understand the relationship of medications to fluid and electrolyte balance are important in their overall care.

Thermoregulation Interventions

Many psychiatric disorders can disturb the body's normal temperature regulation. Thus, patients cannot sense temperature increases or decreases and consequently cannot protect themselves from extremes of hot or cold. This problem is especially difficult for people who are homeless or live outside the protected environments of institutions and boarding homes. In addition, many psychiatric medications affect the ability to regulate body temperature.

Interventions include educating patients about the problem of thermoregulation, identifying potential extremes in temperatures, and developing strategies to protect the patient from the adverse effects of temperature changes. For example, reminding patients to wear coats and sweaters in the winter or to wear loose, lightweight garments in the summer may prevent frostbite or heat exhaustion, respectively.

Pain Management

Psychiatric-mental health nurses are more likely to provide care to patients experiencing chronic pain than acute pain. However, a single intervention is seldom successful for relieving chronic pain. In some instances, pain is managed by medication; in other instances, nonpharmacologic strategies, such as simple relaxation techniques, distraction, or imagery, are used. Indeed, relaxation is one of the most widely used cognitive and behavioral approaches to pain. Education, stress management techniques, hypnosis, and biofeedback are also used in pain management. Physical agents include heat and cold therapy, exercise, and transcutaneous nerve stimulation.

The key to managing pain is identifying how it disrupts the patient's personal, social, professional, and family life. Education focusing on the pain, use of medications for treatment, and development of cognitive skills are important pain management components. In some cases, redefining treatment success as improvement in functioning, rather than alleviation of pain, may be necessary. The interaction between stress and pain is important; that is, increased stress leads to increased pain. Patients can better manage their pain when stress is reduced.

Medication Management

The psychiatric–mental health nurse uses many medication management interventions to help patients maintain therapeutic regimens. Medication management involves more than the actual administration of medications. Nurses also assess medication effectiveness and side effects and consider drug–drug interactions. Monitoring the amount of lethal prescription medication is particularly important. For example, check if patients have old prescriptions of tricyclic antidepressants in their medicine cabinets. Treatment with psychopharmacologic agents can be lengthy because of the chronic nature of many disorders; many patients remain on medication regimens for years, never becoming free of medication. Thus, medication education is an ongoing intervention that requires careful documentation. Medication follow-up may include home visits as well as telephone calls.

Interventions for the Psychological Domain

A major emphasis in psychiatric–mental health nursing is on the psychological domain: emotion, behavior, and cognition. The nurse–patient relationship serves as the basis for interventions directed toward the psychological domain. Because therapeutic interactions and relationships were extensively discussed in Chapters 7 & 8, they are not covered in this chapter. This section does cover counseling, conflict resolution, bibliotherapy and webotherapy, reminiscence, behavior therapy, psychoeducation, health teaching, and spiritual interventions.

Cognitive Interventions

Evidence-based cognitive interventions are used in a variety of practice settings (inpatient and outpatient). The knowledge and skills inherent in cognitively based interventions have been extensively studied and their effectiveness has been demonstrated for a variety of psychiatric disorders, especially depression (see Chapter 19) and anxiety and related disorders (see Chapters 16, 17, & 18).

Cognitive interventions are based on the concept of cognition. **Cognition** can be defined as an internal process of perception, memory, and judgment through which an understanding of self and the world is developed.

Cognitive interventions aim to change or reframe an individual's automatic thought patterns that have developed over time and which interfere with the individual's ability to function optimally. The skills and techniques that were developed on the basis of cognitive theory result in a new view of self and the environment.

Counseling Interventions

Counseling interventions are specific, time-limited interactions between a nurse and a patient, family, or group experiencing immediate or ongoing difficulties related to their health or well-being. Counseling is usually short term and focuses on improving coping abilities, reinforcing healthy behaviors, fostering positive interactions, or preventing illness and disability. Counseling strategies are discussed throughout the text. Psychotherapy, which differs from counseling, is generally a long-term approach aimed at improving or helping patients regain previous health status and functional abilities. Mental health specialists, such as advanced practice nurses, use psychotherapy.

Conflict Resolution and Cultural Brokering

Conflict resolution is a specific type of intervention through which the nurse helps patients resolve disagreements or disputes with family, friends, or other patients. Conflict can be positive if individuals see the problem as solvable and providing an opportunity for growth and interpersonal understanding. The nurse may be in the position of actually resolving a family conflict or teaching family members how to resolve their own conflicts positively. In addition, because nurses are in positions of leadership, they often need conflict resolution skills to settle employee conflicts.

At times, patients who are politically and economically powerless find themselves in conflict with the health care system. Differences in cultural values and languages among patients and health care organizations contribute to feelings of powerlessness. For example, migrant farm workers, people who are homeless, and people who need to make informed decisions under stressful conditions may be unable to navigate the health care system. The nurse can help to resolve such conflicts through **cultural brokering**, the act of bridging, linking, or mediating messages, instructions, and belief systems between groups of people of differing cultural systems to reduce conflict or produce change (Esperat, Inouye, Gonzalez, Owen, & Feng, 2004).

For the "nurse as broker" to be effective, he or she establishes and maintains a sense of connectedness or relationship with the patient. In turn, the nurse also establishes and cultivates networks with other health care facilities and resources. Cultural sensitivity enables the nurse to be aware of and sensitive to the needs of patients from a variety of cultures. Cultural competence is necessary for the brokering process to be effective.

Bibliotherapy and Internet Use

Bibliotherapy, sometimes referred to as bibliocounseling, is the reading of selected written materials to express feelings or gain insight under the guidance of a health care provider. The provider assigns and discusses with the patient a book, story, or article. The provider makes the assignment because he or she believes that the patient can receive therapeutic benefit from the reading. (It is assumed that the provider who assigned the reading has also read it.) The provider needs to consider the patient's reading level before making an assignment. If a patient has limited reading ability, the provider should not use bibliotherapy.

Literary works serve as a projective screen through which people see themselves in the story. Literature can help patients identify with characters and vicariously experience their reality. It can also expose patients to situations that they have not personally experienced—the vicarious experience allows growth in self-knowledge and compassion (Macdonald, Vallance, & McGrath, 2013). Through reading, patients can enrich their lives in the following ways:

- *Catharsis:* expression of feelings stimulated by parallel experiences
- *Problem solving:* development of solutions to problems in the literature from practical ideas about problem solving
- *Insight:* increased self-awareness and understanding as the reader explores personal meaning from what is read
- *Anxiety reduction:* self-help written materials can reduce concerns about a diagnosed problem and treatment.

Using the internet can be helpful to patients, but it also has drawbacks. Some web sites can help patients gain insight into their problems through acquiring new knowledge and interacting with others in the privacy of their own surroundings. Web materials and chat groups are variable in quality and accuracy. Nurses should carefully evaluate the quality of the website when patients are engaging in webotherapy.

Reminiscence

Reminiscence, the thinking about or relating of past experiences, is used as a nursing intervention to enhance life review in older patients. Reminiscence encourages patients, either in individual or group settings, to discuss their past and review their lives. Through reminiscence, individuals can identify past coping strategies that can support them in current stressful situations. Patients can

---

BOX 9.7

Research for Best Practice: Reminiscence Treatment in Older Adults with Dementia

Huang, S., Li., C., Yang, C., & Chen, J. J. (2009). Application of reminiscence treatment on older people with dementia: A case study in Pingtung, Taiwan. Journal of Nursing Research, 17(2), 112–119.

THE QUESTION: Does cognition improve and depression decrease following participation in an eight-week reminiscence social group organized around cooking?

METHODS: A social work group of 10 older adult female residents of a nursing home completed eight sessions of reminiscence cooking lessons consisting of preparing traditional foods. Changes in memory, cognition, brain functioning, and personal interaction were measured pre- and post-session by the mental health status, depression scale, EEG, and feeling of participation scale.

FINDINGS: There were positive changes in all of the measures, but none of these changes were significant.

IMPLICATIONS FOR NURSING: This small study is clinically interesting because the intervention, cooking food as an activity for reminiscence therapy, is unique and rarely reported. The problem with the study is the small sample. The lack of significant findings is predictable with this small group. However, the intervention is logical and deserves further study.

---

also use reminiscence to maintain self-esteem, stimulate thinking, and support the natural healing process of life review. Activities that facilitate reminiscence include writing an account of past events, making a tape recording and playing it back, explaining pictures in old family albums, drawing a family tree, and writing to old friends (Box 9.7).

Behavior Therapy

Behavior therapy interventions focus on reinforcing or promoting desirable behaviors or altering undesirable ones. The basic premise is that because most behaviors are learned, new functional behaviors can also be learned. Behaviors—not internal psychic processes—are the targets of the interventions. The models of behavioral theorists serve as a basis for these interventions (see Chapter 5).

Behavior Modification

Behavior modification is a specific, systematized behavior therapy technique that can be applied to individuals, groups, or systems. The aim of behavior modification is to reinforce desired behaviors and extinguish undesired ones. Desired behavior is rewarded to increase the likelihood that patients will repeat it, and over time, replace the problematic behavior with it. Behavior modification is used for various problematic behaviors, such as dysfunctional eating, addictions, anger management, and

impulse control and often is used in the care of children and adolescents.

Token Economy

Used in inpatient settings and in group homes, a **token economy** applies behavior modification techniques to multiple behaviors. In a token economy, patients are rewarded with tokens for selected desired behaviors. They can use these tokens to purchase meals, leave the unit, watch television, or wear street clothes. In less restrictive environments, patients use tokens to purchase additional privileges, such as attending social events. Token economy systems have been especially effective in reinforcing positive behaviors in people who are developmentally disabled or have severe and persistent mental illnesses. The strategy has been expanded to rehabilitation programs for children (Jones, Webb, Estes, & Dawson, 2013), and cocaine addiction (Farronato, Dursteler-Macfarland, Wiesbeck, & Petitjean, et al., 2013).

> **NCLEXNOTE** Focus on helping patient achieve and maintain self-control of behavior (e.g., contract, behavior modification).

Psychoeducation

Psychoeducation uses educational strategies to teach patients the skills they lack because of a psychiatric disorder. The goal of psychoeducation is a change in knowledge and behavior. Nurses use psychoeducation to meet the educational needs of patients by adapting teaching strategies to their disorder-related deficits (Box 9.8). As patients gain skills, functioning improves. Some patients may need to learn how to maintain their morning hygiene. Others may need to understand their illness and cope with hearing voices that others do not hear.

BOX 9.8

Research for Best Practices: Educational and Self-Management Interventions

Coster, S & Norman, I. (2009). Cochrane reviews of educational and self-management interventions to guide nursing practice: A review. International Journal of Nursing Studies, 46, 508–528.

THE QUESTION: What interventions improve patients' knowledge and skills to manage chronic disease?

METHODS: Thirty Cochrane systematic reviews were identified. Data were extracted and summarized.

FINDINGS: Most of the studies provided inadequate evidence (n = 18, 60%), but of those studies with adequate evidence, mental health is one of the chronic disease states for which patient education makes a difference.

IMPLICATIONS FOR NURSING: Education can be effective in the area of mental health and is a key intervention for patients with emotional problems and mental disorders.

Specific psychoeducation techniques are based on adult learning principles, such as beginning at the point where the learner is currently and building on his or her current experiences. Thus, the nurse assesses the patient's current skills and readiness to learn. From there, the nurse individualizes a teaching plan for each patient. He or she can conduct such teaching in a one-to-one situation or a group format.

Psychoeducation is a continuous process of assessing, setting goals, developing learning activities, and evaluating for changes in knowledge and behavior. Nurses use it with individuals, groups, families, and communities. Psychoeducation serves as a basis for recovery for those with severe and persistent mental illness.

> **NCLEXNOTE** Apply knowledge from social sciences to help patients manage responses to psychiatric disorders and emotional problems.

Health Teaching

Health teaching is one of the standards of care for the psychiatric-mental health nurse. Teaching methods should be appropriate to the patient's development level, learning needs, readiness, ability to learn, language preference, and culture. Based on principles of learning, health teaching involves transmitting new information to the patient and providing constructive feedback and positive rewards, practice sessions, homework, and experimental learning. Health teaching is the integration of principles of teaching and learning with the knowledge of health and illness (Figure 9.2).

Thus, in health teaching, the psychiatric-mental health nurse attends to potential health care problems other than mental disorders and emotional problems. For example, if a person has diabetes mellitus and is taking insulin, the nurse provides health care teaching related to diabetes and the interaction of this problem with the mental disorder.

Spiritual Interventions

Spiritual care is based on an assessment of the patient's spiritual needs. A nonjudgmental relationship and just "being with" (not doing for) the patient are key to providing spiritual intervention. In some instances, patients ask to see a religious leader. Nurses should always respect and never deny these requests. To assist people in spiritual distress, the nurse should know and understand the beliefs and practices of various spiritual groups. **Spiritual support**, assisting patients to feel balance and connection within their relationships, involves listening to expressions of loneliness, using empathy, and providing patients with desired spiritual articles.

Interventions for the Social Domain

The social domain includes the individual's environment and its effect on his or her responses to mental disorders and distress. Interventions within the social domain are geared toward couples, families, friends, and large and small social groups, with special attention given to ethnicity and community interactions. In some instances, nurses design interventions that affect a patient's environment, such as helping a family member decide to admit a loved one to a long-term care facility. In other instances, the nurse actually modifies the environment to promote positive behaviors. Group interventions are discussed in Chapter 11.

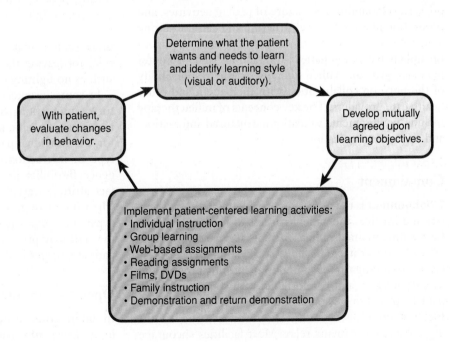

FIGURE 9.2 Teaching evaluation model.

Social Behavior and Privilege Systems in Inpatient Units

In psychiatric units, unrelated strangers who have problems interacting live together in close quarters, sometimes with two to four people sharing bedrooms and bathrooms. For this reason, most psychiatric units develop a list of behavioral expectations called unit rules that staff members post and explain to patients upon admittance. Their purpose is to facilitate a comfortable and safe environment; they have little to do with the patients' reasons for admission. Getting up at certain times, showering before breakfast, making the bed, and not visiting in others' rooms are typical expectations. It is usually the nurse manager who oversees the operation of the unit and implementation of privilege systems.

Most psychiatric facilities use a privilege system to protect patients and to reinforce unit rules and other appropriate behavior (also see the previous section discussing a token economies). The more appropriate the behavior, the more privileges of freedom the person has. Privileges are based on the assessment of a patient's risk to harm himself or herself or others and ability to follow treatment regimens. For example, a patient with few privileges may be required to stay on the unit and eat only with other patients. A patient with full privileges may have freedom to leave the unit and go outside the hospital and into the community for short periods.

Milieu Therapy

Milieu therapy provides a stable and coherent social organization to facilitate an individual's treatment. (The terms *milieu therapy* and *therapeutic environment* are often used interchangeably.) In milieu therapy, the design of the physical surroundings, structure of patient activities, and promotion of a stable social structure and cultural setting enhance the setting's therapeutic potential. A therapeutic milieu facilitates patient interactions and promotes personal growth. Milieu therapy is the responsibility of the nurse in collaboration with the patient and other health care providers. The key concepts of milieu therapy include containment, validation, structured interaction, and open communication.

Containment

Containment is the process of providing safety and security and involves the patient's access to food and shelter. In a well-contained milieu, patients feel safe from their illnesses and protected against social stigma. The physical surroundings are also important in this process and should be clean and comfortable, with special attention paid to promoting a noninstitutionalized environment. Pictures on walls, comfortable furniture, and soothing colors help patients relax. Most facilities encourage patients and nursing staff to wear street clothes, which help decrease the formalized nature of hospital settings and promotes nurse–patient relationships.

Therapeutic milieus emphasize patient involvement in treatment decisions and operation of the unit; nurses should encourage freedom of movement within the contained environment. Patients participate in maintaining the quality of the physical surroundings, assuming responsibility for making their own beds, attending to their own belongings, and keeping an acceptable living area. Families are viewed as a part of the patient's life, and ties are maintained. In most inpatient settings, specific times are set for family interaction, education, and treatment. Family involvement is often a criterion for admission for treatment, and the involvement may include regular family attendance at therapy sessions.

Validation

In a therapeutic environment, **validation** is another process that affirms patient individuality. Staff–patient interactions should constantly reaffirm the patient's humanity and human rights. All interaction a staff member initiates with a patient should reflect his or her respect for that patient. Patients must believe that staff members truly like and respect them.

Structured Interaction

One of the most interesting milieu concepts is **structured interaction**, which is purposeful interaction that allows patients to interact with others in a useful way. For instance, the daily community meeting provides structure to explain unit rules and consequences of violations. Ideally, patients who are either elected or volunteer for the responsibility assume leadership for these meetings. In the meeting, the group discusses behavioral expectations, such as making beds daily, appropriate dress, and rules for leaving the unit. Usually, there are other rules, such as no fighting or name calling.

In some instances, the treatment team assigns structured interactions to specific patients as part of their treatment. Specific attitudes or approaches are directed toward individual patients who benefit from a particular type of interaction. Nurses consistently assume indulgence, flexibility, passive or active friendliness, matter-of-fact attitude, casualness, watchfulness, or kind firmness when interacting with specific patients. For example, if a patient is known to overreact and dramatize events, the staff may provide a matter-of-fact attitude when the patient engages in dramatic behavior.

Open Communication

In **open communication**, the staff and patient willingly share information. Staff members invite patient self-disclosure within the support of a nurse–patient relationship. In addition, they provide a model of effective communication when interacting with one another as well as with patients. They arrange an environment to facilitate optimal interaction and resocialization. Support, attention, praise, and reassurance given to patients improve self-esteem and increase confidence. Patient education is also a part of this support, as are directions to foster coping skills.

Milieu Therapy in Different Settings

Milieu therapy is applied in various settings. In long-term care settings, the therapeutic milieu becomes essential because patients may reside there for months or years. These patients typically have schizophrenia or developmental disabilities. Structure in daily living is important to the successful functioning of the individuals and the overall group but must be applied within the context of individual needs. For example, if a patient cannot get up one morning in time to complete assigned tasks (e.g., showering or making a bed) because of a personal crisis the night before, the nurse should consider the situation compassionately and flexibly, not applying the "consequences" rule or taking away the patient's privileges. In turn, the nurse must weigh individual needs against the collective needs of all the patients. For a patient who is consistently late for treatment activities, the nurse should apply the rules of the unit even if it means taking away privileges.

Recently, concepts of milieu therapy have been applied to short-term inpatient and community settings. In acute-care inpatient settings, nursing actions provide limits to and controls on patient behavior and provide structure and safety for the patients. Milieu treatments are based on the individual needs of the patients and include relaxation groups, discussion groups, and medication groups. Spontaneous and planned activities are possible on a short-term unit as well as in a long-term setting. In the community, it is possible to apply milieu therapy approaches in day treatment centers, group homes, and single dwellings.

Promotion of Patient Safety

Although the use of social rules of conduct and privilege systems can enhance smooth operation of a unit, some potentially serious problems can be associated with these practices. A most critical aspect of psychiatric–mental health nursing is the promotion of patient safety, especially in inpatient units.

Observation

Patient observation is the ongoing assessment of the patient's mental status to identify and subvert any potential problem. An important process in all nursing practice, observation is particularly important in psychiatric-mental health nursing. In psychiatric settings, patients are ambulatory and thus more susceptible to environmental hazards. In addition, judgment and cognition impairment are symptoms of many psychiatric disorders. Often, patients are admitted because they pose a danger to themselves or others. In psychiatric-mental health nursing, observation is more than just "seeing" patients. It means continually monitoring them for any indication of harm to themselves or others.

All patients who are hospitalized for psychiatric reasons are continually monitored. The intensity of the observation depends on their risk to themselves and others. Some patients are merely asked to "check in" at different times of the day, but others have a staff member assigned to only them, such as in instances of potential suicide. Often "sharps," such as razors, are locked up and given to patients at specified times. Mental health facilities and units all have policies that specify levels of observation for patients of varying degrees of risk.

De-escalation

De-escalation is an interactive process of calming and redirecting a patient who has an immediate potential for violence directed toward self or others. This intervention involves assessing the situation and preventing it from escalating to one in which injury occurs to the patient, staff, or other patients. After the nurse has assessed the situation, he or she calmly calls to the patient and asks the individual to leave the situation. The nurse must avoid rushing toward the patient or giving orders (see Chapter 13). Nurses can use various interventions in this situation, including distraction, conflict resolution, and cognitive interventions.

Seclusion

Seclusion is the involuntary confinement of a person in a room or an area where the person is physically prevented from leaving (Centers for Medicare & Medicaid Services [CMS], 2012). A patient is placed in seclusion for purposes of safety or behavioral management. The seclusion room has no furniture except a mattress and a blanket. The walls usually are padded. The room is environmentally safe, with no hanging devices, electrical outlets, or windows from which the patient could jump. When a patient is placed in seclusion, he or she is observed at all times.

There are several types of seclusion arrangements. Some facilities place seclusion rooms next to the nurses' stations. These seclusion rooms have an observation window. Other facilities use a modified patient room and assign a staff member to view the patient at all times. Seclusion is an extremely negative patient

BOX 9.9

Research for Best Practice: Evidence for Seclusion and Restraint Use

Sailas, E., & Fenton, M. (2012). Seclusion and restraint for people with serious mental illnesses. The Cochrane Library (Oxford) (ID 00075320-100000000-00215.

THE QUESTION: How effective are seclusion, restraint, or alternative controls for people with serious mental illness?

METHODS: A meta-analysis of the effectiveness of seclusion and restraint compared with the alternatives for persons with serious mental illnesses was conducted. Randomized controlled trials were included if they focused on the use of restraint or seclusion or strategies designed to reduce the need for restraint or seclusion in the treatment of serious mental illness. The search yielded 2,155 citations. Of these, 35 studies were obtained.

FINDINGS: No controlled studies exist that evaluate the value of seclusion or restraint in those with serious mental illness. There are reports of serious adverse effects for these techniques in qualitative reviews.

IMPLICATIONS FOR NURSING: Alternative ways of dealing with unwanted or harmful behaviors need to be developed. Continuing use of seclusion or restraint must, therefore, be questioned.

experience; consequently, its use is seriously questioned, and many facilities have completely abandoned its practice (Box 9.9). Patient outcomes may actually be worse if seclusion is used.

Restraints

The most restrictive safety intervention is the use of **restraint**, any manual method, physical or mechanical, that immobilizes or reduces the ability of the patient to move. Tucking a patient's sheet in so tightly that the person cannot move is considered a restraint as is the use of leather restraints. **Chemical restraint** is the use of medications for restricting patients' behavior or their freedom of movement. These chemical restraints include drugs that are not a part of their standard psychiatric treatment or that are an inappropriate dosage of their standard medication. If hospitals choose to use any type of restraints for behavioral control, the restraints are applied only after every other intervention is used and the patient continues to be a danger to self or others. Documentation must reflect a careful assessment of the patient that indicates the need for an intervention to protect the patient from harm (CMS, 2012).

The least restrictive type of restraint is selected to keep a patient safe. Wrist restraints restrict arm movement. Walking restraints or ankle restraints are used if a patient cannot resist the impulse to run from a facility but is safe to go outside and to activities. Three- and four-point restraints are applied to the wrist and ankles in bed.

When five-point restraints are used, all extremities are secured, and another restraint is placed across the chest.

The use of both seclusion and restraints must follow the Medicare regulations contained in the *Patients' Rights Condition of Participation* (CMS, 2012). Agencies that do not follow the regulations may lose their Medicare and Medicaid certification and, consequently, their funding. The application of physical restraints should also follow hospital policies. Nurses should document all the previously tried de-escalation interventions before the application of restraints. They should limit use of restraints to times when an individual is judged to be a danger to self or others; they should apply restraints only until the patient regains control over his or her behavior. When a patient is in physical restraints, the nurse should closely observe the patient and protect him or her from self-injury. See Box 9.9.

Home Visits

Patients usually have been hospitalized or have received treatment for acute psychiatric symptoms before being referred to psychiatric home service. The goal of **home visits**, the delivery of nursing care in the patient's living environment, is to maximize the patient's functional ability within the nurse–patient relationship and with the family or partner as appropriate. The psychiatric-mental health nurse who makes home visits needs to be able to work independently, is skilled in teaching patients and families, can administer and monitor medications, and uses community resources for the patient's needs.

Home visits are especially useful in certain situations, including helping reluctant patients enter therapy, conducting a comprehensive assessment, strengthening a support network, and maintaining patients in the community when their condition deteriorates. Home visits are also useful in helping individuals comply with taking medication. The home visit process consists of three steps: the previsit phase, the home visit, and the postvisit phase. During previsit planning, the nurse sets goals for the home visit based on data received from other health care providers or the patient. In addition, the nurse and patient agree on the time of the visit. As the nurse travels to the home, he or she should assess the neighborhood for access to services, socioeconomic factors, and safety.

The actual visit can be divided into four parts. The first is the greeting phase, in which the nurse establishes rapport with family members. Greetings, which are usually brief, establish the communication process and the atmosphere for the visit. Greetings should be friendly but professional. In cultures that consider greetings important, this phase may involve more formal interactions, such as eating food or drinking tea with family members. The next phase establishes the focus of the visit. Sometimes the purpose of the visit is medication administration, health teaching, or counseling. The patient and family must be clear regarding the purpose. The implementation of the service is the next phase and should use most of the visit time. If the purpose of the visit is problem solving or decision making, the family's cultural values may determine the types of interaction and decision-making approaches. Closure is the last phase, the end of the home visit. It is a time to summarize and clarify important points. The nurse should also schedule any additional visits and reiterate patient expectations between visits. Usually, the nurse is the only provider to see the patient regularly. The nurse should acknowledge family members on leaving if they were not a part of the visit.

The postvisit phase includes documentation, reporting, and follow-up planning. This is also when the nurse meets with the supervisor and presents data from the home visit at the team meeting.

Community Action

Nurses have a unique opportunity to promote mental health awareness and support humane treatment for people with mental disorders. Activities range from being an advisor to support groups to participating in the political process through lobbying efforts and serving on community mental health boards. These unpaid activities are usually outside the realm of a particular job. However, an important role of professionals is to provide community service in addition to service through income-generating positions.

EVALUATING OUTCOMES

Evaluation of patient outcomes involves answering the following questions:

- What benefits did the patient receive?
- What was the patient's level of satisfaction?
- Was the outcome diagnosis specific or nonspecific?
- What is the cost effectiveness of the intervention?

Outcomes can be measured immediately after the nursing intervention or after time passes. For example, a patient may be able to resolve the acute depression and demonstrate confidence and improved self-esteem during a hospital stay. In various cases, it may be several months before the person can engage in positive interpersonal relationships.

SUMMARY OF KEY POINTS

- Assessment is the deliberate and systematic collection of biopsychosocial information or data to determine current and past health and functional status and to evaluate present and past coping patterns.

- The biologic assessment includes current and past health status, physical examination with review of body systems, review of physical functions, and pharmacologic assessment.

- The psychological assessment includes the mental status examination, behavioral responses, and risk factor assessment.

  - The mental status examination includes general observation of appearance, psychomotor activity, and attitude; orientations; mood; affect; emotions; speech; and thought processes.

  - Behavioral responses are assessed as are self-concept and current and past coping patterns.

  - Risk factor assessment includes ascertaining whether the patient has any suicidal, assaultive, or homicidal ideation.

- The social assessment includes functional status; social systems; spirituality; occupational, economic, and legal status; and quality of life.

- The biopsychosocial assessment provides the data for nursing diagnoses and planning patient outcomes. Anticipated patient outcomes are the basis for psychiatric–mental health nursing interventions.

- Nursing interventions are implemented for each domain include biologic (self-care, activity and exercise, sleep, nutrition, thermoregulation, and pain and medication management); psychological (counseling, conflict resolution, bibliotherapy and webotherapy, reminiscence, behavior therapy, psychoeducation, health teaching, and spiritual interventions); and social (behavior therapy and modification, milieu therapy, and various home and community interventions).

- Evaluation of patient outcomes involves assessing cost effectiveness of the interventions, benefits to the patient, and the patient's level of satisfaction. Outcomes should be measurable, either immediately after intervention or after some time passes.

CRITICAL THINKING CHALLENGES

1. A 23-year-old white woman is admitted to an acute psychiatric setting for depression and suicidal gestures. This admission is her first, but she has experienced bouts of depression since early adolescence. She and her fiancé have just broken their engagement and moved into separate apartments. She has not yet told anyone that she is pregnant. She said that her mother had told her that she was "living in sin" and that she would "pay for it." The patient wants to "end

it all!" From this scenario, develop three assessment questions for each domain: biologic, psychological, and social.

2. Identify normal laboratory values for sodium, blood urea nitrogen, liver enzymes, leukocyte count and differential, and thyroid functioning. Why are these values important to know?

3. Write a paragraph on your self-concept, including all three components: body image, self-esteem, and personal identity. Explore the type of patient situations in which your self-concept can help your interactions with patients. Explore the types of patient situations in which your self-concept can hinder your interactions with patients.

4. Tom, a 25-year-old man with schizophrenia, lives with his parents, who want to retire to Florida. Tom goes to work each day but relies on his mother for meals, laundry, and reminders to take his medication. Tom believes that he can manage the home, but his mother is concerned. She asks the nurse for advice about leaving her son to manage on his own. Generate a nursing diagnosis, outcomes, and interventions that would meet some of Tom's potential responses to his changing lifestyle.

5. Joan, a 35-year-old married woman, is admitted to an acute psychiatric unit for stabilization of her mood disorder. She is extremely depressed but refuses to consider a recommended medication change. She asks the nurse what to do. Using a nursing intervention, explain how you would approach Joan's problem.

6. A nurse reports to work for the evening shift. The unit is chaotic. The television in the day room is loud; two patients are arguing about the program. Visitors are mingling in patients' rooms. The temperature of the unit is hot. One patient is running up and down the hall yelling, "Help me, help me." Using a milieu therapy approach, what would you do to calm the unit?

REFERENCES

American Nurses Association, American Psychiatric Nurses Association and International Society of Psychiatric-Mental Health Nurses. (2014). *Psychiatric-Mental Health Nursing: Scope and Standards of Practice, 2nd Edition.* Silver spring, MD: Nursebooks.org.

Bulechek, G. M., Butcher, H. K., Dochterman, J., & Wagner, C. (Eds.). (2013). *Nursing interventions classification (NIC)* (6th ed.). St. Louis, MO: Elsevier.

Burkhardt, M. A., & Nagai-Jacobson, M. G. (1997). Spirituality and healing. In B. M. Dossey (Ed.). *Core curriculum for holistic nursing* (pp 42–51). Gaithersburg, MD: Aspen.

Carpenito-Moyet, L. J. (2014). *Nursing diagnosis: Application to clinical practice* (14th ed). Philadelphia: Wolters Kluwer | Lippincott Williams & Wilkins.

Centers for Medicare & Medicaid Services. (2012). *Interpretive guidelines for hospital CoP for patient rights. Quality of care information, quality standards 482.13.* Retrieved May 14, 2014, www.cms.hhs.gov/manuals.

Esperat, M. C., Inouye, J., Gonzalez, E. W., Owen, D. C., & Feng, D. (2004). Health disparities among Asian Americans and Pacific Islanders. *Annual Review of Nursing Research, 22,* 135–159.

Farronato, N. S., Dursteler-Macfarland, K. M., Wiesbeck, G. A., & Petitjean, S. A. (2013). A systematic review comparing cognitive-behavioral therapy and contingency management for cocaine dependence (Review). *Journal of Addictive Diseases, 32*(3), 274–287.

Jones, E. J., Webb, S. J., Estes, A., & Dawson, G. (2013). Rule learning in autism: the role of reward type and social context. *Developmental Neuropsychology, 38*(1), 58–77.

Macdonald, J., Vallance, D., & McGrath, M. (2013). An evaluation of a collaborative bibliotherapy scheme delivered via a library service. *Journal of Psychiatric & Mental Health Nursing, 20*(10), 857–865.

Martin, K. S. (2005). *The Omaha system: A key to practice, documentation, and information management.* (2nd ed). St. Louis: Elsevier Saunders.

Moorhead, S., Johnson, M., Maas, M. L., & Swanson, E. (2008). *Nursing outcomes classification (NOC)* (4th ed). St. Louis: Mosby.

Saba, V. K. (2012). *Clinical care classification (CCC) system (Version 2.1) (User's Guide)* (2nd ed). New York: Springer Publishing Company, LLC.

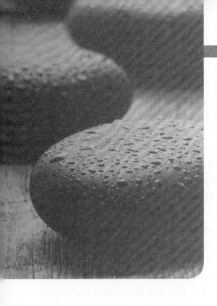

10

Psychopharmacology, Dietary Supplements, and Biologic Interventions

Mary Ann Boyd

KEY CONCEPTS

- agonists
- antagonists
- pharmacokinetics
- pharmacodynamics

LEARNING OBJECTIVES

After studying this chapter, you will be able to:

1. Differentiate target symptoms from side effects.

2. Identify nursing interventions for common side effects of psychiatric medications.

3. Explain the role of the governmental regulatory process in the approval of medication and the use of other biologic interventions.

4. Discuss the pharmacodynamics of psychiatric medications.

5. Discuss the pharmacokinetics of psychiatric medications.

6. Explain the major classifications of psychiatric medications.

7. Identify typical nursing interventions related to the administration of psychiatric medications.

8. Analyze the potential benefits of other forms of somatic treatments, including herbal supplements, nutrition therapies, electroconvulsive therapy, light therapy, transcranial magnetic stimulation, and vagus nerve stimulation.

9. Evaluate the significance of non-adherence and discuss strategies supportive of medication adherence.

KEY TERMS

- absorption • adherence • adverse reactions • affinity • agonists • akathisia • antagonists • atypical antipsychotics
- augmentation • bioavailability • biotransformation • boxed warning • carrier protein • chronic syndromes • clearance
- compliance • conventional antipsychotics • cytochrome P450 (CYP450) system • desensitization • distribution
- dosing • drug–drug interaction • dystonia • efficacy • enzymes • ethnopsychopharmacology • excretion • extrapyramidal symptoms (EPS) • first-pass effect • half-life • hypnotics • inducer • inhibitor • intrinsic activity • metabolism
- metabolites • off-label • partial agonists • pharmacogenomics • phototherapy • polypharmacy • potency • prescribing information • protein binding • pseudoparkinsonism • relapse • repetitive transcranial magnetic stimulation
- sedative–hypnotics • sedatives • selectivity • serotonin syndrome • side effects • solubility • steady state • substrate
- tardive dyskinesia • target symptoms • therapeutic index • tolerance • toxicity • uptake receptors

Recent scientific and technologic developments have opened the door for the development of new medications that treat mental disorders. Although nurses administer these medications, monitor their effectiveness, and manage side effects, they also have an important role in educating patients about their medications. Advanced practice nurses also prescribe medications. Psychiatric medications are increasingly prescribed in primary care settings, and nurses practicing in nonpsychiatric settings now need an in-depth knowledge of them.

This chapter focuses on the pharmacodynamics and pharmacokinetics of psychiatric medications. Included in this chapter is an overview of the major classes of psychopharmacologic drugs used in treating patients with mental disorders and the role of herbal supplements and nutritional therapies. In addition, other biologic treatments are discussed, including electroconvulsive therapy (ECT), light therapy, repetitive transcranial magnetic stimulation (rTMS), and vagus nerve stimulation.

CONSIDERATIONS IN USING PSYCHIATRIC MEDICATIONS

As with any drug, psychiatric medications are designated for use in certain conditions for specific symptoms. The nurse quickly realizes that these symptoms are present in several conditions, leading to medications being prescribed off-label or for other conditions other than those that are approved. Because medications can have both desirable and undesirable effects, it is important for the nurse to consider these factors to help ensure patient safety.

Target Symptoms and Side Effects

Psychiatric medications and other biologic interventions are indicated for **target symptoms**, which are specific measurable symptoms expected to improve with treatment. Standards of care guide nurses in monitoring and documenting the effects of medications and other biologic treatments on target symptoms.

As yet, no drug has been developed that is so specific it affects only its target symptoms; instead, drugs typically act on a number of other organs and sites within the body. Even drugs with a high affinity and selectivity for a specific neurotransmitter will cause some responses in the body that are not related to the target symptoms. These unwanted effects of medications are called **side effects**. If unwanted effects have serious physiologic consequences, they are considered **adverse reactions**. The nurse monitors, documents, and reports the appearance of side effects and adverse reactions and implements nursing interventions for relief of medication side effects (Table 10.1).

Drug Regulation and Use

The U.S. Food and Drug Administration (FDA) is responsible for ensuring the safety, efficacy, and security of human and veterinary drugs, biologic products, medical devices, our nation's food supply, cosmetics, and products that emit radiation (www.FDA.gov). The FDA approves the labeling of medications and other biologic treatments after a thorough review of efficacy and safety data

(Box 10.1). Nurses administering medications are responsible for knowing the labeling content, which is found in each medication's official **Prescribing Information** (PI) or prescribing information and includes approved indications for the medication, side effects, adverse reactions, contraindications, and other important information. If a medication is ordered and administered for a condition that is not approved by the FDA, it is considered **off-label** use. If the FDA identifies serious adverse reactions that can occur with the use of a specific medication, it may issue a warning found in a **boxed warning** in the PI. The nurse should be aware of these boxed warnings and monitor for the appearance of the adverse reactions. If a PI is not readily available, the labeling information is easily found on the FDA's website and in most pharmacy departments.

PSYCHOPHARMACOLOGY

A comparatively small amount of medication can have a significant and large impact on cell function and resulting behavior. When tiny molecules of medication are compared with the vast amount of cell surface in the human body, the fraction seems disproportionate. Yet the drugs used to treat mental disorders often have profound effects on behavior. To understand how this occurs, one needs to understand both where and how drugs work. The following discussion highlights important concepts relevant to psychiatric medications.

Pharmacodynamics: Where Drugs Act

Drug molecules act at specific sites, not on the entire cell surface. Psychiatric medications primarily target the central nervous system (CNS) at the cellular, synaptic level at four sites: receptors, ion channels, enzymes, and carrier proteins.

> **KEYCONCEPT** **Pharmacodynamics** is the action or effects of drugs on living organisms.

Receptors

Receptors are specific proteins intended to respond to a chemical (i.e., neurotransmitter) normally present in blood or tissues (see Chapter 6). Receptors also respond to drugs with similar chemical structures. When drugs attach to a receptor, they can act as **agonists**—substances that initiate the same response as the chemical normally present in the body—or as **antagonists**—substances that block the response of a given receptor. Figure 10.1 illustrates the action of an agonist and an antagonist drug at a receptor site. A drug's ability to interact with a given receptor type may be judged by three properties: selectivity, affinity, and intrinsic activity.

TABLE 10.1	MANAGING COMMON SIDE EFFECTS OF PSYCHIATRIC MEDICATIONS
Side Effect or Discomfort	**Intervention**
Blurred vision	Reassurance (generally subsides in 2 to 6 wk)
Dry eyes	Artificial tears may be required; increased use of wetting solutions for those wearing contact lens
	Alert ophthalmologist; no eye examination for new glasses for at least 3 wk after a stable dose
Dry mouth and lips	Frequent rinsing of mouth, good oral hygiene, sucking sugarless candies or lozenges, lip balm, lemon juice, and glycerin mouth swabs
Constipation	High-fiber diet; encourage bran, fresh fruits, and vegetables
	Metamucil (must consume at least 16 oz of fluid with dose)
	Increase hydration
	Exercise; increase fluids
	Mild laxative
Urinary hesitancy or retention	Monitor frequently for difficulty with urination, including changes in starting or stopping stream
	Notify prescriber if difficulty develops
	A cholinergic agonist, such as bethanechol, may be required
Nasal congestion	Nose drops, moisturizer, *not* nasal spray
Sinus tachycardia	Assess for infections
	Monitor pulse for rate and irregularities
	Withhold medication and notify prescriber if resting rate exceeds 120 bpm
Decreased libido, anorgasmia, ejaculatory inhibition	Reassurance (reversible); change to another medication
Postural hypotension	Frequent monitoring of lying-to-standing blood pressure during dosage adjustment period, immediate changes and accommodation, measure pulse in both positions; consider change to less antiadrenergic drug
	Advise patient to get up slowly, sit for at least 1 min before standing (dangling legs over side of bed), and stand for 1 min before walking or until lightheadedness subsides
	Increase hydration, avoid caffeine
	Elastic stockings if necessary
	Notify prescriber if symptoms persist or significant blood pressure changes are present; medication may have to be changed if patient does not have impulse control to get up slowly
Photosensitivity	Protective clothing
	Dark glasses
	Use of sun block; remember to cover all exposed areas
Dermatitis	Stop medication usage
	Consider medication change; may require a systemic antihistamine
	Initiate comfort measures to decrease itching
Impaired psychomotor functions	Advise patient to avoid dangerous tasks, such as driving
	Avoid alcohol, which increases this impairment
Drowsiness or sedation	Encourage activity during the day to increase accommodation
	Avoid tasks that require mental alertness, such as driving
	May need to adjust dosing schedule or, if possible, give a single daily dose at bedtime
	May need a cholinergic medication if sedation is the problem
	Avoid driving or operating potentially dangerous equipment
	May need change to less-sedating medication
	Provide quiet and decreased stimulation when sedation is the desired effect
Weight gain and metabolic changes	Exercise and diet teaching
	Caloric control
Edema	Check fluid retention
	Reassurance
	May need a diuretic
Irregular menstruation or amenorrhea	Reassurance (reversible)
	May need to change class of drug
	Reassurance and counseling (does not indicate lack of ovulation)
	Instruct patient to continue birth control measures
Vaginal dryness	Instruct in use of lubricants

Testing New Drugs for Safety and Efficacy

PHASES OF NEW DRUG TESTING
- Phase I: Testing defines the range of dosages tolerated in healthy individuals.
- Phase II: Effects of the drug are studied in a limited number of persons with the disorder. This phase defines the range of clinically effective dosage.
- Phase III: Extensive clinical trials are conducted at multiple sites throughout the country with larger numbers of patients. Efforts focus on corroborating the efficacy identified in phase II. Phase III concludes with a new drug application (NDA) being submitted to the U.S. Food and Drug Administration (FDA).
- Phase IV: Drug studies continue after FDA approval to detect new or rare adverse reactions and potentially new indications. During this period, adverse reactions from the new medication should be reported to the FDA.

IMPLICATIONS FOR MENTAL HEALTH NURSES
- Throughout the phases, side effects and adverse reactions are monitored closely. The studies are tightly controlled, and strict regulations are enforced at each step.
- To prove drug effectiveness, diagnoses must be accurate, strict guidelines are followed, and subjects usually are not taking other medications and do not have complicating illnesses.
- A newly approved drug is approved only for the indications for which it has been tested.

KEYCONCEPT *Agonists* (mimic the neurotransmitter) have all three properties: selectivity, affinity, and intrinsic activity. *Antagonists* (block the receptor) have only selectivity and affinity properties; they do not have intrinsic activity because they produce no biologic response by attaching to the receptor.

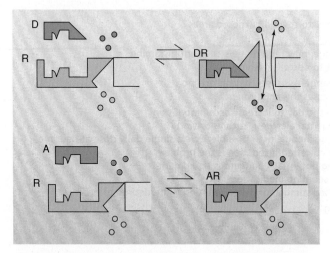

FIGURE 10.1 Agonist and antagonist drug actions at a receptor site. This schematic drawing represents drug–receptor interactions. At the *top*, drug D has the correct shape to fit receptor R, forming a drug–receptor complex, which results in a conformational change in the receptor and the opening of a pore in the adjacent membrane. Drug D is an agonist. At the *bottom*, drug A also has the correct shape to fit the receptor, forming a drug–receptor complex, but in this case, there is no conformational change and therefore no response. Drug A is, therefore, an antagonist.

Some drugs are referred to as **partial agonists** because they have some intrinsic activity (although weak). Because there are no "pure" drugs affecting only one neurotransmitter, most drugs have multiple effects. A drug may act as an agonist for one neurotransmitter and an antagonist for another. Medications that have both agonist and antagonist effects are called *mixed agonist–antagonists*.

Selectivity

Selectivity is the ability of a drug to be specific for a particular receptor. If a drug is highly selective, it will interact only with its specific receptors in the areas of the body where these receptors occur and therefore not affect tissues and organs where its receptors do not occur. Using a "lock-and-key" analogy, only a specific, highly selective key will fit a given lock. The more selective or structurally specific a drug is, the more likely it will affect only the specific receptor for which it is meant. The less selective the drug, the more receptors are affected and the more likely there will be unintended effects or side effects.

Affinity

Affinity is the degree of attraction or strength of the bond between the drug and its biologic target. Affinity is strengthened when a drug has more than one type of chemical bond with its target. If a cell membrane contains several receptors to which a drug will adhere, the affinity is increased. The weaker the chemical bond, the more likely a drug's effects are reversible. Most drugs used in psychiatry adhere to receptors through weak chemical bonds, but some drugs, specifically the monoamine oxidase inhibitors (MAOIs; discussed later), have a different type of bond, called a covalent bond. A covalent bond is formed when two atoms share a pair of electrons. This type of bond is stronger and irreversible at normal temperatures. The effects of the drugs that form covalent bonds are often called "irreversible" because they are long lasting, taking several weeks to resolve. Knowledge of a medication's affinity for receptors and subtypes of receptors may give some indication of the likelihood that specific target symptoms might improve and what side effects might be predicted.

Intrinsic Activity

A drug's ability to interact with a given receptor is its **intrinsic activity**, or the ability to produce a response after it becomes attached to the receptor. Some drugs have selectivity and affinity but produce no response. An important measure of a drug is whether it produces a change in the cell containing the receptor.

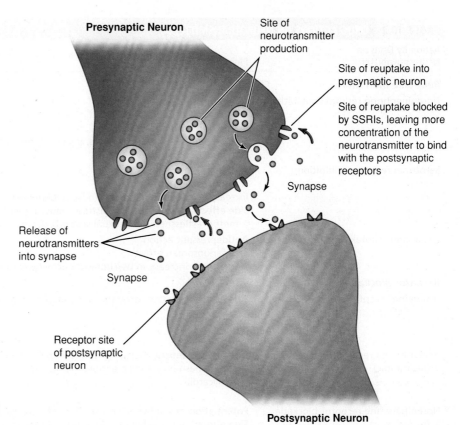

FIGURE 10.2 Reuptake blockade of a carrier molecule for serotonin by a selective serotonin reuptake inhibitor.

Ion Channels

Some drugs directly block the ion channels of the nerve cell membrane. For example, the antianxiety benzodiazepine drugs, such as diazepam (Valium), bind to a region of the gamma-aminobutyric acid (GABA)–receptor chloride channel complex, which helps to open the chloride ion channel. In turn, the activity of GABA is enhanced.

Enzymes

Enzymes are usually proteins that act as catalysts for physiologic reactions and can be targets for drugs. For example, monoamine oxidase is an enzyme required to break down neurotransmitters associated with depression (norepinephrine, serotonin, and dopamine). The MAOI antidepressants inhibit this enzyme, resulting in more neurotransmitter activity.

Carrier Proteins: Uptake Receptors

A **carrier protein** is a membrane protein that transports a specific molecule across the cell membrane. Carrier proteins (also referred to as **uptake receptors**) recognize sites specific for the type of molecule to be transported. When a neurotransmitter is removed from the synapse, specific carrier molecules return it to the presynaptic nerve where

most of it is stored to be used again. Medications specific for this site block or inhibit this transport and therefore increase the activity of the neurotransmitter in the synapse. Figure 10.2 illustrates the reuptake blockade.

Clinical Concepts

Efficacy is the ability of a drug to produce a response and is considered when a drug is selected. The degree of receptor occupancy contributes to the drug's efficacy, but a drug may occupy a large number of receptors and not produce a response. Table 10.2 provides a brief summation of possible physiologic effects from drug actions on specific neurotransmitters. This information should serve only as a guide in predicting side effects because many physical outcomes or behaviors resulting from neural transmission are controlled by multiple receptors and neurotransmitters.

Potency refers to the dose of drug required to produce a specific effect. One drug may be able to achieve the same clinical effect as another drug but at a lower dose, making it more potent. Although the drug given at the lower dose is more potent because both drugs achieve similar effects, they may be considered to have equal efficacy.

In some instances, the effects of medications diminish with time, especially when they are given repeatedly, as in the treatment of chronic psychiatric disorders. This loss of effect is most often a form of physiologic

TABLE 10.2	DRUG ACTIONS ON NEUROTRANSMITTERS	
Action by Drug on Neurotransmitter	**Physiologic Effects**	**Example of Drugs**
Reuptake Inhibition		
Norepinephrine reuptake inhibition	Antidepressant action Potentiation of pressor effects of norepinephrine Interaction with guanethidine Side effects: tachycardia, tremors, insomnia, erectile and ejaculation dysfunction	Desipramine Venlafaxine
Serotonin reuptake inhibition	Antidepressant action Anti-obsessional effect Increase or decrease in anxiety (dose dependent) Side effects: gastrointestinal distress; nausea; headache; nervousness; motor restlessness; and sexual side effects, including anorgasmia	Fluoxetine Fluvoxamine
Dopamine reuptake inhibition	Antidepressant action Antiparkinsonian effect Side effects: increase in psychomotor activity, aggravation of psychosis	Bupropion
Receptor Blockade		
Histamine receptor blockade (H_1)	Side effects: sedation, drowsiness, hypotension, and weight gain	Quetiapine Imipramine Clozapine Olanzapine
Acetylcholine receptor blockade (muscarinic)	Side effects: anticholinergic (dry mouth, blurred vision, constipation, urinary hesitancy and retention, memory dysfunction) and sinus tachycardia	Imipramine Amitriptyline Thioridazine Clozapine
Norepinephrine receptor blockade (α_1 receptor)	Potentiation of antihypertensive effect of prazosin and terazosin Side effects: postural hypotension, dizziness, reflex tachycardia, sedation	Amitriptyline Clomipramine Clozapine
Norepinephrine receptor blockade (α_2 receptor)	Increased sexual desire (yohimbine) Interactions with antihypertensive medications, blockade of the antihypertensive effects of clonidine Side effect: priapism	Amitriptyline Clomipramine Clozapine Trazodone Yohimbine
Norepinephrine receptor blockade (β_1 receptor)	Antihypertensive action (propranolol) Side effects: orthostatic hypotension, sedation, depression, sexual dysfunction (including impotence and decreased ejaculation)	Propranolol
Serotonin receptor blockade (5-HT_{1a})	Antidepressant action Antianxiety effect Possible control of aggression	Trazodone Risperidone Ziprasidone
Serotonin receptor blockade (5-HT_2)	Antipsychotic action Some antimigraine effect Decreased rhinitis Side effects: hypotension, ejaculatory problems	Risperidone Clozapine Olanzapine Ziprasidone
Dopamine receptor blockade (D_2)	Antipsychotic action Side effects: extrapyramidal symptoms, such as tremor, rigidity (especially acute dystonia and parkinsonism); endocrine changes, including elevated prolactin levels	Haloperidol Ziprasidone

adaptation that may develop as the cell attempts to regain homeostatic control to counteract the effects of the drug. There are many reasons for decreased drug effectiveness (Box 10.2).

Desensitization is a rapid decrease in drug effects that may develop in a few minutes of exposure to a drug. This reaction is rare with most psychiatric medications but can occur with some medications used to treat serious side effects (e.g., physostigmine, sometimes used to relieve severe anticholinergic side effects). A rapid decrease can also occur with some drugs because of immediate transformation of the receptor when the drug molecule binds to the receptor. Other drugs cause a decrease in the number of receptors or exhaust the mediators of neurotransmission.

Tolerance is a gradual decrease in the action of a drug at a given dose or concentration in the blood. This decrease may take days or weeks to develop and results in

---

BOX 10.2

Mechanisms Causing Decreases in Medication Effects

- Change in receptors
- Loss of receptors
- Exhaustion of neurotransmitter supply
- Increased metabolism of the drug
- Physiologic adaptation

---

loss of therapeutic effect of a drug. For therapeutic drugs, this loss of effect is often called *treatment refractoriness*. In the abuse of substances such as alcohol or cocaine, tolerance is a part of the addiction (see Chapter 25).

Toxicity generally refers to the point at which concentrations of the drug in the bloodstream are high enough to become harmful or poisonous to the body. Individuals vary widely in their responses to medications. Some patients experience adverse reactions more easily than others. The **therapeutic index** is the ratio of the maximum nontoxic dose to the minimum effective dose. A high therapeutic index means that there is a large range between the dose at which the drug begins to take effect and a dose that would be toxic to the body. Drugs with a low therapeutic index have a narrow range.

This concept of toxicity has some limitations. The range can be affected by drug tolerance. For example, when tolerance develops, the person increases the dosage, which makes him or her more susceptible to an accidental suicide. The therapeutic index of a medication also may be greatly changed by the coadministration of other medications or drugs. For example, alcohol consumed with most CNS-depressant drugs will have added depressant effects, greatly increasing the likelihood of toxicity or death.

Pharmacokinetics: How the Body Acts on the Drugs

The field of pharmacokinetics studies the process of how drugs are acted on by the body through absorption, distribution, metabolism (biotransformation), and excretion. Pharmacokinetics for specific medications are always explained in a drug's PI. Together with the principles of pharmacodynamics, this information is helpful in monitoring drug effects and predicting behavioral response.

> **KEYCONCEPT** **Pharmacokinetics** is the process by which a drug is absorbed, distributed, metabolized and eliminated by the body.

Absorption and Routes of Administration

The first phase of **absorption** is the movement of the drug from the site of administration into the plasma.

The typical routes of administration of psychiatric medications include oral (tablet, capsule, and liquid), deltoid and gluteal intramuscular (IM; short- and long-acting agents), and intravenous (IV; rarely used for treatment of the primary psychiatric disorder but instead for rapid treatment of adverse reactions). A transdermal patch antidepressant and oral inhalation are also available. The advantages and disadvantages of each route and the subsequent effects on absorption are listed in Table 10.3.

Drugs taken orally are usually the most convenient for the patient; however, this route is also the most variable because absorption can be slowed or enhanced by a number of factors. Taking certain drugs orally with food or antacids may slow the rate of absorption or change the amount of the drug absorbed. For example, antacids containing aluminum salts decrease the absorption of most antipsychotic drugs; thus, antacids must be given at least 1 hour before administration or 2 hours after.

Oral preparations are absorbed from the gastrointestinal tract into the bloodstream through the portal vein and then to the liver. They may be metabolized within the gastrointestinal wall or liver before reaching the rest of the body. This is called the **first-pass effect**. The consequence of first-pass effect is that only a fraction of the drug reaches systemic circulation. Oral dosages are adjusted for the first-pass effect. That is, the dose of the oral form is significantly higher than the IM or IV formulations.

Bioavailability describes the amount of the drug that actually reaches systemic circulation unchanged. The route by which a drug is administered significantly affects bioavailability. With some oral drugs, the amount of drug entering the bloodstream is decreased by first-pass metabolism, and bioavailability is lower. On the other hand, some rapidly dissolving oral medications have increased bioavailability.

Distribution

Distribution of a drug is the amount of the drug found in various tissues, particularly the target organ at the site of drug action. Factors that affect distribution include the size of the organ; amount of blood flow or perfusion within the organ; solubility of the drug; plasma **protein binding** (the degree to which the drug binds to plasma proteins); and anatomic barriers, such as the blood–brain barrier, that the drug must cross. A psychiatric drug may have rapid absorption and high bioavailability, but if it does not cross the blood–brain barrier to reach the CNS, it is of little use. Table 10.4 provides a summary of how some significant factors affect distribution. Two of these factors, **solubility** (ability of a drug to dissolve) and protein binding, warrant additional discussion with regard to how they relate to psychiatric medications.

TABLE 10.3	SELECTED FORMS AND ROUTES OF PSYCHIATRIC MEDICATIONS		
Preparation and Route	**Examples**	**Advantages**	**Disadvantages**
Oral tablet	Basic preparation for most psychopharma-cologic agents, including antidepressants, antipsychotics, mood stabilizers, anxiolytics, and so on	Usually most convenient	Variable rate and extent of absorption, depending on the drug May be affected by the contents of the intestines May show first-pass metabolism effects May not be easily swallowed by some individuals
Oral liquid	Also known as concentrates Many antipsychotics, such as haloperidol, chlorpromazine, thioridazine, risperidone The antidepressant fluoxetine Antihistamines, such as diphenhydramine Mood stabilizers, such as lithium citrate	Ease of incremental dosing Easily swallowed In some cases, more quickly absorbed	More difficult to measure accurately Depending on drug: • Possible interactions with other liquids such as juice, forming precipitants • Possible irritation to mucosal lining of mouth if not properly diluted
Rapidly dissolv-ing tablet	Atypical antipsychotics, such as olanzapine, risperidone, asenapine	Dissolves almost instantaneously in mouth	Patient needs to remember to have completely dry hands and to place tablet in mouth immediately Tablet should not linger in the hand Handy for people who have trouble swallowing or for patients who let medication linger in the cheek for later expectoration Can be taken when water or other liquid is unavailable
Intramuscular	Some antipsychotics, such as ziprasidone, haloperidol, and chlorpromazine Anxiolytics, such as lorazepam Anticholinergics, such as benztropine mesylate No antidepressants No mood stabilizers	More rapid acting than oral preparations No first-pass metabolism	Injection-site pain and irritation Some medications may have erratic absorption if heavy muscle tissue at the site of injection is not in use
Intramuscular depot (or long acting)	Risperidone (Risperdal Consta), paliperidone palmitate (Invega Sustenna), olanzapine (Zyprexa Relprevv), aripiprazole (Ability Maintena), haloperidol decanoate, fluphenazine decanoate	May be more convenient for some individuals who have difficulty following medication regimens	Pain at injection site
Intravenous	Anticholinergics, such as diphenhydramine, benztropine mesylate Anxiolytics, such as diazepam, lorazepam, and chlordiazepoxide	Rapid and complete availability to systemic circulation	Inflammation of tissue surrounding site Often inconvenient for patient and uncomfortable Continuous dosage requires use of a constant-rate IV infusion
Transdermal patch	Antidepressant, selegiline	Avoid daily oral ingestion of medication	Skin irritation
Oral inhalation	Conventional antipsychotic, loxapine	Rapidly absorbed to treat psychomotor agitation	Bronchospasm

IV, intravenous.

Solubility

Substances may cross a membrane in a number of ways, but passive diffusion is by far the simplest. To do this, the drug must dissolve in the structure of the cell membrane. Therefore, the solubility of a drug is an important characteristic. Being soluble in lipids allows a drug to cross most of the membranes in the body, and the tissues of the CNS are less permeable to water-soluble drugs than are other areas of the body. Most psychopharmacologic agents are lipid soluble and easily cross the blood–brain barrier. However, this characteristic means that psychopharmacologic agents also cross the placenta; consequently, most are contraindicated during pregnancy.

TABLE 10.4	FACTORS AFFECTING DISTRIBUTION OF A DRUG
Factor	**Effect on Drug Distribution**
Size of the organ	Larger organs require more drug to reach a concentration level equivalent to other organs and tissues.
Blood flow to the organ	The more blood flow to and within an organ (perfusion), the greater the drug concentration. The brain has high perfusion.
Solubility of the drug	The greater the solubility of a drug within a tissue, the greater its concentration.
Plasma protein binding	If a drug binds well to plasma proteins, particularly to albumin, it will stay in the body longer but have a slower distribution.
Anatomic barriers	Both the gastrointestinal tract and the brain are surrounded by layers of cells that control the passage or uptake of substances. Lipid-soluble substances are usually readily absorbed and pass the blood–brain barrier.

Protein Binding

Of considerable importance is the degree to which a drug binds to plasma proteins. Only unbound or "free" drugs act at the receptor sites. High protein binding reduces the concentration of the drug at the receptor sites. However, because the binding is reversible, as the unbound drug is metabolized, more drug is released from the protein bonds. Drugs are also released from storage in the fat depots. These processes can prolong the duration of action of the drug. When patients stop taking their medication, they often do not experience an immediate return of symptoms because they continue to receive the drug as it is released from storage sites in the body.

Metabolism

Metabolism, also called **biotransformation**, is the process by which a drug is altered and broken down into smaller substances, known as metabolites. Most metabolism occurs in the liver, but it can also occur in the kidneys, lungs, and intestines. Lipid-soluble drugs eventually become more water soluble, so they may be readily excreted.

The cytochrome P450 (CYP450) system, a set of microsomal enzymes usually found in the liver is important in the metabolism of a drug. There are more than 50 enzymes, but most of the metabolism occurs in only a few of them. The functioning of these enzymes is influenced by drugs and other chemical substances. Some drugs slow down an enzyme's ability to work and other drugs speed up an enzyme's ability to metabolize drugs. When the enzyme is inhibited from functioning, a drug may not be metabolized as expected, but instead be active longer. That leads to increase in the plasma level which may become toxic. On the other hand, some drugs speed up enzyme metabolism resulting in the drug leaving the body faster than expected with a concentrations below the therapeutic level. A **drug–drug interaction** can occur if one drug inhibits an enzyme system causing another drug to become toxic. The PI will inform the nurse which drugs should not be given together in order to prevent a drug-drug interaction.

Excretion

Excretion refers to the removal of drugs from the body either unchanged or as metabolites. **Clearance** refers to the total volume of blood, serum, or plasma from which a drug is completely removed per unit of time to account for the excretion. The **half-life** of a drug provides a measure of the expected rate of clearance. Half-life refers to the time required for plasma concentrations of the drug to be reduced by 50%. For most drugs, the rate of excretion slows, but the half-life remains unchanged. It usually takes four half-lives or more of a drug in total time for more than 90% of a drug to be eliminated.

Drugs bound to plasma proteins do not cross the glomerular filter freely. These lipid-soluble drugs are passively reabsorbed by diffusion across the renal tubule and thus are not rapidly excreted in the urine. Because many psychiatric medications are protein bound and lipid soluble, most of their excretion occurs through the liver where they are excreted in the bile and delivered into the intestine. Lithium and gabapentin, mood stabilizers, are notable examples of renal excretion. Any impairment in renal function or renal disease may lead to toxic symptoms.

Dosing refers to the administration of medication over time, so that therapeutic levels may be achieved or maintained without reaching toxic levels. In general, it is necessary to give a drug at intervals no greater than the half-life of the medication to avoid excessive fluctuation of concentration in the plasma between doses. With repeated dosing, a certain amount of the drug is accumulated in the body.

Steady-state plasma concentration, or simply **steady state**, occurs when absorption equals excretion and the therapeutic level plateaus. The rate of accumulation is determined by the half-life of the drug. Drugs generally reach steady state in four to five times the elimination half-life. However, because elimination or excretion rates may vary significantly in any individual, fluctuations may still occur, and dose schedules may need to be modified.

Individual Variations in Drug Effects

Many factors affect drug absorption, distribution, metabolism, and excretion. These factors may vary among individuals, depending on their age, genetics, and ethnicity.

Age

Pharmacokinetics are significantly altered at the extremes of the life cycle. Gastric absorption changes as individuals age. Gastric pH increases, and gastric emptying decreases. Gastric motility slows and splanchnic circulation is reduced. Normally, these changes do not significantly impair oral absorption of a medication, but addition of common conditions, such as diarrhea, may significantly alter and reduce absorption. Malnutrition, cancer, and liver disease decrease the production of the primary protein albumin. More free drug is acting in the system, producing higher blood levels of the medication and potentially toxic effects. The activity of hepatic enzymes also slows with age. As a result, the ability of the liver to metabolize medications may slow as much as a fourfold decrease between the ages of 20 and 70 years. Production of albumin by the liver generally declines with age. Changes in the parasympathetic nervous system produce a greater sensitivity in older adults to anticholinergic side effects, which are more severe with this age group.

Renal function also declines with age. Creatinine clearance in a young adult is normally 100 to 120 mL/min, but after age 40 years, this rate declines by about 10% per decade (Glassock, 2009). Medical illnesses, such as diabetes and hypertension, may further the loss of renal function. When creatinine clearance falls below 30 mL/min, the excretion of drugs by the kidneys is significantly impaired, and potentially toxic levels may accumulate.

Ethnopsychopharmacology

Ethnopsychopharmacology investigates cultural variations and differences that influence the effectiveness of pharmacotherapies used in mental health. These differences include genetics and psychosocial factors. Studies of identical and nonidentical twins show that much of the individual variability in elimination half-life of a given drug is genetically determined. For example, some individuals of Asian descent produce higher concentrations of acetaldehyde with alcohol use than do those of European descent, resulting in a higher incidence of adverse reactions such as flushing and palpitations. Asians often require one half to one third the dose of antipsychotic medications and lower doses of antidepressants than whites require (Silva, 2013). More research is needed to understand fully the underlying mechanisms and to identify groups that may require different approaches to medication treatment.

FAME & FORTUNE

Abraham Lincoln (1809–1865)
Civil War President

PUBLIC PERSONA

The 16th president of the United States led a nation through turbulent times during a civil war. Ultimately, his leadership preserved the United States as the republic we know today despite periods of "melancholy" or depression throughout his life. At times, he had strong thoughts of committing suicide. Yet he had an enormous ability to cope with depression, especially in later life. He generally coped with the depression through his work, humor, fatalistic resignation, and even religious feelings. He generally did not let his depression interfere with his work as president. In 1841, he wrote of his ongoing depression, "A tendency to melancholy... let it be observed, is a misfortune, not a fault" (letter to Mary Speed, September 27, 1841).

PERSONAL REALITIES

Lincoln's depression began in early childhood and can be traced to multiple causes. There is evidence that there was a genetic basis because both of his parents had depression. Lincoln was partially isolated from his peers because of his unique interests in politics and reading. Additionally, he suffered through the deaths of his younger brother, mother, and older sister. There is speculation that Lincoln's depression may have dated to Thomas Lincoln's cold treatment of his son. There is also evidence that Abraham Lincoln took a commonly prescribed medication called *blue mass*, which contained mercury. Consequently, some speculate that he had mercury poisoning.

Source: Hirschhorn, N., Feldman, R. G., & Greaves, I. A. (2001). Abraham Lincoln's blue pills: Did our 16th president suffer from mercury poisoning? *Perspectives in Biology and Medicine, 44*(3), 315–322.

PHASES OF DRUG TREATMENT AND THE NURSE'S ROLE

Phases of drug treatment include initiation, stabilization, maintenance, and discontinuation of the medication. The following explains the role of the nurse in these phases.

Initiation Phase

Before the initiation of medications, patients must undergo several assessments.

- A psychiatric evaluation to determine the diagnosis and target symptoms
- A nursing assessment that includes cultural beliefs and practices (see Chapter 9)
- Physical examination and indicated laboratory tests, often including baseline determinations such as a complete blood count (CBC), liver and kidney function tests, electrolyte levels, urinalysis, and possibly

thyroid function tests and electrocardiography (ECG), to determine whether a physical condition may be causing the symptoms and to establish that it is safe to initiate use of a particular medication.

During the initiation of medication, the nurse assesses, observes, and monitors the patient's response to the medication; teaches the patient about the action, dosage, frequency of administration, and side effects; and develops a plan for ongoing contact with clinicians. The first medication dose should be treated as if it were a "test" dose. Patients should be monitored for adverse reactions such as changes in blood pressure, pulse, or temperature; changes in mental status; allergic reactions; dizziness; ataxia; or gastric distress. If any of these symptoms develop, they should be reported to the prescriber.

Stabilization Phase

During stabilization, the prescriber adjusts or titrates the medication dosage to achieve the maximum amount of improvement with a minimum of side effects. Psychiatric–mental health nurses assess for improvements in the target symptoms and for the appearance of side effects. If medications are being increased rapidly, such as in a hospital setting, nurses must closely monitor temperature, blood pressure, pulse, mental status, common side effects, and unusual adverse reactions.

In the outpatient setting, nurses focus on patient education, emphasizing the importance of taking the medication, expected outcomes, and potential side effects. Patients need to know how and when to take their medications, how to minimize any side effects, and which side effects require immediate attention. A plan should be developed for patients and their families to clearly identify what to do if adverse reactions develop. The plan, which should include emergency telephone numbers or available emergency treatment, should be reviewed frequently.

Therapeutic drug monitoring is most important in this phase of treatment. Many medications used in psychiatry improve target symptoms only when a therapeutic level of medication has been obtained in the individual's blood. Some medications, such as lithium, have a narrow therapeutic range and must be monitored frequently and accurately. Nurses must be aware of when and how these levels are to be determined and assist patients in learning these procedures. Because of protein binding and lipid solubility, most medications do not have obtainable plasma levels that are clinically relevant. However, plasma levels of these medications may still be requested to evaluate further such issues as absorption and adverse reactions.

Sometimes the first medication chosen does not adequately improve the patient's target symptoms. In such cases, use of the medication will be discontinued, and treatment with a new medication will be started. Medications may also be changed when adverse reactions or seriously uncomfortable side effects occur or these effects substantially interfere with the individual's quality of life. Nurses should be familiar with the pharmacokinetics of both drugs to be able to monitor side effects and possible drug–drug interactions during this change.

At times, an individual may show only partial improvement from a medication, and the prescriber may try an **augmentation** strategy by adding another medication. For example, a prescriber may add a mood stabilizer, such as lithium, to an antidepressant to improve the effects of the antidepressant. **Polypharmacy**, using more than one group from a class of medications, is increasingly being used as an acceptable strategy with most psychopharmacologic agents to match the drug action to the neurochemical needs of the patient. Nurses must be familiar with the potential effects, side effects, drug interactions, and rationale for the treatment regimen.

Maintenance Phase

After the individual's target symptoms have improved, medications are usually continued to prevent **relapse** or return of the symptoms. In some cases, this may occur despite the patient's continued use of the medication. Patients must be educated about their target symptoms and have a plan of action if the symptoms return. In other cases, the patient may experience medication side effects. The psychiatric–mental health nurse has a central role in assisting individuals to monitor their own symptoms, identify emerging side effects, manage psychosocial stressors, and avoid other factors that may cause the medications to lose effect.

Discontinuation Phase

Some psychiatric medications will be discontinued; others will not. Some require a tapered discontinuation, which involves slowly reducing dosage while monitoring closely for reemergence of the symptoms. Some psychiatric disorders, such as mild depression, respond to treatment and do not recur. Other disorders, such as schizophrenia, usually require lifetime medication. Discontinuance of some medications, such as controlled substances, produces withdrawal symptoms; discontinuance of others does not.

MAJOR PSYCHOPHARMACOLOGIC DRUG CLASSES

Major classes of psychiatric drugs include antipsychotics, mood stabilizers, antidepressants, antianxiety and sedative–hypnotic medications, and stimulants.

Antipsychotic Medications

Antipsychotic medications can be thought of as "newer" and "older" medications. Newer or **atypical antipsychotics** appear to be equally or more effective but have fewer side effects than the traditional older agents. The term *typical or* **conventional antipsychotics** identifies the older antipsychotic drugs. Table 10.5 provides a list of selected antipsychotics.

Indications and Mechanism of Action

Antipsychotic medications are indicated for schizophrenia, mania, and autism and to treat the symptoms of psychosis, such as hallucinations, delusions, bizarre behavior, disorganized thinking, and agitation. (These symptoms are described more fully in later chapters.) These medications also reduce aggressiveness and inappropriate behavior associated with psychosis. Within the typical antipsychotics, haloperidol and pimozide are approved for treating patients with Tourette's syndrome,

reducing the frequency and severity of vocal tics. Some of the typical antipsychotics, particularly chlorpromazine, are used as antiemetics or for postoperative intractable hiccoughs.

The atypical antipsychotic medications differ from the typical antipsychotics in that they block serotonin receptors more potently than the dopamine receptors. The differences between the mechanism of action of the typical and atypical antipsychotic helps to explain their differences in terms of effect on target symptoms and in the degree of side effects they produce.

Pharmacokinetics

Antipsychotic medications administered orally have a variable rate of absorption complicated by the presence of food, antacids, and smoking and even the coadministration of anticholinergics, which slow gastric motility. Clinical effects begin to appear in about 30 to 60 minutes. Absorption after IM administration is less variable because this method avoids the first-pass effects. Therefore, IM

TABLE 10.5	ANTIPSYCHOTIC MEDICATIONS			
Generic (Trade) Drug Name	Usual Dosage Range	Half-Life	Therapeutic Blood Level	Approximate Equivalent Dosage (mg)
Atypical Antipsychotics				
Aripiprazole (Abilify)	5–30 mg/d	75–94 h	Not available	Not available
Aripiprazole (Maintena)	200–400 mg	30–47 days	Not available	Not available
Clozapine (Clozaril)	300–900 mg/d	4–12 h	141–204 ng/mL	50
Risperidone (Risperdal) Oral	2–8 mg/d	20 h	Not available	1
Risperdal Consta	25–50 mg every 2 weeks		Not available	
Olanzapine (Zyprexa)	5–15 mg/d 2.5–10 mg/d IM	21–54 h	Not available	Not available
Olanzapine (Relprevv)	150–300 mg every 2–4 weeks	30 days	Not available	Not available
Paliperidone (Invega Extended Release)	3–12 mg once daily in AM	23 h	Not available	Not available
Paliperidone (Invega Sustenna)	117 mg monthly	29–49 days	Not available	Not available
Paliperidone Invega Trinza	273–819 q 3 months	84–139 days	Not available	Not available
Quetiapine fumarate (Seroquel)	150–750 mg/d	7 h	Not available	Not available
Ziprasidone HCl (Geodon)	40–160 mg/d 10–20 mg/d IM	7 h	Not available	Not available
Iloperidone (Fanapt)	6–12 mg BID	18–33 h	Not available	Not available
Asenapine (Saphris)	5–10 mg BID, (sublingual)	24 h	Not available	Not available
Lurasidone HCL (Latuda)	40–80 mg	18 h	Not available	Not available
Conventional (Typical) Antipsychotics				
Chlorpromazine	50–1200 mg/d	2–30 h	30–100 mg/mL	100
Fluphenazine	2–20 mg/d	4.5–15.3 h	0.2–0.3 ng/mL	2
Perphenazine	12–64 mg/d	Unknown	0.8–12.0 ng/mL	10
Trifluoperazine	5–40 mg/d	47–100 h	1–2.3 ng/mL	5
Thiothixene (Navane)	5–60 mg/d	34 h	2–20 ng/mL	4
Loxapine (Adasuve)	10 mg/d (inhalation)	7 h	Not available	
Haloperidol (Haldol)	2–60 mg/d	21–24 h	5–15 ng/mL	2

BID, twice a day; IM, intramuscular.

administration produces greater bioavailability. It is important to remember that IM medications are absorbed more slowly when patients are immobile because erratic absorption may occur when muscles are not in use, which is especially important to remember when administering IM antipsychotic medication to patients who are restrained. For example, a patient's arm may be more mobile than the buttocks. The deltoid has better blood perfusion, and the medication will be more readily absorbed, especially with use.

Metabolism of these drugs occurs almost entirely in the liver with the exception of paliperidone (Invega Sustenna), which is not extensively metabolized by the liver but is excreted largely unchanged through the kidney and lurasidone (Latuda), which is excreted through the urine and feces. Careful observance of concurrent medication use, including prescribed, over-the-counter, and substances of abuse, is required to avoid drug–drug interactions. Atypical antipsychotic concentrations may be affected by other drugs such as paroxetine and fluoxetine.

Excretion of these substances tends to be slow. Most antipsychotics have a half-life of 24 hours or longer, but many also have active metabolites with longer half-lives. These two effects make it difficult to predict elimination time, and metabolites of some of these agents may be found in the urine months later. When a medication is discontinued, the adverse reactions may not immediately subside. The patient may continue to experience and sometimes need treatment for the adverse reactions for several days. Similarly, patients who discontinue their antipsychotic drugs may still derive therapeutic benefit for several days to weeks after drug discontinuation.

High lipid solubility, accumulation in the body, and other factors have also made it difficult to correlate blood levels with therapeutic effects. Table 10.5 shows the therapeutic ranges available for some of the antipsychotic medications. The potency of the antipsychotics also varies widely and is of specific concern when considering typical antipsychotic drugs. As Table 10.5 indicates, 50 mg of clozapine is roughly equivalent to 1 mg of risperidone and 5 mg of trifluoperazine.

Long-Acting Preparations

Currently, in the United States, atypical and conventional antipsychotics are available in long-acting forms. These antipsychotics are administered by injection once every 2 to 12 weeks. Whereas the long-acting injectable atypical antipsychotics (risperidone, paliperidone, olanzapine, and aripiprazole) are water-based suspensions, the conventional antipsychotics are oil-based solutions. Long-acting injectable medications maintain a fairly constant blood level between injections. Because they bypass problems with gastrointestinal absorption and first-pass metabolism, this method may enhance therapeutic outcomes for the patient. The use of these medications increases the likelihood of adhering to a prescribed medication regimen.

Nurses should be aware that the injection site may become sore and inflamed if certain precautions are not taken. The oil-based injections (fluphenazine and haloperidol) are viscous liquids. For these injections, a large-gauge needle (at least 21 gauge) should be used. Because oil-based medications are meant to remain in the injection site, the needle should be dry, and deep IM injections should be given by the Z-track method. (Note: Do not massage the injection site. Rotate sites and document in the patient's record.) Manufacturer recommendations should be followed.

Side Effects, Adverse Reactions, and Toxicity

Various side effects and interactions can occur with antipsychotics, with the conventional (typical) antipsychotics producing different side effects than the atypical antipsychotics. The side effects vary largely based on their degree of attraction to different neurotransmitter receptors and their subtypes. See Box 10.3 for assessments that should be completed before starting an antipsychotic to reduce the risk of adverse reactions.

Cardiovascular Side Effects

Cardiovascular side effects include orthostatic hypotension and prolongation of the QTc interval. Orthostatic hypotension is very common and depends on the degree of blockade of α-adrenergic receptors. Typical and atypical antipsychotics have been associated with prolonged QTc intervals and should be used cautiously in patients who have increased QTc intervals or are taking other medications that may prolong the QTc interval (Beach,

---

BOX 10.3

Recommended Assessments Before and During Antipsychotic Therapy

- Weigh all patients and track BMI during treatment
  - Determine if overweight (BMI 25–29.9) or obese (BMI ≥30)
  - Monitor BMI monthly for first 3 months; then quarterly
- Obtain baseline personal and family history of diabetes, obesity, dyslipidemia, hypertension, and cardiovascular disease
- Get waist circumference (at umbilicus)
  - Men: >40 inches (102 cm)
  - Women: >35 inches (88)
- Monitor BP, fasting plasma glucose, and fasting lipid profile within 3 months and then annually (more frequently for patients with diabetes or have gained >5% of initial weight)
  - Prediabetes (fasting plasma glucose 100–125 mg/dL)
  - Diabetes (fasting plasma glucose >126 mg/dL)
  - Hypertension (BP >140/90 mm Hg)
  - Dyslipidemia (increased total cholesterol [>200 mg], decreased HDL, and increased LDL)

BMI, body mass index; BP, blood pressure; HDL, high-density lipoprotein; LDL, low-density lipoprotein.

Celano, Noseworthy, Januzzi, & Huffman, 2013). Other cardiovascular side effects from typical antipsychotics have been rare, but occasionally they cause ECG changes that have a benign or undetermined clinical effect.

Anticholinergic Side Effects

Anticholinergic side effects resulting from blockade of acetylcholine are another common side effect associated with antipsychotic drugs. Dry mouth, slowed gastric motility, constipation, urinary hesitancy or retention, vaginal dryness, blurred vision, dry eyes, nasal congestion, and confusion or decreased memory are examples of these side effects. Interventions for decreasing the impact of these side effects are outlined in Table 10.1.

This group of side effects occurs with many of the medications used for psychiatric treatment. Using more than one medication with anticholinergic effects often increases the symptoms. Older patients are often most susceptible to a potential toxicity that results from high blockade of acetylcholine. This toxicity is called an *anticholinergic crisis* and is described more fully, along with its treatment, in Chapter 21.

Weight Gain

Weight gain is a common side effect of the atypical antipsychotics, particularly clozapine and olanzapine (Zyprexa), which can cause a weight gain of up to 20 lb within 1 year. Ziprasidone (Geodon), aripiprazole (Abilify), and lurasidone (Latuda) are associated with little to no weight gain. If a patient becomes overweight or obese, switching to another antipsychotic should be considered and weight control interventions implemented.

Diabetes

One of the more serious side effects is the risk of type II diabetes. The FDA has determined that all atypical antipsychotics increase the risk for type II diabetes. Nurses should routinely assess for emerging symptoms of diabetes and alert the prescriber of these symptoms (see Box 10.3).

Sexual Side Effects

Sexual side effects result primarily from the blockade of dopamine in the tuberoinfundibular pathways of the hypothalamus. As a result, blood levels of prolactin may increase, particularly with risperidone and the typical antipsychotics. Increased prolactin causes breast enlargement and rare but potential galactorrhea (milk production and flow), decreased sexual drive, amenorrhea, menstrual irregularities, and increased risk for growth in preexisting breast cancers. Other sexual side effects include retrograde ejaculation (backward flow of semen), erectile dysfunction, and anorgasmia.

Blood Disorders

Blood dyscrasias are rare but have received renewed attention since the introduction of clozapine. Agranulocytosis is an acute reaction that causes the individual's white blood cell count to drop to very low levels, and concurrent neutropenia, a drop in neutrophils in the blood, develops. In the case of the antipsychotics, the medication suppresses the bone marrow precursors to blood factors. The exact mechanism by which the drugs produce this effect is unknown. The most notable symptoms of this disorder include high fever, sore throat, and mouth sores. Although benign elevations in temperature have been reported in individuals taking clozapine, no fever should go uninvestigated. Untreated agranulocytosis can be life threatening. Although agranulocytosis can occur with any of the antipsychotics, the risk with clozapine is greater than with the other antipsychotics. Therefore, prescription of clozapine requires weekly blood samples for the first 6 months of treatment and then every 2 weeks after that for as long as the drug is taken. Drawing of these samples must continue for 4 weeks after clozapine use has been discontinued. If sore throat or fever develops, medications should be withheld until a leukocyte count can be obtained. Hospitalization, including reverse isolation to prevent infections, is usually required. Agranulocytosis is more likely to develop during the first 18 weeks of treatment. Some research indicates that it is more common in women (Novartis, 2013).

Neuroleptic Malignant Syndrome

Neuroleptic malignant syndrome (NMS) is a serious complication that may result from antipsychotic medications. Characterized by rigidity and high fever, NMS is a rare condition that may occur abruptly with even one dose of medication. Temperature must always be monitored when administering antipsychotics, especially high-potency medications. This condition is discussed more fully in Chapter 21.

Other Side Effects

Photosensitivity reactions to antipsychotics, including severe sunburns or rash, most commonly develop with the use of low-potency typical medications. Sun block must be worn on all areas of exposed skin when taking these drugs. In addition, sun exposure may cause pigmentary deposits to develop, resulting in discoloration of exposed areas, especially the neck and face. This discoloration may progress from a deep orange color to a blue gray. Skin exposure should be limited and skin tone changes reported to the prescriber. Pigmentary deposits, retinitis pigmentosa, may also develop on the retina of the eye.

Antipsychotics may also lower the seizure threshold. Patients with an undetected seizure disorder may experience seizures early in treatment. Those who have a preexisting condition should be monitored closely.

Medication-Related Movement Disorders

Medication-related movement disorders are side effects or adverse reactions that are commonly caused by typical antipsychotic medications but less commonly with atypical antipsychotic drugs. These disorders of abnormal motor movements can be divided into two groups: acute **extrapyramidal symptoms (EPS)**, which develop early in the course of treatment (sometimes after just one dose), and chronic syndromes, which develop from longer exposure to antipsychotic drugs.

Acute Extrapyramidal Symptoms

Acute EPS are acute abnormal movements that include dystonia, pseudoparkinsonism, and akathisia. They develop early in treatment, sometimes from as little as one dose. Although the abnormal movements are treatable, they are at times dramatic and frightening, causing physical and emotional impairments that often prompt patients to stop taking their medication.

Dystonia, sometimes referred to as an *acute dystonic reaction*, is impaired muscle tone that generally is the first EPS to occur, usually within a few days of initiating use of an antipsychotic. Dystonia is characterized by involuntary muscle spasms that lead to abnormal postures, especially of the head and neck muscles. Acute dystonia occurs most often in young men, adolescents, and children. Patients usually first report a thick tongue, tight jaw, or stiff neck. Dystonia can progress to a protruding tongue, oculogyric crisis (eyes rolled up in the head), torticollis (muscle stiffness in the neck, which draws the head to one side with the chin pointing to the other), and laryngopharyngeal constriction. Abnormal postures of the upper limbs and torso may be held briefly or sustained. In severe cases, the spasms may progress to the intercostal muscles, producing more significant breathing difficulty for patients who already have respiratory impairment from asthma or emphysema. The treatment is the administration of a medication such as the anticholinergic agents (Table 10.6).

TABLE 10.6	DRUG THERAPIES FOR ACUTE MEDICATION-RELATED MOVEMENT DISORDERS		
Agents	Typical Dosage Ranges	Routes Available	Common Side Effects
Anticholinergics			
Benztropine (Cogentin)	2–6 mg/d	PO, IM, IV	Dry mouth, blurred vision, slowed gastric motility causing constipation, urinary retention, increased intraocular pressure; overdose produces toxic psychosis
Trihexyphenidyl	4–15 mg/d	PO	Same as benztropine, plus gastrointestinal distress Older adults are most prone to mental confusion and delirium
Biperiden (Akineton)	2–8 mg/d	PO	Fewer peripheral anticholinergic effects Euphoria and increased tremor may occur
Antihistamines			
Diphenhydramine	25–50 mg QID to 400 mg daily	PO, IM, IV	Sedation and confusion, especially in older adults
Dopamine Agonists			
Amantadine	100–400 mg daily	PO	Indigestion, decreased concentration, dizziness, anxiety, ataxia, insomnia, lethargy, tremors, and slurred speech may occur with higher doses Tolerance may develop on fixed dose
β-Blockers			
Propranolol (Inderal)	10 mg TID to 120 mg daily	PO	Hypotension and bradycardia Must monitor pulse and blood pressure Do not stop abruptly because doing so may cause rebound tachycardia
Benzodiazepines			
Lorazepam (Ativan)	1–2 mg IM 0.5–2 mg PO	PO, IM	All may cause drowsiness, lethargy, and general sedation or paradoxical agitation Confusion and disorientation in older adults
Diazepam (Valium)	2–5 mg tid	PO, IV	Most side effects are rare and will disappear if dose is decreased
Clonazepam (Klonopin)	1–4 mg/d	PO	Tolerance and withdrawal are potential problems

IM, intramuscular; IV, intravenous; PO, oral; QID, four times a day; TID, three times a day.

Drug-induced parkinsonism is sometimes referred to as **pseudoparkinsonism** because its presentation is identical to Parkinson's disease. The difference is that the activity of dopamine is blocked in pseudoparkinsonism, and in Parkinson's disease, the cells of the basal ganglia are destroyed. Older patients are at the greatest risk for experiencing pseudoparkinsonism (Lopez et al., 2013). Symptoms include the classic triad of rigidity, slowed movements (akinesia), and tremor. The rigid muscle stiffness is usually seen in the arms. Akinesia can be observed by the loss of spontaneous movements, such as the absence of the usual relaxed swing of the arms while walking. In addition, masklike facies or loss of facial expression and a decrease in the ability to initiate movements also are present. Usually, tremor is more pronounced at rest, but it can also be observed with intentional movements, such as eating. If the tremor becomes severe, it may interfere with the patient's ability to eat or maintain adequate fluid intake. Hypersalivation is possible as well. Pseudoparkinsonism symptoms may occur on one or both sides of the body and develop abruptly or subtly but usually within the first 30 days of treatment. The treatment is the reduction in dosage or a change of antipsychotic that has less affinity for the dopamine receptor. Anticholinergic medication is sometimes given.

Akathisia is characterized by an inability to sit still or restlessness and is more common in middle-aged patients. The person will pace, rock while sitting or standing, march in place, or cross and uncross the legs. All of these repetitive motions have an intensity that is frequently beyond the explanation of the individual. In addition, akathisia may be present as a primarily subjective experience without obvious motor behavior. This subjective experience includes feelings of anxiety, jitteriness, or the inability to relax, which the individual may or may not be able to communicate. It is extremely uncomfortable for a person experiencing akathisia to be forced to sit still or be confined. These symptoms are sometimes misdiagnosed as agitation or an increase in psychotic symptoms. If an antipsychotic medication is given, the symptoms will not abate and will often worsen. Differentiating akathisia from agitation may be aided by knowing the person's symptoms before the introduction of medication. Whereas psychotic agitation does not usually begin abruptly after antipsychotic medication use has been started, akathisia may occur after administration. In addition, the nurse may ask the patient if the experience is felt primarily in the muscles (akathisia) or in the mind or emotions (agitation).

Akathisia is the most difficult acute medication-related movement disorder to relieve. It does not usually respond well to anticholinergic medications. The pathology of akathisia may involve more than just the extrapyramidal motor system. It may include serotonin changes that also affect the dopamine system. The usual approach to treatment is to change or reduce the antipsychotic. A number of medications are used to reduce symptoms, including β-adrenergic blockers, anticholinergics, antihistamines, and low-dose antianxiety agents (Laoutidis & Luckhaus, 2014). The β-adrenergic blockers, such as propranolol (Inderal), given in doses of 30 to 120 mg/d, are the most successful.

A number of nursing interventions reduce the impact of these syndromes. Individuals with acute EPS need frequent reassurance that this is not a worsening of their psychiatric condition but instead is a treatable side effect of the medication. They also need validation that what they are experiencing is real and that the nurse is concerned and will be responsive to changes in these symptoms. Physical and psychological stress appears to increase the symptoms and further frighten the patient; therefore, decreasing stressful situations becomes important. These symptoms are often physically exhausting for the patient, and the nurse should ensure that the patient receives adequate rest and hydration. Because tremors, muscle rigidity, and motor restlessness may interfere with the individual's ability to eat, the nurse may need to assist the patient with eating and drinking fluids to maintain nutrition and hydration.

Risk factors for acute EPS include previous episodes of EPS. The nurse should listen closely when patients say they are "allergic" or have had "bad reactions" to antipsychotic medications. Often, they are describing one of the medication-related movement disorders, particularly dystonia, rather than a rash or other allergic symptoms.

Chronic Syndromes: Tardive Dyskinesia

Chronic syndromes develop from long-term use of antipsychotics. They are serious and affect about 20% of the patients who receive typical antipsychotics for an extended period. These conditions are typically irreversible and cause significant impairment in self-image, social interactions, and occupational functioning. Early symptoms and mild forms may go unnoticed by the person experiencing them.

Tardive dyskinesia, the most well-known of the chronic syndromes, involves irregular, repetitive involuntary movements of the mouth, face, and tongue, including chewing, tongue protrusion, lip smacking, puckering of the lips, and rapid eye blinking. Abnormal finger movements are common as well. In some individuals, the trunk and extremities are also involved, and in rare cases, irregular breathing and swallowing lead to belching and grunting noises. These symptoms usually begin no earlier than after 6 months of treatment or when the medication is reduced or withdrawn. Once thought to be irreversible, considerable controversy now exists as to whether this is true.

Part of the difficulty in determining the irreversibility of tardive dyskinesia is that any movement disorder that persists after discontinuation of antipsychotic medication has been described as tardive dyskinesia. Atypical forms are now receiving more attention because some researchers believe they may have different underlying mechanisms of causation. Some of these forms of the disorder appear to remit spontaneously. Symptoms of what is now called *withdrawal tardive dyskinesia* appear when use of an antipsychotic medication is reduced or discontinued and remit spontaneously in 1 to 3 months. Tardive dystonia and tardive akathisia have also been described. Both appear in a manner similar to the acute syndromes but continue after the antipsychotic medication has been withdrawn. More research is needed to determine whether these syndromes are distinctly different in origin and outcome.

The risk for experiencing tardive dyskinesia increases with age. Although the prevalence of tardive dyskinesia averages 15% to 20%, the rate rises to 50% to 70% in older patients receiving antipsychotic medications; in addition, cumulative incidence of tardive dyskinesia appears to increase 5% per year of continued exposure to antipsychotic medications (Woods et al., 2010). Women are at higher risk than men. Anyone receiving antipsychotic medication can develop tardive dyskinesia. Risk factors are summarized in Box 10.4. The causes of tardive dyskinesia remain unclear. No one medication relieves the symptoms. Dopamine agonists, such as bromocriptine, and many other drugs have been tried with little success. Dietary precursors of acetylcholine, such as lecithin and vitamin E supplements, may prove to be beneficial.

The best approach to treatment remains avoiding the development of the chronic syndromes. Preventive measures include use of atypical antipsychotics, using the lowest possible dose of typical medication, minimizing use of as-needed (PRN) medication, and closely monitoring individuals in high-risk groups for development of the symptoms of tardive dyskinesia. All members of the mental health treatment team who have contact with individuals taking antipsychotics for longer than 3 months must be alert to the risk factors and earliest possible signs of chronic medication-related movement disorders.

Monitoring tools, such as the Abnormal Involuntary Movement Scale (AIMS) (see Appendix B), should be used routinely to standardize assessment and provide the earliest possible recognition of the symptoms. Standardized assessments should be performed at a minimum of 3- to 6-month intervals. The earlier the symptoms are recognized, the more likely they will resolve if the medication can be changed or its use discontinued. Newer, atypical antipsychotic medications have a much lower risk of causing tardive dyskinesia and are increasingly being considered first-line medications for treating patients with schizophrenia. Other medications are under development to provide alternatives that limit the risk for tardive dyskinesia.

Mood Stabilizers (Antimania Medications)

Mood stabilizers, or antimania medications, are psychopharmacologic agents used primarily for stabilizing mood swings, particularly those of mania in bipolar disorders. Lithium, the oldest, is the gold standard of treatment for acute mania and maintenance of bipolar disorders. Not all respond to lithium, and increasingly, other drugs are being used as first-line agents. Anticonvulsants, calcium channel blockers, adrenergic blocking agents, and atypical antipsychotics are used for mood stabilization.

Lithium

Lithium, a naturally occurring element, is effective in only about 40% of patients with bipolar disorder. Although lithium is not a perfect drug, a great deal is known regarding its use—it is inexpensive, it has restored stability to the lives of thousands of people, and it remains the gold standard of bipolar pharmacologic treatment.

Indications and Mechanisms of Action

Lithium is indicated for symptoms of mania characterized by rapid speech, flight of ideas (jumping from topic to topic), irritability, grandiose thinking, impulsiveness, and agitation. Because it has mild antidepressant effects, lithium is used in treating depressive episodes of bipolar illness. It is also used as augmentation in patients experiencing major depression that has only partially responded to antidepressants alone. Lithium also has been shown to be helpful in reducing impulsivity and aggression in certain psychiatric patients.

The exact action by which lithium improves the symptoms of mania is unknown, but it is thought to exert multiple neurotransmitter effects, including enhancing serotonergic transmission, increasing synthesis of norepinephrine, and blocking postsynaptic dopamine. Lithium is actively transported across cell membranes, altering sodium transport in both nerve and muscle cells. It replaces sodium in the sodium–potassium pump and is retained more readily than sodium inside the cells. Conditions that alter sodium content in the body, such

---

BOX 10.4

Risk Factors for Tardive Dyskinesia

- Age older than 50 years
- Female
- Affective disorders, particularly depression
- Brain damage or dysfunction
- Increased duration of treatment
- Standard antipsychotic medication
- Possible—higher doses of antipsychotic medication

as vomiting, diuresis, and diaphoresis, also alter lithium retention (Malhi, Tanious, Das, Coulston, & Berk, 2013).

Pharmacokinetics

Lithium carbonate is available orally in capsule, tablet, and liquid forms. Slow-release preparations are also available. Lithium is readily absorbed in the gastric system and may be taken with food, which does not impair absorption. Peak blood levels are reached in 1 to 4 hours, and the medication is usually completely absorbed in 8 hours. Slow-release preparations are absorbed at a slower, more variable rate.

Lithium is not protein bound, and its distribution into the CNS across the blood–brain barrier is slow. The onset of action is usually 5 to 7 days and may take as long as 2 weeks. The elimination half-life is 8 to 12 hours and is 18 to 36 hours in individuals whose blood levels have reached steady state and whose symptoms are stable. Lithium is almost entirely excreted by the kidneys but is present in all body fluids. Conditions of renal impairment or decreased renal function in older patients decrease lithium clearance and may lead to toxicity. Several medications affect renal function and therefore change lithium clearance. See Chapter 20 for a list of these and other medication interactions with lithium. About 80% of lithium is reabsorbed in the proximal tubule of the kidney along with water and sodium. In conditions that cause sodium depletion, such as dehydration caused by fever, strenuous exercise, hot weather, increased perspiration, and vomiting, the kidneys attempts to conserve sodium. Because lithium is a salt, the kidneys retain lithium as well, leading to increased blood levels and potential toxicity. Significantly increasing sodium intake causes lithium levels to fall.

Lithium is usually administered in doses of 300 mg two to three times daily. Because it is a drug with a narrow therapeutic range or index, blood levels are monitored frequently during acute mania, and the dosage is increased every 3 to 5 days. These increases may be slower in older adult patients or patients who experience uncomfortable side effects. Blood levels should be monitored 12 hours after the last dose of medication. In the hospital setting, nurses should withhold the morning dose of lithium until the serum sample is drawn to avoid falsely elevated levels. Individuals who are at home should be instructed to have their blood drawn in the morning about 12 hours after their last dose and before they take their first dose of medication. During the acute phases of mania, blood levels of 0.8 to 1.4 mEq/L are usually attained and maintained until symptoms are under control. The therapeutic range for lithium is narrow, and patients in the higher end of that range usually experience more uncomfortable side effects. During maintenance, the dosage is reduced, and dosages are adjusted to maintain blood levels of 0.4 to 1 mEq/L.

Lithium clears the body relatively quickly after discontinuation of its use. Withdrawal symptoms are rare, but occasional anxiety and emotional lability have been reported. It is important to remember that almost half of the individuals who discontinue lithium treatment abruptly experience a relapse of symptoms within a few weeks. Some research suggests that discontinuation of the use of lithium for individuals whose symptoms have been stable may lead to lithium's losing its effectiveness when use of the medication is restarted. Patients should be warned of the risks in abruptly discontinuing their medication and should be advised to consider the options carefully in consultation with their prescriber.

Side Effects, Adverse Reactions, and Toxicity

At lower therapeutic blood levels, side effects from lithium are relatively mild. These reactions correspond with peaks in plasma concentrations of the medication after administration, and most subside during the first few weeks of therapy. Frequently, individuals taking lithium complain of excessive thirst and an unpleasant metallic-like taste. Sugarless throat lozenges may be useful in minimizing this side effect. Other common side effects include increased frequency of urination, fine head tremor, drowsiness, and mild diarrhea. Weight gain occurs in about 20% of the individuals taking lithium. Nausea may be minimized by taking the medication with food or by use of a slow-release preparation. However, slow-release forms of lithium increase diarrhea. Muscle weakness, restlessness, headache, acne, rashes, and exacerbation of psoriasis have also been reported. See Chapter 20 for a summary of selected nursing interventions to minimize the impact of common side effects associated with lithium treatment. Patients most frequently discontinued their own medication use because of concerns with mental slowness, poor concentration, and memory problems.

As blood levels of lithium increase, the side effects of lithium become more numerous and severe. Early signs of lithium toxicity include severe diarrhea, vomiting, drowsiness, muscular weakness, and lack of coordination. Lithium should be withheld and the prescriber consulted if these symptoms develop. Lithium toxicity can easily be resolved in 24 to 48 hours by discontinuing the medication, but hemodialysis may be required in severe situations. See Chapter 20 for a summary of the side effects and symptoms of toxicity associated with various blood levels of lithium.

Monitoring of creatinine concentration, thyroid hormones, and CBC every 6 months during maintenance therapy helps to assess the occurrence of other potential adverse reactions. Kidney damage is considered an uncommon but potentially serious risk of long-term lithium treatment. This damage is usually reversible after discontinuation of the lithium use. A gradual rise in serum creatinine and decline in creatinine clearance indicate the development of renal dysfunction. Individuals with preexisting kidney dysfunction are susceptible to lithium toxicity.

Lithium may alter thyroid function, usually after 6 to 18 months of treatment. About 30% of the individuals taking lithium exhibit elevations in thyroid-stimulating hormone (TSH), but most do not show suppression of circulating thyroid hormone. Thyroid dysfunction from lithium treatment is more common in women, and some individuals require the addition of thyroxine to their care. During maintenance, TSH levels may be monitored. Nurses should observe for dry skin, constipation, bradycardia, hair loss, cold intolerance, and other symptoms of hypothyroidism. Other endocrine system effects result from hypoparathyroidism, which increases parathyroid hormone levels and calcium. Clinically, this change is not significant, but elevated calcium levels may cause mood changes, anxiety, lethargy, and sleep disturbances. These symptoms may erroneously be attributed to depression if hypercalcemia is not investigated.

Lithium use must be avoided during pregnancy because it has been associated with birth defects, especially when administered during the first trimester. If lithium is given during the third trimester, toxicity may develop in a newborn, producing signs of hypotonia, cyanosis, bradykinesia, cardiac changes, gastrointestinal bleeding, and shock. Diabetes insipidus may persist for months. Lithium is also present in breast milk, and women should not breastfeed while taking lithium. Women expecting to become pregnant should be advised to consult with a physician before discontinuing use of birth control methods.

Anticonvulsants

In the psychiatric mental health area, anticonvulsants are commonly used to treat patients with bipolar disorder and are considered mood stabilizers. The following discussion highlights the use of anticonvulsants as mood stabilizers in the treatment of bipolar disorder.

Indications and Mechanisms of Action

Valproate (valproic acid; Depakote), carbamazepine (Equetro), and lamotrigine (Lamictal) have FDA approval for the treatment of bipolar disorder, mania, or mixed episodes (see Chapter 20). In general, the anticonvulsant mood stabilizers have many actions, but their effects on ion channels, reducing repetitive firing of action potentials in the nerves, most directly decrease manic symptoms. No one action has successfully accounted for the anticonvulsants' ability to stabilize mood (Bialer, 2012).

Pharmacokinetics

Valproic acid is rapidly absorbed, but the enteric coating of divalproex sodium adds a delay of as long as 1 hour. Peak serum levels occur in about 1 to 4 hours. The liquid form (sodium valproate) is absorbed more rapidly and peaks in 15 minutes to 2 hours. Food appears to slow absorption but does not lower bioavailability of the drug.

Carbamazepine is absorbed in a somewhat variable manner. The liquid suspension is absorbed more quickly than the tablet form, but food does not appear to interfere with absorption. Peak plasma levels occur in 2 to 6 hours. Because high doses influence peak plasma levels and increase the risk for side effects, carbamazepine should be given in divided doses two or three times a day. The suspension, which has higher peak plasma levels and lower trough levels, must be given more frequently than the tablet form.

These medications cross easily into the CNS, move into the placenta as well, and are associated with an increased risk for birth defects. Carbamazepine, valproic acid, and lamotrigine are metabolized in the liver.

Teaching Points

Nurses need to educate patients about potential drug interactions, especially with nonprescription medications. Nurses can also inform other health care practitioners who may be prescribing medication that these patients are taking carbamazepine. It is important to note that oral contraceptives may become ineffective, and female patients should be advised to use other methods of birth control.

Side Effects, Adverse Reactions, and Toxicity of Anticonvulsants

The most common side effects of carbamazepine are dizziness, drowsiness, tremor, visual disturbance, nausea, and vomiting. These side effects may be minimized by initiating treatment in low doses. Patients should be advised that these symptoms will diminish, but care should be taken when changing positions or performing tasks that require visual alertness. Giving the drug with food may diminish nausea. Adverse reactions include rare aplastic anemia, agranulocytosis, severe rash, rare cardiac problems, and SIADH (syndrome of inappropriate secretion of the diuretic hormone) caused by hyponatremia.

Valproic acid also causes gastrointestinal disturbances, tremor, and lethargy. In addition, it can produce weight gain and alopecia (hair loss). These symptoms are transient and should diminish with the course of treatment. Dietary supplements of zinc and selenium may be helpful to patients experiencing hair loss. Constipation and urinary retention occur in some individuals. Nurses should monitor urinary output and assist patients to increase fluid consumption to decrease constipation.

Benign skin rash, sedation, blurred or double vision, dizziness, nausea, vomiting, and other gastrointestinal symptoms are side effects of lamotrigine. In rare cases, lamotrigine (Lamictal) produces severe, life-threatening rashes that usually occur within 2 to 8 weeks of treatment. This risk is highest in children. Use of lamotrigine should be immediately discontinued if a rash is noted.

Transient elevations in liver enzymes occur with both carbamazepine and valproic acid but symptoms of hepatic injury rarely occur. If the patient reports abnormal pain or shows signs of jaundice, the prescriber should be notified immediately. Several blood dyscrasias are associated with carbamazepine, including aplastic anemia, agranulocytosis, and leukopenia. Patients should be advised to report fever, sore throat, rash, petechiae, or bruising immediately. In addition, Patients should be advised of the importance of completing routine blood tests throughout treatment. The risks for aplastic anemia and agranulocytosis with carbamazepine use still require close monitoring of CBCs during treatment. Valproate and its derivatives have had a similar course of development.

Antidepressant Medications

Medications classified as antidepressants are used not only for the treatment of depression but also in the treatment of anxiety disorders, eating disorders, and other mental health states (Table 10.7). They are used very cautiously in persons with bipolar disorder because of the possibility of precipitating a manic episode. The exact neuromechanism for the antidepressant effect is unknown in all of them. The onset of action also varies considerably and appears to depend on factors outside of steady-state plasma levels. Initial improvement with some antidepressants, such as the SSRIs, may appear within 7 days, but complete relief of symptoms may take several weeks. Antidepressants should not be discontinued abruptly because of uncomfortable symptoms that result. Discontinuance of use of these medications requires slow tapering. Individuals taking these medications should be cautioned not to abruptly stop using them without consulting their prescriber. Antidepressant medications are well absorbed from the gastrointestinal system; however, some individual variations exist. Most of the antidepressants are metabolized in the liver, so that other drugs that are metabolized in the liver may decrease or increase antidepressant levels. All of these medications have a "boxed warning" for increased risk of suicidal behavior in children and adolescents compared with placebo.

Serotonin syndrome, or serotonin intoxication syndrome, can occur if there is an overactivity of serotonin or an impairment of the serotonin metabolism. Concomitant medications such as triptans used to treat migraines also can increase the serotonergic activity. With the advent of widely used antidepressants targeting the serotonergic systems, symptoms of this serious side effect should be assessed. Symptoms include mental status changes (hallucinations, agitation, coma), autonomic instability (tachycardia, hyperthermia, changes in blood pressure), neuromuscular problems (hyperreflexia, incoordination), and gastrointestinal disturbance (nausea, vomiting, diarrhea). Serotonin syndrome can be life threatening. The treatment for serotonin syndrome is discontinuation of the medication and symptom management.

Selective Serotonin Reuptake Inhibitors

The serotonergic system is associated with mood, emotion, sleep, and appetite and is implicated in the control of numerous emotional, physical, and behavioral functions (see Chapter 6). Decreased serotonergic neurotransmission has been proposed to play a key role in depression. In 1988, fluoxetine (Prozac) was the first of a class of drugs that acted "selectively" on serotonin, one group of neurotransmitters associated with depression. Other similarly selective medications, sertraline (Zoloft), paroxetine (Paxil), and fluvoxamine (Luvox), soon followed. The newest SSRI is escitalopram oxalate (Lexapro).

All of the SSRIs inhibit the reuptake of serotonin by blocking its transport into the presynaptic neuron, which in turn increases the concentration of synaptic serotonin. The concentration of synaptic serotonin is controlled directly by its reuptake; thus, drugs blocking serotonin transport have been successfully used for the treatment of depression and other conditions associated with serotonergic activity.

The SSRIs also have other properties that account for the common side effects, which include headache, anxiety, insomnia, transient nausea, vomiting, and diarrhea. Sedation may also occur, especially with paroxetine. Most often, these medications are given in the morning, but if daytime sedation occurs, they may be given in the evening. Higher doses, especially of fluoxetine, are more likely to produce sedation. Tolerance develops to the common side effects of nausea and dizziness. These symptoms, along with sexual dysfunction, sedation, diastolic hypertension, and increased perspiration, tend to be dose dependent, occurring more frequently at higher doses. Other common side effects include insomnia, constipation, dry mouth, tremors, blurred vision, and asthenia or muscle weakness.

TABLE 10.7	ANTIDEPRESSANT MEDICATIONS			
Generic (Trade) Drug Name	Usual Dosage Range (mg/d)	Half-Life (h)		Therapeutic Blood Level (ng/mL)
Selective Serotonin Reuptake Inhibitors				
Citalopram (Celexa)	20–50	35		Not available
Escitalopram (Lexapro)	10–20	27–32		Not available
Fluoxetine (Prozac)	20–80	2–9 days		72–300
Fluvoxamine (Luvox)	50–300	17–22		Not available
Paroxetine (Paxil)	10–50	10–24		Not available
Sertraline (Zoloft)	50–200	24		Not available
Serotonin Norepinephrine Reuptake Inhibitors				
Desvenlafaxine (Pristiq Extended Release)	50	11		Not available
Duloxetine (Cymbalta)	40–60	8–17		Not available
Levomilnacipran (Fetzima)	40–120	12		Not available
Nefazodone	100–600	2–4		Not available
Venlafaxine (Effexor)	75–375	5–11		100–500
Norepinephrine Dopamine Reuptake Inhibitor				
Bupropion (Wellbutrin)	200–450	8–24		10–29
α₂ Antagonist				
Mirtazapine (Remeron)	15–45	20–40		Not available
Others				
Trazodone	150–600	4–9		650–1,600
Vilazodone (Viibryd)	10–40	25		Not available
Vortioxetine (Brintellix)	5–20	66		Not available
Tricyclic Antidepressants				
Amitriptyline (Elavil)	50–300	31–46		110–250
Amoxapine	50–600	8		200–500
Clomipramine (Anafranil)	25–250	19–37		80–100
Imipramine (Tofranil)	30–300	11–25		200–350
Desipramine (Norpramin)	25–300	12–24		125–300
Doxepin	25–300	8–24		100–200
Nortriptyline (Aventyl, Pamelor)	30–100	18–44		50–150
Protriptyline (Vivactil)	15–60	67–89		100–200
Tetracyclic				
Maprotiline (Ludiomil)	50–225	21–25		200–300
Monoamine Oxidase Inhibitors				
Isocarboxazid (Marplan)	20–60	Not available		Not available
Phenelzine (Nardil)	15–90	24 (effect lasts 3–4 d)		Not available
Tranylcypromine (Parnate)	10–60	24 (effect lasts 3–10 d)		Not available
Selegiline (Emsam)	6–12 mg/24 h	25%–50% delivered in 24 h		Not available

Sexual dysfunction is a relatively common side effect with most antidepressants. Erectile and ejaculation disturbances occur in men and anorgasmia in women. This side effect is often difficult to assess if the nurse has not obtained a sexual history before initiation of use of the medication. Anorgasmia is particularly common with the SSRIs and often goes unreported, frequently because nurses and other health care providers do not ask.

Serotonin Norepinephrine Reuptake Inhibitors

Decreased activity of the neurotransmitter norepinephrine is also associated with depression and anxiety disorders. Venlafaxine (Effexor), nefazodone, duloxetine (Cymbalta), and desvenlafaxine (Pristiq) prevent the reuptake of both serotonin and norepinephrine at the presynaptic site and are classified as serotonin norepinephrine reuptake inhibitors (SNRIs). Desipramine (Norpramin) is technically a tricyclic antidepressant

(TCA) and is usually categorized as such. It works, however, on both serotonin and norepinephrine, so it can also be considered an SNRI.

The side effects are similar to those of the SSRIs; there is also a risk for an associated increase in blood pressure. Elevations in blood pressure have been described, and nurses should monitor blood pressure, especially in patients who have a history of hypertension. Venlafaxine (Effexor) has little effect on acetylcholine and histamine; thus, it creates only mild sedation and anticholinergic symptoms. This medication is often used if a depressed patient is sleeping excessively and reports little energy. The most common side effects of nefazodone include dry mouth, nausea, dizziness, muscle weakness, constipation, and tremor. It is unlikely to cause sexual disturbance. Nefazodone also has a "boxed warning" for hepatic failure and should not be used in those with acute liver disease.

Norepinephrine Dopamine Reuptake Inhibitors

Bupropion (Wellbutrin, Zyban) inhibits reuptake of norepinephrine, serotonin, and dopamine. Wellbutrin is indicated for depression and Zyban for nicotine addiction. The smoking cessation medication, Zyban, is given at a lower dose than Wellbutrin. Patients should not take Zyban if they are taking Wellbutrin. Bupropion has a chemical structure unlike any of the other antidepressants and somewhat resembles a few of the psychostimulants. Bupropion's activating effects may be experienced as agitation or anxiety by some patients. Others also experience insomnia and appetite suppression. For a few individuals, bupropion has produced psychosis, including hallucinations and delusions. Most likely, this is secondary to overstimulation of the dopamine system. Bupropion is contraindicated for people with seizure disorders and those at risk for seizures. The rate of seizures is similar to that with the SSRIs and mirtazapine but is lower than the rate associated with the older antidepressants. Most important, bupropion has a lower incidence of sexual dysfunction and often is used in individuals who are experiencing these side effects with other antidepressants (GlaxoSmithKline, 2013).

α_2 Antagonist

Mirtazapine (Remeron) boosts norepinephrine or noradrenaline and serotonin by blocking α_2 adrenergic presynaptic receptors on a serotonin receptor ($5HT_{2A}$; $5HT_{2C}$, $5HT_3$). This is a different action than the other antidepressants. A histamine receptor, which is also blocked, may explain its sedative side effect. Mirtazapine is indicated for depression. Side effects include sedation (at lower doses), dizziness, weight gain, dry mouth, constipation, and change in urinary functioning.

Other Antidepressants

Trazodone blocks serotonin 2A receptor potently and blocks the serotonin reuptake pump less potently. It is indicated for depression. Sedation is a very common side effect. Other side effects include weight gain, nausea, vomiting, constipation, dizziness, fatigue, incoordination, and tremor.

Other newly FDA approved antidepressants target other receptor sites. For example, vilazodone (Viibryd) is a serotonin reuptake inhibitor and a partial agonist of $5\text{-}HT_{1A}$; vortioxetine (Brintellix) inhibits reuptake of serotonin and norepinephrine but is also a partial agonist to $5\text{-}HT_{1A}$. These subtle differences translate into subtle clinical effects.

Tricyclic Antidepressants

The TCAs were once the primary medication used for treating depression. With the introduction of the SSRIs and other previously discussed antidepressants, the use of TCAs has significantly declined. In most cases, these medications are as effective as the other drugs, but they have more serious side effects and a higher lethal potential (see Table 10.7). The TCAs act on a variety of neurotransmitter systems, including the norepinephrine and serotonin reuptake systems.

Pharmacokinetics

The TCAs are highly bound to plasma proteins, which make the association between blood levels and therapeutic clinical effects difficult. However, some plasma ranges have been established (see Table 10.7). Most of the TCAs have active metabolites that act in much the same manner as the parent drug. Most of these antidepressants may be given in a once-daily single dose. If the medication causes sedation, this dose should be given at bedtime.

Side Effects, Adverse Reactions, and Toxicity

Because the TCAs act on several neurotransmitters in addition to serotonin and norepinephrine, these drugs have many unwanted effects. With the TCAs, sedation, orthostatic hypotension, and anticholinergic side effects are the most common sources of discomfort for patients receiving these medications. Other side effects of the TCAs include tremors, restlessness, insomnia, nausea and vomiting, confusion, pedal edema, headache, and seizures. Blood dyscrasias may also occur, and any fever, sore throat, malaise, or rash should be reported to the prescriber. Interventions to assist in minimizing these side effects are listed in Table 10.1.

The TCAs have the potential for cardiotoxicity. Symptoms include prolongation of cardiac conduction that may worsen preexisting cardiac conduction problems. The TCAs are contraindicated with second-degree atrioventricular block and should be used cautiously in patients who have other cardiac problems. Occasionally, they may precipitate heart failure, myocardial infarction, arrhythmias, and stroke.

Antidepressants that block the dopamine (D_2) receptor, such as amoxapine, have produced symptoms of NMS. Mild forms of EPS and endocrine changes, including galactorrhea and amenorrhea, may develop.

Monoamine Oxidase Inhibitors

The MAOIs, as their name indicates, inhibit monoamine oxidase (MAO), an enzyme that breaks down the biogenic amine neurotransmitters serotonin, norepinephrine, and others. By inhibiting this enzyme, serotonin and norepinephrine activity is increased in the synapse. In the United States, there are three oral formulations:

phenelzine (Nardil), tranylcypromine (Parnate), and isocarboxazid (Marplan) and one available by a transdermal patch: selegiline (Emsam). These are considered MAOIs because they form strong covalent bonds to block the enzyme monoamine oxidase. This inhibition of this enzyme increases with repeated administration of these medications and takes at least 2 weeks to resolve after discontinuation of use of the medication.

The major problem with the MAOIs is their interaction with tyramine-rich foods and certain medications that can result in a hypertensive crisis. All of the MAOIs have dietary modification except the 6 mg/24 hours dose of selegiline. The enzyme monoamine is important in the breakdown of dietary amines (e.g., tyramine). When the enzyme is inhibited, tyramine, a precursor for dopamine, increases in the nerve cells. Tyramine has a vasopressor action that induces hypertension. If the individual ingests food that contains high levels of tyramine while taking MAOIs, severe headaches, palpitation, neck stiffness and soreness, nausea, vomiting, sweating, hypertension, stroke, and, in rare instances, death may result. Patients who are taking MAOIs are prescribed a low-tyramine diet (Table 10.8).

In addition to food restrictions, many prescription and nonprescription medications that stimulate the

TABLE 10.8	EXAMPLE OF A TYRAMINE-RESTRICTED DIET	
Category of Food	**Foods with Tyramine**	**Food Allowed**
Nonrefrigerated food	Spoiled foods or foods not refrigerated, handled, or stored properly	Food that is handled and stored properly
Cheese	All aged and mature cheeses, especially strong, aged, or processed cheeses such as American processed, cheddar, Colby, blue, brie, mozzarella, and parmesan; yogurt, sour cream	Cottage cheese, cream cheese, ricotta cheese
Meat, fish, and poultry	• Air dried, aged, and fermented meats, sausages, and salamis • Beef or chicken liver • Pepperoni • Dried and pickled herring • Anchovies, meat extracts, meat tenderizers • Meats prepared with tenderizers.	Fresh meat, poultry, and fish, including fresh processed meats (e.g., lunch meats, hot dogs, breakfast sausage, and cooked sliced ham)
Fruits and vegetables	Broad bean pods (Fava bean pods)	All other vegetables
Alcoholic beverages	All tap beers and other beers that have not been pasteurized; red wine, sherry, liqueurs; some alcohol-free and reduced alcohol beer	White wines may not contain tyramine.
Miscellaneous foods	Marmite concentrated yeast extract Sauerkraut Soy sauce and other soybean condiments	Soy milk Pizzas from commercial chain restaurants prepared with cheeses low in tyramine

Source: U.S. Department of Health and Human Services. Food & Drug Administration. Avoid food-drug interactions. A guide from the National Consumers League and U.S. Food and Drug Administration. Publication no. (FDA) CDER 10-1933. www.fda.gov/drugs. Retrieved September 24, 2015; Parke-Davis. (2007). Nardil. http://www.accessdata.fda.gov/Scripts/cder/drugsatfda/index.cfm?fuseaction=Search.Label_ApprovalHistory#labelinfo. Retrieved September 24, 2015.

sympathetic nervous system (sympathomimetic) produce the same risk for hypertensive crisis as do foods containing tyramine. The nonprescription medication interactions involve primarily diet pills and cold remedies. Patients should be advised to check the labels of any nonprescription drugs carefully for a warning against use with antidepressants, especially the MAOIs, and then consult their prescriber before consuming these medications. In addition, symptoms of other serious drug–drug interactions may develop, such as coma, hypertension, and fever, which may occur when patients receive meperidine (Demerol) while taking an MAOI. Patients should notify other health care providers, including dentists, that they are taking an MAOI before being prescribed or given any other medication.

The MAOIs frequently produce dizziness, headache, insomnia, dry mouth, blurred vision, constipation, nausea, peripheral edema, urinary hesitancy, muscle weakness, forgetfulness, and weight gain. Older patients are especially sensitive to the side effect of orthostatic hypotension and require frequent assessment of lying and standing blood pressures. They may be at risk for falls and subsequent bone fractures and require assistance in changing position. Sexual dysfunction, including decreased libido, impotence, and anorgasmia, also is common with MAOIs.

Antianxiety and Sedative–Hypnotic Medications

Sometimes called *anxiolytics*, antianxiety medications, such as buspirone, and sedative–hypnotic medications, such as lorazepam (Ativan), come from various pharmacologic classifications, including barbiturates, benzodiazepines, nonbenzodiazepines, and nonbarbiturate sedative–hypnotic medications, such as chloral hydrate. These drugs represent some of the most widely prescribed medications today for the short-term relief of anxiety or anxiety associated with depression.

Benzodiazepines

Commonly prescribed benzodiazepines include alprazolam (Xanax), lorazepam (Ativan), diazepam (Valium), chlordiazepoxide (Librium), flurazepam, and triazolam (Halcion). Although benzodiazepines are known to enhance the effects of the inhibitory neurotransmitter GABA, their exact mechanisms of action are not well understood. Of the various benzodiazepines in use to relieve anxiety (and treat insomnia), oxazepam (Serax) and lorazepam (Ativan) are often preferred for patients with liver disease and for older patients because of their short half-lives.

Pharmacokinetics

The variable rate of absorption of the benzodiazepines determines the speed of onset. Table 10.9 provides relative indications of the speed of onset, from very fast to slow, for some of the commonly prescribed benzodiazepines. Whereas chlordiazepoxide (Librium) and diazepam (Valium) are slow, erratic, and sometimes incompletely absorbed when given intramuscularly, lorazepam (Ativan) is rapidly and completely absorbed when given intramuscularly.

All of the benzodiazepines are highly lipid soluble and highly protein bound. They are distributed throughout the body and enter the CNS quickly. Other drugs that compete for protein-binding sites may produce drug–drug interactions. The degree to which each of these drugs is lipid soluble affects its duration of action. Most of these drugs have active metabolites, but the degree of activity of each metabolite affects duration of action and elimination half-life. Most of these drugs vary markedly

TABLE 10.9	ANTIANXIETY AND SEDATIVE–HYPNOTIC MEDICATIONS		
Generic (Trade) Drug Name	Usual Dosage Range (mg/d)	Half-Life (h)	Speed of Onset After Single Dose
Benzodiazepines			
Diazepam (Valium)	4–40	30–100	Very fast
Chlordiazepoxide (Librium)	15–100	50–100	Intermediate
Clorazepate (Tranxene)	15–60	30–200	Fast
Lorazepam (Ativan)	2–8	10–20	Slow-intermediate
Oxazepam	30–120	3–21	Slow-intermediate
Alprazolam (Xanax)	0.5–10	12–15	Intermediate
Clonazepam (Klonopin)	1.5–20	18–50	Intermediate
Nonbenzodiazepine			
Buspirone	15–30	3–11	Very slow

in length of half-life. Oxazepam and lorazepam have no active metabolites and thus have shorter half-lives. Elimination half-lives may also be sustained for obese patients when using diazepam, chlordiazepoxide, and halazepam (Paxipam).

Side Effects, Adverse Reactions, and Toxicity

The most commonly reported side effects of benzodiazepines result from the sedative and CNS depression effects of these medications. Drowsiness, intellectual impairment, memory impairment, ataxia, and reduced motor coordination are common adverse reactions. If used for sleep, many of these medications, especially the long-acting benzodiazepines, produce significant "hangover" effects experienced on awakening. Older patients receiving repeated doses of medications such as flurazepam at bedtime may experience paradoxical confusion, agitation, and delirium, sometimes after the first dose. In addition, daytime fatigue, drowsiness, and cognitive impairments may continue while the person is awake. For most patients, the effects subside as tolerance develops; however, alcohol increases all of these symptoms and potentiates the CNS depression. Individuals using these medications should be warned to be cautious when driving or performing other tasks that require mental alertness. If these tasks are part of the person's work requirements, another medication may be chosen. Administered intravenously, benzodiazepines often cause phlebitis and thrombosis at the IV sites, which should be monitored closely and changed if redness or swelling develops.

Because tolerance develops to most of the CNS depressant effects, individuals who wish to experience the feeling of "intoxication" from these medications may be tempted to increase their own dosage. Psychological dependence is more likely to occur when using these medications for a longer period. Abrupt discontinuation of the use of benzodiazepines may result in a recurrence of the target symptoms, such as rebound insomnia or anxiety. Other withdrawal symptoms appear rapidly, including tremors, increased perspiration, palpitations, increased sensitivity to light, abdominal discomfort or pain, and elevations in systolic blood pressure. These symptoms may be more pronounced with the short-acting benzodiazepines, such as lorazepam. Gradual tapering is recommended for discontinuing use of benzodiazepines after long-term treatment. When tapering short-acting medications, the prescriber may switch the patient to a long-acting benzodiazepine before discontinuing use of the short-acting drug.

Individual reactions to the benzodiazepines appear to be associated with sensitivity to their effects. Some patients feel apathy, fatigue, tearfulness, emotional lability, irritability, and nervousness. Symptoms of depression may worsen. The psychiatric–mental health nurse should closely monitor these symptoms when individuals are receiving benzodiazepines as adjunctive treatment for anxiety that coexists with depression. Gastrointestinal disturbances, including nausea, vomiting, anorexia, dry mouth, and constipation, may develop. These medications may be taken with food to ease the gastrointestinal distress.

Older patients are particularly susceptible to incontinence, memory disturbances, dizziness, and increased risk for falls when using benzodiazepines. Pregnant patients should be aware that these medications cross the placenta and are associated with increased risk for birth defects, such as cleft palate, mental retardation, and pyloric stenosis. Infants born addicted to benzodiazepines often exhibit flaccid muscle tone, lethargy, and difficulties sucking. All of the benzodiazepines are excreted in breast milk, and breastfeeding women should avoid using these medications. Infants and children metabolize these medications more slowly; therefore, more drug accumulates in their bodies.

Toxicity develops in overdose or accumulation of the drug in the body from liver dysfunction or disease. Symptoms include worsening of the CNS depression, ataxia, confusion, delirium, agitation, hypotension, diminished reflexes, and lethargy. Rarely do the benzodiazepines cause respiratory depression or death. In overdose, these medications have a high therapeutic index and rarely result in death unless combined with another CNS depressant drug, such as alcohol.

Nonbenzodiazepines: Buspirone

Buspirone, a nonbenzodiazepine, is effective in controlling the symptoms of anxiety but has no effect on panic disorders and little effect on obsessive-compulsive disorder.

Indications and Mechanisms of Actions

Nonbenzodiazepines are effective for treating anxiety disorders without the CNS depressant effects or the potential for abuse and withdrawal syndromes. Buspirone is indicated for treating generalized anxiety disorder; therefore, its target symptoms include anxiety and related symptoms, such as difficulty concentrating, tension, insomnia, restlessness, irritability, and fatigue. Because buspirone does not add to depression symptoms, it has been tried for treating anxiety that coexists with depression. In some instances, it is thought to potentiate the antidepressant actions of other medications.

Buspirone has no effect on the benzodiazepine–GABA complex but instead appears to control anxiety by blocking the serotonin subtype of receptor, 5-HT_{1a}, at both presynaptic reuptake and postsynaptic receptor sites. It has no sedative, muscle relaxant, or anticonvulsant effects. It also lacks potential for abuse.

Pharmacokinetics

Buspirone is rapidly absorbed but undergoes extensive first-pass metabolism. Food slows absorption but appears to reduce first-pass effects, increasing the bioavailability of the medication. Buspirone is given on a continual dosing schedule of three times a day because of its short half-life of 2 to 3 hours. Clinical action depends on reaching steady-state concentrations; taking this medication with food may facilitate this process.

Buspirone is highly protein bound but does not displace most other medications. However, it does displace digoxin and may increase digoxin levels to the point of toxicity. It is metabolized in the liver and excreted predominantly by the kidneys but also via the gastrointestinal tract. Patients with liver or kidney impairment should be given this medication with caution.

Buspirone cannot be used on a PRN basis; rather, it takes 2 to 4 weeks of continual use for symptom relief to occur. It is more effective in reducing anxiety in patients who have never taken a benzodiazepine.

Buspirone does not block the withdrawal of other benzodiazepines. Therefore, a switch to buspirone must be initiated gradually to avoid withdrawal symptoms. Nurses should closely monitor patients who are undergoing this change of medication for emergence of withdrawal symptoms from the benzodiazepines and report such symptoms to the prescriber.

Side Effects, Adverse Reactions, and Toxicity

Common side effects from buspirone include dizziness, drowsiness, nausea, excitement, and headache. Most other side effects occur at an incidence of less than 1%. There have been no reports of death from an overdose of buspirone alone. Older patients, pregnant women, and children have not been adequately studied. For now, buspirone can be assumed to cross the placenta and is present in breast milk; therefore, its use should be avoided in pregnant women, and women who are taking this medication should not breastfeed.

Sedative–Hypnotics

Sedatives reduce activity, nervousness, irritability and excitability without causing sleep, but if given in large enough doses, they have a hypnotic effect. **Hypnotics** cause drowsiness and facilitate the onset and maintenance of sleep. These two classifications are usually referred to as **sedative–hypnotics**—drugs that have a calming effect or depress the CNS. These medications include (1) benzodiazepines (2) GABA enhancers, (3) melatonergic hypnotics, (4) the antihistamines and (5) the orexin receptor antagonists (Table 10.10). The benzodiazepines have been previously discussed. The GABA enhancers modulate GABA-A receptors. They do not cause a high degree of tolerance or dependence and are easier to discontinue than the benzodiazepines. Melatonergic hypnotics are melatonin agonists, and antihistamines are block

TABLE 10.10	HYPNOTICS FOR INSOMNIA		
Generic (Trade) Drug Name	Usual Dosage Range (mg/d)	Elimination Half-Life (h)	Speed of Onset After Single Dose
Benzodiazepine Hypnotics			
Flurazepam	15–30	47–100	Fast
Temazepam (Restoril)	15–30	9.5–20	Moderately fast
Triazolam (Halcion)	0.25–0.5	1.5–5	Fast
Quazepam (Doral)	0.75–15	39	Fast
Estazolam (ProSom)	1	10–24	Fast
Nonbenzodiazepine Hypnotics			
Eszopiclone (Lunesta)	2–3	6	Fast
Zaleplon (Sonata)	10	1	Fast
Zolpidem (Ambien)	5–10	2.6	Fast
Zolpidem CR (Ambien CR)	12.5	2.6	Fast
Melatonergic Hypnotics			
Melatonin	0.1–10	0.5–0.75	Fast
Ramelteon (Rozerem)	8	1–2.6	Fast
Antihistamines			
Hydroxyzine (Vistaril)	50–100	20	Fast
Orexin Receptor Antagonist			
Suvorexan t (Belsomra)	10–20 mg	12	Moderately fast
Doxylamine (Unisom)	25	10	Fast

histamines, causing sedation (Stahl, 2013). The orexin receptor antagonists block the activity of orexins, neurotransmitters involved in wakefulness and arousal. These medications are discussed thoroughly in Chapter 26.

Stimulants and Wakefulness-Promoting Agents

Amphetamines were first synthesized in the late 1800s but were not used for psychiatric disorders until the 1930s. Initially, amphetamines were prescribed for a variety of symptoms and disorders, but their high abuse potential soon became obvious.

Currently among the medications known as stimulants are methylphenidate (Ritalin, Methylin, Metadate), D-amphetamine (Dexedrine), amphetamine/dextroamphetamine (Adderall), dexmethylphenidate (Focalin), lisamphetamine (Vyvanse), and CNS stimulants. Modafinil (Provigil) and armodafinil (Nuvigil) are wakefulness-promoting agents used for narcolepsy and other sleep disorders.

Indications and Mechanisms of Action

Medical use of these stimulants is now restricted to a few disorders, including narcolepsy, attention deficit hyperactivity disorder (ADHD)—particularly in children—and obesity unresponsive to other treatments. However, stimulants are increasingly being used as an adjunctive treatment in depression and other mood disorders to address the fatigue and low energy common to these conditions.

Amphetamines indirectly stimulate the sympathetic nervous system, producing alertness, wakefulness, vasoconstriction, suppressed appetite, and hypothermia. Tolerance develops to some of these effects, such as suppression of appetite, but the CNS stimulation continues. Although the exact mechanism of action is not completely understood, stimulants cause a release of catecholamines, particularly norepinephrine and dopamine, into the synapse from the presynaptic nerve cell. They also block reuptake of these catecholamines. Methylphenidate is structurally similar to the amphetamines but produces a milder CNS stimulation. Psychostimulants should be used very cautiously in individuals who have a history of substance abuse.

Although the stimulant effects of these medications may seem logically indicated for narcolepsy, a disorder in which the individual frequently and abruptly falls asleep, the indications for childhood ADHD seem less obvious. The etiology and neurobiology of ADHD remain unclear, but psychostimulants produce a paradoxic calming of the increased motor activity characteristic of ADHD. Studies show that medication decreases disruptive activity during school hours, reduces noise and verbal activity, improves attention span and short-term memory, improves ability to follow directions, and decreases distractibility and impulsivity. Although these improvements have been well documented in the literature, the diagnosis of ADHD and subsequent use of psychostimulants with children remain matters of controversy (see Chapter 28).

Modafinil (Provigil) and armodafinil (Nuvigil), wake-promoting agents, are used for treating excessive sleepiness associated with narcolepsy, sleep apnea, and residual sleepiness for shift work sleep disorder. Armodafinil is longer acting than modafinil. The mechanism of action is unclear, but it is hypothesized that they increase glutamate and suppress GABA in the hypothalamus, hippocampus, and thalamus. There is no evidence of direct effects on dopamine, but there may be action on a dopamine transport. These drugs may increase the risk of Stevens-Johnson syndrome (Wood, Sage, Shuman, & Anagnostaras, 2013).

Pharmacokinetics

Psychostimulants are rapidly absorbed from the gastrointestinal tract and reach peak plasma levels in 1 to 3 hours. Considerable individual variations occur between the drugs in terms of their bioavailability, plasma levels, and half-lives. Table 10.11 compares the primary psychostimulants used in psychiatry. Some of these differences are age dependent because children metabolize these medications more rapidly, producing shorter elimination half-lives.

TABLE 10.11	PSYCHOSTIMULANT MEDICATIONS	
Generic (Trade) Drug Name	**Usual Dosage Range (mg/d)**	**Elimination Half-Life**
Dextroamphetamine (Dexedrine)	5–40	Highly variable depending on urine pH
Methylphenidate (Ritalin)	10–60	2.4 h (children); 2.1 h (adults)
Amphetamine/dextroamphetamine (Adderall)	2.5 mg (3–5 yr) 5 mg (6 yr) 5–60 mg for narcolepsy	9–11 h
Dexmethylphenidate extended release (Focalin XR)	5–40 mg	3 h
Lisdexamfetamine (Vyvanse)	30 mg	<1 h

The psychostimulants appear to be unaffected by food in the stomach and should be given after meals to reduce the appetite-suppressant effects when indicated. However, changes in urine pH may affect the rates of excretion. Excessive sodium bicarbonate alkalizes the urine and reduces amphetamine secretion. Increased vitamin C or citric acid intake may acidify the urine and increase its excretion. Starvation from appetite suppression may have a similar effect. All of these drugs are highly lipid soluble, crossing easily into the CNS and the placenta. Psychostimulants undergo metabolic changes in the liver where they may affect, or be affected by, other drugs. They are primarily excreted through the kidneys; therefore, renal dysfunction may interfere with excretion.

Psychostimulants are usually begun at a low dose and increased weekly, depending on the improvement of symptoms and occurrence of side effects. Initially, children with ADHD are given a morning dose, so their school performance may be compared from morning to afternoon. Rebound symptoms of excitability and over-talkativeness may occur when use of the medication is withdrawn or after dose reduction. These symptoms also begin about 5 hours after the last dose of medication, which may affect the dosing regimen for some individuals. The return of symptoms in the afternoon for children with ADHD may require that a second dose be given at school. Prescribers should work with parents to implement other interventions after school and on weekends when the psychostimulants are not used. The severity of symptoms may require that the medications be continued during these times, but this dosing schedule should be determined after careful evaluation on an individual basis. Use of these medications should not be stopped abruptly, especially with higher doses, because the rebound effects may last for several days.

Modafinil (Provigil) is absorbed rapidly and reaches peak plasma concentration in 2 to 4 hours. Armodafinil reaches peak plasma concentration later and is maintained for 6 to 14 hours. Absorption of both may be delayed by 1 to 2 hours if taken with food. Modafinil is eliminated via liver metabolism with subsequent excretion of metabolites through renal excretion. They may interact with drugs that inhibit, induce, or are metabolized by CYP450 isoenzymes, including phenytoin, diazepam, and propranolol. Concurrent use of modafinil or armodafinil and other drugs metabolized by the CYP450 isoenzyme system may lead to increased circulating blood levels of the other drugs.

Side Effects, Adverse Reactions, and Toxicity

Side effects associated with psychostimulants typically arise within 2 to 3 weeks after use of the medication begins. From most to least common, these side effects include appetite suppression, insomnia, irritability, weight loss, nausea, headache, palpitations, blurred vision, dry mouth, constipation, and dizziness. Because of the effects on the sympathetic nervous system, some individuals experience blood pressure changes (both hypertension and hypotension), tachycardia, tremors, and irregular heart rates. Blood pressure and pulse should be monitored initially and after each dosage change.

Rarely, psychostimulants suppress growth and development in children. These effects are a matter of controversy, and research has produced conflicting results. Although suppression of height seems unlikely to some researchers, others have indicated that psychostimulants may have an effect on cartilage. Height and weight should be monitored several times annually for children taking these medications and compared with prior history of growth. Weight should be monitored, especially closely during the initial phases of treatment. These effects also may be minimized by drug "holidays," such as during school vacations.

Rarely, individuals may experience mild dysphoria, social withdrawal, or mild to moderate depression. These symptoms are more common at higher doses and may require discontinuation of use of medication. Abnormal movements and motor tics may also increase in individuals who have a history of Tourette's syndrome. Psychostimulants should be avoided by patients with Tourette's symptoms or with a positive family history of the disorder. In addition, dextroamphetamine has been associated with an increased risk for congenital abnormalities. Because there is no compelling reason for a pregnant woman to continue to take these medications, patients should be informed and should advise their prescriber immediately if they plan to become pregnant or if pregnancy is a possibility.

Death is rare from overdose or toxicity of the psychostimulants, but a 10-day supply may be lethal, especially in children. Symptoms of overdose include agitation, chest pain, hallucinations, paranoia, confusion, and dysphoria. Seizures may develop, along with fever, tremor, hypertension or hypotension, aggression, headache, palpitations, rashes, difficulty breathing, leg pain, and abdominal pain. Toxic doses of dextroamphetamine are above 20 mg, with potential death resulting from a 400-mg dose. Parents should be warned regarding the potential lethality of these medications and take preventive measures by keeping the medication in a safe place.

Side effects associated with modafinil and armodafinil include nausea, nervousness, headache, dizziness, and trouble sleeping. If the effects continue or are bothersome, patients should consult the prescriber. Modafinil and armodafinil are generally well tolerated with few clinically significant side effects. It is potentially habit forming and must be used with great caution in individuals with a history of substance abuse or dependence (Cephalon, 2013).

DIETARY SUPPLEMENTS

Herbal Supplements

Many individuals are turning to dietary herbal preparations to address psychiatric symptoms. If these supplements were classified as drugs, their efficacy and safety would have to be approved by the FDA before marketing. However, herbal supplements are regulated like foods, not medications, and thus are exempt from the FDA's efficacy and safety standards. Lack of regulation does not mean that these herbal supplements are effective and safe. These substances often have adverse reactions and interact with prescribed medications. Nurses need to include an assessment of these agents into their overall patient assessment to understand the total picture.

Herbal supplements popular for psychiatric disorders include St. John's Wort (SJW) and kava. SJW, derived from *Hypericum perforatum L.*, is used for depression, pain, anxiety, insomnia, and premenstrual syndrome. SJW is believed to modulate serotonin, dopamine, and norepinephrine. The risk of developing serotonin syndrome is increased when taken with other serotonergic drugs. It is recognized as a potent inducer of CYP3A4 (Sarris, 2013) and has the potential to interact with substrates of this enzyme. It should not be taken with prescribed antidepressants.

Kava, derived from the *Piper methysticum* plant, is used for anxiety reduction. Kava interacts with dopaminergic transmission, inhibits the MAO-B enzyme system, and modulates the GABA receptor. It may also inhibit uptake of noradrenaline. Kava is widely used by Pacific Islanders as a social and ceremonial tranquilizing drink. In 2002, the FDA issued warnings about the risk of severe liver injury associated with kava. Several countries have restricted its use. Thrombocytopenia, leukopenia, and hearing impairment have been reported with the use of kava (Bunchorntavakul & Reddy, 2013).

Valerian, (*Valeriana officinalis*) a member of the Valerianaceae family, is a perennial plant native to Europe and Asia and naturalized to North America. Valerian is a common ingredient in products promoted for insomnia and nervousness. The evidence of its effectiveness is inconclusive. The mechanism of action is unclear but appears to be relatively safe. There are some reports that suggest hepatotoxicity in humans (Modabbernia & Akhondzadeh, 2013).

Vitamin, Mineral, and Other Dietary Supplements

The neurotransmitters necessary for normal healthy functioning are produced from chemical building blocks taken in with the foods we eat. Many nutritional deficiencies may produce symptoms of psychiatric disorders. Fatigue, apathy, and depression are caused by deficiencies in iron, folic acid, pantothenic acid, magnesium, vitamin C, or biotin. Logically, treating these deficiencies with dietary supplements should improve the psychiatric symptoms. The question becomes: Can nutritional supplements improve psychiatric symptoms that are not the result of such deficiencies?

Tryptophan, the dietary precursor for serotonin, has been most extensively investigated as it relates to low serotonin levels and increased aggression. Individuals who have low tryptophan levels are prone to have lower levels of serotonin in the brain, resulting in depressed mood and aggressive behavior (Qureshi & Al-Bedah, 2013).

Dietary supplements such as melatonin, 2-dimethylaminoethanol (DMAE), and lecithin target CNS functioning. Melatonin, a naturally occurring hormone secreted from the pineal gland, is used for treatment of insomnia and prevention of "jet lag" in air travelers. DMAE is promoted for the treatment of ADHD, Alzheimer's disease, Huntington's chorea, and tardive dyskinesia (Copinschi & Caufriez, 2013). DMAE is similar to a former prescription medication removed from the market in 1983 for lack of efficacy. Lecithin, a precursor to acetylcholine, is used to improve memory and treat dementia. The extent to which the level of acetylcholine is raised by ingestion of lecithin is unknown (Tayebati & Amenta, 2013).

Medications may also influence the development of nutritional deficiencies that may worsen psychiatric symptoms. For example, drugs with strong anticholinergic activity often produce impaired or enhanced gastric motility, which may lead to generalized malabsorption of vitamins and minerals. In addition, many vitamin and mineral supplements have toxicities of their own when given in excess. For example, daily ingestion of more than 100 mg of pyridoxine (vitamin B_6) can produce neurotoxic symptoms, photosensitivity, and ataxia. More research is needed to identify the underlying mechanisms and relationships of dietary supplements and dietary precursors of the bioamines to mood and behavior and psychopharmacologic medications. For now, it is important for the psychiatric–mental health nurse to recognize that these issues may be potential factors in improvement of the patient's mental status and target symptoms.

OTHER BIOLOGIC TREATMENTS

Although the primary biologic interventions remain pharmacologic, other somatic treatments have gained acceptance, remain under investigation, or show promise for the future. These include neurosurgery, ECT, phototherapy, and (most recently) **repetitive transcranial magnetic stimulation** (rTMS) and vagus nerve stimulation

(VNS). The use of neurosurgery is very limited and outside the scope of this text.

Electroconvulsive Therapy

For hundreds of years, seizures have been known to produce improvement in some psychiatric symptoms. Camphor-induced seizures were used in the 16th century to reduce psychosis and mania. With time, other substances, such as inhalants, were tried, but most were difficult to control or produced adverse reactions, sometimes even fatalities. ECT was formally introduced in Italy in 1938. It is one of the oldest medical treatments available and remains safely in use today. It is one of the most effective treatments for severe depression but has been used for other disorders, including mania and schizophrenia when other treatments have failed.

With ECT, a brief electrical current is passed through the brain to produce generalized seizures lasting 25 to 150 seconds. The patient does not feel the stimulus or recall the procedure. A short-acting anesthetic and a muscle relaxant are given before induction of the current. A brief pulse stimulus, administered unilaterally on the nondominant side of the head, is associated with less confusion after ECT. However, some individuals require bilateral treatment for effective resolution of depressive symptoms. Induction of a seizure is necessary to produce positive treatment outcomes. Because individual seizure thresholds vary, the electrical impulse and treatment method also may vary. In general, the lowest possible electrical stimulus necessary to produce seizure activity is used. Blood pressure and the ECG are monitored during the procedure. This procedure is repeated two or three times a week, usually for a total of six to 12 treatments. Because there is no particular difference in treatment efficacy and a twice-weekly regimen produces less accumulative memory loss, this treatment course is often chosen. After symptoms have improved, antidepressant medication may be used to prevent relapse. Some patients who cannot take or do not experience response to antidepressant treatment may continue to have ECT treatment. Usually, once-weekly treatments are gradually decreased in frequency to once monthly. The number and frequency vary depending on the individual's response.

Although ECT produces rapid improvement in depressive symptoms, its exact mechanism of antidepressant action remains unclear. It is known to downregulate β-adrenergic receptors in much the same way as antidepressant medications. However, unlike antidepressant therapy, ECT produces an upregulation in serotonin, especially 5-HT$_2$. ECT also has several other actions on neurochemistry, including increased influx of calcium and effects on second messenger systems.

Brief episodes of hypotension or hypertension, bradycardia or tachycardia, and minor arrhythmias are among the adverse reactions that may occur during and immediately after the procedure but usually resolve quickly. Common aftereffects from ECT include headache, nausea, and muscle pain. Memory loss is the most troublesome long-term effect of ECT. Many patients do not experience amnesia, but others report some memory loss for months or even years. Evidence is conflicting on the effects of ECT on the formation of memories after the treatments and on learning, but most patients experience no noticeable change. Memory loss occurring as part of the symptoms of untreated depression presents a confounding factor in determining the exact nature of the memory deficits from ECT. It is important to remember that patient surveys are positive, with most individuals reporting that they were helped by ECT and would have it again (Rajagopal, Chakrabarti, & Grover, 2013).

ECT is contraindicated in patients with increased intracranial pressure. Risk also increases in patients with recent myocardial infarction, recent cerebrovascular accident, retinal detachment, or pheochromocytoma (a tumor on the adrenal cortex) and in patients at high risk for complications from anesthesia. Although ECT should be considered cautiously because of its specific side effects, added risks of general anesthesia, possible contraindications, and substantial social stigma, it is a safe and effective treatment.

Psychiatric–mental health nurses are involved in many aspects of care for individuals undergoing ECT. Informed consent is required, and all treating professionals have a responsibility to ensure that the patient's and family's questions are answered completely. Available treatment options, risks, and consequences must be fully discussed. Sometimes memory difficulties associated with severe depression make it difficult for patients to retain information or ask questions. Nurses should be prepared to restate or explain the procedure as often as necessary. Whenever possible, the individual's family or other support systems should be educated and involved in the consent process. Educational videos are available, but they should not replace direct discussions. Language should be in terms the patient and family members can understand. Other nursing interventions involve preparation of the patient before treatment, monitoring immediately after treatment, and follow-up. Many of these considerations are listed in Box 10.5.

Light Therapy (Phototherapy)

Human circadian rhythms are set by time clues (*Zeitgebers*) inside and outside the body. One of the most powerful regulators of these body patterns is the cycle of daylight and darkness.

Research findings indicate that some individuals with certain types of depression may experience disturbance in these normal body patterns or of circadian rhythms,

BOX 10.5

Interventions for the Patient Receiving Electroconvulsive Therapy

- Discuss treatment alternatives, procedures, risks, and benefits with patient and family. Make sure that informed consent for ECT has been given in writing.
- Provide initial and ongoing patient and family education.
- Assist and monitor the patient who must take NPO after midnight the evening before the procedure.
- Make sure that the patient wears loose, comfortable, non-restrictive clothing to the procedure.
- If the procedure is performed on an outpatient basis, ensure that the patient has someone to accompany him or her home and stay with him or her after the procedure.
- Ensure that pretreatment laboratory tests are complete, including a CBC, serum electrolytes, urinalysis, ECG, chest radiography, and physical examination.
- Teach the patient to create memory helps, such as lists and notepads, before the ECT.
- Explain that no foreign or loose objects can be in the patient's mouth during the procedure. Dentures will be removed, and a bite block may be inserted.
- Insert an IV line and provide oxygen by nasal cannula (usually 100% oxygen at 5 L/min).
- Obtain emergency equipment and be sure it is available and ready if needed.
- Monitor vital signs frequently immediately after the procedure, as in every postanesthesia recovery period.
- When the patient is fully conscious and vital signs are stable, assist him or her to get up slowly, sitting for some time before standing.
- Monitor confusion closely; the patient may need reorientation to the bathroom and other areas.
- Maintain close supervision for at least 12 hours and continue observation for 48 hours after treatment. Advise family members to observe how the patient manages at home, provide assistance as needed, and report any problems.
- Assist the patient to keep or schedule follow-up appointments.

CBC, complete blood count; ECG, electrocardiogram; ECT, electroconvulsive therapy; IV, intravenous; NPO, nothing by mouth.

particularly those who experience a seasonal variation in their depression. These individuals are more depressed during the winter months when there is less light; they improve spontaneously in the spring (see Chapter 20). These individuals usually have symptoms that are somewhat different from classic depression, including fatigue, increased need to sleep, increased appetite and weight gain, irritability, and carbohydrate craving. Sometimes, the symptoms appear in the summer, and some individuals have only subtle changes without developing the full pattern. Administering artificial light to these patients during winter months has reduced these depressive symptoms.

Light therapy, sometimes called **phototherapy**, involves exposing the patient to an artificial light source during winter months to relieve seasonal depression. Artificial light is believed to trigger a shift in the patient's circadian rhythm to an earlier time. Research remains ongoing. The light source must be very bright, full-spectrum light, usually 2,500 lux, which is about 200 times brighter than normal indoor lighting. Harmful ultraviolet light is filtered out. Exposure to this light source has produced improvement and relief of depressive symptoms for significant numbers of seasonally depressed individuals. It produces no change for individuals who are not seasonally depressed.

Studies have shown that morning phototherapy produces a better response than either evening or morning and evening timing of the phototherapy session. Light banks with full-spectrum light may be put together by the individual or obtained from various companies now producing these light sources. Light visors (visors containing small, full-spectrum light bulbs that shine on the eyelids) have also been developed. The patient is instructed to sit in front of the lights at a distance of about 3 feet, engaging in a variety of other activities, but glancing directly into the light every few minutes. This should be done immediately on arising and is most effective before 8 AM. The duration of administration may begin with as little as 30 minutes and increase to 2 to 5 hours. One to 2 hours is usually sufficient, and the antidepressant response begins in 1 to 4 days, with the full effect usually complete after 2 weeks. Full antidepressant effect is usually maintained with daily sessions of 30 minutes (Fisher et al., 2013).

Side effects of phototherapy are rare, but eye strain, headache, and insomnia are possible. An ophthalmologist should be consulted if the patient has a preexisting eye disorder. In rare instances, phototherapy has been reported to produce an episode of mania. Irritability is a more common complaint. Follow-up visits with the prescriber or therapist are needed to help manage side effects and assess positive results. Phototherapy should be implemented only by a provider knowledgeable in its use.

Transcranial Magnetic Stimulation

Transcranial magnetic stimulation was introduced in 1985 as a noninvasive, painless method to stimulate the cerebral cortex. Undergirding this procedure is the hypothesis that a time-varying magnetic field will induce an electrical field, which, in brain tissue, activates inhibitory and excitatory neurons, thereby modulating neuroplasticity in the brain. The low-frequency electrical stimulation from rTMS triggers lasting anticonvulsant effects in rats, and the therapeutic benefits of rTMS in humans are thought to be related to an action similar to that produced by anticonvulsant medication. The rTMS has been used for both clinical and research purposes. The rTMS stimulation of the brain's prefrontal cortex may help some depressed patients in much the same way as ECT but without its side effects (Kirsch & Nichols, 2013). Thus, it has been proposed as an alternative to

ECT in managing symptoms of depression. The rTMS treatment is administered daily for at least 1 week, much like ECT, except that subjects remain awake. Although proven effective for depression, rTMS does have some side effects, including mild headaches.

Vagus Nerve Stimulation

VNS sends electrical impulses to the brain to improve depression. The vagus nerve has traditionally been considered a parasympathetic efferent nerve that was responsible only for regulating autonomic functions, such as heart rate and gastric tone. However, the vagus nerve (cranial X) also carries sensory information to the brain from the head, neck, thorax, and abdomen, and research has identified that the vagus nerve has extensive projections of its sensory afferent connections to many brain areas. Although the basic mechanism of action of VNS is unknown, incoming sensory, or afferent, connections of the left vagus nerve directly project into many of the very same brain regions implicated in neuropsychiatric disorders. These help us to understand how VNS is helpful in treating psychiatric disorders. Vagus nerve stimulation connections change levels of several neurotransmitters implicated in the development of major depression, including serotonin, norepinephrine, GABA, and glutamate, in the same way that antidepressant medications produce their therapeutic effect (Wani, Trevino, Marnell, & Husain, 2013).

Approved by the FDA for the adjunctive treatment of severe depression for adults who are unresponsive to four or more adequate antidepressant treatments, VNS is a permanent implant. VNS is not a cure for depression, and patients must be seen regularly for assessment of mood states and suicidality.

THE ISSUE OF ADHERENCE

Medications and other biologic treatments work only if they are used. On the surface, **adherence**, or **compliance** to a therapeutic routine, seems amazingly simple. However, following therapeutic regimens, self-administering medications as prescribed, and keeping appointments are amazingly complex activities that often prevent successful treatment. Adherence exists on a continuum and can be conceived of as full, partial, or nil. Partial adherence whereby a patient either attempts to take medications but misses doses or takes more than prescribed, is by far the most common. Recent estimates indicate that on the average, 50% or more of the individuals with schizophrenia taking antipsychotic medications stop taking the medications or do not take them as prescribed. It should be remembered that problems with adherence are an issue with many chronic health states, including diabetes and arthritis, not just psychiatric

> **BOX 10.6**
>
> **Common Reasons for Nonadherence to Medication Regimens**
>
> - Uncomfortable side effects and those that interfere with quality of life, such as work performance or intimate relationships
> - Lack of awareness of or denial of illness
> - Stigma
> - Feeling better
> - Confusion about dosage or timing
> - Difficulties in access to treatment
> - Substance abuse

disorders. Box 10.6 lists some of the common reasons for nonadherence. Psychiatric–mental health nurses should be aware that a number of factors influence individuals to stop taking their medications.

The most often cited reasons for noncompliance are related to side effects of the medication. Improved functioning may be observed by health care professionals but not felt by the patient. Side effects may interfere with work performance or other important aspects of the individual's life. For example, a construction worker cannot afford to be drowsy and sedated while operating a crane at a construction site, and a woman in an intimate relationship may find anorgasmia intolerable. Nurses need to be sensitive to the patient's ability to tolerate side effects and to the impact that side effects have on the patient's life. Medication choice, dosing schedules, and prompt treatment of side effects may be crucial factors in helping patients to continue their treatment even if the symptoms for which they initially sought help have improved.

Cognitive deficits associated with some psychiatric disorders may make it difficult for the individual to self-monitor, develop insight, make choices, remember to fill prescriptions, or keep appointments. Forgetfulness, cost, and confusion regarding dosage or timing may also contribute to noncompliance.

Family members may have similar difficulties that influence the individual not to take the medication. They may misunderstand or deny the illness, thinking, for example, "My wife's better, so she doesn't need that medicine anymore." Family members may be distressed when observable side effects occur. Adherence concerns must not be dismissed as the patient's or family's problem. Psychiatric nurses should actively address this issue. A positive therapeutic relationship between the nurse and patient and family must provide a strong sense of trust that side effects and other difficulties in treatment will be addressed and minimized. When individuals report experiencing distressing side effects, the nurse should immediately respond with assessment and interventions to reduce these effects. It is important to assess compliance often, asking questions in a nonthreatening, nonjudgmental manner. It also may be helpful to seek information from others who are involved with the patient.

Adherence can be improved by psychoeducation. This approach is most helpful if it addresses the individual's specific symptoms and concerns. For example, if the patient is having difficulty with understanding the purpose of the medication, it may be helpful to link taking it to reduction of specific unwanted symptoms or improved functioning, such as continuing to work. Family members should also be included in these discussions.

Other factors that interfere with adherence should also be assessed and plans developed to minimize their effect. For example, an individual who is being considered for clozapine therapy may have missed a number of appointments in the past. On assessment, the nurse may discover that it takes the individual 2 hours on three different buses each way to reach the clinic. The nurse can then assist with arranging for a home health nurse to visit the patient's apartment, draw blood samples for analysis, and assess side effects, thus decreasing the number of trips the patient must make to the clinic.

SUMMARY OF KEY POINTS

- Target symptoms and side effects of medications should be clearly identified. The FDA approves the use of medications for specific disorders and symptoms.

- Psychiatric medications primarily act on CNS receptors, ion channels, enzymes, and carrier proteins. Agonists mimic the action of a specific neurotransmitter; antagonists block the response.

- A drug's ability to interact with a given receptor type depends on three qualities: selectivity—the ability to interact with specific receptors while not affecting other tissues and organs; affinity—the degree of strength of the bond between drug and receptor; and intrinsic activity—the ability to produce a certain biologic response.

- Pharmacokinetics refers to how the human body processes the drug, including absorption, distribution, metabolism, and excretion. Bioavailability describes the amount of the drug that actually reaches circulation throughout the body. The wide variations in the way each individual processes any medication often are related to physiologic differences caused by age, genetic makeup, other disease processes, and chemical interactions.

- Antipsychotic medications are drugs used in treating patients with psychotic disorders, such as schizophrenia. They act primarily by blocking dopamine or serotonin postsynaptically. In addition, they have a number of actions on other neurotransmitters. Older typical antipsychotic drugs work on positive symptoms and are inexpensive but produce many side effects. Newer atypical antipsychotic drugs work on positive and negative symptoms and are much more expensive but have far fewer side effects and are better tolerated by patients.

- Medication-related movement disorders are a particularly serious group of side effects that principally occur with the typical antipsychotic medications and that may be acute syndromes, such as dystonia, pseudoparkinsonism, and akathisia, or chronic syndromes, such as tardive dyskinesia.

- The mood stabilizers, or antimania medications, are drugs used to control wide variations in mood related to mania, but these agents may also be used to treat patients with other disorders. Lithium and the anticonvulsants are chemically unrelated and act in different ways to stabilize mood.

- Antidepressant medications are drugs used primarily for treating symptoms of depression. They act by blocking reuptake of one or more of the bioamines, especially serotonin and norepinephrine. These medications vary considerably in their structure and action. Newer antidepressants, such as the SSRIs, have fewer side effects and are less lethal in overdose than the older TCAs.

- Antianxiety medications also include several subgroups of medications, but the benzodiazepines and nonbenzodiazepines are those principally used in psychiatry. The benzodiazepines act by enhancing the effects of GABA, and the nonbenzodiazepine buspirone acts on serotonin. Benzodiazepines can be used on a PRN basis, but buspirone, the one available nonbenzodiazepine, must be taken regularly.

- Psychostimulants enhance neurotransmitter activity, acting at a number of sites in the nerves. These medications are most often used for treating symptoms related to ADHD and narcolepsy.

- ECT uses the application of an electrical pulsation to induce seizures in the brain. These seizures produce a number of effects on neurotransmission that result in the rapid relief of depressive symptoms.

- rTMS and VNS are two emerging somatic treatments for psychiatric disorders. They are both means to directly affect brain function through stimulation of the nerves that are direct extensions of the brain.

- Phototherapy involves the application of full-spectrum light, in the morning hours, which appears to reset circadian rhythm delays related to seasonal affective disorder and other forms of depression. Nutritional therapies are in various stages of investigation.

■ Adherence refers to the ability of an individual to self-administer medications as prescribed and to follow other instructions related to medication treatment. It can be full, partial, or nil. Nonadherence is related to factors such as medication side effects, stigma, and family influences. Nurses play a key role in educating patients and helping them to improve adherence.

CRITICAL THINKING CHALLENGES

1. Discuss how you would go about identifying the target symptoms for a specific patient for the following medications: antipsychotic, antidepressant, and antianxiety drugs.

2. Track the approval process from identification of a potential substance to marketing a medication. Compare at least three psychiatric medications that are in phase III trials (hint: www.FDA.gov).

3. Obtain the PIs for the three atypical antipsychotics, two SSRIs, and one SNRI. Compare their boxed warnings, pharmacodynamics, pharmacokinetics, indications, side effects, and dosages.

4. Compare the oral and IM dose of lorazepam. Why are these doses similar?

5. Mr. J. has schizophrenia and was just prescribed an antipsychotic. His family wants to know the risk–benefits of the medication. How would you answer?

6. Obtain the PI for clozapine, risperidone, quetiapine, and Risperdal Consta. Compare the half-lives of each drug. Discuss the relationship of the drug's half-life to the dosing schedule. When is steady state reached in each of these medications?

7. Explain the health problems associated with anticholinergic side effects of the antipsychotic medications.

8. Compare the type of movements that characterize tardive dyskinesia with those that characterize akathisia and dystonia and explore which one is easier for a patient to experience.

9. One patient is prescribed the MAOI Emsam, 6 mg per day, and another is taking another MAOI, Nardil, 15 mg per day. Are the dietary restrictions different?

10. A patient who is taking an MAOI asks you to explain what will happen if she eats pizza. Prepare a short teaching intervention beginning with the action of the medication and its consequences.

11. Explain how your nursing care would be different for a male patient taking lithium carbonate than for a female patient.

12. Patient A is taking valproic acid (Depakote) for mood stabilization, and patient B is taking lamo-trigine (Lamictal). After comparing notes with each other, they ask you why patient A has to have drug blood levels and patient B does not. How are these two drugs alike? How are they different?

13. Two patients are getting their blood drawn. One patient is getting lithium and the other clozapine. What laboratory tests are being ordered?

14. A patient who is depressed has been started on sertraline. During the assessment, she tells you that she is also taking SJW, lecithin, and a multiple vitamin. What is your next step?

15. Compare different approaches that you might use with a patient with schizophrenia who has decided to stop taking his or her medication because of intolerance to side effects.

REFERENCES

Beach, S. R., Celano, C. M., Noseworthy, P. A., Januzzi, J. L., & Huffman, J. C. (2013). QTc prolongation, torsades de pointes, and psychotropic medications. (Review). *Psychosomatics, 54*(1), 1–13.

Bialer, M. (2012). Why are antiepileptic drugs used for nonepileptic conditions? *Epilepsia, 53*(suppl 7), 26–33.

Bunchorntavakul, C., & Reddy, K. R. (2013). Review article: Herbal and dietary supplement hepatotoxicity. *Alimentary Pharmacology & Therapeutics, 37*(1), 3–17.

Cephalon. (2013). *Nuvigil (armodafinil) tablets.* Retrieved from http://www.nuvigil.com/PDF/Full_Prescribing_Information.pdf

Copinschi, G., & Caufriez, A. (2013). Sleep and hormonal changes in aging. (Review). *Endocrinology and Metabolism Clinics of North America, 42*(2), 371–389.

Fisher, P. M., Madsen, M. K., Mc Mahon, B., Holst, K. K., Andersen, S. B., Laursen, H. R., et al. (2013). Three-Week Bright-Light Intervention Has Dose-Related Effects on Threat-Related Corticolimbic Reactivity and Functional Coupling. *Biological Psychiatry, 19* pii: S0006-3223(13)01102–01105. doi:10.1016/j.biopsych.2013.10.031

Glassock, R. J. (2009). The GFR decline with aging: A sign of normal senescence, not disease. *Nephrology Times, 9*(2), 6–8.

GlaxoSmithKline. (2013). Wellbutrin Prescribing Information. www.wellbutrin.com

Kirsch, D. L., & Nichols, F. (2013). Cranial electrotherapy stimulation for treatment of anxiety, depression, and insomnia. *Psychiatric Clinics of North America, 36*(1), 169–176.

Laoutidis, Z. G., & Luckhaus, C. (2014). 5-HT2A receptor antagonists for the treatment of neuroleptic-induced akathisia: A systematic review and meta-analysis. *International Journal of Neuropsychopharmacology, 17*(5), 823–832.

Lopez, O. L., Becker, J. T., Chang, Y. F., Sweet, R. A., Aizenstein, H., Snitz, B., et al. (2013). The long-term effects of conventional and atypical antipsychotics in patients with probable Alzheimer's Disease. *The American Journal of Psychiatry, 170*(9), 1051–1058.

Malhi, G. S., Tanious, M., Das, P., Coulston, C. M., & Berk, M. (2013). Potential mechanisms of action of lithium in bipolar disorder. Current understanding. *CNS Drugs, 27*(2), 135–153.

Modabbernia, A., & Akhondzadeh, S. (2013). Saffron, passionflower, valerian and sage for mental health. *The Psychiatric Clinics of North America, 36*(1), 85–91.

Novartis. (2013). *Clozaril (prescribing information).* Retrieved from http://www.clozaril.com.

Qureshi, M. A., & Al-Bedah, A. M. (2013). Mood disorders and complementary and alternative medicine: A literature review. *Neuropsychiatric Disease and Treatment, 9*, 639–658. doi:10.2147/NDT.S43419

Rajagopal, R., Chakrabarti, S., & Grover, S. (2013). Satisfaction with electroconvulsive therapy among patients and their relatives. *The Journal of ECT, 29*(4), 283–290.

Sarris, J. (2013). St. John's wort for the treatment of psychiatric disorders. *The Psychiatric Clinics of North America, 36*(1), 65–72.

Silva, H. (2013). Ethnopsychopharmacology and pharmacogenomics. *Advances in Psychosomatic Medicine, 33*, 88–96.

Stahl, S. M. (2013). *Stahl's essential psychopharmacology* (4th ed). New York: Cambridge University Press.

Tayebati, S. K., & Amenta, F. (2013). Choline-containing phospholipids: Relevance to brain functional pathways. (Review). *Clinical Chemistry and Laboratory Medicine, 51*(3), 513–521.

Wani, A., Trevino, K., Marnell, P., & Husain, M. M. (2013). Advances in brain stimulation for depression. *Annals of Clinical Psychiatry, 25*(3), 217–224.

Wood, S., Sage, J. R., Shuman, T., & Anagnostaras, S. G. (2013). Psychostimulants and cognition: A continuum of behavioral and cognitive activation. *Pharmacological Reviews, 66*(1), 193–221.

Woods, S. W., Morgenstern, H., Saksa, J. R., Walsh, B. C., Sullivan, M. C., Money, R., et al. (2010). Incidence of tardive dyskinesia with atypical versus conventional antipsychotic medications: A prospective cohort study. *The Journal of Clinical Psychiatry, 71*(4), 463–474.

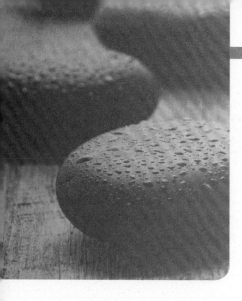

11
Group Interventions

Mary Ann Boyd

KEY CONCEPTS

- group
- group dynamics
- group process

LEARNING OBJECTIVES

After studying this chapter, you will be able to:

1. Discuss concepts used in leading groups.

2. Compare the roles that group members can assume.

3. Identify important aspects of leading a group, such as member selection, leadership skills, seating arrangements, and ways of dealing with challenging behaviors of group members.

4. Identify types of groups: psychoeducation, supportive therapy, psychotherapy, and self-help.

5. Describe common nursing intervention groups.

KEY TERMS

- closed group • cohesion • co-leadership • communications pathways • direct leadership • dyad • formal group roles
- group themes • groupthink • indirect leadership • individual roles • informal group roles • maintenance roles
- open group • task roles • triad

Group interventions are a key nursing strategy in mental health promotion and recovery. A group experience can help an individual enhance self-understanding, conquer unwanted thoughts and feelings, and learn new behaviors. In a group, members learn from each other as well as the leader. Group interventions are efficient because several patients can participate at one time, and they can be used in most settings. Groups can vary in purpose from being a social group attending a local ball game to an intensive psychotherapy group.

> **KEYCONCEPT** A **group** is two or more people who develop interactive relationships and share at least one common goal or issue. *A group is more than the sum of its parts.* A group develops its own personality, patterns of interaction, and rules of behavior.

Nurses in various roles and settings may use group interventions, such as when conducting patient education or leading support groups. This chapter discusses group concepts, considerations in group leadership, and types of groups that nurses commonly lead.

PREPARING TO LEAD A GROUP

Psychiatric nurses lead a wide range of groups (see later discussion of Types of Groups). Some are structured such as a psychoeducation group, and others are unstructured (e.g., a social group). The purpose of the group will dictate the amount of structure and types of activities. In all groups, nurses maintain professional boundaries. Because some group activities are social in nature (unit parties, community trips), it is easy to forget that socialization is a treatment intervention. Nurses should avoid meeting personal social needs within this context.

Thoughtful planning and preparation make for a successful group. The following sections discuss important considerations when planning for a group.

Selecting Members

Individuals can self-refer or be referred to a group by treatment teams or clinicians, but the leader is responsible for assessing each individual's suitability for the group. In instances when a new group is forming, the leader assesses the individual's suitability for the group based on the following criteria:

- Does the purpose of the group match the needs of the potential member?
- Does the potential member have the social skills to function comfortably in the group?
- Will the other group members accept the new group member?
- Can the potential member make a commitment to attending group meetings?

Forming an Open or Closed Group

In planning for a group, one of the early decisions is whether the group will be open or closed. In an **open group**, new members may join, and old members may leave the group at different sessions. Because length of patient hospitalization is relatively short, open groups are typical on inpatient units. For example, a newly admitted patient may join an anger management group that is part of an ongoing program in an inpatient unit.

In a **closed group,** members begin the group at one time, and no new members are admitted. If a member leaves, no replacement member joins. In a closed group, participants get to know one another very well and can develop close relationships. Closed groups are more typical of outpatient groups that have a sequential curriculum or psychotherapy groups. These groups usually meet weekly for a specified period. Outpatient smoking cessation, psychotherapy, and psychoeducation groups are examples.

Determining Composition

Another decision is the group size. The size of a group will depend on the overall group goals and patients' abilities. Patients with challenging behaviors should be carefully screened and may be able to function in smaller rather than larger groups.

Small groups (usually no more than seven to eight members) become more cohesive, are less likely to form subgroups, and can provide a richer interpersonal experience than large groups (Yalom & Leszcz, 2005). A very small group is two people (**dyad**) or three (**triad**). Small groups function nicely with one group leader although many small groups are led by two people. Even though small groups cannot easily withstand the loss of members, they are ideal for patients who are highly motivated to deal with complex emotional problems, such as sexual abuse, eating disorders, or trauma or for those who have cognitive dysfunction and require a more focused group environment with minimal distractions.

In leading a small group, the leader gets to know the members very well but maintains objectivity. The nurse observes for transference of participants toward the leader or other member. If a member becomes a "favorite patient," the leader should reflect upon any underlying personal countertransference issues (see Chapter 8).

> **NCLEXNOTE** Be prepared to select members and plan for a patient or family support group to help deal with the impact of mental illnesses on the family lifestyle.

Large groups (more than eight to 10 members) are effective for specific problems or issues, such as smoking cessation or medication information. Large groups are often used in the workplace (Cahill & Lancaster, 2014). A large group can be ongoing and open ended. Usually, transference and countertransference issues do not develop.

However, leading a large group is challenging because of the number of potential interactions and relationships that can form and the difficulty in determining the feelings and thoughts of the participants (Clark, 2009). As the size of the group increases, the level of engagement decreases and conflict increases (LoCoco, Gullo, LoVerso, & Kivlighan, 2013). It may be difficult to get everyone's attention to begin a group session. Subgroups can form, making it difficult to develop a cohesive group. If subgroups form that are detrimental to the group, the nurse can change the structure and function of communication within the subgroups by rearranging seating and encouraging the subgroup to interact with the rest of the group. Gender mix is also a consideration and can make a difference in the success of the group. For example, research shows that all-female and mixed gender groups rate their groups as more valuable and useful than did members of all-male groups. All-male groups and mixed groups are more task oriented than all-female groups. A high proportion of women in a mixed-gender group might facilitate an early develoment of positive group climate (LoCoco et al., 2013).

Selecting a Leadership Style

A group is led within the context of the group leader's theoretic background and the group's purpose. For example, a leader with training in cognitive-behavioral therapy may focus on treating depression by asking members to think differently about situations, which in turn lead to feeling better. A leader with a psychodynamic orientation may focus on the feelings of depression by examining situations that generate the same feelings. Whatever the leader's theoretic background, his or her leadership behavior can be viewed on a continuum of direct to indirect.

Direct leadership behavior enables the leader to control the interaction by giving directions and information and allowing little discussion. The leader literally tells the members what to do. On the other end of the continuum is **indirect leadership**, in which the leader primarily reflects the group members' discussion and offers little guidance or information to the group. Sometimes the group needs a more direct approach, such as in a psychoeducation class; other times it needs a leader who is indirect. The challenge of providing leadership is to give sufficient direction to help the group meet its goals and develop its own group process but enough freedom to allow members to make mistakes and recover from their thinking errors in a supportive, caring, learning environment.

Co-leadership, when two people share responsibility for leading the group, is useful in most groups as long as the co-leaders attend all sessions and maintain open communication. Co-leadership works well when the co-leaders plan together and meet before and after each session to discuss the group process.

Setting the Stage: Arranging Seating

Group sessions should be held in a quiet, pleasant room with adequate space and privacy. Holding a session in too large or too small a room inhibits communication. The sessions should be held in private rooms that nonmembers cannot access. Interruptions are distracting and can potentially compromise confidentiality. Arrangement of chairs should foster interaction and reduce communication barriers. Communication flows better when no physical barriers, such as tables, are between members. Group members should be able to see and hear each other. Arranging a group in a circle with chairs comfortably close to one another without a table enhances group work. No one should sit outside the group. If a table is necessary, a round table is better than a rectangular one, which implicitly increases the power of those who sit at the ends.

Group members tend to sit in the same places. Those who sit close to the group leader are more likely to have more power in the group than those who sit far away.

Planning the First Meeting

The leader sets the tone of the group at the first meeting. The leader and members introduce themselves. The leader may ask participants to share some introductory information such as why they joined the group and what do they hope to gain from the experience. The leader

---

> **BOX 11.1**
> ### Example of Group Guidelines
> - Group sessions begin and end on time.
> - All views are heard and respected. Cell phones are silenced; there are no side conversations.
> - Only one person speaks at a time. No interrupting.
> - Emotion is acceptable; aggression is not. Disagreements should be expressed calmly and objectively.
> - Everyone is expected to stay for the entire meeting.
> - Who we see and what is said here stay here.

can share name, credentials for leading group, and a brief statement about experience. The leader should avoid self-disclosing personal information.

The first session is the time to explain the structure of group, including the purpose and group rules (Box 11.1). It is important the group starts and ends at scheduled times; otherwise, members who tend to be late will not change their behavior, and those who are on time will resent waiting for the others. The leader also explains when and if new members can join the group.

During the first session, the leader begins to assess the group dynamics or interactions—both verbal and nonverbal. During the course of the group sessions, these interactions will be important in understanding the group process and may determine the success of the group.

> **KEYCONCEPT** **Group dynamics** are the all the verbal and nonverbal interactions that occur in the group.

LEADING A GROUP

A group leader is responsible for monitoring and shaping the group process, as well as focusing on the group content (Puskar, Mazza, Slivka, Westcott, Campbell, & McFadden, 2012). Although models of group development differ, most follow a pattern of a beginning, middle, and ending phase (Corey, Corey, & Corey, 2010) (Table 11.1). These stages should not be viewed as a linear progression with one preceding another but as a dynamic process that is constantly revisiting and reexamining group interactions and behaviors, as well as progressing forward. The group leader needs to be aware of the group's stage of development as well as leadership responsibilities.

> **KEYCONCEPT** **Group process** is the development and culmination of the session-to-session interactions of the members that move the group toward its goals.

Beginning Stage: The Honeymoon

In the beginning, the group leader acknowledges each member; constructs a working environment; develops

TABLE 11.1	COMPARISON OF MODELS OF GROUP DEVELOPMENT		
Phase	Robert Bales (1955)	William Schutz (1960)	Bruce Tuckman (1965)
Beginning	• *Orientation:* What is the problem?	• *Inclusion:* Deal with issues of belonging and being in and out of the group.	• *Forming:* Get to know one another and form a group.
Middle	• *Evaluation:* How do we feel about it?	• *Control:* Deal with issues of authority (who is in charge?), dependence, and autonomy.	• *Storming:* Tension and conflict occur; subgroups form and clash with one another. • *Norming:* Develop norms of how to work together.
Ending	• *Control:* What should we do about it?	• *Affection:* Deal with issues of intimacy, closeness, and caring versus dislike and distancing.	• *Performing:* Reach consensus and develop cooperative relationships.

Sources: Bales, R. (1955). A set of categories for the analysis of small group interaction. *American Sociological Review*, 15, 257–263.

Schutz, W. (1960). *FIRO: A three-dimensional theory of interpersonal behavior*. New York: Holt, Rinehart & Winston.

Tuckman, B. (1965). Developmental sequence in small groups. *Psychological Bulletin*, 63(6), 384–399.

rapport with the members; begins to builds a therapeutic relationship; and clarifies outcomes, processes, and skills related to the group's purpose (Corey et al., 2010). To carry out these functions, the leader processes group interactions by staying objectives and observing members' interactions as well as participating in the group. The leader reflects on, evaluates, and responds to interactions. The use of various techniques enhances the leader's ability to lead the group effectively and to help the group meet its goals (Table 11.2).

During beginning sessions, group members get to know one another and the group leader. The length of the beginning stage depends on the purpose of the group, the number of members, and the skill of the leader. It may last for only a few sessions or several. Members often exhibit polite, congenial behavior typical of those in new social situations. They are "good patients" and often intellectualize their problems; that is, these patients deal with emotional conflict or stress by excessively using abstract thinking or generalizations to minimize disturbing feelings. Members are usually anxious and sometimes display behavior that does not truly represent their feelings.

In this phase, members begin to test whether they can trust one another and the leader. Members may come late to group or try to extend group time. Some time after the initial sessions, group members usually experience a period of conflict, either among themselves or with the leader. This conflict is a normal part of group development, and many believe that conflict is necessary to move into any working phase. Sometimes one or more group members become the scapegoat. Such situations challenge the leader to guide the group during this period by avoiding taking sides and treating all members respectfully.

Working Stage

The working stage of groups involves a real sharing of ideas and the development of closeness. A group personality may emerge that is distinct from the individual personalities of its members. The group develops norms, which are rules and standards that establish acceptable behaviors. Some norms are formalized, such as beginning group on time, but others are never really formalized, such as sitting in the same place each session. These normative standards encourage conformity and discourage behavioral deviations from the established norms. A member quickly learns the norms or is ostracized.

During this stage, the group realizes its purpose. If the purpose is education, the participants engage in learning new content or skills. If the aim of the group is to share feelings and experiences, these activities consume group meetings. During this phase, the group starts on time, and the leader often needs to remind members when it is time to stop.

Facilitating Group Communication

One of the responsibilities of the group leader is to facilitate both verbal and nonverbal communication to meet the treatment goals of the individual members and the entire group. Because of the number of people involved, developing trusting relationships within groups is more complicated than is developing a single relationship with a patient. The communication techniques used in establishing and maintaining individual relationships are the same for groups, but the leader also attends to the communication patterns among the members.

TABLE 11.2	TECHNIQUES IN LEADING GROUPS	
Technique	Purpose	Example
Support: giving feedback that provides a climate of emotional support	Helps a person or group continue with ongoing activities Informs group about what the leader thinks is important Creates a climate for expressing unpopular ideas Helps the more quiet and fearful members speak up	"We really appreciate your sharing that experience with us. It looked like it was quite painful."
Confrontation: challenging a participant (needs to be done in a supportive environment)	Helps individuals learn something about themselves Helps reduce some forms of disruptive behavior Helps members deal more openly and directly with one another	"Tom, this is the third time you have changed the subject when we have talked about spouse abuse. Is something going on?"
Advice and suggestions: sharing expertise and knowledge that the members do not have	Provides information that members can use after they have examined and evaluated it Helps focus the group's task and goals	"The medication you are taking may be causing you to be sleepy."
Summarizing: statements at the end of sessions that highlight the session's discussion, any problem resolution, and unresolved problems	Provides continuity from one session to the next Brings to focus still-unresolved issues Organizes the past in ways that clarify; brings into focus themes and patterns of interaction	"This session, we discussed Sharon's medication problems, and she will be following up with her physicians."
Clarification: restatement of an interaction	Checks on the meanings of the interaction and communication Avoids faulty communication Facilitates focus on substantive issues rather than allowing members to be sidetracked into misunderstandings	"What I heard you say was that you are feeling very sad right now. Is that correct?"
Probing and questioning: a technique for the experienced group leader that asks for more information	Helps members expand on what they were saying (when they are ready to) Gets at more extensive and wider range of information Invites members to explore their ideas in greater detail	"Could you tell us more about your relationship with your parents?"
Repeating, paraphrasing, highlighting: a simple act of repeating what was just said	Facilitates communication among group members Corrects inaccurate communication or emphasizes accurate communication	*Member:* "I forgot about my wife's birthday." *Leader:* "You forgot your wife's birthday."
Reflecting feelings: identifying feelings that are being expressed	Orients members to the feelings that may lie behind what is being said or done Helps members deal with issues they might otherwise avoid or miss	"You sound upset."
Reflecting behavior: identifying behaviors that are occurring	Gives members an opportunity to see how their behavior appears to others and to evaluate its consequences Helps members to understand others' perceptions and responses to them	"I notice that when the topic of sex is brought up, you look down and shift in your chair."

Encouraging Interaction

The nurse leads the group during this phase by encouraging interaction among members and being responsive to their comments. Active listening enables the leader to process events and track interactions. The nurse can then formulate responses based on a true understanding of the discussion. A group leader who listens also models listening behavior for others, helping them improve their skills. Members may need to learn to listen to one another, track discussions without changing the subject, and not speak while others are talking. At the end of the session, the nurse summarizes the work of the session and projects the work for the next meeting.

The leader maintains a neutral, nonjudgmental style and avoids showing preference to one member over another. This may be difficult because some members may naturally seek out the leader's attention or ask for special favors. These behaviors are divisive to the group, and the leader should discourage them. Other important skills include providing everyone with an opportunity to contribute and respecting everyone's ideas. A leader who truly wants group participation and decision making does not reveal his or her beliefs.

Monitoring Verbal Communication

Group interaction can be viewed as a communication network that becomes patterned and predictable. In a group, verbal comments are linked in a chain formation. Monitoring verbal interactions and leading a group at the same time is difficult for one person. If there are two leaders, one may be the active leader of the group, and the other may sit outside the group and observe and record rather than participating. If all members agree, the leader can use an audio or video recorder for reviewing interaction after the group session.

Interesting interaction patterns can be observed and analyzed (Fig. 11.1). By analyzing the content and patterns, the leader can determine the existence of **communications pathways**—who is most liked in the group, who occupies a position of power, what subgroups have formed, and who is isolated from the group. People who sit next to each other tend to communicate among themselves. Usually, those who are well liked or display leadership abilities tend to be chosen for interactions more often than do those who are not. The leader can also determine if there is a change of subject when a sensitive topic is introduced.

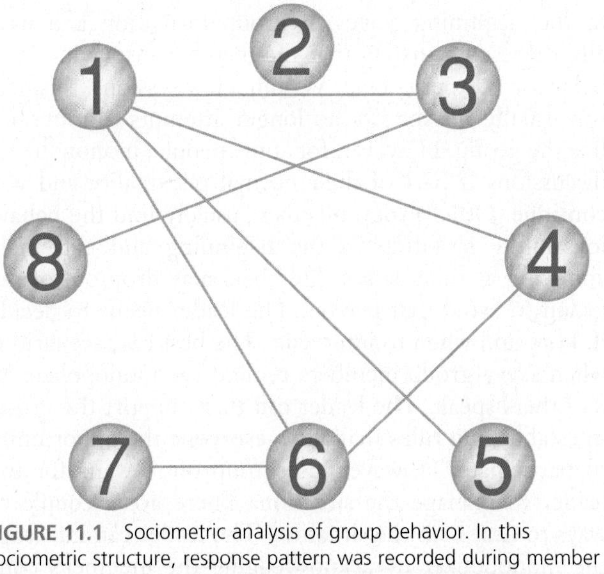

Deciphering Content Themes

Group themes are the collective conceptual underpinnings of a group and express the members' underlying concerns or feelings regardless of the group's purpose. Themes that emerge in groups help members to understand group dynamics. Different groups have different themes. A grief group most likely would have a theme of loss or new beginnings and an adolescent group may have a theme of independence. Although some predictable themes occur in groups, the obvious or assumed themes at the beginning may actually wind up differing from reality as the process continues. In one hospice support group, the members seemed to be focusing on the memories of their loved ones. However, upon examination of the content of their interactions, discussions were revolving around financial planning for the future (Box 11.2).

Monitoring Nonverbal Communication

Observing nonverbal communication contributes to understanding the group dynamics. Members communicate nonverbally with each other, not only the group leader. Eye contact, posture, and body gestures of one

FIGURE 11.1 Sociometric analysis of group behavior. In this sociometric structure, response pattern was recorded during member interaction. Group members interacted with number 1 the most. Therefore, number 1 is the overchosen person. Numbers 5 and 7 are underchosen. Number 2 is never chosen and is determined to be the isolate.

BOX 11.2

Group Themes

A large symptom-management group is ongoing at a psychiatric facility. It is co-led by two nurses who are skilled in directing large groups and knowledgeable about the symptoms of mental disorders. Usually 12 people attend. The usual focus of the group is on identifying symptoms that indicate an impending reemergence of psychotic symptoms, medication side effects, and managing the numerous symptoms that medication is not controlling.

The nurses identified the appearance of the theme of powerlessness based on the following observations:

- **Session 1:** T. L. expressed his frustration at being unable to keep a job because of his symptoms. The rest of the group offered their own experiences of being unable to work.
- **Session 2:** C. R. is late to group and announces that she was late because the bus driver forgot to tell her when to get off, and she missed her stop. She is irritated with the new driver.
- **Session 3:** N. T. is out of medication and says that he cannot get more because he is out of money again. He asks the nurses to lend him some money and make arrangements to get free medication.
- **Session 4:** G. M. relies on his family for all transportation and refuses to use public transportation.

In all of these sessions, participants expressed feelings that are consistent with loss of power.

member impact other members. For example, if one member is explaining a painful experience and another member looks away and tries to engage still another, the self-disclosing member may feel devalued and rejected because the disruptive behavior is interpreted as disinterest. However, if the leader interprets the disruptive behavior as anxiety over the topic, he or she may try to engage the other member in discussing the source of the anxiety.

The leaders should monitor the nonverbal behavior of group members during each session. Often, one or two people can set the overall mood of the group. Someone who comes to a session very sad or angry can set a tone of sadness or anger for the whole group. An astute group leader recognizes the effects of an individual's mood on the total group. If the purpose of the group is to deal with emotions, the group leader may choose to discuss the member's problem at the beginning of the session. The leader, thus, limits the mood to the one person experiencing it. If the group's purpose is inconsistent with self-disclosure of personal problems, the nurse should acknowledge the individual member's distress and offer a private session after the group. In this instance, the nurse would not encourage repeated episodes of self-disclosure from that member or others.

Tracking Group Communication

The leader tracks the verbal and nonverbal interactions throughout the group sessions. Depending on the group's purpose, the leader may or may not share the observations with the group. For example, if the purpose of the group is psychoeducation, the leader may incorporate the information into a lesson plan without identifying any one individual. If the purpose of the group is to improve the self-awareness and interaction skills of members, the leader may point out the observations. The leader needs to be clear about the purpose of the group and tailor leadership strategies accordingly.

Determining Roles of Group Members

There are two official or **formal group roles**, the leader and the members; however, there are also important **informal group roles** or positions with implicit rights and duties that can either help or hinder the group's process. Ideally, one or more members assume **task roles** or functions. These individuals are concerned about the purpose of the group and "keep things on task." For example, *information seeker* is the member who asks for clarification; the *coordinator* spells out relationships among ideas, and the *recorder* keeps the minutes.

Maintenance roles or functions are assumed by those who help keep the group together. Other members assume maintenance roles and make sure that the group members get along with each other and try to make peace if conflict erupts. These individuals are as interested in maintaining the group's cohesiveness as focusing on the group's tasks. The *harmonizer, compromiser*, and *standard setter* are examples of maintenance roles.

Both task and maintenance functions are needed in an effective group. In selecting members and analyzing the progress of the group, the leader pays attention to the balance between the task and maintenance functions. If too many group members assume task functions and too few assume maintenance functions, the group may have difficulty developing **cohesion,** or sticking together. If too many members assume maintenance functions, the group may never finish its work.

Individual roles are played by members to meet personal needs, such as feeling important or being an expert on a subject. These roles have nothing to do with the group's purpose or cohesion and can detract from the group's functioning (Box 11.3). If individual roles predominate, the group may be ineffective.

Dealing with Challenging Group Behaviors

Problematic behaviors occur in all groups. They can be challenging to the most experienced group leaders and frustrating to new leaders. In dealing with any problematic behavior or situation, the leader must remember to support the integrity of the individual members and the group as a whole.

Monopolizer

Some people tend to monopolize a group by constantly talking or interrupting others. This behavior is common in the beginning stages of group formation and usually represents anxiety that the member displaying such behavior is experiencing. Within a few sessions, this person usually relaxes and no longer attempts to monopolize the group. However, for some people, monopolizing discussions is part of their normal personality and will continue. Other group members usually find the behavior mildly irritating in the beginning and extremely annoying as time passes. Members may drop out of the group to avoid that person. The leader needs to decide if, how, and when to intervene. The best case scenario is when savvy group members remind the monopolizer to let others speak. The leader can then support the group in establishing rules that allow everyone the opportunity to participate. However, the group often waits for the leader to manage the situation. There are a couple of ways to deal with the situation. The leader can interrupt the monopolizer by acknowledging the member's contribution but redirecting the discussion to others, or the leader can become more directive and limit the discussion time per member.

BOX 11.3
Roles and Functions of Group Members

TASK ROLES
- *Initiator-contributor* suggests or proposes new ideas or a new view of the problem or goal.
- *Information seeker* asks for clarification of the values pertinent to the group activity.
- *Information giver* offers "authoritative" facts or generalizations or gives own experiences.
- *Opinion giver* states belief or opinions with emphasis on what should be the group's values.
- *Elaborator* spells out suggestions in terms of examples, develops meanings of ideas and rationales and tries to deduce how an idea would work.
- *Coordinator* shows or clarifies the relationships among various ideas and suggestions.
- *Orienter* defines the position of the group with respect to its goals.
- *Evaluator-critic* measures the outcome of the group against some standard.
- *Energizer* attempts to stimulate the group to action or decision.
- *Procedural technician* expedites group movement by doing things for the group such as distributing copies and arranging seating.
- *Recorder* writes suggestions, keeps minutes, and serves as group memory.

MAINTENANCE ROLES
- *Encourager* praises, agrees with, and accepts the contributions of others.
- *Harmonizer* mediates differences among members and relieves tension in conflict situations.
- *Compromiser* operates from within a conflict and may yield status or admit error to maintain group harmony.

- *Gatekeeper* attempts to keep communication channels open by encouraging or facilitating the participation of others or proposes regulation of the flow of communication through limiting time.
- *Standard setter* expresses standards for the group to achieve.
- *Group observer* keeps records of various aspects of group processes and interprets data to group.
- *Follower* goes along with the movement of the group.

INDIVIDUAL ROLES
- *Aggressor* deflates the status of others; expresses disapproval of the values, acts, or feelings of others; attacks the group or problem; jokes aggressively; and tries to take credit for the work.
- *Blocker* tends to be negative and resistant, disagrees and opposes without or beyond "reason," and attempts to bring back an issue after group has rejected it.
- *Recognition seeker* calls attention to self through such activities as boasting, reporting on personal achievements, or acting in unusual ways.
- *Self-confessor* uses group setting to express personal, non–group-oriented feelings or insights.
- *Playboy* makes a display of lack of involvement in group's processes.
- *Dominator* tries to assert authority or superiority in manipulating the group or certain members of the group through flattery, being directive, or interrupting others.
- *Help-seeker* attempts to call forth sympathy from other group members through expressing insecurity, personal confusion, or depreciation of self beyond reason.
- *Special interest pleader* speaks for a special group, such as "grass roots," usually representing personal prejudices or biases.

Adapted with permission from Benne, K., & Sheats, P. (1948). Functional roles of group members. *Journal of Social Issues, 4*(2), 41–49.

"Yes, But …"

Some people have a patterned response to any suggestions from others. Initially, they agree with suggestions others offer them, but then they add "yes, but …" and give several reasons why the suggestions will not work for them. Leaders and members can easily identify this patterned response. In such situations, it is best to avoid problem solving for the member and encourage the person to develop his or her own solutions. The leader can serve as a role model of the problem-solving behavior for the other members and encourage them to let the member develop a solution that would work specifically for him or her.

Disliked Member

In some groups, members clearly dislike one particular member. This situation can be challenging for the leader because it can result in considerable tension and conflict. This person could become the group's scapegoat. The group leader may have made a mistake by placing the person in this particular group, and another group may

be a better match. One solution may be to move the person to a better-matched group. Whether the person stays or leaves, the group leader must stay neutral and avoid displaying negative verbal and nonverbal behaviors that indicate that he or she too dislikes the group member or is displeased with the other members for their behavior. Often, the group leader can manage the situation by showing respect for the disliked member and acknowledging his or her contribution. In some instances, getting supervision from a more experienced group leader is useful. Defusing the situation may be possible by using conflict resolution strategies and discussing the underlying issues.

The Silent Member

The engagement of a member who does not participate in group discussion can be challenging. This member has had a lifetime of being "the quiet one" and is usually comfortable in the silent role. The leader should respect the person's silent nature. Like all the other group members, the silent member often gains a considerable amount of information and support without verbally participating.

It is best for the group leader to get to know the member and understand the meaning of the silence before encouraging interaction.

Group Conflict

Most groups experience periods of conflict. The leader first needs to decide whether the conflict is a natural part of the group process or whether the group needs to address some issues. Member-to-member conflict can be handled through the previously discussed conflict resolution process (see Chapter 9). Leader-to-member conflict is more complicated because the leader has the formal position of power. In this instance, the leader can use conflict resolution strategies but should be sensitive to the power differential between the leader's role and the member's role.

Termination Stage or Saying Good-Bye

Termination can be difficult for a group, especially an effective one. During the final stages, members begin to grieve for the loss of the group's closeness and begin to reestablish themselves as individuals. Individuals terminate from groups as they do from any relationship. One person may not show up at the last session, another person may bring up issues that the group has already addressed, and others may demonstrate anger or hostility. Most members of successful groups are sad as the group terminates. During the last meetings, members may make arrangements for meeting after group. These plans rarely materialize or continue. Leaders should recognize these plans as part of the farewell process—saying good-bye to the group.

In terminating a group, the nurse discusses and summarizes the work of the group, including the accomplishments of members and their future plans. The nurse focuses on ending the group and avoids being pulled into working stage issues. For example, when a patient brings up an issue that was once resolved, the nurse reinforces the skills and then reminds the member of the actions that will be taken after the group has ended.

TYPES OF GROUPS
Psychoeducation Groups

The purposes of psychoeducation groups are to enhance knowledge, improve skills, and solve problems. The intervention strategies used in psychoeducation groups focus on transmission of information necessary for making some type of change and providing a process for making the change (Drum, Becker, & Hess, 2011). Recovery-oriented groups are psychoeducation groups that facilitate consumer involvement in the educational process and build on the recovery principles (see Chapter 1). Learning how to manage a medication regimen or control angry outbursts is an example of a recovery-oriented group.

Psychoeducation groups are formally planned, and members are purposefully selected. The group leader develops a lesson plan for each session that includes objectives, content outline, references, and evaluation tools. These groups are time limited and usually last for only a few sessions. If the group lasts longer than a few sessions, cohesiveness becomes important, especially in those that teach health maintenance behaviors such as exercise and weight control (Brown, 2011).

Task Groups

Task groups focus on completion of specific activities, such as planning a week's menu. When members are strongly committed to completing a task and the leader encourages equal participation, cohesiveness promotes satisfaction and higher performance (de Jong, Curseu, & Leenders, 2014). To complete a task, group cohesiveness is especially important. Leaders can encourage cohesiveness by placing participants in situations that promote social interaction with minimal supervision, such as refreshment periods and team-building exercises.

Without cohesiveness, the group's true existence is questionable. In cohesive groups, members are committed to the existence of the group. In large groups, cohesiveness tends to be decreased, with subsequent poorer performance among group members in completing tasks. However, cohesiveness can be a double-edged sword. In very cohesive groups, members are more likely to transgress personal boundaries. Dysfunctional relationships may develop that are destructive to the group process and ultimately not in the best interests of individual members.

Decision-Making Groups

The psychiatric nurse often leads decision-making groups that plan activities, develop unit rules, and select learning materials. The nurse who is leading a decision-making group should observe the process for any signs of **groupthink,** the tendency of group members to avoid conflict and adopt a normative pattern of thinking that is often consistent with the ideas of the group leader (Janis, 1972, 1982). Group members form opinions consistent with the group consensus rather than critically evaluation the situation. Groupthink is more likely to occur if the leader is respected or persuasive. It can also occur if a closed leadership style is used and external threat is present, particularly with time pressure (Goncalo, Polman, & Maslach, 2010). Many catastrophes, such as the *Challenger* explosion and Bay of Pigs invasion, have been attributed to groupthink.

There may be instances in which groupthink can lead to a reasonable decision: for example, a group decides to arrange a going-away party for another patient. In other situations, groupthink may inhibit individual thinking and problem solving: for example, a team is displaying groupthink if it decides that a patient should lose privileges based on the assumption that the patient is deliberately exhibiting bizarre behaviors. In this case, the team is failing to consider or examine other evidence that suggests the bizarre behavior is really an indication of psychosis.

Supportive Therapy Groups

Supportive therapy groups are usually less intense than psychotherapy groups and focus on helping individuals cope with their illnesses and problems. Implementing supportive therapy groups is one of the basic functions of the psychiatric nurse. In conducting this type of group, the nurse focuses on helping members cope with situations that are common for other group members. Counseling strategies are used. For example, a group of patients with bipolar illness whose illness is stable may discuss at a monthly meeting how to tell other people about the illness or how to cope with a family member who seems insensitive to the illness. Family caregivers of persons with mental illnesses benefit from the support of the group, as well as additional information about providing care for an ill family member.

Psychotherapy Groups

Psychotherapy groups treat individuals' emotional problems and can be implemented from various theoretic perspectives, including psychoanalytic, behavioral, and cognitive. These groups focus on examining emotions and helping individuals face their life situations. At times, these groups can be extremely intense. Psychotherapy groups provide an opportunity for patients to examine and resolve psychological and interpersonal issues within a safe environment. Mental health specialists who have a minimum of a master's degree and are trained in group psychotherapy lead such groups. Patients can be treated in psychotherapy and still be members of other nursing groups. Communication with the therapists is important for continuity of care.

One of the most respected approaches is Irvin D. Yalom's model of group psychotherapy. According to Yalom & Leszcz (2005), there are 11 primary factors through which therapeutic changes occur (Table 11.3). In this model, interpersonal relationships are very important because change occurs through a corrective emotional experience within the context of the group. The group is viewed as a social microcosm of the patients' psychosocial environment (Yalom & Leszcz, 2005).

TABLE 11.3	YALOM'S THERAPEUTIC FACTORS
Therapeutic Factors	**Definition**
Instillation of hope	Hope is required to keep patients in therapy
Universality	Finding out that others have similar problems
Imparting information	Didactic instruction about mental health, mental illness, and so on
Altruism	Learning to give to others
Corrective recapitulation of the primary family group	Reliving and correcting early family conflicts within the group
Development of socializing techniques	Learning basic social skills
Imitative behavior	Assuming some of the behaviors and characteristics of the therapist
Interpersonal learning	Analogue of therapeutic factors in individual therapy, such as insight, working through the transference, and corrective emotional experience
Group cohesiveness	Group members' relationship to therapist and other group members
Catharsis	Open expression of affect to purge or "cleanse" self
Existential factors	Patients' ultimate concerns of existence: death, isolation, freedom, and meaninglessness

Source: Yalom, I., & Leszcz, M. (2005) *The theory and practice of group psychotherapy.* New York: Basic Books.

Self-Help Groups

Self-help groups are led by people who are concerned about coping with a specific problem or life crisis. These groups do not explore psychodynamic issues in depth. Professionals usually do not attend these groups or serve as consultants. Alcoholics Anonymous, Overeaters Anonymous, and One Day at a Time (a grief group) are examples of self-help groups.

Age-Related Groups

Group interventions for specific age groups require attention to the developmental needs of the group members, any physical and mental impairments, social ability, and cognitive level. Children's groups should be structured to accommodate their intellectual and developmental functioning. Groups for older people should be adapted for age-related changes of the members (Box 11.4).

SELF-ASSESSMENT
Because most group leaders do not have personal experience with the issues faced by older adults, the leaders should sensitize themselves to the positive and negative aspects of aging and the developmental issues facing older adults. Leaders need to be aware of their own negative reactions to aging and how this might affect their work.

COHORT EXPERIENCES
There is a wide variation in the experiences and history of older adults. Current 80- to 90-year-old adults grew up in the Great Depression of the 1930s, 65- to 80-year-old adults commonly experienced growing up during World War II, and the Baby Boomers (ages 55 to 65 years) were teenagers or young adults during the political and sexual revolution of the 1960s.

TYPICAL THEMES IN GROUP MEETINGS
- **Continuity with the past:** Older adults enjoy recalling, reliving, and reminiscing about past accomplishments.
- **Understanding the modern world:** They often use groups to understand and adapt to the modern world.
- **Independence:** They worry about becoming dependent. Physical and cognitive impairments are threats to independence. Loss of family members and friends are also threats. Leaders should be familiar with the grieving processes.
- **Changes in family relationships:** Family relationships, especially with children and grandchildren, are increasingly important as social roles change.
- **Changes in resources and environment:** Living on a fixed income focuses older people on the importance of their disposable income. They are more vulnerable to community and neighborhood changes because of their physical and financial limitations.

GROUP LEADERSHIP
- The pace of group meetings should be slowed.
- Greater emphasis should be placed on using wisdom and experience rather than learning new information.
- The group should be encouraged to use life review strategies such as autobiography and reminiscence.
- Teaching new coping skills should be placed within the context of previous attempts to resolve issues and problems (Toseland & Rizzo, 2004).

Family Groups

Families often participate in a psychoeducation, supportive, psychotherapy and self-help group. In some groups, there are multiple families; in others there may be just one family participating. Families are a unique group because the members have already formed a group with established interaction patterns, conflicts, emotional bonds and issues. The leader should identify these family characteristics and determine how they impact the purpose of the group. The leader may choose not to address family conflict when the purpose of the group is to teach the management of a particular symptom. If a family issue is important to the purpose of the group, the leader can include the issue within group discussion.

COMMON NURSING INTERVENTION GROUPS

Nurses lead groups of varying types that are geared toward a specific content area such as medication management, symptom management, anger management, and self-care skills. In addition, nurses groups focus on other issues such as stress management, relaxation, and women's issues. The key to being a good leader is to integrate group leadership, knowledge, and skills with nursing interventions that fit a selected group.

Medication Groups

Nurse-led medication groups are common in psychiatric nursing. Not all medication groups are alike, so the nurse must be clear regarding the purpose of each specific medication group (Box 11.5). A medication group can be used primarily to transmit information about medications, such as action, dosage, and side effects, or it can focus on issues related to medications, such as compliance, management of side effects, and lifestyle adjustments. Many nurses incorporate both perspectives.

Assessing a member's medication knowledge is important before he or she joins the group to determine what the individual would like to learn. People with mental

PURPOSE: Develop strategies that reinforce a self-medication routine.

DESCRIPTION: The medication group is an open, ongoing group that meets once a week to discuss topics germane to self-administration of medication. Members will not be asked to disclose the names of their medications.

MEMBER SELECTION: The group is open to any person taking medication for a mental illness or emotional problem who would like more information about medication, side effects, and staying on a regimen. Referrals from mental health providers are encouraged. Each person will meet with the group leader before attending the group to determine if the group will meet the individual's learning needs.

STRUCTURE: The format is a small group, with no more than eight members and one psychiatric nurse group leader facilitating a discussion about the issues. Topics are rotated.

TIME AND LOCATION: 2:00–3:00 PM, every Wednesday at the Mental Health Center

COST: No charge for attending

TOPICS
- How Do I Know If My Medications Are Working?
- Side Effect Management: Is It Worth It?
- Hints for Taking Medications Without Missing Doses!
- Health Problems That Medications Affect
- (Other topics will be developed to meet the needs of group members.)

EVALUATION: Short pretest and posttest for instructor's use only illness may have difficulty remembering new information, so assessment of cognitive abilities is important. Assessing attention span, memory, and problem-solving skills gives valuable information that nurses can use in designing the group. The nurse should determine the members' reading and writing skills to select effective patient education materials.

An ideal group is one in which all members use the same medication. In reality, this situation is rare. Usually, the group members are using various medications. The nurse should know which medications each member is taking, but to avoid violating patient confidentiality, the nurse needs to be careful not to divulge that information to other patients. If group members choose, they can share the names of their medications with one another. A small group format works best, and the more interaction, the better. Using a lecture method of teaching is less effective than involving the members in the learning process. The nurse should expose the members to various audio and visual educational materials, including workbooks, videotapes, and handouts. The nurse should ask members to write down information to help them remember and learn through various modes. Evaluation of the learning outcomes begins with the first class. Nurses can develop and give pre-tests and post-tests, which in combination can measure learning outcomes.

Symptom Management Groups

Nurses often lead recovery-oriented groups that focus on helping patients deal with a severe and persistent mental illness. Handling hallucinations, being socially appropriate, and staying motivated to complete activities of daily living are a few common topics. In symptom management groups, members also learn when a symptom indicates that relapse is imminent and what to do about it. Within the context of a symptom management group, patients can learn how to avoid relapse.

Anger Management Groups

Anger management is another common topic for a nurse-led group, often in the inpatient setting. The purposes of an anger management group are to discuss the concept of anger, identify antecedents to aggressive behavior, and develop new strategies to deal with anger other than verbal and physical aggression (see Chapter 13). The treatment team refers individuals with histories of being verbally and physically abusive, usually to family members, to these groups to help them better understand their emotions and behavioral responses. Impulsiveness and emotional lability are problems for many of the group members. Anger management usually includes a discussion of associated stressful situations, events that trigger anger, feelings about the situation, and unmet personal needs.

Self-Care Groups

Another common nurse-led recovery-oriented psychiatric group is a self-care group. People with psychiatric illnesses often have self-care deficits and benefit from the structure that a group provides. These groups are challenging because members usually know how to perform these daily tasks (e.g., bathing, grooming, performing personal hygiene), but their illnesses cause them to lose the motivation to complete them. The leader not only reinforces the basic self-care skills but also, more importantly, helps identify strategies that can motivate the patients and provide structure to their daily lives.

Reminiscence Groups

Reminiscence therapy has been shown to be a valuable intervention for older clients. In this type of group, members are encouraged to remember events from past years. Such a group is easily implemented. Usually, a simple question about an important family event will spark memories. Reminiscence groups are usually associated with patients who have dementia who are having difficulty with recent memory. Reminiscence groups can also be used as an intergenerational intervention with healthy older adults and children. Older adults become less lonely and experience an improved quality of life; children's attitudes toward the elderly becomes more positive (Gaggioli et al., 2014; Stinson, 2009).

SUMMARY OF KEY POINTS

- The definition of group can vary according to theoretic orientation. A general definition is that a group is two or more people who have at least one common goal or issue. Group dynamics are the interactions within a group that influence the group's development and process.

- Groups can be open, with new members joining at any time, or closed, with members admitted only once. Either small or large groups can be effective, but dynamics change in different size groups.

- The process of group development occurs in phases: beginning, middle, and termination. These stages are not fixed but dynamic. The process challenges the leader to guide the group. During the working stage, the group addresses its purpose.

- Leading a group involves many different functions, from obtaining and receiving information to testing and evaluating decisions. The leader should explain the rules of the group at the beginning of the group.

- Verbal communication includes the communication network and group themes. Nonverbal communication is more complex and involves eye contact, body posture, and the mood of the group. Decision-making groups can be victims of groupthink, which can have positive or negative outcomes. Groupthink research is ongoing.

- Seating arrangements can affect group interaction. The fewer physical barriers there are, such as tables, the better the communication. Everyone should be a part of the group, and no one should sit outside of it. In the most interactive groups, members face one another in a circle.

- Leadership skills involve listening; tracking verbal and nonverbal behaviors; and maintaining a neutral, nonjudgmental style.

- Although there are only two formal group roles, leader and member, there are many informal group roles. These roles are usually categorized according to purpose—task functions, maintenance functions, and individual roles. Members who assume task functions encourage the group members to stay focused on the group's task. Those who assume maintenance functions worry more about the group working together than the actual task itself. Individual roles can either enhance or detract from the work of the group.

- The leader should address behaviors that challenge the leadership, group process, or other members to determine whether to intervene. In some instances, the leader redirects a monopolizing member; at other times, the leader lets the group deal with the behavior. Group conflict occurs in most groups.

- There are many different types of groups. Psychiatric nurses lead psychoeducation and supportive therapy groups. Mental health specialists who are trained to provide intensive therapy lead psychotherapy groups. Consumers lead self-help groups, and professionals assist only as requested. Leading age-related groups requires attention to the developmental, physical, social, and intellectual abilities of the participants. Themes of older adult groups include continuity with the past, understanding the modern world, independence, and changes in family and resources. Group leadership for older adult groups builds on participants' previous experiences and coping abilities in developing new coping skills.

- Medication, symptom management, anger management, and self-care groups are common nurse-led groups focused on specific interventions.

CRITICAL THINKING CHALLENGES

1. Group members are very polite to one another and are superficially discussing topics. You would assess the group as being in which phase? Explain your answer.

2. After three sessions of a supportive therapy group, two members begin to share their frustration with having a mental illness. The group is moving into which phase of group development? Explain your answer.

3. Define the roles of the task and maintenance functions in groups. Observe your clinical group and identify classmates who are assuming task functions and maintenance functions.

4. Observe a patient group for at least five sessions. Discuss the seating pattern that emerges. Identify the communication network and the group themes. Then identify the group's norms and standards.

5. Discuss the conditions that lead to groupthink. When is groupthink positive? When is groupthink negative? Explain.

6. List at least six behaviors that are important for a group leader, including one for age-related groups. Justify your answers.

7. During the first meeting, one member seems very anxious and tends to monopolize the conversation. Discuss how you would assess the situation and whether you would intervene.

8. At the end of the fourth meeting, one group member angrily accuses another of asking too many questions. The other members look on quietly. How would you assess the situation? Would you intervene? Explain.

 12 Angry Men: 1998. In this excellent film, a young man stands accused of fatally stabbing his father. A jury of his "peers" is deciding his fate. This jury is portrayed by an excellent cast, including Jack Lemmon, George C. Scott, Tony Danza, and Ossie Davis. At first, the case appears to be "open and shut." This film depicts an intense struggle to reach a verdict and is an excellent study of group process and group dynamics.

Viewing Points: Identify the leaders in the group. How does leadership change throughout the film? Do you find any evidence of groupthink? How does the group handle conflict?

REFERENCES

Benne, K., & Sheats, P. (1948). Functional roles of group members. *Journal of Social Issues, 4*(2), 41–49.

Brown, N. W. (2011). *Psychoeducational groups: Process and practice* (3rd ed). New York: Taylor & Frances Group.

Cahill, K., & Lancaster, T. (2014). Workplace interventions for smoking cessation. (Review). *The Cochrane Collaborative, 2 CD003440, doi: 10.1002/14651858.CD003440.pub4*

Clark, C. C. (2009). *Group leadership skills for nurses and health professionals* (5th ed). New York: Springer.

Corey, M. S., Corey, G., & Corey, C. (2010). *Group process and practice.* New York: Brooks Cole.

de Jong, J. P., Curseu, P. L., & Leenders, R. T. (2014). When do bad apples not spoil the barrel? Negative relationships in teams, team performance, and buffering mechanism. *The Journal of Applied Psychology, 99*(3), 514–522.

Drum, D., Becker, M. S., & Hess, E. (2011). Expanding the application of group interventions: Emergence of groups in health care settings. *The Journal for Specialists in Group Work, 36*(4), 247–263.

Gaggioli, A., Morganti, L., Bonfiglio, S., Scaratti, C., Cipresso, P., Serino, S., et al. (2014). Intergenerational group reminiscence: A potentially effective intervention to enhance elderly psychosocial wellbeing and to improve children's perception of aging. *Educational Gerontology, 40*(7), 486–498.

Goncalo, J. A., Polman, E., & Maslach, C. (2010). Can confidence come too soon? collective efficaacy, conflict and group performance over time. *Organizational Behavior & Human Decision Processes, 113*(1), 13–24.

Janis, I. (1972). *Victims of groupthink.* Boston: Houghton Mifflin.

Janis, I. (1982). *Groupthink* (2nd ed). Boston: Houghton Mifflin.

LoCoco, G., Gullo, S., Lo Verso, G., & Kivlighan, D. M. (2013). Sex composition and group climate: A group actor-partner interdependence analysis. *Group Dynamics: Theory, Research, and Practice, 17*(4), 270–280.

Puskar, K., Mazza, G., Slivka, C., Westcott, M., Campbell, F., & McFadden, T. G. (2012). Understanding content and process: Guidelines for group leaders. *Perspectives in Psychiatric care, 48*(4), 225–229.

Stinson, C. K. (2009). Structured group reminiscence: An intervention for older adults. *The Journal of Continuing Education in Nursing, 40*(11), 523–528.

Toseland, R. W., & Rizzo, V. M. (2004). What's different about working with older people in groups? *Journal of Gerontological Social Work, 44*(1/2), 5–23.

Yalom, I., & Leszcz, M. (2005). *The theory and practice of group psychotherapy.* New York: Basic Books.

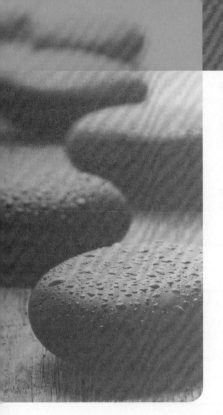

UNIT IV
PREVENTION OF MENTAL DISORDERS

12
Stress and Mental Health

Mary Ann Boyd

KEY CONCEPTS

- allostatic load
- adaptation
- coping
- stress

LEARNING OBJECTIVES

After studying this chapter, you will be able to:

1. Discuss the concept of stress as it relates to mental health and mental illness.

2. Discuss interpersonal and psychological factors affecting the experience of stress, including the person–environment relationship and appraisal.

3. Discuss the variety of stress responses experienced by individuals.

4. Explain the role of coping and adaptation in maintaining and promoting mental health.

5. Apply critical thinking skills to the nursing management process for a person experiencing stress.

KEY TERMS

- allostasis • appraisal • constraints • demands • diathesis • emotion-focused coping • emotions • homeostasis
- life events • person–environment relationship • problem-focused coping • reappraisal • social functioning
- social network • social support • stress response

Stress is a natural part of life, yet it is one of the most complex concepts in health and nursing. Although often thought of as negative, stress can be a positive experience when an individual approaches it with successful coping skills. For example, children learn to cope with stressful situations in preparation for adulthood. During severe stress, some people draw on resources that they never realized they had and grow from those experiences. However, early childhood stress and trauma, unresolved stress, or chronic stress can have negative mental and physical health consequences.

THE ROLE OF STRESS IN MENTAL HEALTH

Stress is a transactional process arising from real or perceived internal or external environmental demands that are appraised as threatening or benign (Lazarus &

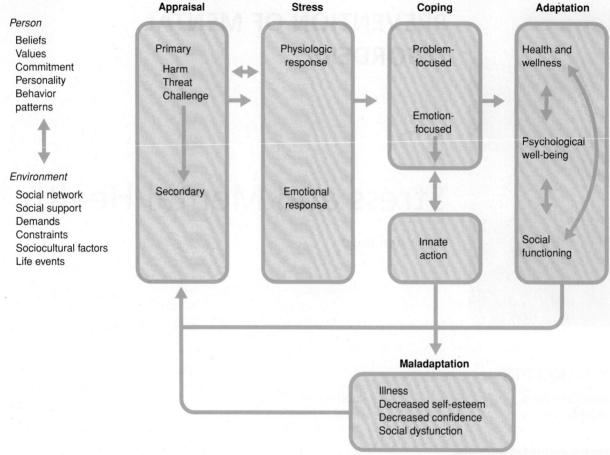

FIGURE 12.1 Stress, coping, and adaptation model.

Folkman, 1984) (Figure 12.1). No one lives in a stress-free environment, yet stress reduction leads to positive mental health. Conversely, many patients attribute their first illness episode to a stressful event such as an assault, rape, or family tragedy.

> **KEYCONCEPT** **Stress** is a transactional process arising from real or perceived internal or external environmental demands that are appraised as threatening or benign (Lazarus & Folkman, 1984).

Stress responses can be acute or chronic. Acute stress can lead to physiologic overload, which in turn can have a negative impact on a person's health. Chronic stress is clearly associated with negative health incomes. Stress is also associated with the development or exacerbation of symptoms of mental illness. For example, psychiatric disorders are prevalent in caregivers of persons with chronic illnesses. Many caregivers of family members with dementia, AIDS, and other long-term illnesses experience severe and chronic stress leading to depression as they continually monitor the family member, cope with illness-related behaviors, and often witness deterioration of their significant other. In addition, the caregiver's own

activities are curtailed (Zegwaard, Aartsen, Cuijpers, & Grypdonck, 2011).

When stress is associated with the development or exacerbation of a mental illness, the diathesis-stress model can be applied. In this model, a **diathesis** or a genetic predisposition increases susceptibility of developing a disorder. For example, in animal models, maternal separation and abandonment demonstrate that early stress experiences alter hypothalamus–pituitary–adrenal (HPA) axis response to stress (discussed later in this chapter). Impaired functioning of the stress response is central to many psychiatric, immune, and physical disorders (Kumari, Badrick, Sacker, Kirschbaum, Marmot, & Chandola, 2010). As a result, adverse events during childhood increase risk of alcohol and drug dependence, eating disorders, affective disorders, posttraumatic stress disorder (PTSD), and suicidal behavior. Another example is the story of a woman whose mother had a long history of depression (indicating a genetic predisposition to mental disorders for the daughter) and who was assaulted as she was leaving work and sustained multiple injuries. Her first manic episode occurred within 2 months (see Chapter 20).

INTERPERSONAL AND PSYCHOSOCIAL ASPECTS OF STRESS

Two important factors determine whether an individual experiences a **stress response**, which is the physiological, behavioral, and cognitive reaction to a perceived threat. They are the person–environment relationship and the person's cognitive appraisal of the risks and benefits of a given situation.

Person–Environment Relationship

The **person–environment relationship** is the interactions between an individual and the environment that change throughout a stress experience. It is based on the values and beliefs people they carry with them in life, as well as personality factors and factors related to the individual's social and physical environment.

Values and Goals

Personal values are developed throughout a lifetime and are shaped by cultural, ethnic, family, and religious beliefs. These values influence the significance of a particular event. What is important to one person may not be to another. For example, one person may value a high-paying salary and another may value the freedom to move around without the boundaries of material things.

If a goal is important, a person is more likely to do what it takes to reach the goal. The more important the goal or the more difficult the goal is to obtain, the greater the likelihood of stress. For example, students who earn mostly or all As often feel more stress about examinations than do students who earn Bs and Cs because the higher grade is more difficult to obtain.

Personality and Behavior Patterns

The association of personality types to health or illness status has been studied for over fifty years (Friedman & Rosenman, 1974). There are four general personality types. Type A personalities are characterized as competitive, aggressive, ambitious, impatient, alert, tense, and restless. They think, speak, and act at an accelerated pace and reflect an aggressive, hostile, and time-urgent style of living that is often associated with increased psychophysiologic arousal (Sogaard, Dalgard, Holme, Roysamb, & Haheim, 2008). In contrast, type B personalities do not exhibit these behaviors and generally are more relaxed, easygoing, and easily satisfied. They have an accepting attitude about trivial mistakes and use a problem-solving approach to major problems. Rarely do type B people push themselves to obtain excesses from the environment or try to accomplish too much in too little time (Tishler, Bartholomae, & Rhodes, 2005).

Type C personalities are described as having difficulty expressing emotion and are introverted, respectful, conforming, compliant, and eager to please and avoid conflict. They respond to stress with depression and hopelessness. This personality type was initially associated with the development of cancer, specifically breast cancer in women, but there has been no clear evidence that the stress associated with this personality type has a role in the etiology of cancer (Bryant-Lukosius, 2003; Lală, Bobîrnac, & Tipa, 2010). The type D (distressed) personalities experience increased negative emotion (depression) and pessimism and are unlikely to show their emotions to others. There is mixed research support for an association between a type D personality and mental health disorders and poor physical health status (Mols & Denollet, 2010; Marchesi et al., 2014; Stevenson & Williams, 2014).

However, overall, research supporting associations between personality types and health status is mixed. Personality characteristics, such as hostility and anger, associated with illnesses continue to be the focus of these studies (Rafanelli, Sirri, Grandi, & Fava, 2013; Shen, Countryman, Spiro, & Niaura, 2008).

Physical and Social Environment

A person has unique interactions daily with the physical and social environments. The external environment includes physical aspects such as air quality, cleanliness of food and water, temperature, and noise. Social aspects include living arrangements and personal contacts.

Social Networks

A **social network** consists of linkages among a defined set of people with whom an individual has personal contacts. A social identity develops within this network (Azmitia, Syed, & Radmacher, 2008). Emotional support, material aid, services, information, and new social contacts increase personal resources, enhance the ability to cope with change, and influence the course of illnesses (Li & Wu, 2010).

A social network may be large, consisting of numerous family and community contacts, or small, consisting of few. Contacts can be categorized according to three levels:

1. Level I consists of six to 12 people with whom the person has close contact.
2. Level II consists of a larger number of contacts, generally 30 to 40 people whom the person sees regularly.
3. Level III consists of the large number of people with whom a person has direct contact, such as the grocer and mail carrier, and can represent several hundred people.

Each person's social network is slightly different. Multiple contacts allow several networks to interact.

Generally, the larger the network, the more support is available. An ideal network structure is fairly dense and interconnected; people within the network are in contact with one another. Dense networks are better able to respond in times of stress and crisis and to provide emotional support to those in distress. For example, residents of a small town are more likely to provide food and shelter to fire victims than neighbors in a large urban area who have little contact with each other.

Ideally, a balance between intense and less intense relationships exists in a social network. When relationships are intense and include only one or two people, the opportunity to interact with other network members is limited. On the other hand, isolation can occur without at least a few intense relationships.

Social networks provide opportunities for give and take. Network members both provide and receive support, aid, services, and information. Reciprocity is particularly important because most friendships do not last without the give and take of support and services. A person who is always on the receiving end eventually becomes isolated from others.

Social Support

One of the important functions of the social network is to provide **social support** in the form of positive interpersonal interactions as part of a dynamic process that is in constant flux and varies with life events and health status (Whatley, Dilorio, & Yeager, 2010). Not all interpersonal interactions within a network are supportive. A person can have a large, complex social network but little social support. Some life events, such as marriage, divorce, and bereavement, actually change the level of social support by adding to or subtracting from a person's social network.

Social support serves three functions:

1. Emotional support contributes to a person's feelings of being cared for or loved.
2. Tangible support provides a person with additional resources.
3. Informational support helps a person view situations in a new light (Table 12.1).

Social support enhances health outcomes and reduces mortality by helping members make needed behavior changes and buffering stressful life events. In a supportive social environment, members feel helped, valued, and in personal control. Healthy people are likely to have strong support systems that help them cope with undesirable life events.

Demands and Constraints

Internal **demands** that pull on an individual's resources are generated by physiologic and psychological needs.

TABLE 12.1	EXAMPLES OF FUNCTIONS OF SOCIAL SUPPORT
Function	**Example**
Emotional support	Attachment, reassurance, being able to rely on and confide in a person
Tangible support	Direct aid such as loans or gifts, services such as taking care of someone who is ill, doing a job or chore
Informational support	Providing information or advice, giving feedback about how a person is doing

From Schaefer, C., Coyne, J., & Lazarus, R. (1982). The health-related functions of social support. *Journal of Behavioral Medicine, 4*(4), 381–406.

External demands are imposed by the physical environment such as crowding, crime, noise, and pollution. The social environment imposes other demands, such as behavioral and role expectations. In contrast to demands, **constraints** are limitations that are both personal and environmental. Personal constraints include internalized cultural values and beliefs and psychological deficits that dictate actions or feelings. Finite resources, such as money and time, are examples of environmental constraints that many people have.

These demands and constraints vary with the individual and contribute to or initiate a stress response (Lazarus, 2001; Segerstrom, 2010). They also interact with one another; for example, work demands, such as changing shifts, may interact with physical demands, such as a need for sleep, creating a high-risk situation in which stress is likely to occur.

Sociocultural Factors

Cultural expectations and role strain serve as both demands and constraints in the experience of stress. If a person violates cultural group values to meet role expectations, stress occurs; for example, a person may stay in an abusive relationship to avoid the stress of violating a cultural norm that values lifelong marriage, no matter what the circumstances. The potential guilt associated with norm violation and the anticipated isolation from being ostracized seem worse than the physical and psychological pain caused by the abusive situation.

Employment is another highly valued cultural norm and provides social, psychological, and financial benefits. In all cultures, work is assigned significance beyond economic compensation. It is often the central focus of adulthood and, for many, a source of personal identity. Even if employment brings little real happiness, being employed implies financial needs are being met. Work offers status, regulates life activities, permits association with others, and provides a meaningful life experience. Although work is demanding, unemployment can actually be more stressful because of the associated isolation and loss of social status.

Gender expectations often become an additional source of demands and constraints for women, who assume multiple roles. In most cultures, women who work outside the home are expected to assume primary responsibility for care of the children and household duties. Most women are adept at separating these roles and can compartmentalize problems at work from those at home. When there is a healthy balance between work and home, women experience a low level of psychological stress. However, when the balance is disturbed, daily stress contributes to health problems (Low, Thurston, & Matthews, 2010).

Life Events

In 1967, Holmes and Rahe presented a psychosocial view of illness by pointing out the complex relationship between life changes and the development of illnesses

(Holmes & Rahe, 1967). They hypothesized that people become ill after they experience major **life events**, such as marriage, divorce, and bereavement. The more frequent the changes, the greater the possibility of becoming sick. The investigators cited the events that they believed partially accounted for the onset of illnesses and began testing whether these life changes were actual precursors to illness. It soon became clear that not all events have the same effects. For example, the death of a spouse is usually much more devastating and stressful than a change in residence. From their research, the investigators were able to assign relative weights to various life events according to the degree of associated stress. Rahe devised the Recent Life Changes Questionnaire (Table 12.2) to evaluate the frequency and significance of life change events (Rahe, 1994). Numerous research studies subsequently demonstrated the relationship between a recent life change and the severity of near-future illness (Rahe, 1994; Rahe, Taylor, Tolles, Newhall, Veach, & Bryson, 2002). Recent studies show that

---

TABLE 12.2   RECENT LIFE CHANGES QUESTIONNAIRE

Directions: Sum the life change units (LCUs) for your life change events during the past 12 months.
250 to 400 LCUs per year: Minor life crisis
Over 400 LCUs per year: Major life crisis

Life Changes	LCU Values*	Life Changes	LCU Values*
Family		Change in sleeping habits	31
Death of spouse	105	Revision of personal habits	31
Marital separation	65	Change in eating habits	29
Death of close family member	65	Change in church activities	29
Divorce	62	Vacation	29
Pregnancy	60	Change in school	28
Change in health of family member	52	Change in recreation	28
Marriage	50	Christmas	26
Gain of new family member	50	***Work***	
Marital reconciliation	42	Fired at work	64
Spouse begins or stops work	37	Retirement from work	49
Son or daughter leaves home	29	Trouble with boss	39
In-law trouble	29	Business readjustment	38
Change in number of family get-togethers	26	Change to different line of work	38
Personal		Change in work responsibilities	33
Jail term	56	Change in work hours or conditions	30
Sex difficulties	49	***Financial***	
Death of a close friend	46	Foreclosure of mortgage or loan	57
Personal injury or illness	42	Change in financial state	43
Change in living conditions	39	Mortgage (e.g., home, car)	39
Outstanding personal achievement	33	Mortgage or loan less than $10,000 (e.g., stereo)	26
Change in residence	33		
Minor violations of the law	32		
Begin or end school	32		

*LCU, life change unit. The number of LCUs reflects the average degree or intensity of the life change.

From Rahe, R. H. (2000). Recent Life Changes Questionnaire (RLCQ).

life changes in older adults that resulted in feeling helpless or fearing for their life reported higher body mass index and more chronic illnesses (Seib et al., 2014). If several life changes occur within a short period, the likelihood that an illness will appear is even greater (Tamers, Okechukwu, Bohl, Gueguen, Goldberg, & Zins, 2014).

Appraisal

All stress responses are affected by the personal meaning of a situation; for example, chest pain is stressful to a person not only because of the immediate pain and incapacitation it causes but also because of the fear that the chest pain may mean that the person is having a heart attack. Thus, the significance of the event actually determines the importance of the person–environment relationship (Lazarus, 2001; Moran, 2001). Stress is initiated not by a single stress but by an unfavorable person–environment relationship that is meaningful in terms of the risks or benefits to that person's well-being.

A given event or situation may be extremely stressful to one person but not to another (Box 12.1). The more important or meaningful the outcome, the more vulnerable the person is to stress. **Appraisal** is the process where all aspects are considered—the demands, constraints, and resources are balanced with personal goals and beliefs.

BOX 12.1 CLINICAL VIGNETTE

Stress Responses to an Examination

Two students are preparing for the same examination. Susan is genuinely interested in the subject, prepares by studying throughout the semester, and reviews the content two days before test day. The night before the examination, she goes to bed early, gets a good night's sleep, and wakes refreshed but is slightly nervous about the test. She wants to do well and expects a difficult test but knows that she can retake it at a later date if she does poorly.

In contrast, Joanne is not interested in the subject matter and does not study throughout the semester. She "crams" 2 days before the test date and does an "all nighter" the night before. This is the last time that Joanne can take the examination, but she believes that she will pass because she has already taken it twice and is familiar with the questions. If she does not pass, she will not be able to return to school. On entering the room, Joanne is physically tired and somewhat fearful of not passing the test. As she looks at the test, she instantly realizes that it is not the examination she expected. The questions are new. She begins hyperventilating and tremoring. After yelling obscenities at the teacher, she storms out of the room. She is very distressed and describes herself as "being in a panic."

What Do You Think?

- How are the students' experiences different? Are there any similarities?
- Are there any nursing diagnoses that apply to Joanne's situation?

A critical factor is the risk involved (Aguilera, 1998; Kendall & Terry, 2009; Lazarus, 2001).

The appraisal process has two levels: primary and secondary. In a primary appraisal, a person evaluates the events occurring in his or her life as a threat, harm, or challenge. During primary appraisal of a goal, the person determines whether (1) the goal is relevant, (2) the goal is consistent with his or her values and beliefs, and (3) whether a personal commitment is present. In the vignette, Susan's commitment to the goal of doing well on the test was consistent with her valuing the content, which in turn motivated her to study regularly and prepare carefully for the examination. She believed that the test would be difficult. Joanne had a commitment to pass the test but did not value the content. Unlike Susan, Joanne believed that the test would be relatively easy because she expected the questions to be the same as those on the previous examination.

In a secondary appraisal, the person explains the outcome of events. There may be blame or credit given for the outcome. In the example, Susan was nervous but took the test. Joanne's secondary appraisal of the test-taking situation began with the realization that she might not pass the test because the questions were different. She acted impulsively by blaming the teacher for giving a different examination and by storming out of the room. She clearly did not cope effectively with a difficult situation.

RESPONSES TO STRESS

After a person–environment relationship is established and an individual appraises a situation as threatening or harmful, an internal stress response occurs. This includes simultaneous physiological and emotional responses.

Physiologic Responses

Physiologic changes in response to stress are automatic and differ based on the type of stress, duration, and intensity, which depend on the appraised risk of the situation. The riskier the situation, the more intense is the physiologic response.

Homeostasis and the Fight or Flight Response

The concept of **homeostasis**, which is the body's tendency to resist physiological change and hold bodily functions relatively consistent, well-coordinated, and usually stable, was introduced by Walter Cannon in the 1930s. The body's internal equilibrium is regulated by physiological processes such as blood glucose, pH, and oxygen. Set points (normal reference ranges of physiological parameters) are maintained (Cannon, 1932).

When the brain (amygdala and hippocampus) interprets an event as a threat, the hypothalamus and autonomic nervous system are signaled to secrete adrenaline,

TABLE 12.3	FLIGHT AND FIGHT: PHYSIOLOGICAL CHANGES	
Sympathetic Nervous System Effect	**Purpose**	**Parasympathetic Nervous System Conservation of Energy**
Increased serum glucose	Increased energy	Decreased sexual and sex hormone activity
Increased cardiac output and blood pressure (increase in renin and angiotensin)	Increased blood flow	Decreased growth, repair, and maturation
Increased oxygen tension and hematocrit	Increased supply of oxygen in blood	Decreased digestion, assimilation, and whole food distribution
Other Physiological Changes		
Effect	*Purpose*	
Increased immune responses	Reduced risk of infections	
Heightened vigilance in the brain	Increased decision-making attention and memory	
Hyperactivation of the hemostatic and coagulation system	Prevention of excessive bleeding from wounds	

Adapted from Diamond, J. W. (2009). Allostatic medicine: Bringing stress, coping, and chronic disease into focus. Part 1. *Integrative Medicine, 8*(6), 40–44.

cortisol, and epinephrine. These hormones activate the sympathetic nervous system, physiological stability is challenged, and a "fight or flight" response occurs. Heart rate, blood pressure, and blood sugar increase. Energy is mobilized for survival. As the sympathetic system is activated, the parasympathic is muted (Table 12.3). After there is no longer a need for more energy and the threat is over, the body returns to a state of homeostasis.

Chronic Stress and Illness

The HPA axis, introduced earlier, is another important part of the stress response. Hans Seyle, who first initiated the study of stress, defined stress as a nonspecific response to an irritant, a perceived danger, or a life threat. He called stress evoked by positive emotions or events *eustress* and stress evoked by negative feelings and events *distress*. He showed that corticosteroid secretion from the pituitary gland increased during stress and contributed to development of illnesses. Seyle described this process as general adaptation syndrome (GAS), which he defined as consisting of three stages: the alarm reaction (a threat is

perceived, and the body responds physiologically), stage of resistance (coping mechanisms are used to try to reestablish homeostasis), and stage of exhaustion (occurs if homeostasis is not achieved) (Selye, 1956, 1974).

We now understand that the sympathetic nervous system activates the HPA axis. When the hypothalamus secretes corticotropin-releasing hormone (CRH), the pituitary gland increases secretion of adrenocorticotropic hormone (corticotropin), which in turn stimulates the adrenocortical secretion of cortisol.

Allostasis and the Allostatic Load

Allostasis is a term used to describe the dynamic regulatory process that maintains homeostasis through a process of adaptation. Physiological stability is achieved when the autonomic nervous system; the HPA; and the cardiovascular, metabolic, and immune systems respond to internal and external stimuli (McEwen, 2005, 2010).

As wear and tear on the brain and body occur, there is a corresponding increase in the number of abnormal biologic parameters called allostatic load (AL) (Figure 12.2).

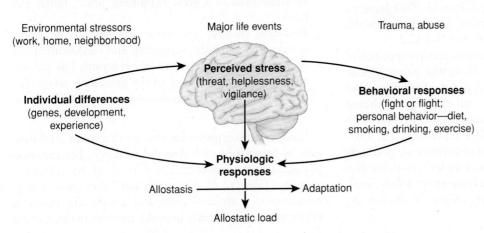

FIGURE 12.2 The development of allostatic load in response to stress. (Redrawn with permission from McEwen, B. S. [1998]. Protective and damaging effects of stress and stress mediators. *New England Journal of Medicine, 3*[38], 171–179.)

AL is measured by the cumulative changes of the biologic regulatory systems as indicated by abnormal laboratory values. The greater the allostatic load, the greater the state of chronic stress and ultimately, the more negative changes in health (McEwen & Gianaros, 2010).

> **KEYCONCEPT** **Allostatic load** is the consequence of the wear and tear on the body and brain and leads to ill health.

Paradoxically, the same systems that are protective in acute stress can damage the body when activated by chronic stress. The benefits of the increase in circulating cortisol to the human body are initially adaptive, but if it continues, it can be quite damaging to both mental (depression) and physical (immune, cardiovascular, and metabolic) health (McVicar, Ravalier, & Greenwood, 2013; Sterling, 2012).

In chronic stress, the immune system is suppressed. Cortisol is primarily immunosuppressive and contributes to reduction in lymphocyte numbers and function (primarily T-lymphocyte and monocyte subsets) and natural killer (NK) activities. The immune cells have receptors for cortisol and catecholamines that can bind with lymphatic cells and suppress the immune system. The continuous sustained activation of the sympathetic nervous system; HPA axis; cardiovascular, metabolic, and immune systems contribute to a hormonal overload, leading to impairment in memory, immunity, cardiovascular, and metabolic function (McEwen, 2000, 2005). Over time, chronic stress compromises health and increases susceptibility to illnesses. For instance, children who have suffered psychological neglect, abuse, or parental loss are more likely to display mood or anxiety disorders during adulthood (Benjet, Borges, & Medina-Mora, 2010).

In addition, health disparities found in lower socioeconomic groups, racial and ethnic minorities, and older adults may be partly explained by the chronic stress they tend to experience. Elevated AL has been shown to exist in these groups and in relatively young women with histories of high stress and especially those with PTSD and depression (Carlson & Chamberlain, 2005; Clark, Bond, & Hecker, 2007; Glover, Stuber, & Poland, 2006; Juruena, 2013; Peek et al., 2010; Seeman, Epel, Gruenewald, Karlamangla, & McEwen, 2010). See Box 12.2.

Elevation of white blood cell counts and lower counts of T, B, and NK cells are found in those who face academic examinations, job strain, caregiving for a family member with dementia, marital conflict, and daily stress. Altered parameters of immune function are present in those with negative moods (chronic hostility, depression, and anxiety), social isolation, and marital disagreement. Antibody titers to Epstein-Barr and herpes simplex viruses are also elevated in stressed populations. If the stress is long term, the immune alteration continues (Kiecolt-Glaser et al., 2005; Segerstrom, 2010).

BOX 12.2

Research for Best Practice: Allostatic Load

de Castro, A. B., Voss, J. G., Ruppin, A., Dominguez, C. F., & Seixas, N. S. (2010). Stressors among Latino day laborers: A pilot study examining allostatic load. AAOHN, 58(5), 185–196.

THE QUESTION: Do participants with higher allostatic load (AL) report greater stress than those with lower AL?

METHODS: For this pilot study, 30 Latino men were recruited from a worker center. Participants completed an interview, and researchers measured six indicators of allostatic load (body mass index, waist-to-hip ration, systolic blood pressure, diastolic blood pressure, C-reactive protein, and cortisol). Percentages and mean scores were calculated for several self-reported stressors in work, economic, and social contexts. Low and high ALs were compared.

FINDINGS: Overall, participants with high ALs reported experiencing more stress than those with low ALs. Latino day laborers experience stress that places them at risk for high AL.

IMPLICATIONS FOR NURSING: Certain cultural and ethnic groups are at high risk for chronic stress. Chronic stress can be assessed by measuring changes in physiological parameters. Nurses need to recognize that the importance of a careful physical assessment as well as a psychosocial assessment.

Emotional Responses

Emotional responses to stress depend on the significance of the event experience. The **emotions** (psychophysiological reactions that define a person's mood) are usually ones of excitement or distress marked by strong feelings and usually accompanied by an impulse toward definite action. If the emotions are intense, a disturbance in intellectual functions occurs. When the situation is viewed as a challenge, emotions are more likely to be positive. If the event is evaluated as threatning or harmful, negative emotions are elicited. Emotions can be categorized as follows:

- *Negative emotions* occur when there is a threat to, delay in, or thwarting of a goal or a conflict between goals: anger, fright, anxiety, guilt, shame, sadness, envy, jealousy, and disgust.
- *Positive emotions* occur when there is movement toward or attainment of a goal: happiness, pride, relief, and love.
- *Borderline emotions* are somewhat ambiguous: hope, compassion, empathy, sympathy, and contentment.
- *Nonemotions* connote emotional reactions but are too ambiguous to fit into any of the preceding categories: confidence, awe, confusion, and excitement (Lazarus, 1999).

Emotions are expressed as themes that summarize dangers or benefits of each stressful situation. For instance, physical danger provokes fear; a loss leads to feelings of sadness (Table 12.4). Emotions have their own innate responses that are automatic and unique; for example, anger may automatically provoke tremors in one person

TABLE 12.4	CORE RELATIONAL THEMES FOR EACH EMOTION
Emotion	Relational Meaning
Anger	A demeaning offense against me and mine
Anxiety	Facing an uncertain, existential threat
Fright	Facing an immediate, concrete, and overwhelming physical danger
Guilt	Having transgressed a moral imperative
Shame	Having failed to live up to an ego ideal
Sadness	Having experienced an irrevocable loss
Envy	Wanting what someone else has
Jealousy	Resenting a third party for the loss of or a threat to another's affection
Disgust	Taking in or being too close to an indigestible object or idea (metaphorically speaking)
Happiness	Making reasonable progress toward the realization of a goal
Pride	Enhancement of one's ego identity by taking credit for a valued object or achievement, either our own or that of someone or a group with whom we identify
Relief	A distressing goal/incongruent condition that has changed for the better or gone away
Hope	Fearing the worst but yearning for better
Love	Desiring or participating in affection, usually but not necessarily reciprocated
Compassion	Being moved by another's suffering and wanting to help

Adapted with permission from Lazarus, R.S. (1991). *Emotion and Adaptation* [table 3.4, p. 122]. Copyright by Oxford University Press.

but both tremors and perspiration in another. Emotions often provoke impulsive behavior. For example, the first impulse of a young musician facing his first performance at Carnegie Hall who experiences stage fright is to run home. As he resists this impulse, he begins coping with his fears in order to perform.

COPING

Coping is a deliberate, planned, and psychological effort to manage stressful demands. The coping process may inhibit or override the innate urge to act. Positive coping leads to adaptation, which is characterized by a balance between health and illness, a sense of well-being, and maximum social functioning. When a person does not cope well, maladaptations occur that can shift the balance toward illness, a diminished self-concept, and deterioration in social functioning.

KEYCONCEPT **Coping** is a deliberate, planned, and psychological effort to manage stressful demands.

There are two types of coping. In **problem-focused coping**, the person attacks the source of stress and solves

---

BOX 12.3

Ways of Coping: Examples of Problem-Focused Versus Emotion-Focused Coping

PROBLEM-FOCUSED COPING
- When noise from the television interrupts a student's studying and causes the student to be stressed, the student turns off the television and eliminates the noise.
- An abused spouse is finally able to leave her husband because she realizes that the abuse will not stop even though he promises never to hit her again.

EMOTION-FOCUSED COPING
- A husband is adamantly opposed to visiting his wife's relatives because they keep dogs in their house. Even though the dogs are well cared for, their presence in the relative's home violates his need for an orderly, clean house and causes the husband sufficient stress that he copes with by refusing to visit. This becomes a source of marital conflict. One holiday, the husband is given a puppy and immediately becomes attached to the dog, who soon becomes a valued family member. The husband then begins to view his wife's relatives differently and willingly visits their house more often.
- A mother is afraid that her teenage daughter has been in an accident because she did not come home after a party. Then the woman remembers that she gave her daughter permission to stay at a friend's house. She immediately feels better.

---

the problem (eliminating it or changing its effects), which changes the person–environment relationship. In **emotion-focused coping**, the person reduces the stress by reinterpreting the situation to change its meaning (Boxes 12.3 and 12.4).

BOX 12.4

Research for Best Practice: Emotion- versus Problem-Focused Coping for Health Threats

Ahmad, M. M., Musil, C. M., Zauszniewski, J. A., & Resnick, M. I. (2005). Prostate cancer: appraisal, coping, and health status. Journal of Gerontological Nursing, 31(10), 34–43.

THE QUESTION: Do men use emotion- or problem-focused coping when appraising a health threat?

METHODS: A convenience sample of 131 men with prostate cancer was surveyed to identify how cognitive appraisal and types of coping affected their health status.

FINDINGS: Men who appraised more harm or loss experienced worse physical and mental health. When the men perceived their diagnosis as posing more harm or loss or greater threat, they were more likely to use emotion-focused coping. When the diagnosis was perceived as a challenge, men were more likely to use problem-focused coping.

IMPLICATIONS FOR NURSING: Patients respond differently to the same medical diagnosis depending on how they appraise the threat of the diagnosis. Problem-focused coping is more likely to be used if the diagnosis is viewed as a challenge ("I can beat it") rather than a threat ("I will die"). Assessing the coping style will provide important assessment data for planning interventions.

No one coping strategy is best for all situations. Coping strategies work best in particular situations. Over time, these strategies become automatic and develop into patterns for each person. Hopefully, the strategies are effective. Some situations require a combination of strategies and activities. Ideally, a stressful situation is matched with the needed resources as the events are unfolding. Social support can be critical in helping people cope with difficult situations. Successful coping with life stresses is linked to quality of life and to physical and mental health (Lazarus, 2001).

As a part of the coping process, reappraisal is important because of the changing nature of the stressful situation. **Reappraisal**, which is the same as appraisal except that it happens after coping, provides feedback about the outcomes and allows for continual adjustment to new information.

ADAPTATION

Adaptation can be conceptualized as a person's capacity to survive and flourish (Lazarus, 1999). Adaptation or lack of it affects three important areas: health, psychological well-being, and social functioning. A period of stress may compromise any or all of these areas. If a person copes successfully with stress, he or she returns to a previous level of adaptation. Successful coping results in an improvement in health, well-being, and social functioning. Unfortunately, at times, maladaptation occurs.

> **KEYCONCEPT** **Adaptation** is a person's capacity to survive and flourish. Adaptation affects three important areas: health, psychological well-being, and social functioning.

It is impossible to separate completely the adaptation areas of health, well-being, and social functioning. A maladaptation in any one area can negatively affect the others. For instance, the appearance of psychiatric symptoms can cause problems in performance in the work environment that in turn elicit a negative self-concept. Although each area will be discussed separately, the reader should realize that when one area is affected, most likely all three areas are affected.

Health

Health can be negatively affected by stress when coping is ineffective and the damaging condition or situation is not ameliorated or the emotional distress is not regulated. Examples of ineffective coping include using emotion-focused coping when a problem-focused approach is appropriate, such as if a woman reinterprets an abusive situation as her fault instead of getting help to remove herself from the environment. In addition, if a coping strategy violates cultural norms and lifestyle, stress is often exaggerated.

Some coping strategies actually increase the risk for mortality and morbidity, such as the excessive use of alcohol, drugs, or tobacco. Many people use overeating, smoking, or drinking to reduce stress. They may feel better temporarily but are actually increasing their risk for illness. For people whose behaviors exacerbate their illnesses, learning new behaviors becomes important. Healthy coping strategies such as exercising and obtaining adequate sleep and nutrition contribute to stress reduction and the promotion of long-term health.

Psychological Well-Being

An ideal outcome to a stress response is feeling good about how stress is handled. Of course, outcome satisfaction for one person does not necessarily represent outcome satisfaction for another. For instance, suppose that two students receive the same passing score on an examination. One may feel a sense of relief, but the other may feel anxious because he appraises the score as too low. Understanding a person's emotional response to an outcome is essential to analyzing its personal meaning. People who consistently have positive outcomes from stressful experiences are more likely to have positive self-esteem and self-confidence. Unsatisfactory outcomes from stressful experiences are associated with negative mood states, such as depression, anger, guilt leading to decreased self-esteem, and feelings of helplessness. Likewise, if the situation was appraised as challenging rather than harmful or threatening, increased self-confidence and a sense of well-being are likely to follow. If the situation was accurately appraised as harmful or threatening but viewed as manageable, the outcome may also be positive.

Social Functioning

Social functioning, the performance of daily activities within the context of interpersonal relations and family and community roles, can be seriously impaired during stressful episodes. For instance, a person who is experiencing the stress of a divorce may not be able to carry out job responsibilities satisfactorily. Social functioning continues to be impaired if the person views the outcome as unsuccessful and experiences negative emotions. If successful coping with a stressful encounter leads to a positive outcome, social functioning returns to normal or is improved.

CARE FOR THE PERSON EXPERIENCING STRESS

Nursing Management: Stress Responses

The overall goals in the nursing care of stress are to resolve the stressful person–environment situation, reduce the stress response, and develop positive coping skills. The goals for those who are at high risk for stress (experiencing recent life changes, vulnerable to stress, or have limited coping mechanisms) are to recognize the potential for stressful situations and strengthen positive coping skills through education and practice.

Stress responses vary from one person to another. Acute stress is easier to recognize than chronic stress. In many instances, living with chronic stress has become a way of life and is no longer recognized. If there are significant emotional or behavioral symptoms in response to an identifiable stressful situation, a diagnosis of adjustment disorder may be made (American Psychiatric Association, 2013). From the assessment data, the nurse can determine any illnesses, the intensity of the stress response, and the effectiveness of coping strategies. Nurses typically identify stress responses in people or family members who are receiving treatment for other health problems.

Biologic Domain

Assessment

An assessment of the biologic domain should include a careful health history, focusing on past and present illnesses and traumas. If a psychiatric disorder is present, psychiatric symptoms may spontaneously reappear even when no alteration has occurred in the patient's medication regimen. Special attention should be paid to disorders of the endocrine system, such as hypothyroidism.

Gender Differences

It is now known that people experience stress differently depending on their gender. Whereas males are more likely to respond to stress with a fight or flight response, females have less aggressive responses; they "tend and befriend." There is a difference in perception of and behavioral response to the stress, as well as a difference in the physiology of the stress response (McEwen, 2005).

Review of Systems

A systems review can elicit the person's own unique physiologic response to stress and can also provide important data on the effect of chronic illnesses. These data are useful for understanding the person–environment situation and the person's stress reactions, coping responses, and adaptation.

Physical Functioning

Physical functioning usually changes during a stress response. Typically, sleep is disturbed, appetite either increases or decreases, body weight fluctuates, and sexual activity changes. Physical appearance may be uncharacteristically disheveled—a projection of the person's feelings. Body language expresses muscle tension, which conveys a state of anxiety not usually present. Because exercise is an important strategy in stress reduction, the nurse should assess the amount of physical activity, tolerance for exercise, and usual exercise patterns. Determining the details of the person's exercise pattern and any recent changes can help in formulating reasonable interventions.

Pharmacologic Assessment

In assessing a person's coping strategies, the nurse needs to ask about the use of alcohol, tobacco, marijuana, and any other addictive substances. Many people begin or increase the frequency of using these substances as a way of coping with stress. In turn, substance abuse contributes to the stress behavior. Knowing details about the person's use of these substances (number of times a day or week, amount, circumstances, side effects) helps in determining the role these substances play in overall stress reduction or management. The more important the substances are in the person's handling of stress, the more difficult it will be to change the addictive behavior.

Stress also often prompts people to use antianxiety medication without supervision. Use of over-the-counter and herbal medications is also common. The nurse should carefully assess the use of any drugs to manage stress symptoms. If drugs are the primary coping strategy, further evaluation is needed with a possible referral to a mental health specialist. If a psychiatric disorder is present, the nurse should assess medication compliance, especially if the psychiatric symptoms are reappearing.

Nursing Diagnoses for the Biologic Domain

Several nursing diagnoses may be generated from an assessment of the biologic domain. For patients with changes in eating, sleeping, or activity, nursing diagnoses of Imbalanced Nutrition, Disturbed Sleep Pattern, and Impaired Mobility may be appropriate. Ineffective Therapeutic Regimen may also be used for patients using excessive over-the-counter medications.

Interventions for the Biologic Domain

People under stress can usually benefit from several biologic interventions. Their activities of daily living are usually interrupted, and they often feel that they have no time for themselves. The stressed patient who is normally fastidiously groomed and dressed may appear disheveled and unkempt. Simply reinstating the daily routine of shaving (for a man) or applying makeup (for a woman) can improve the person's outlook on life and ability to cope with the stress.

Stress is commonly manifested in the areas of nutrition and activity. During stressful periods, a person's eating patterns change. To cope with stress, a person may either overeat or become anorexic. Both are ineffective coping behaviors and actually contribute to stress. Educating the patient about the importance of maintaining an adequate diet during the period of stress will highlight its importance. It will also allow the nurse to help the person decide how eating behaviors can be changed.

Exercise can reduce the emotional and behavioral responses to stress. In addition to the physical benefits of exercise, a regular exercise routine can provide structure to a person's life, enhance self-confidence, and increase feelings of well-being. People who are stressed are often not receptive to the idea of exercise, particularly if it has not been a part of their routine. Exploring the patient's personal beliefs about the value of activity will help to determine whether exercise is a reasonable activity for that person.

The person under stress tends to be tense, nervous, and on edge. Simple relaxation techniques help the person relax and may improve coping skills. If these techniques do not help the patient relax, distraction or guided imagery may be taught to the patient (see Chapter 9). In some instances, spiritually oriented interventions can be used (Box 12.5). Referral to a mental health specialist for hypnosis or biofeedback should be considered for patients who have severe stress responses.

BOX 12.5

Research for Best Practice: Spiritually Based Interventions

Bormann, J. E., Thorp, S., Wetherell, J. L., & Golshan, S. (2008). A spiritually-based group intervention for combat veterans with posttraumatic stress disorder: A feasibility study. Journal of Holistic Nursing, 29(2), 109–116.

THE QUESTION: Is it feasible to use mantram repetition—the spiritual practice of repeating a sacred word or phrase throughout the day—for managing symptoms of posttraumatic stress disorder (PTSD) in veterans?

METHODS: A two group (intervention vs. control) by two time (pre- and postintervention) experimental design was used. Veterans were randomly assigned to intervention ($n = 14$) or delayed-treatment control ($n = 15$). Measures were PTSD symptoms, psychological distress, quality of life, and patient satisfaction. Effect sizes were calculated using Cohen's d.

FINDINGS: Thirty-three male veterans were enrolled, and 29 (88%) completed the study. Large effect sizes were found for reducing PTSD symptom severity ($d = -.72$), psychological distress ($d = -.73$) and increasing quality of life ($d = .70$).

IMPLICATIONS FOR NURSING: A spiritual program may be feasible for reducing symptom severity in PTSD.

Psychological Domain

Assessment

Unlike assessment for other mental health problems, psychological assessment of the person under stress does not ordinarily include a mental status examination. Instead, psychological assessment focuses on the person's emotions and their severity, as well as his or her coping strategies. The assessment elicits the person's appraisal of risks and benefits, the personal meaning of the situation, and the person's commitment to a particular outcome. The nurse can then understand how vulnerable the person is to stress.

Using therapeutic communication techniques, a person's emotional state is assessed in a nurse–patient interview. By beginning the interview with a statement such as, "Let's talk about what you have been feeling," the nurse can elicit the feelings that the person has been experiencing. Identifying the person's emotions can be helpful in assessing the intensity of the stress being experienced. Negative emotions (anger, fright, anxiety, guilt, shame, sadness, envy, jealousy, and disgust) are usually associated with an inability to cope and severe stress.

After identifying the person's emotions, the nurse determines how the person reacts initially to them. For example, does the person who is angry respond by carrying out the innate urge to attack someone whom the person blames for the situation? Or does that person respond by thinking through the situation and overriding the initial innate urge to act? The person who tends to act impulsively has few real coping skills. For the person who can resist the innate urge to act and has developed coping skills, the focus of the assessment becomes determining their effectiveness.

In an assessment interview, it can be determined whether the person uses problem-focused or emotion-focused coping strategies effectively. Problem-focused coping is effective when the person can accurately assess the situation. In this case, the person sets goals, seeks information, masters new skills, and seeks help as needed. Emotion-focused coping is effective when the person has inaccurately assessed the situation and coping corrects the false interpretation.

Nursing Diagnoses for the Psychological Domain

The nurse should consider a nursing diagnosis of Ineffective Coping for patients experiencing stress who do not have the psychological resources to effectively manage the situation. Other useful nursing diagnoses include Disturbed Thought Processes, Disturbed Sensory Perception, Low Self-esteem, Fear, Hopelessness, and Powerlessness.

Interventions for the Psychological Domain

Numerous interventions help reduce stress and support coping efforts. All of the interventions are best carried out within the framework of a supportive nurse–patient relationship. Assisting patients to develop appropriate problem-solving strategies based on personal strengths and previous experiences is important in understanding and coping with stressful situations. Encouraging patients to examine times when coping has been successful and examine aspects of that situation can help in identifying strengths and strategies for the current problem. For example, a young mother was completely overwhelmed with feelings of inadequacy after the birth of her third child. Further assessment revealed that the patient's mother had helped during the 6 weeks after the other children had been born. The patient's mother was not available for the third birth. First, the nurse validated that having three children could be overwhelming for anyone. The nurse also explained the postpartum hormonal changes that were occurring, validating that the patient's feelings were typical of many mothers. Finally, together, the nurse and the patient identified resources in her environment that could support her during the postpartum period.

It is important to have the patient discuss the person–environment situation and develop alternative coping strategies. Some aspects of any situation cannot be changed, such as a family member's illness or a death of a loved one, but usually there are areas within the patient's control that can be changed. For example, a caregiver cannot reverse the family member's disability, but she can arrange for short-term respite.

Social Domain

Assessment

Social assessment data are invaluable in determining the person's resources for positive coping. The ability to make healthy lifestyle changes is strongly influenced by the person's health beliefs and family support system. Even the expression of stress is related to social factors, particularly cultural expectations and values.

Assessment should include use of the Recent Life Changes questionnaire (refer to Table 12.2) to determine the number and importance of life changes that the patient has experienced within the past year. If several recent life changes have occurred, the person–environment relationship has changed. The person is likely to be either at high risk for or already experiencing stress.

Social assessment also includes identification of the person's social network. Because employment is the mainstay of adulthood and the source of many personal contacts, assessment of any recent changes in employment status is important. If a person is unemployed, the nurse should determine the significance of the unemployment and its effects on the person's social network. For children and adolescents, nurses should note any recent changes in their attendance at school. The nurse should elicit the following data:

- Size and extent of the patient's social network, both relatives and nonrelatives, professional and nonprofessional, and how long known
- Functions that the network serves (e.g., intimacy, social integration, nurturance, reassurance of worth, guidance and advice, access to new contacts)
- Degree of reciprocity between the patient and other network members; that is, who provides support to the patient and who the patient supports
- Degree of interconnectedness; that is, how many of the network members know one another and are in contact

Nursing Diagnoses for the Social Domain

The nurse can generate several nursing diagnoses from the social assessment data that involve the person–environment interaction. The challenge of generating nursing diagnoses is to make sure that they are based on the person's appraisal of the situation. Some possible nursing diagnoses include Ineffective Role Performance, Impaired Parenting, Impaired Social Interaction, Social Isolation, and Disabled Family Coping.

Interventions for the Social Domain

Because the experience of stress and the ability to cope are a result of the appraisal of the person–environment relationship, interventions that affect the environment are important. People who are coping with stressful situations can often benefit from interventions that facilitate family unit functioning and promote the health and welfare of all family members. To intervene with the total family, the stressed person must agree for the family members to be involved. If the data gathered from the assessment of supportive and dissupportive factors indicate that the family members are not supportive, the nurse should assist the patient to consider expanding his or her social network. If the family is the major source of support, the nurse should design interventions that support the functioning of the family unit. Parent education can also be effective in supporting family unit functioning. If family therapy is needed, the nurse should refer the family to an advanced practice specialist.

Evaluation and Treatment Outcomes

The treatment outcomes established in the initial plan of care guide the evaluation. Individual outcomes relate to improved health, well-being, and social function. Depending on the level of intervention, there can also be family and network outcomes. Family outcomes may be related to improved communication or social support; for instance, caregiver stress is reduced when other members of the family help in the care of the ill member. Social network outcomes focus on modifying the social network to increase support for the individual.

- Within the social network, social support can help a person cope with stress.

- The overall goals in the nursing management of stress are to resolve the stressful person–environment situation, reduce the stress response, and develop positive coping skills.

SUMMARY OF KEY POINTS

- Stress affects everyone. Coping with stress can produce positive and negative outcomes. The person can learn and grow from the experience or maladaptation can occur.

- Stress is defined as an environmental pressure or force that put's strain on a person's system. Acute stress can lead to physiologic overload, which in turn can have a negative impact on a person's health, well-being, and social functioning. Chronic stress is clearly associated with negative health outcomes.

- Stress responses are determined by the person–environment relationship and the individual's cognitive appraisal of the risks and benefits of a situation. Stress responses are simultaneously emotional and physiologic, leading to an innate tendency to act.

- Many personal factors, such as personality patterns, beliefs, values, and commitment to an outcome, interact with environmental demands and constraints that produce a person–environment relationship.

- The concept of homeostasis is the body's tendency to resist physiological change and hold bodily functions relatively consistent, well-coordinated, and usually stable.

- When the brain interprets an event as a threat, physiological stability is challenged, and a "fight or flight" response occurs.

- Allostasis describes a dynamic regulatory process that maintains homeostasis through a process of adaptation. Physiological stability is achieved when the autonomic nervous system; the HPA; and the cardiovascular, metabolic, and immune systems respond to internal and external stimuli. As wear and tear on the brain and body occur, there is a corresponding increase in the number of abnormal biologic parameters called the allostatic load (AL). AL is an indication of chronic stress.

- Effective coping can be either problem focused or emotion focused. The outcome of successful coping is adaptation through enhanced health, psychological well-being, and social functioning.

CRITICAL THINKING CHALLENGES

1. Compare and contrast the concepts of homeostasis and allostasis.
2. Discuss the impact of acute stress versus chronic stress. Why is chronic stress of more concern than acute stress?
3. Explain why one person may experience the stress of losing a job differently from another.
4. A man is overweight, has hypertension and insomnia, and was recently widowed. The doctor has told him to lose weight and quit smoking. He seeks your advice. Would you recommend a problem-focused or an emotion-focused approach?
5. A woman at the local shelter announced to her group that she was returning to her husband because it was partly her fault that her husband beat her. Is this an example of problem-focused or emotion-focused coping? Justify your answer.
6. Using the Stress Coping and Adaptation Model (Figure 12.1), assess a patient and determine the cognitive appraisal of significant events.

Noise (2007). David Owen (Tim Robbins) copes with the stressful noises of the city, specifically car alarms, by becoming aggressive and destructive. At first the noise is merely an irritant. Later, he interprets the noise as an assault on everyone. He becomes an activist, protecting others and gradually becomes very grandiose. As his grandiosity increases, he becomes more and more driven to damage vehicles with active care alarms.

Viewing Points: What is the relationship between the physiological response to the noise and his eventual grandiose behavior? How would you help his reduce the stressful experience and cope positively? Observe your own feelings throughout the movie. Did you experience stress?

REFERENCES

Aguilera, D. C. (1998). *Crisis intervention: Theory and methodology*, St. Louis: Mosby.

American Psychiatric Association. (2013). *Diagnostic and statistical manual of mental disorders* (5th ed.). Arlington, VA: Author.

Azmitia, M., Syed, M., & Radmacher, K. (2008). On the intersection of personal and social identities: introduction and evidence from a longitudinal study of emerging adults. *New Directions for Child & Adolescent Development, 120,* 1–16.

Benjet, C., Borges, G., & Medina-Mora, M.E. (2010). Chronic childhood adversity and onset of psychopathology during three life stages: Childhood, adolescence and adulthood. *Journal of Psychiatric Research, 44*(11), 732–740.

Bryant-Lukosius, D. (2003). Review: Limited evidence exists on the effect of psychological coping styles on cancer survival or recurrence. *Evidence Based Nursing, 6*(3), 88.

Cannon W. B. (1932). *The wisdom of the body.* New York: Norton.

Carlson, E. D., & Chamberlain, R. M. (2005). Allostatic load and health disparities: A theoretical orientation. *Research in Nursing & Health, 28,* 306–315.

Clark, J. S., Bond, M. F., & Hecker, J. R. (2007). Environmental stress, psychological stress and allostatic load. *Psychology, Health & Medicine, 12*(1), 18–30.

de Castro, A. B., Voss, J. G., Ruppin, A., Dominguez, C. F., & Seixas, N. S (2010). Stressors among Latino day laborers. *American Association of Occupational Health Nurses, 58*(5), 185–196.

Friedman, M., & Rosenman, R. (1974). *Type A and your heart.* New York: Knopf.

Glover, D. A., Stuber, M., & Poland, R. E. (2006). Allostatic load in women with and without PTSD symptoms. *Psychiatry, 69*(3), 191–203.

Holmes, T., & Rahe, R. (1967). The Social Readjustment Patient Scale. *Journal of Psychosomatic Research, 11*(2), 213–218.

Juruena, M. F. (2013). Early-life stress and HPA axis trigger recurrent adulthood depression. *Epilepsy & Behavior.* http://dx.doi.org/10.1016/j.yebeh2013.10.020

Kendall, E., & Terry, D. (2009). Predicting emotional well-being following traumatic brain injury: a test of mediated and moderated models. *Social Science & Medicine, 69*(6), 947–954.

Kiecolt-Glaser, J. K., Loving, T. J., Stowell, J. R., Malarkey, W. B., Lemeshow, S., Dickinson, S. L., et al. (2005). Hostile marital interactions, proinflammatory cytokine production, and wound healing. *Archives of General Psychiatry, 62*(12), 1377–1384.

Kumari, M., Badrick, E., Sacker, A., Kirschbaum, C., Marmot, M., & Chandola, T. (2010). Identifying patterns in cortisol secretionin an older population. Finds from the Whitehall II study. *Psychoneuroendocrinology, 35*(7), 1091–1099.

Lalâ A., Bobîrnac, G., & Tipa, R. (2010). Stress levels, alexithymia, type A and type C personality patterns in undergraduate students. *Journal of Medicine & Life, 3*(2), 200–205.

Lazarus, R., & Folkman, S. (1984). *Stress, appraisal and coping.* New York: Springer.

Lazarus, R. S. (1999). *Stress and emotion: A new synthesis.* New York: Springer.

Lazarus, R. S. (2001). Relational meaning and discrete emotions. In K. R. Scherer, A. Schorr, & T. Johnstone (Eds.), *Appraisal processes in emotion: Theory, methods, research* (pp. 37–67). New York: Oxford University Press.

Li, Y., & Wu, S. (2010). Social networks and health among rural-urban migrants in China: A channel or a constraint? *Health Promotion International, 25*(3), 371–380.

Low, C. A., Thurston, R. C., & Matthews, K. A. (2010). Psychosocial factors in the development of heart disease in women: Current research and future directions. *Psychosomatic Medicine, 72*(9), 842–854.

Marchesi, C., Ossola, P., Scagnelli, F., Paglia, F., Aprile, S., Monici, A., et al. (2014). Type D personality in never-depressed patients and the development of major and minor depression after acute coronary syndrome. *Journal of Affective Disorders, 155,* 194–199.

McEwen, B. S. (2000). Allostasis and allostatic load: Implications for neuropsychopharmacology. *Neuropsychopharmacology, 22,* 108–124.

McEwen, B. S. (2005). Stressed or stressed out: What is the difference? *Journal of Psychiatry Neuroscience, 30*(5), 315–318.

McEwen, B. S., & Bianaros, P. J. (2010). Central role of the brain in stress and adaptation: Links to socioeconomic status, health, and disease. *Annals of the New York Academy of Sciences, 118,* 190–222.

McVicar, A., Ravalier, J. J., & Greenwood, C. (2013). Biology of stress revisited: Intracellular mechanisms and the conceptualization of stress. *Stress & Health.* doi:10.1002/smi.2508

Mols, F., & Denollet, J. (2010). Type D personality in the general population: A systematic review of health status, mechanisms of disease, and work-related problems. *Health and Quality of Life Outcomes, 8,* 9.

Moran, C. C. (2001). Personal predictions of stress and stress reactions in firefighter recruits. *Disaster Prevention & Management, 10*(5), 356–365.

Peek, M. K., Cutchin, M. P., Salinas, J. J., Sheffield, K. M., Eschbach, K., Stowe, R. P., et al. (2010). Allostatic load among non-hispanic whites, non-hispanic blacks, and people of Mexican origin: Effects of ethnicity, nativity, and acculturation. *American Journal of Public Health, 100*(5), 940–946.

Rafanelli, C., Sirri, L., Grandi, S., & Fava, G. A. (2013). Is depression the wrong treatment target for improving outcome in coronary artery disease? *Psychotherapy and Psychosomatics, 82.* doi: 10.1159/000351586

Rahe, R. (1994). The more things change. *Psychosomatic Medicine, 56*(4), 306–307.

Rahe, R. H. (2000). Recent Life Changes Questionnaire (RLCQ).

Rahe, R. H., Taylor, C., Tolles, R. L., Newhall, L. M., Veach, T. L., & Bryson, S. (2002). A novel stress and coping workplace program reduces illness and healthcare utilization. *Psychosomatic Medicine, 64*(2), 278–286.

Seeman, T., Epel, E., Gruenewald, T., Karlamangla, A., & McEwen, B.S. (2010). Soci-economic differentials in peripheral biology: Cumulative allostatic load. *Annals of the New York Academy of Sciences, 1186,* 223–239.

Selye, H. (1956). *The stress of life.* New York: McGraw-Hill.

Selye, H. (1974). *Stress without distress.* Philadelphia: J. B. Lippincott.

Shen, B., Countryman, A. J., Spiro, A., & Niaura, R (2008). The prospective contribution of hostility characteristics to high fasting glucose levels. The moderating role of marital status. *Diabetes Care, 31*(7), 1293–1298.

Segerstrom, S. C. (2010). Resources, stress, and immunity: an ecological perspective on human psychoneuroimmunology [review]. *Annals of Behavioral Medicine, 40*(1), 114–125.

Seib, C., Whiteside, E., Lee, K., Humphreys, J., Tran, T. H., Chopin, L., et al. (2014). Stess, lifestyle, and quality of life in midlife and older Australian women: Results from the Stress and the Health of Women Study. *Women's Health Issues, 24*(1), e43–e52.

Sogaard, A. J., Dalgard, O. S., Holm, I., Roysamb, E., & Haheim, L. L. (2008). Associations between type A behavior pattern and psychological distress: 28 years of follow-up of the Oslo Study 1972/1973. *Social Psychiatry & Psychiatric Epidemiology, 43*(3), 216–223.

Sterling, P. (2012). Allostasis: A model of predictive regulation. *Physiology & Behavior, 106,* 5–15.

Stevenson, C., & Williams, L. (2014). Type D personality, quality of life and physical symptoms in the general population: A dimensional analysis. *Psychology & Health, 29*(3), 365–373.

Tamers, S. L., Okechukwu, C., Bohl, A. A., Gueguen, A., Goldberg, M., & Zins, M. (2014). The impact of stressful life events on excessive alcohol consumption in the French population: Findings from the GAZEL Cohort Study. *PLos One, 9*(1), e87654. www.plosone.org

Tishler, C. L., Bartholomae, S., & Rhodes, A. R. (2005). Personality profiles of normal healthy research volunteers: A potential concern for clinical drug trial investigators? *Medical Hypotheses, 65*(1), 1–7.

Whatley, A. D., Dilorio, C. K., & Yeager, K. (2010). Examining the relationships of depressive symptoms, stigma, social support and regimen-specific support on quality of life in adult patients with epilepsy. *Health Education Research, 25*(4), 575–584.

Zegwaard, M. I., Aartsen, M. J., Cuijpers, P., & Grypdonck, M. H. (2011, in press). Review: A conceptual model of perceived burden of informal caregivers for older persons with a severe functional psychiatric syndrome and concomitant problematic behavior. *Journal of Clinical Nursing.*

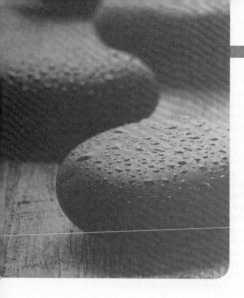

13

Management of Anger, Aggression, and Violence

Sandra P. Thomas

KEY CONCEPTS

- anger
- aggression
- gender, culture, and ethnic differences
- intervention fit
- violence

LEARNING OBJECTIVES

After studying this chapter, you will be able to:

1. Explore difference between healthy and maladaptive styles of anger.

2. Discuss principles of anger management as a psychoeducational intervention.

3. Discuss the factors that influence aggressive and violent behaviors.

4. Discuss theories used to explain anger, aggression, and violence.

5. Identify behaviors or actions that escalate and de-escalate violent behavior.

6. Recognize the risk for verbal and physical attacks on nurses.

7. Generate options for responding to the expression of anger, aggression, and violent behaviors in clinical nursing practice.

8. Apply the nursing process to the management of anger, aggression, and violence in patients.

KEY TERMS

- anger management • catharsis • hostile aggression • instrumental aggression • inwardly directed anger • maladaptive anger • outwardly directed anger

---

Maladaptive anger and potentially lethal violent behavior are increasingly evident in contemporary Western society. Temper tantrums of athletes, episodes of road rage, and school shootings often dominate the evening news. Clearly, mismanagement of angry emotion is a serious social problem.

Language pertaining to anger is imprecise and confusing. Some of the words used interchangeably with anger include *annoyance*, *frustration*, *temper*, *resentment*, *hostility*, *hatred*, and *rage*. To avoid perpetuating the confusion, three key concepts were selected for use in this chapter: *anger*, *aggression*, and *violence*. Anger, aggression, and violence should not be viewed as a continuum because one

does not necessarily lead to another. That is a myth. In fact, cultural myths about anger abound (Table 13.1).

One goal of this chapter is to dispel confusion between anger as a normal, healthy response to violation of one's integrity and maladaptive anger that is detrimental to one's mental and physical health. Understanding this distinction is an important aspect of emotional intelligence.

A second goal of this chapter is to outline risk factors for aggression and violence and describe preventive interventions, particularly as they pertain to the nursing care environment. Assaults by patients toward the staff of hospitals and nursing homes are on the increase, and eight

TABLE 13.1	**CULTURAL MYTHS ABOUT ANGER**
Myth	**Truth**
Anger is a knee-jerk reaction to external events.	Humans can choose to slow down their reactions and to think and behave differently in response to events.
Anger can be uncontrollable, resulting in crimes of passion such as "involuntary manslaughter."	In societies that believe anger can be controlled, there are far fewer violent crimes than in the United States. Compare the statistics of Japan and the United States.
Anger behavior in adulthood is determined by temperament and childhood experiences.	Although temperament and early experiences are important, emotional development continues throughout life. Adults can acquire knowledge and skills to handle emotions more effectively.
Men are angrier than women.	Women experience anger as frequently as men, but societal constraints may inhibit their expression of it.
People have to behave aggressively to get what they want.	Making an assertive request is more likely to lead to the desired outcome.

nurses were fatally injured while on duty during 2003–2009 (American Nurses Association, 2012). Aggression and violence occur across a wide spectrum of health-care settings, requiring all nurses to develop expertise in prevention and management of aggression. Contrary to a popular misconception, patients who have psychiatric problems are not more violent than other patients, but astute clinicians need to know which patients *might* become aggressive given a combination of known risk factors with specific environmental conditions.

ANGER

Anger is an internal affective state, usually temporary rather than an enduring negative attitude. If expressed outwardly, anger behavior can be constructive or destructive. Whereas destructive anger alienates other people and invites retaliation, constructive anger can be a powerful force for asserting one's rights and achieving social justice.

> KEYCONCEPT   **Anger** is "a strong, uncomfortable emotional response to a provocation that is unwanted and incongruent with one's values, beliefs, or rights" (Thomas, 1998).

Anger is a signal that something is wrong in a situation; thus, the angry individual has the urge to take action (Lemay, Overall, & Clark, 2012). The situation is more distressing than a minor annoyance such as a slow grocery line. An interpersonal offense such as unjust or disrespectful treatment (a spouse lying, a coworker taking advantage) often provokes anger. The meaning of an angry episode depends on the relational context. For example, anger is more intense and inter-mingled with considerable hurt when loved ones violate the implicit relational contract ("If he loved me, how could he lie about that? How can I trust him again?") (Thomas, 2006).

Maladaptive anger (excessive outwardly directed anger or suppressed anger) is linked to psychiatric conditions, such as depression (Perugi, Fornaro, & Akiskal, 2011), as well as a plethora of medical conditions. For example, *excessive outwardly directed anger* is linked to coronary heart disease (Ketterer et al., 2011) and myocardial infarction (Mostofsky, Maclure, Tofler, Muller, & Mittleman, 2013). *Suppressed anger* is related to arthritis, breast and colorectal cancer, chronic pain, and hypertension (Burns, Quartana, & Bruehl, 2011; Thomas, 2009). Furthermore, suppressed anger was a predictor of early mortality for both men and women in a large 17-year study (Potpara & Lip, 2011).

In contrast to these maladaptive anger management styles, research shows that anger discussed with other people in a constructive way has a beneficial effect on blood pressure (Everson-Rose & Lewis, 2005; Thomas, 1997a), as well as statistically significant associations with better general health, a higher sense of self-efficacy, less depression, and a lower likelihood of obesity (Thomas, 1997b). Anger controlled through calming strategies is associated with faster wound healing and other health benefits (Gouin, Kiecolt-Glaser, Malarkey, & Glaser, 2008; Gross, Groer, & Thomas, in press). Thus, effective anger management is important in maintenance of holistic health.

Skillful anger control is essential to social and occupational success. People with poor anger control have more conflict at work, change jobs more frequently, take more unwise risks, and have more accidents than people with adaptive anger behavior (Bennett & Lowe, 2008).

The Experience of Anger

When you are angry, your heart pounds, your blood pressure rises, you breathe faster, your muscles tense, and you clench your jaw or fists as you experience an impulse to do something with this physical energy. Some

Self-Awareness Exercise: Personal Experience of Anger

People's reactions differ when they experience anger. Some people report a sense of power, control, and calmness different from their usual experience; others report feeling shaky, tearful, and on the verge of collapse. Still others describe physical sensations of nausea and dizziness.

Think about the last time you felt angry. List the body sensations and other emotions that you experienced. Now ask a friend, colleague, or family member to do the same. Compare lists. What are the similarities and differences between you? How will awareness of these differences help you in your clinical practice?

individuals experience anger arousal as pleasurable, but others find its strong physical manifestations scary and unpleasant. People who were taught that anger is a sin may immediately try to ban it from awareness and deny its existence. However, suppression actually results in greater, more prolonged physiological arousal. A better option is finding a way to safely release the physical energy, either through vigorous physical activity (e.g., jogging) or through a calming activity (e.g., deep breathing). Later, at an opportune time, calmly discussing the incident with the provocateur permits clarification of misunderstandings and resolution of grievances. Box 13.1 invites the reader to explore variations in anger experience.

The physiology of anger involves the cerebral cortex, the sympathetic nervous system, the adrenal medulla (which secretes adrenaline and noradrenaline), the adrenal cortex (which secretes cortisol), the cardiovascular system, and even the immune system. From a biologic viewpoint, angry episodes may partially originate from developmental deficits, anoxia, malnutrition, toxins, tumors, neurodegenerative diseases, or trauma affecting the brain.

The Expression of Anger

While the physiological arousal of anger is similar in all people, ways of expressing anger differ. The most common modes, or styles, of anger expression are listed in Table 13.2.

In Western culture, control of anger was the dominant stance from Greco-Roman times to the 20th century. Anger was viewed as sinful, dangerous, and destructive—an irrational emotion to be contained, controlled, and denied. This pejorative view contributed to the development of a powerful taboo against feeling and expressing anger. People who have accepted this persistent taboo may have difficulty even knowing when they are angry. They may use euphemisms such as "a little upset."

In contrast to the denial or containment of angry emotion, some mental health care providers began to advocate the use of **catharsis** during the early 20th century, based on the animal research of ethologists and on Freud's conceptualization of "strangulated affect"; rather than holding in their anger, people were urged to "vent it," lest there be a dangerous "slush fund" of unexpressed anger building up in the body (Rubin, 1970). The legacy

TABLE 13.2	**STYLES OF ANGER EXPRESSION**	
Style	Characteristic Behaviors	Gender Socialization Issues
Anger suppression	Feeling anxious when anger is aroused Acting as though nothing happened Withdrawing from people when angry Conveying anger nonverbally by body language Sulking, pouting, or ruminating	In North America, girls are often discouraged from openly expressing anger, lest they hurt someone's feelings. Females are more likely than males to engage in passive-aggressive tactics; to ruminate about unresolved conflict; and to have somatic anger symptoms, such as headaches
Unhealthy outward anger expression	Flying off the handle Expressing anger in an attacking or blaming way Yelling, saying nasty things Calling the other person names or using profanity Using fists rather than words to express angry feelings	In North America, boys are encouraged to be aggressive and competitive, to express their anger in "manly" ways. Throughout life, males are more likely to express anger physically than females are.
Constructive anger discussion	Discussing the anger with a friend or family member even if the provocateur cannot be confronted at the time Approaching the person with whom one is angry and discussing the concern directly Using "I" language to describe feelings and request changes in another's behavior	Most research shows that females, more so than males, prefer to talk through anger episodes and restore relationship harmony. Both men and women may benefit from assertiveness training, problem-solving skills training, and conflict resolution workshops.

of the ill-advised "ventilationist movement" is still with us, visible in rude, uncivil behavior in the nation's classrooms, offices, roadways, and other public places, as well as in countless homes where loud arguments are a daily occurrence.

More ideally, the clear expression of honest anger may actually prevent aggression and help to resolve a situation (Thomas, 2009). Suppression of anger, prolonged rumination about the grievance, and malevolent fantasies of revenge do not resolve a problem and may result in negative consequences at a later time. Likewise, antagonistic anger toward an intimate partner or coworker only exacerbates the conflict (Lemay et al., 2012). In contrast, if anger is expressed assertively, beneficial outcomes are possible. In Averill's classic study (1983) of everyday anger, 76% of those who were on the receiving end of someone else's anger reported that they recognized their own faults as a result of the anger incident. Contrary to popular misconception, the relationship with the angry person was strengthened, not weakened.

Special Issues in the Nurse–Patient Relationship

Studies show that nurses often withdraw from angry patients and try to hide their own anger because "good nurses" do not get angry at patients (Farrell, Shafie, & Salmon, 2010). Coldness and distancing on the part of staff are acutely painful to patients (Carlsson, Dahlberg, Ekeburgh, & Dahlberg, 2006). What patients want are steady, dependable, confident caregivers who will remain connected with them when they are angry (Box 13.2).

Nurses' perceptions and beliefs about themselves as individuals and professionals influence their response to aggressive behaviors. For example, a nurse who considers any expression of anger inappropriate will approach an agitated patient differently from a nurse who considers agitated behavior to be meaningful. Understandably, nurses often shrink from patient anger when their own family backgrounds have been characterized by out-of-control anger or abuse. A nurse who has previously been assaulted by a patient is also more likely to have difficulty dealing with subsequent episodes of aggression.

Some patients have an uncanny ability to target a nurse's vulnerable characteristics. Although it is normal to become defensive when feeling vulnerable, maintaining personal control is a must. If not, the potential for punitive interventions is greater. Threatening an agitated patient (e.g., "You are going to get an injection if you don't calm down") will only worsen a volatile situation. Nurses must collaborate with other members of the treatment team when interacting with particularly challenging patients, obtaining consultation from supervisors if necessary.

BOX 13.2

Research for Best Practice: What Do Patients Want from Caregivers?

Carlsson, G., Dahlberg, K., Ekebergh, M., & Dahlberg, H. (2006). Patients longing for authentic personal care: A phenomenological study of violent encounters in psychiatric settings. Issues in Mental Health Nursing, 27(3), 287–305.

THE QUESTION: How does the patient experience violent encounters?

METHODS: This qualitative study is approached from the reflective lifeworld approach. This methodology focuses on the patient experiences of their violent encounters. Seven men and two women, ages 20 to 38 years, agreed to interviews based on the reflective model. The interviews were transcribed verbatim, and the text was analyzed for meaning that was recorded and then transcribed. The goal of the analysis was to describe the essential structure of the phenomenon and its meaning.

FINDINGS: The researchers found that patients wanted steady, dependable, confident caregivers who remained connected with them when they were angry. When caregivers were cold and distant, patients felt a sense of despair, and their aggression increased:

- "My most lasting memory from these moments is the encounter with an expressionless, blank face with expressionless, cold eyes staring back at me" (p. 295).
- "I don't think they [the staff] really care whether I'm dead or alive…nobody is trying to help me to live, to stay alive" (p. 299).

In contrast, when caregivers displayed authentic sensitivity to their suffering, patients' aggression was diffused:

- "I could see in his face then that he liked me, he was not scared.…He was sort of calm and had loving eyes; it was very disarming" (p. 293).
- "You could tell that there is some warmth and authenticity. You can tell that she is serious, that she cares about you…it is authentic, not ingratiating just, so that I will behave" (p. 299).

IMPLICATIONS FOR NURSING: This study helps nurses understand the needs of patients who are violent. Being authentic and sensitive are valued nursing attributes. Demonstration of these attributes can help reduce patients' risk for aggressive behavior.

Assessment of Anger

Both **outwardly directed anger** (particularly the hostile, attacking forms) and **inwardly directed anger** (i.e., anger that is stifled despite strong arousal) produce adverse consequences, indicating a need for anger management intervention. Complicating matters, however, most people's anger styles cannot be neatly categorized as "anger-in" or "anger-out" because they behave differently in different environments (for example, yelling at secretaries in the office, stifling anger at spouse). Therefore, it is necessary to conduct a careful assessment of a patient's behavior pattern across various situations.

The manner of anger expression is not the only important aspect of assessment. The difficulty in regulating the **frequency** and **intensity** of anger must also be assessed along with the extent to which anger is creating problems in work or intimate relationships, and the presence or absence of coping techniques such as calming or diffusion through vigorous exercise. Given the current climate of evidence-based practice, it may be advantageous to administer a questionnaire that has been extensively used with thousands of people, permitting comparison of a particular client with established norms. The Spielberger State-Trait Anger Expression Inventory (STAXI) is one such tool (Spielberger, 1999). This instrument is particularly useful because it measures the general propensity to be angry (trait anger) as well as current feelings (state anger) and several styles of anger expression, including control through calming techniques.

Because anger and aggression can be symptomatic of many underlying psychiatric or medical disorders, from posttraumatic stress disorder (PTSD) and bipolar disorder to toxicities and head injuries, first any underlying disorder must be properly evaluated. At present, only one anger-related disorder, intermittent explosive disorder (IED), appears in the *Diagnostic and Statistical Manual of Mental Disorders (DSM-5)* (American Psychiatric Association [APA], 2013). This diagnosis is used when recurring aggressive outbursts cannot be attributed to any other condition. People with IED display aggressive behavior that is disproportionate to the precipitating event, usually a minor provocation by a family member or other close associate (APA, 2013). Once thought to be rare, new research shows that it is as common as many other psychiatric disorders (Coccaro, 2012). The disorder usually appears during the teen years and persists over the life course. A national study indicates that the average number of lifetime anger attacks per person is large (43 per person). Because the disorder involves inadequate production or functioning of serotonin, IED is commonly treated with selective serotonin reuptake inhibitors (SSRIs). However, behavior therapy should also be included. Only 28.8% of patients with IED ever receive treatment for their anger (Kessler, Coccaro, Fava, Jaeger, Jin, & Walters, 2006) although the IED population is just as responsive to treatment as are non-IED populations (McCloskey, Noblett, Deffenbacher, Gollan, & Coccaro, 2008).

Culture and Gender Considerations in Assessment

Anger is one of the six universal emotions with identifiable facial features and emotionally inflected speech. People across the globe experience the emotion of anger, along with the impulse to take action, but culture is perhaps the most important determinant of what angry individuals actually *do*. Thus, in Japan, a wife might indicate anger to her husband by creating a disorderly flower arrangement. Such a subtle nonverbal cue is unlikely to be understood (or even noticed) by a husband from another culture.

> **KEYCONCEPT** **Gender, culture, and ethnic differences** in the experience and expression of anger must be taken into consideration before planning interventions.

Cultural differences in anger behavior can emanate from the historical trajectories, religions, languages, and customs of a group of people (Thomas, 2006). The same event can provoke very different emotional responses in culturally different persons (e.g., a random act by a stranger could be perceived as insulting by one individual but dismissed with a laugh by someone from another culture).

Gender role socialization influences beliefs about the appropriateness of "owning" angry emotionality and revealing it to others.

Western cultures generally promote more aggressive behavior in males and more conciliatory behavior in females (see Table 13.2). However, these generalizations may not apply to marginalized individuals, such as ethnic minorities. For example, African American mothers often prepare their daughters to mobilize anger to cope with the harsh realities of racist treatment (Thomas & González-Prendes, 2009). Some clients from Eastern cultures disapprove of anger for both genders, particularly cultures emphasizing connectedness rather than individualism (e.g., Japanese). Therefore, clients in such cultures may ruminate for lengthy periods about anger episodes rather than verbalizing their feelings. A more extensive discussion of culture and gender factors can be found in Thomas (2006).

The essential element in a cultural assessment is exploration of what the client learned about anger and its display in his or her culture and family of origin (the primary bearer of that culture). Adult clients can be encouraged to transcend cultural imperatives and childhood admonitions when these no longer serve them well. For example, research has shown that using anger to cope with racism actually has a negative effect on African American well being (Pittman, 2011). Reflecting on negative outcomes of anger behaviors can motivate client adoption of new strategies. Referral to an anger management course or therapy may be useful.

Anger Interventions

Communication techniques that promote the expression of anger in nondestructive ways have been developed and validated through research (Davidson & Mostofsky,

2010; Thomas, 2009). However, most people lack skill in handling anger constructively. Few people have healthy role models to observe while growing up. Therefore, education in anger management can be valuable, both for psychological growth and improved interpersonal relations.

Anger Management: A Psychoeducational Intervention

Anger management is an effective intervention that nurses can deliver to persons whose anger behavior is maladaptive in some way (i.e., interfering with success in work or relationships) but *not violent*. In recent years, there has been an increase in court-mandated "anger management" for persons whose behavior is violent as opposed to angry. When these individuals do not greatly benefit, a conclusion may be drawn that anger management is ineffective. However, psychoeducational anger management courses cannot be expected to modify *violent* behavior (interventions designed for aggressive and violent individuals are presented later in the chapter).

The desired outcomes of any anger management intervention are to teach people to (1) effectively modulate the physiological arousal of anger, (2) alter any irrational thoughts fueling the anger, and (3) modify maladaptive anger behaviors (e.g., blaming, attacking, or suppressing) that prevent problem solving in daily living. Group work is valuable to anger management clients because they need to practice new behaviors in an interpersonal context that offers feedback and support. The leader of an anger management group functions as a teacher and coach, not a therapist. Therefore, potential participants should be screened and referred to individual counseling or psychotherapy if their anger is deep seated and chronic. Exclusion criteria are paranoia, organic disorders, and severe personality disorders (Thomas, 2001). Candidates for psychoeducational anger management classes must have some insight that their behavior is problematic and some desire to enlarge their behavioral repertoire.

Clinicians achieve better outcomes when they follow empirically supported treatment manuals (Goldstein, Kemp, Leff, & Lochman, 2012; Goldstein et al., 2013). Anger management includes both didactic and experiential components. Educational handouts, videos, and workbooks are usually used. Ideally, participants commit to attendance for a series of weekly meetings, ranging from 4 to 10 weeks. Between the group meetings, participants are given homework assignments such as keeping an anger diary and applying the lessons of the class in their homes and work sites. Fresh anger incidents can be brought to the class for role-plays and group discussion. It may be useful to conduct for gender-specific or culturally specific groups (Thomas, 2001). Effectiveness

---

BOX 13.3

Research for Best Practice: Anger Management for Family Members

Son, J. Y., & Choi, Y. J. (2010). The effect of an anger management program for family members of patients with alcohol use disorders. Archives of Psychiatric Nursing, 24(1), 38–45.

THE QUESTION: Can a structured anger management program for family members of patients with alcohol use disorders promote effective anger expression and anger management?

METHODS: Sixty-three family members of patients with alcohol use disorders participated in anger management program of eight sessions with three groups for 2 months. Each session was held once a week for 2 hours by psychiatric–mental health nurse practitioners. Relaxation therapy was conducted at the beginning of each session. The goal of the anger management program was to have the participants express, ventilate, and cope with their anger in appropriate ways by using cognitive-behavioral techniques. The expression of anger was measured before and after the intervention by the Korean Anger Expression Inventory (based on the State-Trait Anger Expression Inventory).

FINDINGS: The total anger expression score of was significantly reduced at the end of the program, indicating that family members had improved their ability to effectively express anger.

IMPLICATIONS FOR NURSING: Anger management classes can be effective in helping family members of patients with substance use disorder learn to understand and modify their experience of anger through cognitive-behavior techniques.

---

of anger management has been demonstrated in studies of college students, angry drivers, angry veterans, various medical and psychiatric outpatients, and parents who have difficulty controlling anger toward their children (Kusmierska, 2012). Family members of patients with alcohol use disorders can also benefit from anger management (Box 13.3).

Studies show that individuals who are comfortable with religious/spiritual anger management strategies can successfully reduce maladaptive anger through prayer for the offender (Bremner, Koole, & Bushman, 2011) or forgiveness (Johnson, 2012; Mefford, Thomas, Callen, & Groer, in press).

Cognitive-Behavioral Therapy for Anger

Individuals who are not suitable candidates for a psychoeducational anger management intervention may benefit from cognitive-behavioral therapy delivered by an APN or psychologist. Deffenbacher (2011) recommends first establishing the therapeutic alliance because some angry individuals are not in a stage of readiness to change their behavior. When clients are more receptive, CBT involves avoidance of provoking stimuli, self-monitoring regarding cues of anger arousal, stimulus control, response disruption, and guided practice of more effective anger behaviors. Relaxation training is often introduced early in the treatment because it strengthens the therapeutic alliance and convinces clients that they can indeed learn to calm themselves when angry. When the body relaxes, there is less physical impetus to act impulsively in a way that one will later regret (Deffenbacher, 2011).

AGGRESSION AND VIOLENCE

Aggression and violence command the attention of the criminal justice system as well as the mental health care system. During periods when people are a danger to others, they may be separated from the larger society and confined in prisons or locked psychiatric units. Because nurses frequently practice in these settings, management of aggressive and violent behavior is an essential skill.

Factors that Influence Aggressive and Violent Behavior

The violent individual may feel trapped, frightened, or desperate, perhaps at the end of his or her rope. The nurse must remember that many violent individuals have experienced childhood abandonment, physical brutality, or sexual abuse. Confinement that replicates earlier experiences of degrading treatment may provoke aggressive response, but humane care may kindle hope of recovery and rehabilitation. The response of the nurse may be critical in determining whether aggression escalates or diminishes. Aggressive or violent behavior does not occur in a vacuum. Both the patient and the context must be considered. Therefore, a multidimensional framework is essential for understanding and responding to these behaviors (Morrison & Love, 2003).

> **KEYCONCEPT** **Aggression** involves overt behavior intended to hurt, belittle, take revenge, or achieve domination and control. Aggression can be verbal (sarcasm, insults, threats) or physical (property damage, slapping, hitting). Mentally healthy people stop themselves from aggression by realizing the negative consequences to themselves or their relationships.

Impulsive aggression occurs in situations of anger and anxiety when the frontal cortex does not rein in the amygdala, resulting in behaviors comparable to "a wild horse." **Instrumental** aggression is premeditated and unrelated to immediate feelings of frustration or threat, as in acts committed "in cold blood" (Audenaert, 2013).

> **KEYCONCEPT** **Violence** is extreme aggression and involves the use of strong force or weapons to inflict bodily harm to another person and in some cases to kill. Violence connotes greater intensity and destruction than aggression. All violence is aggressive, but not all aggression is violent.

Theories of Aggression and Violence

This section discusses some of the main theoretical explanations for aggression and violence. A single model or theory cannot fully explain aggression and violence; instead, choose the most useful theories for explaining a particular patient's experience and for planning interventions.

Biologic Theories

The brain structures most frequently associated with aggressive behavior are the limbic system and the cerebral cortex, particularly the frontal and temporal lobes. Patients with a history of damage to the cerebral cortex are more likely to exhibit increased impulsivity, decreased inhibition, and decreased judgment than are those who have not experienced such damage. The interaction of neurocognitive impairment and social history of abuse or family violence increases the risk for violent behavior (Siever, 2008).

An aggression-related gene (monoamine oxidase A), which affects norepinephrine, serotonin, and dopamine, may play a significant role in the violence enacted by abused children, especially boys (Siever, 2008). Low serotonin levels are also associated with irritability, increased pain sensitivity, impulsiveness, and aggression (Kuepper et al., 2010).

Sex hormones also play a role in some aggressive behavior. Violent male offenders have higher testosterone than control participants, and female offenders are more likely to commit crimes during the low progesterone phase of the menstrual cycle (Glenn & Raine, 2006). The odds of violent behavior also increase when separate risk factors, such as schizophrenia, substance abuse, and not taking prescribed medications, coexist in the same person. Before reading additional research evidence, try the anger exercise in Box 13.4. What does daily experience suggest about biologically based aspects of the experience and expression of anger?

BOX 13.4

***Self-Awareness Exercise:* Intensity of Anger**

Imagine this scene:

You are coming home late at night. You've been at the library studying for midterm examinations and are tired. As you come up the front walk, you trip over a skateboard, probably left by one of the neighborhood children. Before you know it, you are sprawled across the front step.

What emotions threaten to overwhelm you at that moment? What contributes to the intensity of the anger that you feel?

- The pain where you scraped your leg across the cement?
- Your general state of tiredness?
- The fact that you skipped dinner?
- The five cups of coffee you had today?
- The careless children who left a toy in your way?

If the same thing had happened when you were well rested and feeling good, would the feeling and the intensity be the same?

Psychological Theories

Several psychological explanations exist for aggressive and violent behaviors. This section discusses these theories and their treatment approaches.

Psychoanalytic Theories

Psychoanalytic theorists view emotions as instinctual drives. They view suppression of these drives as unhealthy and possible contributors to the development of psychosomatic or psychological disorders. Because the language of hydraulics is evident in Freud's use of terms such as cathexis (filling) and catharsis (release), some psychoanalysts recommended the use of cathartic approaches to release patients' pent-up anger. Following this theoretical formulation, nurses in the mid-20th century often used interventions that directed the patient to "let it out" by pounding a pillow or ripping up telephone books (Thomas, 2009). However, studies did not support the theory that catharsis reduces aggression.

Contemporary psychoanalysts do not adhere to any single explanatory model of aggression, often focusing on patients' tendencies to reenact old childhood conflicts or their defensive attempts to deny vulnerability (Feindler & Byers, 2006). In working with angry patients, they focus on issues such as improved control over outbursts, heightened empathy for others, and repair of deficits in the personality structure. During analytic therapy, patients gradually achieve greater insight into unconscious processes (Feindler & Byers, 2006). Thus, they become aware of the reasons they developed maladaptive anger behaviors.

Behavioral Theories

As behavioral theories came into prominence, anger was viewed as a learned response to a stimulus rather than an instinctual drive. In the 1930s, the frustration-aggression hypothesis was advanced in which a person may experience anger and act violently in response to interference with or blocking of a goal. Laboratory experiments and the reality of everyday experience have proved the limitations of this theory (Thomas, 1990). Not all situations in which one's goal is blocked lead to anger or violence.

Social Learning Theory

In Bandura's social learning theory, he focuses on the role of learning and rewards in the expression of aggression and violence (Bandura, 2001). Children's observations of aggressive behaviors among family members and violence in their communities foster a context for learning that aggressive behavior is an acceptable way of getting what they want. According to this view, people develop aggressive and violent behaviors by participating in an environment that rewards aggression (Palazzolo, Roberto, & Babin, 2010).

General Aggression Model

The general aggression model (GAM) is a framework that accounts for the interaction of cognition, affect, and arousal during an aggressive episode (Anderson & Anderson, 2008) (Figure 13.1). In this model, an episode

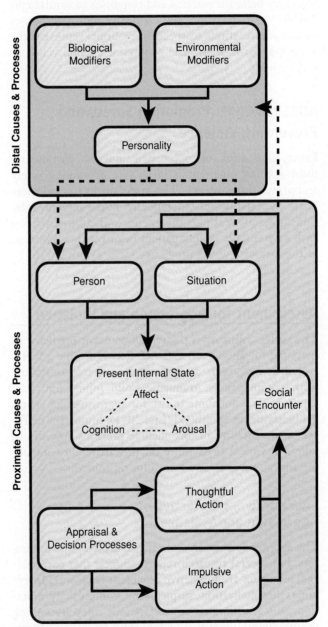

FIGURE 13.1 General aggression model overview. (Redrawn with permission from Anderson, C. A., & Anderson, K. B. [2008]. Men who target women: Specificity of target, generality of aggressive behavior. *Aggressive Behavior, 34*[6], 608.)

consists of *person and situation factors* in an ongoing *social interaction*. The episode is mediated through a person's thoughts, feelings, and intensity of arousal. Within this context, the individual appraises the episode and then makes a decision about a follow-up action. The outcome is either thoughtful or impulsive action. The *person factors* include characteristics such as gender, personality traits, beliefs and attitudes, values, goals, and behavior patterns. *Situational factors* include the actual provocation (insults, slights, verbal and physical aggression, interference with achieving goals) and cues that trigger memories of similar situations. *Cognition* includes hostile thoughts and scripts (previous behavior patterns and responses to similar episodes). Mood, emotion, and expressive motor responses (automatic reactions to specific emotions) represent the *affect component. Arousal* can be physiological, psychological, or both.

NURSING CARE: Promoting Safety and Preventing Violence

Paramount aims of psychiatric nurses, particularly those staffing inpatient facilities, are promoting safety and preventing violence. The nurse works toward these goals by establishing therapeutic nurse–patient relationships and creating a therapeutic milieu. Intervening with a potentially violent patient begins with assessment of the history and the predictive factors outlined in the next section.

Assessment for Aggression and Violence

The patient's history is the most important predictor of potential for aggression and violence. Early life adverse circumstances, such as inadequate maternal nutrition, birth complications, traumatic brain injury, and lead exposure can contribute to risk for aggressive and criminal behaviors in adulthood (Liu, 2011). Important markers in the patient's history include previous episodes of rage and violent behavior, escalating irritability, intruding angry thoughts, and fear of losing control.

Characteristics Predictive of Aggression and Violence

The age, gender, and race of patients are *not* good predictors, but several research reports suggest that particular characteristics are predictive of violent behaviors. Involuntary hospitalization, suspiciousness, impulsivity, agitation, and unwillingness to follow unit rules are among the predictors identified in Johnson's (2004) systematic review of the literature about violence on inpatient psychiatric units. Those with diagnoses such as schizophrenia, bipolar disorder, brain injury, alcohol withdrawal, or

attention deficit hyperactivity disorder are at increased risk for violent episodes (Zuzelo, Curran, & Zeserman, 2012).

Usually, there are some observable precursors to aggression and violence. In a study of aggressive episodes in an emergency department, the following behaviors indicated an impending aggressive episode: (1) *staring and eye contact* or glaring as a way of intimidation; (2) *tone and volume* of voice such as raised voices, sarcastic comments, and urgent or demeaning speech; (3) *anxiety* in patients, family or friends; (4) *mumbling* that shows increasing frustration; and (5) *pacing* that indicates increased agitation (Luck, Jackson, & Usher, 2007). Research by Bowers, James, Quirk, Wright, Williams, and Stewart (2013) points out that the "textbook picture" of gradual escalation of patient behavior does not always occur; aggression can have a sudden onset with no clear precipitant.

Impaired Communication

Impaired communication (including hearing loss and reduced visual acuity), disorientation, and depression have been found to be consistently associated with aggressive behavior among nursing home residents with dementia (Williams & Herman, 2011).

In patients with cognitive impairments, the nurse needs to know when the patient last voided and the pattern of bowel movements. The urge to void can be a powerful stimulus to agitated behavior. Regular toileting routines are not just interventions to prevent incontinence. Similarly, the anticipation of basic needs such as thirst and hunger is important, especially when working with adults and children who cannot readily express their needs. Other discomforts can arise from such conditions as ingrown toenails and adverse medication reactions.

Physical Condition

The patient's physical condition contributes to the likelihood of aggression. Patients with longstanding poor dietary habits (e.g., indigent patients, patients with alcoholism) often have deficiencies of thiamine and niacin. Increased irritability, disorientation, and paranoia may result. Assessing overall dietary intake is relevant, particularly of good tryptophan sources, such as wheat, flour, corn, milk, and eggs. Intake of caffeine, a potent stimulant, should be assessed and limited as necessary (Martin, Cook, Woodring, Burkhardt, Omar, & Kelly, 2008).

Social Factors

The nurse should evaluate social factors, such as crisis conditions in the patient's home, family, or community, that could lead to aggression or violent episodes. If assessment reveals stressful actions by family members, such as evicting the patient from the home, attention must be devoted to mobilizing resources for family and community support and alternative housing.

Are financial or legal troubles placing increased stress on the patient? Is the patient experiencing conflict with other patients on the unit or with certain staff? People reenact in new relationships the same behaviors that created problems in old ones. Thus, behavior in a mental health facility provides important clues to a patient's habitual responses to authority figures, opposite-sex peers, and same-sex peers. Assessment data provide direction for interventions such as reassigning roommates or caregivers.

Milieu and Environmental Factors

Angry or out-of-control behavior is highly influenced by contextual factors. Successful psychiatric stabilization and treatment in a hospital often depend on the nature of the unit itself. A busy, noisy hospital unit can quickly provoke an aggressive episode. A rude comment or staff denial of a patient request can trigger physical assault. Crowding and density during times of high patient census are also associated with patient aggression. Inadequate staffing has been identified as a contributing factor in units with a high incidence of assault.

Many characteristics of the unit culture and staff behavior, such as rigid rules and violation of boundaries, predict patient violence (Box 13.5). In units with a high incidence of violence, nurses should take steps to improve the milieu and staff–patient relationships.

Nursing Diagnoses for Aggression and Violence

The most common nursing diagnoses for patients experiencing intense anger and aggression are Risk for

---

BOX 13.5

Characteristics of Unit Culture and Staff Behavior that Predict Patient Violence

- Rigid unit rules
- Lack of patient privacy or boundary violations
- Lack of patient autonomy (locked doors, restraints)
- Strict hierarchy of authority
- Lack of patient control over the treatment plan
- Denial of patient requests or privileges
- Lack of meaningful and predictable ward activities
- Insufficient help with activities of daily living and other needs from staff
- Patronizing behavior of staff
- Power struggles related to medications
- Failure of staff to listen, convey empathy

Source: Hamrin, V., Iennaco, J., & Olsen, D. (2009). A review of ecological factors affecting inpatient psychiatric unit violence: Implications for relational and unit cultural improvements. *Issues in Mental Health Nursing, 30,* 214–226.

Self-Directed Violence and Risk for Other-Directed Violence (NANDA International, 2012). Outcomes focus on aggression control.

Interventions for Promoting Safety

Both patients and staff have a right to expect safety on a psychiatric unit. Nursing interventions focus on communication and development of the nurse–patient relationship, cognitive interventions, interventions for the milieu and environment, and violence prevention.

Communication and Development of the Therapeutic Nurse–Patient Relationship

Communicating with a patient who has the potential for aggression or violence follows the same principles discussed in Chapter 7. Aggressive behavior can be a patient's way to communicate a need for help (Finfgeld-Connett, 2009). Low self-esteem that has been further eroded during hospitalization or treatment may influence a patient to use force to meet his or her needs or to experience some sense of empowerment. The patient who behaves aggressively may receive rewards such as more frequent observation and more opportunities to discuss concerns with nurses. Clearly, this patient must be taught how to get his or her needs met in a more appropriate way.

Listening to the Patient's Illness Experience and Concerns

Development of the therapeutic nurse–patient relationship begins with listening. Some patient complaints are valid and deserve a respectful hearing. For example, disappointment with "playing little games with staff" or "attending classes" has been expressed by hospitalized psychiatric patients who longed for a deeper connection with nursing staff and more intensive insight-oriented therapies (Thomas, Shattell, & Martin, 2002). While patients and their family members are routinely requested to provide details about past medical treatments, medications, and hospitalizations, what is often overlooked is the subjective experience of the health problem (Thomas & Pollio, 2002). Many patients with persistent mental illness have had frightening medication reactions and unpleasant side effects of treatments (such as memory loss caused by electroconvulsive therapy). Understandably, they may harbor distrust of mental health clinicians and resent being hospitalized again. Inviting patients and families to talk about their experiences with the health care system may highlight both their concerns and resources. Simply listening to patients' concerns and "being with" them is often as significant as "doing for" them (Thomas & Pollio, 2002) (Box 13.6).

BOX 13.6 • THERAPEUTIC DIALOGUE • The Potentially Aggressive Patient

Paul is a 23-year-old patient in the high observation area of an inpatient unit. He is pacing back and forth. He is pounding one fist into his other hand. In the past 24 hours, Paul has been more cooperative and less agitated. The behavior the nurse observes now is more similar to the behavior that Paul displayed 2 days ago. Yesterday the psychiatrist told Paul that he would be granted more freedom in the unit if his behavior improved. The psychiatrist has just seen Paul and refused to change the restrictions on Paul's activities.

INEFFECTIVE APPROACH

Nurse: Paul, I can understand this is frustrating for you.

Paul: How can you understand? Have you ever been held like a prisoner?

Nurse: I do understand, Paul. Now you must calm down or more privileges will be removed.

Paul: [voice gets louder] But I was told that calm behavior would mean more privileges. Now you are telling me calm behavior only gets me what I have got! Can't you talk to the doctor for me?

Nurse: No, Paul, I can't talk to the doctor. [Paul appears more frustrated and agitated as the conversation continues.]

EFFECTIVE APPROACH

Nurse: Paul, you look upset (observation). What happened in your conversation with the psychiatrist? (seeking information)

Paul: Yesterday he said calmer behavior would mean more freedom in the unit. I have tried to be calmer and not to swear. You said you noticed the difference. But today he says "no" to more freedom.

Nurse: Some people might feel cheated if this happened to them. (validation). Is that how you feel?

Paul: Yeah, I feel real cheated. Nothing I do makes a difference. That's the way it is here, and that's the way it is when I am out of the hospital.

Nurse: Sounds like experiences like this leave you feeling pretty powerless. (validation)

Paul: I don't have any power, anywhere. Sometimes when I have no power I get mean. At least then people pay attention to me.

Nurse: In this situation with your doctor, what would help you feel that you had some power? (inviting patient partnership)

Paul: Well, if he would listen to me; if he would read my chart.

Nurse: I am a bit confused by the psychiatrist's decision. I won't make promises that your privileges will change, but would it be okay with you if I talk with him?

Paul: That would make me feel like someone is on my side.

CRITICAL THINKING CHALLENGE

- In the first scenario, how did the nurse escalate the situation?

- Compare the first scenario with the second. How are they different?

Validating

Patients who experience intense anger and rage can feel isolated and anxious. The nurse can acknowledge these intense feelings by reflecting "This must be scary for you." Empathic responding can reduce emotional arousal because the patient feels understood and supported (Jarry & Paivio, 2006). By drawing on past experience with other patients, the nurse can also reassure the patient that others have felt the same way.

Providing Choices

When possible, the nurse should provide the patient with choices, particularly patients who have little control over their situation because of their condition. Offering concrete choices is better than offering open-ended options. For example, a patient who is experiencing a manic episode and is confined to her room may have few options in her daily schedule. However, she may be allowed to make choices about food, personal hygiene, and which pajamas to wear.

Cognitive Interventions to Address Aggression

Cognitive interventions are very useful in interacting with a potentially aggressive patient. These interventions are useful when the patient is in a nonaggressive state and willing to discuss the irrational thought process underlying aggressive episodes. These periods of interaction allow exploration of the patient's beliefs, and provision of reassurance, support, and education.

> **NCLEXNOTE** The best time to teach the patient techniques for managing anger and aggression is when the patient is not experiencing the provoking event. Cognitive therapy approaches are useful and can be prioritized according to responses.

Providing Patient Education

Inpatient hospitalization offers opportunities for education of patients and families about a variety of topics. Nurses can seize "teachable moments" to convey important principles of anger management. For example, after an outburst of loud cursing by John, who mistakenly thought another patient (Jim) had stolen his cigarettes, the nurse helped him consider what he could have done differently in the situation. John was more amenable to learning about calming techniques and problem-solving strategies at this time because his behavior had resulted in adverse consequences (estrangement from Jim, disruption of the dayroom during a popular bingo game, and cancellation of his weekend pass). This incident could also be used for teaching in a subsequent group meeting of inpatients. Many units have daily meetings that permit processing of such conflicts. Jim could be invited to express his feelings about being falsely accused of stealing. Other patients may reveal how distressed they were when John was cursing loudly, providing John useful peer feedback about his outburst. Together, group members could generate ideas for more appropriate behavior.

Developing Prevention Strategies

Although patients are not always aware of it, escalation of feelings, thoughts, and behavior from calmness to violence may follow a particular pattern. Disruption of the pattern can sometimes be a useful means for preventing escalation and helping the patient regain composure. Patients can be actively involved in development of an "early detection plan" based on identification of their own personal warning signs of aggression (Fluttert, Van Meijel, Webster, Nijman, Bartels, & Grypdonck, 2008). Although extant literature continues to focus on staff control of patient behavior, new research shows that aggressive patients would like to learn to handle their impulsive aggressive behavior themselves (deSchutter & Lodewijkx, 2013). Nurses can suggest strategies to interrupt patterns:

- Counting to 10
- Using a relaxation or breathing technique (see Chapter 9)
- Removing oneself from interactions or stimuli that may contribute to increased distress (voluntarily taking "time-out")
- Doing something different (e.g., reading, listening to quiet music, watching television)

Milieu and Environmental Interventions

The inpatient environment can be modified proactively to decrease the potential of aggressive and violent behaviors (Box 13.7).

BOX 13.7

Environmental Management: Violence Prevention

DEFINITION
Monitoring and manipulating the physical environment to decrease the potential of violent behavior directed toward self, others, or environment.

ACTIVITIES
- Remove potential weapons (e.g., sharps, ropelike objects) from the environment.
- Search the environment routinely to maintain it as hazard free.
- Search the patient and his or her belongings for weapons or potential weapons during inpatient admission procedures as appropriate.
- Monitor the safety of items that visitors bring to the environment.
- Instruct visitors and other caregivers about relevant patient safety issues.
- Limit patient use of potential weapons (e.g., sharps, ropelike objects).
- Monitor patient during use of potential weapons (e.g., razors).
- Place the patient with potential for self-harm with a roommate to decrease isolation and opportunity to act on self-harm thoughts, as appropriate.
- Assign a single room to the patient with potential for violence toward others.
- Place the patient in a bedroom located near a nursing station.
- Limit access to windows unless they are locked and shatterproof, as appropriate.
- Lock utility and storage rooms.
- Provide paper dishes and plastic utensils at meals.
- Place the patient in the least restrictive environment that still allows for the necessary level of observation.
- Provide ongoing surveillance of all patient access areas to maintain patient safety and therapeutically intervene, as needed.
- Remove other individuals from the vicinity of a violent or potentially violent patient.
- Maintain a designated safe area (e.g., seclusion room) for patient to be placed when violent.
- Provide plastic, rather than metal, clothes hangers, as appropriate.

Adapted with permission from Bulechek, G., Butcher, H.K., Dochterman, J. M., & Wagner, C. (2012). *Nursing interventions classification (NIC)* (6th ed). St. Louis: Mosby.

Reducing Stimulation

For people whose perceptions or thoughts are disordered from brain damage, degeneration, or other thought-processing difficulties, modification of the environment may be one of the main interventions. The patient with a brain injury, progressive dementia, or distorted vision may be experiencing intense and highly confusing stimulation even though the environment, from the nurse or family's perspective, seems calm and orderly.

Likewise, introducing more structure into a chaotic environment can help decrease the risk for aggressive behavior. It is possible to make stimuli meaningful or to simplify and interpret the environment in many practical ways, such as by identifying people or equipment that may be unfamiliar, providing cues as to what is expected (e.g., posting signs with directions, putting a toothbrush and toothpaste by the sink), and removing or silencing unnecessary stimuli (e.g., turning off paging systems).

Considering the environment from the patient's viewpoint is essential. For instance, if the surroundings are unfamiliar, the patient will need to process more information. Lack of a recognizable pattern or structure further taxes the patient's capacity to encode information. Appropriate interventions include clarifying the meaning and purpose of people and objects in the environment, enhancing the patient's sense of control and the predictability of the environment, and reducing other stimuli as much as possible (Bulechek, Butcher, Dochterman, & Wagner, 2012).

Creating a Culture of Nonviolence

Ultimately, nurses must strive to create cultures of nonviolence. One approach that shows promise is the Violence Prevention Community Meeting (VPCM) pioneered on an acute inpatient psychiatry unit at a veterans' hospital (Lanza, Rierdan, Forester, & Zeiss, 2009). Twice-weekly meetings, lasting 30 minutes, were attended by all patients and staff. Typical topics of discussion were boundary violations, ways of summoning assistance, and ways to air grievances and solve problems. A statistically significant reduction in patient violence resulted from implementation of the VPCM. Another approach illustrating the importance of administrative leadership is the daily interdisciplinary meeting held in the medical director's office at a New Hampshire hospital to review every incident of seclusion and restraint (SR) (Allen, de Nesnera, & Souther, 2009). Direct care staff provide firsthand reports about the incident followed by brainstorming about alternative strategies to be implemented in future incidents of aggressive and violent behavior. Approaches such as these are critical to the achievement of safer and more humane environments for psychiatric care.

Interventions for Managing Imminent Aggression and Violence

De-escalation

Authentic engagement with the patient is the core component in a therapeutic de-escalation by the nurse (Finfgeld-Connett, 2009). Creative, patient-centered strategies, not techniques of physical restraint, are of paramount importance. Individualizing interventions is also emphasized by researchers Johnson and Delaney (2007); astute staff members realized that some patient behaviors (e.g., loudness, pacing) could be ignored and some "escalating" situations would actually subside without any staff intervention.

De-escalating potential aggression is always preferable to challenging or provoking a patient. De-escalating (commonly known as "talking the person down") is a skill that every nurse can develop. Trying to clarify what has upset the patient is important although not all patients are capable of articulating what provoked them, and some analyses will have to take place after a crisis has been diffused. The nurse can use therapeutic communication techniques to prevent a crisis or diffuse a critical situation (see Box 13.6).

The nurse who works with potentially aggressive patients should do so with respect and concern. The goal is to work with patients to find solutions, approaching these patients calmly, empathizing with the patient's perspective, and avoiding a power struggle. In dealing with aggression, as in other aspects of nursing practice, at times the best intervention is silence. It is easy to equate intervention with activity, the sense that "I must do something." But offering quiet calmness may be enough to help a patient regain control of his or her behavior.

> **KEYCONCEPT** **Intervention fit** The nurse who intervenes from within the context of the therapeutic relationship must be cognizant of the fit of a particular intervention.

Interventions that are appropriate in early phases of escalation differ from those used when the patient's agitation is greater. The patient's affective, behavioral, and cognitive response to an intervention provides information about its effects and guides the nurse's next response. The following approaches are important in caring for patients who are aggressive or violent:

- Using nonthreatening body language
- Respecting the patient's personal space and boundaries
- Having immediate access to the door of the room in case you need to leave the room
- Choosing to leave the door open to an office while talking to a patient
- Knowing where colleagues are and making sure those colleagues know where you are

- Removing or not wearing clothing or accessories that could be used to harm you, such as scarves, necklaces, or dangling earrings

Administering and Monitoring PRN Medications

Patients with the potential for aggression and violence usually have a PRN (as-needed) medication order for agitation and aggression. Bowers et al. (2013), after analyzing multiple episodes of aggression, recommended that nurses use PRN medications more frequently although Smith et al. (2013) have cautioned against overexposing patients to psychotropic medications and/or giving medications for staff convenience. Administering a PRN medication is left to the discretion of the nurse, who makes a judgment about the patient after careful assessment.

Avoiding the Use of Seclusion and Restraint

Seclusion and restraint have been used by nurses when patients need to be separated from other patients on the unit. An integrative literature review by Laiho, Kattainen, Astedt-Kurki, Putkonen, Lindberg, and Kylma (2013) revealed that the decision to use SR is a dynamic process involving evaluation of the risk toward the patient, other patients, and the nurses themselves, as well as the need to maintain a therapeutic milieu.

Moylan (2009), an experienced clinician and researcher, reports that some of her patients verbalized positive feelings of safety after restraints were applied. She asserts that restraint can achieve a therapeutic outcome if no excessive force is used and the nurse conveys concern and respect for the patient throughout the period of confinement. Some patients surveyed by Canadian researchers found SR helpful when they felt out-of-control (Larue, Dumais, Boyer, Goulet, Bonin, & Baba, 2013). However, as noted in Chapter 10, SR are controversial interventions to be used judiciously and only when other interventions have failed to control the patient's behavior.

Recently, there has been recognition that SR interventions may be disproportionately applied to certain types of vulnerable patients, such as those who are deaf or hard of hearing. Hartman and Blalock (2011) found greater prevalence of SR interventions in hearing impaired patients than in a matched group of hearing individuals in a state mental hospital setting. SR interventions may cause considerable psychological damage by replicating childhood traumas. For example, seclusion may be extremely painful to a patient who has already experienced abandonment and rejection. Restraint may recreate trauma comparable to a rape ("They held me down, they pulled my drawers down") (Benson, Secker, Balfe, Lipsedge, Robinson, & Walk, 2003). Physical restraint may also produce injury or even death, due to catecholamine hyperstimulation, positional asphyxia, and/ or preexisting medical conditions such as cardiac disease (Duxbury, Aiken, & Dale, 2013). Of 38 restraint-related deaths in the United Kingdom that were analyzed by Duxbury et al., 26 were attributable to asphyxia when the patient was held in a prone position. Supine position can also be problematic. Nurses involved in the physical restraint of patients feel conflicted about having to intervene in this manner, as shown in these excerpts from an interview study: "I felt instantly like a bully. I am awful, you know, look what I have done to this man;" "You kind of feel a bit dirty from the whole experience" (Bigwood & Crowe, 2008).

The controversy over SR interventions and their potential to be applied punitively provided impetus for issuance of federal guidelines for their use. American institutions that receive Medicare or Medicaid reimbursement must adhere to guidelines issued by the Center for Medicare and Medicaid Services. These guidelines specify that a registered nurse must verify the need for restraint or seclusion and then contact the physician or other licensed practitioner; within 1 hour, that practitioner must examine the patient (see Chapter 9). Individual states have also enacted laws to regulate the use of restraints, and professional organizations such as the International Society of Psychiatric-Mental Health Nurses (1999) and the American Psychiatric Nurses Association (2007) have released position statements on restraints as the last resort in an emergency.

Restraint-related injuries and deaths have prompted many facilities to ban their use entirely and train staff in alternative techniques. Examples of restraint-free units can be found in the literature. At one Pennsylvania hospital, the psychiatric unit has been restraint free for 2 years because the staff adopted person-centered, recovery-oriented care principles (Barton, Johnson, & Price, 2009). Although increased use of sedatives might be suspected, there has been a significant decrease in sedative–hypnotic drug administration as well. The old seclusion room was transformed into the Comfort Room and supplied with journaling materials and soothing music. Use of the room is voluntary, unlike staff-mandated "time-outs" or seclusion. Any patient may ask staff to use the room to decrease agitation and anxiety.

Comfort rooms are becoming more widespread, providing an appealing alternative to coercive interventions by unit staff. The majority (92.9%) of patients who used the comfort room at a rural tertiary mental hospital reported that its availability was helpful in reducing their distress (Sivak, 2012). Comfort rooms are more compatible with contemporary philosophies of person-centered, recovery-oriented care (Barton et al., 2009; Sivak, 2012).

Evaluation and Treatment Outcomes

Treatment outcomes can be considered at both individual and aggregate levels. The desired outcome at the individual level is for the patient to regain or maintain control over aggressive or potentially aggressive thoughts, feelings, and actions. The nurse may observe that the patient shows decreased psychomotor activity (e.g., less pacing), has a more relaxed posture, speaks more directly about feelings of anger and personal needs, requires less sedating medication, shows increased tolerance for frustration and the ability to consider alternatives, and makes effective use of other coping strategies.

Evidence of a reduction in risk factors in the treatment setting include decreased noise and confusion in the immediate environment; calmness on the part of nursing staff and others; and a climate of safety, clear expectations, and mutual acceptance and respect. In units, day hospitals, or group home settings, indicators of positive treatment outcomes include a reduction in the number and severity of assaults on staff and other patients, fewer incident reports, and increased staff competency in de-escalating potentially violent situations.

Examination of the interactions of the aggressor, victim, and environment has been proposed by Lanza and colleagues to get a complete picture of the incident (Lanza, Zeiss, & Rierdan, 2009). In the 360-degree interview, the incident becomes the center of a Venn diagram (Figure 13.2), and the victim, the assailant, supervisor, and coworkers are asked by a neutral party for information on the assault. All relevant participants may be asked to provide their perspective. This approach allows for a collaborative, community approach to preventing patient violence and avoids blaming one assailant for incidents that are provoked by a variety of contextual and interpersonal factors.

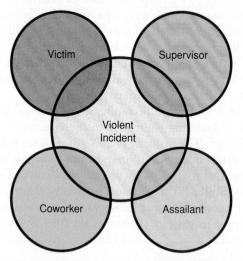

FIGURE 13.2 Application of 360-degree interviewing to a violent incident. (Redrawn with permission from Lanza, M. L., Zeiss, R. A., & Rierdan, J. [2009]. Multiple perspectives on assault: The 360-degree interview. *Journal of the American Psychiatric Nurses Association, 14*[6], 413–420.)

Responding to Assault on Nurses

Because nurses have extended contact with patients during highly stressful circumstances, there is always the risk that they may be the recipients of patient aggression. Nurses and nurses' aides are the targets of patient violence more often than any other health care professionals (Janocha & Smith, 2010), and psychiatric nurses report higher rates of assault than nurses in other specialties (Hartley & Ridenour, 2011).

Assaults on nurses by patients can have both immediate and long-term consequences, as shown in Lanza's seminal research (1992) (Table 13.3). Reported assaults range from verbal abuse or threats and minor altercations to severe injuries, rape, and murder. Any assault can produce severe sequelae for the victim, including PTSD (Jacobowitz, 2013). After a violent incident, nurses struggle with their inclination to avoid the patient, and they watch for any signs of patient remorse; their response differs if the violent behavior was attributable to psychosis versus manipulative or volitional acting out (Zuzelo et al., 2012). Because of their role as caregivers, nurses may suppress the normal range of feelings after an assault, believing that it is wrong to experience strong feelings of anger and fear in this situation. This belief may relate to the conflict nurses experience in having to care for

TABLE 13.3	NURSES' RESPONSES TO ASSAULT	
Response Type	**Personal**	**Professional**
Affective	• Irritability • Depression • Anger • Anxiety • Apathy	• Erosion of feelings of competence, leading to increased anxiety and fear • Feelings of guilt or self-blame • Fear of potentially violent patients
Cognitive	• Suppressed or intrusive thoughts of assault	• Reduced confidence in judgment • Consideration of job change
Behavioral	• Social withdrawal	• Possible hesitation in responding to other violent situations • Possible overcontrolling • Possible hesitation to report future assaults • Possible withdrawal from colleagues • Questioning of capabilities by coworkers
Physiologic	• Disturbed sleep • Headaches • Stomach aches • Tension	• Increased absenteeism because of somatic complaints

patients who have hurt them. The conflict between one's professional role as caregiver and one's own needs as an assault victim has been explored in a support group for nurses and nursing assistants who had been assaulted (Lanza, Demaio, & Benedict, 2005). The support group met twice per week for 6 weeks, allowing expression of anger, blame, and anxiety and concluding with development of personal plans for working with potentially assaultive patients.

Unfortunately, patient aggression directed toward nurses is often minimized or tolerated by nurses as "part of the job" (Poster & Drew, 2006). Nurses seldom report attacks to the police or prosecute their attackers. Aggression by patients must be addressed more vigorously because it can threaten the other patients, other health care professionals, family members, and visitors, as well as the nursing staff. Reporting violent attacks increases public awareness and increases the likelihood that protective legislation will be enacted (Haun, 2013). Steps must be taken by institutions to reduce the incidence of patient assault. The environment should be modified with the addition of security alarms, video monitors, and de-escalation teams.

All nurses must be provided with training programs in the prevention and management of aggressive behavior. These programs, similar to courses on cardiopulmonary resuscitation (CPR), impart both knowledge and skills. Similar to CPR training, the courses need to be made available to nurses regularly, so that they have opportunities to reinforce and update what they have learned. Research shows that nurses who have participated in preventive training programs as students or as professionals become more confident in coping with patient aggression (Jacobowitz, 2013). Jacobowitz recommends resilience-building sessions in which workers meet with a trained facilitator every 4 to 6 weeks. Some states have enacted legislation mandating workplace violence prevention programs, but the curricula vary, and the quality of training lacks systematic evaluation (Peek-Asa et al., 2009). Commercially marketed training programs have been criticized because they fail to consider the predatory aspect of some patients' violence and fail to cite nursing research.

RESEARCH AND POLICY INITIATIVES

Additional understanding of the phenomena of anger, aggression, and violence as they occur in the clinical setting is needed. Research studies that have illuminated this problem from a nursing perspective need to be continued and expanded. The links among biology, neurology, and psychology must be further elucidated. In addition, further explorations of the reciprocal influence of patient interactional style and treatment setting culture assist in the development and management of humane treatment

settings. Finally, and perhaps most importantly, nurses must research the effectiveness of particular anger and aggression management interventions. Interventions aimed at specific populations, such as adolescent girls in residential placements, are being developed; however, outcomes have not yet been evaluated in randomized controlled trials (Goldstein et al., 2013).

Although much of this chapter focused on individuals who need to *down*regulate anger, the reader must remember that anger suppressors have a need to *up*regulate their anger and express it more assertively. Treatments should be tailored accordingly and patients' progress documented by administering questionnaires such as the STAXI both before and after the treatments. Feindler (2006) edited a useful practitioner's guide to comparative treatments of anger-related disorders. However, authors in this edited volume cautioned that research is sparse regarding the efficacy of some treatments, especially for culturally diverse clients whose heritage is quite different from the Euro-American heritage of most mental health clinicians in the United States. Thomas (2006) has pointed out the inadequacy of most training programs in preparing mental health professionals for work with culturally diverse clients. It is unknown what adaptations may be needed to deliver appropriate anger treatments to these individuals. Only by accruing sufficient empirical evidence can we obtain definitive guidance for clinical practice with angry and aggressive individuals.

There is a moral imperative for nurses to be involved in combating violence in the larger community. Lessening anger and violence in the workplace and the home demands involvement of all mental health professionals. Nurses can share their expertise with parents, children, teachers, and community agencies. Nurses are well positioned to teach health-promoting anger management classes in diverse practice settings, such as outpatient clinics, schools, and corporate sites. Classes for children and adolescents can be of great benefit because young people are forming the anger habits that will continue into adulthood (Puskar, Stark, Northcut, Williams, & Haley, 2011; Thomas, 2001).

Compelling scientific evidence is now available to show that violence portrayed in the media is harmful to children. As a result, television networks limit violent programming during hours when children are generally watching programs. However, this gain is offset by the growing availability of violent websites and videogames. Videogames actively involve players in violence and reward them for it. Nurses can add their voices to those of activists who object to the content of these games and to offensive media offerings. As concerned citizens, nurses can advocate for changes in public policy such as those recommended by the World Health Organization (2009) in its *Violence Prevention: The Evidence*.

Finally, nurses can support legislation to make assault on nurses a felony, similar to assault on lifeguards, bus drivers, jurors, umpires, and emergency medical technicians. Such legislation is in place in less than half of the United States. A vital first step is increased reporting of assaults because 80% are never reported (Haun, 2013). Nurses who provide indispensable services in the nation's psychiatric units, emergency rooms, and other settings deserve to be safe from violence in the enactment of their daily work.

SUMMARY OF KEY POINTS

■ Anger is an emotional state, usually temporary, that can be expressed constructively or destructively. Destructive anger alienates other people and invites retaliation.

■ Anger, aggression, and violence should not be viewed as a continuum. The anger of ordinary people seldom progresses to aggression or violence. Anger does not necessarily lead to aggression or violence.

■ Anger management is a useful psychoeducational intervention that is effective with a wide variety of nonviolent individuals. However, anger management is not designed to modify violent behavior.

■ Several theories explain anger, aggression, and violence and include neurobiologic and psychosocial theories. These theories serve as the basis of assessment and interventions.

■ The general aggression model accounts for the interaction of cognition, affect, and arousal during an aggressive episode.

■ There is no one factor that predicts aggression or violence. Factors that have been observed to be precursors are staring and eye contact, tone and volume of voice, anxiety, mumbling, and pacing.

■ Nursing interventions can be affective, cognitive, behavioral, or sociocultural. A therapeutic milieu supports a nonviolent culture.

■ If a violent incident occurs, using a 360-degree evaluation approach will help in understanding the interpersonal and contextual factors that led to the incident.

■ Seclusion or restraints should be used only as a last resort.

■ Patient aggression and violence are serious concerns for nurses in all areas of clinical practice. Training in and policies and procedures for the prevention and management of aggressive episodes should be available in all work settings.

CRITICAL THINKING CHALLENGES

1. Mary Jane, a 24-year-old single woman, has just been admitted to an inpatient psychiatry unit. She was transferred to the unit from the emergency department where she was treated for a drug overdose. She is sullen when she is introduced to her roommate and refuses to answer the questions the nurse has that are part of the admission procedure. The nurse tells Mary Jane that he will come back later to see how she is. A few minutes later, Mary Jane approaches the nursing station and asks in a demanding tone to talk with someone and complains that she has been completely ignored since she came into the unit. What frameworks can the nurse use to understand Mary Jane's behavior? At this point in time, what data does he have to develop a plan of care? What interventions might the nurse choose to use to help Mary Jane behave in a manner that is consistent with the norms of this inpatient unit?

2. Discuss the influence of gender and cultural norms on the expression of anger. When a nurse is caring for a patient from a culture that the nurse is not familiar with, what could the nurse ask to ensure that her or his expectations of the patient's behavior are consistent with the gender and cultural norms of the patient?

3. Under what circumstances should people who are aggressive or violent be held accountable for their behavior? Are there any exceptions?

4. When a nurse minimizes verbally abusive behavior by a patient, family member, or health care colleague, what implicit message does she or he send?

Mandela: Long Walk to Freedom: 2013. South African icon Nelson Mandela displays the gamut of angry behaviors in this biographical epic: (1) righteous anger on behalf of his clients when he was a young lawyer; (2) fiery anger at the cruel persecution of blacks during apartheid; and (3) violence against the government after the failure of nonviolent protests to achieve freedom from oppression. Bomb throwing at government buildings results in 27 years of imprisonment, which could have created lasting bitterness against his oppressors. Yet after his release Mandela forgives those who had imprisoned him, becomes the first black president of his country, and receives the Nobel Peace Prize. This remarkable true story provides many lessons for all of us.

Viewing Points: Although most of us will never be forced to endure such intolerable conditions, we all experience times of unfair or unkind treatment. How can we learn to use our anger productively or learn to let it go by forgiving those who wronged us?

REFERENCES

Allen, D. E., deNesnera, A., & Souther, J. W. (2009). Executive-level reviews of seclusion and restraint promote interdisciplinary collaboration and innovation. *Journal of the American Psychiatric Nurses Association, 15,* 260–264.

American Nurses Association, & Nursing World. (2012). Workplace violence. Retrieved from www.nursingworld.org

American Psychiatric Association (APA). (2013). *Diagnostic and Statistical Manual of Mental Disorders DSM-5.* Arlington, VA: Author.

American Psychiatric Nurses Association. (2007). *2007 Position Statement on the Use of Seclusion and Restraint.* Arlington, VA: Author.

Anderson, C. A., & Anderson, K. B. (2008). Men who target women: specificity of target, generality of aggressive behavior. *Aggressive Behavior, 34*(6), 605–622.

Audenaert, K. (2013). Neurobiology of aggressive behavior: About wild horses and reins. *Proceedings of the 8th European congress on violence in clinical psychiatry* (pp. 44). Amsterdam: Kavanah.

Averill, J. R. (1983). Studies on anger and aggression: Implications for theories of emotion. *American Psychologist, 38,* 1145–1160.

Bandura, A. (2001). Social cognitive theory: An agentic perspective. *Annual Review of Psychology, 52,* 1–26.

Barton, S. A., Johnson, M. R., & Price, L. V. (2009). Achieving restraint-free on an inpatient behavioral health unit. *Journal of Psychosocial Nursing, 47*(1), 35–40.

Bennett, P., & Lowe, R. (2008). Emotions and their cognitive precursors: Responses to spontaneously identify stressful events among hospital nurses. *Journal of Health Psychology, 13*(4), 537–546.

Benson, A., Secker, I., Balfe, E., Lipsedge, M., Robinson, S., & Walker, J. (2003). Discourse of blame: Accounting for aggression and violence on an acute mental health inpatient unit. *Social Science and Medicine, 57,* 917–926.

Bigwood, S., & Crowe, M. (2008). "It's part of the job, but it spoils the job:" A phenomenological study of physical restraint. *International Journal of Mental Health Nursing, 17,* 215–222.

Bowers, L., James, K., Quirk, A., Wright, S., Williams, H., & Stewart, D. (2013). Identification of the "minimal triangle" and other common event-to-event transitions in conflict and containment incidents. *Issues in Mental Health Nursing, 34,* 514–523.

Bremner, R. H., Koole, S. L., & Bushman, B. J. (2011). "Pray for those who mistreat you": Effects of prayer on anger and aggression. *Personality and Social Psychology Bulletin, 37,* 830–837.

Bulechek, G., Butcher, H. K., Dochterman, J. M., & Wagner, C. (2012). *Nursing interventions classification (NIC)* (6th ed). St. Louis: Mosby.

Burns, J. W., Quartana, P., & Bruehl, S. (2011). Anger suppression and subsequent pain behaviors among chronic low back pain patients: Moderating effects of anger regulation style. *Annals of Behavioral Medicine, 42,* 42–54.

Carlsson, G., Dahlberg, K., Ekeburgh, M., & Dahlberg, H. (2006). Patients longing for authentic personal care: A phenomenological study of violent encounters in psychiatric settings. *Issues in Mental Health Nursing, 27,* 287–305.

Coccaro, E. F. (2012). Intermittent explosive disorder as a disorder of impulsive aggression for DSM-5. *American Journal of Psychiatry, 196,* 577–588.

Davidson, K., & Mostofsky, E. (2010). Anger expression and risk of coronary heart disease: Evidence from the Nova Scotia Health survey. *American Heart Journal, 159*(2), 199–206.

Deffenbacher, J. L. (2011). Cognitive-behavioral conceptualization and treatment of anger. *Cognitive and Behavioral Practice, 18,* 212–221.

deSchutter, M., & Lodewijkx, H. (2013). Psychiatric patients need a more active role in managing their own aggression. *Proceedings of the 8th European congress on violence in clinical psychiatry* (pp. 219–223). Amsterdam: Kavanah.

Duxbury, J., Aiken, F., & Dale, C. (2013). A review of theories of restraint-related deaths in the UK. *Proceedings of the 8th European congress on violence in clinical psychiatry* (pp. 46–50). Amsterdam: Kavanah.

Everson-Rose, S. A., & Lewis, T. T. (2005). Psychosocial factors and cardiovascular diseases. *Annual Review of Public Health, 26,* 469–500.

Farrell, G. A., Shafiei, T., & Salmon, P. (2010). Facing up to "challenging behavior": A model for training in staff-client interaction. *Journal of Advanced Nursing, 66*(7), 1644–1655.

Feindler, E. L. (2006). *Anger-related disorders: A practitioner's guide to comparative treatments.* New York: Springer.

Feindler, E. L., & Byers, A. (2006). Multiple perspectives on the conceptualization and treatment of anger-related disorders. In E. L. Feindler (Ed.), *Anger-related disorders: A practitioner's guide to comparative treatments* (pp. 303–320). New York: Springer.

Finfgeld-Connett, D. (2009). Model of therapeutic and non-therapeutic responses to patient aggression. *Issues in Mental Health Nursing, 30*(9), 530–537.

Fluttert, F., Van Meijel, B., Webster, C., Nijman, H., Bartels, A., & Grypdonck, M. (2008). Risk management by early recognition of warning signs in patients in forensic psychiatric care. *Archives of Psychiatric Nursing, 22,* 208–216.

Glenn, A. L., & Raine, A. (2008). The neurobiology of psychopathy. *Psychiatric Clinics of North America, 31*(3), 463–475.

Goldstein, N., Kemp, K., Leff, S., & Lochman, J. (2012). Guidelines for adapting manualized interventions for new target populations: A stepwise approach to using anger management as a model. *Clinical Psychology: Science, Practice, and Culture, 19,* 385–401.

Goldstein, N. E. S., Serico, J. M., Riggs Romaine, C. L., Zelechoski, A., Kalbeitzer, R., Kemp, K., et al. (2013). Development of the juvenile justice anger management treatment for girls. *Cognitive and Behavioral Practice, 20,* 171–188.

Gouin, J., Kiecolt-Glaser, J. K., Malarkey, W. B., & Glaser, R. (2008). The influence of anger expression on wound healing. *Brain, Behavior, and Immunity, 22,* 699–708.

Gross, R., Groer, M., & Thomas, S. P. (in press). Relationship of trait anger and anger expression to C-reactive protein in post-menopausal women. *Health Care for Women International.*

Hamrin, V., Iennaco, J., & Olsen, D. (2009). A review of ecological factors affecting inpatient psychiatric unit violence: Implications for relational and unit cultural improvements. *Issues in Mental Health Nursing, 30,* 214–226.

Harris, D., & Morrison, E. F. (1995). Managing violence without coercion. *Archives of Psychiatric Nursing, 9*(4), 203–210.

Hartley, D., & Ridenour, M. (2011). *Workplace violence in the healthcare setting.* National Institute for Occupational Safety and Health. Retrieved from www.medscape.com/viewarticle/749441

Hartman, B., & Blalock, A. (2011). Comparison of seclusion and restraint prevalence between hearing patients and deaf or hard of hearing patients in a state hospital setting. *Issues in Mental Health Nursing, 32,* 42–45.

Haun, P. (2013). It's time to report workplace violence. *Tennessee Nurse, 76*(4), 12.

International Society of Psychiatric-Mental Health Nurses. (1999). *Position statement on the use of restraint and seclusion.* Philadelphia: Author.

Jacobowitz, W. (2013). PTSD in psychiatric nurses and other mental health providers: A review of the literature. *Issues in Mental Health Nursing, 34,* 787–795.

Jarry, J., & Paivio, S. (2006). Emotion-focused therapy for anger. In E. L. Feindler (Ed.), *Anger-related disorders: A practitioner's guide to comparative treatments* (pp. 203–229). New York: Springer.

Janocha, J. A., & Smith, R. T. (2010). *Workplace safety and health in the health care and social assistance industry, 2003–07.* Washington, DC: U.S. Bureau of Labor Statistics. Retrieved March 25, 2011, from http://www.bls.gov.opub/cwc.sh20100825ar01pl.htm

Johnson, A. (2012). Forgiveness: Moving from anger and shame to self-love. *Psychiatric Services, 63,* 311–312.

Johnson, M. E. (2004). Violence on inpatient psychiatric units: State of the science. *Journal of the American Psychiatric Nurses Association, 10*(3), 113–121.

Johnson, M. E., & Delaney, K. R. (2006). Keeping the unit safe: A grounded theory study. *Journal of the American Psychiatric Nurses Association, 12*(1), 13–21.

Johnson, M. E., & Delaney, K. R. (2007). Keeping the unit safe: The anatomy of escalation. *Journal of the American Psychiatric Nurses Association, 13,* 42–52.

Kessler, R., Coccaro, E., Fava, M., Jaeger, S., Jin, R., & Walters, E. (2006). The prevalence and correlates of DSM-IV intermittent explosive disorder in the National Comorbidity Survey replication. *Archives of General Psychiatry, 63,* 669–678.

Ketterer, M., Rose, B., Knysz, W., Farha, A., Deveshwar, S., Schairer, J., et al. (2011). Is social isolation/alienation confounded with, and non-independent of emotional distress in its association with early onset of coronary artery disease? *Psychology, Health, & Medicine, 16*(2), 238–247.

Kuepper, Y., Alexander, N., Osinsky, R., Kozyra, E., Schmitz, A., Netter, P., et al. (2010). Aggression—interactions of serotonin and testosterone in healthy men and women. *Behavior Brain Research, 206*(1), 93–100.

Kusmierska, G. (2012). Do anger management treatments help angry adults? A meta-analytic answer. *Dissertation Abstracts International; Section B: The Sciences and Engineering, 72*(12B), 7689.

Laiho, T., Kattainen, E., Astedt-Kurki, P., Putkonen, H., Lindberg, N., & Kylma, J. (2013). Clinical decision-making involved in secluding and restraining an adult psychiatric patient: An integrative literature review. *Journal of Psychiatric and Mental Health Nursing, 20,* 830–839.

Lanza, M. L. (1992). Nurses as patient assault victims: An update, synthesis, and recommendations. *Archives of Psychiatric Nursing, 6*(3), 163–171.

Lanza, M. L., Demaio, J., & Benedict, M. A. (2005). Patient assault support group: Achieving educational objectives. *Issues in Mental Health Nursing, 26,* 643–660.

Lanza, M. L., Rierdan, J., Forester, L., & Zeiss, R. A. (2009). Reducing violence against nurses: The Violence Prevention Community Meeting. *Issues in Mental Health Nursing.*

Lanza, M. L., Zeiss, R. A., & Rierdan, J. (2009). Multiple perspectives on assault: The 360-degree interview. *Journal of the American Psychiatric Nurses Association, 14*(6), 413–420.

Larue, C., Dumais, A., Boyer, R., Goulet, M-H., Bonin, J-P., & Baba, N. (2013). The experience of seclusion and restraint in psychiatric settings: Perspectives of patients. *Issues in Mental Health Nursing, 34,* 317–324.

Lemay, E. P., Overall, N. C., & Clark, M. S. (2012). Experiences and interpersonal consequences of hurt feelings and anger. *Journal of Personality and Social Psychology, 103,* 982–1006.

Liu, J. (2011). Early health risk factors for violence: Conceptualization, review of the evidence and implications. *Aggression & Violent Behaviors, 16*(1), 63–73.

Luck, L., Jackson, D., & Usher, K. (2007). STAMP: Components of observable behavior that indicate potential for patient violence in emergency departments. *Journal of Advanced Nursing, 59,* 11–19.

Martin, C. A., Cook, C., Woodring, J. H., Burkhardt, G., Omar, H. A., & Kelly, T. H. (2008). Caffeine use: Association with nicotine use, aggression, and other psychopathology in psychiatric and pediatric outpatient adolescents. *The Scientific World Journal, 8,* 512–516.

McCloskey, M. S., Noblett, K. L., Deffenbacher, J. L., Gollan, J. K., & Coccaro, E. F. (2008). Cognitive-behavioral therapy for intermittent explosive disorder: A pilot randomized trial. *Journal of Consulting and Clinical Psychology, 76,* 876–886.

Mefford, L., Thomas, S. P., Callen, B., & Groer, M. (in press). Religiousness-spirituality and anger management in community-dwelling older persons. *Issues in Mental Health Nursing.*

Mostofsky, E., Maclure, M., Tofler, G., Muller, J., & Mittleman, M. (2013). Relation of outbursts of anger and risk of acute myocardial infarction. *American Journal of Cardiology.* Retrieved from www.ajconline.org

Moylan, L. B. (2009). Physical restraint in acute care psychiatry: A humanistic and realistic nursing approach. *Journal of Psychosocial Nursing, 47*(3), 41–47.

NANDA International. (2012). *Nursing diagnoses: Definitions and classification 2012–2014.* Chichester, UK: Wiley Blackwell.

Palazzolo, K. E., Roberto, A. J., & Babin, E. A. (2010). The relationship between parents' verbal aggression and young adult children's intimate partner violence victimization and perpetration. *Health Communication, 25*(4), 357–364.

Peek-Asa, C., Casteel, C., Allareddy, V., Nocera, M., Goldmacher, S., Ohagan, E., et al. (2009). Workplace prevention programs in psychiatric units and facilities. *Archives of Psychiatric Nursing, 23,* 166–176.

Perugi, G., Fornaro, M., & Akiskal, H. S. (2011). Are atypical depression, borderline personality disorder and bipolar II disorder overlapping manifestations of a common cyclothymic diathesis? *World Psychiatry, 10*(1), 45–51.

Pittman, C. T. (2011). Getting mad but ending up sad: The mental health consequences for African Americans using anger to cope with racism. *Journal of Black Studies, 42,* 1106–1124.

Potpara, T. S., & Lip, G.Y. (2011). Lone atrial fibrillation: What is known and what is to come. *International Journal Clinical Practice, 65*(4), 446–457.

Poster, L., & Drew, B. (2006). Presidents' message. *American Psychiatric Nurses Association News, 18*(4), 2–3.

Puskar, K. R., Stark, K. H., Northcut, T., Williams, R., & Haley, T. (2011). Teaching kids to cope with anger: Peer education. *Journal of Child Health Care, 15*(1):5–13.

Rubin, T. I. (1970). *The angry book.* New York: Collier.

Siever, L. J. (2008). Neurobiology of aggression and violence. *American Journal of Psychiatry, 165*(4), 429–442.

Sivak, K. (2012). Implementation of comfort rooms to reduce seclusion, restraint use, and acting-out behaviors. *Journal of Psychiatric Nursing and Mental Health Services, 50*(2), 24–34.

Smith, G., Davis, R., Altenor, A., Tran, D. P., Wolfe, K. L., Deegan, J. A., et al. (2013). Psychiatric use of unscheduled medications in the Pennsylvania State Hospital System: Effects of discontinuing the use of PRN orders. *Proceedings of the 8th European congress on violence in clinical psychiatry* (pp. 137). Amsterdam: Kavanah.

Spielberger, C. D. (1999). *Manual for the State Trait Anger Expression Inventory-2.* Odessa, FL: Psychological Assessment Resources.

Thomas, S. A., & González-Prendes, A. A. (2009). Powerlessness, anger, and stress in African American women: Implications for physical and emotional health. *Health Care for Women International, 30*(1–2), 93–113.

Thomas, S. P. (1990). Theoretical and empirical perspectives on anger. *Issues in Mental Health Nursing, 11,* 203–216.

Thomas, S. P. (1997a). Women's anger: Relationship of suppression to blood pressure. *Nursing Research, 46,* 324–330.

Thomas, S. P. (1997b). Angry? Let's talk about it! *Applied Nursing Research, 10*(2), 80–85.

Thomas, S. P. (1998). Assessing and intervening with anger disorders. *Nursing Clinics of North America, 33*(1), 121–133.

Thomas, S. P. (2001). Teaching healthy anger management. *Perspectives in Psychiatric Care, 37*(2), 41–48.

Thomas, S. P. (2005). Women's anger, aggression, and violence. *Health Care for Women International, 26,* 504–522.

Thomas, S. P. (2006). Cultural and gender considerations in the assessment and treatment of anger-related disorders. In E. L. Feindler (Ed.), *Anger-related disorders: A practitioner's guide to comparative treatments* (pp. 71–95). New York: Springer.

Thomas, S. P. (2009). *Transforming nurses' stress and anger* (3rd ed) New York: Springer.

Thomas, S. P., & Pollio, H. R. (2002). *Listening to patients.* New York: Springer.

Thomas, S. P., Shattell, M., & Martin, T. (2002). What's therapeutic about the therapeutic milieu? *Archives of Psychiatric Nursing, 16*(3), 99–107.

Williams, K. M., & Herman, R. E. (2011). Linking resident behavior to dementia care communication: Effects of emotional tone. *Behavior Therapy, 42*(1), 42–46.

World Health Organization. (2009). *Preventing violence: The evidence.* Geneva, Switzerland: Author.

Zuzelo, P., Curran, S., & Zeserman, M. (2012). Registered nurses' and behavior health associates' responses to violent inpatient interactions on behavioral health units. *Journal of the American Psychiatric Nurses Association, 18*(2), 112–126.

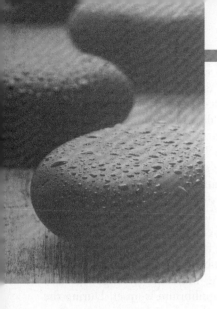

14
Crisis, Grief, and Disaster Management

Mary Ann Boyd

KEY CONCEPTS

- bereavement
- crisis
- grief
- disaster

LEARNING OBJECTIVES

After studying this chapter, you will be able to:

1. Describe the types of crises.

2. Differentiate between grief and bereavement.

3. Compare models of bereavement.

4. Discuss nursing management for persons experiencing crises, grief, and disasters.

5. Evaluate the effects of the crisis or disaster experience on lifestyle and survival.

6. Explain the psychological impact of disaster on victims of catastrophic events.

KEY TERMS

- ABCs of psychological first aid • complicated grief • debriefing • developmental crisis • dual process model
- loss-oriented coping • oscillation • restoration-oriented coping • situational crisis • traumatic crisis • traumatic grief
- uncomplicated grief

Successfully surviving crises and disasters may make a difference between being mentally healthy or mentally ill. This chapter explores the concepts of crisis, grief, and disaster management; broadens the scope and understanding of the responses of persons to crisis, loss, and disaster situations; and describes how the nursing process can be used to care for persons experiencing these events.

CRISIS

Adaptation and coping are a natural part of life. Crisis occurs when there is a perceived challenge or threat that overwhelms the capacity of the individual to cope effectively with the event. Life is disrupted, and unexpected emotional (e.g., depression) and biologic (e.g., nausea, vomiting, diarrhea, headaches) responses occur. Functioning is severely impaired.

> **KEYCONCEPT** **Crisis** is a time-limited event that triggers adaptive or non-adaptive responses to maturational, situational, or traumatic experiences. A crisis results from stressful events for which coping mechanisms fail to provide adequate adaptive skills to address the perceived challenge or threat.

A crisis occurs when an individual is at a breaking point. A crisis is a turning point with either positive or negative outcomes. If positive, there is an opportunity for growth and change as new ways of coping are learned. If negative, suicide, homelessness, or depression can result. A crisis generally lasts no more than

4 to 6 weeks. At the end of that time, the person in crisis should have begun to come to grips with the event and begin to harness resources to cope with its long-term consequences. By definition, there is no such thing as a chronic crisis. People who live in constant turmoil are not in crisis but in chaos.

Many events evoke a crisis, such as natural disasters (e.g., floods, tornadoes, earthquakes) and human-made disasters (e.g., wars, bombings, airplane crashes) as well as traumatic experiences (e.g., rape, sexual abuse, assault). In addition, interpersonal events (divorce, marriage, birth of a child) create crises in the lives of any person.

Feelings of fear, desperation, and being out of control are common during a crisis, but the precipitating event and circumstances are unusual or rare, perceived as a threat, and specific to the individual. For example, a disagreement with a family member may escalate into a crisis for one person, but not another (Lyons, Hopley, Burton, & Horrocks, 2009). If the person is significantly distressed or social functioning is impaired, a diagnosis of acute stress disorder should be considered (American Psychiatric Association [APA], 2013). The person with an acute stress disorder has dissociative symptoms and persistently reexperiences the event (APA; see Chapter 20).

Historical Perspectives of Crisis

The basis of our understanding of a crisis began in the 1940s when Eric Lindemann (1944) studied bereavement reactions among the friends and relatives of the victims of the Cocoanut [sic] Grove nightclub fire in Boston in 1942. That fire, in which 493 people died, was the worst single building fire in the country's history at that time.

Lindemann's goal was to develop prevention approaches at the community level that would maintain good health and prevent emotional disorganization. He described both grief and prolonged reactions as a result of loss of a significant person. He hypothesized that during the course of one's life, some situations, such as the birth of a child, marriage, and death, evoke adaptive mechanisms that lead either to mastery of a new situation (psychological growth) or impaired functioning.

In 1961, psychiatrist Gerald Caplan defined a crisis as occurring when a person faces a problem that cannot be solved by customary problem-solving methods. When the usual problem-solving methods no longer work, a person's life balance or equilibrium is upset. During the period of disequilibrium, there is a rise in inner tension and anxiety followed by emotional upset and an inability to function. This conceptualization of phases of a crisis is used today (Figure 14.1). According to Caplan, during a crisis, a person is open to learning new ways of coping to survive. The outcome of a crisis is governed by the kind of interaction that occurs between the person and available key social support systems.

Types of Crises

Research has focused on categorizing types of crisis events, understanding biopsychosocial responses to a crisis, and developing intervention models that support people through a crisis.

Developmental Crisis

While Lindemann and Caplan were creating their crisis model, Erik Erikson was formulating his ideas about crisis and development. He proposed that maturational

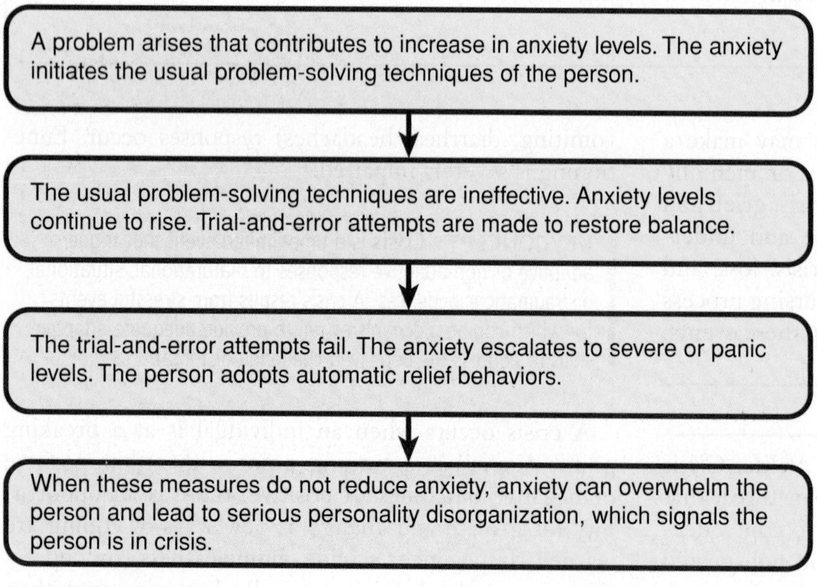

A problem arises that contributes to increase in anxiety levels. The anxiety initiates the usual problem-solving techniques of the person.

↓

The usual problem-solving techniques are ineffective. Anxiety levels continue to rise. Trial-and-error attempts are made to restore balance.

↓

The trial-and-error attempts fail. The anxiety escalates to severe or panic levels. The person adopts automatic relief behaviors.

↓

When these measures do not reduce anxiety, anxiety can overwhelm the person and lead to serious personality disorganization, which signals the person is in crisis.

FIGURE 14.1 Phases of crisis.

crises are a normal part of growth and development and that successfully resolving a crisis at one stage allows the child to move to the next. According to this model, the child develops positive characteristics after experiencing a crisis. If he or she develops less desirable traits, the crisis is not resolved (see Chapter 5). The concept of **developmental crisis** continues to be used today to describe significant maturational events, such as leaving home for the first time, completing school, and accepting the responsibility of adulthood.

Situational Crisis

A **situational crisis** occurs whenever a specific stressful event threatens a person's biopsychosocial integrity and results in some degree of psychological disequilibrium. The event can be an internal one, such as a disease process, or any number of external threats. A move to another city, a job promotion, or graduation from high school can initiate a crisis even though they are positive events. Graduation from high school marks the end of an established routine of going to school, participating in school activities, and doing homework assignments. When starting a new job after graduation, the former student must learn an entirely different routine and acquire new knowledge and skills. If a person enters a new situation without adequate coping skills, a crisis may occur.

Traumatic Crisis

A **traumatic crisis** is initiated by unexpected, unusual events that can affect an individual or a multitude of people. In such situations, people face overwhelmingly hazardous events that entail injury, trauma, destruction, or sacrifice. Examples of events include national disasters (e.g., racial persecutions, riots, war), violent crimes (e.g., rape, murder, kidnappings, and assault and battery), and environmental disasters (e.g., earthquakes, floods, forest fires, hurricanes).

Grief and Bereavement

One of the most common crisis-provoking events is the death of a loved one. Although death is a certainty, much is unknown about the process of death. Fear of the unknown contributes to the mystique of death for the person who is dying, as well as the loved ones. The terms *grief* and *bereavement* are sometimes used interchangeably, but in this text, they are differentiated with grief being an intense biopsychosocial reaction and bereavement being the actual process of mourning and coping. Normally, the death of a loved one produces feelings of grief. Any subsequent loss can also reactivate these feelings.

> **KEYCONCEPT** **Grief** is an intense, emotional reaction to the loss of a loved one. The reaction is a biopsychosocial response that often includes spontaneous expression of pain, sadness, and desolation. **Bereavement** is the process of mourning and coping with the loss of a loved one. It begins immediately after the loss, but it can last months or years. Individual differences and cultural practices influence grieving and bereavement.

Coping with Loss

Stage Theories

There has been wide acceptance that grief and bereavement follow stages (Bowlby & Parkes, 1970; Kubler-Ross, 1969). See Box 14.1. Although over time, the stage theory of grief and bereavement has been challenged and remains unsupported by empirical evidence today, it continues to be used by health care professionals.

Dual Process Model

The **dual process model** (DPM) offers another explanation of how grieving persons come to terms with their loss over time (Stroebe, Schut, & Boerner, 2010). According to DPM, the person adjusts to the loss by oscillating between **loss-oriented coping** (preoccupation with the deceased) and **restoration-oriented coping** (preoccupation with stressful events as a result of the death including financial issues, new identity as a widow[er]). **Oscillation** is the process of confronting (loss-oriented coping) and avoiding (restoration-oriented coping) the stresses associated with bereavement. At times, the bereaved person is confronted with the loss and memories, and at other times, the persons will be distracted and the thoughts and memories will be avoided. The bereaved experiences relief from the intense emotion associated with the loss by focusing on other things. For example, the bereaved person may be recalling a special moment in the relationship such as a wedding or imagining what the person would say about a current event but then switches to thinking about completing tasks that the deceased had

---

BOX 14.1

Stages of Grief and Bereavement

1. *Shock:* denial and disbelief
2. *Acute mourning*
   a. Intense feeling states
   b. Social withdrawal
   c. Identification with the deceased
3. *Resolution:* acceptance of loss, awareness of having grieved, return to well-being, and ability to recall the deceased without subjective pain

Adapted from Zisook, S. (1987). Unresolved grief. In S. Zisook (Ed.), *Biopsychosocial aspects of bereavement* (p. 25). Washington, DC: American Psychiatric Press.

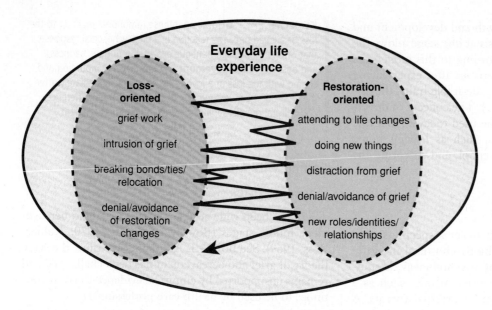

FIGURE 14.2 Dual process model of coping with bereavement. (Redrawn from Stroebe, M., & Schut, H. [1999]. The dual process model of coping with bereavement: Rationale and description. *Death Studies*, 23, 213. Used with permission from Taylor & Francis Group.)

previously undertaken (e.g., paying bills, cooking meals). In the loss-oriented coping mode, emotions relate to the relationship with the deceased person; in the restoration-oriented coping, the bereaved person's emotions relate to the stressful events associated with the responsibilities and changes as a result of the loss. Over time, after repeated confrontation with the loss, there is no longer a need to think about certain aspects of the loss (Caserta, Utz, Lund, Swenson, & de Vries, 2014). See Figure 14.2.

Types of Grief

Uncomplicated Grief

Most bereaved people experience normal or **uncomplicated grief** after the loss of a loved one. Uncomplicated grief is painful and disruptive. At the time of the loss, the grieving person may have a physical response such as tightening in the throat, choking, shortness of breath, a need to sigh, an empty feeling in the abdomen, and a lack of muscular power. A sense of unreality sets in, and there is increased emotional distance from others and an intense preoccupation with the image of the deceased person. Exaggerated feelings of guilt for minor negligence are common. Mourning rites and support from family and friends are helpful.

The most frequent initial reaction in grieving is yearning although disbelief and depression also occur during the first 2 years. Gradually, yearning, disbelief, and depression decline. Within the first 6 months after the loss, there may be signs of limited impairment during adaptation to new situations.

The bereavement process is often applied to other situations in which a loss occurs, not necessarily the death of a person, but has many of the same responses. The "empty nest syndrome" is an example of bereavement for children who have grown up and left home. This bereavement experience is less intense than that triggered by a loss through death, but the bereaved person has many of the same responses.

Most bereaved persons do not need clinical interventions and are able to find meaning and purpose in their lives. Their self-esteem and sense of competency remain intact. They gradually accept the sense of loss as a reality and are able to move on with their lives. There is little evidence that they need or benefit from counseling or therapy. Those who experience suicidal thoughts and gestures should be evaluated for depression and posttraumatic stress disorder (PTSD) (Bennett & Soulsby, 2012; Stroebe, Schut, & Stroebe, 2007; Zhang, El-Jawahri, & Prigerson, 2006).

Traumatic Grief

Traumatic grief is a term that is used for a more difficult and prolonged grief. In traumatic grieving, external factors influence the reactions and potential long-term outcomes. For example, memories of the traumatic death of the deceased may lead to more traumatic memories including the violent death scene (Mutabaruka, Séjourné, Bui, Birmes, & Chabro, 2012). The external circumstances of death associated with traumatic grief include (1) suddenness and lack of anticipation; (2) violence, mutilation and destruction; (3) degree of preventability or randomness of the death; (4) multiple deaths (bereavement overload); and (5) mourner's personal encounter with death involving a significant threat to personal survival or a massive and shocking confrontation with the deaths (or mutilation) of others (Bolton, Michalopoulos, Ahmed, Murray, & Bass, 2013; Reynolds, Stack, & Houle, 2011).

Bereavement of family members for those who committed suicide seems to differ from other sudden deaths. Common experiences during this bereavement process include stigmatization, shame and guilt, and a sense of rejection. The bereaved person may experience self-blame for contributing to the family member's death. Factors that influence bereavement after suicide include age of the deceased, quality of the relationship, the attitude of the bereaved to the loss, and cultural beliefs. These individuals benefit from psychological interventions (McKay & Tighe, 2013).

There is evidence that men experience grief differently than women, who are more likely to confront and express negative emotion (Pilling, Thege, Demetrovics, & Kopp, 2012; Stroebe, Stroebe, & Schut, 2006). Suicide bereavement may be different because of the survivor's questions regarding the family member's suicide and the impact of the suicide on the family (Barlow, Schiff, Chugh, Rawlinson, Hides, Leith, et al., 2010) (see Chapter 15). More research is needed in this area.

Complicated Grief

Complicated grief occurs in about 10% to 20% of bereaved persons (Fujisawa, Miyashita, Nakajima, Ito, Kato, & Kim, 2010). The person is frozen or stuck in a state of chronic mourning. The person feels bitter over the loss and wishes that his or her life could revert to the time they were together. In complicated grief there is an intense longing and yearning for the person who died that lasts for more than 6 months. Additionally, the person may have trouble accepting the death, an inability to trust others since the death, excessive bitterness related to the death, and feeling that life is meaningless without the deceased person (Claxton & Reynolds, 2012).

Nursing Care of Person in Crisis

The goal for people experiencing a crisis is to return to the pre-crisis level of functioning. The role of the nurse is to provide a framework of support systems that guide the patient through the crisis and facilitate the development and use of positive coping skills.

EMERGENCY CARE ALERT ! It is important to be acutely aware that a person in crisis may be at high risk for suicide or homicide. To determine the level of effectiveness of coping capabilities of the person, the nurse should complete a careful assessment for suicidal or homicidal risk. If a person is at high risk for either, the nurse should consider referral for admission to the hospital.

When assessing the coping ability of the client, the nurse should assess for unusual behaviors and determine the level of involvement of the person with the crisis. In addition, assess for evidence of self-mutilation activities that may indicate the use of self-preservation measures to avoid suicide. It is critical to assess the client's perception of the problem and the availability of support mechanisms (emotional and financial) for use by the person (Drenth, Herbst, & Strydom, 2010).

NCLEXNOTE During a crisis, the behaviors and verbalizations of a person may provide data that are indicative of a mental illness. Nursing care should be prioritized according to the severity of responses. After the crisis has been resolved, assess whether the abnormal thoughts or feelings disappear.

During an environmental crisis (e.g., flood, hurricane, forest fire) that affects the well-being of many people, nursing interventions will be a part of the community's efforts to respond to the event. This is covered in more detail in the section of the chapter on disasters. On the other hand, when a personal crisis occurs, the person in crisis may have only the nurse to respond to his or her needs. After the assessment, the nurse must decide whether to provide the care needed or to refer the person to a mental health specialist. Box 14.2 offers guidance in making this decision.

Biologic Domain

Assessment

Biologic assessment focuses on areas that usually undergo initial changes. Eliciting information about changes in health practices provides important data that can be used to determine the severity of the disruption in functioning.

BOX 14.2

Decision Tree for Determining Referral

Situation: A 35-year-old woman is being seen in a clinic because of minor burns she received during a house fire. Her home was completely destroyed. She is tearful and withdrawn, and she complains of a great deal of pain from her minor burns. Biopsychosocial assessment is completed.

ASSESSMENT RESULT	NURSING ACTION
Patient has psychological distress but believes that her social support is adequate. She would like to talk to a nurse when she returns for her follow-up visit.	Provide counseling and support for the patient during her visit. Make an appointment for her return visit to the clinic for follow-up.
The patient is severely distressed. She has no social support. She does not know how she will survive.	Refer the patient to a mental health specialist. The patient will need crisis intervention strategies provided by a mental health specialist.

Biologic functioning is important because a crisis can be physically exhausting. Disturbances in sleep and eating patterns and the reappearance of physical or psychiatric symptoms are common. Changes in body function may include tachycardia, tachypnea, profuse perspiration, nausea, vomiting, dilated pupils, and extreme shakiness. Some individuals may exhibit loss of control and have total disregard for their personal safety. These people are at high risk for injury, which may include infection, trauma, and head injuries (Betancourt et al., 2012). If sleep patterns are disturbed or nutrition is inadequate, the individual may not have the physical resources to deal with the crisis.

Nursing Diagnoses for the Biologic Domain

Biologic responses can be very severe during crises. All body systems can be affected. Possible Nursing Diagnoses may include Risk for Body Temperature Imbalance, Diarrhea, Impaired Urinary Elimination, and Stress Urinary Incontinence. In addition, the person may report a variety of somatic complaints. Implement appropriate nursing interventions to address the nursing diagnoses of assessed needs of the individual and make appropriate referrals.

Interventions for the Biologic Domain

Any negative physiological responses should be treated immediately. Be careful not to give unrealistic or false reassurances of positive outcomes over which you have no control. Other interventions focusing on the biologic domain will be those implemented for nursing diagnoses developed from assessment findings. Make referrals as appropriate (Davidhizar & Shearer, 2005). Pharmacological interventions may be needed to help maintain a high level of psychophysical functioning.

> **NCLEXNOTE** Individual responses to a crisis can be best understood by assessing the usual responses of the person to stressful events. The response to the crisis will also depend on the meaning of the event to the person. The use of therapeutic communication principles is a priority when caring for a person who has experienced a crisis or disaster.

Medication cannot resolve a crisis, but the judicious use of psychopharmacological agents can help reduce its emotional intensity. For example, Mrs. Brown has just learned that both of her parents have perished in an airplane crash. When she arrives at the emergency department to identify their bodies, she is shaking, sobbing, and unable to answer questions. The emergency physician orders lorazepam (Ativan) (Box 14.3). The phases of treatment include initiation of treatment, assessment of stabilization from the treatment, and timeframe for maintenance of treatment.

BOX 14.3
Drug Profile: Lorazepam (Ativan)

DRUG CLASS: Benzodiazepine; antianxiety/sedative hypnotic agent

RECEPTOR AFFINITY: Acts mainly at the subcortical levels of the central nervous system (CNS), leaving the cortex relatively unaffected. Main sites of action may be the limbic system and reticular formation. It potentiates the effects of α-aminobutyric acid, an inhibitory neurotransmitter. The exact mechanism of action is unknown.

INDICATIONS: Management of anxiety disorders or for short-term relief of symptoms of anxiety or anxiety associated with depression (oral forms). Also used as preanesthetic medication in adults to produce sedation, relieve anxiety, and decrease recall of events related to surgery (parenteral form). Unlabeled parenteral uses for management of acute alcohol withdrawal.

ROUTE AND DOSAGE: Available in 0.5-, 1-, and 2-mg tablets; 2 mg/mL concentrated oral solution and 2 mg/mL and 4 mg/mL solutions for injection.

Adults: Usually 2–6 mg/d orally, with a range of 1–10 mg/d in divided doses, with the largest dose given at night. 0.05 mg/kg intramuscularly (IM) up to a maximum of 4 mg administered at least 2 h before surgery. Initially 2 mg total or 0.044 mg/kg intravenously (IV) (whichever is smaller). Doses as high as 0.05 mg/kg up to a total of 4 mg may be given 15–20 min before the procedure to those benefiting by a greater lack of recall.

Geriatric patients: Dosage not to exceed adult IV dose. Orally, 1–2 mg/d in divided doses initially, adjusted as needed and tolerated.

Children: Drug should not be used in children younger than 12 years.

HALF-LIFE (PEAK EFFECT): 10–20 h (1–6 h [oral]; 60–90 min IM; 10–15 min IV).

SELECTED ADVERSE REACTIONS: Transient mild drowsiness, sedation, depression, lethargy, apathy, fatigue, light-headedness, disorientation, anger, hostility, restlessness, confusion, crying, headache, mild paradoxical excitatory reactions during first 2 weeks of treatment, constipation, dry mouth, diarrhea, nausea, bradycardia, hypotension, cardiovascular collapse, urinary retention, and drug dependence with withdrawal symptoms.

WARNINGS: Contraindicated in psychoses; acute narrow angle glaucoma; shock; acute alcoholic intoxication with depression of vital signs; and during pregnancy, labor and delivery, and while breastfeeding. Use cautiously in patients with impaired liver or kidney function and those who are debilitated. When given with theophylline, there is a decreased effect of lorazepam. When using the drug IV, it must be diluted immediately before use and administered by direct injection slowly or infused at a maximum rate of 2 mg/min. When giving narcotic analgesics, reduce its dose by at least half in patients who have received lorazepam.

SPECIFIC PATIENT AND FAMILY EDUCATION
- Take the drug exactly as prescribed; do not stop taking the drug abruptly.
- Avoid alcohol and other CNS depressants.
- Avoid driving and other activities that require alertness.
- Notify the prescriber before taking any other prescription or over-the-counter drug.
- Change your position slowly and sit at the edge of the bed for a few minutes before arising.
- Report to the prescriber any severe dizziness, weakness, drowsiness that persists, rash or skin lesions, palpitations, edema of the extremities, visual changes, or difficulty urinating.

1. **Initiation:** Because Mrs. Brown is overcome by grief and severe anxiety about seeing her parents' bodies, 2 mg of lorazepam is administered intramuscularly as ordered by the doctor. The nurse monitors the patient for onset of action and any side effects. If Mrs. Brown does not have some relief within 20 to 30 minutes, another injection can be given as ordered by the doctor.

2. **Stabilization:** During the next half hour, Mrs. Brown regains some of her composure. She is no longer shaking, and her crying is occasional. She is reluctant to identify her parents but can do so when accompanied by the nurse. After the paperwork is completed, Mrs. Brown is sent home with a prescription for lorazepam, 2 to 4 mg every 12 hours.

3. **Maintenance:** Mrs. Brown takes the medication during the next week as she plans and attends her parents' funeral and manages the affairs surrounding their deaths. The medication keeps her anxiety at a manageable level, enabling her to do the tasks required of her.

4. **Medication cessation:** Two weeks after the death of her parents, Mrs. Brown is no longer taking lorazepam. She is grieving normally and has periods of teariness and sadness about her loss, but she can cope. She visits with friends, reminisces with family members, and reads inspirational poems. All of these activities help her navigate the changes in her life brought about by her parents' sudden death.

This example demonstrates how a medication can be used to assist a person through a crisis. After that crisis has passed, the person can use his or her personal coping mechanisms to adapt.

Psychological Domain

Assessment

Psychological assessment focuses on the individual's emotions and coping strengths. In the beginning of the crisis, the person may report the feeling of numbness and shock. Responses to psychological distress should be differentiated from symptoms of psychiatric illnesses that may be present. Later, as the reality of the crisis sinks in, the person will be able to recognize and describe the felt emotions. The nurse should expect these emotions to be intense and be sure to provide some support during their expression. At the beginning of a crisis, assess the individual for behaviors that indicate a depressed state, the presence of confusion, uncontrolled weeping or screaming, disorientation, or aggression. The person may be suffering from a loss of feelings of well-being and safety. In addition, panic responses, anxiety, and fear may be present (Fischer, Postmes, Koeppl, Conway, & Fredriksson, 2011). The ability to cope by problem solving may be disrupted. By assessing the person's ability to solve problems, the nurse can evaluate whether he or she can cognitively cope with the crisis situation and determine the kind and amount of support needed.

Nursing Diagnoses for the Psychological Domain

Many nursing diagnoses generated from assessment of the psychological domain may be appropriate for the person experiencing the crisis. The nursing diagnoses may include Grieving, Post-Trauma Syndrome, Confusion, Ineffective Coping, Risk for Violence (self-directed or directed toward others), Impaired Communication, Interrupted Family Processes, Anxiety, Powerlessness, and many other diagnoses. The nurse should make sure that the diagnoses are based on the person's appraisal of the situation. In addition, any diagnosis should be determined from the assessment data that have been clustered and prioritized to address identified needs.

Interventions for the Psychological Domain

Safety interventions to protect the person in crisis from harm should include preventing the person from committing suicide or homicide, arranging for food and shelter (if needed), and mobilizing social support. After the person's safety needs have been met, the psychosocial aspects of the crisis can be addressed and the individual can be prepared for recovery. Guidelines for crisis intervention and examples are presented in Table 14.1. Individuals should be encouraged to report any depression, anxiety, or interpersonal difficulties during the recovery period.

Counseling reinforces healthy coping behaviors and interaction patterns. Counseling, which focuses on identifying emotions and positive coping strategies for the corresponding nursing diagnosis, helps the person to integrate the effects of the crisis into a real life experience. Responses to crisis differ with individuals. Some may present with behaviors that indicate transient disruptions in their ability to cope. Others may be totally devastated. At times, telephone counseling may provide the person with enough help that face-to-face counseling is not necessary. If counseling strategies do not work, other stress reduction and coping enhancement interventions can be used (see Chapter 12). The nurse should refer anyone who cannot cope with a crisis to a mental health specialist for an evaluation.

Social Domain

Assessment

Assessment of the impact of the crisis on an individual's social functioning is essential because a crisis usually severely disrupts social proficiencies. The nurse should

TABLE 14.1	GUIDELINES FOR CRISIS INTERVENTION	
Approach	**Rationale**	**Example**
Support the expression (or non-expression) of feelings according to cultural or ethnic practices.	Emotional support helps the person face reality. The emotional expression by the victim may be culturally driven.	Accompany the husband to view the body of his deceased wife.
Help the person think clearly and focus on one implication at a time.	Focusing on all the implications at once can be too overwhelming.	A woman left her husband because of abuse. At first, focus only on her living arrangements and safety. At another time, discuss the other implications of the separation.
Avoid giving false reassurances, such as "It will be all right."	Giving false reassurances blocks communication. It may not be all right.	Patient: "My doctor told me that I have a terminal illness." Nurse: "What does that mean to you?"
Clarify fantasies with facts.	Accurate information is needed to problem solve.	A young mother believes that her comatose child will regain consciousness although the medical evidence contradicts it. Gently clarify the meaning of the medical evidence.
Link the person and family with community resources, as needed.	Strengthening the person's social network so social support can be obtained reduces the effect of the crisis.	Provide information about a meeting of a support group such as that of the American Cancer Society.

Adapted from Lazarus, R. (1991). *Emotion and adaptation* (p. 122). New York: Oxford University Press.

assess the severity of the crisis to determine the capability of the individual or the community to respond in a supportive way.

Nursing Diagnoses for the Social Domain

Nursing diagnoses associated with the social domain include Impaired Adjustment, Impaired Social Interaction, and Impaired Interrupted Family Processes. Other diagnoses may be Ineffective Role Performance and Relocation Stress Syndrome. Any nursing diagnosis generated will depend on the assessment findings related to the needs of the patient.

Interventions for the Social Domain

The nursing interventions for the social domain can focus on the individual, the family, and the community. A crisis often disrupts a person's social network, leading to changes in available social support. Development of a new social support network may help the person cope more effectively with the crisis. Supporting the development of new support contacts within the context of available social networks can be done by contacting available local and state agencies for assistance as well as specific private support groups and religious groups.

Telephone Hotlines

Public and private funding and the efforts of trained volunteers permit most communities to provide crisis services to the public. For example, telephone hotlines for problems ranging from child abuse to suicide are a part of health delivery systems of most communities. Crisis services permit immediate access to the mental health system for people who are experiencing an emergency (such as threatened suicide) or for those who need help with stress or a crisis.

Residential Crisis Services

Many communities provide, as part of the health care network, residential crisis services for people who need short-term housing. The specific residential crisis services available within a community reflect the problems that the community members judge as particularly important. For example, some communities provide shelter for teenage runaways; others offer shelter for abused spouses. Still others provide shelter for people who would otherwise require acute psychiatric hospitalization. These settings provide residents with a place to stay in a supportive, homelike atmosphere. The people who use these services are linked to other community services such as financial aid.

Evaluation and Treatment Outcomes

Outcomes developed in cooperation with the person experiencing the crisis guide the evaluation. Once assessment data are clustered and prioritized the nursing diagnosis and the outcomes are determined. Once interventions are developed and implemented in cooperation with the individual in crisis, the person should come through the crisis with improved health, well-being, and social function. If complications occur, the nurse should make appropriate alterations in the entire nursing process or make appropriate referrals.

DISASTER AND TERRORISM

A disaster is a sudden ecological or human-made phenomenon that is of sufficient magnitude to require external help to address the psychosocial needs as well as the physical needs of the victims. Acts of terrorism present situations that mimic disasters and can be categorized as a type of disaster.

> **KEYCONCEPT**   A **disaster** is a sudden overwhelming catastrophic event that causes great damage and destruction that may involve mass casualties and human suffering requiring assistance from all available resources.

Although crises and disasters are usually viewed as negative experiences, the outcomes can be positive. Some survivors of disasters draw on resources that they never realized they had and grow from those experiences (Osofsky & Osofsky, 2013). However, the survivors of disasters may have severe psychological problems. Fear, anger, and distress elevate severe anxiety to the panic level, which can result in a severe mental illnesses. Unresolved crisis or disastrous events can lead to disorganized thinking and responses that are inappropriate and traumatic for the person experiencing the situation (Wisnivesky et al., 2011). In addition, the victims may experience the development of acute stress disorder (that has a strong emphasis on dissociative symptoms) and PTSD.

Historical Perspectives of Disasters in the United States

Throughout history, disasters have been portrayed from a fatalistic perspective that humans have little control over catastrophic events. Some cultures contend that natural disasters are acts of God. Other cultures express their belief that natural disaster events can be attributed to gods dwelling within such places as volcanoes, with eruptions being an expression of the gods' anger (van Griensven et al., 2006). Although often caused by nature, disasters can have human origins. Wars and civil disturbances that destroy homelands and displace people are included among the causes of disasters. Other causes include a building collapse, blizzard, drought, earthquake, epidemic, explosion, famine, fire, flood, hazardous material or transportation incident (such as a chemical spill), hurricane, nuclear incident, terrorist attack, and tornado. Often, the unpredictability of such disasters causes fear, confusion, and stress that can have lasting effects on the health of affected communities and their sense of well-being (Wisnivesky et al., 2011).

In recent history, we have experienced several attacks of violence and terrorism that are unprecedented in North America. The destruction of the World Trade Center in New York and the attack on the Pentagon in Washington, DC, on September 11, 2001, the dispersal of anthrax spores in the United States mail, the Sandy Hook school tragedy, and the Boston bombing shattered North Americans' sense of safety and security.

Since September 11, 2001, the emergency response planning of federal, state, and local agencies has focused on possible terrorist attacks with chemical, biologic, radiologic, nuclear, or high-yield explosive weapons. Before September 11, 2001, government agencies and public health leaders had not incorporated mental health into their overall response plans to bioterrorism. But in the aftermath of the mass destruction of human life and property in 2001, government and health care leaders are recognizing the need for monumental mental health efforts to be implemented during episodes of terrorism and disaster. The psychological and behavioral consequences of a terrorist attack are now included in most disaster plans.

The earthquake and tsunami in Japan in 2011 and the Hurricane Katrina disaster in the United States in 2005 highlight the importance of government preparedness for natural disasters as well as terrorism. In the United States, the lack of government response and breakdown in communication during Katrina resulted in thousands of hurricane victims being displaced and injured. The Japan disaster became a cascade of disasters, resulting in the death of thousands of residents and contamination from the damaged nuclear site. Consequences of these disasters will still be occurring months and years after the initial events.

Phases of Disaster

Natural and human-made disaster can be conceptualized in three phases:

1. *Prewarning of the disaster*. This phase entails preparing the community for possible evacuation of the environment, mobilization of resources, and review of community disaster plans. In some disasters, such as in the 2011 earthquake in Japan, there is very little warning.
2. *The disaster event occurs*. In this phase, the rescuers provide resources, assistance, and support as needed to preserve the biopsychosocial functioning and survival of the victims. In large disasters, the rescuers and health care professionals also experience the traumatic event as both residents and health care providers. These individuals are more likely to experience greater physical and psychological trauma than those who experience the event solely as a civilian or as a

professional (Leitch, Vanslyke, & Allen, 2009). The victims experience the initial trauma and threats that occur immediately after the disaster such confusion (communication breakdown), lack of safety (no available law enforcement), and lack of health care services.

3. *Recuperative effort.* In the third phase, the focus is on implementing strategies for healing sick and injured people, preventing complications of health problems, repairing damages, and reconstructing the community. The disruption effects can be traumatic to the community residents. The debris, lack of trust of the government, fragmentation of families, financial problems, lack of adequate housing, inadequate temporary housing, and fear of another disaster contribute to the long-term negative effects of disasters.

Long-term mental health consequences are evident in most disasters. For example, in a follow-up study of alcohol use among survivors of 10 disasters, the majority of post-disaster alcohol use disorders represented the continuation or recurrence of preexisting problems. Those with an alcohol abuse disorder were four times more likely to cope by drinking alcohol than those who did not have a substance abuse problem, indicating that this group could benefit from mental health interventions (North, Ringwalt, Downs, Derzon, & Galvin, 2011).

Even though serious mental health problems are known to exist or be exacerbated after a disaster, research has shown few people access mental health services (Noorthoorn, Havenaar, de Haan, van Rood, & van Stiphout, 2010). In a follow-up study of Hurricane Katrina survivors, one-third had evidence of a mood or anxiety disorder, but fewer than 35% of those had used mental health services (Springgate et al., 2011; Wang et al., 2007). Undertreatment of these disorders was evident.

Nursing Care of Person Experiencing a Disaster or Terrorism

Psychiatric nurses encounter three different types of disaster victims. The first category is the victims who may or may not survive. If they survive, the victims often experience severe physical injuries. The more serious the physical injury, the more likely the victim will experience a mental health problem such as PTSD, depression, anxiety, or other mental health problems (Noorthoorn et al., 2010). Victims and families need ongoing health care to prevent complications related to both their physical and mental health (Springgate, et al., 2011).

The second category of victims includes the professional rescuers. These are persons who are less likely to experience physical injury but who often experience psychological stress. The professional rescuers, such as police officers, firefighters, nurses, and so on, have more effective coping skills than do volunteer rescuers who are not

prepared for the emotional impact of a disaster. However, many professional responders report experiencing PTSD for many months after the traumatic event in which they were involved (Haugen, Evces, & Weiss, 2012).

The third category includes everyone else involved in the disaster. Psychological effects may be experienced worldwide by millions of people as they experience terrorism or disaster vicariously or as direct victims of the terrorism/disaster event. After an act of terrorism, most people will experience some psychological stress, including an altered sense of safety, hypervigilance, sadness, anger, fear, decreased concentration, and difficulty sleeping. Others may alter their behavior by traveling less, staying at home, avoiding public events, keeping children out of school, or increasing smoking and alcohol use. In a nationwide interview of 560 adults after September 11, 2001, 90% reported at least one stress symptom and 44% had several symptoms of stress (Schuster et al., 2001). In New York State, almost half a million people reported symptoms that would meet the criteria for acute PTSD (see Chapter 17). In Manhattan, the estimated prevalence of acute PTSD was 11.2%, increasing to 20% in people living close to the World Trade Center (Galea et al., 2002; Schlenger et al., 2002). However, in analysis of suicide rates after September 11, 2001 and the Oklahoma City bombing, there appears to be no support for an increase or decrease in suicides following these events (Pridemore, Trahan, & Chamlin, 2009).

The role of the behavioral health care worker in disasters, specifically a nuclear detonation in a U.S. city is the support of lifesaving activities and the prevention of additional casualties from fallout. There are six broad categories of interventions including promoting appropriate protective actions, discouraging dangerous behaviors, managing patient/survivor flow to facilitate the best use of scarce resources, supporting first responders, assisting with triage, and delivering palliative care when appropriate (Dodgen Norwood, Becker, Perez, & Hansen, 2011).

Victims experiencing head injuries or psychic trauma after a disaster may have to be hospitalized. During a disaster, a victim with a mental illness may experience regression to his or her pretreatment condition. If community mental health facilities are available, they should be directed to seek assistance from mental health care professionals. The victims should receive follow-up care for the disaster response after they are discharged.

Biologic Domain

Assessment

The nurse should assess physical reactions that may involve many changes in body functions, such as tachycardia, tachypnea, profuse perspiration, nausea, vomiting, dilated pupils, and extreme shakiness. Virtually any organ may be involved. Some victims may exhibit panic reactions and loss of control and have a total disregard for their personal safety. The victims may be suicidal or homicidal and are at high risk for injuries that may include infection, trauma, and head injuries. During the rescue, medical care is a priority. Any medical or psychiatric disorders should be assessed and information communicated to the rest of the health care team.

Unexplained physical symptoms such as headache, fatigue, pain, chest pain, and gastrointestinal disturbances have been reported in the aftermath of a disaster in both traumatized and non-traumatized populations. Possible risk factors for the development of unexplained physical symptoms include female gender, high physical damage, and PTSD (Anwar, Mpofu, Matthews, & Brock, 2013; Bonanno et al., 2012).

Nursing Diagnoses for the Biologic Domain

Because the responses to disaster are so varied, almost any nursing diagnosis can be generated from the assessment data. Ineffective Thermoregulation, Ineffective Breathing Patterns, Insomnia, and Risk for Self-harm are examples of possible nursing diagnoses.

Interventions for the Biologic Domain

Any physiological problems or injuries should be treated quickly. During the emergency response, individuals will be triaged to the appropriate level of care. Victims who are primarily distressed and may have somatic symptoms will be treated after those suffering from exposure with critical injuries. The primary public health concern is clean drinking water, food, shelter, and medical care. Natural disasters do not usually cause an increase in infectious disease outbreaks, but contaminated water and food and lack of shelter and medical care may worsen illnesses that already exist (Migl & Powell, 2010). All patients need to be reassured of the caring and commitment of the nurse to their safety, comfort, and well-being throughout the triage process. Ideally, a mental health specialist is an integral member of the triage team. Many of the same interventions used for persons experiencing stress or crisis will be used for these victims. See also Chapter 29 for discussion of somatization.

Psychological Domain

Assessment

Therapeutic communication is key to understanding the extent of the psychological responses to a disaster and to establishing a bridge of trust that communicates respect, commitment, and acceptance. Developing rapport with the victim or victims communicates reassurance and support. The victims should be assessed for behaviors that indicate a depressed state, presence of confusion, uncontrolled weeping or screaming, disorientation, or aggressive behavior. Ideally, the nurse should assess the coping strategies the victim uses to normally manage stressful situations.

During a disaster, fear and hopelessness can immobilize victims. The victims may suffer from loss of feelings of well-being and various psychological problems, including panic responses, anxiety, and fear. Dissociation and fear are predictive of later developing PTSD and depressive symptoms. Victims witnessing others suffer are especially high risk for future mental health problems and should be assessed for the details of the disaster (Rosendal, Salcioğlu, Andersen, & Mortensen, 2011).

The survivors of the disaster may experience traumatic bereavement because of their feelings of guilt that they survived the disaster (Bolton et al., 2013; Viswanath et al., 2012). Responses to psychological distress need to be differentiated from any psychiatric illness that the person may be experiencing. A response to a disaster may leave the person feeling overwhelmed, incapacitated, and disoriented.

Nursing Diagnoses for the Psychological Domain

Initially, fear and hopelessness can be expected. Depending on the long-term impact of the disaster and the type of disaster (e.g., terrorist attack or tsunami), there could be any number of nursing diagnosis such as Grieving, Impaired Resilience, Low Self-Esteem, or Risk for Suicide.

Interventions for the Psychological Domain

The **ABCs of psychological first aid** include focusing on A (arousal), B (behavior), and C (cognition). When arousal is present, the intervention goal is to decrease excitement by providing safety, comfort, and consolation. When abnormal or irrational behavior is present, survivors should be assisted to function more effectively in the disaster, and when cognitive disorientation occurs, reality testing and clear information should be provided. In the initial phases, the nurse should assist the victim in focusing on the reality of problems that are immediate, with specific goals that are consistent with available resources as well as the culture and lifestyle of the victim.

After the initial interventions, the nurse should support the development of resilience, coping, and recovery while providing technical assistance, training, and consultation. During the treatment process, it may become necessary to administer an antianxiety medication or sedative, especially in the early phases of recovery (Centers for Disease Control and Prevention [CDC], 2005). The goals of care include helping the victims prioritize and match available resources with their needs, preventing further complications, monitoring the environment, disseminating information, and implementing disease control strategies (CDC, 2012).

Debriefing (the reconstruction of the traumatic events by the victim) may be helpful for some. Long a common practice, debriefing was believed to be necessary in order for the person to develop a healthy perspective of the event and ultimately prevent PTSD. However, research does not support debriefing as a useful treatment for the prevention of PTSD after traumatic incidents. Additionally, different cultural groups respond differently to traumatic events, and many non-Western ethnic groups present symptoms somatically rather than psychologically. Therefore, compulsory debriefing is not recommended (Hawker, Durkin, & Hawker, 2011).

If the victim has symptoms of PTSD, referral to a mental health clinic for additional evaluation and treatment is important (see Chapter 17). The nurse should prepare the victim for recovery by teaching about the effects of stress and helping the victim identify personal strengths and coping skills. Positive coping skills should be supported. The victims should be encouraged to report any depression, anxiety, or interpersonal difficulty during the recovery period. After most disasters, support groups are established that help victims and their families deal with the psychological effects of the disaster.

Women exhibit higher levels of distress than men after a disaster, especially pregnant women and older women (Tong, Zotti, & Hsia, 2011; Viswanath et al., 2012). Assess the ages of the female victims, their capability to participate in problem-solving activities related to the devastation left by the disaster, and their level of self-confidence or self-esteem that would allow each to participate as a team member or a team leader in addressing the needs of others. This includes encouraging the victims to do necessary chores and participate in decision making and to take advantage of the opportunity to serve as leaders or team members, as dictated by their abilities.

Outreach is especially important because research shows that disaster victims do not access mental health systems. Peer-delivered mental health services are especially effective in identifying and connecting with victims, especially those with pre-disaster psychiatric problems (North & Pfefferbaum, 2013).

Educating the public and emphasizing the natural recovery process is important. Information gaps and rumors add to the anxiety and stress of the situation. Giving information and direction helps the public and victims to use the coping skills they already possess. Initially, the event may leave individuals and families in a stage of ambiguity with frantic, disorganized behavior. In addition, individuals and family members are concerned about their own physical and psychological responses to the disastrous event. Children are especially vulnerable to disasters and respond according to their ages and family experiences. Traumatized children and adolescents are high risk victims of a wide range of behavioral, psychological, and neurologic problems after experiencing various traumatic events (Osofsky & Osofsky, 2013; Pfefferbaum & North, 2013).

When the nurse explains anticipated reactions and behaviors, this helps the victims gain control and improve coping. For example, after a major disaster, they may have excessive worry, preoccupation with the event, and changes in eating and sleeping patterns. With time, counseling, and group work, these symptoms will lessen. Active coping strategies can be presented in multiple media forums, such as television and radio. After the initial shock, victims react by trying to do something to resolve the situation. When victims begin working to remedy the disaster situation, their physical responses become less exaggerated, and they are more able to work with less tension and fear.

Social Domain

Assessment

The nurse should assess the kind and severity of a natural or human-made disaster or terrorist act to determine the capability of individuals and communities to respond in a supportive way. The nurse should maintain a calm demeanor, obtain and distribute information about the disaster and the victims, and reunite victims and their families. In addition, there is a need to monitor the news media's impact on the mental health of the victims of the crisis. Sometimes the persistence of the news media diminishes the ability of the survivors to achieve closure to the crisis (McGinty, Webster, Jarlenski, & Barry, 2014). Constant rehashing of the disaster in the newspapers and on television can increase and prolong the severity or initiate feelings of anxiety and depression.

Cultural values and beliefs help define the significance and meaning of a disaster. In some instances, a disaster can slow development, but usually the customs, beliefs, and value systems remain the same. It is important that first responders and health care teams are sensitive to the cultural and religious beliefs of the community. In many instances, victims' spiritual beliefs and religious faith help them cope with the disaster (Varghese, 2010).

In a disaster, the victims may experience economic distress because of job loss and loss of other resources. This may ultimately lead to psychological distress. In addition, acts of aggression and other mental health problems may emerge (Ozbay, Heyde, Reissman, & Sharma, 2013; Wisnivesky et al., 2011). Again, shelter, money, and food may not be available. The absence of basic human needs such as food, a place to live, or immediate transportation quickly becomes a priority that may precipitate acts of violence.

Nursing Diagnoses for the Social Domain

Nursing diagnoses associated with the social domain include Impaired Adjustment, Impaired Social Interaction, and Interrupted Family Processes. Ineffective Role Performance and Relocation Stress Syndrome are also diagnoses that could be generated during a disaster. Other nursing diagnoses can be generated from the assessment findings according to the needs of the victims.

Interventions for the Social Domain

The focus of nursing interventions for the social domain include the individual, family, and community. The individual should learn about the community resources that can be made available. Family support systems may need to be reestablished. The health care community should actively reach out to the media and keep the press engaged. Direct attention to stories that inform and help the public respond should be encouraged. Some federal agencies assist victims of disasters. This assistance is available for individual, families, and communities. One of these agencies is the Federal Emergency Management Agency (FEMA). When a disaster occurs, FEMA sends a team of specialists who review the devastation of disaster. They provide counseling and mental health services and arrange for many of the victims to access other services needed for survival, including training programs. In addition, the Substance Abuse and Mental Health Services Administration (SAMHSA) of the Department of Health and Human Services is available to assist both victims of and responders to the disaster. When a disaster disrupts the victim's social network, other resources must be made available for social support. The social support system provides an environment in which the victims experience respect and caring from the caregivers, the opportunity to ventilate and examine personal feelings regarding the tragedy, and the opportunity to begin the healing and recovery process. Supporting the development of more contacts within the social network can be done by organizing support groups within the area of the disaster that address grief and loss, trauma, psychoeducational needs, and substance abuse. In addition, the nurse may refer the victims to nearby support groups or religious groups that are appropriate to meet their needs.

Evaluation and Treatment Outcomes

To determine the effectiveness of nursing interventions, the nurse should evaluate the outcomes based on the success of resolution of the disaster. The outcomes will depend on the specific disaster and its meaning (appraisal) to the survivors. For example, are the survivors in a safe place? Are the victims able to cope with the disaster? Were the appropriate supports given, so the victims could draw upon their own strengths?

SUMMARY OF KEY POINTS

- A crisis is a time-limited event that occurs when coping mechanisms fail to provide adaptive skills to address a perceived challenge or threat.

- Grief is an intense emotional response to loss, and bereavement is the process of mourning. There are variations in grief responses that are influenced by the characteristics of the individual and the situation of loss.

- Stage theories of grief although popular, lack evidence. The dual process model explains bereavement as an oscillation between loss-oriented coping and restoration-oriented coping. Over time, there is less of a need to think about the loss.

- Most persons grieve normally and do not need counseling. Complicated grief occurs in about 10% to 20% of bereaved persons. Interventions are required for this group.

- Biopsychosocial assessment reveals changes in domains. Interventions are designed to support people through crises by helping them identify the resources they need and how to get them.

- Disaster is a sudden, overwhelming catastrophic event that causes great damage and may cause mass casualties and human suffering that require assistance from all available resources.

- Depending on the disaster, interventions are provided to individuals, families, and communities.

CRITICAL THINKING CHALLENGES

1. Compare nursing interventions used for crises with those used for disasters. What are the similarities? What are the differences?
2. After the death of his mother, a 24-year-old single man with schizophrenia moves into an apartment. He continues to take his medication but feels sad about his mother's death. He is not adjusting well to living alone and tells his nurse that he no longer wants to go to work. In tears, he admits that he is lonely and can no longer cope with the apartment. The nurse generates the following nursing diagnosis: Ineffective Coping related to inadequate support system. Develop a plan of care for this young man.
3. Compare the evidence for the stage theories of grieving with the dual process model. What are the pros and cons of each?
4. Discuss the role of medication when used in crises.

5. Compare normal grief with complicated grief. How would you recognize the difference? When would it be appropriate to refer a bereaved person to a mental health specialist?

6. There is a terrorist threat in your community. A patient appears in the emergency department convinced that he is going to die. How would you proceed with assessing this patient?

Grace is Gone (2007): Stanley Phillips (John Cusack) is a manager of a home-supply store and parent of two girls, 12-year-old Heidi (Shelan O'Keefe) and 8-year-old Dawn (Gracie Bednarczyk). His wife is a soldier in Iraq, but the viewers know her by her message left on the family answering machine. When an army captain and chaplain deliver the news that Grace had died bravely in combat, Stanley becomes numb. He impulsively takes his girls to wherever they desire—a theme park in Florida. Most of the movie follows the three on the trip and the father's attempt to delay and deny his wife's death.

Viewing Points: Describe Stanley's reaction when he receives the news of his wife's death. What clues are present that Heidi gradually understands that something terrible has happened?

REFERENCES

American Psychiatric Association. (2013). *Diagnostic and statistical manual of mental disorders* (5th ed.). Arlington, VA: Author.

Anwar, J., Mpofu, E., Matthews, L. R., Brock, K. D. (2013). Risk factors of posttraumatic stress disorder after an earthquake disaster. *Journal of Nervous & Mental Disorders, 201*(12), 1045–1052.

Barlow, C. A., Schiff, J. W., Chugh, U., Rawlinson, D., Hides, E., & Leith, J. (2010). An evaluation of a suicide bereavement peer support program. *Death Studies, 34*(10), 915–930.

Bennett, K. M., & Soulsby, L. K. (2012). Wellbeing in bereavement and widowhood illness. *Crisis and Loss, 20*(14), 321–337.

Betancourt, T. S., Newnham, E. A., Layne, C. M., Kim, S., Steinberg, A. M., Ellis, H., et al. (2012). Trauma history and psychopathology in war-affected refugee children referred for trauma-related mental health services in the United States. *Journal of Traumatic Stress, 25*(6), 682–690.

Bolton, P., Michalopoulos, L., Ahmed, A. M., Murray, L. K., & Bass, J. (2013). The mental health and psychosocial problems of survivors of torture and genocide in Kurdistan, Northern Iraq: A brief qualitative study. *Torture, 23*(1), 1–14.

Bonanno, G. A., Mancini, A. D., Horton, J. L., Powell, T. M., Leardmann, C. A., Boyko, E. J., et al. (2012). Trajectories of trauma symptoms and resilience in deployed US military service members: Prospective cohort study. *The British Journal of Psychiatry, 200*(4), 317–323.

Bowlby, J., & Parkes, C. M. (1970). Separation and loss within the family. In E. J. Anthony (Ed.), *The child in his family.* New York: Wiley.

Caffo, E., Forresi, B., & Lievers, L. S. (2005). Impact, psychological sequelae and management of trauma affecting children and adolescents. *Current Opinion in Psychiatry, 18*(4), 422–428.

Caserta, M., Utz, R., Lund, D., Swenson, K. L., & de Vries, B. (2014). Coping processes among bereaved spouses. *Death Studies, 38*(3), 145–155.

Caplan, G. (1961). *An approach to community mental health.* New York: Grune & Stratton.

Centers for Disease Control and Prevention. (2012). Disaster mental health for states: Key principles, issues, and questions. *Emergency Preparedness and Response.* Retrieved from http://emergency.cdc.gov/mental-health/states.asp.

Claxton, R., & Reynolds, C. F. 3rd. (2012). Complicated grief #254. *Journal of Palliative Medicine, 15*(7), 829–830.

Dodgen, D., Norwood, A. D., Becker, S. M., Perez, J. T., & Hansen, C. K. (2011). Social, psychological, and behavioral responses to a nuclear detonation in a U.S. city: Implications for health care planning and delivery. *Disaster Medicine & Public Health Preparedness, 5*(suppl 1), S54–S64.

Drenth, C. M., Herbst, A. F., & Strydom, H. (2010). A complicated grief intervention model. *Health SA Gesondheid, 15*(1), 1–8. doi:10.4102/hsaf.v15i1.415

Fischer, P., Postmes, T., Koeppl, J., Conway, L., & Fredriksson, T. (2011). The meaning of collective terrorist threat: Understanding the subjective causes of terrorism reduces its negative psychological impact. *Journal of Interpersonal Violence, 26*(7), 1432–1445.

Fujisawa, D., Miyashita, M., Nakajima, S., Ito, M., Kato, M., & Kim, Y. (2010). Prevalence and determinants of complicated grief in general population. *Journal of Affective Disorders, 127*(1–3), 352–358.

Galea, S., Ahern, J., Resnick, H., Kilpatrick, D., Bucuvalas, M., Gold, J., & Vlahov, D. (2002). Psychological sequelae of the September 11 terrorist attacks in New York City. *New England Journal of Medicine, 346*(13), 982–987.

Haugen, P. T., Evces, M., & Weiss, D. S. (2012). Treating posttraumatic stress disorder in first responders: A systematic review. *Clinical Psychology Review, 32*(5), 370–380.

Hawker, D. M., Durkin, J., & Hawker, D. S. (2011). To debrief or not to debrief our heroes: That is the question. *Clinical Psychology and Psychotherapy, 18*(6), 453–463.

Kubler-Ross, E. (1969). *On death and dying.* New York: Macmillan Publishing Company.

Lazarus, R. (1991). *Emotion and adaptation* (p. 122). New York: Oxford University Press.

Leitch, M. L., Vanslyke, J., & Allein, M. (2009). Somatic experiencing treatment with social service workers following hurricanes Katrina and Rita. *Social Work, 54*(1), 9–18.

Lindemann, E. (1944). Symptomatology and management of acute grief. *American Journal of Psychiatry, 101*, 141–148.

Lyons, C., Hopley, P., Burton, C. R., & Horrocks, J. (2009). Mental health crisis and respite services: Service user and carer aspirations. *Journal of Psychiatric and Mental Health Nursing, 16*, 424–433.

McGinty, E. E., Webster, D. W., Jarlenski, M., & Barry, C. (2014). News media framing of serious mental illness and gun violence in the United States, 1997–2012. *American Journal of Public Health, 104*(3), 406–413.

McKay, K., & Tighe, J. (2013). Talking through the dead: The impact and interplay of lived grief after suicide. *Omega, 68*(2), 111–121.

Migl, K. S., & Pwell, R. M. (2010). Physical and environmental considerations for first responders. *Critical Care Nursing Clinics of North America, 22*(4), 445–454.

Mutabaruka, J., Séjourné, N., Bui, E., Birmes, P., & Chabro, H. (2012). Traumatic grief and traumatic stress in survivors 12 years after the genocide in Rwanda. *Stress and Health, 28*(4), 289–296.

Noorthoorn, E. O., Havenaar, J. M., de Haan, H.A., van Rood, Y. R., & van Stiphout, W. H. J. (2010). Mental health service use and outcomes after the Enschede Fireworks disaster: A naturalistic follow-up study. *Psychiatric Services, 61*(11), 1138–1143.

North, C. S., & Pfefferbaum, B. (2013). Mental health response to community disasters: A systematic review. *JAMA, 310*(5), 507–518.

North, C. S., Ringwalt, C. L., Downs, D., Derzon, J., & Galvin, D. (2011). Postsidadter course of alcohol use disorders in systematically studied survivors of 10 disasters. *Archives of General Psychiatry, 68*(2), 173–180.

Osofsky, H. J., & Osofsky, J. D. (2013). Hurricane Katrina and the gulf oil spill: Lessons learned. *Psychiatric Clinics of North America, 36*(3), 371–382.

Ozbay, F., Auf der H. T., Reissman, D., Sharma, V. (2013). The enduring mental health impact of the September 11th terrorist attacks: Challenges and lessons learned. *Psychiatric Clinics of North America, 36*(3), 417–429.

Pfefferbaum, B., & North, C. S. (2013). Assessing children's disaster reactions and mental health needs: Screening and clinical evaluation. *Canadian Journal of Psychiatry, 58*(3), 135–142.

Pilling, J., Thege, B. K., Demetrovics, Z., & Kopp, M. S. (2012). Alcohol use in the first three years of bereavement: A national representative survey. *Substance Abuse Treatment, Prevention, and Policy, 7*, 1–5. http://www.substanceabusepolicy.com/content/7/1/3

Pridemore, W. A., Trahan, A., & Chamlin, M. B. (2009). No evidence of suicide increase following terrorist attacks in the United States: An interrupted time-series analysis of September 11 and Oklahoma City. *Suicide & Life-threatening Behavior, 39*(6), 659–670.

Reynolds C. F., Stack J., & Houle J. Healing. (2011). Emotions After Loss (HEAL): Diagnosis and treatment of complicated grief. UPMC Synergies. Available at: http://healstudy.org/wp-content/uploads/2010/10/S270-Synergies_GR_Spring_2011.pdf. Accessed May 21, 2014.

Rosendal, S., Salcioğlu, E., Andersen, H. S., & Mortensen, E. L. (2011). Exposure characteristics and peri-trauma emotional reactions during the 2004 tsunami in Southeast Asia: What predicts posttraumatic stress and depressive symptoms? *Comprehensive Psychiatry*, in press.

Schlenger, W. E., Caddell, J. M., Ebert, L., Jordan, B. K., Rourke, K. M., Wilson, D., et al. (2002). Psychological reactions to terrorist attacks: Findings from the national study of Americans' reactions to September 11. *Journal of the American Medical Association*, *288*(5), 581–588.

Schuster, M. A., Stein, B. D., Jaycox, L., Collins, R. L., Marshall, G. N., Elliott, M. N., et al. (2001). A national survey of stress reactions after September 11, 2001, terrorist attacks. *New England Journal of Medicine*, *345*(20), 1507–1512.

Springgate, B. F., Wennerstrom, A., Meyers, D., Allen, C. E., Vannoy, S. D., Bentham, W., Wells, K. B. (2011). Building community resilience through mental health infrastructure and training in post-Katrina New Orleans. *Ethnicity & Disease*, *21*(3 Suppl 1), S1–20–29.

Stroebe, M., & Schut, H. (1999). The dual process model of coping with bereavement: Rationale and description. *Death Studies*, *23*, 197–224.

Stroebe, M., Schut, H., & Boerner, K. (2010). Continuing bonds in adaptation to bereavement: Toward theoretical integration. *Clinical Psychology Review*, *30*, 259–268.

Stroebe, M., Schut, D., & Stroebe, W. (2007). Health outcomes of bereavement: A review. *Lancet*, *270*(9603), 1960–1973.

Stroebe, M., Stroebe, W., & Schut, D. (2006). Bereavement research: methodological issues and ethical concerns, *Palliative Medicine*, *17*(3), 235–240.

Tong, V. T., Zotti, M. E., & Hsia, J. (2011). Impact of the Red River catastrophic flood on women giving birth in North Dakota, 1994–2000. *Maternal & Child Health Journal*, *15*(3), 281–288.

van Den Berg, B., Grievink, L., Yzermans, J., & Lebret, E. (2005). Medically unexplained physical symptoms in the aftermath of disasters. *Epidemiologic Reviews*, *27*, 92–106.

Varghese, S. B. (2010). Cultural, ethical, and spiritual implications of natural disasters from the survivors' perspective. *Critical Care Nursing Clinics of North America*, *22*(4), 515–522.

Viswanath, B., Maroky, A. S., Math, S. B., John, J. R., Benegal, V., Hamza, A., et al. (2012). Psychological impact of the tsunami on elderly survivors. *American Journal of Geriatric Psychiatry*, *20*(5), 402–407.

Wang, P. S., Gruber, J. J., Powers, R. E., Schoenbaum, M., Speier, A. H., Wells, K. B., & Kessler, R. C. (2007). Mental health service use among Hurricane Katrina survivors in the eight months after the disaster. *Psychiatric Services*, *58*(11), 1403–1411.

Wisnivesky, J. P., Teitelbaum, S. L., Todd, A. C., Boffetta, P., Crane, M., Crowley, L., et al. (2011). Persistence of multiple illnesses in World Trade Center rescue and recovery workers: A cohort study. *Lancet*, *387*(9794), 888–897.

Zhang, B., El-Jawahri, A., & Prigerson, H. G. (2006). Update on bereavement research: Evidence-based guidelines for the diagnosis and treatment of complicated bereavement. *Journal of Palliative Medicine*, *9*(5), 1188–1203.

Zisook, S. (1987). Unresolved grief. In S. Zisook (Ed.), *Biopsychosocial aspects of bereavement* (pp. 21–34). Washington, DC: American Psychiatric Press.

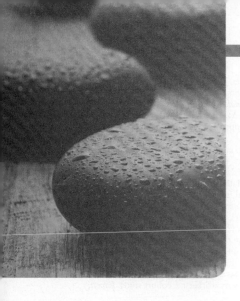

15
Suicide Prevention
Screening, Assessment, and Intervention

Emily J. Hauenstein and Mary Ann Boyd

KEY CONCEPTS

- hopelessness
- lethality
- suicide

LEARNING OBJECTIVES

After studying this chapter, you will be able to:

1. Identify suicide as a major mental health problem in the United States.

2. Define suicide, suicidality, suicide attempt, parasuicide, and suicidal ideation.

3. Describe population groups that have high rates of suicide.

4. Describe risk factors associated with suicide completion.

5. Identify key factors associated with specific suicide acts.

6. Describe evidence-based interventions used to reduce imminent and ongoing suicide risk.

7. Explain the importance of documentation and reporting when caring for patients who may be at risk of suicide.

KEY TERMS

- case finding • commitment to treatment statement • parasuicide • suicidal ideation • suicidality • suicide attempt
- suicide contagion

Suicide is one of the major health problems in the United States, accounting for 38,000 deaths each year. For every suicide death, an additional 25 suicide attempts are made. More than half of people complete suicide in their first attempt, and more than 30% will have a repeat attempt. The public health problem of suicidal behavior is so important that several goals stated in *Healthy People 2010* and retained in *Healthy People 2020* directly target the reduction of deaths by suicide (U.S. Department of Health and Human Services [U.S. DHHS], 2010).

More than 90% of suicides in the United States are associated with mental illness or alcohol and substance abuse (Insel, 2010). The subsequent visibility of the mental disorder discredits the person, leaving him or her open to stigmatization. Suicide is so rejected in contemporary society that people with strong suicidal thoughts do not seek treatment for fear of being stigmatized by others. Reports and portrayals of suicide in the popular media and television further stigmatize those who consider or attempt suicide. Society's unwillingness to talk openly about suicide also contributes to the common misperceptions resulting in many myths regarding suicide (Murphy, Fatoye, & Wibberley, 2013). Box 15.1 presents several myths and facts about suicide.

Suicides are preventable deaths when immediate friends and family and health care providers identify symptoms and use effective interventions. All practicing nurses will come into contact with patients who are thinking about suicide and often can prevent suicides by identifying and intervening with those at risk. Through individual and public education, nurses also can do much to demystify suicide and reduce stigma for those at risk.

BOX 15.1

Myths and Facts about Suicide

Myth: People who talk about suicide do not complete suicide.
Fact: Many people who die by suicide have given definite warnings of their intentions. Always take any comment about suicide seriously.
Myth: Suicide happens without warning.
Fact: Most suicidal people give many clues and warning signs regarding their suicidal intention.
Myth: Suicidal people are fully intent on dying.
Fact: Most suicidal people are undecided about living or dying. A part of them wants to live; however, death seems like the only way out of their pain or situation. They may allow themselves to "gamble" with death, leaving it up to others to save them.
Myth: Suicides occur more frequently during holidays.
Fact: The suicide rate is lowest in December. The rate peaks in the spring and fall.
Myth: Improvement after a suicide crisis means that the risk is over.
Fact: Most suicides occur within 3 months of "improvement" when the individual has the energy and motivation to actually follow through with his or her suicidal thoughts.

Source: Suicide.org. (2011). *Suicide myths. Suicide prevention, awareness and support.* Retrieved July 9, 2012, from http://www.suicide.org/suicide-myths.html.

To reduce the devastating public impact of suicide on those at risk and their families, nurses must be knowledgeable about suicide and be able to implement effective preventive interventions. This chapter contains tools that can be used to reduce the broad effects of suicide and provide appropriate care for suicidal patients.

SUICIDE AND SUICIDE ATTEMPT

KEYCONCEPT **Suicide** is the voluntary act of killing oneself. It is a fatal, self-inflicted destructive act with explicit or inferred intent to die. It is sometimes called suicide completion.

This behavioral definition of suicide is limited and does not consider the complexity of the underlying depressive illness, personal motivations, and situational and family factors that provoke the suicide act. Except for the very young, suicide occurs in all age groups, social classes, and cultures (CDC, 2014a).

The term **suicidality** refers to all suicide-related behaviors and thoughts of completing or attempting suicide and suicide ideation. **Suicidal ideation** is thinking about and planning one's own death. Population studies show that suicidal ideation ranges between 3% and 10% but varies by characteristics of the participants and the way suicidal ideation is measured. Although suicide ideation often does not progress, about 4% to 18% will eventually attempt suicide, with each subsequent attempt associated with greater lethality (Nakagawa Grunebaum, Ocuendo, Burke, Kashima, & Mann, 2009).

A **suicide attempt** is a nonfatal, self-inflicted destructive act with explicit or implicit intent to die. Only recently have data on suicide attempts been compiled. In 2010, 650,000 people visited a hospital for injuries due to self-harm behavior (American Foundation for Suicide Prevention [AFSP], 2014). Adolescents make more attempts than do adults, but they generally are less successful. Suicide ideation, recent psychiatric hospitalization, and a previous attempt are significant predictors of a completed suicide (Selby, Yen, & Spirito, 2013; De Leo, Draper, Snowdon, & Kolves, 2013).

Parasuicide is a voluntary, apparent attempt at suicide, commonly called a suicidal gesture, in which the aim is not death (e.g., taking a sublethal drug). Parasuicidal behavior varies by intent. Some people truly wish to die, but others simply wish to feel nothing for a while. Still others want to send a message about their emotional state. Parasuicide behavior is never normal and should always be taken seriously. Parasuicide occurs frequently in younger age groups but declines after the age of 44 years.

KEYCONCEPT **Lethality** refers to the probability that a person will successfully complete suicide. Lethality is determined by the seriousness of the person's intent and the likelihood that the planned method of death will succeed. A plan to use an accessible firearm to commit suicide has greater lethality than a suicide plan that involves superficial cuts of the wrist.

Suicide is ranked as the 10th leading cause of death and accounts for 12.1 deaths per 100,000 population (Centers for Disease Control and Prevention [CDC], 2014a). A suicide occurs every 13.7 minutes in the United States: a rate of 80 completed successful suicides per day. The suicide rate in the United States has been stable for several years despite a significant increase in the rate of suicide attempts. Mountain regions have the highest rate of suicide (Figure 15.1). Its overall prevalence may be underestimated because suicide can be disguised as vehicular accidents or homicide, especially in young people (CDC, 2014a).

Suicide Across the Life Span

Children, Adolescents, and Young Adults

Among adolescents 15 to 24 years of age, there are approximately 100 to 200 attempts for every completed suicide (CDC, 2014b). Approximately, 15% of high school students have seriously considered suicide and 7% have attempted to take their own life (CDC, 2014a). Among American Indian and Alaskan natives ages 15 to 34 years, suicide is the second leading cause of death (CDC, 2014b).

Mental disorders can lead to school failure, alcohol or other drug abuse, family discord, violence, and suicide. Approximately 20% of U.S. children and adolescents are affected by mental disorders in their lifetime.

Suicide Rate
2000–2006, United States
Age-adjusted Death Rates per 100,000 Population

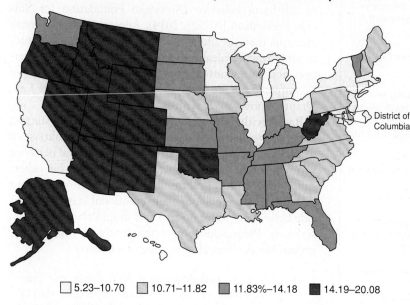

District of
Columbia

□ 5.23–10.70   ▨ 10.71–11.82   ▤ 11.83%–14.18   ■ 14.19–20.08

Note: Reports for All Ages include those of unknown age.   *Data courtesy of CDC*

FIGURE 15.1 Number of deaths attributable to suicide in the United States per 100,000 population, 2007. (From Kaiser Family Foundation, statehealth facts.org. Retrieved from http://www.nimh.nih.gov/statistics/4NAT_MAP.shtml: Centers for Disease Control and Prevention, National Center for Health Statistics, Division of Vital Statistics. (2010, May)

In 2011, 1.8% of youths (grades 9 to 12) reported that they had seriously considered attempting suicide during the preceding 12 months; 12% made a plan, and 7.8% attempted (CDC, 2014a). Suicide attempts vary according to racial and ethnic groups. In 2011 white non-Hispanic adolescents had the lowest rate of suicide attempts in the past 12 months, 1.9% compared to 3.2% Hispanic, 4.5% for Asian and 6.6% for American Indian or Alaska Native. A lower proportion of adolescent males reported suicide attempts in the past 12 months, 1.9% compared to females, 2.9% (U.S. DHHS).

Adults and Older Adults

In adults, death rates from suicide range from 12.3 to 17.2 deaths per 100,000 with the highest rates occurring in the 45- to 54-year age group (CDC, 2014b). Suicide rates peak during middle age, and a second peak occurs in those age 75 years and older. Physical illness and financial difficulties are important precipitants to suicide in older adults (Van Orden & Conwell, 2011).

Suicide death is a leading cause of death among armed service members deployed to Iraq and Afghanistan. Recent studies comparing suicide risk of veterans with the general population show excess risk for firearm suicide deaths. With the repeated deployment of military personnel that occurred, suicide behavior among soldiers remains a significant concern. There are several factors thought to contribute to the suicide rate. Combat

exposure is one of the leading factors for both men and women military members. For women, military sexual trauma also contributes to the suicide ideation and attempts (Boyd, Bradshaw, & Robinson, 2013; Mitchell, Gallaway, Millikan, & Bell, 2012).

Epidemiology and Risk Factors

Mental illness is an important factor contributing to suicide in adults. Most young adults who commit suicide also have a depressive disorder, and many have personality disorders. Adolescents who have panic attacks are particularly at risk for suicide. Auditory hallucinations increase the risk for suicide because of the possibility of individuals impulsively responding to "voices" directing them to kill themselves. Substance abuse increases the likelihood that suicidal ideation will result in both parasuicidal and suicidal behaviors. Box 15.2 identifies risk factors for suicide (Goldston et al., 2009; U.S. DHHS, 2010).

Medical illnesses increase the likelihood of chronic depression, which in turn contributes to the increased suicide rate of those older than the age of 65 years (De Leo et al., 2013; Liu, Kraines, Puzia, Massing-Schaffer, & M. Kleiman, 2013; Kim et al., 2011). Additionally, symptoms of comorbid illnesses often are similar to those of depressive disorder, making recognition of depressive disorder by primary care providers difficult. Patients are often reticent to disclose their suicidal thoughts, further complicating

BOX 15.2
Factors Enhancing Suicide Risk

VULNERABILITY
Primary family member who has completed suicide
Psychiatric disorder
Previous attempt by the patient
Loss (e.g., death of significant other, divorce, job loss)
Unrelenting physical illness

RISK
White or Native American man
Older man
Adolescent non-Hispanic white or Native American male
Gay, lesbian, or bisexual orientation
Access to firearms
Middle-aged woman

INTENT
Suicide plan and means of executing it
Inability to commit to treatment

DISINHIBITION
Impulsivity
Isolation
Psychotic thoughts
Drug or alcohol use

detection. Consequently, health professionals fail to identify many patients who are experiencing suicidal ideation. In one study, 12.4% of persons visiting their primary care physicians for routine medical care had suicidal ideation, yet only 2.1% disclosed that information to their physicians (Bryan, Corso, Rudd, & Cordero, 2008).

Psychological Risk Factors

Internal distress, low self-esteem, and interpersonal distress have long been associated with suicide. Childhood physical and sexual abuse are linked to suicide, suicide ideation, and parasuicide. Cognitive risk factors include problem-solving deficits, impulsivity, rumination, and hopelessness. Impulsivity, anger, and reduced inhibition increase the risk of suicide. Recent purchase of a handgun increases the risk of self-harm (Hawkins & Cougle, 2013; Pompili et al., 2013; Zhang & Li, 2013).

Social Risk Factors

Social isolation is a primary risk factor for suicide. Social distress leads to despair and can be caused by family discord, parental neglect, abuse, parental suicide, and divorce. Social distress can prevent the patient from accessing the support necessary to prevent suicidal acts. Other social factors associated with suicide risk include economic deprivation, unemployment, and poverty, especially among youth. More poorly educated men also have an enhanced risk for suicide (Walsh, Clayton, Liu, & Hodges, 2009; Ando et al., 2013; CDC, 2014).

Gender

Males have a higher suicide completion rate than females. For men, suicide is the eighth leading cause of death, with a rate of 19.9 per 100,000 in 2010, more than four times the rate in women (AFSP, 2014). Men complete 79% of all suicides; 57.5% of these deaths are by firearms. Men are more likely to use means that have a higher rate of success, such as firearms and hanging (U.S. DHHS, 2014). Rural men have a much higher risk of suicide than urban men, and that gap is widening, perhaps attributable to the higher rates of gun ownership in rural areas (McCarthy, Blow, Ignacio, Ilgen, Austin, Valenstein, et al., 2012). Most suicide deaths occur in men with psychiatric disorders, primarily depression, in many cases complicated by substance abuse (Schmutte et al., 2009). Substance abuse, aggression, hopelessness, emotion-focused coping, social isolation, and having little purpose in life have been associated with suicidal behavior in men. Unmarried, unsociable men between the ages of 42 and 77 years with minimal social networks and no close relatives have a significantly increased risk for committing suicide (Walsh et al., 2009). White and American Indian/Alaska native men had the highest rates of any racial/ethnic population in this *older* age group. Suicide attempts are often lethal in this age group because men in this age group and in all racial and ethnic groups except those of Asian descent use firearms to commit suicide (U.S. DHHS, 2014).

Women across age and racial and ethnic groups are less likely to die from suicide than are men but are more likely to attempt suicide. Women make three attempts to every attempt by men. Adolescent girls and women ages 10 to 44 years have the highest rate of suicide attempts. Women are less likely to complete a suicide, partly because they are more likely to choose less lethal methods. For women, whereas current or previous exposure to violence, sexual assault, or both increases a woman's risk for suicidal behavior, having a small child reduces risk (Stack & Wasserman, 2009).

Sexuality

The lesbian, gay, bisexual, and transgender (LGBT) population is at increased risk for suicide (Mustanski & Liu, 2013; Ploderi et al., 2013). Other risk factors include early disclosure of their sexual orientation and early onset of sexual activity (Paul et al., 2002). A cross-national study meta-analysis showed that lifetime suicide ideation was more common among gay men (40%–55%) compared with heterosexual men (18%–30%) as were lifetime suicide attempts (8%–25% for gay men versus 1%–13% in heterosexual men) (Lewis, 2009). Depressive symptoms and suicidality rates in early adolescence are higher among sexual minority youth than among heterosexual youth and these disparities persist into young adulthood. These disparities are largest for females and bisexually-identified youth (Marshal et al., 2013). In lesbian, gay, and bisexual older adults, there are high levels of poor general health disability and depression (Fredriksen-Goldsen et al., 2013).

Race and Ethnicity

There is considerable variation in the profile of suicide rates across racial groups, including the age when rates are at their peak and the duration of high rates across several age groups (Figure 15.2). The suicide rate per 100,000 (both men and women) is 14.1 for whites, 5.1 for African Americans, and 5.9 for Hispanics living in the United States (Wadsworth & Kubrin, 2007).

White adolescents and men have high rates from the age of 15 years onward, but the peak suicide rate is among those older than 75 years. Access to firearms is associated with the risk of completed suicides, particularly for white males. In 2009, 51.8% of deaths from suicide were firearm related and most suicides occur in the victim's home. Firearm ownership in more prevalent in the United States than in any other country—approximately 35% to 39% of households have firearms (Anglemyer, Horvath, & Rutherford, 2014).

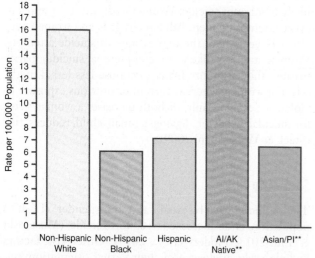

FIGURE 15.2 Suicide rates among persons ages 10 years and older, by race or ethnicity, United States, 2002–2005. During 2005 to 2009, the highest suicide rates were among American Indian or Alaskan natives, and non-Hispanic whites. All rates are age-adjusted to the standard 2000 population. Rates are based on less than 20 deaths are not shown as they are statistically unreliable. AI, American India; AK, Alaskan; PI, Pacific Islander. (From Centers for Disease Control and Prevention. (2014) *Injury prevention & control: Violence prevention.* National Statistics at a Glance. Retrieved from http://www.cdc.gov/violenceprevention/suicide/statistics/rates01.html.)

Although the overall suicide rate for African Americans is low, young African American men take their lives at a rate considerably above that of other age groups. Family cohesion and social support in African American families contribute to the lower rates in this group. Higher rates of suicide in younger men is associated with being in foster care, early aggressive behavior, depression, and dissatisfaction with life (Liu et al., 2013; Wang, Lightsey, Tran, & Bonapart, 2013).

Even though the suicide rate for Hispanics (Latinos) is less than half of the overall U.S. rate, suicide is the 12th leading cause of death for Hispanics of all ages and third leading cause of death for Hispanic males ages 15 to 34. Among Hispanic ethnic subgroups in the United States, Puerto Rican adults have the highest rates of suicide attempts. Hispanics born in the United States have higher rates of suicidal ideation and attempts than Hispanic immigrants (Suicide Prevention Resource Center [SPRC], 2013a).

Suicide is the eighth leading cause of death for American Indians/Alaska Natives of all ages and the second leading cause of death among youth ages 10 to 24. Men and women ages 35 to 64 had a greater percentage increase in suicide rates between 1999 and 2012 than any other racial/ethnic group. Lifetime rates of having attempted suicide reported by adolescents ranged from 15.8% in girls to 11.8% in boys. Adolescent suicide attempts are significantly higher among youth (both sexes) raised on reservations (17.6%) compared to youth raised in urban areas (14.3%). Whereas exposure to suicide and access to alcohol and drugs contribute to suicide rates for Native Americans, family support and cultural and tribal orientation are protective (SPRC, 2013b).

The scant literature on suicide among Asian populations shows that suicide ideation, plans, and attempts are more common than popularly believed and vary within Asian ethnic groups. For example Native Hawaiians living in Hawaii who were between the ages of 15 and 44 had a significantly higher suicide death rate than other racial/ethnic groups, but those over 45 had a much lower rate than Whites, the same rate as Japanese, and a higher rate than Filipinos. Asians who immigrated to the United States as children have higher rates of suicidal ideation and suicide attempts than U.S. born Asians. Cultural identification with the Asian culture (sense of belonging and affiliation with spiritual, material, intellectual, and emotional features) is associated with a 69% reduction in the risk of suicide attempt (SPRC, 2013c).

The reasons for racial and ethnic variations are unclear. The rates of depressive disorder, a major risk factor for suicide, vary across racial group. Cultural stress, perceived discrimination, and vulnerability are thought to contribute to the risk of suicide (Gomez, Miranda, & Polanco, 2011).

Etiology

The convergence of biologic, psychological, and social factors can be directly linked to suicidal behavior. In genetically and physiologically vulnerable individuals, thoughts, feelings, and personality factors can interfere with personal problem solving, promote impulsivity, and support suicidal behavior. Poverty, unemployment, and social conflict also contribute to suicidal behavior in those at risk for suicide.

Biologic Theories

Depression and severe childhood trauma are linked to suicide. Those who complete suicide often have extremely low levels of the neurotransmitter serotonin. Impairments in the serotonergic system contribute to suicidal behavior. Additionally, people who make near-lethal suicide attempts have much lower levels of the neurotransmitter dopamine and noradrenaline (Fernandez-Navarro et al., 2012).

Physiological Effects of Child Abuse

Child abuse has been described as a specific vulnerability for psychopathology and suicide. Enhanced vulnerability to depressive disorder and suicide associated with child abuse apparently is attributable to altered serotonin and dopamine metabolism and subsequent hypothalamic–pituitary–adrenal dysregulation that occurs coincident with the intractable stress of the abuse experience (Guillaume et al., 2013). Twin studies further establish the independent contribution of childhood sexual abuse to biologic alterations that lead to suicidal behavior in adolescence and adults in genetically vulnerability individuals (Roy, Sarchiopone, & Carli, 2009).

Genetic Factors

Suicide runs in families. First-degree relatives of individuals who have completed suicide have a two to eight times higher risk for suicide than do individuals in the general population. Suicide of a first-degree relative is highly predictive of a serious attempt in another first-degree relative. Children of depressed and suicidal parents have higher rates of suicidal behavior themselves. The genetic link to suicide is evident in twin studies. Suicidal behavior has a 50% concordance for completed suicide (Tidemalm et al., 2011).

Psychological Theories

Cognitive Theories

Most evidence on the psychological contributions to suicidal behavior point to cognitive, affective, behavioral, and personality factors that intensify the experience of hopelessness and disconnection from others. Aaron Beck first identified the cognitive triad of hopelessness, helplessness, and worthlessness as integral to the experience of depression (Beck, Rush, Shaw, & Emery, 1979). Since then, a significant evidence base has been established linking hopelessness, loneliness, and other cognitive symptoms to suicide (van Dulmen & Goossens, 2013). Depressed persons who are hopeless are more likely to consider suicide than those who are depressed but hopeful about the future. Furthermore, it appears that lack of positive thoughts about the future is more likely to predict suicidal behavior than negative thoughts even though both contribute to hopelessness (Zhang & Li, 2013). The importance of specific cognitive symptoms to suicide risk varies by age and the suicide attempt history of the individual.

> **KEYCONCEPT** **Hopelessness** is the pervasive belief that undesirable events are likely to occur coupled with the belief that one's situation is unlikely to improve (Ellis & Rutherford, 2008).

Emotional factors and personality traits also play a role in suicidal behavior by enhancing perceptions of helplessness and hopelessness, contributing to poor self-esteem, and interfering with coping efforts. Shame, guilt, despair, and emotion-focused coping have been linked to suicidal behavior (Guerreiro, Cruz, Frasquilho, Santos, Figueira, & Sampaio, 2013; Upthegrove, Ross, Brunet, McCollum, & Jones, 2014). Loss and grief are also important considerations. Emotional distress often is potentiated by personality traits such as in borderline personality disorder (see Chapter 22) that contribute to poor self esteem, impulsivity, and suicidal behavior. Poor self-esteem in turn has been linked to suicide ideation, attempts, and deaths (Capron, Norr, Macatee, & Schmidt, 2013).

Interpersonal–Psychological Theory of Suicidal Behavior

The interpersonal–psychological theory of suicidal behavior (Joiner & Van Orden, 2008; Joiner, et al., 2009) provides a basis for discriminating between those who are thinking about suicide versus those who are likely to engage in suicidal acts. The theory postulates that those most at risk are those who have engaged in previous acts of self-harm, believe they are alienated from social relationships, and perceive themselves to be a burden to those they love. Together these beliefs lead to the misperception that others would be better off without them and the idea that sacrificing themselves is the appropriate action to take. Additionally, recent evidence suggests that over arousal for someone who has developed the capacity for suicide can be particularly significant in identifying potential suicide victims (Ribeiro, Silva, & Joiner, 2014).

Social Theories

Before the turn of the 20th century, Emile Durkheim (1897) linked suicide to the social conditions in which people live. Both a lack of social connectedness and social conditions contribute to suicidal behavior. People who are socially connected are less likely to engage in suicidal behavior. When an individual has others he or she can depend on, suicide can be prevented, even among those at significant risk. Even among people with social bonds, however, lack of community and social resources can interact with physiological and psychological risk to increase the likelihood of suicide.

Social Distress

A lack of social connection contributes to suicide ideation, attempts, and deaths across the age span. Among adults, those who are single, never married, separated, widowed, and homeless without religious affiliation report loneliness or otherwise are socially isolated are also more likely to engage in suicidal behavior (Mezuk, Rock, Lohman, & Choi, 2014; Séquin, Beauchamp, Robert, Dimambro, & Turecki, 2014). Being socially connected, however, does not in itself reduce risk. Interpersonal conflict and being a victim of bullying can contribute to suicidal behavior, especially in adolescents and young adults (Messias, Kindrick, & Castro, 2014).

Suicide Contagion

Social exposure to suicide is associated with an increased personal risk for suicidal behavior, particularly among adolescents. Suicide behavior that occurs after the suicide death of a known other is called **suicide contagion** or cluster suicide. Suicide contagion seems to work through modeling and is more likely to occur when the individual contemplating suicide is of the same age, gender, and background as the person who died. Contagion can be prompted by the suicide of a friend, an acquaintance, online social networking, or an idolized celebrity. Actions of peer groups, media reports of suicide, and even billboards with content about suicide can trigger suicide behavior among adolescents (Robertson, Skegg, Poore, Williams, & Taylor, 2012). In the case of a celebrity suicide, the number of "copycat suicides" is proportional to the amount, duration, and prominence of media coverage (Ju, Young, Seok, & Yip, 2014). Evidence suggests that adolescents also can be influenced by simple individual and community suicide prevention efforts (Robertson et al., 2012).

Economic Disadvantage

Poverty and economic disadvantage are associated with depression, suicide ideation, and suicide mortality. Individuals who are not employed, not married, and with low education and low income have a higher risk of suicide. Suicide risk is greater for low income females in socially deprived areas and males living alone in materially deprived areas (Burrows, Auger, Gamache, & Hamel, 2013). Adolescents from impoverished neighborhoods have more suicidal ideation and attempts, and suicides increase as the percentage of boarded-up buildings in a neighborhood increases, particularly if the individuals have a mental disorder (Page et al., 2014).

In impoverished communities, lack of good schools and employment opportunities lead to unemployment and loss of meaningful social roles. Low-income men are at risk for suicide when they lose their jobs, especially when their wives obtain jobs to support their families (Ying & Chang, 2009). Additionally, access to health care is limited in these communities, and there is an increased exposure to others exhibiting suicidal be- havior that enhances suicide risk (Bernburg, Thorlindsson, & Sigfusdottir, 2009).

Family Response to Suicide

Suicide has devastating effects on everyone it touches, especially family and close friends. One suicide is estimated to leave at least six survivors who are significantly impacted by the loss (Andriessen & Krysinska, 2012). In the aftermath of a family member's suicide, survivors experience more grief, anxiety and depression, guilt, shame, self-blame, and dysfunction than families whose loss was because of other reasons and the personal and familial disruption often lasts for years. Although recovery from a loved one's suicide is an ongoing task, survivors who are emotionally healthy before the suicide act and who have social support are able to manage the psychological trauma associated with suicide. Still, the intensity and duration of the postsuicide grief process for many survivors has led to the development of family intervention programs. Although the evidence base for these interventions is still small, strategies that support a positive sense of self, enhance problem-solving, promote the formation of a suicide story, encourage social reintegration, reduce stigma, use journaling, or permit the survivor to debrief may be effective in reducing subjective distress and to resolve grief (Andriessen & Krysinska, 2012; Buus, Caspersen, Hansen, Stenager, & Fleischer, 2013). These strategies may be most effective delivered in survivor peer help groups.

TREATMENT AND NURSING CARE FOR SUICIDE PREVENTION

Interdisciplinary Treatment and Recovery

The challenges of preventing suicides and promoting healthy coping belong to all disciplines. An interdisciplinary treatment or recovery approach along with peer support is needed for managing the threats of suicide.

Priority Care Issues

| **EMERGENCY CARE ALERT** *!* A true psychiatric emergency exists when an individual presents with one or more symptoms associated with imminent risk for suicidal behavior. Immediate and focused action is needed to prevent the patient's death.

The first priority is to provide for the patient's safety while initiating the *least* restrictive care possible. In contrast, an example of the *most* restrictive care is an outpatient who is admitted to a locked unit with one staff member who is assigned to observe the person at all times. Hospitalization should be reserved for those whose safety cannot be ensured in an outpatient environment.

NURSING CARE: Preventing Suicide and Promoting Mental Health

Suicidal ideation, planning, and acts are not easily predicted and therefore are difficult to study. As a result, few evidence-based treatments exist that are known to prevent suicide and manage suicidal behavior. There is growing consensus that the suicidal act is part of a continuum of behaviors that extend long before and after a specific suicide behavioral incident. The beginning evidence points to four steps in preventing suicide and promoting long-term mental health: identification of those thinking about suicide (case finding), assessment to determine an imminent suicidal threat, intervening to change suicidal behavior associated with a specific suicidal threat, and institution of effective interventions to prevent future episodes of suicidal behavior (Catanese, John, Di Battista, & Clarke, 2009).

Assessment

Case Finding

Case finding refers to identifying people who are at risk for suicide so proper treatment can be initiated. People who are contemplating suicide often do not share their ideation. This lack of disclosure often means that family, friends, and health professionals are unable to intervene until the suicidal ideation and planning have progressed. Yet early identification of suicidal ideation may reduce suicide deaths. Nurses can play important roles in suicide prevention by recognizing the warning signs. See Box 15.3 for the warning signs developed by the American Association of Suicidology (2014); the mnemonic IS PATH WARM can serve as a useful memory aide for these signs.

Case finding requires careful and concerned questioning and listening that make the patient feel valued and cared about (Box 15.4). Most standardized health questionnaires have questions about suicide thoughts.

BOX 15.3

Warning Signs for Suicide

I—Ideation: Talking or writing about death, dying, or suicide
Threatening or talking of wanting to hurt or kill self
Looking for ways to kill self: seeking access to firearms, available pills, or other means
S—Substance abuse: Increased substance (alcohol or drug) use
P—Purposelessness: No perceived reason for living; no sense of purpose in life
A—Anxiety: Anxiety, agitation, unable to sleep or sleeping all the time
T—Trapped: Feeling trapped (like there is no way out)
H—Hopelessness
W—Withdrawal: Withdrawal from friends, family, and society
A—Anger: Rage, uncontrolled anger, seeking revenge
R—Recklessness: Acting reckless or engaging in risky activities, seemingly without thinking
M—Mood change: Dramatic mood changes

Adapted from American Association of Suicidology. (2014). *Know the warning signs.* Retrieved from http://www.suicidology.org/web/guest/stats-and-tools/warning-signs.

Many nurses are concerned that asking patients about their suicidal thoughts will provoke a suicide attempt. This belief simply is not true. The patient expressing suicidal ideation often has had these thoughts for some time and may feel more socially connected when another recognizes the seriousness of the situation. Under no circumstances should a patient be promised secrecy about suicidal thoughts, plans, or acts. Instead, tell patients that disclosure of suicidal intent will be shared with other interdisciplinary team members so the safety of the patient can be ensured.

Assessing Risk

After suicide ideation has been established, the next step is to determine the risk for a suicide attempt. Suicide risk assessment is difficult and whenever possible should proceed only with the assistance of other members of the interdisciplinary treatment team. Assessing for risk includes determining the seriousness of the suicidal ideation, degree of hopelessness, disorders, previous attempt, suicide planning and implementation, and availability and lethality of suicide method. Risk assessment also includes the patient's resources, including coping skills and social supports, that can be used to counter suicidal impulses. Box 15.5 lists some questions that might be asked in assessing the risk for suicide.

The greatest predictor of a future suicide attempt is a previous attempt, partly because the individual already has broken the "taboo" around suicidal behavior. Repeated episodes of self-harm with or without suicidal intent also increase immediate risk because they increase an individual's capacity to complete suicide (Ribeiro et al., 2014). Other important signs of high risk are the presence of

BOX 15.4 • THERAPEUTIC DIALOGUE • Suicide

When Caroline sought medical care for a cold from her nurse practitioner, the nurse observed more than a cough and runny nose. Caroline appeared downcast and unusually sad. As the nurse and patient talked, the subject of family life came up, whereupon Caroline began to cry softly. As words tumbled out, she said she had been unhappy at home for a long time. When she was very young, she recalled being happy, but things changed when her brother was born, 4 years after her. Her father began to abuse her sexually, starting when Caroline was 5 years old and continuing until he moved out of the house when she was 12 years old. Caroline suspects her mother knew of the abuse, although she did nothing about it.

Two years ago, Caroline's father committed suicide. Caroline feels relieved about his death but frustrated that she never got a chance to tell him how angry she was with him. Caroline's relationship with her mother has not improved. Caroline says her mother favors her brother and is always telling her she won't amount to anything. Caroline begins to cry harder.

INEFFECTIVE APPROACH

Nurse: Clearly, many things are troubling you. Don't you think that things seem worse now because you have a cold?

Caroline: Well, that could be. What are you going to do to make me feel better?

Nurse: Give you some medicine to help you sleep and clear your nose. I think you should see a psychiatrist, too.

Caroline: I don't need a psychiatrist. I came here for my cold.

Nurse: I know you did, but you seem to be depressed.

Caroline: What are you, some kind of social worker? I am just tired.

Nurse: I am a nurse, and you seem down to me. Are you thinking about suicide?

Caroline: I don't think you know what you're talking about. I want to go now. Could you give me my medicine?

EFFECTIVE APPROACH

Nurse: It seems as though many things have been piling up on you. Does it seem that way to you, too?

Caroline: It sure does. I've just been trying to get through one day at a time, but now with this cold and no sleep, I feel like I can't go on.

Nurse: When you say you can't go on, what does that mean to you?

Caroline: Lately, I have been thinking about running away to some place where I can't be found and maybe starting over. But then I think, where would I go? Where would I stay? Who would take care of me?

Nurse: When you think that your plan for escape won't work, what happens?

Caroline: (Starting to cry again.) Then I think that maybe it would be better if I just did what my father did. I really don't think anyone would miss me.

Nurse: So you think you might take your life, like your Dad did?

Caroline: Yeah, and what really scares me is lately I have been thinking about that a lot. I keep saying to myself, "You're just tired," but I am so exhausted now that I can't chase the thoughts away.

Nurse: So, do you think about suicide every day?

Caroline: It seems like I never stop thinking about it.

Nurse: Is there anything you can do to make the thoughts go away?

Caroline: Nothing. (Silence.)

Nurse: What would you do?

Caroline: I think I would get as many pills as I could find, drink a lot of alcohol, and maybe smoke some pot and just go to sleep.

Nurse: Do you have enough pills at home to kill yourself?

Caroline (wan smile): I was hoping that the sleeping medicine you would give me might do the job.

Nurse: It sounds like you need some help getting through this time in your life. Would you like some?

Caroline: I honestly don't know—I just want to sleep for a long time.

CRITICAL THINKING CHALLENGE

- In the first interaction, the nurse made two key blunders. What were they? What effect did they have on the patient? How did they interfere with the patient's care?

- What did Caroline do that might have contributed to the nurse's behavior in the first interaction?

- In the second interaction, the nurse did several things that ensured reporting of Caroline's suicidal ideation. What were they? What differences in attitude might differentiate the nurse in the first interaction from the nurse in the second?

BOX 15.5

Assessment of Suicidal Episode

INTENT TO DIE
1. Have you been thinking about hurting or killing yourself?
2. How seriously do you want to die?
3. Have you attempted suicide before?
4. Are there people or things in your life who might keep you from killing yourself?

SEVERITY OF IDEATION
1. How often do you have these thoughts?
2. How long do they last?
3. How much do the thoughts distress you?
4. Can you dismiss them or do they tend to return?
5. Are they increasing in intensity and frequency?

DEGREE OF PLANNING
1. Have you made any plans to kill yourself? If yes, what are they?
2. Do you have access to the materials (e.g., gun, poison, pills) that you plan to use to kill yourself?
3. How likely is it that you could actually carry out the plan?
4. Have you done anything to put the plan into action?
5. Could you stop yourself from killing yourself?

suicide planning behaviors (detailed plan, availability of means, opportunity, and capability) and engaging in final acts such as giving away prized possessions and saying goodbye to loved ones. Although the presence of a specific psychiatric disorder such as depression is an important consideration in risk assessment, anxiety, agitation, alcohol use, and impulsivity may be better indicators of immediate risk. On the other hand, support from important others, religious prohibitions, responsibility for young children, and employment may provide protection from suicidal impulses.

Ideally, an interdisciplinary team conducts suicide risk assessment in an emergency department or outpatient facility with multiple supports. Nurses practicing in more isolated situations should keep a list of contacts in settings that routinely conduct suicide risk assessments so the contacts may be consulted if a seriously suicidal individual appears in the nurse's setting.

NCLEXNOTE Suicide assessment is always considered a priority. Practice by asking patients about suicidal thoughts and plans. Develop a plan with a suicidal patient that focuses on resisting the suicidal impulse. Apply the assessment process that delineates the (1) intent to die, (2) severity of ideation, (3) availability of means, and (4) degree of planning.

Nursing Diagnoses and Outcome Identification

Several nursing diagnoses may be applied when dealing with a suicidal patient, including Risk for Suicide, Interrupted Family Processes, Anxiety, Ineffective Health Maintenance, Risk for Self-Directed Violence, Impaired Social Interaction, Ineffective Coping, Chronic Low Self-Esteem, Insomnia, Social Isolation, and Spiritual Distress.

Interventions for Imminent, Intermediate, and Long-Term Suicide Prevention

Interventions for Those at Imminent Risk

There are three urgent priorities for care of a person who is at imminent risk for suicide: reconnecting the patient to other people and instilling hope, restoring emotional stability and reducing suicidal behavior, and ensuring safety. Reconnecting the patient interpersonally includes listening intently and without judgment to the patient's thoughts and feelings and validating his or her experience and suffering. This intervention directly challenges the patient's belief that no one cares. Using cognitive interventions can help the client to regain hope (see Chapter 9). These actions help reestablish links between the patient's presuicidal past and helps the patient begin establishing goals for the future (Gudmundsdottir & Thome, 2014).

Ensuring Patient Safety

Helping patients develop strategies for making safer choices when distressed is an important goal. Nurses caring for patients who are emerging from the initial hours and days of a suicide attempt can support the patient and focus on managing suicidal urges and developing protective strategies. As the nurse connects with the patient, together they can create a list of personal and professional resources that can be used when the individual is in crisis. With the nurse's help, the patient can visualize "emotional spaces that are safe places to go" when distressed.

Until recently, the no-suicide contract was a staple of psychiatric nursing practice and widely used across disciplines as a means of preventing suicide among those at risk. No-suicide contracts are verbal and written "contracts" between the individual at imminent risk for suicide and a health care provider that contain an agreement that the patient will not commit suicide during a specific time period. Careful evaluation of this practice has not established its efficacy in preventing suicidal behavior and suicide deaths. As a consequence, the nurse should avoid engaging in a no-suicide contract with a patient (Puskar & Urda, 2011).

Inpatient Safety Considerations

When hospitalization is considered the best option to ensure the safety of the patient, the nurse has responsibility for providing a safe, therapeutic environment in which human connection, instilling hope, and changing suicidal behavior can occur. There are no evidence-based guidelines for preventing suicides in hospitals. Inpatient suicides do occur. Between January 1995 and June 30,

2008, 641 of 5,208 sentinel events (12.3%) were inpatient suicides (Janofsky, 2009), a rate that continues to present challenges for the inpatient nursing staff. The vast majority of inpatient suicides take place in psychiatric facilities, and the method used in 75% of these events is hanging (Tishler & Reiss, 2009).

Removal of dangerous items and environmental hazards, continuous or intermittent observation of at-risk patients by hospital personnel trained in observation methods, and limitation of outpatient passes are the mainstays of hospital interventions. Observation procedures vary from facility to facility. For patients who require constant supervision, a staff member will be assigned only to the high-risk patient. For less risky patients, observation may entail close or intermittent observations.

Observation is not, in itself, therapeutic. An observation becomes therapeutic when interaction occurs with the patient. Psychiatric intensive care of this kind and restriction of freedom can be very upsetting to the patient who is withdrawn and isolated. Nurses can help patients reestablish personal control by including them in decisions about their care and restricting their behavior only as necessary. Nurses can also reduce the patient's stress while ensuring the patient's safety by intruding as little as possible on the person's exercise of free will. Observational periods can be used to help patients express a broad range of feelings and strengthen their belief in their own abilities to keep themselves safe. During observation, the nurse can help the patient describe feelings and identify ways to manage safety needs.

Interventions for Intermediate and Long-Term Risk

Patients who are suicidal may need ongoing preventive interventions. The risk varies with the genetic, psychiatric, and psychological profile of the patient and the extent of his or her social support. Discouragement and hopelessness often persist long past the suicidal episode. Episodes of hopelessness should be anticipated and planned for in the patient's care. Patients should be taught to expect setbacks and times when they are unable to see much of a future for themselves. They should be encouraged to think of times in their lives when they were not so hopeless and consider how they may feel similarly in the future. Helping patients review the goals they already have achieved and at the same time set goals that can be achieved in the immediate future can help them manage periods of discouragement and hopelessness.

Interventions for the Biologic Domain

Patients who have survived a suicide attempt often need physical care of their self-inflicted injury. Overdose, gunshot wounds, and skin wounds are common. For both groups, there will be biologic interventions for the underlying psychiatric disorder (see Unit 6).

Medication Management

Medication management focuses on treating the underlying psychiatric disorder. In schizophrenia and schizoaffective disorder, evidence suggests that antipsychotic use is related to decreased mortality compared with those not taking an antipsychotic, but only clozapine has been shown to have a protective effect (De Hert, Corell, & Cohen, 2010). For depression, a nonlethal antidepressant, such as a selective serotonin reuptake inhibitor, usually will be prescribed.

Electroconvulsive Therapy

Electroconvulsive therapy (ECT) has been used in both inpatient and outpatient settings to alleviate severe depression, especially in medically compromised groups such older adults, who may not tolerate conventional pharmacotherapy for depression (see Chapter 10). Rapid reduction in depression often leads to a decreased suicide drive (Fink, 2014). More research is needed to determine the role ECT may play in managing suicidal behavior. At this time, ECT is among several strategies used to decrease suicidal behavior over the long term.

Interventions for the Psychological Domain

The goals of treatment in the psychological domain include reducing the capacity for suicidal behavior, increasing tolerance for distress, expanding coping abilities, and developing effective crisis management strategies. During the early part of a hospitalization, the most important way to reduce stress is to help the patient feel more secure and hopeful. As patients become more comfortable in their environment, the nurse can provide education about emotions, help patients explore and link presuicidal beliefs to a positive and hopeful future, support the application of new skills in managing negative thoughts, and help develop effective problem-solving skills.

Challenging the Suicidal Mindset

Teaching patients to distract themselves when thinking about suicide or engaging in negative self-evaluation can help to diminish suicidal ideation, dysfunctional thinking, and emotional reactivity. Simple distracting techniques such as reminding oneself to think of other things or engaging in other activities such as talking on the telephone, reading, or watching a movie are excellent temporary means of distracting the patient from negative cognitive states. See Boxes 15.6 and 15.7 for additional

Psychoeducation Checklist: Suicide Prevention

When teaching the patient and family about suicide and its prevention, be sure to address the following topics:

- Importance of emotional connections to family and friends
- Importance of instilling hope
- Discouraging suicidal ideation, rumination, self-harming behaviors
- Self-validation
- Emotional distress management
- Finding alternatives to suicidal behavior
- Establishing and using a crisis management plan
- Reestablishing the social network of the patient
- Information about treatment of underlying psychiatric disorders

information for educating patients and their families about suicide prevention.

Validating the patient and teaching the patient to self-validate are powerful means of reducing suicidal thinking. Patients can learn that everyone experiences emotional distress and can begin to recognize it a routine

BOX 15.7
Educational Resources for Suicidal Patients and Families

Biebel, D. B., & Foster, S. L. (2005). *Finding your way after the suicide of someone you love.* Grand Rapids, MI: Zondervan Publishing Company.

Bryson, K. (2006). *Those they left behind: Interviews, stories, essays, and poems by survivors of suicide.* Raleigh, NC: Lulu.com.

Colt, G. (2006). *November of the soul: The enigma of suicide.* New York: Scribner.

Conroy, D. (2006). *Out of the nightmare: Recovery from depression and suicidal pain.* Lincoln, NE: Authors Choice Press.

Crook, M. (2004). *Out of the darkness: Teens talk about suicide.* Vancouver, British Columbia: Arsenal Pulp Press.

Fox, J., & Roldan, M. (2008). *Voices of strength: Sons and daughters of suicide speak out.* Far Hills, NJ: New Horizon Press.

Hays, H. (2005). *Surviving suicide: Help to heal your heart.* Dallas: Brown Books Publishing Group.

Joiner, T. (2005). *Why people die by suicide.* Cambridge: Harvard University Press.

Linn-Gust, M. (2010). *Rocky roads: The journeys of families through suicide grief.* Albuquerque, NM: Chellehead Works.

Lukas, C., & Seiden, H. (2007). *Silent grief: Living in the wake of suicide.* Philadelphia: Jessica Kingsley Publishers.

Myers, M., & Fine, C. (2006). *Touched by suicide: Hope and healing after loss.* New York: Gotham Publishing.

Nelson, R., Galas, J., & Cobain, B. (2006). *The power to prevent suicide: A guide for teens helping teens.* St. Paul, MN: Free Spirit Publishing.

Requarth, M. (2008). *After a parent's suicide: Helping children heal.* Sebastopol, CA: Healing Hearts Press.

Robinson, D. (2008). *Suicide is not a dirty word.* Glasgow, Scotland: SHN publishers.

Rogers, D. (2007). *My child's final act: Suicide.* Frederick, MD: PublishAmerica.

event. To manage emotional distress and increase tolerance for it, patients can be taught simple anxiety management strategies such as relaxation and visualization. The patient can be encouraged to write about his or her emotional experiences.

Patients engage in suicidal behavior because they view it as their only option. When negative thoughts and emotions coexist, they reinforce each other and contribute to hopelessness, which in turn increases the likelihood of a serious suicidal attempt (Catanese et al., 2009). Individuals who are suicidal often believe they are a burden to their family, who would be better off without them. Nurses can challenge negative beliefs, especially the patient's idea that he or she is a burden to others. Ask the patient to describe the events that led to specific suicidal behavior so the patient can be engaged in developing alternative solutions. For each event, work with the patient to identify specific strategies that could be used to manage his or her distress, sense of disconnection, extreme focus on suicidal ideas, and other experiences that led the person to believe he or she had no option other than to die.

Developing New Coping Strategies

Preventing suicidal behavior requires that patients develop crisis management strategies, generate solutions to difficult life circumstances other than suicide, engage in effective interpersonal interactions, and maintain hope. The nurse can help the patient develop a written plan that can be used as a blueprint for action when the patient feels like he or she is losing control. The plan should include strategies that the patient can use to self-soothe; friends and family members that could be called, including multiple phone numbers where they can be reached; self-help groups and services such as suicide hotlines; and professional resources, including emergency departments and outpatient emergency psychiatric services.

Commitment to Treatment

Patients are usually ambivalent about wanting to die. The **commitment to treatment statement** (CTS) directly addresses ambivalence about treatment by asking the patient to engage in treatment by making a commitment to try new approaches. Different from the no-suicide contract, the CTS does not restrict the patient's rights regarding the option of suicide. Instead, the patient agrees to engage in treatment and access emergency service if needed. Underlying the CTS is the expectation that the patient will communicate openly and honestly about all aspects of treatment, including suicide. This commitment is written and signed by the patient. The efficacy of this approach has yet to be established by systematic research. Whether using the CTS or other means, be observant for lapses in the patient's participation in treatment and discuss them with the patient and other members of the interdisciplinary team.

Interventions for the Social Domain

Poor social skills may interfere with the patient's ability to engage others. The nurse should assess the patient's social capability early in treatment and make necessary provisions for social skills training. The interpersonal relationship with the nurse is an ideal place to begin shaping social behaviors that will help the patient to establish a social network that will sustain him or her during periods of discouragement or crisis. Participation in support networks such as recovery groups, clubhouses, drop-in centers, self-help groups, or other therapeutic social engagement will help the patient become connected to others.

Patients need to anticipate that even some of the people closest to them will feel uncomfortable with their suicidal behavior. Helping the patient to anticipate the stigmatizing behavior of others and how to manage it will go far in reintegrating the patient into a supportive social community. The nurse can also explore the patient's participation in specific social activities such as attending church or community activities.

Evaluation and Treatment Outcomes

The most desirable treatment outcome is the patient's recovery with no future suicide attempts. Short-term outcomes include maintaining the patient's safety, averting suicide, and mobilizing the patient's resources. Whether the patient is hospitalized or cared for in the community, his or her emotional distress must be reduced. Long-term outcomes must focus on maintaining the patient in psychiatric treatment, enabling the patient and family to identify and manage suicidal crises effectively, and widening the patient's support network.

Continuum of Care

Whether the suicide prevention plan is instituted in the hospital or in an outpatient setting, the patient cannot be released to home until a workable plan of care is in place. The care plan includes scheduling an appointment for outpatient treatment, providing for continuing somatic treatments until the first outpatient treatment visit, ensuring post-release contact between the patient and significant other, providing for access to emergency psychiatric care, and arranging the patient's environment so it provides both structure and safety.

At the first follow-up visit, the patient and health care provider can establish a plan of care that specifies the intensity of outpatient care. Very unstable patients may need frequent supervision (e.g., telephone or face-to-face meetings or both) in the early days after hospitalization to maintain the patient's safety in the community. These contacts often can be short; their purpose is to convey the ongoing concern and caring of professionals involved in the patient's care. In arranging outpatient care, be certain to refer the patient to a provider who can provide the intensity of care the patient may need.

The patient's outpatient environment should be made as safe as possible before discharge. The nurse must share the care plan with family members so they can remove any objects in the patient's environment that could be used to engage in self-harm. The nurse should explain this measure to the patient to reinforce his or her sense of self-control. It is important to be reasonable in deciding what to remove from the environment. Patients who are truly determined to kill themselves after discharge will succeed in doing so, using whatever means are available.

Documentation and Reporting

The nurse must thoroughly document encounters with suicidal patients. This action is for the patient's ongoing treatment and the nurse's protection. Lawsuits for malpractice in psychiatric settings often involve completed suicides. The medical record must reflect that the nurse took every reasonable action to provide for the patient's safety.

The record should describe the patient's history, assessment, and interventions agreed upon by the patient and nurse. The nurse should document the presence or absence of suicidal thoughts, intent, plan, and available means to illustrate the patient's current and ongoing suicide risk. If the patient denies any suicidal ideation, it is important that the denial is documented. Documentation must include any use of drugs, alcohol, or prescription medications by the patient during the 6 hours before the assessment. It should include the use of antidepressants that are especially lethal (e.g., tricyclics), as well as any medication that might impair the patient's judgment (e.g., a sleep medication). Notes should reflect the level of the patient's judgment and ability to be a partner in treatment.

The documentation should reflect if any medications were prescribed, the dosages, and the number of pills dispensed. Notes should reflect the plan for ongoing treatment, including the time of the next appointment with the provider, instructions given to the patient about obtaining emergency care if needed, and the names of family members and friends who will act as supports if the patient needs them.

NURSES' REFLECTION

Caring for suicidal patients is highly stressful and can lead to secondary trauma for the nurse. Nurses who care for suicidal patients must regularly share their experiences and feelings with one another. Talking about how the situations or actions of patients make them feel will help alleviate symptoms of stress. Some nurses find outpatient therapy helpful because it enhances their understanding of what situations are most likely to trigger secondary trauma. By demonstrating how to manage effectively the stressors in their own lives, nurses can be powerful role models for their patients.

SUMMARY OF KEY POINTS

- Suicide is a common and major public health problem.

- Suicide completion is more common in white men, especially older men.

- Parasuicide is more common among women than men.

- People who attempt suicide and fail are likely to try again without treatment.

- Suicidal behavior has genetic and biologic origins.

- A suicide assessment focuses on the intention to die, hopelessness, available means, previous attempts and self-harm behavior, and degree of planning.

- Patients who are in crisis, depressed, or use substances are at risk for suicide.

- The major objectives of brief hospital care are to maintain the patient's safety, reestablish the patient's biologic equilibrium, help the patient reconnect to others, instill hope, strengthen the patient's cognitive coping skills, and develop an outpatient support system.

- The nurse who cares for suicidal patients is vulnerable to secondary trauma and must take steps to maintain personal mental health.

CRITICAL THINKING CHALLENGES

1. A religious African American woman who lives with her three children, husband, and mother comes to her primary care provider. She is tearful and very depressed. What factors should be investigated to determine her risk for suicide and need for hospitalization?

2. A poor woman with no insurance is hospitalized after her third suicide attempt. Antidepressant medication is prescribed. What kinds of treatment will be most effective in preventing future suicidal behavior?

3. A young man enters his workplace inebriated and carrying a gun. He does not threaten anyone but says that he must end it all. Assuming that he can

be disarmed, what civil rights must be considered in taking further action in managing his suicidal risk?

4. You are a nurse in a large outpatient primary care setting responsible for an impoverished population. You want to implement a case-finding program for suicide prevention. Discuss how you would proceed and some potential problems you might face.

 Daughter of a Suicide: 1996 (Documentary). This personal documentary is the story of a woman whose mother committed suicide when the daughter was 18 years old. The daughter recounts the emotional struggle and depression left as the lifelong legacy of suicide and explores her efforts to heal. Combining digital video, 16-mm, and super-8 film, *Daughter of a Suicide* uses interviews with family and friends to tell the story of both mother and daughter.
Viewing Points: How does this movie show that the effects of suicide do not end with a person's death?

The Virgin Suicides: 1999. After the suicide death of their 13-year-old daughter Cecilia, the Lisbon family becomes recluses. The remaining daughters try to resume their life by defying the withdrawal of their parents. Unsuccessful, the movie climaxes with the suicide deaths of the three remaining teenage girls.
Viewing Points: What conditions in the girls family led the girls to take their lives?

Paradise Now: 2005. This movie traces the motivations of two suicide bombers in Palestine. It explores how the two young men came to the decision to kill themselves and others and their ambivalence about their impending deaths. Ultimately, one decides to live, and the movie ends with an ambiguous fate of the other. This movie provides insight into the background and troubled thoughts that precede a suicidal act.
Viewing Points: Can suicide be a political act? What other factors in these young men's lives might have contributed to their decision to volunteer as suicide bombers?

REFERENCES

American Association of Suicidology. (2014). *Understanding and helping the suicidal individual. Fact sheet.* Retrieved May 28, 2014, from http://www.suicidology.com.

American Foundation for Suicide Prevention. (2014). *Facts and figures. Understanding and preventing suicide through research, education, and advocacy.* Retrieved from http://www.afsp.org/understanding-suicide/facts-and-figures. Retrieved on May 24, 2014.

Ando, S., Kasai, K., Matamura, M., Hasegawa, Y., Hirakawa, H., Asukai, N. (2013). Psychosocial factors associated with suicidal ideation in clinical patients with depression. *Journal of Affective Disorders, 151*(2), 561–565.

Andriessen, K., & Krysinska, K. (2012). Essential questions on suicide bereavement and postvention. *International Journal of Environmental Research and Public Health, 9*(1), 24–32.

Anglemyer, A., Horvath, T., & Rutherford, G. (2014). The accessibility of firearms and risk for suicide and homicide victimization among household members. *Annals of Internal Medicine, 160*(2), 101–110.

Beck, A. T., Rush, A. J., Shaw, B. F., & Emery, G. F. (1979). *Cognitive therapy of depression*. New York: The Guildford Press.

Bernburg, J. G., Thorlindsson, T., & Sigfusdottir, I. D. (2009). The spreading of suicidal behavior: The contextual effect of community household poverty on adolescent suicidal behavior or/and the mediating. *Social Science & Medicine, 68*(2), 380–389.

Boyd, M. A., Bradshaw, W., & Robinson, M. (2013). Mental health issues of women deployed to Iraq and Afghanistan. *Archives of Psychiatric Nursing, 27*(1), 10–22.

Bryan, C. J., Corso, K. A., Rudd, M., & Cordero, L. (2008). Improving detection of suicidal patients in primary care through routine screening. *Primary Care & Community Psychiatry, 13*(4), 143–147.

Burrows, S., Auger, N., Gamache, P., & Hamel, D. (2013). Leading causes of unintentional injury and suicide mortality in Canadian adults across the urban-rural continuum. *Public Health Reports, 128*(6), 443–453.

Buus, N., Caspersen, J., Hansen, R., Stenager, E., & Fleischer, E. (2013). Experiences of parents whose sons or daughters have (had) attempted suicide. *Journal of Advanced Nursing, 70*(4), 823–832.

Capron, D. W., Norr, A. M., Macatee, R. J., & Schmidt, N. B. (2013). Distress tolerance and anxiety sensitivity cognitive concerns: Testing the incremental contributions of affect dysregulation constructs on suicidal ideation and suicide attempt. *Behavior Therapy, 44*(3), 349–358.

Catanese, A. A., John, M. S., Di Battista, J., & Clarke, D.M. (2009). Acute cognitive therapy in reducing suicide risk following a presentation to an emergency department. *Behaviour Change, 26*(1), 16–26.

Centers for Disease Control and Prevention, National Center for Injury Prevention and Control. (2014a). *Suicide facts at a glance* 2012. Retrieved May 25, 2014, from http://www.cdc.gov/violenceprevention/pdf/Suicide_DataSheet-a.pdf.

Center for Disease Control. (2014b). Surveillance for violent deaths - National Violent Death Reporting System, 16 states, 2010. *Morbidity and Mortality Weekly Report, 63*(1), 1–33.

De Hert, M., Correll, C. U., & Cohen, D. (2010). Do antipsychotic medications reduce or increase mortality in schizophrenia? A critical appraisal of the FIN-11 study. *Schizophrenia Research, 117*(1), 68–74.

De Leo, D., Draper, B. M., Snowdon, J., & Kolves, K. (2013). Suicides in older adults: A case-control psychological autopsy study in Australia. *Journal of Psychiatric Research, 47*(7), 980–988.

Durkheim, E. (1951 [1897]). *Suicide*. New York: Free Press.

Ellis, T. E., & Rutherford, B. (2008). Cognition and suicide: Two decades of progress. *International Journal of Cognitive Therapy, 1*(1), 47–68.

Fernández-Navarro, P., Vaquero-Lorenzo, C., Blasco-Fontecilla, H., Díaz-Hernández, M., Gratacòs, M., Estivill, X., et al. (2012). Genetic epistasis in female suicide attempters. *Progress in Neuro-Psychopharmacology & Biological Psychiatry, 38*(2), 294–301.

Fink, M. (2014). What was learned: Studies by the consortium for research in ECT (CORE) 1997-2011. *Acta Psychiatrica Scandinavia, 129*(6), 416–426.

Fredriksen-Goldsen, K. I., Emlet, C. A., Kim, H. J., Muraco, A., Erosheva, E. A., Goldsen, J., et al. (2013). The physical and mental health of lesbian, gay male, and bisexual (LGB) older adults: The role of key health indicators and risk and protective factors. *The Gerontologist, 53*(4), 664–675.

Goldston, D. B., Daniel, S. S., Erkanli, A., Reboussin, B. A., Mayfield, A., Frazier, P. H., & Treadway, S. L. (2009). Psychiatric diagnoses as contemporaneous risk factors for suicide attempts among adolescents and young adults: Developmental changes. *Journal of Consulting & Clinical Psychology, 77*(2), 281–290.

Gomez, J., Miranda, R., & Polanco, L. (2011). Acculturative stress, perceived discrimination, and vulnerability to suicide attempts among emerging adults. *Journal of Youth & Adolescence, 40*(11), 1465–1476.

Gudmundsdottir, R. M., & Thome, M. (2014). Evaluation of the effects of individual and group cognitive behavioural therapy and of psychiatric rehabilitation on hopelessness of depressed adults: A comparative analysis. *Journal of Psychiatric & Mental Health Nursing*, doi:10.1111/jpm.12157

Guerreiro, D. F., Cruz, D., Frasquilho, D., Santos, J. C., Figueira, M. L., & Sampaio, D. (2013). Association between deliberate self-harm and coping in adolescents: A critical review of the last 10 years' literature. *Archives of Suicide Research, 17*(2), 91–105.

Guillaume, S., Perroud, N., Jollant, F., Jaussent, I., Olie, E., Malafosse, A., et al. (2013). HPA axis genes may modulate the effect of childhood adversities on decision-making in suicide attempters. *Journal of Psychiatric Research, 47*(2), 259–265.

Hawkins, K. A., & Cougle, J. R. (2013). A test of the unique and interactive roles of anger experience and expression in suicidality: Findings from a population-based study. *Journal of Nervous & Mental Disease, 201*(11), 959–963.

Insel, T. (2010). The under-recognized public health crisis of suicide. *Director's posts about suicide prevention*. Retrieved September 10, 2010, from http://www.nimh.nih.gov/about/directo/index-suicide-prevention.shtml.

Janofsky, J. S. (2009). Reducing inpatient suicide risk: Using human factors analysis to improve observation practices. *Journal of the American Academy of Psychiatry and the Law, 37*(1), 15–24.

Joe, S., & Niedermeier, D. M. (2008). Social work research on African-Americans and suicidal behavior: A systematic 25 year review. *Health and Social Work, 33*(4), 249–257.

Joiner, T. E., & Van Orden, K. A. (2008). The interpersonal-psychological theory of suicidal behavior indicates specific and crucial psychotherapeutic targets. *International Journal of Cognitive Therapy, 1*(1), 80–89.

Joiner, T. E., Van Orden, K. A., Witte, T. K., Selby, E. garroutte A., Ribeiro, J. D., Lewis, R., & Rudd, M. D. (2009). Main predictions of the interpersonal-psychological theory of suicidal behavior: Empirical tests in two samples of young adults. *Journal of Abnormal Psychology, 118*(3), 634–646.

Ju, J. N., Young, L. W., Seok, N. M., & Yip, P. S. (2014). The impact of indiscriminate media coverage of a celebrity suicide on a society with a high suicide rate: Epidemiological findings on copycat suicides from South Korea. *Journal of Affective Disorders, 156*, 56–61. doi:10.1016/j.ad.2013.11.015

Kim, Y. R., Choi, K. H., Oh, Y., Lee, H. K., Kweon, Y. S., Lee, C.T., et al. (2011). Elderly suicide attempters by self-poisoning in Korea. *International Psychogeriatrics, 23*(6), 979–985.

Lewis, N. M. (2009). Mental health in sexual minorities: Recent indicators, trends, and their relationship to place in North American and Europe. *Health & Place, 15*(4), 1029–1045.

Liu, R. T., Kraines, M. A., Puzia, M. E., Massing-Schaffer, M., & Kleiman, E. M. (2013). Sociodemographic predictors of suicide means in a population-based surveillance system: Findings from the national violent Death Reporting system. *Journal of Affective Disorders, 151*(2), 449–454.

Marshal, M. P., Dermody, S. S., Cheong, J., Burton, C. M., Friedman, M. S., Aranda, F., et al. (2013). Trajectories of depressive symptoms and suicidality among heterosexual and sexual minority youth. *Journal of Youth and Adolescence, 42*(8), 1243–1256.

McCarthy, J. F., Blow, F. X., Ignacio, R. V., Ilgen, M. A., Austin, K. L., & Valenstein, M. (2012). Suicide among patients in the Veterans Affairs health system: Rural-urban differences in rates, risks, and methods. *American Journal of Public Health, 102*(suppl 1), 11–17.

Messias, E., Kindrick, K., & Castro, J. (2014). School bullying, cyberbullying, or both: Correlates of teen suicidality in the 2011 CDC youth risk behavior survey. *Comprehensive Psychiatry, doi:10.1016/comppsych.2014.02.005*

Mezuk, B., Rock, A., Lohman, M. C., & Choi, M. (2014). Suicide risk in long-term care facilities: A systematic review. *International Journal of Geriatric Psychiatry. doi:10.1002/gps.4142*

Mitchell, M. M., Gallaway, M. S., Millikan, A. M., & Bell, M. (2012). Interaction of combat exposure and unit cohesion in predicting suicide-related ideation among post-deployment soldiers. *Suicide & Life threatening Behavior, 42*(5), 486–494.

Mustanski, B., & Liu, R. T. (2013). A longitudinal study of predictors of suicide attempts among lesbian, gay, bisexual, and transgender youth. *Archives of Sexual Behavior, 42*(3), 437–448.

Murphy, N. A., Fatoye, F., & Wibberley, C. (2013). The changing face of newspaper representations of the mentally ill. *Journal of Mental Health, 22*(3), 271–282.

Page, A., Lewis, G., Kidger, J., Heron, J., Chittleborough, C., Evans, J., Gunnell, D. (2014). Parental socio-economic position during childhood as a determinant of self-harm in adolescence. *Social Psychiatry & Psychiatric Epidemiology, 49*(2), 193–203.

Paul, J. P., Catania, J., Pollack, L., Moskowitz, J., Conchola, J., Mills, T., et al. (2002). Suicide attempts among gay and bisexual men: Lifetime prevalence and antecedents. *American Journal of Public Health, 92*(8), 1338–1345.

Ploderi, M., Wagenmakers, E. J., Tremblay, P., Ramsay, R., Kralovec, K., Fartacek, C., et al. (2013). Suicide risk and sexual orientation: A critical review. *Archives of Sexual Behavior, 42*(5), 715–727.

Pompili, M., Innamorati, M., Gonda, X., Serafini, G., Sarno, S., Erbuto, D., et al. (2013). Affective temperaments and hopelessness as predictors of health and social functioning in mood disorder patients: A prospective follow-up study. *Journal of Affective Disorders, 150*(2), 216–222.

Puskar, K., & Urda, B. (2011). Examining the efficacy of no-suicide contracts in inpatient psychiatric settings: Implications for psychiatric nursing. *Issues in Mental Health Nursing, 32*(12), 785–788.

Ribeiro, J. D., Silva, C., & Joiner, T. E. (2014). Overarousal interacts with a sense of fearlessness about death to predict suicide risk in a sample of clinical outpatients. *Psychiatry Research, 218*, 106–112. *doi:10.1016/j.psychres.2014.03.036*

Robertson, L., Skegg, K., Poore, M., Williams, S., & Taylor, B. (2012). An adolescent suicide cluster and the possible role of electronic communication technology. *Crisis, 33*(4), 239–245.

Schmutte, T., O'Connell, M., Weiland, M., Lawless, S., & Davidson, L. (2009). Stemming the tide of suicide in older white men: A call to action. *American Journal of Men's Health, 3*(3), 189–200.

Séquin, M., Beauchamp, G., Robert, M., Dimambro, M., & Turecki, G. (2014). Developmental model of suicide trajectories. *British Journal of Psychiatry*. PMID: 24809398.

Selby, E. A., Yen, S., & Spirito, A. (2013). Time varying prediction of thoughts of death and suicidal ideation in adolescents: Weekly rating over 6-month follow-up. *Journal of Clinical Child & Adolescent Psychology, 42*(4), 481–495.

Stack, S., & Wasserman, I. (2009). Gender and suicide risk: The role of wound site. *Suicide and Life-Threatening Behavior, 39*(1), 13–20.

Suicide Prevention Resource Center (SPRC). (2013a). *Suicide among racial/ethnic populations in the U.S.: Hispanics*. Waltham, MA: Education Development Center, Inc.

Suicide Prevention Resource Center (SPRC). (2013b). *Suicide among racial/ethnic populations in the U.S.: American Indians/Alaska Natives*. Waltham, MA: Education Development Center, Inc.

Suicide Prevention Resource Center (SPRC). (2013c). *Suicide among racial/ethnic populations in the U.S.: Asians, Pacific Islanders, and Native Hawaiians*. Waltham, MA: Education Development Center, Inc.

Tidemalm, D., Runeson, B., Waern, M., Frisell, T., Carlstrom, E., Lichtenstein, P., et al. (2011). Familial clustering of suicide risk: A total population study of 11.4 million individuals. *Psychological Medicine, 41*(12), 2527–2534.

Tishler, C. L., & Reiss, N. S. (2009). Inpatient suicide: preventing a common sentinel event. *General Hospital Psychiatry, 31*(2), 103–109.

Upthegrove, R., Ross, K., Brunet, K., McCollum, R., & Jones, J. (2014). Depression in first episode psychosis: The role of subordination and shame. *Psychiatry Research, 217*(3), 177–184.

Ukrowicz, K. C., Ekblad, A. G. Cheavens, J. S., Rosenthal, M. Z., & Lynch, T. R. (2008). Coping and thought suppression as predictors of suicidal ideation in depressed older adults with personality disorders. *Aging and Mental Health, 12*(1), 149–157.

United States Department of Health and Human Services. (2010). *Healthy people 2020*. Retrieved from http://www.healthypeople.gov. Retrieved on May 25, 2014.

Valentiner, D. P., Gutierrez, P. M., & Blacker, D. (2002). Anxiety measures and their relationship to adolescent suicidal ideation and behavior. *Journal of Anxiety Disorders, 16*(1):11–32.

van Dulmen, M. H., & Goossens, L. (2013). *Loneliness trajectories, Journal of Adolescence, 36*(6), 1247–1249.

van Hooijdonk, C., Droomers, M., Deerenberg, I. M., Mackenbach, J. P., & Kunst, A. E. (2008). The diversity in associations between community social capital and health per health outcome, population group and location studied. *International Journal of Epidemiology, 27*(6), 1384–1392.

Van Orden, K. A., & Conwell, Y. (2011). Suicides in late life. *Current Psychiatry Reports*.

Wadsworth, T., & Kubrin, C. E. (2007). Hispanic suicide in U.S. metropolitan areas: Examining the effects of immigration, assimilation, affluence, and disadvantage. *American Journal of Sociology, 112*(6), 1848–1885.

Walsh, S., Clayton, R., Liu, L., & Hodges, S. (2009). Divergence in contributing factors for suicide among men and women in Kentucky: Recommendations to raise public awareness. *Public Health Reports, 124*(6), 861–867.

Wang, M. C., Lightsey, O. R., Tran, K. K., & Bonaparte, T. S. (2013). Examining suicide protective factors among black college students. *Death Studies, 37*(3), 228–247.

Webb, R. T., Marshall, C. E., & Abel, K. M. (2011). Teenage motherhood and risk of premature death: Long-term follow-up in the ONS longitudinal study. *Psychological Medicine, 41*(9), 1867–1877.

Ying, Y. H., & Chang, K. Y. (2009). A study of suicide and socioeconomic factors. *Suicide and Life-Threatening Behavior, 39*(2), 214–226.

Zhang, J., & Li, Z. (2013). The association between depression and suicide when hopelessness is controlled for. *Comprehensive Psychiatry, 54*(7), 790–796.

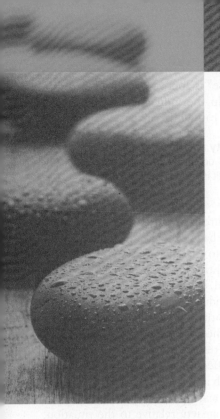

UNIT V
CARE AND RECOVERY FOR PERSONS WITH MENTAL HEALTH DISORDERS

16
Anxiety and Panic Disorders

Nursing Care of Persons with Anxiety and Panic

Judith M. Erickson and Mary Ann Boyd

KEY CONCEPTS

- anxiety
- panic

LEARNING OBJECTIVES

After studying this chapter, you will be able to:

1. Differentiate normal anxiety responses from those suggestive of an anxiety disorder.

2. Identify indicators for the four levels of anxiety and nursing interventions appropriate for each level.

3. Describe the prevalence and incidence of anxiety disorders.

4. Analyze theories of anxiety disorders.

5. Apply nursing process with recovery-oriented interventions for persons with anxiety and anxiety disorders.

KEY TERMS

- agoraphobia • anxiety • depersonalization • exposure therapy • flooding • implosive therapy • interoceptive conditioning • panic • panic attacks • panic control treatment • phobias • positive self-talk • reframing • specific phobia disorder • social anxiety disorder • systematic desensitization

Case Study: Doug

Doug is a 50-year-old man who lives with his wife Norma and two sons, Greg, a sophomore in college and Leon, a high school student. Norma was recently laid off from her job and has been unable to find employment. The family is now experiencing financial and marital problems. Leon was recently expelled from school for drug and alcohol use. Doug had an argument with his boss and is afraid that he will lose his job. He appears at the emergency department for chest pain and is convinced he is having a heart attack. All lab test results are normal. Consider how nurse can help Doug deal with his health issues.

INTRODUCTION

Anxiety is part of many emotional problems and mental disorders. At one time, most mental conditions with anxiety aspects were categorized as "anxiety disorders." Today, trauma–stressor-related disorder and obsessive-compulsive disorder (OCD), both previously identified as anxiety disorders, are now categorized as separate disorders (American Psychiatric Association [APA], 2013). This chapter discusses anxiety and anxiety disorders. Trauma and stressor-related disorders and dissociative disorders are discussed in Chapter 17 and obsessive-compulsive disorders in Chapter 18. In this chapter, panic disorder is also highlighted.

NORMAL VERSUS ABNORMAL ANXIETY RESPONSE

Anxiety is an unavoidable human condition that takes many forms and serves different purposes. Anxiety can be positive and can motivate one to act, or it can produce paralyzing fear, causing inaction. "Normal anxiety" is described as being of realistic intensity and duration for the situation and is followed by relief behaviors intended to reduce or prevent more anxiety (Peplau, 1989). A

"normal anxiety response" is appropriate to the situation and can be used to help the individual identify which underlying problem has caused the anxiety.

> **KEYCONCEPT** **Anxiety** is an uncomfortable feeling of apprehension or dread that occurs in response to internal or external stimuli; it can result in physical, emotional, cognitive, and behavioral symptoms.

During a perceived threat, rising anxiety levels cause physical and emotional changes in all individuals. A normal emotional response to anxiety consists of three parts: physiologic arousal, cognitive processes, and coping strategies. Physiologic arousal, or the fight-or-flight response, is the signal that an individual is facing a threat. Cognitive processes decipher the situation and decide whether the perceived threat should be approached or avoided. Coping strategies are used to resolve the threat. Box 16.1 summarizes many physical, affective, cognitive, and behavioral symptoms associated with anxiety. The factors that determine whether anxiety is a symptom of a mental disorder include the intensity of anxiety relative to the situation, the trigger for the anxiety, and the particular symptom clusters that manifest the anxiety. Table 16.1 describes the four degrees of anxiety and associated perceptual changes

TABLE 16.1 DEGREES OF ANXIETY		
Degree of Anxiety	**Effects on Perceptual Field and on Ability to Focus Attention**	**Observable Behavior**
Mild	Perceptual field widens slightly. Able to observe more than before and to see relationships (make connection among data). Learning is possible.	Is aware, alert; sees, hears, and grasps more than before. Usually able to recognize and identify anxiety easily.
Moderate	Perceptual field narrows slightly. Selective inattention: does not notice what goes on peripheral to the immediate focus but can do so if attention is directed there by another observer.	Sees, hears, and grasps less than previously. Can attend to more if directed to do so. Able to sustain attention on a particular focus; selectively inattentive to contents outside the focal area. Usually able to state, "I am anxious now."
Severe	Perceptual field is greatly reduced. Tendency toward dissociation: to not notice what is going on outside the current reduced focus of attention; largely unable to do so when another observer suggests it.	Sees, hears, and grasps far less than previously. Attention is focused on a small area of a given event. Inferences drawn may be distorted because of inadequacy of observed data. May be unaware of and unable to name anxiety. Relief behaviors generally used.
Panic (e.g., terror, horror, dread, uncanniness, awe)	Perceptual field is reduced to a detail, which is usually "blown up," i.e., elaborated by distortion (exaggeration), or the focus is on scattered details; the speed of the scattering tends to increase. Massive dissociation, especially of contents of self-system. Felt as enormous threat to survival. Learning is impossible.	Says, "I'm in a million pieces," "I'm gone," or "What is happening to me?" Perplexity, self-absorption. Feelings of unreality. Flights of ideas or confusion. Fear. Repeats a detail. Many relief behaviors used automatically (without thought). The enormous energy produced by panic must be used and may be mobilized as rage. May pace, run, or fight violently. With dissociation of contents of self-system, there may be a very rapid reorganization of the self, usually going along pathologic lines (e.g., a "psychotic break" is usually preceded by panic).

Adapted with permission from Peplau, H. (1989). Theoretical constructs: Anxiety, self, and hallucinations. In A. O'Toole & S. Welt (Eds.), *Interpersonal theory in nursing practice: Selected works of Hildegarde E. Peplau*. New York: Springer.

BOX 16.1
Symptoms of Anxiety

PHYSICAL SYMPTOMS
Cardiovascular
Sympathetic
Palpitations
Heart racing
Increased blood pressure

Parasympathetic
Actual fainting
Decreased blood pressure
Decreased pulse rate

Respiratory
Rapid breathing
Difficulty getting air
Shortness of breath
Pressure of chest
Shallow breathing
Lump in throat
Choking sensations
Gasping
Spasm of bronchi

Neuromuscular
Increased reflexes
Startle reaction
Eyelid twitching
Insomnia
Tremors
Rigidity
Spasm
Fidgeting
Pacing
Strained face
Unsteadiness
Generalized weakness
Wobbly legs
Clumsy motions

Skin
Flushed face
Pale face
Localized sweating (palm region)
Generalized sweating
Hot and cold spells
Itching

Gastrointestinal
Loss of appetite
Revulsion about food
Abdominal discomfort
Diarrhea
Abdominal pain
Nausea
Heartburn
Vomiting

Eyes
Dilated pupils

Urinary Tract Parasympathetic
Pressure to urinate
Increased frequency of urination

AFFECTIVE SYMPTOMS
Edgy
Impatient
Uneasy
Nervous
Tense
Wound-up
Anxious
Fearful
Apprehensive
Scared
Frightened
Alarmed
Terrified
Jittery
Jumpy

COGNITIVE SYMPTOMS
Sensory-Perceptual
Mind is hazy, cloudy, foggy, dazed
Objects seem blurred or distant
Environment seems different or unreal
Feelings of unreality
Self-consciousness
Hypervigilance

Thinking Difficulties
Cannot recall important things
Confused
Unable to control thinking
Difficulty concentrating
Difficulty focusing attention
Distractibility
Blocking
Difficulty reasoning
Loss of objectivity and perspective
Tunnel vision

Conceptual
Cognitive distortion
Fear of losing control
Fear of not being able to cope
Fear of physical injury or death
Fear of mental disorder
Fear of negative evaluations
Frightening visual images
Repetitive fearful ideation

BEHAVIORAL SYMPTOMS
Inhibited
Tonic immobility
Flight
Avoidance
Speech dysfluency
Impaired coordination
Restlessness
Postural collapse
Hyperventilation

Adapted from Beck, A. T., & Emery, C. (1985). *Anxiety disorders and phobias: A cognitive perspective* (pp. 23–27). New York: Basic Books.

and patterns of behavior. Anxiety is a component of all the disorders discussed in this chapter.

Defense Mechanisms and Anxiety

Defense mechanisms are used to reduce anxiety by preventing or diminishing unwanted thoughts and feelings. See Chapter 7 for definitions. Defense mechanisms can be helpful in coping with everyday problems, but they become problematic when overused. The first step is identifying a person's use of defense mechanisms. The next step is determining whether the reasons the defense mechanisms are being used support healthy coping or are detrimental to a person's health. What may be healthy for one person may be unhealthy for another. See Box 16.2.

OVERVIEW OF ANXIETY DISORDERS

The primary symptoms of anxiety disorders are fear and anxiety. Even though symptoms of anxiety disorders can be found in healthy individuals, an anxiety disorder is diagnosed when the fear or anxiety is excessive or out of proportion to the situation. An individual's ability to work and interpersonal relationships may be impaired. Anxiety disorders are differentiated by the situation or objects that provoke the fear, anxiety, or avoidance behavior and the reelatedcognitive thoughts (APA, 2013). See Box 16.3 for a list of anxiety disorders.

Anxiety disorders are the most common of the psychiatric illnesses treated by health care providers. Approximately 40 million American adults (older than 18 years old) or about 18.1% of this age group within a given

---

BOX 16.2

Consequences of Decreasing Anxiety by Using Defense Mechanisms

DEFENSE MECHANISM	POSITIVE CONSEQUENCES	NEGATIVE CONSEQUENCES
Altruism	Satisfies internal needs through helping others	Prevents examination of underlying fears or concerns
Denial	Avoids feelings associated with recognizing a problem	Avoidance of major problem that should be addressed
Displacement	By taking out frustrations on an unsuspecting or vulnerable person, animal, or object, anxiety is reduced and the individual is protected from anticipated retaliation from the source of the frustration.	Does not deal with problem and inappropriately expresses feelings towards a more vulnerable person or object.
Intellectualization	Able to analyze events in a distant, objective, analytical way	Inability to acknowledge feelings that may be interfering with relationships
Projection	By assigning unwanted thoughts, feelings or behaviors to another person or object, the individual does not have to acknowledge undesirable or unacceptable thoughts or feelings.	Does not acknowledge undesirable or unwanted feelings or thoughts and can act on inaccurate interpretation of the other person's thoughts and behaviors.
Rationalization	Avoids anxiety by explaining an unacceptable or disappointing behavior or feeling in a logical, rationale way. May protect self-esteem and self-concept.	Avoids the reality of a situation which may be detrimental to the individual.
Reaction Formation	Reduces anxiety by taking the opposite feeling. Hides true feelings, which may be appropriate in many situations.	Unable to acknowledge personal feelings about others, which leads to negative consequences.
Regression	When stressed, abandons effective coping strategies and reverts to behaviors used earlier in development. These strategies are comfortable and may be effective.	May reengage in detrimental behaviors such as smoking, drinking, or inappropriate interpersonal responses leading to ineffective coping.
Repression	Avoids unwanted thoughts and anxiety by blocking thoughts, experiences from conscious awareness.	Cannot recall traumatic events that should be addressed to be healthy, (i.e., rape).
Sublimation	Avoids anxiety and channels maladaptive feelings or impulses into socially acceptable behaviors. Maintains socially acceptable behavior.	By not recognizing maladaptive feelings, the individual cannot address underlying feelings.
Suppression	Reduces anxiety by intentionally avoiding thinking about disturbing problems, wishes, feelings or experiences. Useful in many situations such as test taking situations.	Avoiding problem situation prevents finding a solution to the problem.

BOX 16.3

Anxiety Disorders

DISORDER	DESCRIPTION
Separation anxiety disorder	Fearful, anxious about separation from attachment figures that is developmentally inappropriate
Selective mutism	Consistent failure to speak in social situations when there is an expectation to speak
Specific phobias	Fearful, anxious or avoids a specific object or situations
Social anxiety disorder	Fearful, anxious or avoids social situations that involve possibility of being scrutinized
Panic disorder	Experiences unexpected panic attacks, is worried about having more panic attacks, change in behavior
Agoraphobia	Fearful, anxious about open spaces, being enclosed, or being outside of house
Generalized anxiety disorder	Persistent, excessive anxiety or worry about many aspects of life
Substance/medication-induced anxiety disorder	Anxiety due to excessive substance use, substance withdrawal, and medication use.

(APA, 2013)

year have an anxiety disorder. Direct and indirect costs of treating anxiety disorders amount to tens of billions of dollars. Women experience anxiety disorders more often than men by a 2:1 ratio. Anxiety disorders may also be associated with other mental or physical comorbidities such as heart disease, respiratory disease, and mood disorders (Stein, Aquilar-Gaxiola, Alonso, Bruffaerts, de Jonge, Liu, et al., 2014; Tully & Baune, 2014). The relationship between depression and anxiety disorders is particularly strong. A single patient may concurrently have more than one anxiety disorder or other psychiatric disorders as well.

Anxiety disorders tend to be chronic and persistent, with full recovery more likely among those who do not have other mental or physical disorders (Ayazi, Lien, Eide, Swartz, & Hauff, 2014). Three quarters of those with an anxiety disorder have their first episode by age 21.5 years.

Anxiety Disorders Across the Life-Span

Prompt identification, diagnosis, and treatment of individuals with anxiety disorders may be difficult for special populations such as children and older adult patients. Often, the symptoms suggestive of anxiety disorders may go unnoticed by caregivers or are misdiagnosed because they mimic cardiac or pulmonary pathology rather than

a psychological disturbance. Children and adolescents are discussed in Chapter 28; older adults are discussed in Chapter 29.

Children and Adolescents

Anxiety disorders are among the most common conditions of children and adolescents (Centers for Disease Control and Prevention [CDC], 2013; Kessler, Avenevoli, Costello, Georgiades, Green, Gruber, et al., 2012a). If left untreated, symptoms persist and gradually worsen and sometimes lead to suicidal ideation and suicide attempts, early parenthood, drug and alcohol dependence, and educational underachievement later in life (Kessler, Avenevoli, Costello, Green, Gruber, McLaughlin, et al., 2012b).

Separation anxiety disorder, (i.e., excessive fear or anxiety concerning separation from home or attachment figures), usually first occurs in childhood. Affected children experience extreme distress when separated from home or attachment figures, worry about them when separated from them, and worry about untoward events (i.e., getting lost) and what will happen to them. This disorder is also discussed in Chapter 28.

A rare disorder typically seen in childhood is selective mutism in which children do not initiate speech or respond when spoken to by others (APA, 2013). Children with this disorder are often very anxious when asked to speak in school or read aloud. They may suffer academic impairment because of their inability to communicate with others.

Older Adults

Generally speaking, the prevalence of anxiety disorders declines with age. However, in the older adult population, rates of anxiety disorders are as high as mood disorders, which commonly co-occur. This combination of depressive and anxiety symptoms has been shown to decrease social functioning, increase somatic (physical) symptoms, and increase depressive symptoms (King-Kallimanis, Gum, & Kohn, 2009). In one study, nearly half of primary care patients with chronic pain had at least one attendant anxiety disorder. Detecting and treating anxiety is an important component of pain management (Kroenke, Outcalt, Krebs, Bair, Wu, Chumbler, et al., 2013). Because the older adult population is at risk for suicide, special assessment of anxiety symptoms is essential.

PANIC DISORDER

Panic is an extreme, overwhelming form of anxiety often experienced when an individual is placed in a real or perceived life-threatening situation. Panic is normal during periods of threat but is abnormal when it is continuously experienced in situations that pose no real physical or psychological threat. Some people experience heightened anxiety because they fear experiencing another panic attack. This type of panic interferes with the individual's ability to function in everyday life and is characteristic of panic disorder.

> **KEYCONCEPT** **Panic** is an extremely overwhelming form of anxiety often experienced when an individual is placed in a real or perceived life-threatening situation.

Clinical Course

The onset of panic disorder is typically between 20 to 24 years of age. The disorder usually surfaces in childhood but may not be diagnosed until later. Panic disorder is treatable, but studies have shown that even after years of treatment, many people remain symptomatic. In some cases, symptoms may even worsen (APA, 2013).

Panic Attacks

Panic attacks are a major finding in panic disorder. A panic attack is a sudden, discrete period of intense fear or discomfort that reaches its peak within a few minutes and is accompanied by significant physical discomfort and cognitive distress (APA, 2013). Panic attacks usually peak in about 10 minutes but can last as long as 30 minutes before returning to normal functioning. The physical symptoms include palpitations, chest discomfort, rapid pulse, nausea, dizziness, sweating, paresthesias (burning, tickling, pricking of skin with no apparent reason), trembling or shaking, and a feeling of suffocation or shortness of breath. Cognitive symptoms include disorganized thinking, irrational fears, **depersonalization** (being detached from oneself), and a decreased ability to communicate. Usually, feelings of impending doom or death, fear of going crazy or losing control, and desperation ensue.

The physical symptoms can mimic those of a heart attack. Individuals often seek emergency medical care because they feel as if they are dying, but most have negative cardiac workup results. People experiencing panic attacks may also believe that the attacks stem from an underlying major medical illness (APA, 2013). Even with medical testing and assurance of no underlying disease, they often remain unconvinced.

> In the beginning of the chapter you were introduced to Doug and his family. How can you help Doug recognize that even though he is not having a heart attack, his symptoms are serious and that his panic attack could indicate an underlying anxiety disorder? Why would you not want to tell him that everything is normal?

> **NCLEXNOTE** Physical symptoms of panic attack are similar to cardiac emergencies. These symptoms are physically taxing and psychologically frightening to patients. Recognition of the seriousness of panic attacks should be communicated to the patient.

In a panic disorder, recurrent unexpected panic attacks are followed by persistent concern about experiencing subsequent panic attacks. Because of fear of future attacks, these affected individuals modify normal behaviors to avoid future attacks (APA, 2013). Panic attacks are either expected with an obvious cue or trigger or unexpected with no such obvious cue. The first panic attack is usually associated with an identifiable cue (e.g., anxiety-provoking medical conditions, such as asthma, or in initial trials of illicit substance use) but subsequent attacks are often unexpected without any obvious cue (Box 16.4). Panic attacks not only occur in panic disorder but can also occur in other mental disorders such as depression, bipolar disease, eating disorders, and some medical conditions such as cardiac or respiratory disorders (APA, 2013).

FAME & FORTUNE

Charles Darwin (1809–1882)

Theory of Evolution

PUBLIC PERSONA

Charles Darwin, credited as the first scientist to gain wide acceptance of the theory of natural selection, might never have published his seminal work, *Origin of the Species,* had it not been for his psychiatric illness. Born in England, Charles Darwin, the grandson of a famous poet, inventor, and physician, was expected to accomplish great things. However, his childhood years were troublesome. When he was sent to Cambridge to study medicine, card playing and drinking became his main activities. After meeting a botanist, however, his life changed, and he embarked on a 5-year expedition to the coast of South America.

PERSONAL REALITIES

Darwin described his sensation of fear, accompanied by troubled beating of the heart, sweat, and trembling of muscles. Thought to have panic disorder, he constantly worried about what he thought he knew until he finally published his ideas. In 1859, *The Origin of Species by Means of Natural Selection* was published. In 1882, he died and was buried in Westminster Abbey.

Source: Darwin, C. (1887). *The life and letters of Charles Darwin.* New York: Appleton & Co.

BOX 16.4 CLINICAL VIGNETTE

Panic Disorder

Susan, a 22-year-old female, has experienced several life changes, including a recent engagement, loss of her father to cancer and heart disease, graduation from college, and entrance to the workforce as a computer programmer in a large inner-city company. Because of her active lifestyle, her sleep habits have been poor. She frequently uses sleeping aids at night and now drinks a full pot of coffee to start each day. She continues to smoke to "relieve the stress." While sitting in heavy traffic on the way to work, she suddenly experienced chest tightness, sweating, shortness of breath, feelings of being "trapped," and foreboding that she was going to die. Fearing a heart attack, she went to an emergency department, where her discomfort subsided within a half hour. After several hours of testing, the doctor informed her that her heart was healthy. During the next few weeks, she experienced several episodes of feeling trapped and slight chest discomfort on her drive to work. She fears future "attacks" while sitting in traffic and while in her crowded office cubicle.

What Do You Think?

- What risk factors does Susan have that might contribute to the development of panic attacks?
- What lifestyle changes do you think would help Susan reduce stress?

Diagnostic Criteria

Panic disorder is a chronic condition that has several exacerbations and remissions during the course of the disease. The disabling panic attacks often lead to other symptoms, such as **phobias** (e.g., irrational fear of an object, person, or situation that leads to a compelling avoidance).

Other diagnostic symptoms include palpitations, sweating, shaking, shortness of breath or smothering, sensations of choking, chest pain, nausea or abdominal distress, dizziness, derealization or depersonalization, fear of going crazy, fear of dying, paresthesias, and chills or hot flashes (APA, 2013) (see Key Diagnostic Characteristics 16.1).

Epidemiology and Risk Factors

In the National Epidemiologic Survey on Alcohol and Related Conditions 2001–2002, which had 43,093 participants, 5.1% of those reporting had experienced panic disorder in their lifetimes, and 2.1% had experienced panic disorder in the year preceding the survey. Increased risk is associated with being female; middle aged; of low socioeconomic status; and widowed, separated, or divorced (Grant, Hasin, Stinson, Dawson, Goldstein, Smith, et al., 2006). In another study combining three major epidemiological databases, the authors found significantly higher rates of panic disorder among whites than among African Americans, Asians, and Latinos (Asnaani, Gutner, Hinton, & Hofmann, 2009). The

estimates of isolated panic attacks may affect 22.7% of the population.

Family history, substance and stimulant use or abuse, smoking tobacco, and severe stressors are risk factors for panic disorder. People who have several anxiety symptoms and those who experience separation anxiety during childhood often develop panic disorder later in life. Early life traumas, a history of physical or sexual abuse, socioeconomic or personal disadvantages, and behavioral inhibition by adults have also been associated with an increased risk for anxiety disorders in children (Benjamin, Beidas, Comer, Puliafico, & Kendall, 2011; Jovanovic, Smith, Kamkwalala, Poole, Samples, Norrholm, et al., 2011).

Comorbidity

Patients may experience more than one anxiety disorder, depression, eating disorder, substance use or abuse, or schizophrenia (Torres, Ferrão, Shavitt, Diniz, Costa, do Rosário, et al., 2014). Although people with panic disorder are thought to have more somatic complaints than the general population, panic disorder does correlate with some medical conditions, including vertigo, cardiac disease, gastrointestinal disorders, asthma, and those related to cigarette smoking. In one study, the 12-month prevalence of panic disorder among patients with cardiac disease was found to be significantly higher than among those without cardiac disease (6.0% compared with 3.4%). Furthermore, these patients used emergency departments at a significantly higher rate (Korczak, Goldstein, & Levitt, 2007).

Etiology

Biologic Theories

There appears to be a substantial familial predisposition to panic disorder with an estimated heritability of 48% (Konishi, Tanii, Otowa, Sasaki, Tochigi, Umekage, et al., 2014). Studies show brain abnormalities in the "fear network" (amygdala, hippocampus, thalamus, midbrain, pons, medulla, and cerebellum) and changes in volume in different brain areas (Del Casale, Serata, Rapinesi, Kotzalidis, Angeletti, Tatarelli, et al., 2013).

Serotonin and Norepinephrine

Serotonin and norepinephrine are both implicated in panic disorders. Norepinephrine effects act on those systems most affected by a panic attack—the cardiovascular, respiratory, and gastrointestinal systems. Serotonergic neurons are distributed in central autonomic and emotional motor control systems regulating anxiety states and anxiety-related physiologic and behavioral responses (Ravindran & Stein, 2010).

KEY DIAGNOSTIC CHARACTERISTICS 16.1 • PANIC DISORDER

Diagnostic Criteria

A. Recurrent unexpected panic attacks. A panic attack is an abrupt surge of intense fear or intense discomfort that reaches a peak within minutes, and during which time four (or more) of the following symptoms occur:
   Note: The abrupt surge can occur from a calm state or an anxious state.
   1. Palpitations, pounding heart, or accelerated heart rate.
   2. Sweating.
   3. Trembling or shaking.
   4. Sensations of shortness of breath or smothering.
   5. Feelings of choking.
   6. Chest pain or discomfort.
   7. Nausea or abdominal distress.
   8. Feeling dizzy, unsteady, light-headed, or faint.
   9. Chills or heat sensations.
   10. Paresthesias (numbness or tingling sensations).
   11. Derealization (feelings of unreality) or depersonalization (being detached from oneself).
   12. Fear of losing control or "going crazy."
   13. Fear of dying.
       Note: Culture-specific symptoms (e.g., tinnitus, neck soreness, headache, uncontrollable screaming or crying) may be seen. Such symptoms should not count as one of the four required symptoms.

B. At least one of the attacks has been followed by 1 month (or more) of one or both of the following:
   1. Persistent concern or worry about additional panic attacks or their consequences (e.g., losing control, having a heart attack, "going crazy").
   2. A significant maladaptive change in behavior related to the attacks (e.g., behaviors designed to avoid having panic attacks, such as avoidance of exercise or unfamiliar situations).

C. The disturbance is not attributable to the physiological effects of a substance (e.g., a drug of abuse, a medication) or another medical condition (e.g., hyperthyroidism, cardiopulmonary disorders).

D. The disturbance is not better explained by another mental disorder (e.g., the panic attacks do not occur only in response to feared social situations, as in social anxiety disorder; in response to circumscribed phobic objects or situations, as in specific phobia; in response to obsessions, as in obsessive-compulsive disorder; in response to reminders of traumatic events, as in posttraumatic stress disorder; or in response to separation from attachment figures, as in separation anxiety disorder).

Target Symptoms

• Discrete period of intense fear or discomfort with four (or more) of the following symptoms that develop abruptly and reach a peak within 10 minutes:
   • Palpitations, pounding heart, or accelerated heart rate
   • Sweating
   • Trembling or shaking
   • Sensations of shortness of breath or smothering
   • Feelings of choking
   • Chest pain or discomfort
   • Nausea or vomiting
   • Feeling dizzy, unsteady, lightheaded, or faint
   • Derealization (feeling of unreality) or depersonalization (being detached from oneself)
   • Fear of losing control or going crazy
   • Fear of dying
   • Paresthesias (numbness or tingling sensations)
   • Chills or hot flushes
• Great apprehension about the outcome of routine activities and experiences
• Loss or disruption of important interpersonal relationships
• Demoralization
• Possible major depressive episode

Associated Findings

• Nocturnal panic attack (waking from sleep in a state of panic)
• Constant or intermittent feelings of anxiety related to physical and mental health
• Pervasive concerns about abilities to complete daily tasks or withstand daily stressors
• Excessive use of drugs or other means to control panic attacks

Associated Physical Examination Findings

• Transient tachycardia
• Moderate elevation of systolic blood pressure

Associated Laboratory Findings

• Compensated respiratory alkalosis (decreased carbon dioxide, decreased bicarbonate levels, almost normal pH)

Other Targets for Treatment

• Loss or disruption of important interpersonal or occupational activities
• Demoralization
• Possible major depressive episode

Reprinted with permission from the *Diagnostic and statistical manual of mental disorders, 5th edition* (Copyright ©2013). American Psychiatric Association. All Rights Reserved.

Gamma-Aminobutyric Acid

Gamma-aminobutyric acid (GABA) is the most abundant inhibitory neurotransmitter in the brain. GABA receptor stimulation causes several effects, including neurocognitive effects, reduction of anxiety, and sedation. GABA stimulation also results in increased seizure threshold. Abnormalities in the benzodiazepine–GABA–chloride ion channel complex have been implicated in panic disorder (Stein, Steckler, Lightfoot, Hay, & Goddard, 2010).

Hypothalamic–Pituitary–Adrenal Axis

Research implicates a role of the hypothalamic–pituitary–adrenal axis (HPA) axis in panic disorders (Pace & Heim, 2011). A current explanation is that as stress hormones are activated, anxiety increases, which can lead to a panic attack (See Chapter 12).

Psychosocial Theories

Psychoanalytic and Psychodynamic Theories

Psychodynamic theories examine anxiety that develops after separation and loss. Many patients link their initial panic attack with recent personal losses. However, at this point the empirical evidence remains inadequate for a psychodynamic explanation. It remains unclear why some patients develop panic disorder whereas others with similar experiences develop other disorders (Pilecki, Arentoft, & McKay, 2011).

Cognitive Behavioral Theories

Learning theory underlies most cognitive behavioral explanations of panic disorder. Classic conditioning theory suggests that one learns a fear response by linking an adverse or fear-provoking event, such as a car accident, with a previously neutral event, such as crossing a bridge. One becomes conditioned to associate fear with crossing a bridge. Applying this theory to people with panic disorder has limitations. Phobic avoidance is not always developed secondary to an adverse event.

Further development of this theory led to an understanding of **interoceptive conditioning,** an association between physical discomfort, such as dizziness or palpitations and an impending panic attack. For example, during a car accident, the individual may experience rapid heartbeat, dizziness, shortness of breath, and panic. Subsequent experiences of dizziness or palpitations, unrelated to an anxiety-provoking situation, incite anxiety and panic. Furthermore, people with panic disorder may misinterpret mild physical sensations (e.g., sweating, dizziness) as being catastrophic, causing panic as a result of learned fear (catastrophic interpretation). Some researchers hypothesize that individuals with a low sense of control over their environment or with a particular sensitivity to anxiety are vulnerable to misinterpreting normal stress. Controlled exposure to anxiety-provoking situations and cognitive countering techniques has proven successful in reducing the symptoms of panic.

Family Response to Disorder

Persons with a panic disorder may inadvertently cause excessive fears, phobias, or excessive worry in other family members. Families may limit social functions to prevent a panic attack. Those affected need a tremendous amount of support and encouragement from significant others.

Teamwork and Collaboration: Working Toward Recovery

Nurses are pivotal in providing a safe and therapeutic inpatient environment and teaching patients strategies for managing anxiety and fears. The nurse also administers prescribed medication, monitors its effects, and provides medication education. Advanced practice nurses, licensed clinical social workers, or licensed counselors provide individual psychotherapy sessions as needed. Often, a clinical psychologist gives psychological tests and interprets the results to assist in diagnosing and treating the panic disorder.

Panic Control Treatment

Panic control treatment involves intentional exposure (through exercise) to panic-invoking sensations such as dizziness, hyperventilation, tightness in the chest, and sweating. Identified patterns become targets for treatment. Patients are taught to use breathing training and cognitive restructuring to manage their responses and are instructed to practice these techniques between therapy sessions to adapt the skills to other situations.

Systematic Desensitization

Systematic desensitization, another exposure method used to desensitize patients, exposes the patient to a hierarchy of feared situations that the patient has rated from least to most feared. The patient is taught to use muscle relaxation as levels of anxiety increase through multisituational exposure. Planning and implementing exposure therapy require special training. Because of the multitude of outpatients in treatment for panic disorder and agoraphobia (discussed later in chapter), exposure therapy is a useful tool for home health psychiatric nurses. Outcomes of home-based exposure treatment are similar to clinic-based treatment outcomes.

Implosive Therapy

Implosive therapy is a provocative technique useful in treating panic disorder and agoraphobia in which the therapist identifies phobic stimuli for the patient and then presents highly anxiety-provoking imagery to the patient, describing the feared scene as dramatically and vividly as possible. **Flooding** is a technique used to desensitize the patient to the fear associated with a particular anxiety-provoking stimulus. Desensitizing is done by presenting feared objects or situations repeatedly without session breaks until the anxiety dissipates. For example, a patient with ophidiophobia (i.e., a morbid fear of snakes) might be presented with a real snake repeatedly until the patient's anxiety decreases.

Exposure Therapy

Many of the treatment approaches used for panic disorder are effective for phobias (discussed in later chapters). **Exposure therapy** is the treatment of choice for phobias. The patient is repeatedly exposed to real or simulated anxiety-provoking situations until he or she becomes desensitized and anxiety subsides.

Cognitive Behavioral Therapy

Cognitive behavioral therapy (CBT) is a highly effective tool for treating individuals with panic disorder. It has been considered the first-line treatment for those with panic and other anxiety disorders and is often used in conjunction with medications, including the selective serotonin reuptake inhibitors (SSRIs), in treating those with panic disorder (Ruwaard, Lange, Schrieken, Dolan, & Emmelkamp, 2012). The goals of CBT include helping the patient to manage his or her anxiety and correcting anxiety-provoking thoughts through interventions, including cognitive restructuring, breathing training, and psychoeducation.

Safety Issues

People with panic disorder are often depressed and consequently are at high risk for suicide. Adolescents with panic disorder may be at higher risk for suicidal thoughts or may attempt suicide more often than other adolescents (Katz, Yaseen, Mojtabai, Cohen, & Galynker, 2011). As many as 15% of patients with panic disorder commit suicide; women with both panic disorder and depression or panic disorder and substance abuse are especially at risk (APA, 2013; Katz et al., 2011).

Evidence-based Nursing Care for Persons with Panic Disorder

Individuals often first seek help in the emergency department for their physical symptoms, but they are told that there are no life-threatening cardiac or neurologic causes for the severe physical symptoms. Although no laboratory tests exist to confirm anxiety disorders, a careful clinical assessment will reveal the presence of an anxiety disorder.

Mental Health Nursing Assessment

A comprehensive nursing assessment includes overall physical and mental status, suicidal tendencies and thoughts, cognitive thought patterns, avoidance behavior patterns, and family and cultural factors. Patients can be encouraged to keep a daily log of the severity of anxiety and the frequency, duration, and severity of panic episodes. This log will be a basic tool for monitoring progress as symptoms decrease.

Panic Attack Assessment

If the panic attack occurs in the presence of the nurse, direct assessment of the symptoms should be made and documented. Questions to ask the patient might include the following:

- What were you doing when the panic attack occurred?
- What did you experience before and during the panic episode, including physical symptoms, feelings, and thoughts?
- When did you begin to feel that way? How long did it last?
- Do you have an explanation for what caused you to feel and think that way?
- Have you experienced these symptoms in the past? If so, under what circumstances?
- Has anyone in your family ever had similar experiences?
- What do you do when you have these experiences to help you to feel safe?
- Have the feelings and sensations ever gone away on their own?

Physical Health Assessment

Key assessment areas of physical health include the use of legal or illegal substances that could have precipitated the panic attack, sleep patterns, activity levels, and health conditions.

Substance Use

Caffeine, pseudoephedrine, amphetamines, cocaine, or other stimulants are associated with panic disorder and may stimulate a panic attack. Tobacco use can also contribute to the risk for panic symptoms. Many individuals with panic disorder use alcohol or central nervous system (CNS) depressants in an effort to self-medicate anxiety symptoms; withdrawal from CNS depressants may produce symptoms of panic.

Sleep Patterns

Sleep is often disturbed in patients with panic disorder. In fact, panic attacks can occur during sleep, so the patient may fear sleep for this reason. Nurses should closely assess the impact of sleep disturbance because fatigue may increase anxiety and susceptibility to panic attacks.

Physical Activity

Panic disorder can be improved through active participation in a routine exercise program. If the patient does not exercise routinely, define the barriers to it. If exercise is avoided because of chronic muscle tension, poor muscle tone, muscle cramps, general fatigue, exhaustion, or shortness of breath, the symptoms may indicate poor physical health.

Medications

Several medications can cause anxiety. Bronchodilators, oral contraceptives, amphetamines (i.e., methylphenidate (Ritalin)), steroids, thyroid medication, and several other medications can increase anxiety. Additionally, medicines that contain caffeine such as some pain and anti-inflammatory agents, decongestants (i.e., phenylephrine) and some illegal drugs (cocaine) also increase anxiety.

Other Physical Assessment Areas

Recent changes in physical status should be assessed. For example, pregnant patients should be assessed carefully for an underlying panic disorder. Although pregnancy may actually protect the mother from developing panic symptoms, postpartum onset of panic disorder requires particular attention. During a time that tremendous effort is spent on family, postpartum onset of panic disorder negatively affects lifestyle and decreases self-esteem in affected women, leading to feelings of overwhelming personal disappointment.

Psychosocial Assessment

A psychosocial assessment includes the patient's report of the symptoms and a careful cognitive, behavioral, and social assessment.

Self-Report Scales

Self-evaluation is difficult in panic disorder. Often the memories of the attack and its triggers are irretrievable. Several tools are available to characterize and rate the patient's state of anxiety. Examples of these symptom and behavioral rating scales are provided in Box 16.5. All of these tools are self-report measures and as such are limited by the individual's self-awareness and openness. However, the Hamilton Rating Scale for Anxiety (HAM-A),

---

BOX 16.5

Rating Scales for Assessment of Panic Disorder and Anxiety Disorders

PANIC SYMPTOMS

Panic-Associated Symptom Scale (PASS)
Argyle, N., Delito, J., Allerup, P., Maier, W., Albus, M., Nutzinger, D., et al. (1991). The Panic-Associated Symptom Scale: Measuring the severity of panic disorder. *Acta Psychiatrica Scandinavica, 83,* 20–26.

Acute Panic Inventory
Dillon, D. J., Gorman, J. M., Liebowitz, M. R., Fyer, A. J., & Klein, D. F. (1987). Measurement of lactate-induced panic and anxiety. *Psychiatry Research, 20,* 97–105.

National Institute of Mental Health Panic Questionnaire (NIMH PQ)
Scupi, B. S., Maser, J. D., & Uhde, T. W. (1992). The National Institute of Mental Health Panic Questionnaire: An instrument for assessing clinical characteristics of panic disorder. *Journal of Nervous and Mental Disease, 180,* 566–572.

COGNITIONS

Anxiety Sensitivity Index
Reiss, S., Peterson, R. A., & Gursky, D. M. (1986). Anxiety sensitivity, anxiety frequency, and the prediction of fearfulness. *Behaviour Research and Therapy, 24,* 1–8.

Agoraphobia Cognitions Questionnaire
Chambless, D. L., Caputo, G. C., Bright, P., & Gallagher, R. (1984). Assessment of fear in agoraphobics: The Body Sensations Questionnaire and the Agoraphobic Cognitions Questionnaire. *Journal of Consulting and Clinical Psychology, 52,* 1090–1097.

Body Sensations Questionnaire
Chambless, D. L., Caputo, G. C., Bright, P., & Gallagher, R. (1984). Assessment of fear in agoraphobics: The Body

Sensations Questionnaire and the Agoraphobic Cognitions Questionnaire. *Journal of Consulting and Clinical Psychology, 52,* 1090–1097.

PHOBIAS

Mobility Inventory for Agoraphobia
Chambless, D. L., Caputo, G. C., Jasin, S. E., Gracely, E. J., & Williams, C. (1985). The mobility inventory for agoraphobia. *Behavior Research and Therapy, 23,* 35–44.

Fear Questionnaire
Marks, I. M., & Matthews, A. M. (1979). Brief standard self-rating for phobic patients. *Behaviour Research and Therapy, 17,* 263–267.

ANXIETY

State-Trait Anxiety Inventory (STAI)
Spielberger, C. D., Gorsuch, R. L., & Luchene, R. E. (1976). *Manual for the State-Trait Anxiety Inventory.* Palo Alto, CA: Consulting Psychologists Press.

Penn State Worry Questionnaire (PSWQ)
16 items developed to assess the trait of worry
Meyer, T., Miller, M., Metzger, R., & Borkovec, T. (1990). Development and validation of the Penn State Worry Questionnaire. *Behaviour Research and Therapy, 28*(6), 487–495.

Beck Anxiety Inventory
21 items rating the severity of symptoms on a 4-point scale
Beck, A., Epstein, N., Brown, G., & Steer, R. (1988). An inventory for measuring clinical anxiety: The Beck Anxiety Inventory. *Journal of Consulting and Clinical Psychology, 56,* 893–897.

TABLE 16.2	HAMILTON RATING SCALE FOR ANXIETY	

Max Hamilton designed this scale to help clinicians gather information about anxiety states. The symptom inventory provides scaled information that classifies anxiety behavior and assists the clinician in targeting behaviors and achieving outcome measures. Provide a rating for each indicator based on the following scale:

0 = None
1 = Mild
2 = Moderate
3 = Severe
4 = Severe, grossly disabling

Item	Symptoms	Rating
Anxious mood	Worries, anticipation of the worst, fearful anticipation, irritability	
Tension	Feelings of tension, fatigability, startle response, moved to tears easily, trembling, feelings of restlessness, inability to relax	
Fear	Of dark, strangers, being left alone, animals, traffic, crowds	
Insomnia	Difficulty in falling asleep, broken sleep, unsatisfying sleep and fatigue on waking; dreams, nightmares, night terrors	
Intellectual (cognitive)	Difficulty concentrating, poor memory	
Depressed mood	Loss of interest, lack of pleasure in hobbies, depression, early waking, diurnal swings	
Somatic (sensory)	Tinnitus, blurring of vision, hot and cold flushes, feelings of weakness, prickly sensation	
Somatic (muscular)	Pains and aches, twitching, stiffness, myoclonic jerks, grinding of teeth, unsteady voice, increased muscular tone	
Cardiovascular symptoms	Tachycardia, palpitations, pain in chest, throbbing of vessels, fainting feelings, missing beat	
Respiratory symptoms	Pressure or constriction in chest, choking feelings, sighing, dyspnea	
Gastrointestinal symptoms	Difficulty in swallowing, gas, abdominal pain, burning sensation, abdominal fullness, nausea, vomiting, looseness of bowels, loss of weight, constipation	
Genitourinary symptoms	Frequency of micturition, urgency of micturition, amenorrhea, menorrhagia, development of frigidity, premature ejaculation, loss of libido, impotence	
Autonomic symptoms	Dry mouth, flushing, pallor, tendency to sweat, giddiness, tension headache, raising of hair	
Behavior at interview	Fidgeting, restlessness or pacing, tremor of hands, furrowed brow, strained face, sighing or rapid respiration, facial pallor, swallowing, belching, brisk tendon jerks, dilated pupils, exophthalmos	

From Hamilton, M. (1959). The assessment of anxiety states by rating. *British Journal of Medical Psychology*, (32), 54.

provided in Table 16.2, is an example of a scale rated by the clinician (Hamilton, 1959). This 14-item scale reflects both psychological and somatic aspects of anxiety.

Mental Status Examination

During a mental status examination, individuals with panic disorder may exhibit anxiety symptoms, including restlessness, irritability, poor concentration, and apprehensive behavior. Disorganized thinking, irrational fears, and a decreased ability to communicate often occur during a panic attack. Assess by direct questioning whether the patient is experiencing suicidal thoughts, especially if he or she is abusing substances or is taking antidepressant medications.

Cognitive Thought Patterns

Catastrophic misinterpretations of trivial physical symptoms can trigger panic symptoms. After they have been identified, these thoughts should serve as a basis for individualizing patient education to counter such false beliefs. Table 16.3 presents a scale to assess catastrophic misinterpretations of the symptoms of panic.

Several studies have found that individuals who feel a sense of control have less severe panic attacks. Individuals who fear loss of control during a panic attack often make the following type of statements:

- "I feel trapped."
- "I'm afraid others will know or that I'll hurt someone."
- "I feel alone. I can't help myself."
- "I'm losing control."

These individuals also tend to show low self-esteem, feelings of helplessness, demoralization, and overwhelming fears of experiencing panic attacks. They may have difficulty with assertiveness or expressing their feelings.

TABLE 16.3	PANIC ATTACK COGNITIONS QUESTIONNAIRE

Rate each of the following thoughts according to the degree to which you believe each thought contributes to your panic attack.

1 = Not at all
2 = Somewhat

3 = Quite a lot
4 = Very much

	1	2	3	4
1. I'm going to die.	1	2	3	4
2. I'm going insane.	1	2	3	4
3. I'm losing control.	1	2	3	4
4. This will never end.	1	2	3	4
5. I'm really scared.	1	2	3	4
6. I'm having a heart attack.	1	2	3	4
7. I'm going to pass out.	1	2	3	4
8. I don't know what people will think.	1	2	3	4
9. I won't be able to get out of here.	1	2	3	4
10. I don't understand what is happening to me.	1	2	3	4
11. People will think I am crazy.	1	2	3	4
12. I'll always be this way.	1	2	3	4
13. I am going to throw up.	1	2	3	4
14. I must have a brain tumor.	1	2	3	4
15. I'll choke to death.	1	2	3	4
16. I'm going to act foolish.	1	2	3	4
17. I'm going blind.	1	2	3	4
18. I'll hurt someone.	1	2	3	4
19. I'm going to have a stroke.	1	2	3	4
20. I'm going to scream.	1	2	3	4
21. I'm going to babble or talk funny.	1	2	3	4
22. I'll be paralyzed by fear.	1	2	3	4
23. Something is physically wrong with me.	1	2	3	4
24. I won't be able to breathe.	1	2	3	4
25. Something terrible will happen.	1	2	3	4
26. I'm going to make a scene.	1	2	3	4

Adapted from Clum, G. A. (1990). Panic attack cognitions questionnaire. *Coping with panic: A drug-free approach to dealing with anxiety attacks.* Pacific Grove, CA: Brooks/Cole.

Family Factors

Marital and parental functioning can be adversely affected by panic disorder. During the assessment, the nurse should try to grasp the patient's understanding of how panic disorder with or without severe avoidance behavior has affected his or her life along with that of the family. Pertinent questions include the following:

• How has the disorder affected your family's social life?
• What limitations related to travel has the disorder placed on you or your family?
• What coping strategies have you used to manage symptoms?
• How has the disorder affected your family members or others?

Cultural Factors

Cultural competence calls for the understanding of cultural knowledge, cultural awareness, cultural assessment skills, and cultural practice. Therefore, cultural differences must be considered in the assessment of panic disorder. Different cultures interpret sensations, feelings, or understandings differently. For example, symptoms of anxiety might be seen as witchcraft or magic (APA, 2013). Several cultures do not have a word to describe "anxiety" or "anxious" and instead may use words or meanings to suggest physical complaints. In addition, showing anxiety may be a sign of weakness in some cultures (Roberts, 2010). Many Asian over-the-counter (OTC) herbal remedies contain substances that may induce panic by increasing the heart rate, basal metabolic rate, blood pressure, and sweating (see Chapter 10).

Identifying Strengths

During the assessment, the patient's strengths will emerge. For example, a patient may tell you that he does not drink alcohol or use tobacco. Another may relate that he would like to exercise. Still another patient has a supportive partner or family member. The nurse can support these positive behaviors as the care plan is established.

Nursing Diagnoses

There are several nursing diagnoses for the individual with panic disorder including Anxiety, Risk for Self-Harm, Social Isolation, Powerlessness, and Ineffective Family Coping. Other possible diagnoses include Risk for Self-Harm, Social Isolation, Powerlessness, Ineffective Family Coping, Social Isolation, Impaired Social Interaction, and Risk for Loneliness. Diagnoses specific to physical panic symptoms such as dizziness, hyperventilation, and other findings are likely. Because the whole family is affected by one member's symptoms, Interrupted Family Processes may also occur. Outcomes will depend upon the particular nursing diagnosis and the interventions that are agreed upon by the patient and nurse.

Biologic Interventions

The course of panic disorder culminates in phobic avoidance as the affected person attempts to avoid situations that increase panic. Because identifying and avoiding anxiety-provoking situations are important during therapy, drastically changing lifestyle to avoid situations does not aid recovery. Interventions that focus on the physical aspects of anxiety and panic are particularly helpful in reducing the number and severity of the attacks, giving patients a rapid sense of accomplishment and control.

Teaching Breathing Control

Hyperventilation is common. Often, people are unaware that they take rapid shallow breaths when they become anxious.

Teaching patients breathing control can be helpful. Focus on the breathing and help them to identify the rate, pattern, and depth. If the breathing is rapid and shallow, reassure the patient that exercise and breathing practice can help change this breathing pattern. Then, assist the patient in practicing abdominal breathing by performing the following exercises:

- Instruct the patient to breathe deeply by inhaling slowly through the nose. Have him or her place a hand on the abdomen just beneath the rib cage.
- Instruct the patient to observe that when one is breathing deeply, the hand on the abdomen will actually rise.
- After the patient understands this process, ask him or her to inhale slowly through the nose while counting to five, pause, and then exhale slowly through pursed lips.
- While the patient exhales, direct attention to feeling the muscles relax, focusing on "letting go."

- Have the patient repeat the deep abdominal breathing for 10 breaths, pausing between each inhalation and exhalation. Count slowly. If the patient complains of light-headedness, reassure him or her that this is a normal feeling while deep breathing. Instruct the patient to stop for 30 seconds, breathe normally, and then start again.
- The patient should stop between each cycle of 10 breaths and monitor normal breathing for 30 seconds.
- This series of 10 slow abdominal breaths followed by 30 seconds of normal breathing should be repeated for 3 to 5 minutes.
- Help the patient to establish a time for daily practice of abdominal breathing.

Abdominal breathing may also be used to interrupt an episode of panic as it begins. After patients have learned to identify their own early signs of panic, they can learn the four-square method of breathing, which helps divert or decrease the severity of the attack. Patients should be instructed as follows:

- Advise the patient to practice during calm periods and to begin by inhaling slowly through the nose, count to four, and then hold the breath for a count of four.
- Direct the patient to exhale slowly through pursed lips to a count of four and then rest for a count of four (no breath).
- Finally, the patient may take two normal breaths and repeat the sequence.

After patients practice the skill, the nurse should assist them in identifying the physical cues that will alert them to use this calming technique.

Teaching Nutritional Planning

Maintaining regular and balanced eating habits reduces the likelihood of hypoglycemic episodes, light-headedness, and fatigue. To help teach the patient about healthful eating and ways to minimize physical factors contributing to anxiety:

- Advise the patient to reduce or eliminate substances in the diet that promote anxiety and panic, such as food coloring, monosodium glutamate, and caffeine (withdrawal from which may stimulate panic). Patients need to plan to reduce caffeine consumption and then eliminate it from their diet. Many OTC remedies are now used to boost energy or increase mental performance; some of these contain caffeine. A thorough assessment should be made of all OTC products used to assess the potential of anxiety-provoking ingredients.
- Instruct the patient to check each substance consumed and note whether symptoms of anxiety occur and whether the symptoms are relieved by not consuming the product.

Teaching Relaxation Techniques

Teaching the patient relaxation techniques is another way to help individuals with panic and anxiety disorders. Some are unaware of the tension in their bodies and first need to learn to monitor their own tension. Isometric exercises and progressive muscle relaxation are helpful methods to learn to differentiate muscle tension from muscle relaxation. This method of relaxation is also useful when patients have difficulty clearing the mind, focusing, or visualizing a scene, which are often required in other forms of relaxation, such as meditation. Box 16.6 provides one method of progressive muscle relaxation.

Promoting Increased Physical Activity

Physical exercise can effectively decrease the occurrence of panic attacks by reducing muscle tension, increasing metabolism, increasing serotonin levels, and relieving stress. Exercise programs reduce many of the precipitants of anxiety by improving circulation, digestion, endorphin stimulation, and tissue oxygenation. In addition, exercise lowers cholesterol levels, blood pressure, and weight. After assessing for contraindications to physical exercise, assist the patient in establishing a routine exercise program. Engaging in 10- to 20-minute sessions on treadmills or stationary bicycles two to three times weekly is ideal during the winter months. Casual walking or bike riding during warmer weather promotes health. Help the patient to identify community resources that promote exercise.

Pharmacologic Interventions

Some antidepressants (e.g., SSRIs and SNRIs), and antianxiety medication (e.g., benzodiazepines) are FDA approved for treating people with panic disorders (see Table 16.4).

Selective Serotonin Reuptake Inhibitors

The SSRIs are recommended as the first drug option in the treatment of patients with panic disorder. They have the best safety profile, and if side effects occur, they tend to be present early in treatment before the therapeutic effect takes place. Hence, the SSRIs should be started at low doses and titrated every 5 to 7 days. Antidepressant therapy is recommended for long-term treatment of the disorder and antianxiety as adjunctive treatment (Andrisano, Chiesa, & Serretti, 2013).

The SSRIs produce anxiolytic effects by increasing the transmission of serotonin by blocking serotonin reuptake at the presynaptic cleft. The initial increase in serotonergic activity with SSRIs may cause temporary increases in panic symptoms and even panic attacks. After 4 to 6 weeks of treatment, anxiety subsides, and the antianxiety effect of the medications begins (see Chapter 10). Increased serotonin activity in the brain is believed to decrease norepinephrine activity. This decrease lessens cardiovascular symptoms of tachycardia and increased blood pressure that are associated with panic attacks. See Chapter 19 for administration and monitoring side effects.

> **NCLEXNOTE** Psychopharmacologic treatment is almost always needed. Antidepressants are the medications of choice. Antianxiety medication is used only for short periods of time.

Serotonin–Norepinephrine Reuptake Inhibitors

The SNRIs increase levels of both serotonin and norepinephrine by blocking their reuptake presynaptically. Classified as antidepressants, the SNRIs are also used in

---

BOX 16.6

Teaching Progressive Muscle Relaxation

Choose a quiet, comfortable location where you will not be disturbed for 20 to 30 minutes. Your position may be lying or sitting, but all parts of your body should be supported, including your head. Wear loose clothing, taking off restrictive items, such as glasses and shoes.

Begin by closing your eyes and clearing your mind. Moving from head to toe, focus on each part or your body and assess the level of tension. Visualize each group of muscles as heavy and relaxed.

Take two or three slow abdominal breaths, pausing briefly between each breath. Imagine the tension flowing from your body.

Each muscle group listed below should be tightened (or tensed isometrically) for 5 to 10 seconds and then abruptly released; visualize this group of muscles as heavy, limp, and relaxed for 15 to 20 seconds before tightening the next group of muscles. There are several methods to tighten each muscle group and suggestions are provided below. Each muscle group may be tightened two to three times until relaxed. Do not overtighten or strain. You should not experience pain.

- Hands: tighten by making fists
- Biceps: tighten by drawing forearms up and "making a muscle"
- Triceps: extend forearms straight, locking elbows
- Face: grimace, tightly shutting mouth and eyes
- Face: open mouth wide and raise eyebrows
- Neck: pull head forward to chest and tighten neck muscles
- Shoulders: raise shoulders toward ears
- Shoulders: push shoulders back as if touching them together
- Chest: take a deep breath and hold for 10 seconds
- Stomach: suck in your abdominal muscles
- Buttocks: pull buttocks together
- Thighs: straighten legs and squeeze muscles in thighs and hips
- Calves: pull toes carefully toward you, avoid cramps
- Feet: curl toes downward and point toes away from your body

Finally, repeat several deep abdominal breaths and mentally check your body for tension. Rest comfortably for several minutes, breathing normally, and visualize your body as warm and relaxed. Get up slowly when you are finished.

TABLE 16.4	MEDICATION FOR PANIC DISORDER			
Medication	Starting Dose (mg/day)	Therapeutic Dose	Side Effects	
Selective serotonin reuptake inhibitors (SSRIs)			Class effects: nausea, anorexia, tremors, anxiety, sexual dysfunction, jitteriness, insomnia, suicidality	
Fluoxetine (Prozac)	10	20–60	Class effects	
Sertraline (Zoloft)	25	50–200	Class effects, loose stools	
Paroxetine (Paxil)	10	10–60	Class effects, drowsiness, fatigue	
Paroxetine (controlled release) (Paxil CR)	12.5	12.5–75	Class effects	
Serotonin–norepinephrine reuptake inhibitors (SNRIs)			Class effects: nausea, sweating, dry mouth, dizziness, insomnia, somnolence, sexual dysfunction, hypertension	
Venlafaxine (extended release)	37.5	75–300	Class effects	
Benzodiazepines			Class effects: sedation, cognitive slowing, physical dependence	
Clonazepam (Klonopin)	0.25 tid	0.5–2.0 bid	Class effects	
Alprazolam (Xanax)	0.25 tid	0.5–1.5 tid	Class effects	

tid, three times a day.

anxiety disorders. Venlafaxine (Effexor) is the most commonly used SNRI (see Table 16.4). These medications have been shown to reduce the severity of panic and anticipatory anxiety. Similar to the SSRIs, they should not be abruptly discontinued (see Chapter 10).

Benzodiazepine Therapy

The high-potency benzodiazepines have produced antipanic effects; their therapeutic onset is much faster than that of antidepressants (see Table 16.4). Therefore, benzodiazepines are tremendously useful in treating intensely distressed patients. Alprazolam (Xanax), lorazepam (Ativan), and clonazepam (Klonopin) are widely used for panic disorder. They are well tolerated but carry the risk for withdrawal symptoms upon discontinuation of use (see Box 16.7). The benzodiazepines are still commonly used for panic disorder even though the SSRIs are recommended for first-line treatment of panic disorder (Stein et al., 2010).

BOX 16.7

Drug Profile: Alprazolam (Xanax)

DRUG CLASS: Antianxiety agent

RECEPTOR AFFINITY: Exact mechanism of action is unknown; believed to increase the effects of γ-aminobutyrate

INDICATIONS: Management of anxiety disorders, short-term relief of anxiety symptoms or depression-related anxiety, panic attacks with or without agoraphobia.

ROUTES AND DOSAGES: Available in 0.25-, 0.5-, 1-, and 2-mg scored tablets.

Adults: For anxiety: Initially, 0.25 to 0.5 mg PO tid titrated to a maximum daily dose of 4 mg in divided doses. For panic disorder: Initially, 0.5 mg PO tid increased at 3- to 4-d intervals in increments of no more than 1 mg/d.

Geriatric patients: Initially, 0.25 mg bid to tid, increased gradually as needed and tolerated

HALF-LIFE (PEAK EFFECT): 12 to 15 h (1–2 h)

SELECTED ADVERSE REACTIONS: Transient mild drowsiness, initially; sedation, depression, lethargy, apathy, fatigue, light-headedness, disorientation, anger, hostility, restlessness, headache, confusion, crying, constipation, diarrhea, dry mouth, nausea, and possible drug dependence

WARNINGS: Contraindicated in patients with psychosis, acute narrow-angle glaucoma, shock, acute alcoholic intoxication with depressed vital signs, pregnancy, labor and delivery, and breastfeeding. Use cautiously in patients with impaired hepatic or renal function and severe debilitating conditions. Risk for digitalis toxicity if given concurrently with digoxin. Increased CNS depression if taken with alcohol, other CNS depressants, and propoxyphene (Darvon).

SPECIFIC PATIENT AND FAMILY EDUCATION
- Avoid using alcohol, sleep-inducing drugs, and other OTC drugs.
- Take the drug exactly as prescribed and do not stop taking the drug without consulting your primary health care provider.
- Take the drug with food if gastrointestinal upset occurs.
- Avoid driving a car or performing tasks that require alertness if drowsiness or dizziness occurs.
- Report any signs and symptoms of adverse reactions.
- Notify your primary health care provider if severe dizziness, weakness, or drowsiness persists or if rash or skin lesions, difficulty voiding, palpitations, or swelling of the extremities occurs.

CNS, central nervous system; OTC, over the counter; PO, oral; tid, three times a day.

Administering and Monitoring Benzodiazepines. Treatment may include administering benzodiazepines concurrently with antidepressants for the first 4 weeks and then tapering the benzodiazepine to a maintenance dose. This strategy provides rapid symptom relief but avoids the complications of long-term benzodiazepine use. Benzodiazepines with short half-lives do not accumulate in the body, but benzodiazepines with half-lives of longer than 24 hours tend to accumulate with long-term treatment, are removed more slowly, and produce less intense symptoms on discontinuation of use (see Chapter 10).

Short-acting benzodiazepines, such as alprazolam, are associated with rebound anxiety, or anxiety that increases after the peak effects of the medication have decreased. Medications with short half-lives (alprazolam, lorazepam) should be given in three or four doses spaced throughout the day, with a higher dose at bedtime to allay anxiety-related insomnia. Clonazepam, a longer-acting benzodiazepine, requires less frequent dosing and has a lower risk for rebound anxiety.

Because of their depressive CNS effects, benzodiazepines should not be used to treat patients with comorbid sleep apnea. In fact, these drugs may actually decrease the rate and depth of respirations. Exercise caution in older adult patients for these reasons. Discontinuing medication use requires a slow taper during a period of several weeks to avoid rebound anxiety and serious withdrawal symptoms. Benzodiazepines are not indicated in the chronic treatment of patients with substance abuse but can be useful in quickly treating anxiety symptoms until other medications take effect.

Symptoms associated with withdrawal of benzodiazepine therapy are more likely to occur after high doses and long-term therapy. They can also occur after short-term therapy. Withdrawal symptoms manifest in several ways, including psychological (e.g., apprehension, irritability; agitation).

Monitoring for Drug Interactions. SSRIs should not be given with MAOIs because of potential drug interaction. Drugs that interact with benzodiazepines include the TCAs and digoxin; interaction may result in increased serum TCA or digoxin levels. Alcohol and other CNS depressants, when used with benzodiazepines, increase CNS depression. Their concomitant use is contraindicated. Histamine-2 blockers (e.g., cimetidine) used with benzodiazepines may potentiate sedative effects. Monitor closely for effectiveness in patients who smoke; cigarette smoking may increase the clearance of benzodiazepines.

Managing Side Effects. The side effects of benzodiazepine medications generally include headache, confusion, dizziness, disorientation, sedation, and visual disturbances. Sedation should be monitored after beginning medication use or increasing the dose. The patient should avoid operating heavy machinery until the sedative effects are known.

Drugs that interact with benzodiazepines include the TCAs and digoxin; interaction may result in increased serum TCA or digoxin levels. Alcohol and other CNS depressants, when used with benzodiazepines, increase CNS depression. Their concomitant use is contraindicated. Histamine-2 blockers (e.g., cimetidine) used with benzodiazepines may potentiate sedative effects. Monitor closely for effectiveness in patients who smoke; cigarette smoking may increase the clearance of benzodiazepines. Concurrent use of SSRIs and the MAOIs is contraindicated. These antidepressants should not be given together.

Teaching Points. Warn patients to avoid alcohol because of the chance of CNS depression. In addition, warn them not to operate heavy machinery until the sedative effects of the medication are known.

Psychosocial Interventions

Reaction to Stimuli

Peplau (1989) devised general guidelines for nursing interventions that might be successful in treating patients with anxiety. These interventions help the patient attend to and react to input other than the subjective experience of anxiety. They are designed to help the patient focus on other stimuli and cope with anxiety in any form (Table 16.5). These general interventions apply to all anxiety disorders and therefore are not reiterated in subsequent sections

Distraction

After patients can identify the early symptoms of panic, they may learn to implement distraction behaviors that take the focus off the physical sensations. Some activities include initiating conversation with a nearby person or engaging in physical activity (e.g., walking, gardening, or housecleaning). Performing simple repetitive activities such as snapping a rubber band against the wrist, counting backward from 100 by 3s, or counting objects along the roadway might also deter an attack.

Reframing is a cognitive technique that can change the way a situation, event, or person is viewed and reduce the impact of anxiety provoking thoughts. People with anxiety disorders often view themselves negatively and use "should statements" and "negative labels." Should statements lead to rigid rules and unrealistic expectations. By encouraging patients to avoid the use of should statements and reframe their views, they can change their beliefs to be more realistic. For example, if a patient says "I should be a better parent" or "I'm a useless failure,"

Degree of Anxiety	Nursing Interventions
TABLE 16.5	**NURSING INTERVENTIONS BASED ON DEGREES OF ANXIETY**
Mild	Assist patient to use the energy anxiety provides to encourage learning.
Moderate	Encourage patient to talk: to focus on one experience, to describe it fully, and then to formulate the patient's generalizations about that experience.
Severe	Allow relief behaviors to be used but do not ask about them. Encourage the patient to talk: ventilation of random ideas is likely to reduce anxiety to a moderate level.
Panic	Stay with the patient. Allow pacing and walk with the patient. No content inputs to the patient's thinking should be made by the nurse. (They burden the patient, who will distort them.) Be direct with the fewest number of words: e.g., "Drink this" (give liquids to replace lost fluids and to relieve dry mouth); "Say what's happening to you," "Talk about yourself," or "Tell what you feel now" (to encourage ventilation and externalization of inner, frightening experience). Pick up on what the patient says, e.g., Patient: "What's happening to me—how did I get here?" Nurse: "Say what you notice." Use short phrases to the point of the patient's comment. Do not touch the patient; patients experiencing panic are very concerned about survival, are experiencing a grave threat to self, and usually distort intentions of all invasions of their personal space.

Adapted from Peplau, H. (1989). Theoretical constructs: Anxiety, self, and hallucinations. In A. O'Toole & S. Welt (Eds.), *Interpersonal theory in nursing practice: Selected works of Hildegarde E. Peplau.* New York: Springer.

the nurse could ask the person to identify the positive aspects of parenting and other successes.

> **Remember Doug?**
> What interventions would be helpful for him to reduce his anxiety and frequency of his panic attacks?

Positive Self-Talk

During states of increased anxiety and panic, individuals can learn to counter fearful or negative thoughts by using another cognitive approach. **Positive self-talk** involves planning and rehearsing positive coping statements "This is only anxiety, and it will pass," "I can handle these symptoms," and "I'll get through this" are examples of positive self-talk. These types of positive statements can give the individual a focal point and reduce fear when panic symptoms begin. Handheld cards that offer positive statements can be carried in a purse or wallet so the person can retrieve them quickly when panic symptoms are felt (Box 16.8).

NCLEXNOTE Cognitive interventions give patients with anxiety a sense of control over the recurring threats of panic and obsessions.

Psychoeducation

Psychoeducation programs help to teach patients and families about the symptoms of panic. Individuals with panic disorder legitimately fear going crazy, losing control, or dying because of their physical symptoms.

Attempting to convince a patient that such fears are groundless only heightens anxiety and impedes communication. Information and physical evidence (e.g., electrocardiogram results, laboratory test results), should be presented in a caring and open manner that demonstrates acceptance and understanding of his or her situation.

Box 16.9 suggests topics for individual or small-group discussion. It is especially important to cover such topics as the differences between panic attacks and heart attacks, the difference between panic disorder and other psychiatric disorders, and the effectiveness of various treatment methods.

Lifestyle Changes

Individuals with panic disorder, especially those with significant anxiety sensitivity, may need assistance in reevaluating their lifestyle. Time management can be a useful tool. In the workplace or at home, underestimating the time needed to complete a chore or being overly involved in several activities at once increases stress and anxiety. Procrastination, lack of assertiveness, and difficulties with prioritizing or delegating tasks intensify these problems.

Writing a list of chores to be completed and estimating time to complete them provides concrete feedback to the individual. Crossing out each activity as it is completed helps the patient to regain a sense of control and accomplishment. Large tasks should be broken into a series of smaller tasks to minimize stress and maximize sense of achievement. Rest, relaxation, and family time—frequently omitted from the daily schedule—must be included.

BOX16.8 • THERAPEUTIC DIALOGUE • Panic Disorder

Doug is admitted to an inpatient unit following another severe panic attack. He had an argument with his high school son who continues to use alcohol and marijuana. Financial problems are also escalating.

INEFFECTIVE APPROACH

Nurse: Oh…. Why are you crying?

Doug: (Looks up, gives a nervous chuckle.) Obviously, because I'm upset. I am tired of living this way. I just want to be normal again. I can't even remember what that feels like.

Nurse: You look normal to me. Everyone has bad days. It'll pass.

Doug: I've felt this way longer than you've been alive. I've tried everything, and nothing works.

Nurse: You're not the first depressed person that I've taken care of. You just need to go to groups and stay out of your room more. You'll start feeling better.

Doug: (Angrily) Oh, it's just that easy. You have no idea what I'm going through! You don't know me! You're just a kid.

Nurse: I can help you if you help yourself. A group starts in 5 minutes, and I'd like to see you there.

Doug: I'm not going to no damn group! I want to be alone so I can think!

Nurse: (Looks about anxiously.) Maybe I should come back after you've calmed down a little.

EFFECTIVE APPROACH

Nurse: Doug, I noticed that you are staying in your room more today. What's troubling you?

Doug: (Looks up) I feel like I've lost complete control of my life. I'm so anxious, and nothing helps. I'm tired of it.

Nurse: I see. That must be difficult. Can you tell me more about what you are feeling right now?

Doug: I feel like I'm going crazy. I worry all the time about having panic attacks. They make me scared I'm going to die. Sometimes I think I'd be better off dead.

Nurse: (Remains silent, continues to give eye contact.)

Doug: Do you know what it's like to be a prisoner to your emotions? I can't even go to work sometimes, and when I do, it's terrifying. I don't know what to think anymore.

Nurse: Doug, you have lived with this disorder for a long time. You say that the medications do not work to your liking, but what has helped you in the past?

Doug: Well, I learned in relaxation group that panic symptoms are probably caused by chemicals in my brain that are not working correctly. I learned that medications can help, but they don't work well for me. I tried an exposure plan and relaxation techniques to deal with my fears of leaving the house and my chronic anxiety. That did help some, but it's scary to do.

Nurse: It sounds like you have learned a lot about your illness, one that can be treated, so that you don't always have to feel this way.

Doug: This is easier to say right now when I'm here and can get help if I need it. It's hard to remember this when I'm in the middle of a panic attack and think I'm dying.

Nurse: It's harder when you're alone?

Doug: Much harder! And I'm alone so much of the time.

Nurse: Let's talk about some ways you can manage your panics when you're alone. Tell me some of the techniques you've learned.

CRITICAL THINKING CHALLENGE

- What tone is established by the nurse's opening question in the first scenario?

- Which therapeutic communication techniques did the nurse use in the second scenario to avoid the pitfalls encountered in the first scenario?

- What information was uncovered in the second scenario that was not touched on in the first?

- What predictions can you make about the interpersonal relationship likely to develop between the nurse and the patient in each scenario?

BOX 16.9

Psychoeducation Checklist: Panic Disorder

When caring for the patient with panic disorder, be sure to include the following topic areas in the teaching plan:

- Psychopharmacologic agents (anxiolytics or antidepressants) if ordered, including drug action, dosage, frequency, and possible adverse effects
- Breathing control measures
- Nutrition
- Exercise
- Progressive muscle relaxation
- Distraction behaviors
- Exposure therapy
- Time management
- Positive coping strategies

Evaluation and Treatment Outcomes.

Although many researchers consider panic disorder a chronic, long-term condition, the positive results from outcome studies should be shared with patients to provide encouragement and optimism that patients can learn to manage these symptoms. Outcome studies have demonstrated success with panic control treatment, CBT therapy, exposure therapy, and various medications specific to certain symptoms.

Continuum of Care

As with any disorder, a continuum of patient care across multiple settings is crucial. Patients are treated in the least restrictive environment that will meet their safety needs. As the patient progresses through treatment, the environment of care changes from an emergency or inpatient setting to outpatient clinics or individual therapy sessions.

Inpatient-Focused Care

Inpatient settings provide control for the stabilization of the acute panic symptoms and initiation of recovery-oriented strategies. Medication use often is initiated here because patients who show initial panic symptoms require in-depth assessment to determine the cause. As recovery begins, crisis stabilization, medication management, milieu therapy, psychotherapies are introduced, and outpatient discharge linkage appointments are set. See Nursing Care Plan 16.1, available at http://thepoint. lww.com/BoydEssentials.

Emergency Care

Because individuals with panic disorder are likely to first present for treatment in an emergency department or primary care setting, nurses working in these settings should be involved in early recognition and referral. Consultation with a psychiatrist or mental health professional by the primary care physician can decrease both costs and overall patient symptoms. Several interventions may be useful in reducing the number of emergency department visits related to panic symptoms. Psychiatric consultation and nursing education can be provided in the emergency department to explore other avenues of treatment. Remembering that the patient experiencing a panic attack is in crisis, nurses can take several measures to help alleviate symptoms, including the following:

- Stay with the patient and maintain a calm demeanor. (Anxiety often produces more anxiety and a calm presence will help calm the patient.)
- Reassure the patient that you will not leave, that this episode will pass, and that he or she is in a safe place. (The patient often fears dying and cannot see beyond the panic attack.)
- Give clear concise directions using short sentences. Do not use medical jargon.
- Walk or pace with the patient to an environment with minimal stimulation. (The patient in panic has excessive energy.)
- Administer PRN (i.e., as-needed) anxiolytic medications as ordered and appropriate. (Pharmacotherapy is effective in treating those patients with acute panic attack.)

After the panic attack has resolved, allow the patient to vent his or her feelings. This often helps the patient in clarifying his or her feelings.

Family Interventions

In addition to learning the symptoms of panic disorder, nurses should have information sheets or pamphlets available concerning the disorder and any medications prescribed. Parents, especially single parents, will need assistance in child-rearing and may benefit from services designed to provide some respite. Moreover, the entire family will need support in adjusting to the disorder. A referral for family therapy is indicated, because involving the entire family in the therapy process is imperative. Families experience the symptoms, treatments, clinical setbacks, and recovery from chronic mental illnesses as a unit. Misunderstandings, misconceptions, false information, and the stigma of mental illness, singly or collectively, impede recovery efforts.

Community Treatment

Most individuals with panic disorder are treated on an outpatient basis. Referral lists of community resources and support groups are useful in this setting. A discussion about the recovery and the importance of the 10 components help healing to begin (see Chapter 1). Nurses are more directly involved in treatment, conducting psychoeducation groups on relaxation and breathing techniques, symptom management, and anger management. Advanced practice nurses conduct CBT and individual and family psychotherapy. In addition, medication monitoring groups reemphasize the role of medications, monitor for side effects, and enhance treatment compliance overall.

GENERALIZED ANXIETY DISORDER

Generally speaking, patients with generalized anxiety disorder (GAD) feel frustrated, disgusted with life, demoralized, and hopeless. They may state that they cannot remember a time that they did not feel anxious. They experience a sense of ill-being and uneasiness and a fear of imminent disaster. Over time, they may recognize that their chronic tension and anxiety are unreasonable.

Clinical Course

The onset of GAD is insidious. Many patients complain of being chronic worriers. GAD affects individuals of all ages. About half of individuals with GAD report an onset in childhood or adolescence, although onset after 20 years of age is also common. Adults with GAD often worry about matters such as their job, household finances, health of family members, or simple matters (e.g., household chores or being late for appointments). The intensity of the worry fluctuates and stress tends to intensify the worry and anxiety symptoms (APA, 2013).

Patients with GAD may exhibit mild depressive symptoms, such as dysphoria. They are also highly somatic, with complaints of multiple clusters of physical symptoms, including muscle aches, soreness, and gastrointestinal ailments. In addition to physical complaints, patients with GAD often experience poor sleep habits, irritability, trembling, twitching, poor concentration, and an exaggerated startle response. People with this disorder often are seen in a primary care setting with somatic symptoms (Kroenke et al., 2013).

Diagnostic Criteria

GAD is characterized by excessive worry and anxiety (apprehensive expectation) for at least 6 months. The anxiety does not usually pertain to a specific situation; rather, it concerns several real-life activities or events. Ultimately, excessive worry and anxiety cause great distress and interfere with the patient's daily personal or social life.

Nursing Care

Nursing care for the person with GAD is similar to the care of the individual with a panic disorder. In many instances, antidepressants and an antianxiety agent will

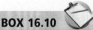

BOX 16.10

Psychoeducation Checklist: Generalized Anxiety Disorder

When caring for the patient with generalized anxiety disorder, be sure to include the following topic areas in the teaching plan:

- Psychopharmacologic agents (benzodiazepines, antidepressants, nonbenzodiazepine anxiolytics, β-blockers) if ordered, including drug action, dosage, frequency, and possible adverse effects
- Breathing control
- Nutrition and diet restriction
- Sleep measures
- Progressive muscle relaxation
- Time management
- Positive coping strategies

be prescribed. Nursing interventions should focus on helping the person target specific areas of anxiety and reducing the impact of the anxiety. See Box 16.10.

Other Anxiety Disorders

Other disorders exist that have anxiety as their defining feature. These include generalized phobia, agoraphobia, specific phobias, and social anxiety disorder.

Agoraphobia

Agoraphobia is fear or anxiety triggered by about two or more situations such as using public transportation, being in open spaces, being in enclosed places, standing in line, being in a crowd, or being outside of the home alone (APA, 2013). When these situations occur, the individual believes that something terrible might happen and that escape may be difficult. The individual may experience panic-like symptoms or other embarrassing symptoms (e.g., vomiting, diarrhea) (APA, 2013). Agoraphobia leads to avoidance behaviors. Such avoidance interferes with routine functioning and eventually renders the person afraid to leave the safety of home. Some affected individuals continue to face feared situations but with significant trepidation (i.e., going in public only to pay bills or to take children to school). Agoraphobia may occur with panic disorder but is considered a separate disorder.

Specific Phobia

Specific phobia disorder is marked by persistent fear of clearly discernible, circumscribed objects or situations, which often leads to avoidance behaviors. Phobic objects can include animals (e.g., spiders, snakes), natural environment (e.g., heights, storms), blood injection injury (e.g., fear of blood, injections), and situational (e.g., elevators, enclosed spaces). The lifetime prevalence rates range from 7% to 9%, and the disorder generally affects women twice as much as men (APA, 2013). It has a bimodal distribution, peaking in childhood and then again in the 20s. The focus of the fear in specific phobia may result from the anticipation of being harmed by the phobic object. For example, dogs are feared because of the chance of being bitten or automobiles are feared because of the potential of crashing. The focus of fear may likewise be associated with concerns about losing control, panicking, or fainting on exposure to the phobic object.

Anxiety is usually felt immediately on exposure to the phobic object; the level of anxiety is usually related to both the proximity of the object and the degree to which escape is possible. For example, anxiety heightens as a cat approaches a person who fears cats and lessens when the cat moves away. At times, the level of anxiety escalates to a full panic attack, particularly when the person must remain in a situation from which escape is deemed to be impossible. Fear of specific objects is fairly common and the diagnosis of specific phobia is not made unless the fear significantly interferes with functioning or causes marked distress. Assessment differentiates simple phobia from other diagnoses with overlapping symptoms. Box 16.11 lists a number of specific phobias. Among adult patients who are seen in clinical settings, the most-to-least common phobias are situational phobias, natural environment phobias, blood injection, injury phobia, and animal phobias (APA, 2013).

Blood injection injury phobia merits special consideration because the phobia involves medical treatments. The physiologic processes that are exhibited during phobic exposure include a strong vasovagal response, which significantly increases blood pressure and pulse, followed by deceleration of the pulse and lowering of blood pressure in the patient. Monitor closely when giving required injections or medical treatments.

About 75% of patients with blood injection injury phobia report fainting on exposure. Factors that may predispose individuals to specific phobias may include traumatic events; unexpected panic attacks in the presence of the phobic object or situation; observation of others experiencing a trauma; or repeated exposure to information warning of dangers, such as parents repeatedly warning young children that dogs bite.

Phobic content must be evaluated from an ethnic or cultural background. In many cultures, fears of spirits or magic are common. They should be considered part of a disorder only if the fear is excessive in the context of the culture, causes the individual significant distress, or impairs the ability to function.

Psychotropic drugs have not been effective in the treatment of specific phobia. Anxiolytics may give short-term relief of phobic anxiety, but no evidence confirms that they affect the course of the disorder. The treatment of choice for specific phobia is exposure therapy. Patients who are highly motivated can experience success with treatment (Peñalba, McGuire, & Leite, 2008).

Social Anxiety Disorder (Social Phobia)

Social anxiety disorder involves a persistent fear of social or performance situations in which embarrassment may occur. Exposure to a feared social or performance situation nearly always provokes immediate anxiety and may trigger panic attacks. People with social anxiety disorder fear that others will scrutinize their behavior and judge them negatively. They often do not speak up in crowds out of fear of embarrassment. They go to great lengths to avoid feared situations. If avoidance is not possible, they suffer through the situation with visible anxiety (APA, 2013).

People with social anxiety disorder appear to be highly sensitive to disapproval or criticism, tend to evaluate themselves negatively, and have poor self-esteem and a distorted view of their personal strengths and weaknesses. They may magnify their personal flaws and underrate any talents. They often believe others would act with more assertiveness in a given social situation. Men and women with social anxiety disorder tend to have difficulties with dating and with sexual relationships (Xu, Schneier, Heimberg, Princisvalle, Liebowitz, Wang, et al., 2012). Children tend to underachieve in school because of test-taking anxiety. This is an important area that should be assessed in all patients.

Generalized social anxiety disorder is diagnosed when the individual experiences fears related to most social situations, including public performances and social interactions. These individuals are likely to demonstrate

---

BOX 16.11

Common Phobias

- Acrophobia: fear of heights
- Agoraphobia: fear of open spaces
- Ailurophobia: fear of cats
- Algophobia: fear of pain
- Arachnophobia: fear of spiders
- Brontophobia: fear of thunder
- Claustrophobia: fear of closed spaces
- Cynophobia: fear of dogs
- Entomophobia: fear of insects
- Hematophobia: fear of blood
- Microphobia: fear of germs
- Nyctophobia: fear of night or dark places
- Ophidiophobia: fear of snakes
- Phonophobia: fear of loud noises
- Photophobia: fear of light
- Pyrophobia: fear of fire
- Topophobia: fear of a place, like a stage
- Xenophobia: fear of strangers
- Zoophobia: fear of animal or animals

deficiencies in social skills and their phobias interfere with their ability to function (MacKenzie & Fowler, 2013). Generalized social anxiety disorder may be linked to low dopamine receptor binding, as suggested by recent research (Cervenka, Hedman, Ikoma, Djurfeldt, Rück, Halldin, et al., 2012).

People with social anxiety disorder fear and avoid only one or two social situations. Classic examples of such situations are eating, writing, or speaking in public or using public bathrooms. The most common fears for individuals with social anxiety disorder are public speaking, fear of meeting strangers, eating in public, writing in public, using public restrooms, and being stared at or being the center of attention.

Pharmacotherapy is a relatively new area of research in treating patients with social anxiety disorder. SSRIs are used to treat those with social anxiety disorder because they significantly reduce social anxiety and phobic avoidance. Benzodiazepines are also used to reduce anxiety caused by phobias. Providing referrals for appropriate psychiatric treatment is a critical nursing intervention.

SUMMARY OF KEY POINTS

- Anxiety-related disorders are the most common of all psychiatric disorders and comprise several disorders, including panic disorder.

- The anxiety disorders share the common symptom of recurring anxiety but differ in symptom profiles. Panic attacks can occur in many different disorders.

- Those experiencing anxiety disorders have a high level of physical and emotional illness and often experience dual diagnoses with other anxiety disorders, substance abuse, or depression. These disorders often render individuals unable to function effectively at home or at a job.

- Patients with panic disorder are often seen in various health care settings, frequently in hospital emergency departments or clinics, presenting with a confusing array of physical and emotional symptoms. Skillful assessment is required to eliminate possible life-threatening causes.

- Treatment approaches for all anxiety-related disorders are somewhat similar, including pharmacotherapy, psychological treatments, or often a combination of both.

- Nursing interventions include helping patients manage a panic attack, promoting healthy diet, exercise and sleep hygiene habits, medication administration and monitoring, psychoeducation, and cognitive interventions.

CRITICAL THINKING CHALLENGES

1. A patient is unable to focus on your directions. He does not seem to notice others in the room; instead he is intent on cutting his food into small pieces. Applying Peplau's stages of anxiety, what level of anxiety is he experiencing?

2. Compare and contrast the following treatment modalities for anxiety disorders: systematic desensitization, implosive therapy, exposure therapy, and cognitive behavioral therapy.

3. Identify the major nursing assessment areas for a person experiencing a panic disorder.

4. A patient asks you how to prevent hyperventilation. How would you answer her question?

5. Delineate the differences in treatment effects of antidepressants vs. antianxiety medication in the treatment of panic disorder.

6. Compare the various phobias that people experience. What interventions should a nurse use for a person who has a blood injection injury phobia?

7. How might one differentiate shyness from social anxiety disorder?

 A related Psychiatric-Mental Health Nursing video on the topic of Anxiety is available at http://thepoint.lww.com/BoydEssentials.

 A Psychiatric-Mental Health Nursing Practice and Learn Activity related to the video on the topic of Anxiety is available at http://thepoint.lww.com/BoydEssentials.

REFERENCES

American Psychiatric Association. (2013). *Diagnostic and statistical manual of mental disorders DSM-5* (5th ed.). Arlington, VA: Author.

Andrisano, C., Chiesa, A., & Serretti, A. (2013). Newer antidepressants and panic disorder: A meta-analysis. (Review). *International Clinical Psychopharmacology, 28*(1), 33–45.

Asnaani, A., Gutner, C., Hinton, D., & Hofmann, S. (2009). Panic disorder, panic attacks and panic attack symptoms across race-ethnic groups: Results of the collaborative psychiatric epidemiology studies. *CNS Neuroscience & Therapeutics, 15*(3), 249–254.

Ayazi, T., Lien, L., Eide, A., Swartz, L., & Hauff, E. (2014). Association between exposure to traumatic events and anxiety disorders in a post-conflict setting: A cross-sectional community study in South Sudan. *BMC Psychiatry, 14*, 6. doi:10.1186/1471-244X-14-6

Beck, A., & Emery, G. (1985). *Anxiety disorders and phobias: A cognitive perspective.* New York: Basic Books.

Benjamin, C. L., Beidas, R. S., Comer, J. S., Puliafico, A. C., & Kendall, P. C. (2011). Generalized anxiety disorder in youth: Diagnostic considerations. *Depression and Anxiety, 28*(2), 173–182.

Centers for Disease Control and Prevention. (2013). Mental health surveillance among children–United States, 2005–2011. *Morbidity and Mortality Weekly Report, 62*(suppl 2), 1–35.

Cervenka, S., Hedman, E., Ikoma, Y., Djurfeldt, D. R., Rück, C., Halldin, C., et al. (2012). Changes in dopamine D2-receptor binding are associated to symptom reduction after psychotherapy in social anxiety disorder. *Translational Psychiatry, 2*, e120. doi:10.1038/tp.2012.40

Clum, G. A. (1990). Panic attack cognitions questionnaire. *Coping with panic: A drug-free approach to dealing with anxiety attacks.* Pacific Grove, CA: Brooks/Cole.

Del Casale, A., Serata, D., Rapinesi, C., Kotzalidis, G. D., Angeletti, G., Tatarelli, R., et al. (2013). Structural neuroimaging in patients with panic disorder: Findings and limitations of recent studies. *Psychiatria Danubina*, 25(2), 108–114.

Grant, B. F., Hasin, D. S., Stinson, F. S., Dawson, D. A., Goldstein, R. B., Smith, S., et al. (2006). The epidemiology of DSM-IV panic disorder and agoraphobia in the United States: Results from the National Epidemiologic Survey on Alcohol and Related Conditions. *The Journal of Clinical Psychiatry*, 67(3), 363–374.

Hamilton, M. (1959). The assessment of anxiety states by rating. *British Journal of Medical Psychology*, 32, 54.

Jovanovic, T., Smith, A., Kamkwalala, A., Poole, J., Samples, T., Norrholm, S. D., et al. (2011). Physiological markers of anxiety are increased in children of abused mothers. *Journal of Child Psychology and Psychiatry, and Allied Disciplines*, 52(8): 844–852.

Katz, C., Yaseen, Z. S., Mojtabai, R., Cohen, L. J., & Galynker II. (2011). Panic an independent risk factor for suicide attempt in depressive illness: Findings from the National Epidemiological survey on Alcohol and Related Conditions (NESARC). *Journal of Clinical Psychiatry*, 72(12), 1628–1635.

Kessler, R. C., Avenevoli, S., Costello, E. J., Georgiades, K., Green, J. G., Gruber, M. J., et al. (2012a). Prevalence, persistence, and sociodemographic correlates of DSM-IV disorders in the national Comorbidity survey Replication Adolescent Supplement. *Archives of General Psychiatry*, 69(4), 372–380.

Kessler, R. C., Avenevoli, S., Costello, J., Green, J. G., Gruber, M. J., McLaughlin, K. A., et al. (2012b). Severity of 12-month DSM-IV disorders in the National Comorbidity Survey Replication Adolescent Supplement. *Archives of General Psychiatry*, 69(4), 381–389.

King-Kallimanis, B., Gum, A., & Kohn, R. (2009). Comorbidity of depressive and anxiety disorders for older Americans in the national comorbidity survey replication. *American Journal of Geriatric Psychiatry*, 17(9), 782–792.

Konishi, Y., Tanii, H., Otowa, T., Sasaki, T., Tochigi, M., Umekage, T., et al. (2014). Gene x gene x gender interaction of BDNF and COMT genotypes associated with panic disorder. *Progress in Neuro-Psychopharmacology & Biological Psychiatry*. doi:10.1016/j.pnpbp.2014.01.020

Korczak, D., Goldstein, B., & Levitt, A. (2007). Panic disorder, cardiac diagnosis and emergency department utilization in an epidemiologic community sample. *General Hospital Psychiatry*, 29(4), 335–339.

Kroenke, K., Outcalt, S., Krebs, E., Bair, M. J., Wu, J., Chumbler, N., et al. (2013). Association between anxiety, health-related quality of life and functional impairment in primary care patients with chronic pain. *General Hospital Psychiatry*, 35(4), 359–365.

MacKenzie, M. B., & Fowler, K. F. (2013). Social anxiety disorder in the Canadian population: Exploring gender differences in sociodemographic profile. *Journal of Anxiety Disorders*, 27(4), 427–434.

Pace, T. W., & Heim, C. M. (2011). A short review on the psychoneuroimmunology of posttraumatic stress disorder: From risk factors to medical comorbidities. *Brain Behavior and Immunity*, 25(1), 6–13.

Peñalba, V., McGuire, H., & Leite, J. R. (2008). Psychosocial interventions for prevention of psychological disorders in law enforcement officers. *The Cochrane Database of Systematic Reviews*, (3), CD005601

Peplau, H. (1989). Theoretic constructs: Anxiety, self, and hallucinations. In A. O'Toole & S. Welt (Eds.), *Interpersonal theory in nursing practice: Selected works of Hildegarde E. Peplau*. New York: Springer.

Pilecki, B., Arentoft, A., & McKay, D. (2011). An evidence-based causal model of panic disorder. *Journal of Anxiety Disorders*, 25(3), 381–388.

Ravindran, L. N., & Stein, M. B. (2010). The pharmacologic treatment of anxiety disorders: A review of progress. *Journal of Clinical Psychiatry*, 71(7), 839–854.

Roberts, L. W. (2010). Stigma, hope, and challenge in psychiatry: Trainee perspectives from five countries on four continents. *Academic Psychiatry*, 34(1), 1–4.

Ruwaard, J., Lange, A., Schrieken, B., Dolan, C. V., & Emmelkamp, P. (2012). The effectiveness of online cognitive behavioral treatment in routine clinical practice. *PLoS One*, 7(7), e40089.

Stein, D. J., Aquilar-Gaxiola, S., Alonso, J., Bruffaerts, R., de Jonge, P., Liu, Z., et al. (2014). Associations between mental disorders and subsequent onset of hypertension. *General Hospital Psychiatry*, 36(2), 142–149.

Stein, M., Steckler, T., Lightfoot, J. D., Hay, E., & Goddard, A. W. (2010). Pharmacologic treatment of panic disorder. *Current Topics in Behavioral Neurosciences*, 2, 469–485.

Torres, A. R., Ferrão, Y. A., Shavitt, R. G., Diniz, J. B., Costa, D. L., do Rosário, M. C., et al. (2014). Panic disorder and agoraphobia, in OCD patients: Clinical profile and possible treatment implications. *Comprehensive Psychiatry*, 55(3), 588–97. doi:10.1016/j.comppsych.2013.11.017

Tully, P. J., & Baune, B. T. (2014). Comorbid anxiety disorders alter the association between cardiovascular diseases and depression: The German National Health Interview and Examination Survey. *Social Psychiatry and Psychiatric Epidemiology*, 49(5), 683–691. doi:10.1007/s00127-013-0784-x

Xu, Y., Schneier, R., Heimberg, R. G., Princisvalle, K., Liebowitz, M. R., Wang, S., et al. (2012). Gender differences in social anxiety disorder: Results from the national epidemiologic sample on alcohol and related conditions. *Journal of Anxiety Disorders*, 26(1), 12–19.

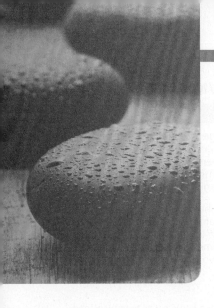

17

Trauma- and Stressor-Related Disorders

Nursing Care of Persons with Trauma-Related Stress

Mary Ann Boyd

KEY CONCEPTS

- resilience
- psychological trauma
- traumatic event

LEARNING OBJECTIVES

After studying this chapter, you will be able to:

1. Discuss the role of psychological trauma in mental disorders.

2. Discuss the importance of resilience in prevention of mental disorders.

3. Describe the prevalence and incidence of trauma–stressor-related disorders.

4. Delineate clinical symptoms and course of trauma–stressor-related disorders.

5. Analyze theories of trauma–stressor-related disorders.

6. Apply nursing process with recovery-oriented interventions for persons with trauma–stressor-related disorders.

7. Describe dissociation and dissociative disorders.

KEY TERMS

- depersonalization • derealization • dissociation • emotional reactions • hyperarousal • intrusion • kindling • numbing
- posttraumatic stress disorder • psychological trauma • resilience • traumatic events

Case Study: Susan

Thirty-year-old Susan is admitted to an inpatient mental health unit following a suicide attempt. Her relationship with her husband has deteriorated since she returned from Iraq 6 months ago. She is overwhelmed by her responsibilities as a parent and wife. She has been diagnosed with posttraumatic stress disorder.

INTRODUCTION

All of us experience stress in our daily lives, but our responses vary from person to person. One person may develop a severe **emotional reaction** (strong agitation of feelings) and another resilient individual is hardly aware of a traumatic event. While most stressful events do not lead to mental disorders, sometimes, emotional problems and mental disorders develop as the response to trauma. This chapter explains the role of resilience in buffering the mental health consequences of psychological trauma and the nursing care for those who develop trauma and stressor-related disorders. **Posttraumatic stress disorder** (PTSD) is highlighted in this chapter.

TRAUMA AND RESILIENCE

Trauma can be viewed from several different perspectives. Physical trauma may result from bodily injury resulting from an accident, self-inflicted damage, or violence perpetrated by others. Falls are a leading cause of accidents in the home. Automobile accidents are a major threat to adolescents. Self-inflicted physical trauma is often associated with mental disorders. Physical abuse of intimate partners and elder abuse are nation-wide health problems. Rape and sexual abuse, although physically traumatic, may also produce psychological trauma.

| **KEYCONCEPT** **Psychological trauma** is an emotional injury caused by an overwhelmingly stressful event that threatens one's survival and sense of security.

Harassment, embarrassment, child abuse, sexual abuse, employment discrimination, police brutality, bullying, and domestic violence are examples of events that can lead to psychological trauma. Family violence, loss of family members, acts of terrorism and natural disasters are all traumatic events. Exposure to war, natural disasters, and witnessing catastrophic events also may cause psychological trauma.

Not everyone who experiences a traumatic event will be emotionally injured. One explanation for the variability in experiencing psychological trauma is resilience.

FAME & FORTUNE

Tyler Perry (1969–)

PUBLIC PERSONA

Tyler Perry, born Emmitt Perry, Jr. is a well-known American actor, filmmaker, author, director, and composer. His highly successful career includes stage plays, films, and television shows. His movies include *Diary of a Mad Black Woman*, *Madea's Family Reunion*, and *Daddy's Little Girls*. He also teamed up with Oprah Winfrey to produce the film *Precious*.

PERSONAL REALITIES

Tyler Perry grew up in New Orleans, Louisiana with his mother, Willie Maxine Perry and his abusive father, Emmitt Perry, Sr., who frequently beat him and other family members. He was sexually abused by trusted adults. Perry did not tell anyone but later reported feeling guilty and betrayed. As a child, Perry attempted suicide. In an attempt to distance himself from his father, he changed his name to Tyler from Emmitt. Tyler did not complete high school, but did earn a GED. He began his writing career after watching an episode of the *Oprah Winfrey Show* when the therapeutic effects of writing were discussed. His early writings became a basis for the play *I Know I've Been Changed*.

Source: Tyler Perry Biography – Inspired by Oprah, Perseverance Paid Off, concentrated on Madea character. http://biography.jrank.org/pages/2872/Perry-Tyler.html retrieved April 24, 2015. Oprah Talks to Tyler Perry. http://www.oprah.com/entertainment/Oprah-Interviews-Tyler-Perry_1 Retrieved April 25, 2015.

BOX 17.1 CLINICAL VIGNETTE

Resilience

Joe, a 22-year-old college student, was a victim of an armed robbery. His companion was shot and killed when Joe refused give the robbers his money. After the incident, he was preoccupied with thoughts of the murder and felt personally responsible for his friend's death.

Joe sought psychological help from the college counseling center. During weekly counseling sessions, Joe was able to reframe his experience. Although he still has brief periods of sadness, he no longer blames himself for his friend's death. He is now resuming his normal activities and is no longer having intrusive thoughts.

| **KEYCONCEPT** **Resilience** is the capacity to withstand stress and catastrophe. It develops over time and is the culmination of multiple internal and external factors.

Resilience reduces the impact of risk factors and enhances the ability to "bounce back" and recover from stressful experiences. The stronger the resilience, the less likely the individual will experience reactions that lead to maladaptive behaviors and outcomes (Ursano, Colpe, Heeringa, Kessler, Shoenbaum, Stein, et al., 2014). An important mental health promotion nursing strategy is enhancing resilience, especially for persons with mental and/or substance abuse problems. See Box 17.1.

Resilience develops when a positive self-concept and self-worth, a feeling of being in control one's life, and a feeling of power exists. Resilience is acquired over time, beginning in early childhood, as positive problem-solving, communication, and coping skills are learned. Some children seem more resilient to trauma and are able to cope quite well with traumatic events (Weems & Graham, 2014). Positive family and community support also play a role in developing resilience.

OVERVIEW OF TRAUMA- AND STRESSOR-RELATED DISORDERS

Exposure to a traumatic or otherwise stressful event can lead to a trauma- and stressor-related disorders such as reactive attachment disorder, disinhibited social engagement disorder, PTSD, acute stress disorder, and adjustment disorder. See Table 17.1 for descriptions of these disorders.

Trauma- and Stressor-Related Disorders Across the Lifespan

Trauma- and stressor-related disorders can develop at any time throughout a lifespan. In children, exposure to trauma can cause enduring emotional problems that lead to any one of these disorders. One of the most traumatic losses for children is an unexpected death of a loved one

TABLE 17.1	TRAUMA- AND STRESSOR-RELATED DISORDERS
Disorder	**Description**
Acute stress disorder	Development PTSD symptoms 3 days to 1 month after exposure to a traumatic event. Acute stress disorder may progress to PTSD.
Adjustment disorder	Emotional or behavior symptoms in response to a stressful event that does not, however, meet criteria for PTSD.
Disinhibited social engagement disorder (children)	Child is culturally inappropriate and overly familiar with strangers. Condition usually diagnosed in childhood.
Posttraumatic stress disorder	Development of intrusive, dissociative, mood, cognitive, or hyperarousal symptoms following exposure to a traumatic event.
Reactive attachment disorder (children)	Inability to develop positive attachments to caregivers because of prior social neglect

BOX 17.2

PTSD Symptoms in Children and Adolescents

PTSD SYMPTOMS IN CHILDREN
- Bedwetting, after they had learned how to use a toilet
- Forgetting how or being unable to talk
- Acting out the scary event during playtime
- Being unusually clingy with a parent or other adult

PTSD SYMPTOMS IN ADOLESCENTS
- May show symptoms similar to adult
- Develop disruptive, disrespectful, or destructive behaviors
- Feel guilty for not preventing injury or death
- Thoughts of revenge

Source: U.S. Department of Health & Human Services (retrieved 4/21/2015). www.nimh.nih.gov

KEYCONCEPT   Traumatic events include those that are directly experienced, witnessed, learned about from others, or repeated exposure to adverse events.

which can lead to multiple psychiatric disorders (Keyes, Pratt, Galea, McLaughlin, Koenen, & Hear, 2014). Childhood psychological and physical abuse including sexual abuse can lead to a life-long struggle with a trauma- and stressor-related disorder. See Chapter 30.

Military violence is responsible for life-long effects for deployed service members. There are many reports of older adults who served in World War II developing symptoms of PTSD in later life. There is a growing number of research studies that demonstrate the traumatic impact on children during military deployment and reintegration of their parents (Creech, Hadley, & Borsari, 2014).

When an older adult experiences trauma, memories of a lifetime of previous traumas and abuse influence the current experience. Loss of partners, friends, and family members through death, marriage, or relocation can add to the trauma. Elder abuse is discussed in Chapter 30.

Posttraumatic Stress Disorder

Posttraumatic Stress Disorder occurs following exposure to an actual or threatened traumatic event such as death, serious injury, or sexual violence (American Psychiatric Association [APA], 2013). Traumatic events include those that are directly experienced, witnessed, learned about from others, or repeated exposure to aversive events. Examples of traumatic events are violent personal assault, rape, military combat, natural disasters, terrorist attacks, being taken hostage, incarceration as a prisoner of war, torture, an automobile accident, or being diagnosed with a life-threatening illness.

Clinical Course

Most people who experience a traumatic event do not develop PTSD. However, for those who do, the symptoms often develop 3 to 6 months after the event. About one third of the persons diagnosed with PTSD develop chronic symptoms. For these individuals, symptoms fluctuate in intensity with time and usually are worse during periods of stress. Children with PTSD may react differently than adults. See Box 17.2.

Diagnostic Criteria

PTSD is diagnosed following exposure to a traumatic event when symptoms in four general areas appear: 1) intrusive symptoms, avoidance of person(s), places or objects that are a reminder of the traumatic event, 2) negative mood and cognitions or negative thoughts associated with the event, and 3) hyperarousal characterized by aggressive, reckless or self-destructive behavior, 4) sleep disturbances or hypervigilance for at least 1 month (APA, 2013).

Intrusion

In PTSD, **intrusion** is defined as involuntary appearance of thoughts, memories, or dreams of traumatic events that cause psychological and sometimes physiologic distress. Often the intrusive thoughts are associated with cues that symbolize or resemble the original event. Sometimes, the traumatic images, thoughts, or perceptions are re-experienced. Nightmares are common. Intrusive symptoms also include dissociative reactions (i.e., feeling or acting as if the event is re-occurring). Sleeping is difficult. Terrifying flashbacks and nightmares often include fragments of traumatic events exactly as they happened. Many stimuli (e.g., loud noises, odors) associated with the trauma cause flashbacks and dreams. Consequently, affected individuals avoid such stimuli (Heir, Piatigorsky, & Weisaeth, 2010).

Remember Susan?
She suffers from flashbacks of exploding helicopters when she hears loud noises. Her husband tells her she screams while sleeping. She reports frightening nightmares.

Avoidance and Numbing (Dissociative Symptoms)

Individuals with PTSD **avoid** reminders of the event including people, places, or activities associated with the event (e.g., fireworks may bring back memories of war). Many persons suffering with this disorder escape situations by altering their state of consciousness or **numbing,** by dissociating. **Dissociation** is a disruption in the normally occurring linkages among subjective awareness, feelings, thoughts, behavior, and memories (APA, 2013). A person who dissociates is making him- or herself "disappear." That is, the person has the feeling of leaving his or her body and observing what happens to him or her from a distance. During trauma, dissociation enables a person to observe the event while experiencing no pain or only limited pain and to protect him- or herself from awareness of the full impact of the traumatic event. See Box 17.3. Examples of dissociation include (1) **derealization** (feelings of unreality) and **depersonalization** (the experience of self or the environment as strange or unreal); (2) periods of disengagement from the immediate environment during stress, such as "spacing out"; (3) alterations in bodily perceptions; (4) emotional numbing; (5) out-of-body experiences; and (6) amnesia about abuse-related memories.

Mood and Cognition

After a traumatic event, moods often become more irritable with episodes of explosive anger, fear, guilt, or shame. Individuals with PTSD often have difficulty experiencing

BOX 17.3 CLINICAL VIGNETTE

Dissociation

Carol, a 14-year-old high school student was brutally raped by an older man. When the accused man was arrested, Carol could not recall any part of the attack. Her last memory was walking home after school and seeing a strange man parked on the street.

positive emotions such as happiness or love. Consequently, they become estranged from loved ones who become frustrated with their family member's unpredictable moods and lack of emotional connection. In PTSD, the thought process becomes distorted with exaggerated negative beliefs or expectations about oneself, others, and the world. They may believe that no one can be trusted or that they are terrible people (APA, 2013).

Hyperarousal

After a traumatic experience, the stress system seems to go on permanent alert, as if the danger might return at any time. In this state of physiologic **hyperarousal,** the traumatized person is hypervigilant for signs of danger, startles easily, reacts irritably to small annoyances, and sleeps poorly. The state of hyperarousal causes other problems for family members. The affected individual is irritable and overreacts to others which cause others to avoid the person who in turn maintains a state of continual arousal (Lanius, Vermetten, Loewenstein, Brand, Schmal, Bremner, et al., 2010).

Susan and her family
Susan feels she does not fit into the family and no longer believes she has a role as a wife and mother. She is extremely irritable and argues with her husband constantly. She is suspicious of her neighbors and fearful that her children will be kidnapped.

Epidemiology and Risk Factors

PTSD affects approximately 8% of men and 20% of women who are exposed to traumatic events, but is variable among different groups (Warner, Warner, Appenzeller, & Hogue, 2013). Risk factors for PTSD include a prior diagnosis of acute stress disorder; the extent, duration, and intensity of trauma involved; and environmental factors. High levels of anxiety, low self-esteem, and existing personality difficulties may increase the likelihood that PTSD will develop.

PTSD varies among both genders. Women are approximately twice as likely as men to experience PTSD; the median time from onset to remission for women is 4 years compared with 1 year for men. Several factors may contribute to these differences. Men and women experience different types of traumatic events. More men report exposure to events such as fires or disasters, life-threatening accidents, physical assault, combat, being threatened with a weapon, and being held captive. More women report anxiety and depressive disorders, child abuse, sexual molestation, sexual assault, and traumatic events before the age of 18 years. Sexual violence is associated with a high risk for the development of PTSD (Masho & Ahmed, 2007; Roth, Geisser, & Bates, 2008).

> **Consider this:**
> Susan was exposed to exploding IEDs (improvised explosive devices) while serving in Iraq. Between the ages of 6 to 9 years old, she was sexually abused by an uncle. She never told anyone.

PTSD symptoms in women who were sexually assaulted were found to vary based on their age at the time of the first sexual assault. In one study, the prevalence among women who had never experienced sexual assault was 8%, but rates for those who were sexually assaulted ranged from 30% (older than 18 years of age) to 35% (younger than 18 years of age) (Masho & Ahmed, 2007). Women who experienced intimate partner violence had a rate of 74% to 92% compared with 6% to 13% among non-abused women (Scott-Tilley, Tilton, & Sandel, 2010). See Box 17.4.

Childhood cancer survivors have been found to have four times the risk of developing PTSD as their siblings (Stuber, Meeske, Krull, Leisenring, Stratton, Kazak, et al., 2010). In another study of childhood cancer survivors, nearly 16% had PTSD (Rourke, Hobbie, Schwartz, & Katz, 2007). Similarly, high rates of PTSD have been reported among patients with alcohol and drug dependence who have experienced childhood abuse (Driessen, Schulte, Luedecke, Schaefer, Sutmann, Ohlmeier, et al., 2008; Moselhy, 2009).

BOX 17.4

Research for Best Practices: PTSD and Sexual Revictimization

Walsh, K. Resnick, H. S., Danielson, C .K., McCauley, J. L., Saunders, B. E., & Kilpatrick, D. G. (2014). Patterns of drug and alcohol use associated with lifetime sexual revictimization and current posttraumatic stress disorder among three national samples of adolescent, college, and household-residing women. Addictive behaviors, 39(3), 684–689.

THE QUESTION: What is the association among substance use (alcohol, marijuana, other illicit drugs, and nonmedical prescription drugs), PTSD, and sexual revictimization in women.

METHODS: Participants were 1763 adolescent girls, 2000 college women, and 3001 household-residing women. Rape history, PTSD, and use of substances were assessed in the past year during structured telephone interviews in 2005–2006.

FINDINGS: Revictimization was associated with more substance use across all groups. Prescription drugs were associated with the college women. For adolescents, PTSD was associated with an increased risk of drug use.

IMPLICATIONS FOR NURSING: Early intervention in primary care and school settings for girls and women who are victims of sexual assault may prevent future revictimization and PTSD.

However, high rates of PTSD in veterans returning from Iraq and Afghanistan are unprecedented in modern times. Approximately 27% of women and 35% of men have been diagnosed with PTSD. These veterans have more medical conditions than those veterans without mental disorders (Kimerling, 2010).

Etiology

A growing body of research postulates that biologic factors, including neurobiology and genetics, interact with environmental factors, such as childhood experiences, and the severity and extent of the traumatic exposure, to affect susceptibility to PTSD. The amygdala and hippocampus also appear to be important players in fear conditioning along with the thalamus, locus ceruleus, and sensory cortex. Interaction between the cortex and the amygdala may be necessary for specific stimuli to elicit traumatic memories (Lanius, et al., 2010).

Several neurochemical systems are involved in regulating fear conditioning, including norepinephrine, dopamine, opiate, and corticotropin-releasing systems. In addition, N-methyl-D-aspartate (NMDA), one of the major excitatory neurotransmitters in the brain, appears necessary for this type of learning to occur. NMDA antagonists applied to the amygdala prevent the development of fear-conditioned responses (Heim & Nemeroff, 2009; Jovanovic & Ressler, 2010). Hyperarousal symptoms are characteristic of increased noradrenergic function, particularly in the locus ceruleus and in the limbic system (hypothalamus, hippocampus, and amygdala), and of increased dopamine activity, particularly in the prefrontal cortical dopamine system (Jovanovic & Ressler, 2010; Lanius, et al., 2010).

Behavioral sensitization may be one mechanism underlying the hyperarousal seen in PTSD. This phenomenon, sometimes referred to as **kindling,** occurs after exposure to severe, uncontrollable stressors. The sensitized person reacts with a magnified stress response to later, milder stressors Research shows that a single or repeated exposure to a severe stressor potentiates the capacity of a subsequent stressor to increase synaptic levels of norepinephrine and dopamine in the forebrain (Heim & Nemeroff, 2009). This finding would account for the fact that some individuals with PTSD experience intense fear, anxiety, and panic in response to minor stimuli. One example of behavioral sensitization is that PTSD after combat exposure is more likely to develop in veterans who are survivors of childhood abuse than in those who have not experienced prior trauma (Jovanovic & Ressler, 2010; Heim & Nemeroff, 2009).

Teamwork & Collaboration: Working toward Recovery

Major approaches to the treatment of PTSD include pharmacotherapy and psychotherapy. The selective serotonin reuptake inhibitors (SSRIs), benzodiazepines, and β-blockers have been shown to be effective in reducing the symptoms of PTSD (Bastien, 2010). When prescribed in conjunction with psychotherapy, pharmacotherapy can minimize the excessive fear and anxiety of PTSD (Ellen, Olver, Norman, & Burrows, 2008).

Psychotherapeutic approaches to the treatment of patients with PTSD include psychodynamic psychotherapy; cognitive behavioral therapy (CBT); and eye movement, desensitization, and reprocessing (EMDR). *Psychodynamic psychotherapy* focuses on different factors that may influence current PTSD symptoms such as early childhood experience and current relationships. There is emphasis on the unconscious mind. *Cognitive behavioral therapies* focus on the evaluation of situations, thoughts, feelings and the problematic ways these evaluations cause a person to act. See Box 17.5.

EDMR is a process of reviewing and visualizing disturbing memories of traumatic or distressing experiences to reduce the long-term impact of the events. The patient is guided through images of the trauma, allowing for progressive desensitization. Under deep relaxation, the patient maintains an image of the traumatic event while focusing on the lateral movement of the clinician's finger. This recent approach has been successful in minimizing the fear response and avoidance pattern of those with PTSD (Beevers, Lee, Wells, Ellis, & Telch, 2011).

Group therapy and family therapy should also be considered in the treatment of those with PTSD. Sharing the traumatic experiences with family or with others who have experienced trauma can be both supportive and therapeutic. PTSD disrupts both the life of the patient and his or her significant others. Social support is a protective factor in the development of the disorder, and patients who have PTSD can benefit from tangible social support they receive from spouses, family, and friends (Pietrzak & Southwick, 2011).

Although few studies have explored the neurobiologic effects of psychotherapy, growing evidence indicates that psychotherapeutic approaches, such as CBT and meditation, improve the synaptic links with the amygdala, and thus effect the processing of emotion and anxiety (Mayo, 2010).

Safety Issues

PTSD is associated with an increased risk of suicide, suicide attempts, aggression, and substance abuse (Ramchand, Rudavsky, Grant, Tanielian, Jaycox, 2015). The first contact the nurse often has with the patient is after a suicide attempt or an aggressive episode. A careful assessment should include determination of the risk for self-injury or aggression towards others. These individuals are at high risk for substance abuse and suicide, so that a suicide risk assessment should be included in the nursing assessment. Safety measures such as suicide precautions may be needed, particularly if the person is hospitalized.

Evidence-Based Nursing Care of the Person with PTSD

Patients with PTSD receive nursing services in a variety of settings throughout the continuum of care. Many will access care through a primary care setting and others will seek out services in a mental health or primary health clinic. In many instances, the patient is reluctant to disclose information and has a difficult time trusting others. Distrust is especially common in persons whose trauma is associated with a violation of trust such as a rape. Gaining the patient's trust through a warm, empathic interaction can lead to a meaningful therapeutic relationship. See Nursing Care Plan 17.1, available at http://thepoint.lww.com/BoydEssentials.

Mental Health Nursing Assessment

After the physical health needs are met and suicidal/aggressive safety measures are established, the mental health nursing assessment targets specific areas. These include identification of the original trauma, specific physical symptoms, and the emotional and behavioral consequences of the patient's PTSD. The nursing assessment is best conducted through an interview to identify

---

BOX 17.5

Cognitive Behavioral Therapies

Exposure Therapy	Helps people face and control their fear by exposing them to the trauma in a safe way. Strategies are mental imagery, writing, or visits to the place where the event happened.
Cognitive Restructuring	Helps people make sense of the bad memories by reframing their experiences in a more realistic way. They may feel guilt or shame about what is not their fault.
Cognitive Processing Therapy	Helps people understand why recovery from traumatic events has been difficult and how symptoms of PTSD affect daily life. Focus is on identifying how traumatic experiences changed thoughts and beliefs and influenced current feelings and behaviors.
Stress Inoculation Training	Teaches a person how to reduce anxiety. Like cognitive restructuring, this treatment helps people look at their memories in a healthy way.

the impact of the trauma and the individual's physical and psychological strengths.

Trauma

Identifying the original trauma establishes the nature of the trauma and the length of time that the patient's PTSD has been present. The following questions can be used in the assessment:

- What happened that led to the PTSD? When?
- How did you respond?
- Did anyone help you?
- How did that experience change your life?
- How did you respond to the incident?
- Were you a victim of trauma or abuse prior to the trauma associated with PTSD?

Physical Health Assessment

The assessment should not only focus on the physical problems, but also on healthy aspects. For example, nutrition, exercise and self-care may be the individual's strengths. The assessment process should be similar to the one described in Chapter 16.

Sleep: In PTSD, sleep is often disrupted or practically nonexistent. Disturbing nightmares are common. The nurse should compare sleep patterns before and after the trauma. Insomnia is typically characterized by difficulty falling asleep, fragmented sleep, or panic-like awakenings. The nurse should also assess for nightmares including frequency and intensity. Family members may be able to provide detailed information that is out of the patient's awareness.

Substance Use: Commonly, individuals with PTSD self-medicate to relieve the discomfort, anxiety, or pain caused by the trauma. The use of alcohol or other drugs is common. Assessment of the use of substances and the frequency will give direction for interventions.

> **Consider this:**
> Susan started drinking alcohol regularly in Iraq. After returning home, she continued to drink 6 to 8 cans of beer every day.

Pain: The original trauma may result in chronic pain. For example, physical abuse or wartime injury may result in long-term physical treatment and pain. Prescribed pain medication is often used for reasons other other than those for which it was prescribed. For example, a cooccurring traumatic brain injury may be present.

Other Somatic Responses: Patients with PTSD often have multiple unexplained physical problems (e.g., gastrointestinal, cardiovascular, neurologic, and musculoskeletal symptoms). Sometimes the patient is reluctant to admit a trauma such as a rape or domestic assault and instead seeks out medical care for physical problems. Obtaining a trauma history becomes very important when multiple physical symptoms are present.

Psychosocial Assessment

The focus of the psychosocial assessment is identifying the severity of the PTSD symptoms and the disruptions that these symptoms cause the affected individual and family. The patient should be asked about intrusive thoughts, irritable moods, negative thoughts, avoidance behaviors, and arousal behaviors and what impact they have on their their daily lives.

In PTSD, guilt, shame, and depression are often present. Guilt may relate to feeling responsible for the events that led up to the trauma. Survivor guilt occurs when one person survives a traumatic event when others do not. See Box 17.6. Assessing self-esteem and self-concept will provide clues to the patient's resilience. See Chapter 9. A family assessment focusing on any changes in family dynamics that has occurred since the traumatic event should also be included.

Strength Assessment

Throughout the assessment, the nurse should be listening for evidence of individual physical and psychosocial strengths. Was the patient physically healthy before the traumatic event occurred? Does the patient have family or friends who can support the individual? Is the patient motivated to deal with PTSD symptoms? Are there financial or social resources available? This information can be used in helping patient develop a safety and recovery plan.

Nursing Diagnoses

Several nursing diagnoses can be generated from the assessment data. Depending on the trauma, post-trauma syndrome, rape trauma syndrome, risk for suicide, anxiety, defensive coping, hopelessness, ineffective impulse

BOX 17.6 **CLINICAL VIGNETTE**

Survivor Guilt

A 92-year-old survivor of World War II concentration camps has suffered from depression most of his adult life. When admitted to a long-term care facility, his daughter told the nurse that her dad often had bouts of depression where he would bemoan the fact that he had lived and his parents and siblings had not. He often told his daughter that he felt guilty because he had survived the holocaust.

BOX 17.7 • THERAPEUTIC DIALOGUE • Approaching Susan

Susan did not want to be admitted to the inpatient unit and reported that she did not want to live. Her husband wants Susan to forget about Iraq and return to her former self. When she arrived on the unit, she was asked several assessment questions. She did not want to tell her story again to the nurse. The nurse needed to complete the admission assessment.

INEFFECTIVE APPROACH

Nurse: Susan, I need to ask you some questions.

Susan: Can't it wait?

Nurse: Oh – unfortunately I have to ask questions.

Susan: I am tired of talking. Everyone is asking the same questions. For the record, I do not have a problem, I do not drink too much, and I wish my husband would go away.

Nurse: Your husband is a nice guy and is only trying to help.

Susan: You do not know what you are talking about. He wants to control me.

Nurse: If you just answer some questions, I can finish my assessment.

Susan: Not now. Go away.

EFFECTIVE APPROACH

Nurse: Hi Susan, my name is Jane, and I am your nurse today.

Susan: What do you want? I don't need a nurse.

Nurse: Well, we can just talk. What brought you here?

Susan: I am tired of talking. Everyone is asking the same questions. For the record, I do not have a problem, I do not drink too much, and I wish my husband would go away.

Nurse: Talking can be tiring. What questions have you been asked?

Susan: My whole life story – where I grew up, when I got married, how do I get along with my husband and children, what happened in Iraq?

Nurse: You have had a lot of questions since you have been here. How were you able to answer all those questions?

Susan: The worst questions were about abuse and Iraq. I don't think I can talk about that yet.

Nurse: Why don't we stick to the easier ones for now?

Susan: OK, I can try.

CRITICAL THINKING CHALLENGE

- What ineffective techniques did the nurse use in the first scenario? Whose needs was the nurse meeting?

- What effective techniques did the nurse use in the second scenario?

control and powerlessness, are examples of nursing diagnoses generated by assessment of a person with PTSD.

Therapeutic Relationship

Establishing a trusting relationship with a person with PTSD is the basis of nurse-patient collaboration. This may take time because many victims have also experienced their trust being violated during the traumatic event. See Box 17.7.

Nursing Interventions

Physical Health Interventions

Many of the same nursing interventions discussed in Chapter 16 are used with the person with PTSD. Proper nutrition and regular exercise can help fortify the resilience.

Sleep Enhancement

Sleep hygiene is also an important strategy because sleep disruption is common in PTSD. See Chapter 26. Nurses should collaborate with the patient in finding a strategy that will help the person sleep and manage nightmares. For example, the individual may want to sleep with the lights on because of the nightmares. However, light interferes with nighttime sleep for some people. It may be possible to go to sleep with the lights on, but to ask a family member to turn off the lights later. Some persons with PTSD find that they cannot sleep in their bed, but can sleep in a chair. Some of the following strategies may be helpful:

- Establish and maintain a regular bedtime and rising time.
- Avoid naps.
- Abstain from alcohol. Although alcohol may assist with sleep onset, an alerting effect occurs when it wears off.

- Refrain from caffeine after midafternoon. Avoid nicotine before bedtime and during the night. Caffeine and nicotine are strong stimulants and cause fragmented sleep.
- Exercise regularly, avoiding the 3 hours before bedtime.

Medications: Two SSRI antidepressants, sertraline (Zoloft) and paroxetine (Paxil), are approved for PTSD and are used to treat symptoms such as sadness, worry, anger, and feeling numb inside. See Box 17.8.

Because the person with PTSD may take many different types of medication, the nurse needs to monitor for any drug interactions and teach the person about all the medications including expected therapeutic effect(s) and side effects. These individuals often take prescribed or over-the-counter (OTC) pain medications that may interact with mood stabilizers, antidepressants, antianxiety agents, or antipsychotic agents.

Substance Abuse Interventions: If the person has been using substances to dull the feelings associated with the trauma, the nurse should educate the individual about the addiction and make a referral to a substance abuse treatment team. It is important for the nurse to use a nonjudgmental approach, recognizing the person is suffering from the trauma and is trying to cope with intrusive thoughts and pain. The nurse should emphasize that there are more effective coping mechanisms and offer hope that the person can find other means of alleviating the PTSD symptoms.

Psychosocial Interventions

Many of the same psychosocial interventions discussed in Chapter 16 can be used for persons with PTSD. Relaxation strategies and stress reduction techniques are particularly helpful for these individuals. Encouraging the person to participate in a support group can decrease the isolation that may be present and learn how others deal with their symptoms. Service and companion dogs are also helpful in helping the person address the stress of PTSD.

Evaluation and Treatment Outcomes

The treatment of PTSD may last several years with changing goals. Early in treatment, the goals may be to reduce the intrusive thoughts and regulate sleep; later goals may include being able to establish a trusting relationship with a partner. The evaluation will be modified as the goals and interventions change.

Continuum of Care

The person with PTSD is primarily treated in the community rather than a medical facility as an inpatient. Short-term hospitalization for safety may be needed if suicidal or homicidal thoughts are strong or for an adjustment of medication.

Inpatient-Focused Care

Inpatient settings provide a safe environment for the person who is tormented with frequent flashbacks, has become depressed and potentially suicidal, or is harboring thoughts about hurting others. Medications may be initiated or adjusted.

Emergency Care

When individuals with PTSD need emergency care, they are usually having suicidal ideation or thoughts to hurt others. Safety interventions should be implemented.

BOX 17.8

Drug Profile: Sertraline (Zoloft)

DRUG CLASS: Antidepressant (selective serotonin reuptake inhibitor – SSRI)

RECEPTOR AFFINITY: blocks the reuptake of serotonin

INDICATIONS: major depressive disorder, obsessive-compulsive disorder, panic disorder, posttraumatic stress disorder, premenstrual dysphoric disorder, social anxiety disorder

ROUTES AND DOSAGES: Available in 25-mg, 50-mg, 100-mg tablets, 20 mg/mL

Adults: 50–200 mg PO once daily; Start 50 mg PO once daily, may increase by 50 mg/day

HALF-LIFE (PEAK EFFECT): 62–104 hours

SELECTED ADVERSE REACTIONS: nausea, headache, insomnia, diarrhea, dry mouth, ejaculatory dysfunction, somnolence, weakness, lack of energy, tremor, dyspepsia, anorexia, constipation, decrease in libido, nervousness, anxiety, rash, visual disturbance

WARNINGS: Increase suicidality risk in children, adolescents, and young adults with major depressive or other psychiatric disorders. Contradicted in persons being treated with monoamine oxidase inhibitors and pimozide, an antipsychotic. Risk for serotonin syndrome.

SPECIFIC PATIENT & FAMILY EDUCATION
- Take exactly as prescribed.
- Can be taken with or without food
- If a dose is missed, take missed dose as soon as patient remembers unless time for next dose; then skip missed dose.
- Can cause sleepiness or may affect ability to make decisions, think clearly or react quickly
- Do not drive, operate heavy machinery until patient knows how medication will affect him or her.
- Do not drink alcohol while taking medication.
- Report any signs and symptoms of adverse reactions, suicidal thoughts, or actions.
- Notify your health care provider if severe agitation, hallucinations, coordination problems, muscle twitching, racing heartbeat, high or low blood pressure, muscle rigidity, sweating or fever, nausea, vomiting, diarrhea occur.

It is important for the nurse to know the nature of the trauma to be able to approach the patient. For example, a person previously exposed to combat may be sensitive to loud noises and is more likely to become aggressive when doors slam, whereas a woman who has been raped may not tolerate anyone touching her.

Family Interventions

Families need support as they learn to cope with their family member with PTSD. Family members often feel hopeless in trying to understand the changes that their loved one is undergoing. In many instances, the member with PTSD is unable to share information about the trauma and the symptoms. If alcohol or other drugs are used to self-medicate, the family has additional challenges in dealing with the substance use. Support groups, education about PTSD, and family therapy are helpful.

Community Treatment

Treatment mostly occurs in the community with the individual attending group therapy, support groups, individual therapy, and medication management. Most appointments will occur after working hours. Nursing care can be delivered in all settings. The community setting is an excellent opportunity for patient and family education. See Box 17.9.

OTHER TRAUMA- AND STRESSOR-RELATED DISORDERS

Acute stress disorder is similar to PTSD except that it is resolved within 1 month of the traumatic event. Acute stress disorder can develop into PTSD if the symptoms last longer than 1 month. Two trauma- and stressor-related disorders typically occurring in childhood are reactive attachment disorder and disinhibited social engagement disorder. *Reactive attachment disorder* is characterized by inhibited, emotionally withdrawn behavior toward an adult caregiver. These children rarely seek or respond to comfort when distressed. This disorder usually occurs when the primary caregiver frequently changes. In *disinhibited social engagement disorder*, the child is overly familiar with others in ways uncharacteristic of cultural norms. For instance, the child does not hesitate to go somewhere with an unfamiliar adult.

One of the most common diagnoses for hospitalized persons is adjustment disorder (APA, 2013). These disorders occur within 3 months of the stressor. Affected individuals experience distress that seems out of proportion to the severity of the stressor and may be unable to function socially. After the situation is resolved, the symptoms subside.

Dissociative Disorders

Dissociative disorders are thought to be responses to extreme external or internal events or stressors where dissociation, or a splitting from the self, occurs as a way of coping with severe anxiety. Prevalence is higher among people who experience childhood physical or sexual abuse than among others. The onset of these disorders may be sudden or may occur gradually; the course of each may be long-term or transient.

The essential feature of these disorders involves a failure to integrate identity, memory, and consciousness. That is, unwanted intrusive thoughts disrupts one's contact with the here and now or memories that are normally accessible are lost. These disorders are closely related to the trauma- and stressor-related disorders but are categorized separately. They are described in Table 17.2. Persons with dissociative disorders may also have comorbid substance abuse, mood disorders, personality disorders, or PTSD (APA, 2013).

BOX 17.9

Psychoeducation Checklist: Posttraumatic Stress Disorder

When caring for a person with a PTSD, be sure to include the following topic areas in the teaching plan:

- Identification of individual triggers and cues that lead to reexperiencing trauma
- Safety plans for stressful periods
- Recovery plans that focus on personal strengths
- Risk factors for reoccurrence of symptoms
- Various treatment options: if one does not help, others exist
- Avoid substances such as alcohol and drugs
- Nutrition
- Exercise
- Sleep hygiene
- Follow-up appointments
- Community services

TABLE 17.2	DISSOCIATIVE DISORDERS
Disorder	**Description**
Dissociative amnesia	The inability to recall important yet stressful information
Depersonalization/derealization disorder	The feeling of being detached from one's mental processes
Dissociative identity disorder (formerly called multiple personality disorder)	Presence of at least two distinct personality or identity states

Treatment options include the use of antidepressants to treat the patient's underlying mood and anxiety. Psychotherapy options include hypnotherapy, cognitive behavioral therapy (CBT), and psychoanalytic psychotherapy to determine the triggers that lead to heightened anxiety and dissociation.

SUMMARY OF KEY POINTS

- The development of psychological trauma depends on the meaning of the event and the resilience of the individual. The stronger the resilience, the more likely the individual will be able to withstand the negative impact of a potentially traumatic event.

- Resilience develops over time when there are a positive self-concept and measured self-worth, and when problem-solving, communication, and coping skills have been learned.

- PTSD occurs after a traumatic event and is characterized by involuntary intrusive thoughts, avoidance and numbing, negative moods and thoughts, and hyperarousal.

- Women are twice as likely as men to experience PTSD. Service members retirning from Iraq and Afghanistan have high rates of PTSD.

- There are several approaches to the treatment of PTSD including CBT, traditional psychotherapy, and medications.

- Nursing care focuses on asssessing symptoms of PTSD, building strengths, and collaborating with the patient in counseling interventions, administration of medication, psychoeducation, and family support.

CRITICAL THINKING CHALLENGES

1. What are the various traumatic events that can lead to PTSD? Why do some people develop PTSD and others, who have experienced the same trauma, do not?

2. Identify strategies the nurse can use to support the development of resilience.

3. Differentiate intrusive thoughts from dissociative symptoms.

4. Give examples of derealization and depersonalization.

5. Compare trauma- and stressor related disorders with dissociative disorders. How are they similar? How are they different?

6. How should a nurse approach a military veteran who is having intrusive thoughts, nightmares, and is unable to sleep?

The Dry Land (2010)

James (Ryan O'Nan), an Iraq war veteran, returns to his small-town life in Texas. His family quickly realizes that he has changed and has PTSD. He is irritable, anxious, and considers suicide. He keeps a gun at his bedside. He drinks with his friends and is easily provoked into fights. His family cannot truly understand the pain he feels. An award-winning movie, it depicts a veteran's struggle with regaining his life.

Viewing Points: Identify the behaviors that are characteristic of PTSD. Identify the strengths that he demonstrated that represented resilience. Develop a plan of care that includes his family, friends, and community support.

M●**VIE** viewing**GUIDES**   related to this chapter are available at http://thepoint.lww.com/BoydEssentials.

REFERENCES

American Psychiatric Association. (2013). *Diagnostic and statistical manual of mental disorders DSM-5 (5th ed.).* Arlington, VA: Author.

Bastien, D. (2010). Pharmacological treatment of combat-induced PTSD: A literature review. *British Journal of Nursing, 19*(5), 318–321.

Beevers, C. G., Lee, H., Wells, T. T., Ellis, A. J., & Telch, M. J. (2011). Association of predeployment gaze bias for emotion stimuli with later symptoms of PTSD and depression in soldiers deployed in Iraq. *American Journal of Psychiatry, 168*:735–741. doi:10.1176/appi.ajp.2011.10091309.

Creech, S. K., Hadley, W., & Borsari, B. (2014). The impact of military deployment and reintegration on children and parenting: A systematic review. *Professional Psychology Research & Practice, 45*(6), 452–464. doi: 10.1037/a0035055.

Driessen, M., Schulte, S., Luedecke, C., Schaefer, I., Sutmann, F., Ohlmeier, M., et al. (2008). Trauma and PTSD in patients with alcohol, drug, or dual dependence: A multi-center study. *Alcoholism, Clinical & Experimental Research, 32*(3), 481–488.

Ellen, S., Olver, J., Norman, T., & Burrows, G. (2008). The neurobiology of benzodiazepine receptors in panic disorder and post-traumatic stress disorder. *Stress and Health, 24*, 13–21.

Green, B. (2014). Prazosin in the treatment of PTSD (Review). *Journal of Psychiatric Practice, 20*(4), 253–259.

Heim, C., & Nemeroff, C. (2009). Neurobiology of posttraumatic stress disorder. *International Journal of Neuropsychiatric Medicine, 14*(1 suppl 1), 13–14.

Heir, T., Piatigorsky, A., & Weisaeth, L. (2010). Posttraumatic stress symptoms clusters associations with psychopathology and functional impairment. *Journal of Anxiety Disorders, 24*(8), 936–940.

Jovanovic, T., & Ressler, K. (2010). How the neurocircuitry and genetics of fear inhibition may inform our understanding of PTSD. *American Journal of Psychiatry, 167*(6), 648–662.

Keyes, K. M., Pratt, C., Galea, S., McLaughlin, K. A., Koenen, K. C., & Hear, M. K. (2014). The burden of loss: Unexpected death of a loved one and psychiatric disorders across the life course in a national study. *American Journal of Psychiatry, 171*(8), 864-871.

Kimerling, R. (2010). Gender and medical needs of OEF/OIF veterans with PTSD II. HSR&D study. Retrieved from http://www.hsrd.research.va.gov July 21, 2015.

Lanius, R. A., Vermetten, E., Loewenstein, R. J., Brand, B., Schmal, C., Bremner, J. D., et al. (2010). Emotion modulation in PTSD: Clinical and neurobiological evidence for a dissociative subtype. *The American Journal of Psychiatry, 167*(6), 640–647.

Masho, S., & Ahmed, G. (2007). Age at sexual assault and posttraumatic stress disorder among women: Prevalence, correlates, and implications for prevention. *Journal of Women's Health, 16*(2), 262–267.

Mayo, K. (2010). Support from neurobiology for spiritual techniques for anxiety: A brief review. *Journal of Healthcare Chaplaincy, 16*(1–2), 53–57.

Moselhy, H. (2009). Co-morbid post-traumatic stress disorder and opioid dependence syndrome. *Journal of Dual Diagnosis, 5*, 30–40.

Pietrzak, R. H., & Southwick, S. M. (2011). Psychological resilience in OEF-OIF Veterans: Application of a novel classification approach and examination of demographic and psychosocial correlates. *Journal of Affective Disorders, 133*(3), 560–568.

Ramchand, R., Rudavsky, R., Grant, S., Tanielian, T., & Jaycox, L. (2015). Prevalence of, risk factors for, and consequences of posttraumatic stress disorder and other mental health problems in military populations deployed to Iraq and Afghanistan. *Current Psychiatry Reports, 17*(5):37. doi: 10.1007/s11920-015-0575-z.

Roth, R., Geisser, M., & Bates, R. (2008). The relation of post-traumatic stress symptoms to depression and pain in patients with accident-related chronic pain. *Journal of Pain, 9*(7), 588–596.

Rourke, M., Hobbie, W., Schwartz, L., & Kazak, A. (2007). Posttraumatic stress disorder (PTSD) in young adult survivors of childhood cancer. *Pediatric Blood and Cancer, 49*(2), 177–182.

Scott-Tilley, D., Tilton, A., & Sandel, M. (2010). Biologic correlates to the development of post-traumatic stress disorder in female victims of intimate partner violence: Implications for practice. *Perspectives in Psychiatric Care, 46*(1), 26–31.

Stuber, M., Meeske, K. A., Krull, K. R., Leisenring, W., Stratton, K., Kazak, A. E., et al. (2010). Prevalence and predictors of posttraumatic stress disorder in adult survivors of childhood cancer. *Pediatrics, 125*(5), e1124–e1134.

Ursano, R. J., Colpe, L .J., Heeringa, S. G., Kessler, R. C., Shoenbaum, M., Stein, M. B., & Army STARRS collaborators. (2014). The Army study to assess risk and resilience in servicemembers (Army STARRS). *Psychiatry, 77*(2), 107–119.

U.S. Department of Health and Human Services. Post-Traumatic Stress Disorder (PTSD). National Institute of Mental Health. NIH Publication No. 08 6388. Retrieved 4/21/15. www.nimh.nih.gov/health/publications/post-traumatic-stress-disorder-ptsd/index.shtml.

Walsh, K. Resnick, H. S., Danielson, C. K., McCauley, J. L., Saunders, B. E., & Kilpatrick, D. G. (2014). Patterns of drug and alcohol use associated with lifetime sexual revictimization and current posttraumatic stress disorder among three national samples of adolescent, college, and household-residing women. *Addictive Behaviors, 39*(3), 684–689.

Warner, C. H., Warner, C. M., Appenzeller, G. N., & Hoge, C. W. (2013). Identifying and managing posttraumatic stress disorder. *American Family Physician, 88*(12), 827–834.

Weems, C. F., & Graham, R. A. (2014). Resilience and trajectories of posttraumtic stress among youth exposed to disaster. *Journal of Child and Adolescent Psychopharmacology, 24*(1), 2–8. Doi: 10.1089/cap.2013.0042.

Xu, Y., Schneier, R., Heimberg, R. G., Princisvalle, K., Liebowitz, M. R., Wang, S., et al. (2012). Gender differences in social anxiety disorder: Results from the national epidemiologic sample on alcohol and related conditions. *Journal of Anxiety Disorders, 26*(1), 12–19.

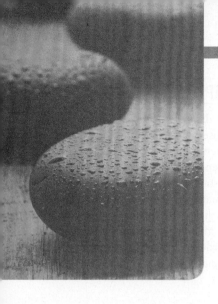

18
Obsessive-Compulsive and Related Disorders

Nursing Care of Persons with Obsessions and Compulsions

Mary Ann Boyd and Judith M. Erickson

KEY CONCEPTS

- compulsions
- obsessions

LEARNING OBJECTIVES

After studying this chapter, you will be able to:

1. Discuss the role of obsessions and compulsions in mental disorders.

2. Describe the prevalence and incidence of obsessive-compulsive disorders.

3. Delineate clinical symptoms and course of obsessive-compulsive disorders.

4. Analyze theories of obsessive-compulsive disorders.

5. Apply nursing process with recovery-oriented interventions for persons with obsessive-compulsive disorders.

6. Differentiate other obsessive-compulsive disorders.

KEY TERMS

- Conditioned stimuli • Isolation • Obsessive-compulsive disorder • Reaction formation • Undoing

Case Study: Tim

Tim, a 32-year-old engineer, was diagnosed with OCD as a teenager when his obsession with cleanliness and compulsively washing his hands interfered with his friendships and school work.

INTRODUCTION

Most of us experience times when we are preoccupied with specific thoughts or ideas. Many also find that routines or rituals are important in organizing our work and home life. When these preoccupations and rituals interfere with daily life, they become abnormal and may represent symptoms of a mental disorder. This chapter explains obsessions and compulsions and their role in obsessive-compulsive disorders. **Obsessive-compulsive disorder** is highlighted in this chapter.

OBSESSIONS AND COMPULSIONS

When preoccupied thoughts become excessive, intrusive or unwanted, such thoughts are considered to be obsessions.

> **KEY CONCEPT** **Obsessions** are excessive, unwanted, intrusive, and persistent thoughts, impulses, or images that cause anxiety and distress.
> Obsessions are not under the person's control and are inconsistent with the person's usual thought patterns.

Common obsessions include fears of contamination, pathologic doubt, the need for symmetry and completion, thoughts of hurting someone, and thoughts of sexual images.

Routines are a part of everyday life. Getting up in the morning at the same time and going to work or school structures our lives and helps us be productive. When routines become ritualistic and interfere with normal daily activity, they become compulsions.

| KEY CONCEPT **Compulsions** are repetitive behaviors performed in a ritualistic fashion with the goal of preventing or relieving anxiety and distress caused by obsessions.

For example, making sure a stove is turned off before leaving the house can be a safety routine, but being late for work because of making several trips to the stove before leaving the house is a compulsion. Common compulsions include handwashing, excessive cleaning, checking, arranging things, counting, ordering, and hoarding.

OVERVIEW OF OBSESSIVE-COMPULSIVE AND RELATED DISORDERS

Obsessions and compulsions are characteristic of obsessive-compulsive and related disorders. These disorders include obsessive-compulsive disorder (OCD), body dysmorphic disorder, hoarding disorder, trichotillomania (i.e., compulsively pulling out one's hair), excoriation disorder, and substance/medication-induced OCD. See Table 18.1 for description of these disorders. These disorders are closely related to anxiety disorders (American Psychiatric Association [APA], 2013).

TABLE 18.1	OBSESSIVE-COMPULSIVE AND RELATED DISORDERS
Disorder	**Description**
Obsessive-Compulsive Disorder	Distressful obsessions and compulsions that interfere with daily living and quality of life
Body Dysmorphic Disorder	Preoccupation with slight or imagined physical defects that are not apparent to others
Hoarding Disorder	Difficulty discarding or parting with possessions with a strong need to save
Trichotillomania (hair pulling disorder)	Inability to stop recurrent pulling out of hair with hair loss that is related to emotional release or anxiety release.
Excoriation Disorder (skin picking)	Inability to stop recurrent picking at skin for emotional release or anxiety release
Substance/medication-induced obsessive-compulsive disorder	OCD symptoms related to intoxication or withdrawal of substances

(APA, 2013).

OBSESSIVE-COMPULSIVE DISORDER

In obsessive-compulsive disorder (OCD), affected persons may have both obsessions and compulsions and believe that they have no control over them, which results in devastating consequences for affected individuals. Because of the nature of the disorder, nurses who work in settings other than psychiatric settings or in home health care may be among the first to identify an individual's symptoms as OCD and make the appropriate referrals. OCD is a separate disorder from obsessive-compulsive personality disorder discussed in Chapter 22.

Clinical Course

The average age of onset of OCD is 19 years, but can occur into the 20s to mid-30s (National Institute of Mental Health [NIMH], 2014). Although symptoms of OCD often begin in childhood, many persons receive treatment only after the disorder has significantly affected their lives. The astute parent may notice that the child spends great amounts of time on trivial tasks or has falling grades because of poor concentration. Symptom onset of the disorder is gradual, with some individuals showing a progressive decline in social and occupational functioning (APA, 2013). Men are affected more often as children and are most commonly affected by obsessions. Women have a higher incidence of checking-and-cleaning rituals, with onset typically in the early 20s. This chronic disorder is characterized by episodes of symptom diminution and exacerbation (APA, 2013).

Obsessions create tremendous anxiety; individuals perform compulsions to relieve the anxiety temporarily. If the compensatory ritual is not performed, the person feels increased anxiety and distress. Compulsions are necessary, not pleasurable. They are often recognized as odd or strange to the individual. Initially, attempts are made to resist the compulsive behavior, but eventually, resistance fails, and the repetitive behaviors are incorporated into daily routines.

The most common obsession is fear of contamination and results in compulsive handwashing. Fear of contamination usually focuses on dirt or germs, but other materials may be feared as well, such as toxic chemicals, poison, radiation, and heavy metals. Individuals with contamination obsessions report anxiety as their most common effect, but shame and disgust, linked with embarrassment and guilt, also are experienced.

Remember Tim?

When Tim was in high school, he was unable to eat at the school cafeteria because he was afraid the other students' germs would contaminate his food. He avoided touching doorknobs, and would wash his hands for 3 minutes if he inadvertently touched a doorknob.

Persons with OCD may become incapacitated by their symptoms and spend most of their waking hours locked in a cycle of obsessions and compulsions. They may even become unable to complete a task as simple as walking through a door without performing rituals. Interpersonal relationships suffer, and the person may actively isolate him- or herself. Individuals with OCD may use dissociation (disruption in among subjective awareness, feelings, thoughts, behavior, and memories) as a defense mechanism.

Diagnostic Criteria

OCD is diagnosed when recurrent obsessions or compulsions (or both) take up more than one hour a day or cause considerable stress to the individual. These obsessions or compulsions are not caused by substance or medication use or other disorders. Some individuals recognize that these obsessions or compulsions are excessive and unrealistic; others have limited insight and are unsure whether the obsessive thoughts are true, but continue to have the thoughts and feel compelled to perform the actions.

Another group of individuals are convinced that their obsessive thoughts are true. These thoughts and compulsive behaviors are stressful and interfere with normal daily routines (APA, 2013).

Obsessions

Some individuals have obsessions surrounding aggressive acts of hurting someone or themselves. After hitting a bump in the road, for example, they may obsess for hours over whether they have hit someone. Parents may have recurrent intrusive thoughts that they may hurt their child. Others obsess over the meaning of sins or whether they have followed the letter of the law. They tend to be hypermoral and have the need to confess. Their obsessions are seen as a form of religious suffering. These patients are often resistant to treatment. Religious obsessions are most common where severe religious restrictions exist. Diagnosis is not made unless the thoughts or rituals clearly exceed cultural or religious norms, occur at inappropriate times as described by members of the same religion or culture, or interfere with social obligations (APA, 2013).

Compulsions

Rituals are common compulsions in which objects must be in a certain order, motor activities are performed in a rigid fashion, or things are arranged in perfect symmetry. A ritual consumes a great deal of time to complete even the simplest task. Some individuals experience discontent, rather than anxiety, when things are not symmetrical or perfect. Others think magically and perform compulsive rituals to ward off an imagined disaster such as repeatedly turning on and off the alarm clock to prevent disaster. Those who hoard are compelled to check their belongings repeatedly to see that all is accounted for and check the garbage to make sure that nothing of value has been discarded.

Obsessive-Compulsive Disorder Across the Life-Span

OCD affects people of all ages. Identification, diagnosis, and treatment of OCD are necessary for recovery and optimal functioning.

Children and Adolescents

OCD affects between 1% and 3% or more of children and adolescents (Jacob & Storch, 2013). Because children subscribe to myths, superstition, and magical thinking, obsessive and ritualistic behaviors may go unnoticed. Behaviors such as touching every third tree, avoiding cracks in the sidewalk, or consistently verbalizing fears of losing a parent in an accident may have some underlying pathology but are common behaviors in childhood. Typically, parents notice that a child's grades begin to fall as a result of decreased concentration and great amounts of time spent performing rituals.

Older Adults

OCD typically manifests in childhood and the second decade of life and can be a lifelong illness, lasting more than 30 years (Lochner & Stein, 2010). One large population survey of older adults found a 1-year prevalence rate of 1.5% (Grenier, Preville, Boyer, & O'Connor, 2009). Late onset OCD is more likely to occur in females with a history of subclinical obsessive-compulsive symptoms, cooccurrence of PTSD after age 40, and a history of recent pregnancy herself or significant others (Frydman, do Brasil, Torres, Shavitt, Ferrão, Rosário, et al., 2014). See Box 18.1. Predictors of poor outcomes during life-long treatment include initial symptom onset during childhood, low social functioning, and the presence of both obsessions and compulsions (Ruscio, Stein, Chiu, & Kessler, 2010).

Epidemiology and Risk Factors

OCD has a lifetime prevalence rate of 1.2% with females having a slightly higher rate than males (APA, 2013). First-degree relatives of people with OCD have a higher prevalence rate than the general population. Early-onset OCD increases the chances of OCD in relatives and predicts poorer treatment outcomes (Ruscio, et al., 2010).

Studies provide some support for a link between infection with β-hemolytic streptococci and OCD (Hachiya, Miyata, Tanuma, Hongou, Tanaka, Shimoda, et al., 2013). High rates of OCD are found among individuals who are young, divorced or separated, and unemployed. OCD appears to be less common among African Americans than among non-Hispanic whites.

Comorbidity

It is estimated that one third of persons with OCD experience depression because of OCD's effects on their lifestyle. Bipolar, cyclothymic, panic, mood, eating, and impulse control disorders also commonly occur in those with OCD. A significant number of older depressed persons have OCD. Tourette syndrome and OCD frequently occur together (Grados, 2010).

Many individuals self-medicate to relieve the anxiety produced by obsessive thoughts. About one third experience substance abuse or dependence in their lifetime. In addition, some individuals may abuse benzodiazepines and other prescription medication. Personality disorders are also prevalent in those with OCD, occurring in more than 80% of patients. Dependent personality disorder most frequently coexists with OCD and is diagnosed in about half of affected individuals (see Chapter 22).

People with OCD are highly somatic and frequently seek medical treatment for physical symptoms, often just to get reassurance. Acquired immunodeficiency syndrome, cancer, heart attacks, and sexually transmitted infections are some of the most common obsessional fears.

> **Consider this:**
> As a child, Tim frequently went to the school nurse about multiple physical symptoms. Later, he was reluctant to engage in sexual relations with a long-time girlfriend because of fear of acquiring a sexually transmitted disease.

BOX 18.1 CLINICAL VIGNETTE

Older Adult

Louise, a 76-year-old retired accountant, resides in an assisted living complex with her husband. Always very neat and organized, she recently began cleaning excessively, sometimes in the middle of the night. She developed a routine where she had to have everything cleaned before she could eat. Her husband expressed his concern to their primary care provider who referred them to a geriatric psychiatrist. A diagnosis of late onset OCD was made. Louise recognizes that she her behavior has changed and is interfering with her life but says she gets too nervous if she doesn't carry out her routine.

What Do You Think?
- Are there indications that she may have had subclinical OCD symptoms?
- What symptoms of OCD is Louise experiencing?

Etiology

During the 1990s, research evidence from neuroimaging studies, neurochemical studies, and treatment advances substantiated a predominantly neurobiologic basis for OCD. The following sections provide a brief overview of these findings and evidence pointing to genetic vulnerability. Psychological factors are also discussed because of their contributions to the disorder. Because no single explanation accounts for all aspects of OCD, a combination of factors will probably be found to produce the disorder.

Biologic Theories

Genetic, neuropathologic, and biochemical research, reviewed in this section, suggests that OCD has a biologic basis involving several neuroanatomic structures.

Genetic Factors

OCD occurs more often in people who have first-degree relatives with OCD or with Tourette syndrome than it does in the general population. Some studies show an increased prevalence of anxiety and mood disorders in relatives of individuals who have OCD. Twin studies indicate that OCD occurs more frequently in siblings of twins. Further studies implicate specific genes and associate them with OCD (Shaw, Sharp, Sudre, Wharton, Greenstein, Raznahan, et al., 2014). These discoveries may lead to breakthroughs in pharmacologic treatments of OCD.

Neuropathologic Theories

Recent neuroimaging studies of individuals with OCD show hyperactivity in the orbitofrontal cortex, anterior cingulated cortex, and caudate nucleus, suggesting a causal role in the etiology of OCD (Shaw, et al., 2014).

Increased cerebral glucose metabolism is identified in various studies. The most replicated results demonstrate increased glucose metabolism in the caudate nucleus (part of the basal ganglia), the orbitofrontal gyri (the gyri directly above the orbit of the eye), and the cingulate gyri (considered to be part of the limbic system) (Whiteside, Port & Abramowitz, 2004). Studies measuring cerebral blood flow and glucose metabolism in individuals with OCD during exposure to feared stimuli and during relaxation further implicate these regions of the brain (Shaw, et al., 2014).

Biochemical Theories

Serotonin plays a role in OCD. It has been studied through challenge tests in which serotonin agonists were administered to persons with OCD and with control subjects. The most convincing evidence for serotonin's role is that serotonin-specific antidepressants relieve the symptoms of OCD for most persons. A single neurotransmitter is unlikely to be entirely responsible for OCD, but to date, serotonin is the only neurotransmitter to have been implicated. Conventional and novel antipsychotic medications and mood stabilizers are used in conjunction with serotonin-targeting medications to treat refractory symptoms, indicating that other biochemical processes exist (Ravindran & Stein, 2010).

Psychological Theories

Although psychological theories of OCD have not been scientifically tested, the rich literature describing clinical examples and case histories help us understand the symptoms and behaviors related to OCD. In addition, behavioral treatment of individuals with severe compulsions improves symptoms.

Psychodynamic Factors

The psychodynamic theory hypothesizes that OCD symptoms and character traits arise from three unconscious defense mechanisms: **isolation** (separation of affect from a thought or impulse), **undoing** (an act performed with the goal of preventing consequences of a thought or impulse), and **reaction formation** (behavior and consciously stated attitudes that oppose underlying impulses). Classic psychoanalytic theory describes OCD as regression from the oedipal phase to the anal phase of development, which includes preoccupations with anger and dirt (see Chapter 5). This regression occurs when the patient becomes anxious about retaliation or loss of love.

Behavioral Factors

Behavioral explanations for OCD stem from learning theory. From this viewpoint, obsessions are seen as **conditioned stimuli.** Through being associated with noxious events, stimuli that are usually considered neutral become anxiety provoking. The individual then engages in activities to escape or avoid the anxiety. Compulsions develop as the individual discovers behaviors that successfully reduce the obsessional anxiety. As the principles of operant conditioning indicate, the more the behaviors decrease the anxiety, the more likely the individual is to continue using them. However, the rituals or behaviors preserve the fear response because the person avoids the initial stimuli and thus never extinguishes the compulsion. Interrupting this cycle is the focus of behavioral therapy in treating an individual with OCD.

Family Response to Disorder

Marital status appears to be affected by OCD. Patients with OCD tend to remain single more often than people without the disorder. They also have higher rates of celibacy, possibly because they fear being dirty or becoming contaminated. The divorce rate is lower than would be expected, given the stress of living with this disorder; individuals with OCD are able to gradually draw their families into accommodating abnormal behavior. For example, the families of patients with cleaning compulsions may forego normal family and social activities to "help" the individual complete compulsive cleaning of the family home and decrease the anxiety level in the household.

Family assessment will reveal the amount of education and support needed and will begin the partnership among the individual, family, and treatment team. Evaluate the family's understanding of the disorder and of proposed treatments. Are they able and willing to help the individual practice cognitive and behavioral techniques? Are they knowledgeable about prescribed medicines? These questions offer a wonderful opportunity for individual and family education.

Family members offer a perspective on the severity of the individual's illness. Family members are experts in the patient's rituals and may observe subtle changes. Evaluate the family's response to changes in the individual's behavior as treatment progresses. You may have to discuss how the family will manage the changes brought about by a decrease in rituals. If obsessions and compulsions make it difficult for the individual to leave the home or function at work, financial difficulties may result. These factors should be assessed and appropriate assistance obtained through social services when necessary.

Tim's Family

Tim's parents recognized their son had unusual behaviors that interfered with his normal growth and development. When he was in high school, his parents took him to a psychiatrist who prescribed medication and offered brief counseling. Tim was able to successfully complete high school with honors and was accepted into a highly respected college. He was able to function when taking medications.

Teamwork and Collaboration: Working Toward Recovery

OCD can be difficult to treat because obsessions and compulsions consistently interfere with recovery efforts. OCD is treated with medications, cognitive behavioral therapy (CBT), and supportive therapy. If medications and therapy are not successful, electroconvulsive therapy (ECT) can be considered. In very severe instances, psychosurgery may be a treatment option. The overall goal is for the patient to recover and to decrease the symptoms. Staff may have differing opinions about the amount of control the individual has over the behavior, but these differences of opinion must be resolved. All staff must be consistent in their expectations and acceptance of the patient's behaviors to keep these patients from becoming frustrated or confused regarding expectations during treatment (Box 18.2).

Electroconvulsive Therapy

The effect of ECT on decreasing obsessions and compulsions has not been extensively studied. However, it may be helpful in treating symptoms that occur in association with depression. It also may be used to treat depressive symptoms in patients who have not responded to other treatments and who are at risk for suicide. Nursing's role in caring for the individual undergoing ECT is outlined in Chapter 10.

BOX 18.2 CLINICAL VIGNETTE

More Teamwork Needed

Robert, a 32-year-old man, is a new patient at a local psychiatric unit. He admitted himself to have his medicines evaluated because his obsessive thoughts and depression have worsened since his recent divorce. While in the hospital, he has quickly become viewed as a "problem patient" because he hoards linens and demands a new bar of soap for each of his five daily showers. He is compelled to open and close his door five times when he leaves or enters his room but does not know why. This behavior has led to arguments with his roommate. In an effort to "help him," the psychiatric technicians locked his bathroom door to prevent him from showering so frequently. He tried to enter his bathroom to shower and panicked when the technicians refused to allow him to shower, telling him, "You can live without it." After receiving PRN medication for extreme anxiety, Robert signed out of the hospital against medical advice because of embarrassment and anger toward the nursing staff.

What Do You Think?
- How could the technicians have handled the situation differently so as to not disrupt Robert's or the unit's clinical care?
- What nursing interventions might be appropriate in providing Robert's care?

Psychosurgery

Psychosurgery is sometimes used to treat extremely severe OCD that has not responded to prolonged and intensive drug treatment, behavioral therapy, or a combination of the two. Modern stereotactic surgical techniques that produce lesions of the cingulum bundle (a bundle of connective tissue) or anterior limb of the internal capsule (a region near the thalamus and part of the circuit connecting to the cortex) may bring about substantial clinical benefit in some individuals without causing significant morbidity (Csigó, Harsányi, Demeter, Rajkai, Németh, & Racacsmány, 2010). Other treatment options include radiotherapy and deep brain stimulation in which electrical current is applied through an electrode inserted into the brain (Robinson, Taghva, Liu, & Apuzzo, 2013).

Safety Issues

As with any individual with a mental disorder, a suicide assessment must be completed. Although individuals with OCD do not usually become suicidal as a direct result of anxiety, the disorder greatly distresses the person, who realizes the pointlessness and absurdity of the behaviors. Often, the person has tolerated symptoms for quite some time before seeking treatment. The person may feel a sense of hopelessness and helplessness and may contemplate suicide to end the suffering. An additional risk for suicide is created by the high probability of major depression, which often accompanies OCD. Patients may feel a need to punish themselves for their intrusive thoughts (e.g., religious coupled with sexual obsessions). Some persons have aggressive obsessions, so that external limits may have to be imposed for the protection of others.

Evidence-Based Nursing Care of Persons with OCD

Persons with OCD may be any age; many have other disorders. Nursing care involves a careful assessment of the impact of the mental health disorder on individual and family. Nursing Care Plan 18.1 is available at http://thepoint.lww.com/BoydEssentials.

Mental Health Nursing Assessment

The nurse should assess the type and severity of the person's obsessions and compulsions. If the assessment occurs in a hospital, remember that some individuals with OCD experience a transient decrease in symptoms when admitted to a hospital; therefore, sufficient time must be allowed for an accurate assessment. If that time is unavailable, family members or significant others may provide an important source of information, with the individual's permission.

Physical Health Assessment

Individuals with OCD do not have a higher prevalence of physical disease than others. However, they may report multiple physical symptoms. With late-onset OCD (i.e., after 35 years of age) and with symptoms that occur with a febrile illness, cerebral pathology should be considered. Each person with OCD should be assessed for dermatologic lesions caused by repetitive handwashing, excessive cleaning with caustic agents, or bathing. Osteoarthritic joint damage secondary to cleaning rituals may also be observed.

Most individuals appear neatly dressed and groomed, cooperative, and eager to answer questions. Speech will be at normal rate and volume, but often, individuals with an obsessional style of thinking exhibit circumferential speech. This speech, loaded with irrelevant details, eventually addresses the question. Listening may be frustrating and require considerable patience, but you must remember that such speech is part of the disorder and may be beyond the person's awareness. Continually interrupting and redirecting them can interfere with establishing a therapeutic relationship, especially in the initial assessment. Redirection should be done in a gentle and noncritical manner to allow the patient time to refocus.

Psychosocial Assessment

Identifying the degree to which the OCD symptoms interfere with the patient's daily functioning is important.

BOX 18.3

Rating Scales for Assessing Obsessive-Compulsive Symptoms

YALE-BROWN OBSESSIVE COMPULSIVE SCALE (Y-BOCS)
Goodman, W., Price, L., Rasmussen, S., Mazure, C., Fleischmann, R. L., Hill, C. L., et al. (1989). The Yale-Brown Obsessive Compulsive Scale (Y-BOCS): Part I. Development, use and reliability. *Archives of General Psychiatry, 46*, 1006–1011.

THE MAUDSLEY OBSESSIONAL-COMPULSIVE INVENTORY (MOC)
Rachman, S. & Hodgson, R. (1980). *Obsessions and compulsions*. New York: Prentice-Hall.

THE LEYTON OBSESSIONAL INVENTORY
Cooper, J. (1970). The Leyton Obsessional Inventory. *Psychiatric Medicine, 1*, 48.

Several rating scales can be used to identify symptoms and monitor improvement. Examples of these scales are provided in Box 18.3. Some of these scales are to be used by the nurse; others are self-rating scales. The Yale-Brown Obsessive Compulsive Scale (Y-BOCS) is a popular clinician-rated 16-item scale that obtains separate subtotals for severity of obsessions and compulsions. The Maudsley Obsessive-Compulsive Inventory is a 30-item, true–false, self-assessment tool that may help the individual to recognize individual symptoms.

Sociocultural factors are very important. At times, cultural or religious beliefs may be misunderstood and mistaken for obsessions or compulsions. These beliefs and actions must be evaluated in the context of the individual's culture. If these beliefs are consistent with the patient's social or cultural environment, are not harmful to the individual or others, and do not interfere with individual functioning in that environment, they should not be considered symptoms of OCD.

Strength Assessment

The personal and social strengths of the person should emerge during the assessment interview. Does the child or adult enjoy good physical health? Is the person motivated for treatment? Does the person recognize that obsessions or compulsions are unusual or abnormal? Are there social supports? This information will be useful in establishing a recovery plan.

Nursing Diagnoses

Patients with OCD may present with various symptoms, depending on the particular obsession and the compulsions that have evolved to cope with that obsession. As a result, the nursing diagnoses applied to patients with this disorder can run the gamut from the primary diagnosis of Anxiety to other physiologic

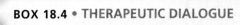

BOX 18.4 • THERAPEUTIC DIALOGUE

Tim is admitted to an inpatient unit; an initial assessment is currently being conducted.

INEFFECTIVE APPROACH

Nurse: Could you tell me what brings you here?

Tim: My car.

Nurse: Excuse me. No, why are you here? What do you hope to accomplish while you are here.

Tim: Well, this is how I see it. We need to make sure everyone is healthy and I want to make sure.

Nurse: No, you don't understand what I am asking. WHY are you here.

Tim: Forget it. I want to see my wife.

EFFECTIVE APPROACH

Nurse: Tim, how can we help you?

Tim: Well, I am not sure. My wife thinks I am doing strange things. See, I want everyone to be protected and I think that it is important to stay healthy. There is an outbreak of staph infections and I want to make sure that my family is safe and I am just trying to figure things out.

Nurse: OK, it sounds like you are concerned about your family and you are trying to protect them.

Tim: Yes, it is all of the germs. They are everywhere.

Nurse: And you are trying to get rid of them?

Tim: Yes, my wife thinks I am going overboard and wants me to take my medication.

Nurse: Your medication?

Tim: Yes, I used to take medication when I felt like this.

Nurse: You don't take your medication anymore?

Tim: No, I don't need it.

Nurse: I see. But your wife thinks you do?

Tim: Yes, but I don't like the side effects.

Nurse: Such as?

Tim: Well, to tell you the truth, I'd rather not talk about it.

Nurse: OK. While you are here, we can look at different options to help you feel more comfortable.

CRITICAL THINKING CHALLENGE

- How did the first nurse's interaction block communication and increase Tim's frustration?

- What effective communication techniques did the nurse use in the second scenario?

---

disturbances of the compulsion, such as Impaired Skin Integrity, which may result from continuous hand washing. Hopelessness, Loneliness, Powerlessness, Self-Concept, Readiness for Enhanced Coping, Role Conflict, and Sedentary Lifestyle are possible nursing diagnoses. Outcomes are determined collaboratively with the person and directed by the nursing diagnoses and interventions selected.

Nursing Interventions

Establishing a therapeutic relationship with a person with OCD requires patience and active listening. The individual may go to great lengths to explain some minute aspect of her or his life. It is important not to interrupt or rush these explanations. Being unable to finish thoughts increases the patient's anxiety and frustration. See Box 18.4

The nurse's interpersonal skills are crucial to successful intervention with the patient who has OCD. Nurses must control their own anxiety. The nurse should interact with the individual in a calm, nonauthoritarian fashion without exhibiting any disapproval of the patient or the patient's behaviors while demonstrating empathy about the distress that the disorder has caused (See Box 18.4). This approach is one of the most effective means available for communicating appreciation for the individual as separate from the illness.

Interventions focus on the physical consequences of the compulsion as well as the psychosocial aspects. The next section provides an overview of biopsychosocial interventions including medications.

BOX 18.5

Antidepressants FDA Approved for Obsessive-Compulsive Disorder

MEDICATIONS	CLASSIFICATION	DOSAGE	SIDE EFFECTS
Sertraline (Zoloft)	SSRI	Children (6–12yrs old) 25mg per day (13–17) 50 mg per day Adults 50 mg titrated to 200 mg/day	Sedation, dizziness, somnolence or insomnia, headache, sexual dysfunction, can cause excitability when initiated, weight gain (rare)
Fluvoxamine	SSRI	Children (8–17) 25–200 mg per day Adults 50–300 mg per day	
Fluoxetine (Prozac)	SSRI	Adolescents 20–60 mg per day Adults 20–60 mg per day	
Paroxetine (Paxil)	SSRI	Adults 20–60 mg per day	
Clomipramine (Anafranil)	TCA	Children (6–17) 25 mg per day Adults Starting dose 25 mg; titrated to150–250 mg per day	Significant sedation, anticholinergic effects, increased risk for seizures, dizziness, tremulousness, headache

Maintaining Skin Integrity

For the patient with cleaning or handwashing compulsions, attention to skin condition is necessary. Encourage the individual to use tepid water when washing and hand cream after washing. Remove harsh abrasive soaps and replace them with moisturizing soaps. Attempt to decrease the frequency of washing by agreeing on a time schedule and time-limited washing.

Medications

Selective serotonin reuptake inhibitors (SSRIs), including fluoxetine, fluvoxamine, paroxetine, and sertraline are recommended medications. Clomipramine (a tricyclic antidepressant) is also frequently prescribed and was the first drug to produce significant advances in treating OCD (U.S. Department of Health and Human Services [HHS], 2012). See Box 18.5.

Administering and Monitoring Medications

Antidepressants used to treat persons with OCD are often given in higher doses than those normally used to treat depressed patients. See Box 18.5. Aggressive treatment may be indicated to bring the symptoms under control. Thus, medication effects must be closely monitored, including signs of toxicity, to provide safe and adequate care. All antidepressants have a black box warning for suicidality in children, adolescents, and young adults. These medications often take several weeks or months to relieve compulsions and may take even longer to decrease obsessions. One of the older antidepressants, clomipramine, is commonly used in the treatment of OCD. See Box 18.6.

Monitoring for Drug Interactions

All antidepressant medications interact with the monoamine oxidase inhibitors (MAOIs), causing hypertensive crises; interaction with tryptophan may cause serotonin syndrome. Therefore, concomitant use should be avoided. Because of the extensive list of drug–drug interactions associated with these medications, a prudent nurse will consult a drug reference handbook before administering any medications. Quick recognition of signs and symptoms of interactions or toxic symptoms is imperative for safe care.

Exposure and Response Prevention

An effective behavioral intervention for individuals with OCD who perform rituals is exposure and response prevention (ERP) (McGuire, Lewin, & Storch, 2014). The person is exposed to situations or objects that are known to induce anxiety but is asked to refrain from performing the ritualistic behaviors. One goal of this procedure is to help the person understand that resisting the rituals while exposed to the object of anxiety is less stressful and time-consuming than performing the rituals. Another goal is to confound the expectation of distressing outcomes and eventually extinguish the compulsive behaviors. Most individuals improve with ERP, but few become completely asymptomatic.

Thought Stopping

Thought stopping is used with individuals who have obsessional thoughts (Abramowitz, et al, 2010). The person is taught to interrupt obsessional thoughts by saying, "Stop!" either aloud or silently. This activity interrupts and delays

---

BOX 18.6

Drug Profile: Clomipramine (Anafranil)

DRUG CLASS: Tricyclic Antidepressant

RECEPTOR AFFINITY: Exact mechanism of action unknown: inhibits norepinephrine and serotonin reuptake

ROUTES AND DOSAGE: Available in 25 mg, 50 mg, and 75 mg capsules

Adults: 150–250 mg at bedtime. PO Initial dose 25 mg PO daily, increase by 25 mg/day every 4 to 7 days; Maximum 100 mg/day in first 2 weeks, 250 mg/day for maintenance. Give in divided doses with food during initial titrate increase taper dose gradually to discontinue.

Children: Approved for children over the age of 10. 100–200 mg PO at bedtime. Start: 25 mg PO every day, increase by 25 mg q4–7 days; Maximum 3 mg/kg/day up to 100 mg/day in first 2 weeks and up to 200 mg/day maintenance. Give in divided doses with food during initial titration; taper dose gradually.

HALF-LIFE (PEAK EFFECT): 32 hours (2 hours)

SELECTED SIDE EFFECTS: Suicidality, sedation, seizures, orthostatic hypotension, hypertension, syncope, ventricular arrhythmias, QT prolongation, torsade de pointe, atrioventricular block, myocardial infarction, stroke, extrapyramidal symptoms ataxia, tardive dyskinesia, anticholinergic effects, fatigue, ejaculatory dysfunction, nausea/vomiting, appetite changes, and weight changes

WARNINGS: Suicidality risk in children, adolescents, and young adults with major depressive disorder, dose selection for an elderly patient should be cautious, usually starting at the low end of the dosing range, reflecting the greater frequency of decreased hepatic, renal, or cardiac function and of concomitant disease or other drug therapy.. Should not be giving in conjunction with or within 14 days before or after treatment with monoamine oxidase inhibitor.

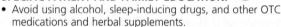

SPECIFIC PATIENT AND FAMILY EDUCATION:
- Avoid using alcohol, sleep-inducing drugs, and other OTC medications and herbal supplements.
- Take the drug exactly as prescribed and do not stop taking the drug without consulting your health care provider.
- Take the drug with food.
- Avoid driving a car or performing tasks that require alertness if drowsiness or dizziness occurs.
- Report any signs and symptoms of side effects.
- Notify your health care provider of severe drowsiness, ataxia, vomiting, cyanosis, agitation, severe perspiration, muscle rigidity, or heart palpitations.

---

the uncontrollable spiral of obsessional thoughts. Research supporting this technique is scant; however, practitioners have found it useful in multimodal treatment with ERP, relaxation, and cognitive restructuring.

Relaxation Techniques

Individuals with OCD experience insomnia because of heightened anxiety levels. Relaxation exercises may be helpful in improving sleep patterns. These exercises do not affect OCD symptoms but they may be used to decrease anxiety. The nurse may also teach the person other relaxation measures, such as deep breathing, taking warm baths, practicing meditation, and music therapy, or other quiet activities.

Cognitive Restructuring

Cognitive restructuring is a method of teaching the person to restructure dysfunctional thought processes by defining and testing them (Beck & Emery, 1985). Its goal is to alter the person's immediate, dysfunctional appraisal of a situation and perception of long-term consequences. The individual is taught to monitor automatic thoughts and then to recognize the connection between thoughts, emotional response, and behaviors. The distorted thoughts are examined and tested by for-or-against evidence presented by the therapist, which helps the individual to realistically assess the likelihood that the feared event will happen if the compulsive behavior is not performed. The person begins to analyze his or her thoughts as incongruent with reality. For example, even if the alarm clock is not checked 30 times before going to bed, it will still go off in the morning, and the person will not be disciplined for tardiness at work. Maybe it needs to be checked only once or twice.

Cue Cards

Cue cards are tools used to help the individual restructure thought patterns. They contain statements that are positively oriented and pertain to the person's specific obsessions and compulsions. Cue cards use information from the individual's symptom hierarchy, an organizational system that breaks down the obsessions and compulsions from least to most anxiety provoking. These cards can help reinforce the belief that the person is safe and can tolerate the anxiety caused by delaying or controlling compulsive rituals. Examples of cue cards are shown in Box 18.7.

Interventions for the Social Domain

- For a hospitalized individual, unit routines must be carefully and clearly explained to decrease fear of the unknown.

BOX 18.7

Examples of Cue Card Statements

- It's the OCD, not me.
- These are only OC thoughts. OC thoughts don't mean action; I will not act on the thoughts.
- My anxiety level goes up but will always go down.
- I never sat with the anxiety long enough to see that it would not harm me.
- Trust myself.
- I did it right the first time.
- Checking the locks again won't keep me safe. I really am safe in the world.

- At least initially, do not prevent the individual from engaging in rituals because the person's anxiety level will increase.
- Recognize the significance of the rituals to the person and empathize with the person's need to perform them.
- Assist the individual in arranging a schedule of activities that incorporates some private time but also integrates the person into normal unit activities.

Psychoeducation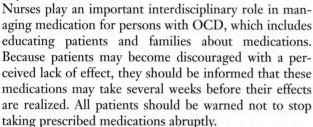

Nurses play an important interdisciplinary role in managing medication for persons with OCD, which includes educating patients and families about medications. Because patients may become discouraged with a perceived lack of effect, they should be informed that these medications may take several weeks before their effects are realized. All patients should be warned not to stop taking prescribed medications abruptly.

Individuals should be instructed to avoid alcohol and not to operate heavy machinery while taking these medications until the sedative effects are known. Instruct patients to inform their providers about any over-the-counter (OTC) medications and herbal supplements they are taking because some will interact with these medications.

Psychoeducation is a crucial nursing intervention for the person with OCD. Knowledge is power; the more the person knows about his or her disorder, the more control he or she will have over symptoms. The individual should be instructed not only about the biologic components of OCD but also about its treatments and disease course. Treatment is a shared responsibility between the individual and the health care provider; the individual should be included in the medication and treatment decision-making processes. If local support groups are available, the person should be referred to reduce feelings of uniqueness and embarrassment about the disease. Family education is also important so the individual will have help in practicing behavioral homework (Box 18.8).

Evaluation and Treatment Outcomes

Several methods can be used to measure the response to treatment (including nursing care): changes in Y-BOCS scores or other rating scales, remission of presenting symptoms, and the ability to complete activities of daily living. The individual should be able to participate in social or group activities with a degree of comfort and without self-harm or aggressive intent. He or she should also be able to demonstrate common knowledge of OCD by describing its symptoms, biologic basis, and treatments.

BOX 18.8

Psychoeducation Checklist: Obsessive-Compulsive Disorder

When caring for the patient with OCD, be sure to include the patient's primary caregiver, if appropriate, and address the following topic areas in the teaching plan:

- Psychopharmacologic agents if ordered, including drug action, dosage, frequency, and possible side effects
- Skin care measures
- Ritualistic behaviors and alternative activities
- Thought stopping
- Relaxation techniques
- Cognitive restructuring
- Recovery strategies
- Community resources

MAOI, monoamine oxidase inhibitor; SSRI, selective serotonin reuptake inhibitor.

Continuum of Care

The symptoms of OCD can become debilitating. The symptoms wax and wane throughout treatment. As the focus of treatment shifts from inpatient to outpatient environments, individuals must be assessed continually to ensure favorable outcomes through early intervention if symptoms resurface.

Inpatient-Focused Care

In an inpatient setting, the presence of a person with severe OCD may present a nursing management challenge. These individuals require a significant amount of staff time. They may monopolize bathrooms or showers or have disruptive rituals involving eating. Nurses play an integral role in treating the person with OCD. The nurse should help the individual perform activities of daily living to ensure that they are completed. Monitoring medication effects, teaching psychoeducation groups, ensuring adequate caloric intake, and providing individual patient counseling are additional inpatient interventions.

Emergency Care

Individuals with OCD frequently use medical services long before they seek specialized psychiatric treatment. Therefore, early recognition of symptoms and referral are important concerns for nurses working in primary care and other medical settings. After individuals are referred, most psychiatric treatment of OCD occurs on an outpatient basis. Although only individuals with severely debilitating symptoms or self-harming thoughts and actions are hospitalized, patients may experience intense anxiety symptoms to the point of panic. In such an emergency, benzodiazepines and other anxiolytics can be used.

Family Interventions

The families of persons with OCD need to be educated about the causes of the disorder. Understanding the biologic basis of the disorder should decrease some of the stigma and embarrassment they may feel about the bizarre nature of the patient's obsessions and compulsions. Education about both biologic and psychological treatment approaches should be provided.

Family assistance in monitoring symptom remission and side effects of the medication is invaluable. Family members can also assist the person with behavioral and cognitive interventions.

When caring for the person with OCD, be sure to include the individual's caregiver, if appropriate, and address the following topic areas in the teaching plan:

- Medications, including drug action, dosage, frequency, and possible side effects
- Skin care measures
- Ritualistic behaviors and alternative activities
- Thought stopping
- Relaxation techniques
- Cognitive restructuring
- Community resources

Community Treatment

Partial hospitalization programs and day treatment programs help individuals in their quest for recovery. These programs can support independence while individuals begin medications and behavioral therapies. Some patients require outpatient treatment daily when symptoms increase. Maintenance outpatient therapy may be scheduled weekly or twice weekly for several weeks until the symptoms are well controlled. Community agency visits are recommended to monitor medication.

TRICHOTILLOMANIA AND EXCORIATION DISORDER

Trichotillomania is chronic self-destructive hair pulling that results in noticeable hair loss, usually in the crown, occipital, or parietal areas of the head, although sometimes also involve the eyebrows and eyelashes. The individual has an increase in tension immediately before pulling out the hair or while attempting to resist the behavior. After the hair has been pulled, the person feels a sense of relief. Some would classify this disorder as one of self-mutilation. It becomes a problem when accompanied by significant distress or impairment in other areas of function. A hair-pulling session can last several hours, and the individual may either ritualistically eat the hairs or discard them. Hair ingestion

may result in the development of a hair ball, which can lead to anorexia, stomach pain, anemia, intestinal obstruction, and peritonitis. Other medical complications include infection at the hair-pulling site. Hair pulling is done alone, and usually patients deny it. Instead of pain, these persons experience pleasure and tension release (Duke, Keeley, Geffken, & Storch, 2010).

Clinical Course

The onset of trichotillomania occurs among children before the age of 5 years and in adolescents. For the young child, distraction or redirection may successfully eliminate the behavior. The behavior in adolescents may begin a chronic course that may last well into adulthood.

Diagnostic Criteria

Trichotillomania is diagnosed when recurrent pulling out of hair with hair loss occurs. The individual is unable to decrease of stop such hair pulling, which causes considerable distress (APA, 2013).

Etiology and Treatment

This disorder is poorly understood. An etiologic relationship to OCD has not been established, but support is present for a familial connection (Keuthen, Altenburger, & Pauls, 2014). The prevalence of trichotillomania is estimated at 1% to 2% of the population (APA, 2013). No particular medication class demonstrates effectiveness in treatment. Studies of individual medications including olanzapine (antipsychotic) and clomipramine (tricyclic antidepressant) show treatment effectiveness (Rothbart, Amos, Siegfried, Ipser, Fineberg, Chamberlain, et al., 2013). Cognitive behavior therapy and habit reversal training, a behavioral intervention, can improve the symptoms (Duke, et al., 2010; Rogers, Banis, Falkenstein, Malloy, McDonough, Nelson, et al., 2014).

Evidenced-Based Nursing Care of Persons with Trichotillomania

The assessment includes a review of current problems, developmental history (especially school conflicts and learning difficulties), family and social history, identification of support systems, previous psychiatric treatment, and general health history. The cultural context in which the trichotillomania occurs must be taken into consideration because in some cultures, this behavior may be viewed as socially acceptable. The hair-pulling history and pattern are also used to determine the duration and severity of the disorder. Typical nursing diagnoses include Self-mutilation, Low Self-esteem, Hopelessness, Impaired

Skin Integrity, and Ineffective Denial. Within the therapeutic relationship, a cognitive behavioral approach can be used to help the person identify when hair pulling occurs, the precipitating events, and the details of the episode.

Individuals with trichotillomania report that anxiety, loneliness, anger, fatigue, guilt, frustration, and boredom can all trigger the hair-pulling behaviors. Current research has also shown that persons with chronic hair pulling typically avoid social activities and events (Tung, Flessner, Grant, Keuthen, 2015). In addition, the economic impact of trichotillomania can be significant in relation to lost work or school days. Teaching about the disorder will help affected individuals understand that they are not alone and that others have also had this problem. The goal of treatment is to help the individual learn to substitute positive behaviors for the hair-pulling behavior through self-monitoring of events that precipitate the episodes.

Excoriation (Skin-Picking) Disorder

Repetitive and compulsive picking of skin causing tissue damage characterizes **excoriation or skin-picking isorder** (APA, 2013). Although face, arms, or hands are the most common sites for picking, it can occur at other body sites. Most affected people pick with their fingers, but tweezers or pins are also sometimes used. Similar to other disorders, skin picking causes significant distress to individuals. Prevalence is estimated at 1.4%; it occurs more frequently in persons with OCD (APA, 2013). Treatment data are limited, but lamotrigine (mood stabilizer/anticonvulsant agent) has been shown to be successful in one study (Grant, Odluag, Chamberlain, & Kim, 2010). Nursing care is similar to caring for a person with trichotillomania.

Body Dysmorphic Disorder

Individuals with body dysmorphic disorder (BDD) focus on real (but slight) or imagined defects in appearance, such as a large nose, thinning hair, or small genitals. Preoccupation with the perceived defect causes significant distress and interferes with their ability to function socially. They feel so self-conscious that they avoid work or public situations. Some fear that their "ugly" body part will malfunction. Surgical correction of the problem by a plastic surgeon or a dermatologist does not correct their preoccupation and distress. BDD is an extremely debilitating disorder and can significantly impair an individual's quality of life. BDD usually begins in adolescence and continues throughout adulthood. These individuals are not usually seen in psychiatric settings unless they have a coexisting psychiatric disorder or a family member insists on psychiatric attention.

BOX 18.9 CLINICAL VIGNETTE

Body Dysmorphic Disorder

K, a 16-year-old girl, for about 6 months has believed that her pubic bone is becoming increasingly dislocated and prominent. She believes that everyone stares at it and talks about it. She does not remember a particular event related to the appearance of the symptom but is absolutely convinced that she can be helped only by a surgical correction of her pubic bone.

She was treated recently for anorexia nervosa with marginal success. Although her weight is nearly normal, she continues to be preoccupied with the looks of her body. She spends almost the entire day in her bedroom, wearing excessively large pajamas and she refuses to leave the house. Once or twice a day, she lowers herself to the ground and measures, with her fingers, the distance between her pelvic girdle and the ground in order to check the position of the pubic bone.

In desperation, her parents called the clinic for help.

The family was referred to a home health agency and a psychiatric home health nurse who arranged for an assessment visit.

What Do You Think?
- How should the nurse approach K? Should an assessment begin immediately?
- From the vignette, identify nursing diagnoses, outcomes, and interventions.

Adapted from Sobanski, E. & Schmidt, M. H. (2000). "Everybody looks at my pubic bone"—a case report of an adolescent patient with body dysmorphic disorder. *Acta Psychiatrica Scandinavica, 101,* 80–82.

This disorder occurs in men and women, with a prevalence of 2.4% in the United States (APA, 2013). Sixty percent of the persons with BDD also have an anxiety disorder (Mufaddel, Osman, Almugaddam, & Jafferany, 2013). The risk of depression, suicide ideation, and suicide is high. The lifetime suicide attempt rate is estimated at 22% to 24% (Bjornsson, Didie, & Phillips, 2010). No single theory explains the cause of BDD. Unrealistic cultural expectations and genetic predisposition most likely underlie this disorder. See Box 18.9.

Hoarding Disorder

Difficulty parting with or discarding possessions, regardless of actual value, characterize hoarding disorder. Individuals with this disorder have a need to save items and experience distress if their items are discarded. Most affected individuals with hoarding disorder also exhibit excessive acquisition (excessive purchasing of items or collecting free items).

The prevalence of this disorder is estimated 2% to 6% (APA, 2013). Hoarding may begin in childhood with an increase in severity throughout a lifespan. This disorder tends to be familial and present in different generations. Being Native American, being born in the United States;

over the age of 45 years; high school educated; widowed, separated, or divorced; living in a rural community increases the likelihood of having difficulty discarding items. Being African American, Asian, and Hispanic, and earning more than $35,000 per year, and never married decrease the likelihood of having difficulty discarding items (Rodriguez, Simpson, Liu, Levinson, & Blanco, 2013). These individuals seek mental health care, with depression being the most common reason (Hall, Tolin, Frost, & Steketee, 2013).

Hoarding poses public health and safety risks for individuals, families, and communities (Fleury, Gaudette, & Moran, 2012). Excessive collection of items not only clutters living areas but can lead to being trapped in an inaccessible environment and one that is high risk for fire. Home health nurses are often the first health care providers that recognize the problem and so are a valuable resource in determining the safety hazards and helping the individual become aware of the problem and seek treatment. The nurse can also contact community agencies (Sorrell, 2012). Currently, treatment outcomes with medication and CBT are limited. More research is needed to understand the disorder and treatment (Singh & Jones, 2013). See Box 18.10.

BOX 18.10

Research for Best Practice: Compulsive Hoarding Syndrome

Singh, S. & Jones, C. (2013). Compulsive hoarding syndrome: Engaging the patients in treatment. Mental Health Practice, 17(4), 16–20.

THE QUESTION: How can persons with hoarding disorder be engaged in treatment?

METHODS: A CBT treatment approach is described that has been adapted to include visual methods (photographs, videos) and imagery. The group approach encourages the individuals to be "in the moment" and experience the discomfort of their difficulties. Participants photographed cluttered areas in their home and determined what they would like to overcome, imagined life without all of the clutter, and identified how their life and relationships are affected by the problem. Then they identified what they would like to do about the problem. This exercise helped them recognize the problem and what to do about it. Psychoeducation is included in the group and is based on themes that emerge in the session.

FINDINGS: Using group processes, the group members became supportive of each other when undertaking changes. The group developed a buddy system where members supported each other outside the group. Through using the visual methods, the individuals were able to distance themselves from the problem and decrease the feeling of being overwhelmed. They were able to be more objective and develop an action plan.

IMPLICATIONS FOR NURSING: Helping individuals with this disorder will require creative, eclectic approaches using a combination of modalities.

SUMMARY OF KEY POINTS

- Obsessions are excessive, intrusive, or unwanted thoughts. Compulsions are repetitive behaviors performed in a ritualistic manner.

- The most common obsession is the fear of contamination.

- Compulsions relieve anxiety and should not be interrupted unless the behavior jeopardizes the safety of the person or others. Interrupting compulsive behavior increases the person's anxiety.

- OCD is characterized by obsessions, compulsion, or both. OCD can occur in children and adults.

- Medications and cognitive behavior therapy can help affected individuals to get through episodes and reduce the compulsive behavior.

- Nursing care focuses on motivating the person for change, administering and monitoring medication, providing psychoeducation, and supporting positive new behaviors.

- The primary characteristics of trichotillomania and excoriation disorders are compulsive behaviors that damage the hair or skin. Compulsive behaviors of both disorders cause significant distress to the person who cannot stop or decrease the behaviors. Medications and psychotherapy can reduce these behaviors.

- BDD involves excessive focus on slight or imagined defects in appearance. The person with these extremely distressing defects seeks treatment by plastic surgeons or dermatologists. Correction does not relieve the patient's preoccupation, which continues to interfere with his or her quality of life. These individuals are high risk for depression and suicide.

- Hoarding disorder can begin in childhood and last a lifetime. Individuals with this disorder need to save things and become very upset if items are removed. When excessive collection leads to extreme clutter, it becomes a safety issue.

CRITICAL THINKING CHALLENGES

1. Differentiate an obsession from a compulsion.

2. List common obsessions and their consequences to the individual and family.

3. Jane, a 35-year-old single mother, has been unable go to work because she fears her apartment will burn down. She is constantly checking the stove and furnace. Her family convinced her to be admitted to a

mental health unit. Discuss how you would prioritize her assessment and develop a plan of care.

4. Jon, a 25-year-old man, is admitted to an inpatient unit for depression and extreme anxiety. He was diagnosed with OCD as a child and had been able to function with medication. He recently married and decided to stop taking his medication. When his symptoms recurred, his wife tried to prevent Jon's compulsive behaviors by removing the knobs from the stove. He became more anxious. As Jon's nurse, develop a teaching plan about OCD for his wife.

5. Explain the behaviors associated with trichotillomania, excoriation disorder, BDD, and hoarding disorder. What are the similarities and differences?

 Aviator: 2004. The movie starring Leonardo DiCapri depicts the earlier years of film producer, industrialist, and aviator Howard Hughes who suffered from OCD. Hughes' perfectionism in his film making and his need for order related to his food and cleanliness eventually contributed to his functional decline. Several scenes illustrate his obsession and compulsion. Hughes' symptoms eventually take over his life and he retreats to a self-imposed solitary confinement.

Viewing Points: How does his early life contribute to the development of his OCD symptoms? Identify his obsessions and compulsions. If Howard Hughes were your patient, what nursing diagnoses and interventions would you want to implement? Identify teaching needs related to medication and the obsessions and compulsions.

MOVIE viewing **GUIDES** related to this chapter are available at http://thepoint.lww.com/BoydEssentials.

REFERENCES

Abramowitz, J.S., Meltzer-Brody, S., Leserman, J., Killenberg, S., Rinaldi, K., Mahaffey, B.L., & Pedersen, C. (2010). Obsessional thoughts and compulsive behaviors in a sample of women with postpartum mood symptoms. *Archives of Women's Mental Health*, 13(6), 523–530.

American Psychiatric Association. (2013). *Diagnostic and statistical manual of mental disorders* (5th ed.) (DSM-5). Arlington, VA: Author.

Beck, A., & Emery, G. (1985). *Anxiety disorders and phobias: A cognitive perspective*. New York: Basic Books.

Bjornsson, A. S., Didie, E. R., & Phillips, K. A. (2010). Body dysmorphic disorder. *Dialogues in Clinical Neuroscience*, 12(2), 221–232.

Cooper, J. (1970). The Leyton obsessional inventory. *Psychological Medicine*, 1, 48–64.

Csigó, K., Harsányi, A., Demeter, G., Rajkai, C., Németh, A., & Racacsmány, M. (2010). Long-term follow-up of patients with obsessive-compulsive disorder treated by anterior capsulotomy: A neuropsychological study. *Journal of Affective Disorders*, 126(1–2), 198–205.

Duke, D. C., Keeley, J. L., Geffken, G. R., & Storch, E. A. (2010). Trichotillomania: A current review. *Clinical Psychology Review*, 30(2), 181–93.

Fleury, G., Gaudette, L., & Moran, P. (2012). Compulsive hoarding: Overview and implications for community health nurses. *Journal of Community Health Nursing*, 29(3), 154–162.

Frydman, I., do Brasil, P. E., Torres, A. R., Shavitt, R. G., Ferrão, Y. A., Rosário, M. C., et al. (2014). Late-onset obsessive-compulsive disorder: Risk factors and correlates. *Journal of Psychiatric Research*, 49, 68–74.

Goodman, W., Price, L., Rasmussen, S., Mazure, C., Fleischmann, R. L., Hill, C. L., et al. (1989). The Yale-Brown Obsessive Compulsive Scale (Y-BOCS): Part 1. Development, use and reliability. *Archives of General Psychiatry*, 46, 1006–1011.

Grados, M. A. (2010). The genetics of obsessive-compulsive disorder and Tourette syndrome: An epidemiological and pathway-based approach for gene discovery. *Journal of the American Academy of Child and Adolescent Psychiatry*, 49(8), 810–819.

Grant, J. E., Odlaug, B. L., Chamberlain, M. D., & Kim, S. W. (2010). A double-blind, placebo-controlled trial of lamotrigine for pathologic skin picking: Treatment efficacy and neurocognitive predictors of response. *Journal of Clinical Psychopharmacology*, 30(4), 396–403.

Grenier, S., Preville, M., Boyer, R., & O'Connor, K. (2009). Prevalence and correlates of obsessive-compulsive disorder among older adults living in the community. *Journal of Anxiety Disorders*, 23(7), 858–865.

Hachiya, Y., Miyata, R., Tanuma, N., Hongou, K., Tanaka, K., Shimoda, K., et al. (2013). Autoimmune neurological disorders associated with group-A beta-hemolytic streptococcal infection. *Brain & Development*, 35(7), 670–674.

Hall, B. J., Tolin, D. F., Frost, R. O., & Steketee, F. (2013). An exploration of comorbid symptoms and clinical correlates of clinically significant hoarding symptoms. *Depression & Anxiety*, 30(1), 67–76.

Jacob, M. L., & Storch, E. A. (2013). Pediatric obsessive-compulsive disorder: A review for nursing professionals. *Journal of Child and Adolescent Psychiatric Nursing*, 26, 138–148.

Keuthen, N. J., Altenburger, E. M., & Pauls, D. (2014). A family study of trichotillomania and chronic hair pulling. *American Journal of Medical Genetics. Part B: Neuropsychiatric Genetics*, 165(2), 167–174.

Lochner, C., & Stein, D. J. (2010). Obsessive-compulsive spectrum disorders in obsessive-compulsive disorder and other anxiety disorders. *Psychopathology*, 43(6), 389–396.

McGuire, J. F., Lewin, A.B., & Storch, E.Q. (2014). Enhancing exposure therapy for anxiety disorders, obsessive-compulsive disorder and post-traumatic stress disorder. (Review). *Expert Review of Neurotherapeutics*, 14(8), 893–910.

Mufaddel, A., Osman, O. T., Almugaddam, F., & Jafferany, M. (2013). A review of body dysmorphic disorder and its presentation in different clinical setting. *dymd Primary Care Companion CNS Disorders; 15*(4): PCC.12r01464. doi: 10.4088/PCC.12r01464. Retrieved August 2, 2015.

Ravindran, L. N., & Stein, M. B. (2010). The pharmacologic treatment of anxiety disorders: A review of progress. *Journal of Clinical Psychiatry*, 71(7), 839–854.

Rodriguez, C. I., Simpson, H. B., Liu, S. Levinson, A., & Blanco, C. (2013). Prevalence and correlates of difficulty discarding: Results from a national sample of the US population. *The Journal of Nervous and Mental Disease*, 201(9), 795–801.

Robinson, R. A., Taghva, A., Liu, C. Y., & Apuzzo, M. L. (2013). Surgery of the mind, mood, and conscious state: An idea in evolution. *World Neurosurgery*, 80(3), S2–S26.

Rogers, K., Banis, M., Falkenstein, M. F., Malloy, E. J., McDonough, L., Nelson, S. O., et al. (2014). Stepped care in the treatment of trichotillomania. *Journal of Consulting and Clinical Psychology*, 82(2), 361–367.

Rothbart, R., Amos, T., Siegfried, N., Ipser, J. C., Fineberg, N., Chamberlain, S. R., et al. (2013). Pharmacotherapy for trichotillomania. *The Cochrane Database of Systematic Reviews*.

Ruscio, A. M., Stein, D. J., Chiu, W. T., & Kessler, R. C. (2010). The epidemiology of obsessive-compulsive disorder in the National Comorbidity Survey Replication. *Molecular Psychiatry*, 15(1), 53–63.

Shaw, P., Sharp, W., Sudre, G., Wharton, A., Greenstein, D., Raznahan, A., et al. (2014). Subcortical and cortical morphological anomalies as an endophenotype in obsessive-compulsive disorder. *Molecular Psychiatry.*, 20(2), 224–231.doi:10.1038/mp.2014.3

Singh, S., & Jones, C. (2013). Compulsive hoarding syndrome: Engaging the patients in treatment. *Mental Health Practice*, 17(4), 16–20.

Sorrell, J. M. (2012). Understanding hoarding in older adults. *Journal of Psychosocial Nursing & Mental Health Services*, 50(3), 17–21.

Tung, E.S., Flessner, C.A., Grant, J.E., Keuthen, N.J. (2015). Predictors of life disability in trichotillomania. *Comprehensive Psychiatry*, 56, 239–244.

Whiteside, S.P., Port, J. D., & Abramowitz, J.S. (2004). A meta-analysis of functional neuroimaging in obsessive-compulsive disorder. *Psychiatry Research Neuroimaging*, 132(1), 69–79.

U.S. Department of Health and Human Services (2012). *Practice guideline for the treatment of patients with obsessive-compulsive disorder*. Guideline Summary NGC-5841. National Guideline Clearing House. Agency for Healthcare Research and Quality. Retrieved from http://www.guideline.gov/content.aspx?id = 11078 on April 30, 2015.

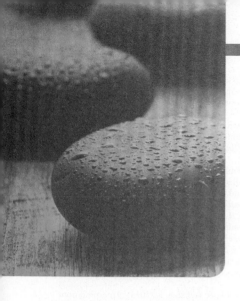

19
Depression

Nursing Care of Persons with Depressive Moods and Suicidal Behavior

Barbara Jones Warren

KEY CONCEPTS

- mood
- depression
- suicidal behavior

LEARNING OBJECTIVES

After studying this chapter, you will be able to:

1. Discuss the role of mood and depression in mental disorders.

2. Describe the prevalence and incidence of major depressive disorder.

3. Delineate the clinical symptoms and course of major depressive disorder including suicidal behavior.

4. Discuss the primary theories of major depressive disorder and their relationship to suicidal behavior.

5. Apply the nursing process with recovery-oriented interventions for persons with major depressive disorder including those with suicidal behavior.

6. Describe other depressive disorders.

KEY TERMS

- affect • anhedonia • depression • depressive disorders • disruptive mood dysregulation disorder • persistent depressive disorder • premenstrual dysphoric disorder • major depressive disorder • major depressive episodes • mood • serotonin syndrome • suicidal behavior • suicidality

Case Study: Louise

Louise is a 31-year-old woman who was admitted voluntarily to an inpatient mental health unit with depression with suicidal ideation. Louise and her husband Brian have three children ages 9, 5, and 3 years old.

INTRODUCTION

Most people have bad days or times of feeling sad and overwhelmed. When depressed feelings interfere with daily activities and relationships, however, this mood can impair judgment and contribute to negative views of the world. In some instances, depression is a symptom of a depressive disorder. This chapter discusses mood and depression, depressive disorders, and the related serious issue of suicidal behavior. **Major depressive disorder** is highlighted.

MOOD AND DEPRESSION

Normal variations in mood occur in response to life events. Normal mood variations (e.g., sadness, euphoria, and anxiety) are time-limited and are not usually associated with significant functional impairment. Normal range of mood or affect, the expression of mood, varies considerably both within and among different cultures (Pedersen, Draguus, Lonner, & Trimble, 2008; Purnell, 2012; Rosenquist, Fowler, & Christakis, 2011; Warren, 2012; 2011a; Warren & Broome, 2011).

KEYCONCEPT   **Mood** is a pervasive and sustained emotion that influences one's perception of the world and how one functions.

Affect, or outward emotional expression, is related to the concept of mood. Affect provides clues to the person's mood. For example, in depression, people often have limited facial expression. Several terms are used to describe affect, including the following:

- *Blunted:* significantly reduced intensity of emotional expression
- *Bright:* smiling, projection of a positive attitude
- *Flat:* absent or nearly absent affective expression
- *Inappropriate:* discordant affective expression accompanying the content of speech or ideation
- *Labile:* varied, rapid, and abrupt shifts in affective expression
- *Restricted or constricted:* mildly reduced in the range and intensity of emotional expression

Depression is the primary mood of depressive disorders. Depression can be overwhelming. Unless appropriately treated, depression persists over time, has a significant negative effect on quality of life, and increases the risk of suicide.

KEYCONCEPT   **Depression** is a common mental state characterized by sadness, loss of interest or pleasure, feelings of guilt or low self-worth, disturbed sleep or appetite, low energy, and poor concentration (American Psychiatric Association [APA], 2013; McEnany, 2011; World Health Organization [WHO], 2014).

OVERVIEW OF DEPRESSIVE DISORDERS

When a sad mood interferes with daily life, a **depressive disorder** may exist that will benefit from treatment. In depressive disorders, a sad, irritable, or empty mood is present with somatic and cognitive changes that interfere with functioning. Several depressive disorders vary according to duration, timing, or cause (APA, 2013). These include disruptive mood dysregulation, major depressive disorder, persistent depressive (dysthymia), premenstrual dysphoric, substance/medication-induced, other specified depressive and unspecified depressive disorders (APA, 2013). Disruptive mood dysregulation disorder is a new depressive disorder diagnostic category in the DSM-5. See Table 19.1.

The clinical symptoms and course of depressive phenomena are complex, dynamic, biopsychosocial processes involving life-span and cultural aspects. Persons with depressive disorders experience a lower quality of life and are at greater risk for development of physical health problems than those who are not depressed. Depressive disorders are so widespread that they are generally

TABLE 19.1	DEPRESSIVE DISORDERS
Disorder	**Description**
Disruptive Mood Dysregulation	Persistent irritability and frequent episodes of extreme verbal and behavior outburst (children)
Major Depressive disorder	Episodes of depressed mood that impact functioning
Persistent Depressive (Dysthymia) Disorder	Mood disturbance last more than 2 years with a depressed mood daily
Premenstrual Dysphoric Disorders	Depressed mood following ovulation until a few days after menses
Substance/Medication-induced Disorder or medical condition	Depressed mood associated with substance use, medication, or a medical disorder

(APA, 2013)

diagnosed and treated in the primary care setting. Every nurse will have an opportunity to impact this pandemic health concern (WHO, 2014).

Depressive disorders are characterized by severe and debilitating depressive episodes and are associated with high levels of impairment in occupational, social, and physical functioning. They cause as much disability and distress to patients as chronic medical disorders. Frequently, they are undetected and untreated. Because suicide is a significant risk, these disorders are associated with premature death (Tsai, Lin, Chang W.L., Chang H.C., & Chou, 2010).

Depressive Disorders Across the Life-Span

Children and Adolescents

Children with depressive disorders have symptoms similar to those seen in adults with a few exceptions. They are more likely to have anxiety symptoms, such as fear of separation, and somatic symptoms, such as stomach aches and headaches. They may have less interaction with their peers and avoid play and recreational activities that they previously enjoyed. Mood may be irritable, rather than sad, especially in adolescents. See Chapter 28 for discussion of mental health disorders in children.

The risk of suicide, which peaks during the midadolescent years, is very real in children and adolescents. Mortality from suicide, which increases steadily through the teens, is the third leading cause of death for that age group. Findings from research indicate that deaths caused by illegal drug use and automobile crashes may be the outcome of adolescent depression and suicidal ideation (Brière, Rohde, Seeley, Klein, & Lewinsohn, 2015; Dulcan & Lake, 2012; Liehr & Diaz, 2010). See

Chapter 15 for further discussion of suicide in children and adolescents.

Older Adults

Most older patients with symptoms of depression do not meet the full criteria for major depression. However, it is estimated that 8% to 20% of older adults in the community and as many as 37% in primary care settings experience depressive symptoms (Blazer & Steffens, 2015). Treatment is successful in 60% to 80%, but response to treatment is slower than in younger adults. Depression in older adults is often associated with chronic illnesses, such as heart disease, stroke, and cancer; symptoms may have a more somatic focus. Depressive symptomatology in this group may be confused with symptoms of dementia or cerebrovascular accidents. Hence, differential diagnosis may be required to ascertain the root and cause of symptoms. See Chapter 29 for further discussion of mental health disorders in older adults.

Suicide is a very serious risk for older adults, especially men. Suicide rates peak during middle age, but a second peak occurs in those age 75 years and older. See Chapter 15.

Death is more likely during or after a suicide attempt in older adults. Suicide rates for men are highest among those aged 75 and older (36 per 100,000) (Centers for Disease Control and Prevention [CDC], 2015). See Box 19.1.

MAJOR DEPRESSIVE DISORDER

Clinical Course

Major depressive disorder is commonly a progressively recurrent illness. With time, episodes tend to occur more frequently, become more severe, and are of a longer duration. Onset of depression may occur at any age. However, the initial onset may occur in puberty; the highest onset occurs within persons in their 20s (APA, 2013).

Rcurrences of depression are related to age of onset, increased intensity and severity of symptoms, and presence of psychosis, anxiety, and/or personality features. The risk for relapse is higher in persons who have experienced initial symptoms at a younger age and incur other mental disorders (Brière, et al., 2015).

Diagnostic Criteria

The primary diagnostic criterion for major depressive disorder is one or more **major depressive episodes,** which is either a depressed mood or a loss of interest or pleasure in nearly all activities for at least 2 weeks. Four of seven additional symptoms must be present: disruption in sleep, appetite (or weight), concentration, or energy; psychomotor agitation or retardation; excessive guilt or feelings of worthlessness; and suicidal ideation (Key Diagnostic Characteristics 19.1).

The incidence of misdiagnosis is often greater for persons who are treated by someone from culturally and ethnically different populations because their explanation of their symptomatology may be expressed using different terminology. (Munoz, Primm, Ananth, & Ruiz, 2007; Tusaie, 2013)

Epidemiology and Risk Factors

The prevalence of major depressive disorder within the United States population is approximately 7% within a 12-month time period. Individuals between the ages of 18 and 29 years have a three times higher prevalence rate of major depressive disorder than those persons aged 60 and older (APA, 2013). The prevalence rates for females and males differ with females experiencing "a 1.5- to 3-fold higher rate than males beginning in early adolescence" (APA, 2013, p. 165). The recurrence of major depressive disorder is contingent on the severity and persistence of symptoms, younger age of initial occurrence, and presence of comorbid psychiatric illness (APA, 2013; Josey & Neidert, 2013; Tarraza, 2013). An estimated 17 million Americans experience a depressive disorder on an annual basis.

Data from the WHO indicate that depression is the leading cause of years lost because of disability. More than 50% of persons who recover from an initial episode of depression experience another episode within 5 to 10 years (WHO, 2014).

Risk factors for the development of depression include the following:

• Prior episode of depression
• Family history of depressive disorder
• Lack of social support
• Lack of coping abilities
• Presence of life and environmental stressors
• Current substance use or abuse
• Medical and/or mental illness comorbidity

KEY DIAGNOSTIC CHARACTERSTICS 19.1 • MAJOR DEPRESSIVE DISORDER 296.XX

296.2X MAJOR DEPRESSIVE DISORDER, SINGLE EPISODE
296.3X MAJOR DEPRESSIVE DISORDER, RECURRENT

Diagnostic Criteria

A. Five (or more) of the following symptoms have been present during the same 2-week period and represent a change from previous functioning; at least one of the symptoms is either (1) depressed mood or (2) loss of interest or pleasure.

Note: Do not include symptoms that are clearly attributable to another medical condition.

1. Depressed mood most of the day, nearly every day, as indicated by either subjective report (e.g., feels sad, empty, hopeless) or observation made by others (e.g., appears tearful). (**Note:** In children and adolescents, can be irritable mood.)

2. Markedly diminished interest or pleasure in all, or almost all, activities most of the day, nearly every day (as indicated by either subjective account or observation).

3. Significant weight loss when not dieting or weight gain (e.g., a change of more than 5% of body weight in a month), or decrease or increase in appetite nearly every day. (**Note:** In children, consider failure to make expected weight gain.)

4. Insomnia or hypersomnia nearly every day.

5. Psychomotor agitation or retardation nearly every day (observable by others, not merely subjective feelings of restlessness or being slowed down).

6. Fatigue or loss of energy nearly every day.

7. Feelings of worthlessness or excessive or inappropriate guilt (which may be delusional) nearly every day (not merely self-reproach or guilt about being sick).

8. Diminished ability to think or concentrate, or indecisiveness, nearly every day (either by subjective account or as observed by others).

9. Recurrent thoughts of death (not just fear of dying), recurrent suicidal ideation without a specific plan, or a suicide attempt or a specific plan for committing suicide.

The symptoms cause clinically significant distress or impairment in social, occupational, or other important areas of functioning.

The episode is not attributable to the physiological effects of a substance or to another medical condition.

B. The symptoms cause clinically significant distress or impairment in social, occupational, or other important areas of functioning.

C. The episode is not attributable to the physiological effects of a substance or to another medical condition.

Note: Criteria A–C represent a major depressive episode.

Note: Responses to a significant loss (e.g., bereavement, financial ruin, losses from a natural disaster, a serious medical illness or disability) may include the feelings of intense sadness, rumination about the loss, insomnia, poor appetite, and weight loss noted in Criterion A, which may resemble a depressive episode. Although such symptoms may be understandable or considered appropriate to the loss, the presence of a major depressive episode in addition to the normal response to a significant loss should also be carefully considered. This decision inevitably requires the exercise of clinical judgment based on the individual's history and the cultural norms for the expression of distress in the context of loss.

The occurrence of the major depressive episode is not better explained by schizoaffective disorder, schizophrenia, schizophreniform disorder, delusional disorder, or other specified and unspecified schizophrenia spectrum and other psychotic disorders.

There has never been a manic episode or a hypomanic episode.

Note: This exclusion does not apply if all of the manic-like or hypomanic-like episodes are substance-induced or are attributable to the physiological effects of another medical condition.

Consider this:

Louise's sister died as a result of drowning 2 months ago. She has been telling her husband that she just wants to go to sleep and not wake up.

Age of Onset and Gender

The mean age of onset for major depressive disorder is about 30 years; 50% of all patients have an onset between the ages of 20 and 50 years. During a 20-year period, the mean number of episodes is five or six. Symptoms usually develop during a period of days to months. About 50% of patients have significant depressive symptoms before the first identified episode. An untreated episode typically lasts 6 to 13 months, regardless of the age of onset (Kessler et al., 2005).

It appears that the chances of experiencing major depressive disorder are increasing in progressively younger age groups. Major depressive disorder is twice as common in adolescent and adult women as in adolescent and adult men. (Rawana & Morgan, 2014).

Ethnicity and Culture

Prevalence rates of depressive disorders are unrelated to race. Culture can influence the experience and communication of symptoms of depression. Persons from culturally and ethnically diverse populations may formulate and describe their depressive symptomatology differently than in the clinical language used for diagnosis. For example, expressions such as "heartbrokenness" (Native American and Middle Eastern), "brain fog" (persons from the West Indies), "zar," and "running amok" may be used in place of such terms as "depressed," "sad," "hopeless," and "discouraged" (Beeber, Lewis, Cooper, Maxwell, & Sandelowski, 2010; Warren, 2013a; 2013b; 2013c; Warren & Lutz, 2007).

In some cultures, somatic symptoms, rather than sadness or guilt, may predominate. Individuals from various Asian cultural groups may have complaints of weakness, tiredness, or imbalance. "Problems of the heart" (in Middle Eastern cultures) or of being "heartbroken" (among Native Americans of the Hopi tribe) may be the way that persons from these cultural groups express their depressive experiences. Culturally distinctive experiences need to be assessed to ascertain any presence of depressive disorder from a "normal" cultural emotional response (Munoz, et al., 2007; Pedersen, et al., 2008).

Comorbidity

Major depressive disorders often co-occur with other psychiatric disorders including those that are substance related. Depression often is associated with a variety of medical conditions, particularly endocrine disorders, cardiovascular disease, neurologic disorders, autoimmune conditions, viral or other infectious diseases, certain cancers, and nutritional deficiencies, or as a direct physiologic effect of a substance (e.g., a drug of abuse, a medication, other somatic treatment for depression, or toxin exposure) (Gonzales, Vega, Williams, Tarraf, West, & Neighbors, 2010).

Etiology

Biologic Theories

Genetic

Family, twin, and adoption studies demonstrate that genetic influences undoubtedly play a substantial role in the etiology of mood disorders. Major depressive disorder is more common among first-degree biologic relatives of people with this disorder than among the general population (McInnis, Riba, Greden, 2014). Currently, a major research effort is focusing on developing a more accurate paradigm regarding the contribution of genetic factors to the development of mood disorders (Shi, Potash, Knowles, Weissman, Coryell, Lawson, et al., 2011).

Neurobiologic Hypotheses

Neurobiologic theories of the etiology of depression emerged in the 1950s. These theories posit that major depression is caused by a deficiency or dysregulation in central nervous system (CNS) concentrations of the neurotransmitters norepinephrine, dopamine, and serotonin or in their receptor functions. These hypotheses arose in part from observations that some pharmacologic agents elevated mood; subsequent studies identified their mechanisms of action. All antidepressants currently available have their therapeutic effects on these neurotransmitters or receptors. Current research focuses on the synthesis, storage, release, and uptake of these neurotransmitters, as well as on postsynaptic events (e.g., second-messenger systems) (Stahl, 2013a; 2013b).

Neuroendocrine and Neuropeptide Hypotheses

Major depressive disorder is associated with multiple endocrine alterations, specifically of the hypothalamic–pituitary–adrenal axis, the hypothalamic–pituitary–thyroid axis, the hypothalamic–growth hormone axis, and the hypothalamic–pituitary–gonadal axis. In addition, mounting evidence indicates that components of neuroendocrine axes (e.g., neuromodulatory peptides such as corticotropin-releasing factor) may themselves contribute to depressive symptoms. Evidence also suggests that the secretion of these hypothalamic and growth hormones is controlled by many of the neurotransmitters implicated in the pathophysiology of depression (Stahl, 2013a).

Psychoneuroimmunology

Psychoneuroimmunology is a recent area of research into a diverse group of proteins known as *chemical messengers* between immune cells. These messengers, called cytokines, signal the brain and serve as mediators between immune and nerve cells. The brain is capable of influencing immune processes, and conversely, immunologic response can result in changes in brain activity (Shi, Potash, Knowles, Weissman, Coryell, Lawson, et al., 2011). The specific role of these mechanisms in psychiatric disease pathogenesis remains unknown.

Psychological Theories

Psychological theories that serve as a basis for nursing practice for persons with a mental health disorder are explained in Chapter 5. Depression is one of the disorders that is treated from a psychological perspective. The following discussion identifies theoretical models often used in nursing care.

Psychodynamic Factors

Most psychodynamic theorists acknowledge some debt to Freud's original conceptualization of the psychodynamics of depression, which ascribes the cause to an early lack of love, care, warmth, and protection and resultant anger, guilt, helplessness, and fear regarding the loss of love. The ensuing conflict between wanting to be loved and fear of rejection engenders pathologic self-punishment (also conceptualized as aggression turned inward), self-rejection, low self-esteem, and depressive symptoms (see Chapter 5).

Behavioral Factors

The behavioral psychologists hold that depression primarily result from a severe reduction in rewarding activities or an increase in unpleasant events in one's life. The subsequent depression then leads to further restriction of activity, thereby decreasing the likelihood of experiencing pleasurable activities, which, in turn, intensifies the mood disturbance. Affected individuals often self-criticize and believe that they do not have the coping skills to deal with life's stresses. If family members believe that the person is "sick" and so lacks the necessary coping skills, they inadvertently reinforce the hopeless self-view of the depressed person.

Cognitive Factors

The cognitive approach maintains that irrational beliefs and negative distortions of thought about the self, the environment, and the future engender and perpetuate depressive effects (see Chapter 5). These depressive cognitions can be learned socially from family members or lack of experience in developing coping skills. These individuals think differently than nondepressed individuals and view their environment and themselves in negative ways. They blame themselves for any misfortunes that occur and see situations as being much worse than they are.

Developmental Factors

Developmental theorists posit that depression may result from the loss of a parent through death or separation or lack of emotionally adequate parenting. These factors may delay or prohibit the realization of appropriate developmental milestones.

Social Theories
Family Factors

Family theorists ascribe maladaptive patterns in family interactions as contributing to the onset of depression, particularly in the onset and occurrence of depression in younger individuals. A family becomes dysfunctional when interactions, decisions, or behaviors interfere with the positive development of the family and its individual members. Most families have periods of dysfunction, such as during a crisis or stressful situation when coping skills are not available. Unhealthy interactions within a family system can have a negative impact on one or more family members who do not have the coping skills to deal with the situation.

Environmental Factors

Depression has long been understood as a multifactorial disorder that occurs when environmental factors (e.g., death of family member) interact with the biologic and psychological makeup of the individual. Major depression may follow adverse or traumatic life events, especially those that involve the loss of an important human relationship or role in life. Social isolation, deprivation, and financial deprivation are risk factors (APA, 2013). Recent evidence suggests that depression in one person is associated with similar symptoms in friends, coworkers, siblings, spouses, and neighbors. Female friends seem to be especially influential in the spread of depression from one friend to another (Rosenquist, et al., 2011).

Family Response to Disorder

Depression in one family member affects the whole family. Spouses, children, parents, siblings, and friends experience frustration, guilt, and anger when a family member is immobilized and cannot function. It is often hard for others to understand the depth of the mood and how disabling it can be. Financial hardship can occur when the affected family member cannot work and instead spends days in bed. The lack of understanding and difficulty of living with a depressed person can lead to abuse. Women between the ages of 18 and 45 years constitute the majority of those experiencing depression. This incidence may affect women's ability to not only have productive lives and take care of themselves but to also take care of their children or other family members for whom they may have responsibility. Moreover, research indicates that the incidence of depression may be higher in children whose mothers experience depression (Lutz & Warren, 2007; Warren & Lutz, 2007).

> ### Remember Louise?
> According to her husband, Louise has neglected her self-care and that of her children since her sister's death. Brian is very understanding and supportive of Louise's need to grieve, but he is concerned that this is more than grief. Brian says that he is afraid to leave her alone and the children are suffering.

Teamwork and Collaboration: Working Toward Recovery

Although depressive disorders are the most commonly occurring mental disorders, they are usually treated within the primary care setting, rather than psychiatric setting. Nursing practice requires a coordinated ongoing interaction among patients, families, and health care providers to deliver comprehensive services. This includes using the complementary skills of both psychiatric and medical care colleagues for forming overall goals, plans, and decisions and for providing continuity of care as needed. Collaborative care between the primary care provider and mental health specialist is also key to achieving remission of symptoms and physical well-being, restoring baseline occupational and psychosocial functioning, and reducing the likelihood of relapse or recurrence.

Individuals with depression enter mental health settings when their symptoms become so severe that hospitalization is needed, usually after suicide attempts, or if they self-refer because of incapacitation. Antidepressants are indicated for depression and are discussed later in this chapter. Interdisciplinary treatment of these disorders, which is often lifelong, needs to include a wide array of health professionals in all areas. The specific goals of treatment are:

- Reduce or control symptoms and, if possible, eliminate signs and symptoms of the depressive syndrome.
- Improve occupational and psychosocial function as much as possible.
- Reduce the likelihood of relapse and recurrence through recovery-oriented strategies.

Cognitive and Interpersonal Therapies

Recent studies suggest that short-term cognitive and interpersonal therapies may be as effective as pharmacotherapy in milder depressions. In many instances, cognitive behavioral therapy (CBT) is an effective strategy for preventing relapse in patients who have had only a partial response to pharmacotherapy alone (APA, 2013). CBT is implemented in individual or group therapy by a trained clinician.

Interpersonal therapy seeks to recognize, explore, and resolve the interpersonal losses, role confusion and transitions, social isolation, and deficits in social skills that may precipitate depressive states. It maintains that losses must be mourned and related affects appreciated, role confusion and transitions must be recognized and resolved, and social skills deficits must be overcome to acquire social supports. Some evidence in controlled studies suggests that interpersonal therapy is more effective in reducing depressive symptoms with certain populations, such as depressed patients with human immunodeficiency virus infection, and less successful with patients who have concurrent personality disorders (Abbass, et al, 2014) (see Chapter 22).

Combination Therapies

For patients with severe or recurrent major depressive disorder, the combination of psychotherapy (including interpersonal, cognitive behavioral, behavior, brief dynamic, or dialectical behavioral therapies) and pharmacotherapy has been found to be superior to treatment using a single modality. Clinical practice guidelines suggest that the combination of medication and psychotherapy is particularly useful in more complex situations (e.g., depression in the context of concurrent, chronic general-medical or other psychiatric disorders, or in patients who fail to experience complete response to either treatment alone). Psychotherapy in combination with medication is also used to address collateral issues, such as medication adherence or secondary psychosocial problems (Clarke, Mayo-Wilson, Kenny, & Pilling, 2015). If medications and psychotherapy are not effective, other options are available: electroconvulsive therapy (ECT), light therapy, and repetitive transcranial magnetic stimulation discussed later in the chapter.

Alternative Therapies

Alternative or complementary therapies are often used in the treatment of depression. Acupuncture, yoga or tai chi, meditation, guided imagery and massage therapy are a few therapies that may be helpful palliate depression. Music or art therapy is also used often in conjunction with medication or psychotherapy.

Safety Issues

The overriding concern for people with mood disorders is safety because these individuals may experience self-destructive thoughts and suicidal ideation. Hence, the assessment of possible suicide risk should be routinely conducted in any depressed person (see Chapter 15).

Evidence-Based Nursing Care of Persons with Depressive Disorder

An awareness of the risk factors for depression, a comprehensive and culturally competent mental health nursing assessment, history of illness, and past treatment are key to formulating a treatment or recovery plan and to evaluating outcomes. Interviewing a family member or close friend about the patient's day-to-day functioning and specific symptoms may help determine the course of the illness, current symptoms, and level of functioning. The family's level of support and understanding of the disorder also need to be assessed. Nursing Care Plan 19.1 is available at http://thepoint.lww.com/BoydEssentials.

Mental Health Nursing Assessment

The mental health nursing assessment focuses on the physical consequences of the depression as well as the psychosocial aspects. The symptoms of depression are similar to those of some medical problems or medication side effects. Often, the mental health nurse is the only clinician who provides holistic care to a person with depression who is often treated by other disciplines.

Physical Health Assessment

The nursing assessment should include a physical systems review and thorough history of medical problems, with special attention to CNS function, endocrine function, anemia, chronic pain, autoimmune illness, diabetes mellitus, or menopause. Additional medical history includes surgeries; medical hospitalizations; head injuries; episodes of loss of consciousness; and pregnancies, childbirths, miscarriages, and abortions. A complete list of prescribed and over-the-counter (OTC) medications and herbal supplements should be compiled, including the reason a medication was prescribed or its use discontinued. A physical examination is recommended with baseline vital signs and baseline laboratory tests, including a comprehensive blood chemistry panel, complete blood counts, liver function tests, thyroid function tests, urinalysis, and electrocardiograms (see Chapter 9).

The following symptoms are characteristic of depression:

- *Appetite and weight changes:* In major depression, changes from baseline include a decrease or increase in appetite with or without significant weight loss or gain (i.e., a change of more than 5% of body weight in 1 month). Weight loss occurs when the person not dieting. Older adults with moderate-to-severe depression need to be assessed for dehydration as well as weight changes.
- *Sleep disturbance:* The most common sleep disturbance associated with major depression is insomnia, which is broken into three categories: initial insomnia (difficulty falling asleep), middle insomnia (waking up during the night and having difficulty returning to sleep), and terminal insomnia (waking too early and being unable to return to sleep). Less frequently, the sleep disturbance is hypersomnia (i.e., prolonged sleep episodes at night or increased daytime sleep). The individual with either insomnia or hypersomnia complains of not feeling rested on awakening.
- *Tiredness, decreased energy, and fatigue:* Fatigue associated with depression is a subjective experience of feeling tired regardless of how much sleep or physical activity a person has had. Even the smallest tasks require substantial effort.

NCLEXNOTE In determining severity of depressive symptoms, nursing assessment should explore physical changes in appetite and sleep patterns and decreased energy. Remember these three major assessment categories. A question in the test may state several patient symptoms and expect the student to recognize that the patient being described is depressed.

Louise's Physical Changes
Louise has not been eating because she is not hungry and has lost 15 pounds over the last 6 weeks. She is also not sleeping well. She wakes up during the middle of the night and cannot go back to sleep.

Medication Assessment

In addition to a physical assessment, an assessment of current medications should be completed. The frequency and dosage of prescribed medications, OTC medications, and use of herbal or culturally related medication treatments should be explored. In depression, the nurse must always assess the possible lethality of the medication the patient is taking. For example, if a patient has sleeping medications at home, the individual should be further queried about the number of pills in the bottle. Patients also need to be assessed for their use of alcohol, marijuana, and other mood-altering medications, as well as herbal substances because of the potential for drug–drug interactions. For example, patients taking antidepressants that affect serotonin regulation could also be taking St. John's wort (*Hypericum perforatum*) to fight depression. The combined drug and herb could interact to cause serotonin syndrome (altered mental status, autonomic dysfunction, and neuromuscular abnormalities). SAMe (S-adenosy-L-methionine) is another herbal preparation that patients may be taking. Patients need to be advised of possible adverse side effects of SAMe taken with any prescribed antidepressant because the exact action of this herb remains unclear.

Psychosocial Assessment

The psychosocial assessment for persons who have major depressive disorder includes the mental status (mood and affect, thought processes and content, cognition, memory, and attention), coping skills, developmental history, family psychiatric history, patterns of relationships, quality of support system, education, work history, and impact of physical or sexual abuse on interpersonal function. See Chapter 9. The nurse should be identifying the individual's strengths, as well as problem areas, by asking the patient to describe their thoughts, feelings and behaviors before the current depressive episode. Including a family member or close friend in the assessment process can be helpful. The following discussion identifies key assessment areas for a depressed person.

Mood and Affect

The person with major depressive disorder has a sustained period of feeling depressed, sad, or hopeless and may experience **anhedonia** (loss of interest or pleasure). The patient may report "not caring any more" or not

FAME & FORTUNE

Wilbur Wright (1867–1912)
Genius Inventor

PUBLIC PERSONA

Of the Wright brothers, Wilbur and Orville, Wilbur Wright is viewed as the real genius and the one who developed intellectual control over the problem of flight. Although his brother, Orville, had inventive skills and was an ideal counterpart, Wilbur was the one who envisioned things that others could not see. Together, the brothers had the skill to build what they imagined. They once built a wagon that reduced the wheel friction so it could haul 10 times as much as before. In his early teens, Wilbur invented a machine to fold newspapers, and Orville built a small printing press for a newspaper he started.

PERSONAL REALITIES

Wilbur Wright had depression that started after a childhood injury he sustained when he was hit in the face with a bat during a game. Complications followed from the medication he received, which affected his heart. He then developed an intestinal disorder, which caused him to abandon his college plans and remain secluded for 4 years. He thought he could never realize his goal of becoming a clergyman. During his period of poor health and seclusion, he cared for his mother, who was ill with tuberculosis, which eventually caused her death. After his mother died, Wilbur emerged from his depression, and he and his brother went into the printing business together. Later, they focused on airplanes and flying.

Source: Crouch, T. D. (1990). *The bishop's boys: A life of Wilbur and Orville Wright.* New York: W.W. Norton & Company.

feeling any enjoyment in activities that were previously considered pleasurable. In some individuals, this may include a decrease in or loss of libido (i.e., sexual interest or desire) and sexual function. In others, irritability and anger are signs of depression, especially in those who deny being depressed. Individuals often describe themselves as depressed, sad, hopeless, discouraged, or "down in the dumps." If individuals complain of feeling "blah," having no feelings, constantly tired, or feeling anxious, a depressed mood can sometimes be inferred from their facial expression and demeanor (APA, 2013).

Numerous assessment scales are available for assessing depression. Easily administered self-report questionnaires can be valuable detection tools. These questionnaires cannot be the sole basis for making a diagnosis of major depressive episode, but they are sensitive to depressive symptoms. The following are five commonly used self-report scales:

* General Health Questionnaire (GHQ)
* Center for Epidemiological Studies Depression Scale (CES-D)
* Beck Depression Inventory (BDI)
* Zung Self-Rating Depression Scale (SDS)
* PRIME-MD

Clinician-completed rating scales may be more sensitive to improvement in the course of treatment, can assess symptoms in relationship to the depressive diagnostic criteria, and may have a slightly greater specificity than do self-report questionnaires in detecting depression. These include the following:

* Hamilton Rating Scale for Depression (HAM-D)
* Montgomery-Asberg Depression Rating Scale (MADRS)
* National Institute of Mental Health Diagnostic Interview Schedule (DIS)

Thought Content

Depressed individuals often have an unrealistic negative evaluation of their worth or have guilty preoccupations or ruminations about minor past failings. Such individuals often misinterpret neutral or trivial day-to-day events as evidence of personal defects. They may also have an exaggerated sense of responsibility for untoward events. As a result, they feel hopeless, helpless, worthless, and powerless. The possibility of disorganized thought processes (e.g., tangential or circumstantial thinking) and perceptual disturbances (e.g., hallucinations, delusions) should also be included in the assessment.

Cognition and Memory

Many individuals with depression report an impaired ability to think, concentrate, or make decisions. They may appear easily distracted or complain of memory difficulties. In older adults with major depression, memory difficulties may be the chief complaint and may be mistaken for early signs of dementia (pseudodementia) (APA, 2013). When the depression is fully treated, the memory problem often improves or fully resolves.

Behavior

Changes in patterns of relating (especially social withdrawal) and changes in level of occupational functioning are commonly reported and may represent a significant deterioration from baseline behavior. Increased use of "sick days" may occur. For people who are depressed, special attention should be given to the individual's spiritual dimension and religious background.

Suicidal Behavior

Patients with major depressive disorder are at increased risk for suicide. The development of suicide behavior is a complex phenomenon because symptoms are often hidden or veiled by somatic symptoms.

KEYCONCEPT **Suicidal behavior** is the occurrence of persistent thought patterns and actions that indicate a person is thinking about, planning, or enacting suicide.

Suicidal ideation includes thoughts that range from a belief that others would be better off if the person were dead or thoughts of death (passive suicidal ideation) to actual specific plans for committing suicide (active suicidal ideation). See Chapter 15. The frequency, intensity, and lethality of these thoughts can vary and can help to determine the seriousness of intent. The more specific the plan and the more accessible the means, the more serious becomes the intent. The risk for suicide needs to be initially assessed in patients who incur depressive disorders as well as reassessed throughout the course of treatment.

Suicidal ideation is not a normal reaction to stress. Persons who express any suicidal ideation need immediate mental health assessment regarding the depth of their thoughts and intentions. More than 90% of persons who complete suicide have one or more of the following risk factors: lack of availability and inadequacy of social supports; family violence, including physical or sexual abuse; past history of suicidal ideation or behavior; presence of psychosis or substance use or abuse; and decreased ability to control suicidal impulses (NIMH, 2015).

Ethnic and cultural differences exist regarding suicidal behavior. Men often use firearms. Women often use pills or other poisonous substances to commit suicide. Children often use suffocation. Data on suicide completion rates are reported highest in persons from Native Americans, Alaskan Natives, and those of non-Hispanic white descent. These rates are lowest for persons from Hispanic, non-Hispanic black, and Asian and Pacific Islander descent. Ongoing research regarding suicide in veterans indicates that they have a higher risk than persons in the general population (Dobscha, et al., 2014). Psychological stress and previously diagnosed psychiatric disorders are chief risk factors for veterans. Counseling and supportive services need to be provided to family and friends of persons who attempt or commit suicide because family and friends may experience feelings of grief, guilt, anger, and confusion (Cerel, Jordan, & Duberstien, 2008).

NCLEXNOTE The possibility of suicide should always be a priority with patients who are depressed. Assessment and documentation of suicide risk should always be included in patient care.

Strength Assessment

Throughout the assessment, the nurse should be observing for strengths such as positive physical health status, coping skills, and social support. The following questions may be used to determine a person's strength

• When you have been depressed before, how did you cope with the feelings?

• What do you do to relax?
• Do you reach out to anyone when you are feeling down?
• When you are not depressed, what makes you feel good?

Nursing Diagnoses

Several nursing diagnoses are possible including Insomnia, Imbalanced Nutrition, Fatigue, Self-Care Deficit, Nausea, Disturbed Thought Processes, Sexual Dysfunction, Hopelessness, Low Self-Esteem, Ineffective Individual Coping, Decisional Conflict, Spiritual Distress, Dysfunctional Grieving. Ineffective Family Coping, Ineffective Role Performance, Interrupted Family Processes, and Caregiver Role Strain are also possibilities. If patient data lead to the diagnosis of Risk for Suicide, the patient should be further assessed for plan, intent, and accessibility of means. The nursing assessment should also generate strength-based nursing diagnoses such as Readiness for Hope, Readiness for Enhanced Coping, or Readiness for Enhanced Sleep.

Therapeutic Relationship

One of the most effective tools for caring for any person with a mental disorder is the therapeutic relationship. For a person who is depressed, there are a number of effective approaches:

• Establishment and maintenance of a supportive relationship based on the incorporation of culturally competent interventions and strategies
• Availability in times of crisis
• Vigilance regarding danger to self and others
• Education about the illness and treatment goals
• Encouragement and feedback concerning progress
• Guidance regarding the patient's interactions with the personal and work environment
• Realistic goal setting and monitoring
• Support of individual strengths in treatment choices.

Interacting with depressed individuals is challenging because they tend to be withdrawn and have difficulty expressing feelings and engaging in interpersonal interactions. The therapeutic relationship can be strengthened through the use of cognitive interventions as well as the nurse's ability to win the patient's trust through the use of culturally competent strategies in the context of empathy (Box 19.2).

Cheerleading, or being overly cheerful to a person who is depressed, blocks communication and can be quite irritating to depressed patients. Nurses should avoid approaching patients with depression with an overly cheerful attitude. Instead, a calm, supportive empathic approach helps keep communication open.

> **BOX 19.2 • THERAPEUTIC DIALOGUE • Approaching the Depressed Patient**

Louise is severely depressed and has not left her hospital room since admission to the mental health unit. She has missed breakfast and is not interested in taking a shower or getting dressed.

INEFFECTIVE APPROACH

Nurse: Hello, Louise. My name is Sally. How are you feeling today?

Louise: I didn't sleep last night and need to rest. Please go away.

Nurse: Sorry, but it is time to get up. You have already missed breakfast. You have to take a quick shower now to get to group on time.

Louise: I have no interest in taking a shower or going to group.

Nurse: Why are you here if you don't want to be treated?

Louise: Go away. I don't want you in this room.

EFFECTIVE APPROACH

Nurse: Good morning. My name is Sally. I am your nurse today.

Louise: I didn't sleep last night and need to rest. Please go away.

Nurse: You didn't sleep well last night?

Louise: No, I can't remember when I was able to sleep through the night.

Nurse: Oh, I see. Is that why you missed breakfast?

Louise: I'm just not hungry. I have no energy.

Nurse: Lack of appetite and lack of energy are very common when people are depressed.

Louise: Really?

Nurse: Yes, so let's take one step at time. I'd like to help you get up.

Louise: Ok, I might be able to sit up.

Nurse: (Helps her sit up.) Now, let's walk to the bathroom.

Louise: (Walks to the bathroom.) Now what?

Nurse: Let's work on your AM care.

CRITICAL THINKING CHALLENGE

- What ineffective techniques did the nurse use in the first scenario and how did they impair communication?

- What effective techniques did the nurse use in the second scenario and how did they facilitate communication?

NCLEXNOTE Establishing the patient–nurse relationship with a person who is depressed requires an empathic quiet approach that is grounded in the nurse's understanding of the cultural needs of the patient.

Mental Health Nursing Interventions

Nursing intervention selection is a collaborative process between the patient and nurse. As goals and interventions are agreed by both the nurse and the patient, the person's strengths (e.g., motivation to get better, resources, family support) should be emphasized in making treatment choices.

Physical Care

Because weeks or months of disturbed sleep patterns and nutritional imbalance only worsen depression, one of the first nursing interventions is helping the person re-establish normal sleep patterns and healthy nutrition. Supporting self-care management by encouraging patients to practice positive sleep hygiene and eat well-balanced meals regularly helps the patient move toward remission or recovery.

Deep-breathing exercises three times a day have been shown to reduce self-reported depressive symptoms within 4 weeks in patients with coronary heart disease (Box 19.3). Activity and exercise are also important for improving depressed mood state. Most people find that regular exercise is hard to maintain. People who are depressed may find it impossible. When teaching about exercise, it is important to start with the current level of patient activity and increase it slowly. For example, if the patient is spending most of the time in bed, encouraging the patient to get dressed every day and walk for 5 or 10 minutes may be all that patient can tolerate. Gradually, patients should be encouraged to have a regular exercise program and to slowly increase their food intake.

BOX 19.3

Research for Best Practice: Home-based Deep Breathing for Depression in Patients with Coronary Heart Disease

Chung, L. J., Tsai, P. S., Liu, B. Y., Kuei-Ru, C., Wei-Hsiang, L., Yuh-Kae, S., & Mei-Yeh, W. (2010). Home-based deep breathing for depression in patients with coronary heart disease: a randomized controlled trial. International Journal of Nursing Studies, 47(11), 1346–1353.

THE QUESTION: How effective is a home-based deep-breathing training program compared with weekly telephone support in patients with coronary heart disease (CHD)?

METHODS: In a controlled trial, 62 patients with CHD with Beck Depression Inventory-II (BDI-II) scores above 10 were randomized to receive either home-based deep breathing training (*n* = 28) or weekly telephone support (*n* = 34). The deep breathing exercise consisted of diaphragmatic breathing with four to six slow and deep breaths per minute, three times per day. Participants and raters were blinded to the study hypothesis. Depressive symptoms were assessed with the BDI-II and the Patient Health Questionnaire-9 (PHQ-9) at baseline and 2 weeks after the test.

FINDINGS: The group using the deep breathing exercise has significantly lower depression scores than the control group.

IMPLICATIONS FOR NURSING: Nurses should consider teaching patients who are depressed deep breathing exercises to their improve mood and reduce their depressive symptoms.

Medications

Antidepressant medications have proved effective in all forms of major depression. To date, controlled trials have shown no single antidepressant drug to have greater efficacy in the treatment of major depressive disorder. See Chapter 10 for a list of antidepressant medications, usual dosage range, half-life, and therapeutic blood levels.

An antidepressant is selected based primarily on an individual patient's target symptoms; genetic factors; responses related to cultural, racial, and ethnic influences; and the medication's side effect profile (Posmontier, 2013; Warren, 2011a). Other factors that may influence choice include prior medication response, drug interactions and contraindications, concurrent medical and psychiatric disorders, patient age, and cost of medication. Failure to consider these influences may increase the risk of aversive and injurious side effects (Dollard, 2013).

The newer antidepressants, selective serotonin reuptake inhibitors (SSRIs), serotonin-norepinephrine reuptake inhibitors (SNRIs), and the norepinephrine dopamine reuptake inhibitor (NDRI) are used most often because these drugs selectively target the neurotransmitters and receptors thought to be associated with depression and minimize side effects. See Box 19.4 Individualizing dosages is usually done by fine-tuning medication dosage based on patient feedback. The tricyclic antidepressants (TCAs) and monoamine oxidase inhibitors (MAOIs) are being used less often than the

BOX 19.4

Drug Profile: Escitalopram Oxalate (Lexapro)

DRUG CLASS: Antidepressant

RECEPTOR AFFINITY: A highly selective serotonin reuptake inhibitor with low affinity for 5HT 1–7 or α- and β-adrenergic, dopamine D1–5, histamine H1–3, muscarinic M1–5, and benzodiazepine receptors or for Na^+, K^+, Cl^-, and Ca^{++} ion channels that have been associated with various anticholinergic, sedative, and cardiovascular side effects

INDICATIONS: Treatment of major depressive disorder, generalized anxiety disorder

ROUTES AND DOSAGES: Available as 5-, 10-, and 20-mg oral tablets

Adults: Initially 10 mg once a day. May increase to 20 mg after a minimum of 1 week. Trials have not shown greater benefit at the 20-mg dose

Geriatric: The 10-mg dose is recommended. Adjust dosage related to the drug's longer half-life and the slower liver metabolism of older adult patients

Renal impairment: No dosage adjustment is necessary for mild to moderate renal impairment

Children: Safety and efficacy have not been established in this population

HALF LIFE (PEAK EFFECT): 27–32 h (4–7 h)

SELECTED ADVERSE REACTIONS: Most common adverse events include insomnia, ejaculation disorder, diarrhea, nausea, fatigue, increased sweating, dry mouth, somnolence, dizziness, and constipation. Most serious adverse events include ejaculation disorder in men; fetal abnormalities and decreased fetal weight in pregnant patients; and serotonin syndrome if coadministered with MAOIs, St. John's wort, or SSRIs, including citalopram (Celexa), of which escitalopram (Lexapro) is the active isomer.

BOXED WARNING: Suicidality in children, adolescents, and young adults

WARNING: There is potential for interaction with MAOIs. Lexapro should not be used in combination with an MAOI or within 14 days of discontinuing an MAOI.

SPECIFIC PATIENT AND FAMILY EDUCATION
- Do not take in combination with citalopram (Celexa) or other SSRIs or MAOIs. A 2-week washout period between escitalopram and SSRIs or MAOIs is recommended to avoid serotonin syndrome.
- Families and caregivers should be advised of the need for close observation and communication with the prescriber.
- Notify your prescriber if pregnancy is possible or being planned. Do not breast-feed while taking this medication.
- Use caution driving or operating machinery until you are certain that escitalopram does not alter your physical abilities or mental alertness.
- Notify your prescriber of any OTC medications, herbal supplements, and home remedies being used in combination with escitalopram.
- Ingestion of alcohol in combination with escitalopram is not recommended, although escitalopram does not seem to potentiate mental and motor impairments associated with alcohol.

MAOI, monoamine oxidase inhibitor; OTC, over the counter; SSRI, selective serotonin reuptake inhibitor.

Source: http://www.accessdata.fda.gov/drugsatfda_docs/label/2014/021323s044,021365s032lbl.pdf

---

BOX 19.5

Drug Profile: Mirtazapine (Remeron)

DRUG CLASS: Antidepressant

RECEPTOR AFFINITY: Believed to enhance central noradrenergic and serotonergic activity antagonizing central presynaptic α_2-adrenergic receptors. Mechanism of action is unknown

INDICATIONS: Treatment of depression

ROUTES AND DOSAGE: Available as 15- and 30-mg tablets

Adults: Initially, 15 mg/d as a single dose preferably in the evening before sleeping. Maximum dosage is 45 mg/d

Geriatric: Use with caution; reduced dosage may be needed.

Children: Safety and efficacy have not been established.

HALF-LIFE (PEAK EFFECT): 20–40 h (2 h)

SELECTED ADVERSE REACTIONS: Somnolence, increased appetite, dizziness, weight gain, elevated cholesterol or triglyceride and transaminase levels, malaise, abdominal pain, hypertension, vasodilation, vomiting, anorexia, thirst, myasthenia, arthralgia, hypoesthesia, apathy, depression, vertigo, twitching, agitation, anxiety, amnesia, increased cough, sinusitis, pruritus, rash, urinary tract infection, mania (rare), agranulocytosis (rare)

BOXED WARNING: Suicidality in children, adolescents, and young adults

WARNING: Contraindicated in patients with known hypersensitivity. Use with caution in older adults, patients who are breast-feeding, and patients with impaired hepatic function. Avoid concomitant use with alcohol or diazepam, which can cause additive impairment of cognitive and motor skills.

SPECIFIC PATIENT AND FAMILY EDUCATION
- Take the dose once a day in the evening before sleep.
- Families and caregivers should be advised of the need for dose observation and communication with the prescriber.
- Avoid driving and performing other tasks requiring alertness.
- Notify your prescriber before taking any OTC or other prescription drugs.
- Avoid alcohol and other CNS depressants.
- Notify your prescriber if pregnancy is possible or planned.
- Monitor temperature and report any fever, lethargy, weakness, sore throat, malaise, or other "flu-like" symptoms.
- Maintain medical follow-up, including any appointments for blood counts and liver studies.

CNS, central nervous system; OTC, over the counter.

---

other agents. See Box 19.5. Given their dietary restrictions, MAOIs usually are reserved for patients whose depression fails to respond to other antidepressants or patients who cannot tolerate typical antidepressants.

> **NCLEXNOTE**   Patients may be reluctant to take prescribed antidepressant medications or may self-treat depression based on their cultural beliefs and values (Institute of Medicine [IOM], 2003); (Munoz et al., 2007); (Warren, 2013a), (2013b), (2013c). A culturally competent nursing care and teaching plan needs to address the importance for adherence to a medication regimen and emphasize any potential drug–drug interactions.

Administering Medications

Antidepressants are available in oral form and should be taken as prescribed. See Box 19.6. Even after the first episode of major depression, medication should be continued for at least 6 months to 1 year after the patient achieves complete remission of symptoms. If the patient experiences a recurrence after tapering the first course of treatment, the regimen should be reinstituted for at least another year, and if the illness reoccurs, medication should be continued indefinitely (Schatzberg & DeBattista, 2015).

Monitoring Medications

Patients should be carefully observed for therapeutic and side effects of the antidepressants. In the depths of depression, saving medication for a later suicide attempt is quite common. During antidepressant treatment, the nurse should monitor and document vital signs, plasma drug levels (as appropriate), liver and thyroid function

---

BOX 19.6

Guidelines for Administering and Monitoring Antidepressant Medications

Nurses should do the following in administering and monitoring antidepressant medications:
- Observe the patient for cheeking or saving medications for a later suicide attempt.
- Monitor vital signs (such as orthostatic vital signs and temperature): obtain baseline data before the initiation of medications.
- Monitor periodically results of liver and thyroid function tests, blood chemistry, and complete blood count as appropriate and compare with baseline values.
- Monitor the patient symptoms for therapeutic response and report inadequate response to prescriber.

- Monitor the patient for side effects and report to the prescriber serious side effects or those that are chronic and problematic for the patient. (Table 19.2 indicates pharmacologic and nonpharmacologic interventions for common side effects.)
- Monitor drug levels as appropriate. (Therapeutic drug levels for antidepressants are listed in Chapter 10.)
- Monitor dietary intake as appropriate, especially with regard to MAOI antidepressants.
- Inquire about patient use of other medications, alcohol, "street" drugs, OTC medications, and herbal supplements that might alter the desired effects of prescribed antidepressants.

MAOI, monoamine oxidase inhibitor; OTC, over the counter.

tests, complete blood counts, and blood chemistry to make sure that patients are receiving a therapeutic dosage and are adherent to the prescribed regimen. Results of these tests also help evaluate for toxicity (see Chapter 10 for therapeutic blood levels).

Baseline orthostatic vital signs should be obtained before initiation of any medication, and in the case of medications known to have an impact on vital signs, such as TCAs, MAOIs, or SNRIs, they should be monitored on a regular basis. If these medications are administered to children or older adults, the dosage should be lowered to accommodate the physiologic state of the individual.

Managing Side Effects

Many people stop taking the prescribed antidepressants because of the side effects. (See Box 19.7.) Ideally, side effects are minimal and can be alleviated by nonpharmacologic interventions. For example, if patient is having difficulty going to sleep, avoiding caffeinated products may help (Table 19.2). SSRIs tend to be safer and have fewer side effects than the older medications. The most common reason individuals stop taking their SSRIs are gastrointestinal side effects including diarrhea, cramping, and heartburn. The most common side effects associated with TCAs are the antihistaminic side effects (e.g., sedation weight gain) and anticholinergic side effects (potentiation of CNS drugs, blurred vision, dry mouth, constipation, urinary retention, sinus tachycardia, and decreased memory).

For the MAOIs, the most common side effects of are headache, drowsiness, dry mouth and throat, constipation, blurred vision, and orthostatic hypotension. Additional selected adverse effects of MAOIs include

---

BOX 19.7

Antidepressants and Common Side Effects in Treating Depression

MEDICATIONS	COMMON SIDE EFFECTS	MEDICATIONS	COMMON SIDE EFFECTS
Selective Serotonin Reuptake Inhibitors (SSRIs)		**Other Antidepressants**	
Fluoxetine (Prozac) Sertraline (Zoloft) Paroxetine (Paxil) Fluvoxamine (Luvox) Citalopram (Celexa) Escitalopram (Lexapro)	Gastrointestinal distress Sedation Anticholinergic effects Weight gain or loss in some people Sexual dysfunction Dizziness Diaphoresis	Trazadone (Oleptro)	Sedation Anticholinergic effects Headache Dizziness Nausea/vomiting
		Vilazodone (Viibryd)	Diarrhea Nausea Dizziness Dry mouth Insomnia Abnormal dreams
Serotonin Norepinephrine Reuptake Inhibitors (SNRIs)			
Desvenlafaxine (Pristiq Extended Release) Duloxetine (Cymbalta) Levomilnacipran (Fetzima) Venlafaxine (Effexor XR)	Gastrointestinal Distress Anticholinergic effects Insomnia or sedation Decreased appetite Sexual dysfunction Abnormal dreams Dizziness Jitteriness Hypertension Irritability Photosensitivity	Vortioxetine (Brintellix)	Nausea Diarrhea Dizziness Dry mouth Constipation Vomiting
Norepinephrine Dopamine Reuptake Inhibitor (NDRI)		**Tricyclic Antidepressants**	
Bupropion (Wellbutrin)	Anticholinergic effects Headache Agitation Gastrointestinal distress Insomnia Anorexia Anxiety Weight loss Diarrhea and flatulence	Amitriptyline Amoxapine Clomipramine (Anafranil) Imipramine (Torfanil) Desipramine (Norpramin) Doxepin Nortriptypline (Aventyl, Pamelor) Protriptyline (Vivactil)	Drowsiness Anticholinergic effects Orthostatic hypotension Palpitations Tachycardia Impaired coordination Increase appetite Diaphoresis Weakness Disorientation Sexual side effects (impotence, changes in libido)
apha$_2$ Antagonist		**Tetracyclic Antidepressants**	
Mirtazapine (Remeron)	Sedation Anticholinergic effects Appetite increase Weight gain Hypercholesterolemia Weakness and lack of energy Dizziness Hypertriglyceridemia	Maprotiline	Blurred vision Dizziness Lightheadedness Sedation Dry mouth Libido changes Impotence Weight changes

(Continued)

BOX 19.7

Antidepressants and Common Side Effects in Treating Depression *(Continued)*

MEDICATIONS	COMMON SIDE EFFECTS	MEDICATIONS	COMMON SIDE EFFECTS
Monoamine Oxidase Inhibitors		Tranylcypromine (Parnate)	Orthostatic hypotension
Isocarboxazid (Marplan)	Dizziness		Dizziness
	Headache		Headache
	Nausea		Drowsiness
	Dry mouth		Sleep disturbance
	Constipation		Restlessness
	Drowsiness		Central nervous system
	Sleep disturbance		stimulation
	Orthostatic hypotension	Selegiline (Emsam)	Application site reaction
Phenelzine (Nardil)	Orthostatic hypotension		Headache
	Edema		Insomnia
	Dizziness		Diarrhea
	Headache		Dry mouth
	Drowsiness		Orthostatic hypotension
	Sleep disturbance		Dyspepsia

TABLE 19.2 INTERVENTIONS TO RELIEVE SIDE EFFECTS OF ANTIDEPRESSANTS

Side Effect	Pharmacologic Intervention	Nonpharmacologic Intervention
Dry mouth, caries, inflammation of the mouth	Bethanechol 10–30 mg tid Pilocarpine drops	Sugarless gum Sugarless lozenges 6–8 cups of water per day Toothpaste for dry mouth
Nausea, vomiting	Change medication	Take medication with food Soda crackers, toast, tea
Weight gain	Change medication	Nutritionally balanced diet Daily exercise
Urinary hesitation Constipation	Bethanechol 10–30 mg tid Stool softener	6–8 cups of water per day Bulk laxative Daily exercise 6–8 cups of water per day Diet rich in fresh fruits, vegetables, and whole grains
Diarrhea	OTC antidiarrheal	Maintain fluid intake
Orthostatic hypotension		Increase hydration Sit or stand up slowly
Drowsiness	Shift dosing time Lower medication dose Change medication	One caffeinated beverage at strategic time Do not drive when drowsy No alcohol or other recreational drugs Plan for rest time
Fatigue	Lower medication dose Change medication	Daily exercise
Blurred vision	Bethanechol 10–30 mg tid Pilocarpine eye drops	Temporary use of magnifying lenses until body adjusts to medication
Flushing, sweating	Terazosin 1 mg once daily Lower medication dose Change medication	Frequent bathing Lightweight clothing
Tremor	-blockers Lower medication dose	Reassure the patient that tremor may decrease as the patient adjusts to medication. Notify the caregiver if tremor interferes with daily functioning.

OTC, over the counter; tid, three times a day.

insomnia, nausea, agitation, dizziness, asthenia, weight loss, and postural hypotension. Although priapism was not reported during clinical trials, the MAOIs are structurally similar to trazodone, which has been associated with priapism (prolonged painful erection). For those taking, MAOIs, close attention to dietary restrictions should be given. See Chapter 10 for tyramine-restricted diets.

> **EMERGENCY CARE ALERT** ❗ If coadministered with food or other substances containing tyramine (e.g., aged cheese, beer, red wine), MAOIs can trigger a hypertensive crisis that may be life threatening. Symptoms include a sudden, severe pounding or explosive headache in the back of the head or temples, racing pulse, flushing, stiff neck, chest pain, nausea and vomiting, and profuse sweating.

Managing Adverse Events
Suicidality
Suicidality is included in a "boxed warning" on all antidepressants indicating an increased risk of suicide exists in children, adolescents, and young adults with major depressive or other psychiatric disorders. After the age of 24 years, the suicidality risk does not increase and after 65, the risk of suicide actually decreases when taking an antidepressant. The SSRIs are the least lethal of the antidepressants, but fatalities have been reported (Schatzberg & DeBattisa, 2015).

> **EMERGENCY CARE ALERT** ❗ If possible, TCAs should not be prescribed for patients at risk for suicide. Lethal doses of TCAs are only three to five times the therapeutic dose, and more than 1 g of a TCA is often toxic and may be fatal. Death may result from cardiac arrhythmia, hypotension, or uncontrollable seizures.

Serum TCA levels should be evaluated when overdose is suspected. In acute overdose, almost all symptoms develop within 12 hours. Anticholinergic effects are prominent and include dry mucous membranes, warm and dry skin, blurred vision, decreased bowel motility, and urinary retention. CNS suppression (ranging from drowsiness to coma) or an agitated delirium may occur. Basic overdose treatment includes induction of emesis, gastric lavage, and cardiorespiratory supportive care.

MAOIs are more lethal in overdose than are the newer antidepressants and thus should be prescribed with caution if the patient's suicide potential is elevated (see Chapter 10). An MAOI generally is given in divided doses to minimize side effects.

Serotonin Syndrome
Serotonin syndrome is a potentially serious side effect caused by drug-induced excess of intrasynaptic serotonin, 5-hydroxytryptamine [5-HT]). See Box 19.8. First reported in the 1950s, it was relatively rare until the introduction of the SSRIs. Serotonin syndrome is most often reported in patients taking two or more medications that increase CNS serotonin levels by different mechanisms

---

> ### BOX 19.8 ❗
> ## Serotonin Syndrome
>
> **CAUSE:** Excessive intrasynaptic serotonin
>
> **HOW IT HAPPENS:** Combining medications that increase CNS serotonin levels, such as SSRIs + MAOIs; SSRIs + St. John's wort; or SSRIs + diet pills; dextromethorphan or alcohol, especially red wine; or SSRI + street drugs, such as LSD, MMDA, or Ecstasy
>
> **SYMPTOMS:** Mental status changes, agitation, ataxia, myoclonus, hyperreflexia, fever, shivering, diaphoresis, diarrhea
>
> **TREATMENT**
> - Assess all medications, supplements, foods, and recreational drugs ingested to determine the offending substances.
> - Discontinue any substances that may be causative factors. If symptoms are mild, treat supportively on an outpatient basis with propranolol and lorazepam and follow-up with the prescriber.
> - If symptoms are moderate to severe, hospitalization may be needed with monitoring of vital signs and treatment with intravenous fluids, antipyretics, and cooling blankets.
>
> **FURTHER USE:** Assess on a case-by-case basis and minimize risk factors for further medication therapy.
>
> CNS, central nervous system; LSD, lysergic acid diethylamide; MAOI, monoamine oxidase inhibitor; MMDA, 3-methoxy-4,5-methylenedioxyamphetamine; SSRI, selective serotonin reuptake inhibitor.

(Stahl, 2013a). The most common drug combinations associated with serotonin syndrome involve the MAOIs, the SSRIs, and the TCAs.

Although serotonin syndrome can cause death, it is mild in most patients, who usually recover with supportive care alone. Unlike neuroleptic malignant syndrome, which develops within 3 to 9 days after the introduction of antipsychotic medications (see Chapter 21), serotonin syndrome tends to develop within hours or days after starting or increasing the dose of serotonergic medication. Symptoms include altered mental status, autonomic dysfunction, and neuromuscular abnormalities. At least three of the following findings must be present for a diagnosis: mental status changes, agitation, myoclonus, hyperreflexia, fever, shivering, diaphoresis, ataxia, and diarrhea. In patients who also have peripheral vascular disease or atherosclerosis, severe vasospasm and hypertension may occur in the presence of elevated serotonin levels. In addition, in a patient who is a slow metabolizer of SSRIs, higher-than-normal levels of these antidepressants may circulate in the blood. Medications that are not usually considered serotonergic, such as dextromethorphan (Pertussin) and meperidine (Demerol), have been associated with the syndrome (Alpern & Henretig, 2010).

> **EMERGENCY CARE ALERT** ❗ The most important emergency interventions are stopping use of the offending drug, notifying the prescriber, and providing necessary supportive care (e.g., intravenous fluids, antipyretics, cooling blanket). Severe symptoms have been successfully treated with antiserotonergic agents, such as cyproheptadine (Alusik, Kalatova, & Paluch, 2014).

Monitoring for Drug Interactions

Several potential drug interactions are associated with antidepressants. Alcohol consumption should be avoided when taking any antidepressant because SSRIs are metabolized in the liver, other medications that are also metabolized by the same enzyme can cause an increase in drug levels leading to toxicity and serotonin syndrome. For example, if migraine medications known as "triptans" are given with the SSRIs, serotonin syndrome can occur. Bupropion cannot be given at the same time as an MAOI. Grapefruit should not be consumed while taking trazodone. It is beyond the scope of this text to review drug-drug interactions in detail. Nurses should check with pharmacy resources for any drug-drug interactions when administering medications. See Table 19.3.

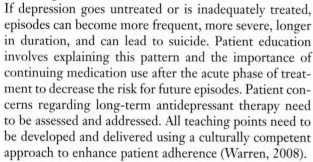

Teaching Points

If depression goes untreated or is inadequately treated, episodes can become more frequent, more severe, longer in duration, and can lead to suicide. Patient education involves explaining this pattern and the importance of continuing medication use after the acute phase of treatment to decrease the risk for future episodes. Patient concerns regarding long-term antidepressant therapy need to be assessed and addressed. All teaching points need to be developed and delivered using a culturally competent approach to enhance patient adherence (Warren, 2008).

Patients should also be advised not to take herbal substances such as St. John's wort or SAMe if they are also taking prescribed antidepressants. St. John's wort also should not be taken if the patient is taking nasal decongestants, hay fever and asthma medications containing monoamines, amino acid supplements containing phenylalanine, or tyrosine. The combination may cause hypertension.

Other Somatic Therapies

Electroconvulsive Therapy

Although its therapeutic mechanism of action is unknown, ECT is an effective treatment for patients with severe depression. It is generally reserved for patients whose disorder is refractory or intolerant to initial drug treatments and who are so severely ill that rapid treatment is required (e.g., patients with malnutrition, catatonia, or suicidality).

ECT is contraindicated for patients with increased intracranial pressure. Other high-risk patients include those with recent myocardial infarction, recent cerebrovascular accident, retinal detachment, or pheochromocytoma (a tumor in the cellsof the adrenal gland) and those at risk for complications of anesthesia. Older age has been associated with a favorable response to ECT, but the effectiveness and safety in this group have not been shown. Because depression can increase the mortality risk for older adults, in particular, and some older adults

TABLE 19.3	DRUG–DRUG INTERACTIONS: ANTIDEPRESSANTS	
Antidepressant	**Other Drug**	**Effect of Interaction or Treatment**
Fluvoxamine	Theophylline	Increased theophylline level: seizures. Tx: Reduce theophylline levels when administering with fluvoxamine.
Fluoxetine Paroxetine	TCAs Benzodiazepines Phenothiazines	Increased in plasma levels of TCA. Tx: Reduce TCA levels when giving with fluoxetine or paroxetine.
Fluoxetine Fluvoxamine Nefazodone	Alprazolam Benzodiazepines	Increased plasma levels of alprazolam. Tx: Reduce dose of alprazolam when administered with benzodiazepines.
Nefazodone	Digoxin Phenothiazines Antihistamines	Increased levels of digoxin, antihistamines, and benzodiazepines. Tx: Reduce dose of nefazodone when giving with these medications.
Fluvoxamine	Caffeine Nicotine	Lowered levels of fluvoxamine. Tx: Increase dose of fluvoxamine in smokers or patients whose coffee, tea, or caffeinated drink intake is high.
SSRIs	Warfarin	Increased prothrombin time, bleeding. Tx: Monitor closely; decrease dose of warfarin if giving with SSRIs.
SSRIs	Lithium TCAs Barbiturates	Increased CNS effects of SSRIs. Tx: Adjust dosage of SSRI.
SSRIs	Phenytoin	Increased serum levels of phenytoin. Tx: Adjust dosage of phenytoin.

CNS, central nervous system; SSRI, selective serotonin reuptake inhibitor; TCA, tricyclic antidepressant; Tx, treatment.

Source: Stahl, S. M. (2013a). *Stahl's essential psychopharmacology: Neuroscientific basis and practical applications* (4th ed.). New York: Cambridge University Press.

do not respond well to medication, effective treatment is especially important for this age group (Van der Wurff, Stek, Hoogendijk, & Beekman, 2009).

The role of the nurse in the care of the patient undergoing ECT is to provide educational and emotional support for the patient and family, assess baseline or pretreatment levels of function, prepare the patient for the ECT process, monitor and evaluate the patient's response to ECT, provide assessment data with the ECT team, and modify treatment as needed (see Chapter 10 for more information). The actual procedure, possible therapeutic mechanisms of action, potential adverse effects, contraindications, and nursing interventions are described in detail in Chapter 10.

Light Therapy (Phototherapy)

Light therapy is described in Chapter 10. Given current research, light therapy is an option for well-documented mild-to-moderate seasonal, nonpsychotic, winter depressive episodes in patients with recurrent major depressive disorders, including children and adolescents. Evidence also indicates that light therapy can modestly improve symptoms in nonseasonal depression, especially when administered during the first week of treatment in the morning for those experiencing sleep deprivation (Lewy, Lefler, Emens, & Bauer, 2006).

Repetitive Transcranial Magnetic Stimulation

In 2008, the U.S. Food and Drug Administration approved repetitive transcranial magnetic stimulation (rTMS) for the treatment of patients with mild treatment-resistant depression. In rTMS, a magnetic coil placed on the scalp at the site of the left motor cortex releases small electrical pulses that stimulate the site of the left dorsolateral prefrontal cortex in the superficial cortex. This rapidly changing magnetic field stimulates the brain sufficiently to depolarize neurons and exert effects across synapses. These pulses (similar in type and strength as a magnetic resonance imaging machine) easily pass through the hair, skin, and skull, requiring much less electricity than ECT. The patient is awake, reclining in an rTMS chair during the procedure, and can resume normal activities immediately after the procedure. Because anesthesia is not required, no risks are associated with sedation. Treatment of depression typically consists of 20 to 30 sessions, lasting 37 minutes each over 4 to 6 weeks. Depending on the level of practice and training, the nurse's role the use of the rTMS varies from education, preparation, and postprocedure care to performing the procedure (Bernard, Westmand, Dutton, & Lanocha, 2009).

Psychosocial Interventions

Individuals experiencing depression are often withdrawn from daily activities, such as engaging in family activities, attending work, and participating in community functions.

During hospitalization, patients often withdraw to their rooms and refuse to participate in unit activity. Nurses help the patient balance the need for privacy with the need to return to normal social functioning. Even though depressed patients should not be approached in an overly enthusiastic manner, they should be encouraged to set realistic goals to reconnect with their families and communities. Explain to patients that attending social activities, even though they do not feel like it, will promote the recovery process and help them achieve their goals

Cognitive Interventions

Cognitive interventions such as thought stopping and positive self-talk can dispel irrational beliefs and distorted attitudes and in turn reduce depressive symptoms during the acute phase of major depression (see Chapter 9). Nurses should consider using cognitive approaches when caring for persons who are depressed. The use of cognitive interventions in the acute phase of treatment combined with medication is now considered first-line treatment for mildly to moderately depressed outpatients.

NCLEXNOTE A cognitive therapy approach is recommended for helping persons restructure the negative thinking processes related to a person's concept of self, others, and the future. This approach should be included in most nursing care plans for patients with depression.

Behavioral Interventions

Behavioral interventions are effective in the acute treatment of patients with mildly to moderately severe depression, especially when combined with pharmacotherapy. Therapeutic techniques include activity scheduling, social skills training, and problem solving. Behavioral therapy techniques are described in Chapter 5.

Group Interventions

Individuals who are depressed can receive emotional support in groups and learn how others deal with similar problems and issues. As group members serve as role models for new group members, they also benefit as their self-esteem increases, which strengthens their ability to address their issues (see Chapter 11). Group interventions are often used to help an individual cope with depression associated with bereavement or chronic medical illness. Group interventions are also commonly used to educate patients and families about their disorder and medications.

Psychoeducation

Patients with depression and their significant others often incorrectly believe that their illness is their own fault and

---

BOX 19.9

Major Depressive Disorder

When caring for the patient with a major depressive disorder, be sure to include the following topic areas in the teaching plan:

- Psychopharmacologic agents, including drug action, dosing frequency, and possible side effects
- Risk factors for recurrence; signs of recurrence
- Adherence to therapy and treatment program
- Recovery strategies
- Nutrition
- Sleep measures
- Self-care management
- Goal setting and problem solving
- Social interaction skills
- Follow-up appointments
- Community support services

---

that they should be able to "pull themselves up by their bootstraps and snap out of it." Persons from some cultural groups believe that the symptoms of depression may be a result of someone placing a hex on the affected person because the person has done something evil (Warren, 2008). It is vital to be culturally competent to be effective in teaching patients and their families about the treatment modalities for depression.

Patients need to know the full range of suitable treatment options before consenting to participate in treatment. Information empowers patients to ask questions, weigh risks and benefits, and make the best treatment choices. The nurse can provide opportunities for patients to question, discuss, and explore their feelings about past, current, and planned use of medications and other treatments. Developing strategies to enhance adherence and to raise awareness of early signs of relapse can be important aids to increasing treatment efficacy and promoting recovery (Box 19.9).

The family needs education and support during and after the treatment of family members. Because major depressive disorder is a recurring disorder, the family needs information about specific antecedents to a family member's depression and what therapeutic steps to take. For example, one patient may routinely become depressed during the fall of each year, with one of the first symptoms being excessive sleepiness. For another patient, a major loss, such as a child going to college or the death of a pet, may precipitate a depressive episode. Families of older adults need to be aware of the possibility of depression and related symptoms, which often occur after the deaths of friends and relatives. Families of children who are depressed often misinterpret depression as behavioral problems.

Milieu Therapy

While hospitalized, milieu therapy (see Chapter 9) helps depressed patients maintain socialization skills and continue

to interact with others. When depressed, people are often unaware of the environment and withdraw into themselves. On a psychiatric unit, depressed patients should be encouraged to attend and participate in unit activities. These individuals have decreased energy levels and thus may be moving more slowly than others; however, their efforts should be praised.

Safety

In many cases, patients are admitted to the psychiatric hospital because of a suicide attempt. Suicidality should continually be evaluated, and the patient should be protected from self-harm (see Chapter 15). During the depths of depression, patients may not have the energy to complete a suicide. As patients begin to feel better and have increased energy, they therefore may be at a greater risk for suicide. If a previously depressed patient appears to have become energized overnight, he or she may have made a decision to commit suicide and thus may be relieved that the decision is finally made. The nurse may misinterpret the mood improvement as a positive move toward recovery; however, this patient may be very intent on suicide. These individuals should be carefully monitored to maintain their safety.

Family Interventions

Patients who perceive high family stress are at risk for greater future severity of illness, higher use of health services, and higher health care expense. Marital and family problems are common among patients with mood disorders; comprehensive treatment requires that these problems be assessed and addressed. They may be a consequence of the major depression but may also predispose persons to develop depressive symptoms or inhibit recovery and resilience processes. Research suggests that marital and family therapy may reduce depressive symptoms and the risk for relapse in patients with marital and family problems (Whisman & Beach, 2012). The depressed spouse's depression has marked impact on the marital adjustment of the nondepressed spouse. It is recommended that treatment approaches be designed to help couples be supportive of each other, to adapt, and to cope with the depressive symptoms within the framework of their ongoing marital relations. Many family nursing interventions may be used by the psychiatric nurse in providing targeted family-centered care. These include:

- Monitoring patient and family for indicators of stress
- Teaching stress management techniques
- Counseling family members on coping skills for their own use
- Providing necessary knowledge of options and support services
- Facilitating family routines and rituals

- Assisting the family to resolve feelings of guilt
- Assisting the family with conflict resolution
- Identifying family strengths and resources with family members
- Facilitating communication among family members

Support Groups

Nurses are exceptionally well positioned to engage patients and their families in the active process of improving daily functioning, increasing knowledge and skill acquisition, and increasing independent living. Consumer-oriented support groups can help to enhance the self-esteem and the support network of participating patients and their families. Advice, encouragement, and the sense of group camaraderie may make an important contribution to recovery (APA, 2013). Organizations providing support and information include the Depression and Bipolar Support Network (DBSA), National Alliance on Mental Illness (NAMI), and the Mental Health Association and Recovery, Inc. (a self-help group).

Evaluation and Treatment Outcomes

The major goals of treatment are to help the patient to be as independent as possible and to achieve stability, remission, and recovery from major depression. It is often a lifelong struggle for the individual. Ongoing evaluation of the patient's symptoms, functioning, and quality of life should be carefully documented in the patient's record in order to monitor outcomes of treatment.

Continuum of Care

Mild to moderate depression is often first recognized in primary care settings. Primary care nurses should be able to recognize depression in these patients and make appropriate interventions or referrals. Those with more severe depressive symptoms may be directly admitted to inpatient and outpatient mental health settings or emergency departments. The continuum of care beyond these settings may include partial hospitalization or day treatment programs; individual, family, or group psychotherapy; and home visits. Although most patients with major depression are treated in outpatient settings, brief hospitalization may be required if the patient is suicidal or psychotic (Dollard, 2013; Mitchell, Kane, Kameg, Spino, & Hong, 2013).

Nurses working on inpatient units provide a wide range of direct services, including administering and monitoring medications and target symptoms; conducting psychoeducational groups; and more generally, structuring and maintaining a therapeutic environment. Nurses providing home care have an excellent opportunity to detect undiagnosed depressive disorders and make appropriate referrals.

OTHER DEPRESSIVE DISORDERS

Other depressive disorders with similar symptoms are treated similarly to the major depressive disorders. Nursing care should be individualized and based on their patients' mental health needs and strengths. A diagnosis of **persistent depressive disorder** (*dysthymia*) is made if major depressive disorder symptoms last for 2 years for an adult and 1 year for children and adolescents. These individuals are depressed for most of each day (APA, 2013). A major depressive disorder may precede the persistent depressive disorder or co-occur with it.

Premenstrual dysphoric disorder is characterized by recurring mood swings, feelings of sadness, or sensitivity to rejection in the final week before the onset of menses. The mood begins to improve a few days after menses begins. Stress, history of interpersonal trauma, seasonal changes are associated with this disorder (APA, 2013).

Disruptive mood dysregulation disorder is characterized by severe irritability and outbursts of temper. The onset of disruptive mood dysregulation disorder begins before the age of 10 when children have verbal rages and/or are physically aggressive toward others or property. These outbursts are outside of the normal temper tantrums children display. They are more severe than what would be expected developmentally and occur frequently (i.e., two or three times a week). The behavior disrupts family functioning as well as the child's ability to succeed in school and social activities. This disorder can co-occur with attention-deficit/hyperactivity disorder. See Chapter 28.

Disruptive mood dysregulation disorder is similar to pediatric bipolar disorder, but the DSM-5 differentiates it from bipolar disorder. Children with this disorder have similar deficits in recognition of emotion through facial expression, decision-making, and control as those with bipolar disorder. More research is needed in understanding this disorder.

SUMMARY OF KEY POINTS

- Moods influence perception of life events and functioning. Depressive disorders are characterized by persistent or recurring disturbances in mood that cause significant psychological distress and functional impairment (typified by feelings of sadness, hopelessness, loss of interest, and fatigue).

- Depressive disorders include both major depressive disorder, persistent depressive disorder (dysthymia), premenstrual dysphoric disorder, disruptive mood dysregulation disorder, and other related to medical conditions, medications, or substance use.

- Risk factors include a family history of depressive disorders, prior depressive episodes; lack of social support; stressful life events; substance use; and medical problems, particularly chronic or terminal illnesses.

■ Treatment of major depressive disorder primarily includes antidepressant medication, psychotherapy or a combination of both. ECT, light therapy, and repetitive transcranial magnetic stimulation are also used.

■ Nurses must be knowledgeable regarding culturally competent strategies related to the use of antidepressant medications, pharmacologic therapeutic effects and associated side effects, toxicity, dosage ranges, and contraindications. Nurses must also be familiar with ECT protocols and associated interventions. Patient education and the provision of emotional support during the course of treatment are also nursing responsibilities.

■ Many symptoms of depression (e.g., weight and appetite changes, sleep disturbance, decreased energy, fatigue) are similar to those of medical illnesses. Assessment includes a thorough medical history and physical examination to detect or rule out medical or psychiatric comorbidity.

■ Mental health nursing assessment includes assessing mood; speech patterns; thought processes and content; suicidal or homicidal thoughts; cognition and memory; and social factors, such as patterns of relationships, quality of support systems, and changes in occupational functioning. Several self-report scales are helpful in evaluating depressive symptoms.

■ Establishing and maintaining a therapeutic culturally competent nurse–patient relationship is key to successful outcomes. Nursing interventions that foster the therapeutic relationship include being available in times of crisis, providing understanding and education to patients and their families regarding goals of treatment, providing encouragement and feedback concerning the patient's progress, providing guidance in the patient's interpersonal interactions with others and work environment, and helping to set and monitor realistic goals.

■ Psychosocial interventions for depressive disorders include self-care management, cognitive therapy, behavior therapy, interpersonal therapy, patient and family education regarding the nature of the disorder and treatment goals, marital and family interventions, and group interventions that include medication maintenance support groups and other consumer-oriented support groups.

CRITICAL THINKING CHALLENGES

1. Describe how you would do a suicide assessment on a patient who comes into a primary care office and is distraught and expressing concerns about her ability to cope with her current situation.

2. Describe how you would approach the patient who does not want to talk with you?

3. Describe how you would approach a patient who is expressing concern that the diagnosis of depressive disorder will negatively affect her social and work relationships.

4. Your depressed patient does not seem inclined to talk about his depression. Describe the measures you would take to initiate a therapeutic relationship with him.

5. Compare the side effects of the SSRIs, TCAs, and MAOIs.

6. Think about all the above situations and relate them to persons from culturally and ethnically diverse populations (e.g., African, Latino, or Asian descent; Jewish or Jehovah's Witness religions; across the life-span of individuals from children to older adult populations).

About Schmidt: (2002). This movie is about a 67-year-old man, Warren Schmidt, played by Jack Nicholson, who retires from his job as an insurance company executive. He experiences work withdrawal and a lack of direction for his retirement. His wife, Helen, irritates him, and he has no idea what to do to fill his days. While watching television one day, he is moved to sponsor a child in Africa with whom he begins a long, one-sided correspondence. When his wife dies unexpectedly, he is initially numb, then sad, and finally angry when he discovers that she had an affair with his best friend many years ago. He is estranged from his only daughter, Jeanie, whose wedding to Randall, a man he thinks is beneath her, is imminent. The movie follows Warren as he searches for connection and meaning in his life.

Significance: Warren Schmidt demonstrates a common phenomenon among older adults when they retire. He also shows the impact of grief superimposed on initial dysthymia or depression.

Viewing Points: Look for the changes in Schmidt's manifestations of depression in different situations. Note how he experiences the various stages of grieving. What do you think about Schmidt's search for significance and meaning in his life?

Dead Poet's Society: (1989). This classic film portrays John Keating, played by Robin Williams, as a charismatic English teacher in a conservative New England prep school for boys in 1959. John brings his love of poetry to the students and encourages them to follow their dreams and talents and make the most of every day. His efforts put him at odds with the administration of the school, particularly the headmaster, played by Norman Lloyd, as well as Tom Perry, the father of one of his students, played by Kurtwood Smith. Tom's son, Neil, played by Robert Sean Leonard, chooses to act in a school play despite the objection of his father to any extracurricular activities. When Neil cannot reconcile his love of theater and his father's expectations that he pursue a career in medicine, he kills himself. John Keating blames himself for the death, as does the school administration. He is fired by the administration but has a moment of pride when his students demonstrate their ability to think and act for themselves.

Significance: This film accurately portrays the sensitivity of adolescents and their longing for worthwhile role models. It also shows adolescent growth and development in a realistic manner. It demonstrates the combination of factors that accompany a decision to commit suicide. We can see how Neil feels caught between his desires and the demands of his father. In the cultural context of the late 1950s, few children or adolescents dared to challenge or defy their parents, especially such a domineering man as Tom Perry.

Viewing Points: Look for the differences in Neil's behavior with his peers and his father or other adults besides Mr. Keating. What, if any, clues do you get that Neil might attempt suicide? What actions by any of the main characters might have prevented his suicide?

M VIE viewing **GUIDES** related to this chapter are available at http://thepoint.lww.com/BoydEssentials.

 A related Psychiatric-Mental Health Nursing video on the topic of Depression is available at http://thepoint.lww.com/BoydEssentials.

 A Psychiatric-Mental Health Nursing Practice and Learn Activity related to the video on the topic of Depression is available at http://thepoint.lww.com/BoydEssentials.

REFERENCES

Abbass, A.A., Kisely, S.R., Town, J.M., Leichsenring, F., Driessen, E., DeMaat, S., Gerber, A., Dekker, J., Rabung, S., Rusalovska, S., & Crowe, E. (2014). Short-term psychodynamic psychotherapies for common mental disorders (Review). *Cochrane Database of systematic Reviews 2014, 7*, CD004687. doi: 10.1002/14651858.CD004687.pub4.

Alpern, E. R., & Henretig, F. M. (2010). Fever. In G. R. Fleisher & S. Ludwig (Eds.). *Textbook of pediatric emergency* (pp. 273–274). Philadelphia: Wolters Kluwer.

Alusik, S., Kalatova, D., & Paluch, Z. (2014). Serotonin syndrome. *Neuroendocrinology Letters, 35*(4), 265-273.

American Psychiatric Association (APA). (2013). *Diagnostic and statistical manual of mental disorders DSM-5 (5th ed.).* Arlington, VA: Author.

Beeber, L. S., Lewis, V. S., Cooper, C., Maxwell, L., & Sandelowski, M. (2010). Meeting the "now" need: PMH-APRN- Interpreter teams provide in-home mental health intervention for depressed Latina mothers with limited English proficiency. *Journal of the American Psychiatric Nurses Association, 15*(4), 249–259.

Bernard, S., Westmand, G., Dutton, P. R., & Lanocha, K. (2009). A psychiatric nurse's perspective: Helping patients undergo repetitive

transcranial magnetic stimulation (rTMS) for depression. *Journal of the American Psychiatric Nurses Association, 15*(5), 325–337.

Blazer, D.G., & Steffens, D.C. (2015). Depressive Disorders. In D.G. Blazer, D.C. Steffens, & M. Thakur, (Eds.). *The American Psychiatric Publishing Textbook of Geriatric Psychiatry* 5th ed. Arlington, VA: American Psychiatric Association. http://dx.doi.org/10.1176/appi.books.9781615370054.ds09

Brière, F.N., Rohde, P., Seeley, J.R., Klein, D., Lewinsohn, P.M. (2015). Adolescent suicide attempts and adult adjustment. *Depression & Anxiety, 32*(4), 270-6.

Centers for Disease Control and Prevention. National Center for Injury Prevention and Control (2015). *Suicide facts at a glance 2012.* Retrieved May 11, 2015. http://www.cdc.gov/violenceprevention/pdf/suicide-datasheet-a.pdf

Cerel, J., Jordan, J. R., & Duberstein, P. R. (2008). The impact of suicide on the family. *Crisis, 29*, 38–44.

Clarke, K., Mayo-Wilson, E., Kenny, J., & Pilling, S. (2015). Can non-pharmacological interventions prevent relapse in adults who have recovered from depression? A systematic review and meta-analysis of randomized controlled trials. *Clinical Psychology Review, 39*, 58–70. doi: 10.1016/j.cpr.2015.04.002.

Dobscha, S.K., Denneson, L.M., Kovas, A.E., Teo, A., Forsberg, C.W., Kaplan, M.S., Bossarte, R., & McFarland, B.H. (2014). Correlates of suicide among veterans treated in primary care: Case-control study of a nationally representative sample. *Journal of General Internal Medicine, 29*(Suppl 4, issue 4), 853–60.

Dollard, M. K. (2013). Psychopharmacology in psychiatric emergency. In L. G. Leahy & C. G. Kohler (Eds.), *Manual of clinical psychopharmacology for nurses* (Chapter 11, pp. 301–329). Washington, DC: American Psychiatric Publishing.

Dulcan, M. K., & Lake, M. (2012). *Concise guide to child and adolescent psychiatry* (4th ed.). Washington, DC: American Psychiatric Publishing.

Gonzalez, H. M., Vega, W. A., Williams, D. R., Tarraf, W., West, B. T., & Neighbors, H. (2010). Depression care in the United States. *Archives of General Psychiatry, 67*(1), 37–46.

Institute of Medicine. (2003). *Unequal treatment: Confronting racial and ethnic disparities in health care.* Washington, DC: National Academies Press.

Josey, L. M., & Neidert, E. M. (2013). Depressive disorders. In L. G. Leahy & C. G. Kohler (Eds.), *Manual of clinical psychopharmacology for nurses* (Chapter 3, pp. 59–84). Washington, DC: American Psychiatric Publishing.

Kessler, R.C., Berglund, P., Demler, Ol, Jin, R., Merikangas, K.R., & Walters, E.E. (2005). Lifetime prevalence and age-of-onset distributions of DSM-IV disorders in the National comorbidity Survey Replication. *Archives of General Psychiatry, 62*(6), 593–602.

Lewy, A. J., Lefler, B. J., Emens, J. S., & Bauer, V. K. (2006). The circadian basis of winter depression. Retrieved from http://www.pnas.org/cgi/doi/10.1073/pnas.0602425103. Retrieved August 3, 2015.

Liehr, P., & Diaz, N. (2010). A pilot study examining the effect of mindfulness on depression and anxiety for minority children. *Archives of Psychiatric Nursing, 24*(1), 69–71.

Lutz, W. J., & Warren, B. J. (2007). The state of nursing science: Cultural and lifespan issues depression part II: Focus on children and adolescents. *Issues in Mental Health Nursing, 28*(7), 749–764.

McEnany, G. P. (2011). Sleep in psychiatric mental health settings. In N. S. Redeker & G. P. McEnany (Eds.), *Sleep disorders and sleep promotion in nursing practice*, (Chapter 19, pp. 309–320). Washington, DC: American Psychiatric Publishing.

McInnis, M.G., Riba, M., & Greden, J.F. (2014). Depressive disorders. In R.E. Hales, S.C. Yudofsky, & L.W. Roberts (Eds.). *The American Psychiatric Publishing Textbook of Psychiatry* 6th ed. Arlington, VA: American Psychiatric Association. http://dx.doi.org/10.1176/appi.books.9781585625031.rh11

Mitchell, A. M., Kane, I., Kameg, K. M., Spino, E. R., & Hong, B. (2013). Integrated management of self-directed injury. In K. R. Tusaie & J. J. Fitzpatrick (Eds.), *Advanced practice psychiatric nursing: Integrating psychotherapy, psychopharmacology, and complementary and alternative approaches* (Chapter 15, pp. 362–387). New York: Springer Publishing Company.

Munoz, R., Primm, A., Ananth, J., & Ruiz, P. (2007). *Life in color: Culture in American psychiatry.* Chicago, IL: Hilton Publishing.

National Institutes of Mental Health. (2015). *Suicide in the U.S: Statistics and prevention.* Retrieved from http://www.nimh.nih.gov/health/publications/suicide-in-the-us-statistics-and-prevention/index.shtml. Retrieved May 16, 2015.

Pedersen, C. A., Draguus, J. G., Lonner, W. J., & Trimble, J. E. (2008). *Counseling across cultures* (6th ed.). Thousand Oaks, CA: Sage Publishing.

Posmontier, B. (2013). Complementary and alternative pharmacotherapies. In L. G. Leahy & C. G. Kohler (Eds.), *Manual of clinical psychopharmacology for nurses* (Chapter 13, pp. 353–377). Washington, DC: American Psychiatric Publishing.

Purnell, L. D. (2012). *Transcultural health care (4th ed.).* Philadelphia: F. A. Davis.

Rawana, J.S., & Morgan, A.S. (2014). Trajectories of depressive symptoms from adolescence to young adulthood: the role of self-esteem and body-related predictors. *Journal of Youth & Adolescence, 43*(4), 597–611.

Rosenquist, J. N., Fowler, J. H., & Christakis, N. A. (2011). Social network determinants of depression. *Molecular Psychiatry, 16*(3), 273–281.

Schatzberg, A. F., & DeBattista, C. (2015). *Manual of Clinical Psychopharmacology (8th ed).* Arlington, VA: American Psychiatric Publishing.

Shi, J., Potash, S. J., Knowles, J. A., Weissman, M. M., Coryell, W., Lawson, W. B., et al. (2011). Genome-wide association study of recurrent early-onset major depressive disorder. *Molecular Psychiatry, 16*(2), 193–201.

Stahl, S. M. (2013a). *Stahl's essential psychopharmacology: Neuroscientific basis and practical applications (4th ed.).* New York: Cambridge University Press.

Stahl, S. M. (2013b). *Stahl's essential psychopharmacology: The prescriber's guide (4th ed.).* New York: Cambridge University Press.

Tarraza, M. (2013). Medical problems and psychiatric syndromes. In K. R. Tusaie & J. J. Fitzpatrick (Eds.), *Advanced practice psychiatric nursing: Integrating psychotherapy, psychopharmacology, and complementary and alternative approaches* (Chapter 18, pp. 468–485). New York: Springer Publishing Company.

Tsai, W. P., Lin, L. Y., Chang, W. L., Chang, H. C., & Chou, M. C. (2010). The effects of suicide awareness program in enhancing community volunteers' of suicide warning signs. *Archives of Psychiatric Nursing, 24*(1), 63–68.

Tusaie, K. R. (2013). Integrative management of disordered mood. In K. R. Tusaie & J. J. Fitzpatrick (Eds.), *Advanced practice psychiatric nursing: Integrating psychotherapy, psychopharmacology, and complementary and alternative approaches* (Chapter 8, pp. 122–157). New York: Springer Publishing Company.

United States Department of Health and Human Services (USDHHS). (1999). *Mental health: A report of the Surgeon General.* Rockville, MD: United States Department of Health and Human Services, Substance Abuse and Mental Health Services Administration, Center for Mental Health Services, National Institutes of Health, National Institute of Mental Health.

Van der Wurff, F. B., Stek, M., Hoogendijk W., & Beekman A. (2009). Electroconvulsive therapy for the depressed elderly. *Cochrane Database of Systematic Reviews,* (2), CD003593.

Warren, B. J. (2008). Cultural and ethnic considerations. In D. Antai-Otong (Ed.), *Psychiatric nursing: Biological and behavioral concepts* (2nd ed., pp. 174–193). Clifton Park, NJ: Thomson Delmar Learning.

Warren, B. J. (2011a). Guest Editor. CNE Series: Two sides of the coin: The bully and the bullied. *Journal of Psychosocial Nursing and Mental Health Services, 49*(10), 22–29.

Warren, B. J. (2011b). Cultural competence in psychiatric nursing. In N. L. Keltner, C. E. Bostrom, & T. McGuinness (Eds.), *Psychiatric nursing* (6th ed.) Chapter 14, pp. 164–172). St. Louis, MO: Mosby.

Warren, B. J., & Broome, B. (2011). CNE Series: The culture of adolescents with urologic dysfunction: Mental health, wellness, and illness awareness. *Urologic Nursing, 31*(2), 95–104.

Warren, B. J. (2012). Depression: Management of depressive disorders and suicidal behavior. In M. A. Boyd (Ed.), *Psychiatric nursing: Contemporary practice* (5th ed.enhanced update) (Chapter 24, pp. 401–425). Philadelphia: Wolters Kluwer.

Warren, B. J. (2013a). How culture is assessed in the DSM-5. *Journal of Psychosocial Nursing, 51*(4), 40–45.

Warren, B. J. (2013b). Culturally sensitive psychopharmacology. In L. G. Leahy C. G. Kohler (Eds.), *Clinical manual of psychopharmacology for nurses* (Chapter 14, pp. 379–402). Washington, DC: American Psychiatric Publishing, Inc.

Warren, B. J. (2013c) *Ethnopharmacology.* In B. Cockerman (Ed.), Blackwell encyclopaedia health and society medical anthropology. Somerset, NJ: Wiley.

Warren, B. J., & Lutz, W. J. (2007). The state of nursing science: Cultural and lifespan issues depression Part II: Focus on adults. *Issues in Mental Health Nursing, 28*(7), 707–748.

Whisman, M.A., & Beach, S.R.H. (2012). Couple therapy for depression. *Journal of Clinical Psychology: In Session, 68*(5), 526-535..

World Health Organization (WHO). (2014). *Evidence-based recommendations for management of depression in non-specialized health settings.* Retrieved from http://www.who.int/mental_health/mhgap/evidence/depression/en/index.html

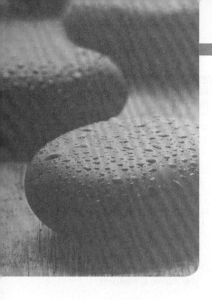

20
Bipolar Disorders
Nursing Care of Persons with Mood Lability

Mary Ann Boyd

KEY CONCEPTS

- bipolar disorder
- mania
- mood lability

LEARNING OBJECTIVES

After studying this chapter, you will be able to:

1. Discuss the role of mania in mental disorders.

2. Describe the prevalence and incidence of bipolar disorders.

3. Delineate the clinical symptoms of bipolar disorders with emphasis on mood lability.

4. Describe the theories explaining bipolar disorder and mood lability.

5. Identify evidence-based interventions for patients diagnosed with bipolar disorders and for those who exhibit mood lability.

6. Develop recovery-oriented strategies that address the needs of persons diagnosed with bipolar disorders and for those who exhibit mood lability.

7. Differentiate other bipolar and related disorders.

KEY TERMS

- bipolar I disorder • bipolar II disorder • cyclothymic disorder • elation • elevated mood • euphoria • expansive mood • grandiosity • hypomania • mania • mood lability • rapid cycling

Case Study: Christine

Christine is a 34-year old female woman has a history of Bipolar I disorder. She is brought to emergency room by the police from the airport where she was demanding a plane ticket to Hawaii. She became very belligerent when she did not get her ticket. She is wearing an evening dress with several pieces of expensive jewelry.

INTRODUCTION

Everyone has ups and downs. Mood changes are a part of everyday life; expression of feeling is integral to communication. But when moods are so pervasive that they cloud reasoning and judgment, they become problematic and interfere with interpersonal relationships. In some instances, extreme moods such as mania are symptoms of mental disorders. This chapter discusses bipolar disorders that are characterized by severe mood changes with **bipolar I disorder** highlighted.

MANIA

Mania is one of the primary symptoms of bipolar disorders. It is recognized by an elevated, expansive, or irritable mood. Mania is easily recognized by the cognitive changes that occur. Elevated self-esteem is expressed as **grandiosity** (exaggerating personal importance) and may range from unusual self-confidence to grandiose delusions. Speech is pressured; the person is more talkative than usual and at times is difficult to interrupt. There is often a flight of ideas (illogical connections between thoughts) or racing thoughts. Distractibility increases.

> **KEYCONCEPT** **Mania** is primarily characterized by an abnormally and persistently elevated, expansive, or irritable mood.

In mania, the need for sleep is decreased and energy is increased. The individual often remains awake for long periods or wakes up several times at night full of energy. Initially, there is an increase in goal-directed activity that is purposeful (e.g., cleaning the house), but it deteriorates into hyperactivity, agitation, and disorganized behavior. Social activities, occupational functioning, and interpersonal relationships are eventually impaired. There can be excessive involvement in pleasurable activities with little regard for painful consequences (e.g., excessive spending, risky sexual behavior, drug or alcohol abuse) (Box 20.1). Persons with mania are often hospitalized to prevent self-harm.

Even though mania is primarily associated with bipolar disorders, other psychiatric disorders, including schizophrenia, schizoaffective disorder, anxiety disorders, some personality disorders (borderline personality disorder and histrionic personality disorder), substance abuse involving stimulants, and adolescent conduct disorders, may have symptoms that mimic a manic episode. Mania can also be caused by medical disorders or their treatments, certain metabolic abnormalities, neurologic disorders, central nervous system (CNS) tumors, and medications.

Mood lability is the term used for the rapid shifts in moods that often occur in bipolar disorder. One month a person is happy and the next he or she is in the depths of depression. These mood shifts leave everyone around the person confused and interfere with social interaction.

BOX 20.1 CLINICAL VIGNETTE

The Patient with Mania

George was a day trader on the stock market. Initially, he was quite successful and, as a result, upgraded his lifestyle with a more expensive car; a larger, more luxurious house; and a boat. When the stock market declined dramatically, George continued to trade, saying that if he could just find the "right" stock he could earn back all of the money he had lost. He spent his days and nights in front of his computer screen, taking little or no time to eat or sleep. He defaulted on his mortgage and car and boat payments and was talking nonstop to his wife. She brought him to the hospital for evaluation.

What Do You Think?
- What behavioral symptoms of mania does George exhibit?
- What cognitive symptoms of mania does George exhibit?

TABLE 20.1	BIPOLAR AND RELATED DISORDERS
Disorder	**Description**
Bipolar I	Manic episode that may be followed by or preceded by a depressive or hypomanic state.
Bipolar II	Lifetime experience of at least one episode of major depression and one hypomanic episode.
Cyclothymic	Hypomanic and depressive periods for at least 2 years (children, 1 year) without meeting criteria of bipolar I or II disorder.
Substance abuse, prescription/medical associated with manic-like symptoms	Other conditions that might cause the manic symptoms

> **KEYCONCEPT** Mood lability is alterations in moods with little or no change in external events.

Rapid cycling is an extreme form of mood lability that can occur in bipolar disorders. In its most severe form, rapid cycling includes continuous cycling between subthreshold mania and depression or hypomania and depression.

BIPOLAR DISORDERS

Bipolar and related disorders are characterized by periods of mania or hypomania that alternate with depression. These disorders are further classified as bipolar I, bipolar II, and cyclothymic disorder, depending on the severity of the manic and depressive symptoms. Bipolar disorder may also be related to substance abuse, prescription use, or a medical condition. See Table 20.1.

BIPOLAR I DISORDER

Bipolar I disorder is the classic manic-depressive disorder with mood swings alternating from depressed to manic. Although the depression component is similar to that experienced in a major depressive disorder, in this disorder there is also a distinct period (of at least 1 week or less if hospitalized) of abnormally and persistently elevated, expansive, or irritable mood with abnormally increased goal-directed behavior or energy (American Psychiatric Association [APA], 2013). An **elevated mood** can be expressed as **euphoria** (exaggerated feelings of well-being) or **elation** (feeling "high," "ecstatic," "on top of the world," or "up in the clouds"). An **expansive mood** is characterized by lack of restraint in expressing feelings; an overvalued sense of self-importance; and a constant and indiscriminate enthusiasm for interpersonal, sexual, or occupational interactions.

For some people, an irritable mood instead of an elevated mood is pervasive during mania. Such individuals are easily annoyed and provoked to anger, particularly when their wishes are challenged or thwarted. Maintaining social relationships during these episodes is difficult.

> ### Consider Christine
> When Christine is brought to the hospital, she is experiencing grandiose delusions. She believes that she is starting a business. She has spent a large amount of money over a short period of time on clothes and jewelry. Her neighbors report that she has been selling household goods in her yard. Her mood is labile. She is loud and condescending toward staff members. She has push of speech and flight of ideas.

Clinical Course

Bipolar I disorder is a chronic cyclic disorder. Those with an earlier onset have more frequent episodes than persons who develop the illness later in life. An early onset and a family history of illness are associated with multiple episodes or continuous symptoms. Symptoms of the illness can be unpredictable and variable. Bipolar I disorder can lead to severe functional impairment such as alienation from family, friends, and coworkers; indebtedness; job

> ## FAME & FORTUNE
>
> ### Vincent Van Gogh (1853–1890)
> *Post-Impressionist Artist*
>
> **PUBLIC PERSONA**
> Vincent Van Gogh, born in Holland, was the son of a pastor and grew up to be one of the most important artists in Western culture. His works are found in museums worldwide.
>
> **PERSONAL REALITIES**
> As a child, Van Gogh lacked self-confidence and was described as highly emotional. As an adult, he was unsuccessful in relationships and was unable to maintain friendships. His moods vacillated between high-energy periods, when he would produce his multiple works, followed by exhaustion and then depression. Because of his mood lability, many believe that he had bipolar disorder. He also had episodes of psychosis, delusions, and seizures. During one of his episodes, he cut off a lobe of his left ear. Ultimately, he committed suicide at a young age.

loss; divorce; and other problems of living (Lee, Tsang, Kessler, Jin, Sampson, Andrade et al., 2010).

Diagnostic Criteria

To be diagnosed with bipolar I diorder, at least one manic episode or mixed episode and a depressive episode have to occur. See Key Diagnostic Characteristics 20.1. The

---

KEY DIAGNOSTIC CRITERIA 20.1 • BIPOLAR I DISORDER 296.XX

296.4X—BIPOLAR I, CURRENT OR MOST RECENT EPISODE MANIC
296.4X—BIPOLAR I, CURRENT OR MOST RECENT EPISODE HYPOMANIC
296.4X—BIPOLAR I, CURRENT OR MOST RECENT EPISODE DEPRESSED

Diagnostic Criteria

The essential feature of a manic episode is a distinct period during which there is an abnormally, persistently elevated, expansive, or irritable mood and persistently increased activity or energy that is present for most of the day, nearly every day, for a period of at least 1 week (or any duration if hospitalization is necessary), accompanied by at least three additional symptoms from Criterion B. If the mood is irritable rather than elevated or expansive, at least four Criterion B symptoms must be present.

Manic Episode

A. A distinct period of abnormally and persistently elevated, expansive, or irritable mood and abnormally and persistently increased goal-directed activity or energy, lasting at least 1 week and present most of the day, nearly every day (or any duration if hospitalization is necessary).

B. During the period of mood disturbance and increased energy or activity, three (or more) of the following symptoms (four if the mood is only irritable) are present to a

significant degree and represent a noticeable change from usual behavior:

1. Inflated self-esteem or grandiosity.
2. Decreased need for sleep (e.g., feels rested after only 3 hours of sleep).
3. More talkative than usual or pressure to keep talking.
4. Flight of ideas or subjective experience that thoughts are racing.
5. Distractibility (i.e., attention too easily drawn to unimportant or irrelevant external stimuli), as reported or observed.
6. Increase in goal-directed activity (either socially, at work or school, or sexually) or psychomotor agitation (i.e., purposeless non-goal-directed activity).
7. Excessive involvement in activities that have a high potential for painful consequences (e.g., engaging in unrestrained buying sprees, sexual indiscretions, or foolish business investments).

term mixed episode is used when mania and depression occur at the same time, which leads to extreme anxiety, agitation, and irritability. These individuals are clearly miserable and are at high risk for suicide.

Bipolar I Disorder Across the Life-Span

Children and Adolescents

Bipolar disorder in children has been recognized only recently. Although it has not been well studied, depression usually appears first. Somewhat different than in adults, the hallmark of childhood bipolar disorder is intense rage. Children may display seemingly unprovoked rage episodes for as long as 2 to 3 hours. The symptoms of bipolar disorder reflect the developmental level of the child. Children younger than 9 years exhibit more irritability and emotional lability; older children exhibit more classic symptoms, such as euphoria and grandiosity. The first contact with the mental health system often occurs when the behavior becomes disruptive, possibly 5 to 10 years after its onset. These children often have other psychiatric disorders, such as attention deficit hyperactivity disorder or conduct disorder (Chen, M. H., Sun, Chen, Y. S., Chang, et al., 2013; Wozniak, Faraone, Mick, Monuteaux, Coville, & Biederman, 2010). See Chapter 28.

Older Adults

Older adults with bipolar disorder have more neurologic abnormalities and cognitive disturbances (confusion and disorientation) than do younger patients. The incidence of mania decreases with age, but the onset of bipolar disorder can also occur in older adults. Symptoms are similar to the earlier onset bipolar disorder (Forester, Ajilore, Spino, & Lehmann, 2015). See Chapter 29.

Epidemiology and Risk Factors

Risk factors for bipolar disorders include a family history of mood disorders; prior mood episodes; lack of social support; stressful life events; substance use; and medical problems, particularly chronic or terminal illnesses (Theodoridou, Heckeren, Dvorsky, Metzler, Franscini, Hoker, et al., 2014).

Age of Onset

Bipolar disorder has a lifetime prevalence of 1.1% for bipolar I and 1.4% for bipolar II (Kessler, Petukhova, Sampson, Zaslavsky, & Wittchen, 2012). Most patients with bipolar disorder experience significant symptoms before age 25 years. The estimated mean age of onset is between 21 and 30 years. Nearly 20% of those with bipolar disorder, however, have symptoms before the age of 19 years. Estimates of the prevalence of bipolar disorder

in older adults decline with age (Byers, Yaffe, Covinsky, Friedman, & Bruce, 2010).

Gender

Although no significant gender differences have been found in the incidence of bipolar I and II disorders diagnoses, gender differences have been reported in phenomenology, course, and treatment response. In addition, some data show that female patients with bipolar disorder are at greater risk for depression and rapid cycling than are male patients, but male patients are at greater risk for manic episodes.

Ethnicity and Culture

No significant differences have been found based on race or ethnicity (Perron, Fries, Kilbourne, Vaughn, & Bauer, 2010).

Comorbidity

The two most common comorbid conditions are anxiety disorders (panic disorder and social phobia are the most prevalent) and substance use (most commonly alcohol and marijuana). Individuals with a comorbid anxiety disorder are more likely to experience a more severe course. A history of substance use further complicates the course of illness and results in less chance for remission and poorer treatment compliance (Kessler et al., 2012; Kenneson, Fundeburk, & Maisto, 2013).

Etiology

The etiology of mood disorders is unknown, but the current thinking is that bipolar disorder results when an interaction exists between the genetic predisposition and psychosocial stress such as abuse or trauma (Hashimoto, 2010; Liu, 2010).

Biologic Theories

Chronobiologic Theories

Sleep disturbance is common in individuals with bipolar disorder, especially mania. Sleep patterns appear to be regulated by an internal biologic clock center in the hypothalamus. Artificially induced sleep deprivation is known to precipitate mania in some patients with bipolar disorder. It is possible that circadian dysregulation underlies the sleep–wake disturbances of bipolar disorder. Seasonal changes in light exposure also trigger affective episodes in some patients, typically depression in winter and hypomania in the summer in the northern hemisphere (Salvatore, Indic, Murray, & Baldessarini, 2012).

Genetic Factors

Results from family, adoption, and twin studies indicate that bipolar disorder is highly heritable. Studies of monozygotic twins show risks from 40% to 90% of acquiring the illness if their identical twin has the disorder range (Craddock & Sklar, 2009). No one gene or sequence of genes is responsible for the pathology of bipolar disorder. Evidence suggests that the genetic etiologies of schizophrenia and bipolar disorders overlap (Lee, Ripke, Faraone, Purcell, Purcell, S. M., and the members of the Cross-Border Disorder Group of the Pschiatric Genomics Consortium, 2013).

Chronic Stress and Kindling

The role of an allostatic load or wear and tear on the body (see Chapter 12) is thought to contribute to cognitive impairment, comorbidity, and eventual mortality of those with bipolar disorder (Vieta, Popovic, Rosa, Sole, Grande, Frey, et al., 2013). In this model, bipolar disorder is viewed as a disorder where the allostatic load increases as the number of mood episodes increases, which increases physical and mental health problems. An interaction between stress and brain development is viewed as dynamic; individuals have different kinds of stress adaptation depending on their neurobiologic responses (Brietzke, Mansur, Soczynska, Powell, & McIntyre, 2012).

A closely related concept is the kindling theory that posits that as genetically predisposed individuals experience repetitive subthreshold stressors at vulnerable times, mood symptoms of increasing intensity and duration occur. Eventually, a full-blown depressive or manic episode erupts. Each episode leaves a trace and increases the person's vulnerability or sensitizes the person to have another episode with less stimulation. In later episodes, there may be little or no stress may occur before the depression or mania. The disorder takes on a life of its own, and over time, the time between episodes decreases (Bender & Alloy, 2011).

Psychological and Social Theories

Psychosocial theories are useful in planning recovery-oriented interventions that focus on reducing environmental stress and trauma in genetically vulnerable individuals. It is now generally accepted that psychosocial and environmental events contribute to the severity of the disorder and the frequency of the mood episodes (Bender & Alloy, 2011). Two promising theories are currently receiving research support.

The *behavioral approach system dysregulation* theory proposed that individuals with bipolar disorder are overly sensitive and overreact to relevant cues when approaching a reward. That is, the intensity of the goal-motivated behavior can lead to manic symptoms such as euphoria, decreased need for sleep, and excessive self-confidence. Conversely, the system can be deactivated and lead to depressive symptoms such as decreased energy, hopelessness, and sadness (Bender & Alloy, 2011).

The *social rhythm disruption theory* is consistent with the research on the impact of the circadian rhythm dysregulation previously discussed. In our society, usually patterned social events occur, such as meal times, exercise times, and regular companionship. Individuals with bipolar disorder have fewer regular social rhythms than those without bipolar disorder. This theory suggests that when patterned social events are disrupted, mood swings are more likely to appear (Bender & Alloy, 2011).

Family Response to Disorder

Bipolar disorder can devastate families, who often feel that they are on an emotional merry-go-round, particularly if they have difficulty understanding the mood shifts. A major problem for family members is dealing with the consequences of impulsive behavior during manic episodes, such as taking on excessive debt, assault charges, and sexual infidelities.

> ### Remember Christine?
> Christine has been married for 2 years to Karl, who was unaware of her bipolar disorder. He believed that she used to take antidepressants, but that she no longer needed them. Her episode at the airport occurred when he was out of town. He is concerned about her health and their new financial obligations.

Teamwork and Collaboration: Working toward Recovery

An important recovery goal is to minimize or prevent both manic and depressive episodes, which tend to accelerate over time. The fewer the episodes, the more likely the person can live a fully productive life. Patients with bipolar disorder have a complex set of issues and have the best chance of recovery by working with an interdisciplinary team. Nurses, physicians, social workers, psychologists, and activity therapists all have valuable expertise. For children with bipolar disorder, schoolteachers and counselors are included in the team. For older adult patients, the primary care physician becomes part of the team. Helping the patient and family to learn about the disorder and manage it throughout a lifetime is critical for recovery.

The primary treatment modalities are medications, psychotherapy, education, and support. Mood stabilizers and antipsychotics are the mainstay medications in the treatment of bipolar disorders. Mood stabilizers are discussed later in this chapter. Antipsychotics are discussed in Chapter 21. Long-term psychotherapy may help prevent symptoms by reducing the stresses that trigger episodes and increasing the patient's acceptance of the need for medication. Patients should be encouraged to keep their appointments with the therapist, be honest and open, do the assigned homework, and give the therapist feedback on whether the treatment is effective.

Safety Issues

During a manic episode, patient safety is a priority. Risk of suicide is always present for those having a depressive or manic episode. During a depressive episode, the patient may believe that life is not worth living. During a manic episode, the patient may believe that he or she has supernatural powers, such as the ability to fly.

During a manic episode, poor judgment and impulsivity lead to risk-taking behaviors that can have dire consequences for the patient and family. For example, when one patient gambled all of his family's money away, he blamed his partner for letting him have access to the money. A physical confrontation with the partner resulted.

As patients recover from a manic episode, they may be so devastated by the consequences of their impulsive behavior and poor judgment during the episode that suicide seems like the only option.

Consider Christine's history of poor judgment during a manic episode:

Christine has a history of bipolar disorder. She left her first husband and their two children during her third manic episode. At that time, Christine went to Hawaii and stayed there for several months without informing her family of her whereabouts. She was homeless most of the time.

Evidence-Based Nursing Care of Persons with Bipolar Disorder

The nursing care of patients with a bipolar disorder is one of the most interesting yet greatest challenges in psychiatric nursing. In general, the behavior of patients with bipolar disorder is normal between mood episodes. The nurse's first contact with the patient is usually during a manic or depressive episode (see Nursing Care Plan 20.1, available at http://thepoint.lww.com/BoydEssentials).

Mental Health Nursing Assessment

Recovery-oriented nursing care begins with the initial assessment through engaging the patient in a partnership

---

BOX 20.2

Research for Best Practice: Promoting Choice for People with Bipolar Disorder

Jones, M., & Jones, A. (2008). Promotion of choice in the care of people with bipolar disorder: A mental health nursing perspective. Journal of Psychiatric & Mental Health Nursing, 15(2), 87–92.

THE QUESTION: What key issues arise with persons diagnosed with bipolar disorder?

METHODS: This case study was a detailed account of interviews with a person who was hospitalized for 4 weeks for bipolar mania.

FINDINGS: The nurse and the patient have negotiated throughout the 4 weeks to reach the best medication regimen. The nurse has found that partnering with the patient and promoting a shared decision-making approach was important in reducing the symptoms and focusing on recovery. A multidisciplinary approach is recommended.

IMPLICATIONS FOR NURSING: Promoting patient choice in treatment selection results in the successful reduction of symptoms and helps the patient learn to manage the illness.

---

and empowering the person to make decisions in setting overall goals of care (Box 20.2). During acute episodes, the patient's judgment may be impaired, but as the manic or depressive symptoms subside, the person will be able to participate in care decisions.

Physical Health Assessment

The physical health assessment should follow the process explained in Chapter 9. Target assessment symptoms include the changes and severity of activity, eating, and sleep patterns. The patient may not sleep, resulting in irritability and physical exhaustion. Diet and body weight usually change during a manic or depressive episode. Laboratory studies, such as thyroid function and electrolytes, should be completed to detect evidence of malnutrition and fluid imbalance. Abnormal thyroid functioning can be responsible for the mood and behavioral disturbances. In mania, patients often become hypersexual and engage in risky sexual practices. Changes in sexual practices should be included in the assessment.

A careful assessment of current medications is important in determining physical status. Many times, manic or depressive episodes occur after patients stop taking their medication. Exploring reasons for discontinuing the medication will help in planning adherence strategies in the future. Some stop taking their medications because of side effects; others do not believe they have a mental disorder. The use of alcohol and other substances should be carefully assessed. Usually, a drug screen is ordered. In some instances, patients have been taking an antidepressant as prescribed for depression without realizing that a bipolar disorder existed.

Psychosocial Assessment

The psychosocial assessment should follow the process explained in Chapter 9. Individuals with bipolar disorder can usually participate fully in this part of the assessment.

Mood

By definition, bipolar disorder is a disturbance of mood. If the patient is depressed, using an assessment tool for depression may help determine the severity of depression. If mania predominates, evaluating the quality of the mood (e.g., elated, grandiose, irritated, or agitated) becomes important. Usually, mania is diagnosed by clinical observation.

Cognition

In a depressive episode, an individual may not be able to concentrate enough to complete cognitive tasks, such as those called for in a mental status assessment. During the acute phase of a manic or depressive episode, mental status may be abnormal, and in a manic phase, judgment is impaired by extremely rapid, disjointed, and distorted thinking. Moreover, feelings such as grandiosity can interfere with executive functioning. See Box 20.3.

Thought Disturbances

Psychosis commonly occurs in patients with bipolar disorder, especially during acute episodes of mania. Auditory hallucinations and delusional thinking are part of the clinical picture. In children and adolescents, however, psychosis is not so easily disclosed.

Stress and Coping

Stress and coping are critical assessment areas for a person with bipolar disorder. A stressful event often triggers a manic or depressive episode. In some instances, no particular stressors had preceded the episode, although it is important to discuss the possibility. Determining the patient's usual coping skills for stresses lays the groundwork for developing interventional strategies. Negative coping skills, such as substance use or aggression, should be identified because these skills need to be replaced with positive coping skills.

Risk Assessment

Persons with bipolar disorder are at high risk for injury to themselves and others, with 23-26% attempting suicide. People with bipolar disorder account for 3.4–14% of all suicide deaths with self-poisoning and hanging being the most common methods (Schaffer et al., 2015). Child abuse, spouse abuse, or other violent behaviors may occur during severe manic or depressive episodes; thus, patients should be assessed for suicidal or homicidal risk. Additionally, they are high risk for comorbid mental disorders such as substance abuse and anxiety disorders. Significant risks for cardiovascular and metabolic disease are found in this group (Vancampfort, Vansteelandt, Correll, Mitchell, D Heerdt, Sienart, et al., 2013). Smoking is also a major health hazard (Thomson, Berle, Dodd, Rapado-Cantro, Quirk, Ellegaard, et al., 2015).

Social and Occupational Functioning

One of the tragedies of bipolar disorder is its effect on social and occupational functioning. Cultural views of mental illness influence the patient's acceptance of the disorder. During illness episodes, patients often behave in ways that jeopardize their social relationships. Losing a job and going through a divorce are common events. When performing an assessment of social function, the nurse should identify changes resulting from a manic or depressive episode.

Strength Assessment

The nurse should always be listening for thoughts, feelings or behaviors that could be identified as strengths. For example, one patient recognized an increase in drinking alcohol as a sign that he was beginning a manic episode and made an appointment with a health care provider.

BOX 20.3

The Personal Experience of Mania

Sam is a 35 year-old man who was diagnosed with bipolar disorder 10 years ago. He is now being successfully treated and has insight into his disorder. In a recent discussion with his close friend, he describes his personal experience of mania.

At first, I started having more energy and felt happy most of the time. I decided to date a couple of women because I thought my girlfriend Jill was rather boring. Within a couple of weeks, I started sleeping less, but I thought that meant I could do more things. I decided to go back to school to be a scientist— thought I could save the world. I started to apply to graduate school and became very upset when I was told that I did not have the prerequisites for biochemistry. I was so mad that I started threatening the admissions counselor who in turn called the police. My family was called. They convinced the police that I would not bother the school again. After that I started drinking and smoking pot. I had periods of confusion and my family said I became disoriented. There is a lot I don't remember. Eventually, I was hospitalized and started on medication.

WHAT DO YOU THINK?

- At what point could have an early intervention prevented Sam from progressing to a major manic episode?
- Why does Sam not remember the complete manic episode?

The following questions may be used to determine a person's strength.

- What healthy behaviors do you routinely practice?
- Are there any cues that a manic or depressive episode will occur?
- Who provides emotional support to you?
- What do you do to relax? Manage stress?
- What makes you feel good when you are on medication?
- How do you remember to take your medications?

Nursing Diagnoses

Potential nursing diagnoses for persons with bipolar disorder include Sleep Deprivation; Imbalanced Nutrition; Hypothermia, Deficient Fluid Volume; and Non-adherence if patients have stopped taking their medication. Disturbed Personal Identity, Disturbed Sensory Perception, Disturbed Thought Processes, Defensive Coping, Risk for Suicide, Risk for Violence, Ineffective Coping are also potential nursing diagnoses. If patients are in the depressive phase of illness, the previously discussed diagnoses for depression should be considered. If the disorder has had an impact on social and occupational functioning, other diagnoses might be Ineffective Role Performance, Interrupted Family Processes, Impaired Social Interaction, Impaired Parenting, and Compromised Family Coping.

Therapeutic Relationship

Interacting with a person with mania is interesting and, at times, exhausting. The individual often quickly jumps from subject to subject and is usually unable to sit still. When in a manic state, the individual can be very engaging and intense. Their stories may be very grandiose. The nurse should acknowledge the verbal content but recognize that many of the thoughts, feelings, and behaviors are symptomatic of mania and then try to re-focus the patient. If a person is in a depressive state, the nurse should use the same approach as when caring for a person with a depressed disorder as discussed in Chapter 19.

People with mania are typically impatient with others and may express irritability at someone's perceived incompetence and lack of understanding of their special powers. When interacting with a person with bipolar disorder, the nurse should remain calm and avoid any arguments. This is not the time to confront the person about his or her unrealistic perceptions of his or her status. For example, one agitated person was convinced that he owned a hotel. The nurse acknowledged how difficult it must be to have such responsibilities. He agreed with her and subsequently became less agitated. See Box 20.4.

BOX 20.4

Interacting with a Person with Mania

- Use a calm nonthreatening approach.
- Be direct and use simple commands (e.g., time for lunch, let's go to group).
- Avoid open-ended sentences; redirect conversation if flight of ideas occur
- Avoid confrontation and arguments.
- Limit interaction time and recognize the patient's need for space and movement.
- Do not place demands on patient that may be interpreted as excessive.

In some instances, a person who has mania cannot sit still long enough to have a meaningful interaction. The nurse can initiate a conversation while walking with the patient, but there will be times when the nurse needs to give the patient space to avoid increasing agitation.

A therapeutic relationship can actually be instrumental in preventing a relapse. When a person is in the depths of a depression or the height of mania, therapeutic interaction is critical in helping the person take steps in recovery from either the depression or mania. However often long periods of time pass when the affected person is living comfortably with bipolar disorder and attending to other issues. The periods of stable mental health are perfect times to focus on stress reduction, illness management, and relapse prevention.

Nursing Interventions

Self-Care

In a state of mania, the patient's physical needs are rest, adequate hydration and nutrition, and reestablishment of physical well-being. Self-care has usually deteriorated. For a patient unable to sit long enough to eat, snacks and high-energy foods that can be eaten while moving should be provided. Consumption of alcohol should be avoided. Sleep hygiene is a priority but may not be realistic until medications have taken effect. Limiting stimuli can be helpful in decreasing agitation and promoting sleep.

> **NCLEXNOTE** Protection of patients with mania is always a priority. Ongoing assessment should focus on irritability, fatigue, and the potential for harming self or others.

After the patient's mood stabilizes, the nurse should focus on monitoring changes in physical functioning in sleep or eating behavior and teaching patients to identify antecedents to mood episodes such as a family argument or a financial problem. Strategies for dealing with future events can then be identified. The patient can begin to problem solve the best approach for future episodes.

A regular sleep routine should be maintained if possible. High-risk times for manic episodes, such as changes

BOX 20.5 • THERAPEUTIC DIALOGUE • Instilling Hope

Christine is sitting in the dayroom of an inpatient unit with tears in her eyes. She is acknowledges that she has bipolar disorder and wishes that she had been taking her medication and told her husband about her previous relapses.

INEFFECTIVE APPROACH

Nurse: Christine, I am glad that you realize that you have bipolar disorder and want to take your medication. You must commit to staying on your medicine.

Christine: No one understands what it is like to have this problem. I don't quite understand how this little pill and seeing a shrink will help.

Nurse: Well, medication and therapy will help.

Christine: You don't know what I am talking about.

EFFECTIVE APPROACH

Nurse: Christine, I hope that you are feeling better.

Christine: No one understands what it is like to have this problem. I don't quite understand how this little pill and seeing a shrink will help.

Nurse: Let's talk about it. What does it feel like to have bipolar disorder?

Christine: Sometimes it is wonderful—on top of the world, but after the mood goes away, having this problem is terrible. The bad times outweigh the good feelings.

Nurse: Other people have said the same thing. Many people decide to take their medication and "check in" with a mental health provider in order to stay on track and avoid the bad times that can happen after a manic period.

Christine: Really?

Nurse: There are many successful people who have bipolar disorder who find that taking medication helps keep order in their life. I can give you information about a support group.

Christine: Ok, I'm willing to try.

Nurse: Now, what about this medication. Are you willing to try it also? This medication is an effective treatment for bipolar disorder and has helped others to control moods.

Christine: Okay, but I want to know more about this medication.

Nurse: It's a deal. We can spend some time talking about your medications after dinner.

CRITICAL THINKING CHALLENGE

- How did the nurse block communication with Christine in the first scenario? Did she seem hopeful after the interaction?

- How did the nurse instill hope in Christine in the second scenario?

in work schedule (day to night), should be avoided if possible. Patients should be encouraged to monitor the amount of their sleep each night and report decreases in sleep of longer than 1 hour per night because this may be a precursor to a manic episode.

Highlighting the recovery concept of hope will support the person who has had multiple episodes and is frustrated with the impact of several episodes (Box 20.5). In educating persons with bipolar disorder, the nonlongitudinal nature of the disorders should be emphasized.

Medications

Medications are essential in bipolar disorder to achieve two goals: rapid control of symptoms and prevention of future episodes or, at least, reduction in their severity and frequency.

Mood-Stabilizing Drugs

The mainstays of pharmacotherapy are the mood-stabilizing drugs, including lithium carbonate (Lithium), divalproex sodium (Depakote), and lamotrigine (Lamictal). Equetro (an extended release formulation of carbamazepine) is the only formulation of this medication FDA approved for acute mania and mixed episodes. Antidepressant therapy is not recommended in persons with bipolar depression because of a risk of switching from depression to mania.

Lithium Carbonate. Lithium is the most widely used mood stabilizer (Box 20.6). Combined response rates from five studies demonstrate that 70% of patients experienced at least partial improvement with lithium therapy. However, for many patients, lithium is not a fully adequate treatment for all phases of the illness, and particularly during the acute phase, supplemental use of

BOX 20.6
Drug Profile: Lithium Carbonate

DRUG CLASS: Mood stabilizer

RECEPTOR AFFINITY: Alters sodium transport in nerve and muscle cells, increases norepinephrine uptake and serotonin receptor sensitivity, slightly increases intraneuronal stores of catecholamines, and delays some second messenger systems. Mechanism of action is unknown.

INDICATIONS: Treatment and prevention of manic episodes in bipolar affective disorder

ROUTES AND DOSAGE: 150-, 300-, and 600-mg capsules. Lithobid, 300-mg slow-release tablets; Eskalith CR, 450-mg controlled-release tablets; lithium citrate, 300-mg/5 mL liquid form

Adult: In acute mania, optimal response is usually 600 mg tid or 900 mg bid. Obtain serum levels twice weekly in acute phase. Do not rely on serum levels alone. Maintenance: Use lowest possible dose to alleviate symptoms and maintain serum level of 0.6–1.2 mEq/L. In uncomplicated maintenance, obtain serum levels every 2–3 months. Monitor patient's side effects.

Geriatric: Increased risk for toxic effects; use lower doses; monitor frequently.

Children: 6 to 12 years:15 to 60 mg/kg/day in 3 to 4 divided doses.

HALF-LIFE (PEAK EFFECT): Mean, 24 h (peak serum levels in 1–4 h). Steady state reached in 5–7 d.

SELECTED ADVERSE REACTIONS: Weight gain

WARNING: Avoid use during pregnancy or while breastfeeding. Hepatic or renal impairments increase plasma concentration.

SPECIFIC PATIENT/FAMILY EDUCATION
- Avoid alcohol and other CNS depressant drugs.
- Notify your prescriber if pregnancy is possible or planned. Do not breastfeed while taking this medication.
- Notify your prescriber before taking any other prescriptions, OTC medications, or herbal supplements.
- May impair judgment, thinking, or motor skills; avoid driving or other hazardous tasks.
- Do not abruptly discontinue use.

bid, twice a day; CNS, central nervous system; OTC, over the counter; tid, three times a day.

TABLE 20.2	LITHIUM BLOOD LEVELS AND ASSOCIATED SIDE EFFECTS
Plasma Level	**Side Effects or Symptoms of Toxicity**
<1.5 mEq/L Mild side effects	Metallic taste in mouth
	Fine hand tremor (resting)
	Nausea
	Polyuria
	Polydipsia
	Diarrhea or loose stools
	Muscular weakness or fatigue
	Weight gain
	Edema
	Memory impairments
1.5–2.5 mEq/L Moderate toxicity	Severe diarrhea
	Dry mouth
	Nausea and vomiting
	Mild-to-moderate ataxia
	Incoordination
	Dizziness, sluggishness, giddiness, vertigo
	Slurred speech
	Tinnitus
	Blurred vision
	Increasing tremor
	Muscle irritability or twitching
	Asymmetric deep tendon reflexes
	Increased muscle tone
>2.5 mEq/L Severe toxicity	Cardiac arrhythmias
	Blackouts
	Nystagmus
	Coarse tremor
	Fasciculations
	Visual or tactile hallucinations
	Oliguria, renal failure
	Peripheral vascular collapse
	Confusion
	Seizures
	Coma and death

antipsychotics and benzodiazepines is often beneficial. Lithium is poorly tolerated in at least one third of treated patients and has a narrow gap between therapeutic and toxic concentrations (Freeman, Wiegand, & Gelenberg, 2011) (Table 20.2). Response to lithium is associated with genome variations (Chen, Lee, C. S., Lee, M. T., Ouyang, Chen, Chong, et al., 2014).

NCLEXNOTE Monitoring blood levels of lithium carbonate and divalproex sodium is an ongoing nursing assessment for patients receiving these medications. Side effects of mood stabilizers vary.

Lithium is a salt; the interaction between lithium levels and sodium levels in the body and the relationship between lithium levels and fluid volume in the body remain crucial issues in its safe, effective use. The higher the sodium levels, the lower the lithium level will be and vice versa. Thus, changes in dietary sodium intake can affect lithium blood levels that, in turn, may affect therapeutic results or increase the incidence and severity of side effects. The same principle applies to fluid volume. If body fluid decreases significantly because of hot weather, strenuous exercise, vomiting, diarrhea, or drastic reduction in fluid intake for any reason, then lithium levels can rise sharply, causing an increase in side effects, progressing to lethal lithium toxicity. The key is to start with a lower dose and then increase it slowly to maximize the therapeutic response and avoid overshooting the therapeutic window. See Table 20.3 for lithium interactions with other drugs. See Chapter 10 for further discussion of lithium's possible mechanisms of action, pharmacokinetics, side effects, and toxicity.

EMERGENCY CARE ALERT ❗ If symptoms of moderate or severe toxicity (e.g., cardiac arrhythmias, blackouts, tremors, seizures) are noted, withhold additional doses of lithium, immediately obtain a blood sample to analyze the lithium level, and push fluids if the patient can take fluids. Contact the physician for further direction about relieving the symptoms.

TABLE 20.3	LITHIUM INTERACTIONS WITH MEDICATIONS AND OTHER SUBSTANCES
Substance	Effect of Interaction
ACE inhibitors, such as: • Captopril • Lisinopril • Quinapril	Increase serum lithium; may cause toxicity and impaired kidney function
Acetazolamide	Increases renal excretion of lithium; decreases lithium levels
Alcohol	May increase serum lithium level
Caffeine	Increases lithium excretion; increases lithium tremor
Carbamazepine	Increases neurotoxicity despite normal serum levels and dosage
Fluoxetine	Increases serum lithium levels
Haloperidol	Increases neurotoxicity despite normal serum levels and dosage
Loop diuretics, such as furosemide	Increase lithium serum levels but may be safer than thiazide diuretics; potassium-sparing diuretics (e.g., amiloride, spirolactone) are safest
Methyldopa	Increases neurotoxicity without increasing serum lithium levels
NSAIDs, such as: • Diclofenac • Ibuprofen • Indomethacin • Piroxicam	Decrease renal clearance of lithium Increase serum lithium levels by 30%–60% in 3–10 days Aspirin and sulindac do not appear to have the same effect
Osmotic diuretics, such as: • Urea • Mannitol • Isosorbide	Increases renal excretion of lithium and decreases lithium levels
Sodium chloride	High sodium intake decreases lithium levels; low sodium diets may increase lithium levels and lead to toxicity
Thiazide diuretics, such as: • Chlorothiazide • Hydrochlorothiazide	Promote sodium and potassium excretion; increase lithium serum levels; may produce cardiotoxicity and neurotoxicity
TCAs	Increases tremor; potentiates pharmacologic effects of tricyclic antidepressants

ACE, angiotensin-converting enzyme; NSAID, nonsteroidal anti-inflammatory drug; TCA, tricyclic antidepressant.

Mild side effects tend to subside or can be managed by nursing measures (Table 20.4).

Divalproex Sodium. Divalproex sodium (Depakote), an anticonvulsant, has a broader spectrum of efficacy and has about equal benefit for patients with pure mania as for those with other forms of bipolar disorder (i.e., mixed mania, rapid cycling, comorbid substance abuse, and secondary mania) (Box 20.7). The recommended initial dose in 750 mg daily, increase as rapidly as possible to achieve therapeutic response or desired plasma level. The maximum recommended dosage is 60 mg/kg/day (Depakote Prescribing Information, 2015). Divalproex is usually initiated at 250 mg twice a day or lower. In the inpatient setting, it can be initiated in Baseline liver function tests and a complete blood count with platelets should be obtained before starting therapy, and patients with known liver disease should not be given divalproex sodium. The black box warns of hepatotoxicity. Optimal blood levels appear to be in the range of 50 to 150 ng/mL. Levels should be obtained weekly until the patient is stable and then every 6 months.

Divalproex sodium is associated with increased risk for birth defects. Cases of life-threatening pancreatitis have been reported in adults and children receiving valproate, both initially and after several years of use. Some cases were described as hemorrhagic, with a rapid progression from onset to death. If pancreatitis is diagnosed, valproate use should be discontinued (Depakote Prescribing Information, 2015).

Carbamazepine (Equetro). Carbamazepine, an anticonvulsant, also has mood-stabilizing effects. Data from various studies suggest that it may be effective in patients who experience no response to lithium. The most common side effects of carbamazepine are dizziness, drowsiness, nausea, and vomiting, which may be avoided with slow incremental dosing. Carbamazepine has a boxed warning for aplastic anemia and agranulocytosis, but frequent clinically unimportant decreases in white blood cell counts also occur. Estimates of the rate of severe blood dyscrasias vary from one 1 in 10,000 patients treated to a more recent estimate of one 1 in 125,000 (Schatzberg & DeBattista, 2015). Mild, nonprogressive elevations of

TABLE 20.4 INTERVENTIONS FOR LITHIUM SIDE EFFECTS

Side Effect	Intervention
Edema of feet or hands	Monitor intake and output of water; check for possible decreased urinary output. Monitor sodium intake. Patient should elevate legs when sitting or lying. Monitor weight.
Fine hand tremor	Provide support and reassurance if it does not interfere with daily activities. Tremor worsens with anxiety and intentional movements; minimize stressors. Notify prescriber if tremor interferes with patient's work so that compliance may be an issue. More frequent smaller doses of lithium may also help.
Mild diarrhea	Take lithium with meals. Provide for fluid replacement. Notify prescriber if it worsens; may need a change in medication preparation or may be early sign of toxicity.
Muscle weakness, fatigue, or memory and concentration difficulties	Provide support and reassurance; this side effect will usually pass after a few weeks of treatment. Short-term memory aids such as lists or reminder calls may be helpful. Notify prescriber if side effect becomes severe or interferes with the patient's desire to continue treatment.
Metallic taste	Suggest sugarless candies or throat lozenges. Encourage frequent oral hygiene.
Nausea or abdominal discomfort	Consider dividing the medication into smaller doses or giving it at more frequent intervals. Give medication with meals.
Polydipsia	Reassure patient that this is a normal mechanism to cope with polyuria.
Polyuria	Monitor intake and output. Provide reassurance and explain the nature of this side effect. Explain that this side effect causes no physical damage to the kidneys.
Toxicity	Withhold medication. Notify prescriber. Use symptomatic treatments.

liver function test results are relatively common. Carbamazepine is associated with increased risk for birth defects.

In patients older than 12 years, carbamazepine is begun at 200 mg once or twice a day. The dosage is increased by no more than 200 mg every 2 to 4 days, to 800 to 1,000 mg a day or until therapeutic levels or effects are achieved. It is important to monitor for blood dyscrasias and liver damage. Liver function tests and complete blood counts with differential are the minimal pretreatment

BOX 20.7

Drug Profile: Divalproex Sodium (Depakote)

DRUG CLASS: Antimania agent

RECEPTOR AFFINITY: Thought to increase level of inhibitory neurotransmitter, GABA, to brain neurons. Mechanism of action is unknown.

INDICATIONS: Mania, epilepsy, migraine.

ROUTES AND DOSAGE: Available in 125-mg delayed-release capsules, and 125-, 250-, and 500-mg enteric-coated tablets.

Adult Dosage: Dosage depends on symptoms and clinical picture presented; initially, the dosage is low and gradually increased depending on the clinical presentation

HALF-LIFE (PEAK EFFECT): 6–16 h (1–4 h)

SELECTED ADVERSE REACTIONS: Sedation, tremor (may be dose related), nausea, vomiting, indigestion, abdominal cramps, anorexia with weight loss, slight elevations in liver enzymes, hepatic failure, thrombocytopenia, transient increases in hair loss

BOXED WARNING: Hepatotoxicity, teratogenicity, pancreatitis

WARNING: Use cautiously during pregnancy and lactation. Contraindicated in patients with hepatic disease or significant hepatic dysfunction. Administer cautiously with salicylates; may increase serum levels and result in toxicity.

SPECIFIC PATIENT AND FAMILY EDUCATION
- Take with food if gastrointestinal upset occurs.
- Swallow tablets or capsules whole to prevent local irritation of mouth and throat.
- Notify your prescriber before taking any other prescription or OTC medications or herbal supplements.
- Avoid alcohol and sleep-inducing OTC products.
- Avoid driving or performing activities that require alertness.
- Do not abruptly discontinue use.
- Keep appointments for follow-up, including blood tests to monitor response.

GABA, gamma-aminobutyric acid; OTC, over the counter.

TABLE 20.5	SELECTED MEDICATION INTERACTIONS WITH CARBAMAZEPINE
Interaction	Drug Interacting With Carbamazepine
Increased carbamazepine levels	Erythromycin Cimetidine Propoxyphene Isoniazid Calcium channel blockers (verapamil) Fluoxetine Danazol Diltiazem Nicotinamide
Decreased carbamazepine levels	Phenobarbital Primidone Phenytoin
Drugs whose levels are decreased by carbamazepine	Oral contraceptives Warfarin, oral anticoagulants Doxycycline Theophylline Haloperidol Divalproex sodium Tricyclic antidepressants Acetaminophen: increased metabolism but also increased risk for hepatotoxicity

laboratory tests and they should be repeated about 1 month after initiating treatment and at 3 months, 6 months, and yearly. Other yearly tests assessments should include electrolytes, blood urea nitrogen, thyroid function tests, urinalysis, and eye examinations. Carbamazepine levels are measured monthly until the patient is on a stable dosage. Studies suggest that blood levels in the range of 8 to 12 ng/mL correspond to therapeutic efficacy. See Table 20.5 for carbamazepine's interactions with other drugs. See Chapter 10 for further discussion of carbamazepine's possible mechanisms of action, pharmacokinetics, side effects, and toxicity.

EMERGENCY CARE ALERT ! Both valproate and carbamazepine may be lethal if high doses are ingested. Toxic symptoms appear in 1 to 3 hours and include neuromuscular disturbances, dizziness, stupor, agitation, disorientation, nystagmus, urinary retention, nausea and vomiting, tachycardia, hypotension or hypertension, cardiovascular shock, coma, and respiratory depression.

Lamotrigine. For a depressive episode, mood stabilizers such as lamotrigine (Lamictal), which requires a dose titration are frequently prescribed (Box 20.8). Lamotrigine is approved by the U.S. Food and Drug Administration (FDA) for the maintenance treatment of bipolar disorder. It may be particularly effective for rapid cycling and in the depressed phase of bipolar illness. If lamotrigine is given with valproic acid (Depakote), the dose should be reduced. Valproic acid decreases the clearance of lam-

otrigine. Lamotrigine does have a "boxed warning" for rash. Nurses should be especially vigilant for the appearance of any rash. If a rash does appear, it is most likely benign. However, it is not possible to predict whether the rash is benign or serious (Stevens-Johnson syndrome).

Antipsychotics
Several atypical antipsychotics that were primarily developed for the treatment of schizophrenia are also FDA approved for treatment of various symptoms of bipolar disorder. See Table 20.6. The dosages for the treatment of patients with bipolar disorder are generally lower than for those for schizophrenia. Recently, these agents have become a mainstay of treatment because they provide some of the broadest efficacy and are more likely used as the only medication to treat bipolar disorder than the mood stabilizers (Stahl, 2013). An overview of antipsychotics is presented in Chapter 10 and they are discussed in detail in Chapter 21.

Administering and Monitoring Medications
During acute mania, patients may not believe that they have a psychiatric disorder and may refuse to take

TABLE 20.6	FDA-APPROVED ANTIPSYCHOTICS FOR THE TREATMENT OF SYMPTOMS OF BIPOLAR DISORDER	
Antipsychotic Agent	FDA Indication for Bipolar Disorder	Adult Dosage
Aripiprazole (Abilify)	Acute treatment of manic and mixed episodes associated with bipolar disorder	10–30 mg per day
Asenapine (Saphris)	Acute treatment of manic or mixed episodes associated with bipolar 1 disorder as monotherapy or adjunctive treatment to lithium or valproate	5–10 mg twice daily
Lurasidone (Latuda)	Depressive episodes associated with Bipolar I disorder as monotherapy or as adjunctive treatment to lithium or valproate	20–120 mg daily with food (comprising 350 calories)
Olanzapine (Zyprexa)	Acute treatment of manic or mixed episodes associated with Bipolar I disorder (monotherapy and in combination with lithium or valproate) and maintenance treatment of Bipolar I disorder	10–15 mg daily
Quetiapine (Seroquel)	Bipolar 1 disorder, manic or mixed episodes; bipolar disorder, depressive episodes	300–800 mg daily
Risperidone (Risperdal)	Bipolar mania, combination of risperiodone with lithium or valproate for short-term treatment of acute manic or mixed episodes associated with Bipolar I disorder	2–6 mg daily
Ziprasidone (Geodon)	Acute manic or mixed episodes associated with bipolar disorder, with or without psychotic features	40–80 mg with food (comprising 500 calories)

FDSA U.S. Food and Drug Administration

medication. Because their energy level is still high, they can be very creative in avoiding medication. Through patience and the development of a trusting relationships, patients will be more likely begin to participate in a shared decision-making process. It is important for patients to have a sense of empowerment and participation in treatment even during the most acute episodes. After patients begin to take medications, symptom improvement should be evident. If a patient is very agitated, a benzodiazepine may be given for a short period.

Managing Side Effects

Patients with bipolar disorder order are usually treated with several medications. Additionally, patients may be taking other "nonpsychiatric" medications. In some instances, one agent is used to augment the effects of another, such as supplemental thyroid hormone to boost antidepressant response in depression. Possible side effects for each medication should be listed and cross-referenced. When a side effect appears, the nurse should document the side effect and notify the prescriber, so that further evaluation can be made. In some instances, medications should be changed.

Monitoring for Drug Interactions

It is a well-established practice to combine mood stabilizers with antidepressants or antipsychotics. The previously discussed drug interactions should be considered when caring for a person with bipolar disorder. One big challenge is monitoring alcohol, drugs, over-the-counter (OTC) medications, and herbal supplements. A complete list of all medications should be maintained and evaluated for any potential interaction.

Promoting Adherence

Adherence to a complex medication regimen over months to years is difficult. Yet, one of the primary reasons that acute symptoms reappear is because of discontinuation of medications. It is important to recognize that taking medication as prescribed over time is difficult. Nurses can help patients and families incorporate taking medications into their lifestyles by developing realistic plans. The use of pill boxes, reminders, and other cues will increase the likelihood of adherence.

Teaching Points

For patients who are taking lithium, it is important to explain that a change in dietary salt intake can affect the therapeutic blood level. If salt intake is reduced, the body will naturally retain lithium to maintain homeostasis. This increase in lithium retention can lead to toxicity. After the patient has been stabilized on a lithium dose, salt intake should remain constant. This is fairly easy to do except during the summer, when excessive perspiration can occur. Patients should increase salt intake during periods of perspiration, increased exercise, and dehydration. Most mood stabilizers and antidepressants can cause weight gain. Patients should be alerted to this potential side effect and should be instructed to monitor any changes in eating, appetite, or weight. Weight reduction techniques may need to be instituted. Patients also should be clearly instructed to check with the nurse or physician before taking any over-the-counter medications, herbal supplements, or any other complementary and alternative treatment approaches.

Other Somatic Therapies

Electroconvulsive therapy (ECT) may be a treatment alternative for patients with severe mania who exhibit unremitting, frenzied physical activity. Other indications for ECT are acute mania that is unresponsive to antimanic agents or high suicide risk. ECT is safe and effective in patients receiving antipsychotic drugs. Use of valproate or carbamazepine will elevate the seizure threshold, requiring some adjustments in treatment.

Psychosocial Interventions

Medications are necessary for treatment of bipolar disorder, but it is only one aspect of recovery. Psychosocial strategies are critical in successful treatment and prevention of relapse. Psychoeducation, individual cognitive behavioral therapy, individual interpersonal therapy, and adjunctive therapies (such as those for substance use) are all recommended psychotherapeutic approaches (Crowe, Whitehead, Wilson, Carlyle, O'Brien, Linder et al., 2010; Hoberg, Vickers, Ericksen, Bauer, Kung, Stone, et al., 2013) (Box 20.9).

Several risk factors associated with bipolar disorders make patients more vulnerable to relapses and resistant to recovery. Among these are high rates of nonadherence to medication therapy, obesity, marital conflict, separation, divorce, unemployment, and underemployment. Even those who take their medication regularly are likely to experience recurrences and have difficulty keeping jobs and maintaining significant relationships.

Important goals of psychosocial interventions are identifying risk factors and developing strategies to address them. It is also important to help the patient understand the disorder and manage the mood lability and dysfunctional thoughts that are often precursors to a manic or depressive episode. The nurse partners with the patient in developing strategies to remember to take medications, identify therapeutic and side effects, and know when and how to contact a clinician. Particularly important are enhancing social and occupational functioning, improving quality of life, increasing the patient and family's acceptance of the disorder, and reducing the suicide risk (Crowe et al., 2010).

Teaching Patients and Family

Psychoeducation is designed to provide information on bipolar disorder and its successful treatment and recovery. The nurse can provide information about the illness and obstacles to recovery. Helping the patient recognize warning signs and symptoms of relapse and to cope with residual symptoms and functional impairment are important interventions. Watching for early warning signs and triggers can mean early treatment. Family members should be included in developing an emergency plan for recognizing and intervening if relapse symptoms occur (Box 20.10).

BOX 20.9

Research for Best Practice: Psychosocial Interventions for People with Bipolar Disorder

Crowe, Whitehead, L., Wilson, L., Carlyle, D., O'Brien, A., Inder, M., et al. (2010). Disorder-specific psychosocial interventions for bipolar disorder—A systematic review of the evidence for mental health nursing practice. International Journal of Nursing Studies, 47(896–908).

THE QUESTION: Are psychosocial interventions for bipolar disorder efficacious for medication adherence?

METHODS: An extensive review of literature using Medline, CINAHL and PsycINFO databases resulted in the selection of 35 relevant research studies.

FINDINGS: Psychopharmacologic-only interventions are not effective for the management of bipolar disorder because of high rates of nonadherence. Group psychoeducation, interpersonal social rhythm therapy, family interventions, and cognitive behavioral therapy are all effective when used as an adjunct to psychotherapy. The common factors of these interventions were that they were all structured and adhered to protocols for up to 2 years.

IMPLICATIONS FOR NURSING: Psychiatric mental health nurses are in excellent position to integrate psychosocial interventions into their clinical practice settings. These interventions require about 2 years to teach the patients the skills that are needed to manage bipolar disorder.

BOX 20.10

Relapse Prevention and Emergency Plan

COMMON INDICATORS FOR RELAPSE

Mania
Reading several books or newspapers at once
Cannot concentrate on one topic
Talking faster than usual
Feeling irritable
Hungry all the time
Friends remark on changes in mood
More energy than usual

Depression
Quit cooking, cleaning, daily chores
Avoid people
Crave foods (e.g., chocolate)
Headaches
Do not care about other people
Sleeping more or restless sleep
People are irritating to be around

EMERGENCY PLAN
Keep a list of emergency contacts (primary health care provider, close family members).
Keep a current list of all medications, including their dosages.
Information about other health problems.
Symptoms that indicate others need to take responsibility for care.
Treatment preferences (who, where, medications, advanced directive location).

In the interest of improved medication adherence, listening carefully to the patient's concerns about the medication, dosing schedules and dose changes, and side effects is helpful. Resistance to accepting the illness and to taking medication, the symbolic meaning of medication taking, and worries about the future can be discussed openly. Health teaching and weight management should be components of any psychoeducation program. In addition to individual variations in body weight, many of the medications (divalproex sodium, lithium, antidepressants, and atypical antipsychotics) are associated with weight gain. Monitoring weight and developing individual weight management plans can reduce the risk of relapse and increase the possibility of medication adherence. Box 20.11 provides a checklist for psychoeducation.

Support Groups

Support groups are helpful for people with this disorder. Participating in groups allows the person to meet others with the same disorder and to learn management and preventive strategies. Support groups also are helpful in dealing with the stigma associated with mental illness.

Interventions for Family Members

Marital and family interventions are often needed at different periods in the life of a person with bipolar disorder. For the family with a child with this disorder, additional parenting skills are needed to manage the behaviors. The goals of family interventions are to help the family understand and cope with the disorder. Interventions may range from occasional counseling sessions to intensive family therapy.

Family psychoeducation strategies have been shown to be particularly useful in decreasing the risk of relapse and hospitalization. The sooner the education is begun, the more effective this approach is (Popovic, Reinares, Scott, Nivoli, Muren, Pacchiarotti, et al., 2013); (Reinares, Sánchez-Moreno, & Fountoulakis, 2014).

Evaluation and Treatment Outcomes

Desired treatment outcomes are stabilization of mood and enhanced quality of life. Primary tools for evaluating outcomes are nursing observation and patient self-report.

Continuum of Care

Inpatient-Focused Care

Inpatient admission is the treatment setting of choice for patients who are severely psychotic or who are an immediate threat to themselves or others. In acute mania, nursing interventions focus on patient safety because patients are prone to injury because of hyperactivity and are often are unaware of injuries they sustain. Distraction may also be effective when a patient is talking or acting inappropriately. Removal to a quieter environment may be necessary if other interventions have not been successful, but the patient should be carefully monitored. During acute mania, patients are often impulsive, disinhibited, and interpersonally inappropriate, so the nurse should avoid direct confrontations or challenges.

During manic phases, patients usually violate others' boundaries. For example, roommate selection for patients requiring hospital admittance needs to be carefully considered. If possible, a private room is ideal because patients with bipolar disorder tend to irritate others, who quickly tire of the intrusiveness. These patients may miss the cues indicating anger and aggression from others. The nurse should protect the patient who is manic from self-harm, as well as harm from other patients.

The length of stay in an inpatient unit will be relatively short, 3 to 5 days. The plan of care will focus on medication management, including control of side effects, initiation or revision of a recovery plan, psychoeducation, and promotion of self-care. Nurses should be familiar with drug–drug interactions and with interventions to help control side effects.

Intensive Outpatient Programs

Intensive outpatient programs for several weeks of acute-phase care during a manic or depressive episode are used when hospitalization is not necessary or to prevent or shorten hospitalization. These programs are usually called partial hospitalization. Close medication monitoring and milieu therapies that foster restoration of a patient's previous adaptive abilities are the major nursing responsibilities in these settings.

Setting up frequent office visits and crisis telephone calls are additional nursing interventions that can help to shorten or prevent hospitalization during the acute phase of a manic episode. Family sessions or psycho-education that includes the patient are alternatives. Severely and persistently ill patients may need ongoing intensive treatment, but the frequency of visits can be decreased for patients whose conditions stabilize and who enter the continuation or the maintenance phase of treatment.

Spectrum of Care

In today's health care climate, with efforts to reduce hospitalization, most patients with bipolar disorder are treated in a community setting. Hospitalizations are usually brief; recovery is emphasized. Medication regimens that promote adherence. Psychoeducation helps in understanding and managing the disorder, and supportive psychotherapy helps these individuals move towards recovery. Patients need extended and continued follow-up to monitor medication trials and side effects, reinforce self-care management, and provide continued psychosocial support.

Mental Health Promotion

Mental health promotion activities should be the focus during remissions. During this period, patients have an opportunity to learn new coping skills that promote positive mental health. Stress management and relaxation techniques can be practiced for use when needed. A plan for managing emerging symptoms can also be developed during this period.

OTHER BIPOLAR AND RELATED DISORDERS

In **bipolar II disorder**, the individual is mostly depressed that this disorder can severely affect their social and occupational life. They have brief periods of elevated, expansive, or irritable moods, but bipolar II disorder is not as easily recognized as bipolar I disorder because the symptoms are less dramatic. **Hypomania**, a mild form of mania, is characteristic of bipolar II disorder. Judgment remains fundamentally intact.

In a **cyclothymic disorder**, hypomanic symptoms occur alternating with numerous periods of depressive symptoms. However, these symptoms are less severe than the bipolar disorders. To be diagnosed with this disorder, the symptoms have to be present for at least 2 years of numerous periods of hypomanic symptoms.

Illicit drug, prescription medications, and some medical conditions such as changes in thyroid functioning can be responsible for manic-like behavior. These symptoms cause significant distress and impairment in social functioning.

SUMMARY OF KEY POINTS

- Bipolar and related disorders are characterized by one or more manic episodes or mixed mania (co-occurrence of manic and depressive states) that cause marked impairment in social activities, occupational functioning, and interpersonal relationships and may require hospitalization to prevent self-harm.

- Bipolar and related disorders are characterized by periods of mania or hypomania that alternate with depression. These disorders are classified as bipolar I disorder, bipolar II disorder, or cyclothymic disorder, depending on the severity of the manic and depressive symptoms. Bipolar disorder may also be related to substance abuse, prescription drug use, or a medical condition.

- Manic episodes are periods in which the individual experiences abnormally and persistently elevated, expansive, or irritable mood characterized by inflated self-esteem, decreased need to sleep, excessive energy or hyperactivity, racing thoughts, easy distractibility, and an inability to stay focused. Other symptoms can include hypersexuality and impulsivity.

- Bipolar disorders are underreported and are often misdiagnosed. Bipolar I disorder is more dramatic than bipolar II disorder so it is easier to diagnosis.

- Genetics plays a role in the etiology of bipolar disorders. Risk factors include a family history of mood disorders; prior mood episodes; lack of social support; stressful life events; substance use; and medical problems, particularly chronic or terminal illnesses.

- Mental health nursing assessment includes assessing mood; speech patterns; thought processes and thought content; suicidal or homicidal thoughts; cognition and memory; and social factors, such as patterns of relationships, quality of support systems, and changes in occupational functioning. Several self-report scales are helpful in evaluating depressive symptoms.

- Many symptoms of bipolar depression, such as weight gain and appetite changes, sleep disturbance, decreased energy, and fatigue, are similar to those of medical illnesses. Assessment includes a thorough medical history and physical examination to detect or rule out medical or psychiatric comorbidity.

- Establishing and maintaining a therapeutic nurse–patient relationship is key to successful outcomes. Shared decision-making with the patient leads to positive outcomes. Recovery-oriented nursing interventions that foster the therapeutic relationship include being available in times of crisis, providing understanding and education to patients and their families regarding goals of treatment and recovery, providing encouragement and feedback concerning the patient's progress, providing guidance in the patient's interpersonal interactions with others and work environment, and helping to set and monitor realistic goals.

■ Pharmacotherapy includes mood stabilizers used alone or in combination with antipsychotics or benzodiazepines to treat psychosis, agitation, or insomnia. Electroconvulsive therapy is a valuable alternative for patients with severe mania that does not respond to other treatment.

■ Recent major advances in bipolar disorder treatment research validate the efficacy of integrated psychosocial and pharmacologic treatment involving family or couples therapies, psychoeducational programs, and individual cognitive behavioral or interpersonal therapies.

■ Psychosocial interventions for bipolar disorders include self-care management, cognitive therapy, behavior therapy, interpersonal therapy, patient and family education regarding the nature of the disorder and treatment goals, marital and family therapy, and group therapy that includes medication maintenance support groups and other consumer-oriented support groups.

CRITICAL THINKING CHALLENGES

1. A patient tells you that he no longer needs medication because he has special powers that protect him from evil forces. He no longer needs sleep and can see things that others do not see. What approaches would you use to help the patient decide to take his medication?

2. Describe how you would approach a patient who is expressing concern that the diagnosis of bipolar disorder will negatively affect her social and work relationships.

3. Your patient with mania is experiencing physical hyperactivity that is interfering with his sleep and nutrition. Describe the actions you would take to meet the patient's needs for rest and nutrition.

4. Prepare a hypothetical discussion with a patient with potential bipolar disorder concerning the advantages and disadvantages of lithium versus divalproex sodium for treatment of bipolar disorder.

5. Think about all of the above situations and relate them to persons from culturally and ethnically diverse populations (e.g., African American, Latino, or Asian descent; Jewish or Jehovah's Witness religions; across the life-span of individuals from children to older adult populations).

Michael Clayton (2007). Arthur Edens (Tom Wilkinson), a successful corporate lawyer, is experiencing the stress of a high-profile legal case and stops taking his medication. Consequently, he has a manic episode with delusions about one of the jurors, who he eventually contacts. The story traces the attempts by his colleague and friend Michael Clayton (George Clooney) to repair the damage Arthur's behavior has caused to the lawsuit and to get his friend treated before his mania further damages his life.

Significance: Viewers can gain insight into the devastating impact of mental illness on the successful career of a well-respected attorney. This film depicts the poor judgment, impulsivity, and consequences of a full-blown mania episode.

Viewing Points: Identify the mania symptoms that Arthur displays. What feelings are evoked when you see the strange behavior that he exhibits? If Arthur were your patient, how would you approach him, and what medication would you expect him to be prescribed?

M●VIE viewing **GUIDES** related to this chapter are available at http://thepoint.lww.com/BoydEssentials.

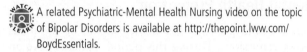 A related Psychiatric-Mental Health Nursing video on the topic of Bipolar Disorders is available at http://thepoint.lww.com/BoydEssentials.

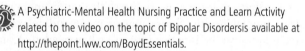 A Psychiatric-Mental Health Nursing Practice and Learn Activity related to the video on the topic of Bipolar Disordersis available at http://thepoint.lww.com/BoydEssentials.

REFERENCES

American Psychiatric Association. (2013). *Diagnostic and statistical manual of mental disorders (5th ed.).* Arlington, VA: Author.

Bender, R. E., & Alloy, L. B. (2011). Life stress and kindling in bipolar disorder: Review of the evidence and integration with emerging biopsychosocial theories. *Clinical Psychology Review, 31*(3), 383–398.

Brietzke, E., Mansur, R. B., Soczynska, J., Powell, A. M., & McIntyre, R. S. (2012). A theoretical framework informing research about the role of stress in the pathophysiology of bipolar disorder. *Progress in Neuro-Psychopharmacology & Biological Psychiatry, 39*(1), 1–8.

Byers, A. L., Yaffe, K., Covinsky, K. E., Friedman, M. B., & Bruce, J. L. (2010). The occurrence of mood and anxiety disorders among older adults. *Archives of General Psychiatry, 67*(5), 489–496.

Chen, C. H., Lee, C. S., Lee, M. T., Ouyang, W. C., Chen, C. C., Chong, M. Y., et al. (2014). Variant GADL1 and response to lithium therapy in bipolar I disorder. *The New England Journal of Medicine, 370*(2), 119–128.

Chen, M. H., Su, T. P., Chen, Y. S., Hsu, J. W., Huang, K. L., Chang, W. H., et al. (2013). Higher risk of developing mood disorders among adolescents with comorbidity of attention deficit hyperactivity disorder and disruptive behavior disorder: A nationwide study. *Journal of Psychiatric Research, 47*(8), 1019–1023.

Craddock, N., & Sklar, P. (2009). Genetics of bipolar disorder: Successful start to a long journey. *Trends in Genetics, 25*(2), 99–105.

Crowe, M., Whitehead, L., Wilson, L., Carlyle, D., O'Brien, A., Inder, M., et al. (2010). Disorder-specific psychosocial interventions for bipolar disorder—A systematic review of the evidence for mental health nursing practice. *International Journal of Nursing Studies, 47*(7), 896–908.

Depakote Presribing Information. (March 2015) http://www.accessdata.fda.gov/drugsatfda_docs/label/2015/018723s054,019680s041lbl.pdf

Forester, B.P., Ajiilore, O., Spino, C., & Lehmann, S. W. (2015). Clinical characteristics of patients with late life bipolar disorder in the community:

Data from the NNDC registry. *American Journal of Geriatric Psychiatry.* doi: 10.1016/j.jagp.2015.01.001

Freeman, M. P., Wiegand, C. B., & Gelenberg, A. J. (2011). Lithium. In A. F. Schatzberg & C. B. Nemeroff (Eds.), *The American Psychiatric Publishing textbook of psychopharmacology* (4th ed). Washington, DC: American Psychiatric Publishing.

Hashimoto, K. (2010). Brain-derived neurotrophic factor as a biomarker for mood disorders: An historical overview and future directions. *Psychiatry and Clinical Neurosciences, 64*(4), 341–357.

Hoberg, A. A., Vickers, K. S., Ericksen, J., Bauer, G., Kung, S., Stone, R., et al. (2013). Feasibility evaluation of and interpersonal and social rhythm therapy group delivery model. *Archives of Psychiatric Nursing, 27*(6), 271–277.

Kenneson, A., Funderburk, F. S., & Maisto, S. A. (2013). Risk factors for secondary substance use disorders in people with childhood and adolescent-onset bipolar disorder. Opportunities for prevention. *Comprehensive Psychiatry, 54*(5), 439–446.

Kessler, R. C., Petukhova, M., Sampson, N. A., Zaslavsky, A. M., & Wittchen, H. (2012). Twelve-month and lifetime prevalence and lifetime morbid risk of anxiety and mood disorders in the United States. *International Journal of Methods in Psychiatric Research, 21*(3), 169–184.

Lee, S. H., Ripke, S., Neale, B. M., Faraone, S. V., Purcell, S. M., and members of the Cross-Disorder Group of the Psychiatric Genomics Consortium, et al. (2013). Genetic relationship between five psychiatric disorders estimated from genome-wide SNPs. *Nature Genetics, 45*(9), 984–994.

Lee, S., Tsang, A., Kessler, R. C., Jin, R., Sampson, N., Andrade, L., et al. (2010). Rapid-cycling bipolar disorders: Cross-national community study. *British Journal of Psychiatry, 196*, 217–225.

Liu, R. T. (2010). Early life stressors and genetic influences on the development of bipolar disorder: The roles of childhood abuse and brain-derived neurotrophic factor. *Child Abuse & Neglect, 34*(7), 516–522.

Perron, B. D., Fries, L. E., Kilbourne, A. M., Vaughn, M. G., & Bauer, M. (2010). Racial/ethnic group differences in bipolar symptomatology in a community sample of persons with bipolar I disorder. *The Journal of Nervous and Mental Disease, 198*(1), 16–21.

Popovic, D., Reinares, M., Scott, J., Nivoli, A., Murru, A., Pacchiarotti, I., et al. (2013). Polarity index of psychological interventions in maintenance treatment of bipolar disorder. *Psychotherapy and Psychosomatics, 82*(5), 292–298.

Reinares, M., Sánchez-Moreno, J., & Fountoulakis, K. N. (2014). Psychosocial interventions in bipolar disorder: What, for whom, and when. *Journal of Affective Disorders, 156*, 46–55.

Salvatore, P., Indic, P., Murray, G., & Baldessarini, R. J. (2012). Biological rhythms and mood disorders. *Dialogues in Clinical Neuroscience, 14*(4), 369–379.

Schaffer, A., Isometsä, E.T., Tondo, L., Moreno, D.H., Sinyor, M., Kessing, L.V., Turecki, G.,…Yatham, L. (2015). Epidemiology, neurobiology and pharmacological interventions related to suicide deaths and suicide attempts in bipolar disorder: Part I of a report of the International Society for Bipolar Disorders Tasks Force on Suicide in Bipolar Disorder. *Australian & New Zealand Journal of Psychiatry*, 1–18. Doi:10.1177/0004867415594427.

Schatzberg, A. F., & DeBattista, C. (2015). *Manual of Clinical Psychopharmacology (8th ed).* Arlington, VA: American Psychiatric Publishing. http://psychiatryonline.org/doi/full/10.1176/appi.books.9781615370047.AS03

Stahl, S. M. (2013). *Stahl's essential psychopharmacology* (4th ed). New York: Cambridge University Press.

Theodoridou, A., Heekeren, K., Dvorsky, D., Metzler, S., Franscini, M., Haker, H, et al. (2014). Early recognition of high risk of bipolar disorder and psychosis: an overview of the ZInEP "early recognition" study. *Frontiers in Public Health, 2*(166), 1–8.

Thomson, D., Berk, M., Dodd, S., Rapado-Castro, M., Quirk, S.E., Ellegaard, P.K., et al. (2015) Tobacco use in bipolar disorder. *Clinical Psychopharmacology & Neuroscience, 13*(1), 1–11.

Vancampfort, D., Vansteelandt, K., Correll, C.U., Mitchell, A.J., DeHerdt, A., Sienaert, P., et al. (2013). Metabolic syndrome and metabolic abnormalities in bipolar disorder: A meta-analysis of prevalence rates and moderations. *American Journal of Psychiatry, 170*(3), 265–74.

Vieta, E., Popovic, D., Rosa, A. R., Solé, B., Grande, I., Frey, B. N., et al. (2013). The clinical implications of cognitive impairment and allostatic load in bipolar disorder. *European Psychiatry, 28*(1), 21–29.

Wozniak, J., Faraone, S. V., Mick, E., Monuteaux, C., Coville, A., & Biederman, J. (2010). A controlled family study of children with DSM: Bipolar-I disorder and psychiatric co-morbidity. *Psychological Medicine, 40*(7), 1079–1088.

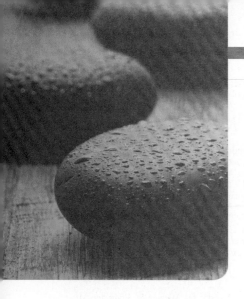

21
Schizophrenia and Related Disorders

Nursing Care of Persons with Thought Disorders

Andrea C. Bostrom and Mary Ann Boyd

KEY CONCEPTS

- disorganized symptoms
- delusions
- hallucinations
- negative symptoms
- neurocognitive symptoms
- positive symptoms
- psychosis

LEARNING OBJECTIVES

After studying this chapter, you will be able to:

1. Identify key symptoms of schizophrenia.

2. Describe theories relevant to schizophrenia.

3. Develop strategies to establish a patient-centered, recovery-oriented therapeutic relationship with a person with schizophrenia.

4. Develop recovery-oriented nursing interventions for patients with schizophrenia.

5. Discuss medications used to treat people with schizophrenia and the evaluate their effectiveness.

6. Identify and evaluate expected outcomes of nursing care for persons with schizophrenia.

7. Discuss other common schizophrenia spectrum disorders.

KEY TERMS

- affective lability • aggression • agitation • agranulocytosis • akathisia • alogia • ambivalence • anhedonia • apathy • autistic thinking • avolition • catatonia • catatonic excitement • circumstantiality • clang association • command hallucinations • cholinergic rebound • concrete thinking • confused speech and thinking • delusions • diminished emotional expression • echolalia • echopraxia • extrapyramidal side effects • flight of ideas • hallucinations • hypervigilance • hypofrontality • illusions • loose associations • metonymic speech • neologisms • neuroleptic malignant syndrome • oculogyric crisis • paranoia • polyuria • pressured speech • prodromal • psychosis • referential thinking • regressed behavior • retrocollis • stereotypy • stilted language • tangentiality • tardive dyskinesia • torticollis • verbigeration • waxy flexibility • word salad

Case Study: Arnold

Arnold, a 53-year-old man, who was diagnosed with paranoid schizophrenia at an early age, had been living on the family farm for the last thirty years with his mother. After his mother's death, the farm was to be sold and divided among the siblings, who arranged for Arnold to move to town. Arnold became agitated and threatening and refused to believe that his parents had died and that he would have to leave the farm.

INTRODUCTION

These fascinating schizophrenia spectrum disorders have confounded scientists and philosophers for centuries. Schizophrenia spectrum disorders are among the most severe mental illnesses; they are found in all cultures, races, and socioeconomic groups. Their symptoms have been attributed to possession by demons, considered punishment by gods for evils done, or accepted as evidence of the inhumanity of its sufferers. These explanations have resulted in enduring stigma for people diagnosed with these disorders. Today, the stigma persists, although it has less to do with demonic possession than with society's unwillingness to shoulder the costs associated with housing, treatment, and rehabilitation. All nurses need to understand these disorders.

SCHIZOPHRENIA SPECTRUM DISORDER

The schizophrenia spectrum disorders include schizophrenia, schizoaffective, delusional, and schizotypal disorders, brief psychotic disorder, schizophreniform disorder, and substance/medication-induced psychotic disorder (American Psychiatric Association [APA], 2013). Schizophrenia is the highlighted disorder in this chapter because it has a broad range of symptoms that are found in the other schizophrenia spectrum disorders. See Table 21.1. A discussion of the other disorders follows the content on schizophrenia. Schizotypal disorders will be discussed in the Personality Disorders chapter (see Chapter 22).

Central to understanding the problems of persons with schizophrenia spectrum disorders is the concept of **psychosis**, a term used to describe a state in which an individual experiences positive symptoms of schizophrenia, also known as psychotic symptoms (e.g., hallucinations; delusions; disorganized thoughts, speech, or behavior).

> **KEYCONCEPT**   **Psychosis**, a state in which a person experiences hallucinations, delusions, or disorganized thoughts, speech, or behavior, is the key diagnostic factor in schizophrenia spectrum disorders.

SCHIZOPHRENIA

In the late 1800s, Emil Kraepelin first described the course of the disorder he called *dementia praecox* because of its early onset and notable changes in an individual's cognitive functioning. In the early 1900s, Eugen Bleuler renamed the disorder *schizophrenia*, meaning *split minds*, and began to determine that there was not just one type of schizophrenia but rather a group of schizophrenias. More recently, Kurt Schneider differentiated behaviors associated with schizophrenia as "first rank" symptoms (e.g., psychotic delusions, hallucinations) and "second rank" symptoms (i.e., all other experiences and behaviors associated with the disorder). These pioneering physicians had a great influence on the current diagnostic conceptualizations of schizophrenia that emphasize the heterogeneity of the disorder in terms of symptoms, course of illness, and positive and negative symptoms.

Clinical Course

Schizophrenia robs people of mental health and imposes social stigma. People with schizophrenia struggle to maintain control of their symptoms, which affect every aspect of their lives. The person with schizophrenia displays various interrelated symptoms and experiences and cognitive deficits in several areas.

Because schizophrenia is a disorder of thoughts, perceptions, and behavior, it is sometimes not recognized as an illness by the person experiencing the symptoms. Many people with thought disorders do not believe that they have a mental illness. Their denial of mental illness and the need for treatment poses problems for the family and clinicians. Ideally, in lucid moments, patients recognize that their thoughts are really delusions, that their perceptions are hallucinations, and that their behavior is disorganized. In reality, many patients do not believe that they have a mental illness but agree to treatment to please family and clinicians.

The natural progression of schizophrenia is usually described as a chronic illness that deteriorates over time and with an eventual plateau in the symptoms. Only for older adults with schizophrenia has it been suggested that improvement might occur. In reality, no one really knows what the course of schizophrenia would be if patients

TABLE 21.1	SCHIZOPHRENIA SPECTRUM DISORDERS
Disorders	**Description**
Schizophrenia	Psychotic symptoms that last for at least 6 months
Schizoaffective Disorder	Mood-related symptoms and symptoms of schizophrenia occur simultaneously
Delusional Disorder	Delusions only, no other psychotic symptoms
Brief Psychotic Disorder	Symptoms similar to schizophrenia, but only lasts one month
Schizophreniform Disorder	Symptoms equivalent to those of schizophrenia except for the duration (less than 6 months) and the absence of a decline in functioning
Substance/Medication–Induced Psychotic Disorder	Psychotic symptoms caused by a substance or medication
Schizotypal Personality Disorder	Pervasive pattern of deficits including social and interpersonal (i.e., impaired capacity for close relationship), cognitive or perceptual distortion, and eccentricities

(APA, 2013)

were able to adhere to a treatment regimen throughout their lives. Only recently have medications become relatively effective, with manageable side effects. The clinical picture of schizophrenia is complex; individuals differ from one another, and the experience for a single individual may vary from episode to episode.

Prodromal Period

A **prodromal period** (stage of early changes that are a precursor to the disorder) may begin in early childhood. More than half of patients report the following prodromal symptoms: tension and nervousness, lack of interest in eating, difficulty concentrating, disturbed sleep, decreased enjoyment and loss of interest, restlessness, forgetfulness, depression, social withdrawal from friends, feeling laughed at, more thinking about religion, feeling bad for no reason, feeling too excited, and hearing voices or seeing things (Barajas, Usall, Baños, Dolz, Villalta-Gil, Vilaplana, et al., 2013; Tarbox, Addington, Cadenhead, Cannon, Cornblatt, Perkins, et al., 2013). The benefit of discovering the presence of symptoms early, before they have solidified into a major disorder, is that treatment might be initiated earlier.

Acute Illness

Initially, the behaviors of this illness may be both confusing and frightening to the individual and the family. The symptoms of acute illness usually occur in late adolescence or early adulthood. The behaviors may be subtle; however, at some point they become so disruptive or bizarre that they can no longer be overlooked. These might include episodes of staying up all night for several nights, incoherent conversations, or aggressive acts against oneself or others. For example, one patient's parents reported their son walking around the apartment for several days holding his arms and hands as if they were a machine gun, pointing them at his parents and siblings, and saying "rat-a-tat-tat, you're dead." Another father described his son's first delusional–hallucinatory episode as so convincing that it was frightening. His son began visiting cemeteries and making "mind contact" with the deceased. He saw his deceased grandmother walking around in the home and was certain that pipe bombs were hidden in objects in his home.

As symptoms worsen, patients are less and less able to care for their basic needs (e.g., eating, sleeping, bathing). Substance use is common. Functioning at school or work deteriorates. Dependence on family and friends increases, so those individuals recognize the patients' need for treatment. In the acute phase, individuals afflicted by schizophrenia are at high risk for suicide. Patients may be hospitalized to protect themselves or others.

Initial treatment focuses on alleviation of symptoms through beginning therapy with medications, decreasing the risk of suicide through safety measures, normalizing sleep, and reducing substance use. Functional deficits persist during this period, so the patient and family must begin to learn to cope with these deficits. Emotional blunting diminishes the ability and desire to engage in hobbies, vocational activities, and relationships. Limited participation in social activities spirals into numerous skill deficits, such as difficulty engaging others interpersonally. Cognitive deficits lead to problems recognizing patterns in situations and transferring learning and behaviors from one circumstance to a similar one.

Stabilization

After the initial diagnosis of schizophrenia and initiation of treatment, stabilization of symptoms becomes the focus. Symptoms become less acute but may still be present. Treatment is intense during this period as medication regimens are established and patients and their families begin to adjust to the idea of a family member having a long-term severe mental illness. Ideally, the use of substances is eliminated. Socialization with others begins to increase, so that rehabilitation begins.

Recovery

The ultimate goal is recovery. Medication generally diminishes the symptoms and allows the person to work towards recovery. However, no medication will cure schizophrenia. As with any chronic illness, following a therapeutic regime, maintaining a healthy lifestyle, managing the stresses of life, and developing meaningful interpersonal relationships are important parts of the recovery. Family support and involvement are extremely important at this time. After the initial diagnosis has been made, patients and families must be educated to anticipate and expect relapse and know how to cope with it.

Relapses

Relapses can occur at any time during treatment and recovery. They are very detrimental to the successful management of this disorder. Relapse is not inevitable; however, it occurs with sufficient regularity to be a major concern in the treatment of schizophrenia. With each relapse, there is a longer period of time is needed to recover. Combining medications and psychosocial treatment greatly diminishes the severity and frequency of recurrent relapses (Guo, Zhai, Liu, Fang, Wang, B., Wang, C., et al., 2010).

One major reason for relapse is failure to take medication consistently. Even with newer medications, adherence continues to be a challenge (Kaplan, Casoy, &

Zummo, 2013). Discontinuing medications will almost certainly lead to a relapse (Acosta, Hernández, Pereira, Herrera, & Rodríguez, 2012). Lower relapse rates are found, for the most part, among groups who carefully follow a treatment regimen.

Many other factors trigger relapse. Impairment in cognition and coping leaves patients vulnerable to stressors. Limited accessibility of community resources, such as public transportation, housing, entry-level and low-stress employment, and limited social services leaves individuals without access to social support. Income supports that can buffer the day-to-day stressors of living may be inadequate. The degree of stigmatization that the community holds for mental illness attacks the self-concept of patients. The level of responsiveness from family members, friends, and supportive others (e.g., peers and professionals) when patients need assistance also has an impact.

> Recall that Arnold's relapse was triggered by his mother's death and being forced to leave the family farm.

Diagnostic Criteria

Schizophrenia is characterized by positive and negative symptoms that are present for a significant portion of a 1-month period but with continuous signs of disturbance persisting for at least 6 months (APA, 2013). We define **positive symptoms** as hallucinations and delusions and **negative symptoms** as diminished emotional expression and avolition (lack of interest or motivation in goal-directed behavior, such as getting dressed, going to work or to school). See Key Diagnostic Characteristics 21.1.

KEY DIAGNOSTIC CHARACTERISTICS 21.1 • SCHIZOPHRENIA

Diagnostic Criteria

A. Two (or more) of the following, each present for a significant portion of time during a 1-month period (or less if successfully treated). At least one of these must be (1), (2), or (3):
   1. Delusions.
   2. Hallucinations.
   3. Disorganized speech (e.g., frequent derailment or incoherence).
   4. Grossly disorganized or catatonic behavior.
   5. Negative symptoms (i.e., diminished emotional expression or avolition).

B. For a significant portion of the time since the onset of the disturbance, level of functioning in one or more major areas, such as work, interpersonal relations, or self-care, is markedly below the level achieved prior to the onset (or when the onset is in childhood or adolescence, there is failure to achieve expected level of interpersonal, academic, or occupational functioning).

C. Continuous signs of the disturbance persist for at least 6 months. This 6-month period must include at least 1 month of symptoms (or less if successfully treated) that meet Criterion A (i.e., active-phase symptoms) and may include periods of prodromal or residual symptoms. During these prodromal or residual periods, the signs of the disturbance may be manifested by only negative symptoms or by two or more symptoms listed in Criterion A present in an attenuated form (e.g., odd beliefs, unusual perceptual experiences).

D. Schizoaffective disorder and depressive or bipolar disorder with psychotic features have been ruled out because either 1) no major depressive or manic episodes have occurred concurrently with the active-phase symptoms, or 2) if mood episodes have occurred during active-phase symptoms, they have been present for a minority of the total duration of the active and residual periods of the illness.

E. The disturbance is not attributable to the physiological effects of a substance (e.g., a drug of abuse, a medication) or another medical condition.

F. If there is a history of autism spectrum disorder or a communication disorder of childhood onset, the additional diagnosis of schizophrenia is made only if prominent delusions or hallucinations, in addition to the other required symptoms of schizophrenia, are also present for at least 1 month (or less if successfully treated).

Target Symptoms and Associated Findings

- Inappropriate affect
- Loss of interest or pleasure
- Dysphoric mood (anger, anxiety, or depression)
- Disturbed sleep patterns
- Lack of interest in eating or refusal of food
- Difficulty concentrating
- Some cognitive dysfunction, such as confusion, disorientation, or memory impairment
- Lack of insight
- Depersonalization, derealization, and somatic concerns
- Motor abnormalities

Associated Physical Examination Findings

- Physically awkward
- Poor coordination or mirroring
- Motor abnormalities
- Cigarette-related pathologies, such as emphysema and other pulmonary and cardiac problems

Associated Laboratory Findings

- Enlarged ventricular system and prominent sulci in the brain cortex
- Decreased temporal and hippocampal size
- Increased size of basal ganglia
- Decreased cerebral size
- Slowed reaction times
- Abnormalities in eye tracking

Positive Symptoms of Schizophrenia

Positive symptoms can be thought of as excessive or distorted thoughts and perceptions that occur within the individual but are not experienced by others. Hallucinations and delusions are positive symptoms of schizophrenia. An easy way to remember the difference between hallucinations and delusions is that hallucinations involve one or more of the five senses. Delusions involve only thoughts.

A fairly common hallucination is a **command hallucination**, that is, an auditory hallucination instructing the patient to act in a certain way, because, voices are telling the person to do something. Command hallucinations range from innocuous (eat all of your dinner) to very serious (hurt someone or jump in front of a bus).

KEYCONCEPT **Positive symptoms** reflect an excess or distortion of normal functions, including delusions and hallucinations. (APA), 2013).

KEYCONCEPT **Hallucinations** are perceptual experiences that occur without actual external sensory stimuli. They can involve any of the five senses, but they are usually *visual* or *auditory*. Auditory hallucinations are more common than visual ones. For example, the patient may hear voices carrying on a discussion about his or her own thoughts or behaviors.

KEYCONCEPT Delusions are erroneous, fixed, false beliefs that cannot be changed by reasonable argument. They usually involve a misinterpretation of experience. For example, the patient believes someone is reading his or her thoughts or

plotting against him or her. Various types of delusions include the following:

- *Grandiose:* the belief that one has exceptional powers, wealth, skill, influence, or destiny
- *Nihilistic:* the belief that one is dead or a calamity is impending
- *Persecutory:* the belief that one is being watched, ridiculed, harmed, or plotted against
- *Somatic:* beliefs about abnormalities in bodily functions or structures

Negative Symptoms of Schizophrenia

The term "negative symptoms" is used to describe emotions and behaviors that should be present, but are diminished in persons with schizophrenia. Negative symptoms are not as dramatic as positive symptoms, but they can interfere greatly with the patient's ability to function day to day. Because expressing emotion is difficult for them, people with schizophrenia laugh, cry, and get angry less often. Their affect is flat; they show little or no emotion when personal loss occurs. They also experience ambivalence, which is the concurrent experience of equally strong opposing feelings so that it is impossible to make a decision. Avolition may be so profound that simple activities of daily living (ADLs), such as dressing or combing hair, may not get done. Anhedonia prevents the person with schizophrenia from enjoying activities. People with schizophrenia may have limited speech and difficulty saying anything new or carrying on a conversation. These negative symptoms cause the person with schizophrenia to withdraw and experience feelings of severe isolation.

KEYCONCEPT **Negative symptoms** reflect a lessening or loss of normal functions, such as restriction or flattening in the range and intensity of emotion (**diminished emotional expression**), reduced fluency and productivity of thought and speech (**alogia**), withdrawal and inability to initiate and persist in goal-directed activity (**avolition**), and inability to experience pleasure (**anhedonia**).

Neurocognitive Impairment

Neurocognitive impairment exists in people with schizophrenia and may be independent of positive and negative symptoms. Neurocognition includes memory (short- and long-term); vigilance or sustained attention; verbal fluency or the ability to generate new words; and executive functioning, which includes volition, planning, purposeful action, and self-monitoring behavior. Working memory is a concept that includes short-term memory and the ability to store and process information.

KEYCONCEPT **Neurocognitive impairment** in memory, vigilance, and executive functioning is related to poor functional outcomes in schizophrenia (Fanning, Bell, & Fiszdon, 2012).

This impairment is independent of the positive symptoms. That is, cognitive dysfunction can exist even if the positive symptoms are in remission. Not all areas of cognitive functioning are impaired. Long-term memory and intellectual functioning are not necessarily affected. However, low intellectual functioning is common and may be related to a lack of educational opportunities. Neurocognitive dysfunction is often manifested in disorganized symptoms.

> **KEYCONCEPT** **Disorganized symptoms** of schizophrenia are findings that make it difficult for the person to understand and respond to the ordinary sights and sounds of daily living. These include confused speech and thinking, and disorganized behavior.

Disorganized Thinking

The following are examples of **confused speech and thinking** patterns:

- **Echolalia**—repetition of another's words that is parrot-like and inappropriate
- **Circumstantiality**—extremely detailed and lengthy discourse about a topic
- **Loose associations**—absence of the normal connectedness of thoughts, ideas, and topics; sudden shifts without apparent relationship to preceding topics
- **Tangentiality**—the topic of conversation is changed to an entirely different topic that is a logical progression but causes a permanent detour from the original focus
- **Flight of ideas**—the topic of conversation changes repeatedly and rapidly, generally after just one sentence or phrase
- **Word salad**—stringing together words that are not connected in any way
- **Neologisms**—words that are made up that have no common meaning and are not recognizable
- **Paranoia**—suspiciousness and guardedness that are unrealistic and often accompanied by grandiosity
- **Referential thinking**—a belief that neutral stimuli have special meaning to the individual, such as a television commentator who is speaking directly to the individual
- **Autistic thinking**—restricts thinking to the literal and immediate so that the individual has private rules of logic and reasoning that make no sense to anyone else
- **Concrete thinking**—lack of abstraction in thinking; inability to understand punch lines, metaphors, and analogies
- **Verbigeration**—purposeless repetition of words or phrases
- **Metonymic speech**—use of words with similar meanings interchangeably

- **Clang association**—repetition of words or phrases that are similar in sound but in no other way, for example, "right, light, sight, might"
- **Stilted language**—overly and inappropriately artificial formal language
- **Pressured speech**—speaking as if the words are being forced out

Disorganized perceptions often create oversensitivity to colors, shapes, and background activities. **Illusions** occur when the person misperceives or exaggerates stimuli that actually exist in the external environment. This is in contrast to hallucinations, which are perceptions in the absence of environmental stimuli. Ancillary symptoms that may accompany schizophrenia include anxiety, depression, and hostility.

Disorganized Behavior

Disorganized behavior (which may manifest as very slow, rhythmic, or ritualistic movement) coupled with disorganized speech make it difficult for the person to partake in daily activities. Examples of disorganized behavior include the following:

- **Aggression**—behaviors or attitudes that reflect rage, hostility, and the potential for physical or verbal destructiveness (usually comes about if the person believes someone is going to do him or her harm)
- **Agitation**—inability to sit still or attend to others, accompanied by heightened emotions and tension
- **Catatonia**—psychomotor disturbances such as stupor, mutism, posturing or repetitive behavior
- **Catatonic excitement**—a hyperactivity characterized by purposeless activity and abnormal movements, such as grimacing and posturing
- **Echopraxia**—involuntary imitation of another person's movements and gestures
- **Regressed behavior**—behaving in a manner of a less mature life stage; childlike and immature behavior
- **Stereotypy**—repetitive purposeless movements that are idiosyncratic to the individual and to some degree outside of the individual's control
- **Hypervigilance**—sustained attention to external stimuli as if expecting something important or frightening to happen
- **Waxy flexibility**—posture held in an odd or unusual fixed position for extended periods of time

Schizophrenia Across the Life-Span
Children

The diagnosis of schizophrenia is rare in children before adolescence. When it does occur in children ages 5 or 6 years, the symptoms are essentially the same as in adults.

In this age group, hallucinations tend to be visual and delusions less developed. Because disorganized speech and behavior may be explained better by other disorders that are more common in childhood, those disorders should be considered before applying the diagnosis of schizophrenia to a child.

However, new studies suggest that the likelihood of children later experiencing schizophrenia can be predicted. Developmental abnormalities in childhood, including delays in attainment of speech and motor development, problems in social adjustment, and poorer academic and cognitive performance have been found to be present in individuals who experience schizophrenia in adulthood. Specific factors that appear to predict schizophrenia in adulthood include problems in motor and neurologic development, deficits in attention and verbal short-term memory, poor social competence, positive formal thought disorder-like symptoms, and severe instability of early home environment (Meier, Caspi, Reichenberg, Keefe, Fisher, Harrington, et al., 2013).

Older Adults

People with schizophrenia usually get older and some people develop schizophrenia in late life. For older patients who have had schizophrenia since young adulthood, this may be a time in which they experience some improvement in symptoms or decrease in relapse fluctuations. There is some evidence that suggests that older adults with schizophrenia may be more likely to develop cognitive impairment than those without mental disorders (Loewenstein, Czaja, Bowie, & Harvey, 2012). However, their lifestyle is probably dependent on the effectiveness of earlier treatment, the support systems that are in place (including relationships with family members and professionals), and the interaction between environmental stressors and the patient's functional impairments. The cost of caring for older patients with schizophrenia remains high because many are no longer cared for in institutions and because community-based treatment has developed more slowly for this age group than for younger adults.

Epidemiology

Schizophrenia is found in all cultures and countries. It is prevalent in about 0.7% of the worldwide population and is listed within the top 20 illnesses for life lost resulting from premature death and years lived in less than full health (Department of Health Statistics and Information Systems, 2013). Its economic costs are enormous. Direct costs include treatment expenses; indirect costs include lost wages, premature death, and involuntary commitment. In addition, employment among people with schizophrenia is one of the lowest of any group with disabilities. The costs of schizophrenia in terms of individual and family suffering are probably inestimable.

People with schizophrenia tend to cluster in the lowest social classes in industrialized countries and urban communities. The symptoms of the illness are so pervasive that it is difficult for these individuals to maintain any type of gainful employment. Homelessness is a problem for people with severe mental illness (e.g., schizophrenia or bipolar illness). People with schizophrenia are more likely to remain homeless with few opportunities for employment (Auquier, Tinland, Fortanier, Loundou, Baumstarck, Lanson, et al., 2013).

Risk Factors

Genetic factors related to cognitive and brain function and brain structure are known risks for schizophrenia. Early neurologic problems, stressful life events, and nonhereditary genetic factors also contribute to the likelihood of developing the disorder. Environmental factors include migrant status, having an older father, *Toxoplasma gondii* antibodies, prenatal famine, lifetime cannabis use, obstetric complications, urban rearing, and winter or spring birth (Brown, 2011).

Age of Onset

Schizophrenia is usually diagnosed in late adolescence and early adulthood. Men tend to be diagnosed between the ages of 18 and 25 years and women between the ages of 25 and 35 years. The earlier the diagnosis and the longer the psychosis remains untreated, the more severe the disorder becomes (Fraguas, Del Rey-Mejias, Morenos, Castro-Fornieles, Graell, Otero, et al., 2013).

Gender Differences

Men tend to be diagnosed earlier and have a poorer prognosis than women. This may be a sex-linked outcome, but it may also reflect the poorer prognosis for any individual who develops the disorder at an early age (Goldstein, Cherkerzian, Tsuang, & Petryshen, 2013).

Ethnic and Cultural Differences

Increasingly, efforts are being made to consider culture and ethnic origin when diagnosing and treating individuals with schizophrenia. Racial groups may have varying diagnostic rates of schizophrenia. However, it is not clear whether these findings represent correct diagnosis or misdiagnosis of the disorder based on the cultural bias of the clinician. For instance, schizophrenia has been consistently overdiagnosed among African Americans. African American and Hispanic individuals with bipolar disorder are more likely to have misdiagnoses of schizophrenia than are white individuals. Serious mental disorders may remain unrecognized in Asian Americans because of stereotypical beliefs that they are "problem free" (Cohen & Marino, 2013).

Familial Differences

First-degree biologic relatives (e.g., children, siblings, parents) of an individual with schizophrenia have a 10 times estimated greater risk for schizophrenia than the general population. Other relatives may have an increased risk for related disorders such as schizoaffective disorder and schizotypal personality disorder (Boshes, Manschreck, & Konigsberg, 2012).

Comorbidity

Several somatic and psychological disorders coexist with schizophrenia. This results in significant morbidity and mortality for people with schizophrenia, with individuals who have this diagnosis dying up to 20 years earlier than the general population. Physical health conditions and illnesses to which people with schizophrenia are particularly susceptible include tuberculosis, human immuno-deficiency disease, hepatitis B and C, osteoporosis, poor dentition, impaired lung function, altered (reduced) pain sensitivity, sexual dysfunction, obstetric complications, cardiovascular problems, hyperpigmentation, obesity, diabetes mellitus (DM), metabolic syndrome with hyperlipidemia, polydipsia, thyroid dysfunction, and hyperprolactinemia (Laursen, Nordentoft, & Mortensen, 2013; Carliner, Collins, Cabassa, McNallen, Joestl, Lewis-Fernández, 2013). Several health system factors contribute to this, including barriers to obtaining primary care, the insufficient preparation of mental health practitioners in managing physical illness, the tendency for mental health providers to fail to ask about physical health, and the absence of standards of care that include screening and monitoring medical issues.

Substance Abuse and Depression

Among the behavioral comorbidities, substance use is common. Depression may also be observed in patients with schizophrenia. This is an important symptom for several reasons. First, depression may be evidence that the diagnosis of a mood disorder is more appropriate. Second, depression is not unusual in chronic stages of schizophrenia and deserves attention. Third, the suicide rate (4.9%) among individuals with schizophrenia is higher than that of the general population. Risk factors for suicide are untreated psychosis, history of suicide attempt, age younger than 28 years, severity of depression, and substance abuse (Austad, Joa, Johannessen, & Larsen, 2015; Challis, Nielssen, Harris, & Large, 2013).

Diabetes Mellitus and Obesity

Interest has been renewed in the relationship between DM and schizophrenia. Years ago, an association was established between glucose regulation and psychiatric disorders, suggesting that people with schizophrenia may be more prone to Type II DM than the general public (Franzen, 1970; Schimmelbusch, Mueller, & Sheps, 1971). Evidence that supports this view includes a higher rate of type II diabetes in first-degree relatives of people with schizophrenia and higher rates of impaired glucose tolerance and insulin resistance among people with schizophrenia. However, obesity, which is associated with type II diabetes, is a growing problem in the United States in general and is complicated in schizophrenia treatment by the tendency of individuals to gain weight after their disease is managed with medications. Weight gain in some individuals may be attributed to a return to a healthier living situation in which regular meals are available and symptoms that interfere with obtaining food regularly (e.g., delusions) are decreased. For others, weight gain may be a medication side effect (McDaid & Smyth, 2015).

Etiology

Schizophrenia is believed to be caused by the interaction of a biologic predisposition or vulnerability and environmental stressors (see the diathesis-stress model discussed in Chapter 12). See Box 21.1 for deficits related to vulnerability in schizophrenia. Environmental risk factors

---

BOX 21.1

Deficits That Cause Vulnerability in Schizophrenia

COGNITIVE DEFICITS
- Deficits in processing complex information
- Deficits in maintaining a steady focus of attention
- Inability to distinguish between relevant and irrelevant stimuli
- Difficulty forming consistent abstractions
- Impaired memory

PSYCHOPHYSIOLOGIC DEFICITS
- Deficits in sensory inhibition
- Poor control of autonomic responsiveness

SOCIAL SKILLS DEFICITS
- Impairments in processing interpersonal stimuli, such as eye contact or assertiveness
- Deficits in conversational capacity
- Deficits in initiating activities
- Deficits in experiencing pleasure

COPING SKILLS DEFICITS
- Overassessment of threat
- Underassessment of personal resources
- Overuse of denial

Source: McGlashan, T. H. (1994). Psychosocial treatments of schizophrenia: The potential relationships. In N. C. Andreasen (Ed.), *Schizophrenia: From mind to molecule* (pp. 189–215). Washington, DC: American Psychiatric Press.

include pregnancy or obstetric complications and social adversity such as migration, unemployment, urban living, childhood abuse, and social isolation or absence of close friends (Goff, 2013).

Biologic Theories

Neuroanatomic Findings

The lateral and third ventricles are somewhat larger and total brain volume is somewhat less in persons with schizophrenia compared with those without schizophrenia. The thalamus and the medial temporal lobe structures, including the hippocampus, and superior temporal and prefrontal cortices, tend to be smaller also (Birnbaum & Weinberger, 2013; Johnson, Wang, Alpert, Greenstein, Clasen, Lalonde, et al., 2013).

Familial Patterns

The likelihood of first-degree relatives (including siblings and children) developing schizophrenia has long been recognized as 10 times more likely than in individuals in the general population. Although this likelihood clearly suggests a strong genetic factor, the concordance for schizophrenia among monozygotic (i.e., identical) twins is 50%, suggesting that environmental factors may also be involved (Bonsch, Wunschel, Lenz, Janssen, Weisbrod, & Sauer, 2012).

Genetic Associations

Genetic associations have been identified in a number of regions of the brain, and some have already been tied to altered dopamine transmission. However, these associations are more likely related to the susceptibility of developing the schizophrenia disorder rather than the cause of it. (Birnbaum & Weinberger, 2013).

Neurodevelopment

The neurodevelopmental hypothesis explains the etiology of schizophrenia as pathologic processes caused by genetic and environmental factors that begin before the brain reaches its adult state. Evidence suggests that in utero during the first or second trimester, genes involved with cell migration, cell proliferation, axonal outgrowth, and myelination may be affected by neurologic insults such as viral infections. That is, early neurodevelopmental insults may lead to dysfunction of specific networks that become obvious at adolescence during the normal loss of some plasticity and synapse (Goff, 2013).

Neurotransmitters, Pathways, and Receptors

Positron emission tomography (PET) scan findings suggest that in schizophrenia, brain metabolism is generally reduced, with a relative hypermetabolism in the left side of the brain and in the left temporal lobe. Abnormalities exist in specific areas of the brain in the frontal, temporal, and cingulate regions (Smieskova, Marmy, Schmidt, Bendfeldt, Riecher-Rossler, Walter, et al., 2013). These findings support further exploration of differential brain hemisphere function in people with schizophrenia (Figure 21.1). Other PET studies show **hypofrontality**, or a reduced cerebral blood flow and glucose metabolism in the prefrontal cortex of people with schizophrenia and hyperactivity in the limbic area (Buchsbaum, 1990) (Figures 21.2 and 21.3).

Dopamine Dysregulation

Positive symptoms of schizophrenia, specifically, hallucinations and delusions, are thought to be related to dopamine *hyperactivity* in the mesolimbic tract at the D2 receptor site in the striatal area where memory and emotion are regulated. Dopamine dysfunction is thought to be involved not only in schizophrenia, but also in psychosis in other disorders. If no psychosis is present, it is unlikely that there is an overactivity of dopamine in the striatal region.

Conversely, chronic low levels of dopamine in the prefrontal cortex are thought to underlie cognitive dysfunction in schizophrenia. Cognitive and negative symptoms of schizophrenia, previously thought to be related to dopamine dysfunction on a single pathway, are now thought to be associated with transmitter or neural connectivity systems. In many cases, these dysfunctions precede the onset of psychosis (Lau, Wang, Hsu, & Liu, 2013).

Role of Other Receptors

Other receptors are also involved in dopamine neurotransmission, especially serotonergic receptors. It is becoming clear that schizophrenia does not result from dysregulation of a single neurotransmitter or biogenic amine (e.g., norepinephrine, dopamine, or serotonin). Investigators are also hypothesizing a role for glutamate and gamma-aminobutyric acid (GABA) because of the complex interconnections of neuronal transmission and the complexity and heterogeneity of schizophrenia symptoms. The N-methyl-D-aspartate (NMDA) class of glutamate receptors is being studied because of the actions of phencyclidine (PCP) at these sites and because of the similarity of the psychotic behaviors that are produced when someone takes PCP (Goff, 2013) (see Figures 21.1, 21.2, and 21.3).

Psychosocial Theories

Social factors can contribute to the changes in brain function that result in schizophrenia and add to the day-to-day challenges of living with a mental illness. Childhood trauma, living in an urban environment, and being

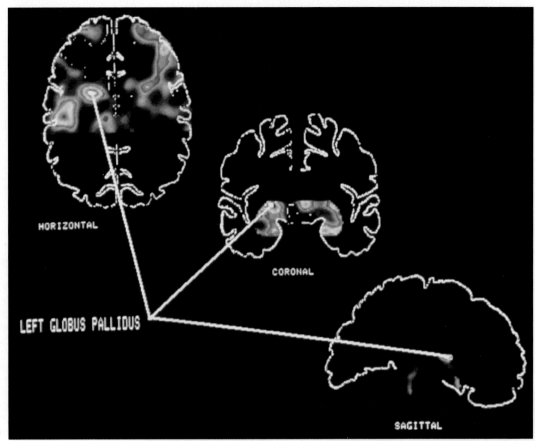

FIGURE 21.1 Area of abnormal functioning in a person with schizophrenia. These three views show the excessive neuronal activity in the left globus pallidus (portion of the basal ganglia next to the putamen). (Courtesy of John W. Haller, PhD, Departments of Psychiatry and Radiology, Washington University, St. Louis.)

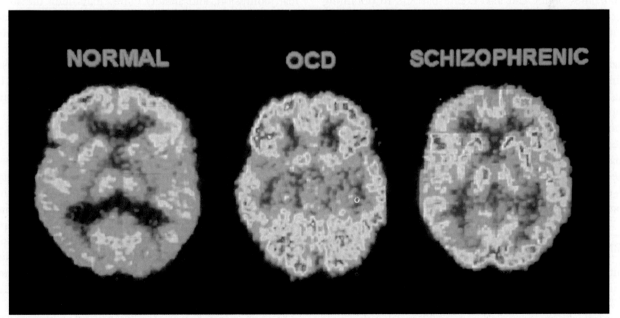

FIGURE 21.2 Metabolic activity in a control subject (*left*), a subject with obsessive-compulsive disorder (*center*), and a subject with schizophrenia (*right*). (Courtesy of Monte S. Buchsbaum, MD, The Mount Sinai Medical Center and School of Medicine, New York.)

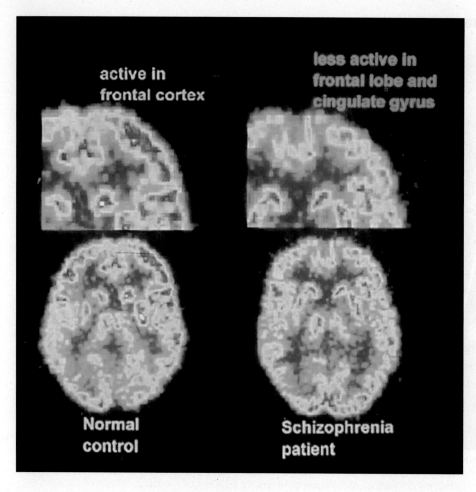

FIGURE 21.3 Positron emission tomography scan with 18F-deoxyglucose shows metabolic activity in a horizontal section of the brain in a control subject (*left*) and in an unmedicated patient with schizophrenia (*right*). *Red* and *yellow* indicate areas of high metabolic activity in the cortex; *green* and *blue* indicate lower activity in the white matter areas of the brain. The frontal lobe is magnified to show reduced frontal activity in the prefrontal cortex of the patient with schizophrenia. (Courtesy of Monte S. Buchsbaum, MD, The Mount Sinai Medical Center and School of Medicine, New York.)

a member of a minority are all associated with psychotic syndromes. They can also create barriers to obtaining necessary treatment and recovery (van Os, Kenis, & Rutten, 2010).

One of the major social stressors is the social stigma that surrounds all mental illnesses (see Chapter 1). The clinical vignette in Box 21.2 describes the impact of living with a stigmatizing illness. Another is the absence of good, affordable, and supportive housing in many communities. With 2010's enactment of insurance parity for mental illness in the Affordable Care Act, it is hoped that quality and continuity of care will be enhanced. Finally, the mental health service delivery system is fragmented; its quality and types of services vary from community to community (National Alliance on Mental Illness, 2013).

Family Response to Disorder

Initially, families usually experience disbelief, shock, and fear along with concern for the family member. Families may attribute the episode to taking illicit drugs or to extraordinary stress or fatigue and hope that this is an isolated or transient event. They may be fearful of the behaviors and respond to patient anger and hostility with fear, confusion, and anxiety. They may deny the severity and chronicity of the illness and only partially engage in treatment. As families begin to acknowledge the disorder and the long-term care nature of recovery, they themselves may feel overwhelmed, angry, and depressed (McAuliffe, O'Connor, & Meagher, 2015). See Box 21.3 for discussion of recovery-oriented family interventions.

Teamwork and Collaboration: Working Toward Recovery

The most effective approach to treatment for individuals with schizophrenia involves various disciplines, including nursing (both generalist and advanced practice psychiatric nurses), psychiatry, psychology, social work, occupational and recreational therapy, and pastoral counseling. Individuals with general education in psychology, sociology, and social work often serve as case managers, nursing aides, technicians, and other support personnel in hospitals and community treatment agencies.

Patients need help in accepting and understanding their illness, setting goals, and developing a support

BOX 21.2 CLINICAL VIGNETTE

Graduate Student in Peril

BGW, born in 1973, spent most of his teenage years using drugs and alcohol, behavior that started when he was 11 years old. He and his small group of friends spent their teenage years outside of school riding around on bicycles. He failed 8th grade, repeated it, and made it to 10th grade. He was removed permanently from school at the age of 16 years. His dress included a dirty denim jacket or Army fatigues, torn tee shirts with rock band logos, and tight-fitting jeans. At age 16, he was hospitalized for a psychotic episode initiated by lysergic acid diethylamide (LSD); it was the scariest moment of his life. His mind had been getting fuzzier every day; he had dabbled with black magic and Satanism. Later, he admitted that for years he had been trapped in a fantasy land, only partially explained by his drug use.

Years of treatment followed; even with abstinence from drugs, his mental status fluctuated. After antipsychotic agents were prescribed, he began to feel like himself. He was motivated to complete his GED and entered college. He kept his mental illness a secret. While in graduate school, his thoughts, feelings, and behaviors began to change. His thinking became delusional, his moods unpredictable, and his behaviors illogical. Finally, he was hospitalized again, and his condition was stabilized with medication. Currently, he is reapplying to graduate school and this time he vows to keep people close to him aware of his mental status.

What Do You Think?

- What role did stigma play in the treatment process?
- What information should BGW share with his social network about his mental illness and treatment?

Adapted from Graduate student in peril: a first person account of schizophrenia. (2002). *Schizophrenia Bulletin, 28*(4), 745–755.

BOX 21.3

Research for Best Practice: Recovery for People with Schizophrenia and Their Families

Nilsen, L., Grich, J. C., Friis, S. & Røssberg, J .I. (2014). Patients' and family members' experiences of a psychoeducational family intervention after a first episode psychosis: A qualitative study. Issues in Mental Health Nursing, 35(1), 58–68.

THE QUESTION: What are the patients' and family members' experiences of the different elements of a psychoeducational family intervention?

METHODS: A qualitative, explorative study was performed with 12 patients and 14 family members. The interviews were transcribed in a slightly modified verbatim mode.

FINDINGS: Patients and family members identified several themes as important: alliance, support, anxiety and tension, knowledge and learning, time and structure. A good relationship between the leader and the group is essential in preventing patient dropout. Meeting other people with the same issues increased hope for the future. Hearing real life stories was more important for gaining knowledge than lectures and workshops. New patients experienced anxiety during the first sessions.

IMPLICATIONS FOR NURSING: Nurses should recognize the anxiety and tension of new group members. Teaching strategies should focus on encouraging group members to share personal experiences within the structure of the group.

---

system that encourages their recovery. Recovery-oriented strategies can address any hopelessness associated with suicide attempts and encourage an independent lifestyle. Medication management is central to the treatment of schizophrenia and is the responsibility of the patient, physicians, nurses, and pharmacists. Psychosocial interventions can be implemented by all members of the mental health team and may include cognitive behavioral, music, vocational, and support therapies. These varied professionals and paraprofessionals are important because of the complex nature of the symptoms, the long-term nature of the disorder, and the need for health promotion support. Complementary and alternative therapies such as yoga, breathing exercises, relaxation, meditation, and aerobic exercise may be helpful as adjunctive to the usual care.

Safety Issues

Several special concerns exist when working with people with schizophrenia. A suicide assessment always should be completed when a person is experiencing a psychotic episode. In an inpatient unit, patient safety concerns extend to potentially aggressive actions toward staff and other patients during episodes of psychosis. During times of acute illness, a priority of care is treatment with antipsychotic medications and, in some instances, hospitalization.

Nurses should assess the person's risk for suicide because of the high suicide and attempted suicide rates among persons with schizophrenia. See Chapter 15. Does the patient speak of suicide, have delusional thinking that could lead to dangerous behavior, or have command hallucinations telling him or her to harm self or others? Does the patient have homicidal ideations? Does the patient lack social support and the skills to be meaningfully engaged with other people or a vocation? Substance-related disorders are also common among patients with schizophrenia, so that nurses should assess for substance use.

EVIDENCE-BASED NURSING CARE OF PERSONS WITH SCHIZOPHRENIA

Recovery is a long-term journey requiring various nursing interventions at different times. During exacerbation of symptoms, many patients are hospitalized for safety and medication adjustment. During periods of relative stability, the nurse and patient collaborate in developing recovery-oriented strategies that include maintaining a healthy lifestyle, developing positive coping skills, and seeking meaningful relationships. Schizophrenia research is ongoing and the results are leading to new treatment approaches. It is critical that nurses continually seek out evidence-based strategies through accessing the best possible sources of evidence and formulating clinical questions. Nursing Care Plan 21.1 is available at http://thepoint.lww.com/BoydEssentials.

Mental Health Nursing Assessment

The nursing assessment should include the biologic, psychological, and social aspects because schizophrenia affects all aspects of the person's life. Not only are symptoms assessed, but strengths are also important in the assessment process.

Physical Health

The nurse should first determine whether any underlying medical disorders are present, particularly those associated with schizophrenia such as DM, hypertension, and cardiac disease, or a family history of such disorders. Usually a medical examination is conducted by primary care providers prior to initiation of mental health care. People with schizophrenia have a higher mortality rate from physical illness and often have smoking-related illnesses, such as emphysema as well as other pulmonary and cardiac problems (Gimblett, 2015).

Physical Functioning

Physical abilities can be a strength; the potential to maintain optimal physical health should be assessed. Self-care often deteriorates in schizophrenia; sleep may be nonexistent during acute phases. Information regarding physical functioning may best be collected from family members.

Nutrition

A nutritional history should be completed to determine baseline eating habits and preferences. A healthy diet is important in managing the illness. Medications can alter normal nutrition leading to excessive consumption of calories.

Medication

The nurse should obtain a complete list of medications that the patient is taking including over-the-counter (OTC) agents and herbal supplements. Before initiation of psychiatric medications, standardized assessment of abnormal motor movements should be conducted using one of several assessment tools designed for that purpose, such as the Abnormal Involuntary Movement Scale (AIMS) (see Appendix B), the Dyskinesia Identification System (DISCUS) (Sprague & Kalachnik, 1991) (Box 21.4), or the Simpson-Angus

Rating Scale (Simpson & Angus, 1970), which is designed for Parkinson's symptoms.

Substance Use (Alcohol, Illicit Drugs, Tobacco)

The nurse should asked specific questions about alcohol, drug, and tobacco use. The use of these substances is quite common with people with schizophrenia and will significantly influence the treatment approach.

Psychosocial Assessment

The individual who is in an acute phase may be unable to provide an accurate history of early psychosocial issues. Family members' reports help in detailing occurrences of psychotic symptoms of delusions and hallucinations; however, onset of negative symptoms may be more difficult to date. In fact, negative symptoms vary from a slight deviation from normal to a clear impairment. Negative symptoms probably occur earlier than positive symptoms but are less easily recognized. Several assessment scales have been developed to help evaluate clusters of positive and negative symptoms. See Box 21.5.

Mental Status and Appearance

The patient may look eccentric or disheveled or have poor hygiene and bizarre dress. The patient's posture may suggest lethargy or stupor.

Mood and Affect

Patients with schizophrenia often display altered mood states. In some cases, they may show heightened emotional activity; others may display severely limited emotional responses. Affect, the outward expression of mood, is categorized on a continuum: flat (i.e., emotional expression entirely absent), blunted (i.e., expression of emotions present but greatly diminished), and full range of expression. Inappropriate affect is marked by incongruence between the emotional expression and the thoughts expressed (e.g., laughing when telling a sad story). Other common emotional symptoms include the following:

- **Affective lability**—abrupt, dramatic, unprovoked changes in type of emotions expressed
- **Ambivalence**—the presence and expression of two opposing feelings, leading to inaction
- **Apathy**—little emotional expression; diminished interest and desire

Speech

Thought content and other mental processes are expressed in speech. Both content and speech patterns should be

BOX 21.4

The Dyskinesia Identification System: Condensed User Scale (DISCUS)

NAME	I.D.

(facility)

Dyskinesia Identification System: Condensed User Scale (DISCUS)

CURRENT PSYCHOTROPICS/ANTI-CHOLINERGIC AND TOTAL MG/DAY

_____ _____mg
_____ _____mg
_____ _____mg
_____ _____mg

See Instructions on Other Side

EXAM TYPE (check one)
- ☐ 1. Baseline
- ☐ 2. Annual
- ☐ 3. Semi annual
- ☐ 4. D/C—1 mo
- ☐ 5. D/C—2 mo
- ☐ 6. D/C—3 mo
- ☐ 7. Admission
- ☐ 8. Other

COOPERATION (check one)
- ☐ 1. None
- ☐ 2. Partial
- ☐ 3. Full

SCORING

0—**Not present** (movements not observed or some movements observed but not considered abnormal)

1—**Minimal** (abnormal movements are difficult to detect or movements are easy to detect but occur only once or twice in a short nonrepetitive manner)

2—**Mild** (abnormal movements occur infrequently and are easy to detect)

3—**Moderate** (abnormal movements occur frequently and are easy to detect)

4—**Severe** (abnormal movements occur almost continuously **and** are easy to detect)

NA—**Not assessed** (an assessment for an item is not able to be made)

ASSESSMENT
DISCUS Item and Score (circle one score for each item)

1. Tics .... 0 1 2 3 4 NA
2. Grimaces .... 0 1 2 3 4 NA

3. Blinking .... 0 1 2 3 4 NA

4. Chewing/Lip Smacking .... 0 1 2 3 4 NA
5. Puckering/Sucking/
   Thrusting Lower Lip. .... 0 1 2 3 4 NA

6. Tongue Thrusting/
   Tongue in Cheek .... 0 1 2 3 4 NA
7. Tonic Tongue .... 0 1 2 3 4 NA
8. Tongue Tremor .... 0 1 2 3 4 NA
9. Athetoid/Myokymic/
   Lateral Tongue .... 0 1 2 3 4 NA

10. Retrocollis/Torticollis .... 0 1 2 3 4 NA
11. Shoulder/Hip Torsion .... 0 1 2 3 4 NA

12. Athetoid/Myokymic
    Finger–Wrist–Arm .... 0 1 2 3 4 NA
13. Pill Rolling .... 0 1 2 3 4 NA

14. Ankle Flexion/Foot
    Tapping .... 0 1 2 3 4 NA
15. Toe Movement .... 0 1 2 3 4 NA

EVALUATION (see Appendix C)

1. Greater than 90 days neuroleptic exposure?	:	YES	NO
2. Scoring/intensity level met?	:	YES	NO
3. Other diagnostic conditions? (if yes, specify)	:	YES	NO

_____
_____
_____

4. Last exam date: _____
   Last total score: _____
   Last conclusion: _____

Preparer signature and title for items 1–4 (if different from physician):

5. Conclusion (circle one):
   A. No TD (if scoring prerequisite met, list other diagnostic condition or explain in comments)
   B. Probable TD
   C. Masked TD
   D. Withdrawal TD
   E. Persistent TD
   F. Remitted TD
   G. Other (specify in comments)

6. Comments:

_____
_____
_____
_____
_____
_____
_____

COMMENTS/OTHER

_____
_____
_____
_____
_____

TOTAL SCORE
(items 1–21 only)

EXAM DATE

RATER SIGNATURE AND TITLE	NET EXAM DATE	CLINICIAN SIGNATURE	DATE

From Sprague, R. L., & Kalachnik, J. E. (1991). Reliability, validity, and a total score cutoff for the Dyskinesia Identification System, Condensed User Scale (DISCUS) with mentally ill and mentally retarded populations. *Psychopharmacology Bulletin, 27*(1), 51–58.

BOX 21.5

Rating Scales for Use With Schizophrenia

SCALE FOR THE ASSESSMENT OF NEGATIVE SYMPTOMS (SANS)
Available from Nancy C. Andreasen, MD, PhD, Department of Psychiatry, College of Medicine, The University of Iowa, Iowa City, IA 52242. Copyright 1984.

SCALE FOR THE ASSESSMENT OF POSITIVE SYMPTOMS (SAPS)
Available from Nancy C. Andreasen (see above).

POSITIVE AND NEGATIVE SYNDROME SCALE (PANSS)
Kay, S. R., Fiszbein, A., & Opler, L. A. (1987). The Positive and Negative Syndrome Scale (PANSS) for Schizophrenia. *Schizophrenia Bulletin, 13,* 261–276. Available from first author.

ABNORMAL INVOLUNTARY MOVEMENT SCALE (AIMS)
Guy, W. (1976), *ECDEU: Assessment manual for psychopharmacology* (DHEW Publication No. 76–338). Washington, DC: Department of Health, Education, and Welfare, Psychopharmacology Branch.

BRIEF PSYCHIATRIC RATING SCALE (BPRS)
Overall, J. E., & Gorham, D. R. (1988). The Brief Psychiatric Rating Scale (BPRS): Recent developments in ascertainment and scaling. *Psychopharmacology Bulletin, 24,* 97–99.

DYSKINESIA IDENTIFICATION SYSTEM: CONDENSED USER SCALE (DISCUS)
Sprague, R. L., & Kalachnik, J. E. (1991). Reliability, validity, and a total score cutoff for the Dyskinesia Identification Scale System: Condensed User Scale (DISCUS) with mentally ill and mentally retarded populations. *Psychopharmacology Bulletin, 27*(1), 51–58. See Box 21.4.

SIMPSON-ANGUS RATING SCALE
Simpson, G. M., & Angus, J. W. S. L. (1970). A rating scale for extrapyramidal side effects. *Acta Psychiatrica Scandinavica, 212*(suppl), 11–19. Copyright 1970 Munksgaard International Publishers, Ltd.

---

assessed by the nurse. Speech content may include obvious obsessions or delusions, loose associations, or flight of ideas. In some instances, as already noted, patients make up their own words (neologisms). Speech may be pressured (words seem to rapidly jump out without pauses) or slow. The nurse should note any difficulty in articulating words (dysarthria) or difficulty in swallowing (dysphagia) as indicators of medication-related side effects.

Thought Process Assessment

Thought process assessment includes determining if any hallucinations, delusions, disorganized communication, or cognitive impairments are present. Because thought process assessment is critical in the nursing assessment, each area is discussed separately below.

Hallucinations

Hallucinations are the most common example of disturbed sensory perception observed in patients with schizophrenia. Hallucinations are experienced in the sensory modalities (visual, auditory, gustatory, tactile, olfactory); however, auditory hallucinations are the most common type in schizophrenia. Some specific hallucinations may be sufficient to diagnose schizophrenia, such as hearing voices conversing with each other or carrying on a discussion with someone who is not there. Because most individuals will not spontaneously share their hallucinatory experiences with an interviewer, the nurse may need to rely on indirect evidence in the patient's behavior, such as (1) pauses during conversations in which the individual seems preoccupied or appears to be listening to someone other than the interviewer, (2) looking toward the perceived source of a voice, or (3) responding to the voices in some manner. Although patients may not spontaneously share their hallucinations, many validate observations of the examiner or admit to a history of hallucinations when asked. See Box 21.6. If a patient has command hallucinations, it is important for the safety of the person and others to know what the voices are telling the patient to do.

Delusions

Delusions are different from strongly held beliefs. Delusions do not change even though strong evidence contradicts the belief. The person continues to hold the belief despite contradictory evidence (APA, 2013). The person's culture must be considered when evaluating delusions. Delusional beliefs are those not sanctioned or held by a cultural or religious subgroup.

Bizarre delusions alone are sufficient to diagnose schizophrenia (APA, 2013). Bizarre delusions are those beliefs that are impossible, illogical, and not derived from ordinary life experiences. Bizarre delusions often include delusions of control (that some outside force controls thoughts and actions), thought broadcasting (that others can read or hear one's thoughts), thought insertion (that someone has placed thoughts into one's mind), and thought withdrawal (that someone is removing thoughts from one's mind). For example, a patient who has been seeing a hypnotist for 2 months reports that the hypnotist continued to read his mind and was "picking his brain away piece by piece." Another patient was convinced that a computer chip was placed in her vagina during a gynecologic examination and that this somehow directly influenced her physical movements and her thoughts.

> Remember Arnold? He believes that his parents were still alive and that they would return. He refuses to leave the farm and insists that everything be left as it is.

Nonbizarre delusions generally have themes of jealousy and persecution and are derived from plausible life experiences. For example, a woman believes that her husband,

BOX 21.6 • THERAPEUTIC DIALOGUE • The Patient With Hallucinations

The following conversation took place in Arnold's room during the night checks. The nurse observed that Arnold was talking with someone, but no one else was in the room.

INEFFECTIVE APPROACH

Nurse: Arnold?

Arnold: Yeah?

Nurse: Who are you talking to?

Arnold: My mother visits me at night. I am telling her about my day.

Nurse: You know, Arnold, you are having an hallucination. Your mother died a few weeks ago.

Arnold: She did not. She is away for a while, but she will be back soon.

Nurse: Arnold. (Looks at nurse.) You are going to have to accept that your mother is gone.

Arnold: Oh yeah? What do you know?

Nurse: Well, we can talk about it in the morning.

Arnold: You don't know what you are talking about.

EFFECTIVE APPROACH

Nurse: Arnold?

Arnold: Yeah?

Nurse: Are you talking to someone?

Arnold: Yes, she visits me at night?

Nurse: Oh, does she talk to you?

Arnold: Yes, she asks me about my day. She visits in the evening?

Nurse: Is there anything else you talk about?

Arnold: No, she leaves after I tell her.

Nurse: OK, how do you feel when she visits you?

Arnold: A little sad, but I like to tell her about my day.

Nurse: A little sad?

Arnold: Yeah, I wish I could see her more.

Nurse: Sounds like you are lonely?

Arnold: Yea, it's nice when you talk with me.

Nurse: I can do that. If you are not asleep when I finish rounds, we can talk more.

CRITICAL THINKING CHALLENGE

- How did the nurse's impatience translate into Arnold's response in the first scenario?

- What effective communicating techniques did the nurse use in the second scenario?

from whom she has recently separated, is trying to poison her, or a man who believes that members of the Mafia are trying to kill him because, when he was in high school, he reported to the principal that several of his classmates were selling drugs at school (APA, 2013).

Assessing and judging the content of the delusion and exploring other aspects of the delusional experience are helpful in understanding the significance of these false beliefs. The underlying feeling that accompanies the delusion (i.e, fear or inflated self-esteem) should be explored. Other aspects to consider include the conviction with which the delusion is held; the extent to which other aspects of the individual's life are incorporated or affected by the delusion; the degree of internal consistency, organization, and logic evidenced in the delusion; and evaluating the amount of pressure (in terms of preoccupation and concern) individuals feel in their lives as a result of the delusion (Box 21.7).

Disorganized Communication

Abrupt shifts in the focus of conversation, which are often altered in schizophrenia, are typically symptomatic of disorganized thinking. Impaired verbal fluency (i.e., ability to produce spontaneous speech) is commonly present. The most severe shifts in focus may occur after only one or two words (i.e., word salad), after one or two phrases or sentences (i.e., flight of ideas or loose associations), or somewhat less severely as a shift that occurs when a new

BOX 21.7 • THERAPEUTIC DIALOGUE • The Patient With Delusions

John joined the nurse in a game of pool. The following conversation occurred as they played.

INEFFECTIVE APPROACH

John: The CIA put a transmitter in my molar, here (points to his right cheek).

Nurse: No one would put a transmitter in your tooth; come on, the CIA isn't looking for you.

John: Yeah, they want to monitor me while I'm here. I know that they have the real Osama bin Laden here in the hospital. They are trying to get the President to intervene with the Michigan Militia. Mark from Michigan told me that.

Nurse: Osama bin Laden can't possibly be here; he died years ago.

John: Maybe—but that was an imposter. They're just trying to keep people from knowing what they're doing.

Nurse: John, Osama bin Laden isn't in the hospital; if he were, I would know it because I work here.

John: (With anger) You don't know anything! You are probably working for the CIA too. I have nothing else to say to you.

EFFECTIVE APPROACH

John: The CIA put a transmitter in my molar, here (points to his right cheek).

Nurse: Oh. Which balls are mine?

John: You get the striped ones. Yeah, they want to monitor me while I'm here. I know that they have the real Osama bin Laden here in the hospital. They are trying to get the President to intervene with the Michigan Militia. Mark from Michigan told me that.

Nurse: Well, I don't know anything about that, but I want you to know that we will keep you safe.

John: Maybe…

Nurse: You sound a little overwhelmed with all the information you have.

John: No, no. I can handle it. The CIA can't do anything to me. I'll never talk.

Nurse: I thought they could hear you when you talk to me.

John: Huh? Oh, that transmitter is so that they can send me misinformation. They send a tower of babble to my brain. They are trying to confuse me so that I stay away from Osama Bin Laden. They all think they can keep me from my mission.

Nurse: Who are they?

John: Everyone in the government. The CIA, FBI, ATF, IRS—all those alphabets.

Nurse: So everyone in the government is trying to get to you?

John: Well, maybe not everybody. Just the ones that care about money and the militia. I don't think they care about me much in Commerce or Health and Human Services. Although they'd care too if they knew.

Nurse: I would think that's pretty frightening to have all these people out looking for you. You must be scared a lot.

John: It's scary, but I can handle it. I've handled it all my life.

Nurse: You've been in scary situations all your life?

John: Yeah. I don't know. Maybe not scary, just hard. I never seemed to be able to do as well as my parents wanted—or as I wanted.

CRITICAL THINKING CHALLENGE

- How did the nurse's argumentative responses cause the patient to react in the first scenario?

- What effective communication techniques did the nurse use in the second scenario?

topic is repeatedly suggested and pursued from the current topic (i.e., tangentiality).

Cognitive Impairments

Mental status assessment focuses on eliciting indications of cognitive impairments associated with schizophrenia.

Although these impairments vary widely from patient to patient, several primary problems have been identified:

- Attention may be increased and sustained on external stimuli over a period of time (hypervigilance).
- The ability to distinguish and focus on relevant stimuli may be diminished.

- Familiar cues may go unrecognized or be improperly interpreted.
- Information processing may be diminished, leading to inappropriate or illogical conclusions from available observations and information (Baker, Holmes, Masters, Yeo, Krienen, Buckner, et al., 2014; Lepage, Bodnar, & Bowie, 2014).

Cognitive impairments are not easy to recognize. By relying only on clinical assessment, the nurse can miss the extent of the impairment. Using a standardized instrument can provide a screening measurement of cognitive function. See Chapter 9. If impairment exists, neuropsychological testing by a qualified psychologist may be necessary.

Memory and Orientation

Impairment in orientation, memory, and abstract thinking is often present. Orientation to time, place, and person may remain relatively intact unless the patient is particularly preoccupied with delusions and hallucinations. Although all aspects of memory may be affected in schizophrenia, registration or the recall within seconds of newly learned information may be particularly diminished. This affects the individual's short- and long-term memory. The ability to engage in abstract thinking may be impaired. See Box 21.8.

BOX 21.8

Arnold's Cognitive Symptoms

Arnold's symptoms of schizophrenia began long before he was actually diagnosed. Throughout school he had difficulty learning new material. His teachers would describe him as being "slow" or "inattentive." Because he appeared to be functioning normally, his teachers and family attributed his poor academic behavior to lack of interest. His father would often get frustrated with him because he would spend many hours in his bedroom and would not help out on the farm. When prodded to complete school work or a household task, he would often get distracted before finishing the tasks. Family members and teachers quickly learned to provide several prompts for Arnold to complete a task. As he progressed to high school, he was labeled as a "slow learner" and assigned to less demanding classes.

The reality was that Arnold was experiencing unrecognized prodromal cognitive symptoms of schizophrenia. He was having difficulty remembering his assignments. He was having difficulty grasping concepts that other students seemed to easily understand. He was becoming frustrated with his difficulty and retreated to his room. He waited for specific directions that he could easily process. His thinking was concrete and he had difficulty expressing himself. When he was bombarded with several directions at once, he could not process any of the directions. In his frustration, he would throw objects, frightening others. His family was very concerned with the changes that were occurring with their once easy-going son.

Insight and Judgment

Insight and judgment are closely related to each other. Individuals display insight when they recognize that their hallucinations or delusions are symptoms of a mental disorder. Judgment is the ability to decide or act about a situation. If judgment is poor, the person may not recognize personal vulnerabilities and consequently engages in detrimental behavior. For example, the individual may be taken advantage by others or fail to realize a potentially dangerous situation.

Behavioral Responses

During periods of psychosis, unusual or bizarre behavior often occurs. These behaviors can usually be understood within the context of the patient's disturbed thinking. The nurse needs to understand the significance of the behavior to the individual. For example, one patient moved the family furniture into the yard because he thought that evil spirits were hiding in the furniture. His bizarre behavior was an attempt to protect his family. Another patient painted a sequence of numbers on his bedroom walls. He said that the numbers were the language of the angels. His delusional thoughts were the basis of his behavior.

Because of the negative symptoms, specifically avolition, patients may not seem interested or organized enough to complete normal daily activities. They may stay in bed most of the day or refuse to take a shower. Many times, they agree to get up in the morning and go to work, but they never get around to it. Several specific behaviors are associated with schizophrenia, including stereotypy (i.e., idiosyncratic, repetitive, purposeless movements), echopraxia (i.e., involuntary imitation of others' movements), and waxy flexibility (i.e., posture held in odd or unusual fixed positions for extended periods). In some cases, certain behaviors need to be evaluated carefully to distinguish them from movements that are associated with medication-related side effects, such as grimacing, stereotypical behavior, or agitation.

Self-Concept

In schizophrenia, self-concept is usually poor. Patients often are aware that they are hearing voices others do not hear. They recognize that they are different from others and are often scared of "going crazy." Many are aware of the loss of expectations for their future achievements. The pervasive stigma associated with having a mental illness contributes to the poor self-concept. Body image can be disturbed, especially during periods of hallucinations or delusions. For example, one patient believed that her body was infected with germs and she could feel them eating away her insides.

Stress and Coping Patterns

Stressful events are often linked to psychiatric symptoms. It is important to determine stresses from the patient's perspective because a stressful event for one may not be stressful for another. It is also important to determine typical coping patterns, especially negative coping strategies, such as the use of substances or showing aggressive behavior.

> Recall Arnold's symptoms? They appeared after the stress of his parents' death.

Social Network

Several difficulties involving social functioning occur in schizophrenia. As the disorder progresses, individuals can become increasingly socially isolated. On a one-to-one basis, this occurs as the individual seems unable to connect with people in his or her environment. Several aspects of symptoms already discussed can contribute to this. For example, emotional blunting and anhedonia (the inability to experience pleasure) result in an experience of not being engaged in activities and relationships.

Interpretation of facial expressions and affect is often problematic for people with schizophrenia. These cognitive deficits are related to recall of past interactions and problems with decision making and judgment, and with poverty of speech and language. Poor functioning and the inability to complete ADLs are manifested in poor hygiene, malnutrition, and social isolation.

Functional Status

Functional status of patients with schizophrenia should be assessed initially and at regular intervals. Level of independence, ability to work, ability to maintain an independent living environment, and self-care should be evaluated.

Support Systems

In schizophrenia, support systems become very important in maintaining the patient in the community. The individual may become socially isolated if the treatment and management occur in long-term care facilities and group homes away from family and friends. One challenge is to identify and maintain the patient's links with family and significant others. Assessment of the formal support (e.g., family, health care providers) and informal support (e.g., neighbors, friends) should be conducted.

Quality of Life

People with schizophrenia often have a poor quality of life, especially older people, who may have spent many years in long-term hospitals. The nurse should assess the patient's quality of life and how it could be improved. Simple changes, such as arranging for a different roommate or improving access to social activities by meeting transportation needs, can greatly improve a patient's quality of life.

Strength Assessment

An important part of recovery is identification of personal and family strengths. Because schizophrenia is usually diagnosed at a young age, the person may be physically fit with little evidence of chronic illness. As the assessment is completed, strengths will emerge. Family support is critical for a person with schizophrenia. Intellectual ability and coping with stress are areas that can be strengths. The following questions are examples that can be used in assessing strengths.

- What do you do for relaxation, fun?
- How do you manage stressful events?
- How do you cope with the voices, thoughts, or impulses?
- Who do you talk with when you are upset?
- Are you hopeful about the future?

NURSING DIAGNOSES

There are many nursing diagnoses generated from the assessment data. Typical nursing diagnoses focusing on the physical aspects include Self-Care Deficit and Disturbed Sleep Pattern. During a relapse, Ineffective Therapeutic Regimen Management, Imbalanced Nutrition, Excess Fluid Volume, and Sexual Dysfunction are possible diagnoses. For psychological aspects, Disturbed Thought Processes can be used for delusions, confusion, and disorganized thinking. Disturbed Sensory Perception is appropriate for hallucinations or illusions. Other examples of diagnoses include Chronic Low Self-esteem, Personal Identity Disturbance, Risk for Violence, Ineffective Coping, and Knowledge Deficit. The nursing diagnoses generated from the assessment of the social domain are typically Impaired Social Interaction, Ineffective Role Performance, Disabled Family Coping, or Interrupted Family Processes. Outcomes depend on the specific diagnostic area. Several strength-based nursing diagnoses can be generated from the assessment data, such as Readiness for Enhanced Coping and Readiness for Enhanced Hope.

> **NCLEXNOTE** When assessing a patient with schizophrenia, the nurse should prioritize the severity of the current responses to the disorder. If hallucinations are impairing function, then managing hallucinations is a priority and medications are needed immediately. If hallucinations are not a problem, however, coping with negative symptoms becomes a priority.

THERAPEUTIC RELATIONSHIP

Development of the therapeutic nurse-patient relationship centers on developing trust, accepting the person as a worthy human being, and infusing the relationship with hope. People with schizophrenia are often reluctant to engage in any relationship because of previous rejection and, in some instances, an underlying suspiciousness, which is a part of the illness. They are often trying to trust their own thoughts and perceptions, so interactions with another human being may prove to be too overwhelming. If they are having hallucinations, their images of other people may be distorted and frightening as they struggle to trust their own thoughts and perceptions.

The nurse should approach the patient in a calm and caring manner. Engaging the patient in a relationship may take time but it begins with the first encounter. Short time-limited interactions are best for a patient who is experiencing psychosis. Being consistent in interactions and following through on promises will help establish trust within the relationship.

Establishing a therapeutic relationship is crucial, especially with patients who deny that they are ill. Patients are more likely to agree to and continue treatment if these recommendations are made within the context of a safe, trusting relationship. Even if some patients deny having mental illness, they may take medication and attend treatment activities because they trust the nurse (Jaeger, Seißhaupt, Flammer, Steinert, 2014).

Furthermore, for long-term care and outcomes, recovery-oriented relationships are important. Using the recovery model, all efforts should be made to individualize treatment. Care should be person-centered through partnering with the patient in all aspects of care and encourage self-direction. Treatment should be focused on strengths and the empowerment of the individual. Patients need encouragement to see that although their diagnosis may seem devastating, recovery is possible (Pandya & Myrick, 2013).

MENTAL HEALTH NURSING INTERVENTIONS

Self-Care

For many people with schizophrenia, the plan of care will include specific interventions to enhance self-care, nutrition, and overall health knowledge. Negative symptoms commonly leave patients unable to initiate these seemingly simple activities. Developing a daily schedule of routine activities (e.g., showering, shaving) can help the patient structure the day. Most patients actually know how to perform self-care activities (e.g., hygiene, grooming) but lack motivation (avolition) to carry them out consistently. Interventions include developing a schedule with the patient for various hygiene-related activities and emphasizing the importance of maintaining appropriate self-care activities. Given the problems related to attention and memory in people with schizophrenia, education about these areas requires careful planning.

Activity, Exercise, and Nutritional Interventions

Encouraging activity and exercise is necessary, not only to maintain a healthy lifestyle but also to counteract the side effects of psychiatric medications that cause weight gain. Because the diagnosis is usually made in late adolescence or early adulthood, it is possible to establish solid exercise patterns early.

During episodes of acute psychosis, patients are sometimes unable to focus on eating. Often when patients begin antipsychotic medication, normal satiety and hunger responses change, and overeating or weight gain can become a problem. Promoting healthy nutrition is a key intervention. Maintaining healthy nutrition and monitoring calorie intake also become important because of the effect many medications have on eating habits. Patients report that their appetites increase and cravings for food develop when some medications are initiated.

Weight gain is one of the reasons some patients stop taking their medications. Increased weight places patients at greater risk for several health problems, such as type II DM and early death. Monitoring for DM and managing weight are important activities for all health care providers. Patients should be screened for risk factors of DM, such as family history, obesity as indicated by a body mass index (BMI) exceeding or equal to 27, and age older than 45 years. Patients' weight should be measured at regular intervals and the BMI calculated. Blood pressure readings should be taken regularly. Laboratory findings for triglycerides, high-density lipoprotein cholesterol, and glucose level should be monitored and reviewed regularly. All health care providers should be alert to the development of hyperglycemia, particularly in patients known to have DM who begin taking second-generation antipsychotic agents. A program to address weight gain should be initiated at the earliest sign of weight gain (probably between 5 and 10 pounds over desired body weight). Reduced caloric intake may be accomplished by increasing the patient's access to affordable, healthful, and easy-to-prepare foods. Behavioral management of weight gain includes keeping a food diary, diet teaching, and support groups (Koch & Scott, 2012; Soundy, Muhamed, Stubbs, Probst, & Vancampfort, 2014).

Thermoregulation Interventions

Patients with schizophrenia may have disturbed body temperature regulation. In winter, they may seem to be oblivious to cold weather. In the heat of summer, they may dress for winter. Observing patients' responses to temperatures helps in identifying problems in this area. In patients who are taking psychiatric medications, body temperature needs to be monitored, and the patient needs to be protected from extremes in temperature.

Fluid Balance

Some persons with schizophrenia develop disturbed fluid and electrolyte balance. Nurses should observe for polydipsia (frequently drinking an excessive amount of fluids) or frequent incontinence. These individuals are obsessed with drinking water and compulsively consume fluids. For persons with schizophrenia who demonstrate polydipsia, regulation of their fluid intake is disturbed, resulting in an abnormally low serum sodium level, which can lead to severe water intoxication, a medical emergency.

Nursing interventions include teaching and assisting the patient to develop self-monitoring skills. Fluid intake and weight gain should be monitored to control fluid intake and reduce the likelihood of developing water intoxication. Patients with mild polydipsia are easily treated in outpatient settings and benefit from educational programs that teach them to monitor their own urine's specific gravity and daily weight gains. Patients with moderate polydipsia may respond well to education but still have a more difficult time controlling their own fluid intake, which requires more careful monitoring of intake and weight throughout the day. Patients with severe polydipsia require considerable assistance, probably in an inpatient unit, to restrict their continual water-seeking behavior. These patients may create disruption on the unit, so they are best managed by one-on-one observation to redirect their behavior.

Medication Interventions: Antipsychotics

Antipsychotic medications are the treatment of choice for patients with psychosis. Antipsychotic drugs are used because they have the general effect of blocking dopamine transmission leading to a decrease in psychotic symptoms (see Chapter 10). Some medications also block other receptors of other neurotransmitters to varying degrees. See Table 21.2.

The prescription of first-generation antipsychotics (e.g., haloperidol, chlorpromazine) decreased dramatically with the introduction of second-generation antipsychotics. However, it is important that medication choice be individualized based on each patient's experience and preference as well as the side effect profiles of selected drugs rather than to limit drug selection to one type or class of antipsychotic medication. This is particularly true during the acute phase of the illness for

TABLE 21.2	SELECTED ANTIPSYCHOTIC DRUGS	
Generic Name	Trade Name	Dosage Range for Adults (mg/d)
Second-Generation Antipsychotics		
aripiprazole	Abilify	10–15
asenapine	Saphris	10–20
clozapine	Clozaril	200–600
risperidone	Risperdal	4–16
olanzapine	Zyprexa	10–20
paliperidone	Invega	3–12
quetiapine	Seroquel	300–400
ziprasidone	Geodon	40–160
lurasidone	Latuda	40–80 mg
Selected First-Generation Antipsychotic Drugs Used to Treat Psychosis in the United States		
chlorpromazine	NA*	30–800
fluphenazine	NA	0.5–20
haloperidol	Haldol	1–15
loxapine	Loxitane	20–250
perphenazine	NA	4–32
pimozide	NA	1–10
thiothixene	Navane	5–25
trifluoperazine	NA	5–25

*Not Applicable. No longer available as proprietary formulations.

people with schizophrenia who are known to respond to treatment.

Second-generation antipsychotic drugs including risperidone (Risperdal), olanzapine (Zyprexa), quetiapine (Seroquel), paliperidone (Invega), ziprasidone (Geodon), aripiprazole (Abilify), iloperidone (Fanapt), asenapine (Saphris), and lurasidone (Latuda) are available in a variety of formulations. See Box 21.9 for more information about risperidone. They are effective in treating both negative and positive symptoms. These newer drugs also target other neurotransmitter systems, such as serotonin. This is believed to contribute to their antipsychotic effectiveness.

Administering Medications

Nursing interventions during the initial acute phase of schizophrenia include prompt, safe, and informed administration of antipsychotic medications. Generally, it takes about 1 to 2 weeks for antipsychotic drugs to effect a change in symptoms. During the stabilization period, the selected drug should be given an adequate trial, generally 6 to 12 weeks, before considering a change in the drug prescription. For maximum absorption, ziprasidone and lurasidone should be given with food. Ziprasidone should be taken with a high-fat meal of 500 calories. For lurasidone, 350 calories should be eaten when administering this medication (Lincoln,

BOX 21.9

Drug Profile: Risperidone (Risperdal)

DRUG CLASS: Atypical antipsychotic

RECEPTOR AFFINITY: Antagonist with high affinity for D2 and 5-HT2, also histamine (H1) and α_1-, α_2-adrenergic receptors, weak affinity for D1 and other serotonin receptor subtypes; no affinity for acetylcholine or β-adrenergic receptors

INDICATIONS: Treatment of schizophrenia; short-term treatment of acute manic or mixed episodes associated with bipolar I disorder; and irritability associated with autistic disorder in children and adolescents, including symptoms of aggression towards others, deliberate self-injuriousness, temper tantrums, and quickly changing moods

ROUTES AND DOSAGE: 0.25-, 0.5-, 1-, 2-, 3-, and 4-mg tablets and liquid concentrate (1 mg/mL); orally disintegrating tablets, 0.5-, 1-, 2-, 3-, and 4-mg

Adult: Schizophrenia: Initial dose: typically 1 mg bid. Maximal effect at 6 mg/d. Safety not established above 16 mg/d. Use lowest possible dose to alleviate symptoms.

Bipolar mania: 2 to 3 mg/d

Geriatric: Initial dose, 0.5 mg/d; increase slowly as tolerated

Children: 0.25 mg per day for patients <20 kg and 0.5 mg per day for patients >20 kg

HALF-LIFE (PEAK EFFECT): Mean, 20 h (1 h; peak active metabolite = 3–17 h)

SELECT SIDE EFFECTS: Insomnia, agitation, anxiety, extrapyramidal symptoms, headache, rhinitis, somnolence, dizziness, headache, constipation, nausea, dyspepsia, vomiting, abdominal pain, hypersalivation, tachycardia, orthostatic hypotension, fever, chest pain, coughing, photosensitivity, weight gain

BOXED WARNING: Increased mortality in elderly patients with dementia-related psychosis

WARNING: Rare development of neuroleptic malignant syndrome. Observe frequently for early signs of tardive dyskinesia. Use caution with individuals who have cardiovascular disease; risperidone can cause electrocardiographic changes. Avoid use during pregnancy or while breast-feeding. Hepatic or renal impairments increase plasma concentration.

SPECIFIC PATIENT/FAMILY EDUCATION
- Notify your prescriber if tremor, motor restlessness, abnormal movements, chest pain, or other unusual symptoms develop.
- Avoid alcohol and other CNS depressant drugs.
- Notify your prescriber if pregnancy is possible or if planning to become pregnant. Do not breastfeed while taking this medication.
- Notify your prescriber before taking any other prescription or OTC medication.
- May impair judgment, thinking, or motor skills; avoid driving or potentially other hazardous tasks.
- During titration, the individual may experience orthostatic hypotension and should change positions slowly.
- Do not abruptly discontinue.

bid, twice a day; CNS, central nervous system; OTC, over-the-counter.

Steward, & Preskorn, 2010; Pfizer, 2014; Sunovion, 2013). If treatment effects are not seen, a different antipsychotic agent may be tried. Clozapine is used when no other second-generation antipsychotic is effective; see Box 21.10 for more information about clozapine.

Adherence to a prescribed medication regimen is the best approach to prevent relapse. Unfortunately, adherence to the second-generation antipsychotic agents is not improved from the first-generation antipsychotic agents (Guo, Fang, Zhai, Wang, B., Wang, C., Hu, et al., 2011). The use of long-acting injectables is expected to improve compliance outcomes (Altamura, Aguglia, Bassi, Bogetto, Cappellari, & De Giorgi, et al., 2012). Box 21.11 provides evidence related to interventions that promote medication adherence for patients with schizophrenia.

Patients with schizophrenia generally face a lifetime of taking antipsychotic medications. Rarely is discontinuation of medications prescribed; however, many patients stop taking medications on their own. Some conditions do require the cessation of medication use such as neuroleptic malignant syndrome (see later discussion), agranulocytosis (i.e., dangerously low level of circulating neutrophils), or drug reaction with eosinophilia and systemic symptoms (i.e., fever with a rash and/or swollen lymph glands). Discontinuation is an option when tardive dyskinesia develops. Discontinuation of medications, other than in the circumstances of a medical emergency, should be achieved by gradually lowering the dose over time. This diminishes the likelihood of withdrawal symptoms.

Monitoring Extrapyramidal Side Effects

Parkinsonism caused by antipsychotic drugs is identical in appearance to Parkinson disease and tends to occur in older patients. The symptoms are believed to be caused by the blockade of dopamine D_2 receptors in the basal ganglia, which throws off the normal balance between acetylcholine and dopamine in this area of the brain and effectively increases acetylcholine transmission. The symptoms are managed by reducing dosage and thereby increasing dopamine activity or adding an anticholinergic drug, thus decreasing acetylcholine activity, such as benztropine or trihexyphenidyl.

Dystonic reactions are also believed to result from the imbalance of dopamine and acetylcholine, with the latter dominant. Young men seem to be more vulnerable to this particular extrapyramidal side effect. This side effect, which develops rapidly and dramatically and can be very frightening for patients as their muscles tense and their body contorts. The experience often starts with **oculogyric crisis**, in which the muscles that control eye movements tense and pull the eyeball so that the patient is looking toward the ceiling. This may be followed rapidly by **torticollis**, in which the neck muscles pull the head to the side, or **retrocollis**, in which the head is pulled back, or orolaryngeal–pharyngeal hypertonus, in which the patient has extreme difficulty in swallowing. The patient may also experience contorted limbs. These symptoms

---

BOX 21.10

Drug Profile: Clozapine (Clozaril)

DRUG CLASS: Atypical antipsychotic

RECEPTOR AFFINITY: D1 and D2 blockade, antagonist for 5-HT2, histamine (H1), α-adrenergic, and acetylcholine. These additional antagonist effects may contribute to some of its therapeutic effects. Produces fewer extrapyramidal effects than standard antipsychotics with lower risk for tardive dyskinesia.

INDICATIONS: Severely ill individuals who have schizophrenia and have not responded to standard antipsychotic treatment; reduction in risk of recurrent suicidal behavior in schizophrenia or schizoaffective disorders.

ROUTES AND DOSAGE: Available only in tablet form, 25- and 100-mg doses.

Adult Dosage: Initial dose 25 mg PO twice or 4 times daily, may gradually increase in 25–50 mg/d increments, if tolerated, to a dose of 300–450 mg/d by the end of the second week. Additional increases should occur no more than once or twice weekly. Do not exceed 900 mg/d. For maintenance, reduce dosage to lowest effective level.

Children: Safety and efficacy with children younger than age 16 years have not been established.

HALF-LIFE (PEAK EFFECT): 12 h (1–6 h)

SELECT ADVERSE REACTIONS: Drowsiness, dizziness, headache, hypersalivation, tachycardia, hypo- or hypertension, constipation, dry mouth, heartburn, nausea or vomiting, blurred vision, diaphoresis, fever, weight gain, hematologic changes, seizures, tremor, akathisia

BOXED WARNING: Agranulocytosis, defined as a granulocyte count of <500 mm3, occurs at about a cumulative 1-year incidence of 1.3%, most often within 4–10 weeks of exposure, but may occur at any time; WBC count before initiation, and weekly WBC counts while taking the drug and for 4 weeks after discontinuation.

Seizures, myocarditis, and other adverse cardiovascular and respiratory side effects (i.e., orthostatic hypotension).

WARNING: Increased mortality in elderly patients with dementia-related psychosis; rare development of NMS; *hyperglycemia and DM, tardive dyskinesia,* cases of sudden, unexplained death have been reported; avoid use during pregnancy and while breast-feeding.

PRECAUTIONS: Fever, pulmonary embolism, hepatitis, anticholinergic toxicity, and interference with cognitive and motor functions.

SPECIFIC PATIENT/FAMILY EDUCATION

• Need informed consent regarding risk for agranulocytosis. Weekly or biweekly blood draws are required. Notify your prescriber immediately if lethargy, weakness, sore throat, malaise, or other flu-like symptoms develop.

• You should not take clozapine if you are taking other medicines that may cause the same serious bone marrow side effects.

• Inform the patient of risk of seizures, hyperglycemia and diabetes, and orthostatic hypotension. It may potentiate the hypotensive effects of antihypertensive drugs and anticholinergic effects of atropine-like drugs.

• Administration of epinephrine should be avoided in the treatment of drug-induced hypotension.

• Notify your prescriber if pregnancy is possible or if you are planning to become pregnant. Do not breastfeed while taking this medication.

• Notify your prescriber before taking any other prescription or OTC medication. Avoid alcohol or other CNS depressant drugs.

• May cause drowsiness and seizures; avoid driving or other hazardous tasks.

• During titration, the individual may experience orthostatic hypotension and so should change positions slowly.

• Do not abruptly discontinue.

CNS, central nervous system; NMS, neuroleptic malignant syndrome; OTC, over-the-counter; WBC, white blood cell.

---

occur early in antipsychotic drug treatment, when the patient may still be enduring psychotic symptoms, which compounds the patient's fear and anxiety and requires a quick response. The immediate treatment is to administer benztropine 1 to 2 mg, or diphenhydramine (Benadryl), 25 to 50 mg, intramuscularly or intravenously. This is followed by daily administration of anticholinergic drugs and, possibly, by a decrease

---

BOX 21.11

Research for Best Practice: Medication Adherence in People With Schizophrenia

Gray, R., White, J., Schulz, M., & Abderhalden, C. (2010). Enhancing medication adherence in people with schizophrenia: An international programme of research. International Journal of Mental Health Nursing, 19 (1), 36–44.

THE QUESTION: Do adherence therapy interventions improve adherence?

METHODS: Adherence therapy facilitates shared decision-making between patients and clinicians. This paper reviewed the results of four adherence therapy trials that had mixed results. The authors then developed an adherence intervention based on six adherence-modifying factors: efficacy of medication, side effect management, clinician characteristics, medication side effects, experiences of medication and illness, and beliefs and attitudes about medications.

FINDINGS: Two studies showed improvement in symptoms and quality of life through implementing adherence therapy session over 8 weeks starting in the inpatient unit before discharge to the community. In adherence therapy, the five key exercises broadly follow this sequence: structured medication problem-solving (e.g., practical problems, such as side effects), looking back (e.g., reviewing past experiences of illness and treatment), exploring ambivalence, discussing beliefs and concerns, and looking forward (e.g., life goals).

IMPLICATIONS FOR NURSING: The authors confirm that people with schizophrenia need to be more involved in decision-making and in control of their own medications. Future studies are needed to evaluate the effectiveness of interventions that enhance the feeling of being in control over medication.

in dosage antipsychotic medication. See Box 21.12 for more information about benztropine.

Akathisia appears to be caused by the same biologic mechanism as other **extrapyramidal side effects**. Patients are restless and report they feel driven to keep moving. They are extremely uncomfortable. Frequently, this response is misinterpreted as anxiety or increased psychotic symptoms, so that the patient may inappropriately be given increased dosages of an antipsychotic drug, which only perpetuates the side effect. If possible, the dose of antipsychotic drug should be reduced. A beta-adrenergic blocker such as propranolol (Inderal), 20 to 120 mg, may be required. An anticholinergic medication may not be helpful. Failure to manage this side effect is a leading cause of patients ceasing to take antipsychotic medications (see Chapter 10).

Tardive dyskinesia, tardive dystonia, and tardive akathisia are less likely but still possible to appear in individuals taking second-generation, rather than first-generation, antipsychotics. Table 21.3 describes these and associated motor abnormalities. **Tardive dyskinesia** is late-appearing abnormal involuntary movements It can be viewed as the opposite of parkinsonism both in observable movements and in etiology. Whereas muscle rigidity and absence of movement characterize parkinsonism, constant movement characterizes tardive dyskinesia. Typical movements involve the mouth, tongue, and jaw and include lip smacking, sucking, puckering, tongue protrusion, the "bonbon sign" (where the tongue rolls around in the mouth and protrudes into the cheek as if the patient is sucking on a piece of hard candy), athetoid (worm-like) movements of the tongue and chewing. Other facial movements, such as grimacing and eye blinking, may also be present.

Movements in the trunk and limbs are frequently observable. These include rocking from the hips, athetoid movements of the fingers and toes, jerking movements of the fingers and toes, guitar strumming movements of the fingers, and foot tapping. The long-term health problems for people with tardive dyskinesia are choking associated with loss of control of muscles used for swallowing and compromised respiratory function leading to infections and possibly respiratory alkalosis.

Because the movements resemble the dyskinetic movements of some patients who have idiopathic Parkinson disease and who have received long-term treatment with L-DOPA (a direct-acting dopamine agonist that crosses the blood–brain barrier), the suggested hypothesis for tardive dyskinesia includes the supersensitivity of the dopamine receptors in the basal ganglia.

No consistently effective treatment yet exists; however, antipsychotic drugs mask the movements of tardive dyskinesia and have periodically been suggested as a treatment. This is counterintuitive because these are drugs cause the disorder. Second-generation antipsychotic

---

BOX 21.12

Drug Profile: Benztropine Mesylate

DRUG CLASS: Antiparkinsonism agent

RECEPTOR AFFINITY: Blocks cholinergic (acetylcholine) activity, which is believed to restore the balance of acetylcholine and dopamine in the basal ganglia.

INDICATIONS: Used in psychiatry to reduce extrapyramidal symptoms (acute medication-related movement disorders), including pseudoparkinsonism, dystonia, and akathisia (but not tardive syndromes) caused by neuroleptic drugs such as haloperidol. Most effective with acute dystonia.

ROUTES AND DOSAGE: Available in tablet form, 0.5-, 1-, and 2-mg doses, also injectable 1 mg/mL

Adult Dosage: For acute dystonia, 1–2 mg IM or IV usually provides rapid relief. No significant difference in onset of action after IM or IV injection. Treatment of emergent symptoms may be relieved in 1 or 2 days, with 1–2 mg PO 2–3 times/d. Maximum daily dose is 6 mg/d. After 1–2 weeks, withdraw drug to see if continued treatment is needed. Medication-related movement disorders that develop slowly may not respond to this treatment.

Geriatric: Older adults and very thin patients cannot tolerate large doses.

Children: Do not use in children younger than 3 years of age. Use with caution in older children.

HALF-LIFE: 12–24 h; very little pharmacokinetic information is available.

SELECT SIDE EFFECTS: Dry mouth, blurred vision, tachycardia, nausea, constipation, flushing or elevated temperature, decreased sweating, muscular weakness or cramping, urinary retention, urinary hesitancy, dizziness, headache, disorientation, confusion, memory loss, hallucinations, psychoses, and agitation in toxic reactions, which are more pronounced in elderly adults and occur at smaller doses

WARNING: Avoid use during pregnancy and while breastfeeding. Give with caution in hot weather because of possible heatstroke. Contraindicated with angle-closure glaucoma, pyloric or duodenal obstruction, stenosing peptic ulcers, prostatic hypertrophy or bladder neck obstructions, myasthenia gravis, megacolon, and megaesophagus. May aggravate the symptoms of tardive dyskinesia and other chronic forms of medication-related movement disorder. Concomitant use of other anticholinergic drugs may increase side effects and risk for toxicity. Coadministration of haloperidol or phenothiazines may reduce serum levels of these drugs.

SPECIFIC PATIENT/FAMILY EDUCATION
- Take with meals to reduce dry mouth and gastric irritation.
- Dry mouth may also be alleviated by sucking sugarless candies, maintaining adequate fluid intake, and good oral hygiene; increase fiber and fluids in diet to avoid constipation; stool softeners may be required. Notify your prescriber if urinary hesitancy or constipation persists.
- Notify your prescriber if rapid or pounding heartbeat, confusion, eye pain, rash, or other side effects develop.
- May cause drowsiness, dizziness, or blurred vision; use caution driving or performing other hazardous tasks requiring alertness. Avoid alcohol and other CNS depressants.
- Do not abruptly stop this medication because a flu-like syndrome may develop.
- Use with caution in hot weather. Ensure adequate hydration. May increase susceptibility to heat stroke.

CNS, central nervous system; IM, intramuscular; IV, intravenous; PO, oral.

TABLE 21.3	EXTRAPYRAMIDAL SIDE EFFECTS OF ANTIPSYCHOTIC DRUGS	
Side Effect	Period of Onset	Symptoms
Acute Motor Abnormalities		
Parkinsonism or pseudoparkinsonism	5–30 d	Resting tremor, rigidity, bradykinesia or akinesia, masklike face, shuffling gait, decreased arm swing
Acute dystonia	1–5 d	Intermittent or fixed abnormal postures of the eyes, face, tongue, neck, trunk, and limbs
Akathisia	1–30 d	Obvious motor restlessness evidenced by pacing, rocking, shifting from foot to foot; subjective sense of not being able to sit or be still; these symptoms may occur together or separately
Late-Appearing Motor Abnormalities		
Tardive dyskinesia	Months to years	Abnormal dyskinetic movements of the face, mouth, and jaw; choreoathetoid movements of the legs, arms, and trunk
Tardive dystonia	Months to years	Persistent sustained abnormal postures in the face, eyes, tongue, neck, trunk, and limbs
Tardive akathisia	Months to years	Persistent unabating sense of subjective and objective restlessness

Ferrando, S.J., Owen, J.A., Levenson, J.L. (2014). Psychopharmcology. In R.E. Hales, S.C. Ydofsky, & L.W. Roberts (Eds). *The American Psychiatric Publishing Textbook of Psychiatry* 6th ed. Arlington, VA: American Psychiatric Association. http://psychiatryonline.org/doi/full/10.1176/appi.books.9781585625031.rh27

drugs, such as clozapine, may be less likely to cause it. The best management remains prevention through using the lowest possible dose of an antipsychotic drug over time that minimizes the symptoms of schizophrenia.

Monitoring Other Side Effects

Orthostatic hypotension is a common side effect of antipsychotic drugs. Primarily an antiadrenergic effect, decreased blood pressure may be generalized or orthostatic. Patients may be protected from falls by teaching them to rise slowly and by monitoring blood pressure before giving the medication. The nurse should monitor and document lying, sitting, and standing blood pressures when any antipsychotic drug therapy begins.

Hyperprolactinemia can occur. When dopamine is blocked in the tuberoinfundibular tract, it can no longer repress prolactin, the neurohormone that regulates lactation and mammary function. The prolactin level increases and, in some individuals, side effects appear. Gynecomastia (i.e., enlarged breasts) can occur in people of both sexes and is understandably distressing to individuals who may be experiencing delusional or hallucinatory body image disturbances. Galactorrhea (i.e., lactation) may also occur. Menstrual irregularities and sexual dysfunction are possible. If these symptoms appear, the medication should be reduced or changed to another antipsychotic agent. Hyperprolactinemia is associated with the use of haloperidol and risperidone.

Sedation is another possible side effect of antipsychotic medication. Patients should be monitored for the sedating effects of antipsychotic agents. In elderly patients, sedation can be associated with falls.

Weight gain is related to antipsychotic agents, especially olanzapine and clozapine. Patients may gain as much as 20 or 30 pounds within 1 year. Such increased appetite and weight gain are distressing to patients. Diet teaching and monitoring may have some effect. Another solution is to increase the accessibility of healthful easy-to-prepare food.

New-onset DM should be assessed in patients taking antipsychotic drugs. An association has been found between new-onset DM and the administration of second-generation antipsychotic agents, especially after weight gain. Patients should be monitored for clinical symptoms of diabetes. Fasting blood glucose tests are commonly ordered for these individuals.

Cardiac arrhythmias may also occur. Prolongation of the QTc interval is associated with torsade de pointe (polymorphic ventricular tachycardia) or ventricular fibrillation. The potential for drug-induced prolonged QT interval is associated with many drugs. Ziprasidone (Geodon) is more likely than other second-generation antipsychotics to prolong the QT interval and thus change the heart rhythm. For these patients, baseline electrocardiograms may be ordered. Nurses should observe these patients for cardiac arrhythmias.

Agranulocytosis is a reduction in the number of circulating granulocytes and decreased production of granulocytes in the bone marrow, which limits one's ability to fight infection. Agranulocytosis can develop with the use of all antipsychotic drugs, but it is most likely to develop with clozapine use. Although laboratory values below 500 cells/mm^3 are indicative of agranulocytosis, often granulocyte counts drop to below 200 cells/mm^3 with this syndrome.

Patients taking clozapine should have regular blood tests. White blood cell and granulocyte counts should be measured before treatment is initiated and at least weekly or twice weekly after treatment begins. Initial white blood cell counts should be above 3,500 cells/mm^3 before treatment initiation; in patients with counts of 3,500 and 5,000 cells/mm^3, cell counts should be monitored three times a week if clozapine is prescribed. Any time the white blood cell count drops below 3,500 cells/mm^3 or granulocytes drop below 1,500 cells/mm^3, use of clozapine should be stopped, and the patient should be monitored for infection.

However, a faithfully implemented program of blood monitoring should not replace careful observation of the patient. It is not unusual for blood cell counts to drop precipitously over a period of 2 to 3 days. This may not be discovered when the patient is on a strict weekly blood monitoring schedule. Any reported symptoms that suggest a bacterial infection (e.g., fever, pharyngitis, weakness) should be cause for concern, so immediate evaluation of blood count status should be undertaken. Because patients are frequently discharged before the critical period of risk for agranulocytosis, patient education about these symptoms is also essential so that they will report these symptoms and obtain blood monitoring. In general, granulocyte levels return to normal within 2 to 4 weeks after discontinuation of use of the medication.

Drug Reaction with Eosinophilia and Systemic Symptoms (DRESS) is a very rare, potentially life-threatening, drug-induced hypersensitivity reaction recently associated with ziprasidone therapy (Geodon). The FDA recently published a safety announcement related to ziprasidone's association to. Symptoms include skin eruption, hematologic abnormalities (e.g., eosinophilia, atypical lymphocytosis), lymphadenopathy, and internal organ involvement (e.g., liver, kidney, lung). DRESS has a mortality rate of 10% (U.S. Food and Drug Administration, 2014).

Preventing Drug–Drug Interactions

Antipsychotic medications have the potential to interact with other medications, nicotine, and grapefruit juice. For example, olanzapine and clozapine have the potential to interact with some antidepressants. Some antipsychotics are metabolized faster in smokers than nonsmokers (Stahl, 2013). Before giving a medication, the nurse should check all medications for potential interactions.

Teaching Points

Non-adherence to the medication regimen is an important factor in relapse; the family must be made aware of the importance of the patient's taking medications consistently. Medication education should cover the association between medications and the amelioration of symptoms, side effects and their management, and interpersonal skills that help the patient and family report medication effects.

Management of Complications
Neuroleptic Malignant Syndrome

Neuroleptic malignant syndrome (NMS) is a life-threatening condition that can develop in reaction to antipsychotic medications. The primary symptoms of NMS are: *mental status changes, severe muscle rigidity*, and *autonomic changes* including elevated temperature (usually between 101° and 103° F), tachycardia, and blood pressure lability. Mental status changes and severe muscle rigidity occur usually within the first week of initiation of antipsychotic therapy and can include two or more of the following: hypertension, tachycardia, tachypnea, prominent diaphoresis, incontinence, mutism, leukocytosis, and laboratory evidence of muscle injury (e.g., elevated creatinine phosphokinase). The incidence of NMS has decreased recently from 3% to 0.2% probably because of increased awareness of symptoms and earlier interventions such as stopping the offending medication (Margetić & Aukst-Margetić, 2010). As many as one third of affected patients may die as a result of the syndrome. NMS is probably underreported and may account for unexplained emergency department deaths of patients taking these drugs because their symptoms do not seem serious.

The most important aspects of nursing care for patients with NMS relate to recognizing symptoms early, withholding any antipsychotic or any other dopamine antagonist (e.g., gastric reflux medications), and initiating supportive nursing care (Figure 21.4). In any patient with muscle rigidity, fluctuating vital signs, abrupt changes in levels of consciousness, or any of the symptoms presented in Box 21.13, NMS should be suspected. The nurse should be especially alert for early signs and symptoms of NMS in high-risk patients, such as those who are agitated, physically exhausted, or dehydrated or who have an existing medical or neurologic illness. Patients receiving parenteral or higher doses of neuroleptic drugs or lithium concurrently must also be carefully assessed. The nurse should carefully monitor fluid intake, and fluid and electrolyte status.

NCLEXNOTE Recognition of side effects, including movement disorders, tardive dyskinesia, and weight gain, should lead to interventions. NMS is a medical emergency.

Medical treatment includes administering dopamine agonist drugs, such as bromocriptine (modest success), and muscle relaxants, such as dantrolene or benzodiazepine. Antiparkinsonism drugs are not particularly useful.

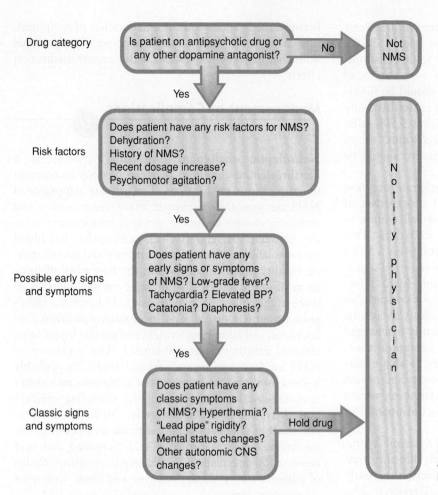

Drug category

Is patient on antipsychotic drug or any other dopamine antagonist? — No → Not NMS

Yes ↓

Risk factors

Does patient have any risk factors for NMS? Dehydration? History of NMS? Recent dosage increase? Psychomotor agitation?

Yes ↓

Possible early signs and symptoms

Does patient have any early signs or symptoms of NMS? Low-grade fever? Tachycardia? Elevated BP? Catatonia? Diaphoresis?

Yes ↓

Classic signs and symptoms

Does patient have any classic symptoms of NMS? Hyperthermia? "Lead pipe" rigidity? Mental status changes? Other autonomic CNS changes? — Hold drug →

Notify physician

FIGURE 21.4 Action tree for "holding" an antipsychotic drug because of suspected neuroleptic malignant syndrome.

BOX 21.13

Recognizing Neuroleptic Malignant Syndrome

Onset: 2 weeks after initiation of antipsychotic treatment or change in dosage
Risk factors: Male gender, preexisting medical or neurologic disorders, depot injection administration, and high ambient temperature

IMMINENT INDICATORS
- Mental status changes
- Muscle rigidity
- Hyperthermia
- Tachycardia
- Hypertension or hypotension
- Tachypnea or hypoxia
- Diaphoresis or sialorrhea
- Tremor
- Incontinence
- Creatinine phosphokinase elevation or myoglobinuria
- Leukocytosis
- Metabolic acidosis

Sources: Agar, L. (2010). Recognizing neuroleptic malignant syndrome in the emergency department: A case study. *Perspectives in Psychiatric Care, 46*(2), 143–151.

Gillman, P. K. (2010). Neuroleptic malignant syndrome: Mechanisms, interactions, and causality. *Movement Disorders, 25*(12), 1780–1790.

Trollor, J. N., Chen, X., & Sachdev, P. S. (2009). Neuroleptic malignant syndrome associated with atypical antipsychotic drugs. *CNS Drugs, 23*(6), 477–492.

Some patients experience improvement with electroconvulsive therapy (ECT).

The nurse must frequently monitor vital signs of the patient with symptoms of NMS. In addition, it is important to check the results of the patient's laboratory tests for increased creatine phosphokinase, an elevated white blood cell count, elevated liver enzymes, or myoglobinuria. The nurse must be prepared to initiate supportive measures or anticipate emergency transfer of the patient to a medical-surgical or an intensive care unit.

Treating fever (which frequently exceeds 103°F) is an important priority for these patients. High body temperature may be reduced with a cooling blanket and acetaminophen therapy. Because many of these patients experience diaphoresis, temperature elevation, or dysphagia, it is important to monitor hydration. Another important aspect of care for patients with NMS is safety. Joints and extremities that are rigid or spastic must be protected from injury. The treatment of these patients depends on the facility and availability of medical support services. In general, patients in psychiatric inpatient units that are separated from general hospitals are transferred to medical-surgical settings for treatment.

TABLE 21.4	NURSING INTERVENTIONS FOR ANTICHOLINERGIC SIDE EFFECTS
Effect	**Intervention**
Dry mouth	Provide sips of water, hard candies, and chewing gum (preferably sugar free).
Blurred vision	Avoid dangerous tasks; teach patient that this side effect will diminish in a few weeks.
Decreased lacrimation	Use artificial tears if necessary.
Mydriasis	May aggravate glaucoma; teach patient to report eye pain.
Photophobia	Wear sunglasses.
Constipation	High-fiber diet; increased fluid intake; take laxatives as prescribed.
Urinary hesitancy	Privacy; run water in sink; warm water over perineum
Urinary retention	Regular voiding (at least every 2–3 h) and whenever urge is present; catheterize for residual urine; record intake and output; evaluate for benign prostatic hypertrophy.
Tachycardia	Evaluate for preexisting cardiovascular disease.

Cholinergic Rebound

If patients are prescribed an anticholinergic agent, such as benztropine, for movement disorders and they abruptly stop taking it, they could experience **cholinergic rebound** symptoms including vomiting, excessive sweating, and altered dreams and nightmares. Cholinergic rebound can be especially problematic if patients discontinue other medications with anticholinergic properties (e.g., antipsychotics, antidepressants, antibiotics) at the same time. Medications with anticholinergic properties should be reduced gradually (tapered) over several days. Table 21.4 lists anticholinergic side effects and several antipsychotic medications and interventions to manage them.

Anticholinergic Medication Abuse

The potential exists for abuse of anticholinergic drugs. Some patients may find the anticholinergic effects of these drugs on mood, memory, and perception pleasurable. Although at toxic dosages, patients may experience disorientation and hallucinations, lesser doses may cause patients to experience greater sociability and euphoria.

Anticholinergic Crisis

An **anticholinergic crisis** is a potentially life-threatening medical emergency caused by an overdose of or sensitivity to drugs with anticholinergic properties. This syndrome (also called anticholinergic delirium) may

> **BOX 21.14**
> ### Signs and Symptoms of Anticholinergic Crisis
> - **Neuropsychiatric signs:** confusion; recent memory loss; agitation; dysarthria; incoherent speech; pressured speech; delusions; ataxia; periods of hyperactivity alternating with somnolence, paranoia, anxiety, or coma
> - **Hallucinations:** accompanied by "picking," plucking, or grasping motions; delusions; or disorientation
> - **Physical signs:** nonreactive dilated pupils; blurred vision; hot, dry, flushed skin; facial flushing; dry mucous membranes; difficulty swallowing; fever; tachycardia; hypertension; decreased bowel sounds; urinary retention; nausea; vomiting; seizures; or coma

result from an accidental or intentional overdose of anticholinergic drugs, including atropine, scopolamine, or belladonna alkaloids, which are present in numerous prescription drugs and OTC medicines. The syndrome may also occur in psychiatric patients who are receiving therapeutic doses of anticholinergic drugs but who are also taking other drugs with anticholinergic properties. As a result of either drug overdose or sensitivity, these anticholinergic substances may produce acute delirium or a psychotic reaction resembling schizophrenia. Severe anticholinergic effects may occur in older patients, even at therapeutic levels (Stahl, 2013).

The signs and symptoms of anticholinergic crisis are dramatic and physically uncomfortable (Box 21.14). This disorder is characterized by fever; parched mouth; burning thirst; hot dry skin; decreased salivation; decreased bronchial and nasal secretions; widely dilated eyes (because bright light becomes painful painful); decreased ability to accommodate visually; increased heart rate; constipation; difficulty urinating; and hypertension or hypotension. The face, neck, and upper arms may become flushed because of a reflexive blood vessel dilation. In addition to peripheral symptoms, patients with anticholinergic psychosis may experience neuropsychiatric symptoms of anxiety, agitation, delirium, hyperactivity, confusion, hallucinations (especially visual), speech difficulties, psychotic symptoms, or seizures. The acute psychotic reaction that is produced resembles schizophrenia. The classic description of anticholinergic crisis is summarized in the following mnemonic: "Hot as a hare, blind as a bat, mad as a hatter, dry as a bone."

In general, episodes of anticholinergic crisis are self-limiting, usually subsiding in 3 days. However, if left untreated, the associated fever and delirium may progress to coma or cardiac and respiratory depression. Although rare, death is generally caused by hyperpyrexia and brain stem depression. After use of the offending drug is discontinued, improvement usually occurs within 24 to 36 hours.

A specific and effective antidote, physostigmine, an inhibitor of anticholinesterase, is frequently used to treat and diagnoeg anticholinergic crisis. Administration of this drug rapidly reduces both behavioral and physiologic symptoms. However, the usual adult dose of physostigmine is 1 to 2 mg intravenously given slowly during a period of 5 minutes because rapid injection of physostigmine may cause seizures, profound bradycardia, or heart block. Physostigmine is relatively short acting, so it may need to be given several times during the course of treatment. This drug provides relief from symptoms for a period of 2 to 3 hours. In addition to receiving physostigmine, patients who intentionally overdose on large amounts of anticholinergic drugs are treated by gastric lavage, administration of charcoal, and catharsis. The dose may be given again after 20 or 30 minutes.

It is important for the nurse to be alert for signs and symptoms of anticholinergic crisis, especially in elderly and pediatric patients, who are much more sensitive to the anticholinergic effects of drugs, and in patients who are receiving multiple medications with anticholinergic effects. If signs and symptoms of the syndrome occur, the nurse should discontinue use of the offending drug and notify the physician immediately.

Electroconvulsive Therapy

ECT is suggested as a possible alternative when the patient's schizophrenia is not being successfully treated by medication alone. For the most part, this modality is not indicated unless the patient is catatonic or has depression that is not treatable by other means. In general, ECT is not used often for the treatment of schizophrenia, but it may be useful for those persons who are medication resistant, assaultive, and psychotic (Kristensen, Brandt-Christensen, Ockelmann, & Jørgensen, 2012).

Psychosocial Interventions

Psychosocial interventions, such as counseling, conflict resolution, behavior therapy, and cognitive interventions, are appropriate for patients with schizophrenia. The following discussion focuses on applying these interventions.

Therapeutic Interactions

Although antipsychotic medications may relieve positive symptoms, they do not always eliminate hallucinations and delusions. The nurse must continue helping the patient develop creative strategies for dealing with these sensory and thought disturbances. Information about the content of the hallucinations and delusions is necessary, not only to determine whether the medications are effective but also to assess safety and the meaning of these thoughts and perceptions to the patient. In caring for a patient who is experiencing hallucinations or delusions, nursing actions should be guided by three general patient outcomes:

- Decrease the frequency and intensity of hallucinations and delusions.
- Recognize that hallucinations and delusions are symptoms of a brain disorder.
- Develop strategies to manage the recurrence of hallucinations or delusions.

When interacting with a patient who is experiencing hallucinations or delusions, the nurse must remember that these experiences are real to the patient. It is important for the nurse to understand the content and meaning of the hallucinations, particularly those involving command hallucinations.

The nurse should never tell a patient that these experiences are not real. Discounting the experiences blocks communication. It is also dishonest to tell the patient that you are having the same hallucinatory experience. It is best to validate the patient's experiences and identify the meaning of these thoughts and feelings to the patient. For example, a patient who believes that he or she is under surveillance by the Federal Bureau of Investigation probably feels frightened and suspicious of everyone. By acknowledging how frightening it must be to always feel like you are being watched, the nurse focuses on the feelings that are generated by the delusion, not the delusion itself. The nurse can then offer to help the patient feel safe within this environment. The patient, in turn, begins to feel that someone understands him or her.

Enhancing Cognitive Functioning

After identifying deficits in cognitive functioning, the nurse and patient can develop interventions that target specific deficits. The most effective interventions usually involve the whole treatment team. If the ability to focus or maintain attention is an issue, patients can be encouraged to select activities that improve attention, such as computer games. For memory problems, patients can be encouraged to make lists and to write down important information.

Executive functioning problems are the most challenging for these patients. Patients who cannot manage daily problems may have planning and problem-solving impairments. For these patients, developing interventions that closely simulate real-world problems may help. Through coaching, the nurse can teach and support the development of problem-solving skills. For example, during hospitalizations, patients are given medications and reminded to take them on time. They are often instructed in a classroom setting but rarely have an opportunity to practice self-medication and figure out what to do if their prescription expires, the medications are lost, or they forget to take their medications. Even so, when discharged, patients are expected to take medication at the prescribed dose at the prescribed time. Interventions designed to have patients actively engage in problem-solving behavior with real problems are needed.

Other approaches to helping patients solve problems and learn new strategies for dealing with problems include solution-focused therapy, which focuses on the strengths and positive attributes that exist within each person, and cognitive behavioral therapy (Mueser, Deavers, Penn, & Cassisi, 2013), which focuses directly on collaboratively determined symptoms and strategies to address them. These therapies involve years of training to master, but certain techniques can be used. For example, the nurse can ask patients to identify the most important problem from their perspective. This focuses the patient on an important issue for him or her.

Using Behavioral Interventions

Behavioral interventions can be very effective in helping patients improve motivation and organize routine, daily activities, such as maintaining a regular schedule and completing activities. Reinforcement of positive behaviors (getting up on time, completing hygiene, going to treatment activities) can easily be included in a treatment plan. In the hospital, patients gain unit privileges by following an agreed-on treatment plan. A social learning intervention called a token economy, which is built on positive reinforcement principles, has a large supportive base of evidence for its success (McDonnell, Strebnik, Angelo, McPherson, Lowe, Sugar, et al., 2013). Unfortunately, behavioral interventions have fallen out of favor because of practitioner attitudes and some problematic past implementations. Their use should be reconsidered.

Psychoeducation

Teaching Strategies

Cognitive deficits (e.g., difficulty in processing complex information, maintaining steady focus of attention, distinguishing between relevant and irrelevant stimuli, and forming abstractions), may challenge the nurse planning educational activities. Evidence indicates that people with schizophrenia may learn best in an errorless learning environment (Leshner, Tom, & Kern, 2013). That is, they are directly given correct information and then encouraged to write it down. Errorless learning is an educational intervention based on the principle of operant conditioning that learning is stronger and more likely to last if it occurs in the absence of errors. Asking questions that encourage guessing is not as effective in helping patients retain information. Trial-and-error learning is avoided.

Teaching and explaining should occur in an environment with minimal distractions. Terminology should be clear and unambiguous. Visual aids can supplement verbal information, but these materials should have simple information stated in simple language. The nurse takes care not to overcrowd the visual material or incorporate images that draw attention away from important content. Teaching should occur in small segments with frequent reinforcement. Most importantly, teaching should occur when the patient is ready. Regular assessments of cognitive abilities with standardized instruments can help determine this readiness. These suggestions can be adapted for teaching during any phase of the illness.

Teaching About Symptoms

Teaching patients that hallucinations and delusions are part of the disorder becomes easier after the medication begins working. When patients believe and acknowledge that they have a mental illness and that some of their thoughts are delusions and some of their perceptions are hallucinations, they can develop strategies to manage their symptoms.

Patients benefit greatly by learning recovery strategies of self-regulation, symptom monitoring, and relapse prevention. By monitoring events, time, place, and stimuli surrounding the appearance of symptoms, the patient can begin to predict high-risk times for symptom recurrence. Cognitive behavioral therapy is often used in helping patients monitor and identify their emerging symptoms to prevent relapse (Mueser, et al., 2013).

Another important nursing intervention is to help the patient identify to whom and where to talk about delusional or hallucinatory material. Because self-disclosure of these symptoms immediately labels someone as having a mental illness, patients should be encouraged to evaluate the environment for negative consequences of disclosing these symptoms. For example, it may be fine to talk about it at home but not at the grocery store.

Teaching How to Cope With Stress

Developing skills to cope with personal, social, and environmental stresses is important to everyone but particularly to those with a severe mental illness. Stresses can easily trigger symptoms that patients are trying to avoid. Establishing regular counseling sessions to support the development of positive coping skills is helpful for both hospitalized patients and those living in the community.

Social Skills Training

Social skills training, provided either individually or in groups, is also useful when working with patients who have schizophrenia (Mueser, et al., 2013). This training teaches patients specific behaviors needed for social interactions. The skills are taught by lecture, demonstration, role-playing, and homework assignments. Nurses may be team members and be involved in case management or provision of services. Furthermore, efforts to offer supportive employment experiences (Mueser, et al., 2013) that incorporate patient preferences, rapid job search and employment, and ongoing job supports have shown effectiveness. Although long-term self-sufficiency has not necessarily been achieved, supportive employment has been the most effective vocational rehabilitation method.

Skill-training interventions should be designed to compensate for cognitive deficits. To help patients learn to process complex activities, such as catching a bus, preparing a meal, or shopping for food or clothing, nurses should break the activity into small parts or steps and list them for the patient's reference, for example:

- Leave your apartment with your keys in hand.
- Make sure you have correct bus fare in your pocket.
- Close the door.
- Walk to the corner.
- Turn right and walk three blocks to the bus stop.

Providing Family Education

Because having a family member with schizophrenia is a life-changing event for the family and friends who provide care and support, educating patients and their families is crucial. It is a primary concern for the psychiatric–mental health nurse. Family support is crucial to help patients maintain treatment. Education should include information about the disease course, treatment regimens, support systems, and life management skills (Box 21.15). The most important factor to stress during patient and family education is the consistent taking of medication.

Promoting Patient Safety

Although violence is not a consistent behavior of people with schizophrenia, it is always a concern during the initial phase when hallucinations or delusions may put patients at risk for harming themselves or others. Nonviolent patients who are experiencing hallucinations and delusions can also be at risk for victimization by more aggressive patients. The patient who is hallucinating needs to be protection, which may include increased staff monitoring and, if necessary, a safer environment in a secluded area.

Identifying patient risk factors for violence, such as a history of violence can alert the nursing staff of a potential for engaging in aggressive behavior, but careful assessment and management of the immediate environment and treating the psychiatric symptoms are more important in avoiding aggression (Chu, Thomas, Ogloff & Daffern, 2013). The nurse's best approach to avoiding violence or aggression is to demonstrate respect for the patient and the patient's personal space, assess and monitor for signs of fear and agitation, and use preventive interventions before the patient loses control. Patients should be encouraged to discuss their anger and to be involved in their treatment decisions. Medications should be administered as ordered. Because most antipsychotic and antidepressant medications take 1 to 2 weeks to begin moderating behavior, the nurse must be vigilant during the acute illness.

If the patient loses control and is a danger to self or others, restraints and seclusion may be used as a last resort. Health Care Financing Administration (HCFA) guidelines and hospital policy must be followed (see Chapter 4), and staff should be trained in the proper use of seclusion and restraints. In addition, staff need to have planned sessions after all incidents of violence or physical management to analyze the event. These sessions allow clinicians to learn how better to manage these situations and evaluate patients' cues. With sensitive leadership, these sessions can help health care workers to learn more about the interaction of patient and staff characteristics that can contribute to these incidents.

Convening Support Groups

People with mental illness benefit from support groups that focus on daily problems and the stress of dealing with a mental illness. These groups are useful throughout the continuum of care and help reduce the risk of suicide. In the hospital setting, the focus of the group can be simply sharing the experience of living with a mental illness. In the community, a regular support group can provide interaction with people with similar problems and issues. Friendships often develop from these groups. Using peer counseling and support groups is also supported within the recovery model of care (Pratt, MacGregor, Reid, & Given, 2012).

BOX 21.15

Psychoeducation Checklist: Schizophrenia

When caring for the patient with schizophrenia, be sure to include the caregiver during planning as appropriate and address the following topic areas in the teaching plan:

- Psychopharmacologic agents, including drug action, dosage, frequency, and possible side effects; stress the importance of adherence to the prescribed regimen
- Management of hallucinations
- Recovery strategies
- Coping strategies (e.g., self-talk, getting busy with something)
- Management of the environment
- Community resources

Implementing Milieu Therapy

Individuals with schizophrenia may be hospitalized or may live in group homes for a long period of time. The challenge is helping people who are unable to live with family members to live harmoniously with strangers who have similar interpersonal difficulties. Arranging the treatment environment to maximize therapy is crucial to the rehabilitation of the patient.

Developing Recovery-Oriented Rehabilitation Strategies

Rehabilitation strategies are used to support the individual's recovery and integration into the community. See Box 21.16. Factors that have been shown to promote recovery include:

- Adjustment, coping, and reappraisal
- Responding to the illness
- Social support, close relationships, and belonging

Factors that have a negative impact on the process of recovery include 1) negative interactions and isolation, 2) internal barriers, and 3) uncertainty and hopelessness (Soundy, Stubbs, Roskell, Williams, Fox, & Vancampfort, et al., 2015).

Community-based psychosocial rehabilitation programs usually offer long-term intensive case management services to adults with schizophrenia. Programs provide a continuum of services to meet the changing needs of people with psychiatric disabilities. Patients set rehabilitation goals and services are then provided to help "clients" (most programs do not use the term "patients") reach their goals. Services range from daily home visits to providing transportation, occupational training, and group support. Assertive community treatment (ACT) is one example of these types of services and has a solid base of evidence to support its use (Mueser, et al., 2013).

Evaluation and Treatment Outcomes

Outcome research related to schizophrenia has redefined previous ways of thinking about the course of the disorder. Schizophrenia was formerly considered to have a progressively long-term and downward course, but it is now known that schizophrenia can be successfully treated and managed. In one older but significant study, the researchers interviewed patients 20 to 25 years after diagnosis and found that 50% to 66% experienced significant improvement or recovery (Harding, Zubin, & Strauss, 1987). This study is important because it occurred before the development of second-generation antipsychotic agents. Today, we can be hopeful that even more people can experience improvement or recover from schizophrenia.

BOX 21.16
A Brother's Perspective

A sibling describes his brother with schizophrenia and the importance of both medications and relationships.

In 1998, at the age of 40 years, Robert was admitted to a psychiatric hospital. His brother was told at the time that he would never be able to live independently, and even if discharged, would only be repeatedly hospitalized. Robert had a long history of treatment and in 1998 he had received various types of antipsychotic medications, but he had not received any of the "new atypical variety." He was prescribed one of these drugs, and within months, the staff who had predicted the most discouraging of outcomes told Robert's brother that he was in the midst of a miraculous recovery—his thinking was clear and free from delusions and they were preparing Robert's discharge.

A few weeks into the discharge planning, Robert called his brother; Robert was distressed because his social worker, whom Robert had known for years from a prior hospitalization, was leaving. The social worker had been abruptly transferred to another hospital. Robert deteriorated rapidly into tantrums, hallucinations, and dangerous behaviors. His discharge was put on hold. Robert's brother's rhetorical question was, "What was the difference between Robert on the same medication on Monday, when he was all right, and Tuesday, when he no longer was?" His answer to Robert's condition caused the loss of an important relationship.

Robert is now living in a community-based home where the dedicated staff members have shown that they can maintain rehospitalization rates below 3%.

Robert's brother has interviewed many former psychiatric patients for a book. He found that every one of his interviewees, while attributing their recovery to medications or finding God, or a particular program, also identified an important relationship with one human being who believed in their ability to recover. Most of the time, this person was a professional, such as a social worker, a nurse, or a doctor. Sometimes, however, it was a member of the clergy or family member.... A believing relationship....

Robert's brother concluded, "Let's provide a range of medications, and let's study their effectiveness, but let's remember that the pill is the ultimate downsizing. Let's find resources to give people afflicted with mental illness what all of us need: fellow human beings upon whom we can depend to help us through our dark times and, once through, to emerge into gloriously imperfect lives."

For nurses, it is important to remember that it is not what we do *to* people, but rather, what we do *with* people: give hope, listen to their dreams, help them find ways to get as close as they can.

Adapted from Neugeboren, J. (2006). Meds alone couldn't bring Robert back. *Newsweek*, from http://www.power2u.org/articles/recovery/meds.html. Retrieved August 3, 2015.

Continuum of Care

Continuity of care has been identified as a primary strategy for recovery because individuals with schizophrenia are at risk for becoming "lost" to services if left alone after discharge. Discharge planning encourages follow-up care in the community. In fact, many state mental health systems require an outpatient appointment before discharge. Treatment of people with schizophrenia occurs across a variety of settings. Not only inpatient hospitalization but also partial hospitalization, day treatment, and crisis stabilization can be used effectively.

Emergency Care

Emergency care ideally takes place in a hospital emergency department, but often the crisis occurs in the home. Patients are usually relapsing and do not recognize their bizarre or aggressive behaviors as symptoms. A specially trained crisis team is sent to assess the emergency and recommend further treatment. In the emergency department, patients are brought not only because of relapse but also because of medication side effects or water intoxication. Nurses should refer to the previous discussion for nursing management.

Inpatient-Focused Care

Inpatient hospitalizations are brief and focus on stabilization. Many times, patients are involuntarily admitted for a short period (see Chapter 3). During the stabilization period, the status is changed to voluntary admission, whereby the patient agrees to treatment.

Community Care

Most of the care of persons with schizophrenia is provided in the community through publicly supported recovery-oriented mental health delivery systems. The recovery journey can be long and require a variety of services such as ACT; outpatient therapy; case management; and psychosocial rehabilitation, including clubhouse programs (Box 21.17). While the patient is in the community, his or her health care should be integrated with physical health care. Nurses should be especially vigilant that patients with mental illnesses receive proper primary and medical health care.

> NCLEXNOTE Priorities in the patient with acute symptoms of schizophrenia include managing psychosis and keeping the patient safe and free from harming him- or herself or others. In the community, the priorities are preventing relapse, maintaining psychosocial functioning, engaging in psychoeducation, improving quality of life, and instilling hope.

In some cases, it is not the disorder itself that threatens the mental health of the person with schizophrenia but the stresses of trying to receive care and services. Health care systems are complex and are often at the mercy of a outdated policies. Development of assertiveness and conflict resolution skills can help the person in negotiating access to systems that will provide services. Developing a positive support system for stressful periods helps promote a positive outcome.

SCHIZOAFFECTIVE DISORDER

Schizoaffective disorder (SAD), a complex and persistent psychiatric illness, is one of the schizophrenia spectrum disorders. SAD is characterized by periods of

---

BOX 21.17

Research for Best Practice: The Process of Self-Recovery

Shea, J. M. (2010). Coming back normal: The process of self-recovery in those with schizophrenia. Journal of the American Psychiatric Nurses Association, 16 *(1), 43–51.*

THE QUESTION: How is the process of self-identity (important for recovery) reconstructed in people with schizophrenia?

METHODS: A grounded theory study was conducted with 10 participants representing 3 categories of community adjustment and 4 significant others. Nineteen semistructured interviews were completed.

FINDINGS: The final results supported the use of the term *recovery* rather than *reconstruction of self* because the process involved more than simply putting the pieces together. The self-recovery process included 6 stages: entering the territory, struggling for control, active self-care, finding a social fit, checking out the self, and coming back to normal.

IMPLICATIONS FOR NURSING: This process has a direct impact on the daily struggles of those with schizophrenia. Using this model, the nurse can determine at which stage the person with schizophrenia is in the recovery journeys.

---

intense symptom exacerbation alternating with periods of adequate psychosocial functioning. This disorder is at times marked by psychosis; at other times, by mood disturbance. When psychosis and mood disturbance occur at the same time, a diagnosis of SAD is made (APA, 2013). Patients with SAD are more likely to exhibit persistent psychosis than are patients with a mood disorder. They feel that they are on a "chronic roller coaster ride" of symptoms that are often difficult to manage.

The long-term outcome of SAD is generally better than that of schizophrenia but worse than that of mood disorder (Möller, Jäger, Riedel, Obermeier, Strauss, & Bottlender, 2010). These patients resemble the mood disorder group in work function (see Chapter 19) and the schizophrenia group in social function. Persons with SAD usually have higher functioning than those with schizophrenia with severe negative symptoms and early onset of illness (Bora, Yucel, & Pantelis, 2009).

Patients with SAD are at risk for suicide. The risk for suicide in patients with psychosis is increased by the presence of depression. Risk factors for suicide increase with the use of alcohol or substances, cigarette smoking, previous suicide attempts and hospitalizations (Bolton & Robinson, 2010).

Lack of regular social contact may be a factor that confers a long-term risk for suicidal behavior, which may be reduced by treatments designed to enhance social networks and contact and help patients to protect themselves against environmental stressors (Reutfors, Bahmanyar, Jönsson, Ekbom, Nordström, Brandt, et al., 2010).

DELUSIONAL DISORDER

Delusional disorder is another schizophrenia spectrum disorder that is characterized by stable and well-systematized delusions that occur in the absence of other psychiatric disorders. A diagnosis of delusional disorder is based on the presence of one or more delusions for at least 1 month (APA, 2013). Delusions are the primary symptom of this disorder. Apart from the direct impact of the delusion, psychosocial functioning is not markedly impaired. Examples of delusions include being followed, poisoned, infected, loved at a distance, or deceived by a spouse or lover.

The course of delusional disorder varies. The onset can be acute, or the disorder can occur gradually and become chronic. Patients usually live with delusions for years, rarely receiving psychiatric treatment unless their delusion relates to their health (somatic delusion), or they act on the basis of their delusion and violate legal or social rules. Full remissions can be followed by relapses. Behavior is remarkably normal except when the patient focuses on the delusion. At that time, thinking, attitudes, and mood may change abruptly. Personality does not usually change, but the patient is gradually and progressively involved with the delusional concern (APA, 2013). Delusional disorder is relatively uncommon in clinical settings.

OTHER PSYCHOTIC DISORDERS

Schizophreniform Disorder

The essential features of schizophreniform disorder are identical to those of schizophrenia, with the exception of the duration of the illness, which can be less than 6 months. Symptoms must be present for at least 1 month to be classified as a schizophreniform disorder. About one third of the individuals recover with the other two thirds developing schizophrenia (APA, 2013).

Brief Psychotic Disorder

In brief psychotic disorder, the length of the episode is at least 1 day but less than 1 month. The onset is sudden and includes at least one of the positive symptoms of schizophrenia. The person generally experiences emotional turmoil or overwhelming confusion and rapid, intense shifts of affect (APA, 2013). Although episodes are brief, impairment can be severe, and supervision may be required to protect the person. Suicide is a risk, especially in younger patients.

Psychotic Disorders Attributable to a Substance

Patients with a psychotic disorder attributable to a substance present with prominent hallucinations or delusions that are the direct physiologic effects of a substance (e.g.,

drug use, toxin exposure) (APA, 2013). During intoxication, symptoms continue as long as the use of the substance continues. Withdrawal symptoms can last for as long as 4 weeks. Differential diagnosis is recommended.

SUMMARY OF KEY POINTS

- The schizophrenia spectrum disorders include schizophrenia, schizoaffective, delusional, and schizotypal disorders, brief psychotic disorder, schizophreniform disorder, and substance/medication–induced psychotic disorder (APA, 2013). Schizophrenia displays a complex of symptoms typically categorized as positive symptoms (i.e., those that exist but should not), such as delusions or hallucinations and disorganized thinking and behavior, and negative symptoms (characteristics that should be there but are lacking), such as alogia, avolition, anhedonia, and diminished emotional expression.

- The clinical course of schizophrenia begins with a prodromal period in childhood but is usually not recognized as a precursor to schizophrenia. An acute illness usually occurs in late adolescence and may require hospitalization when medication and recovery-oriented care are initiated. Recovery-oriented care is initiated, the nurse instills hope, partners with the person with schizophrenia in developing strategies to recover and lead a meaningful life.

- The cause of schizophrenia is thought to be related to genetic, neurodevelopmental, and neurotransmission dysfunction. Environmental stress can trigger acute episodes.

- Nursing assessment begins with the development of the therapeutic relationship and includes biologic, psychological and social areas.

- Risk for self-injury or injury to others should always be included in the assessment. Establishment of baseline health information should be done before any medications are administered. Several standardized assessment tools are available to help assess characteristic abnormal motor movements.

- In general, the antipsychotic drugs used to treat patients with schizophrenia block dopamine transmission in the brain but also cause some troublesome and sometimes serious side effects, primarily anticholinergic side effects and extrapyramidal side effects (i.e., motor abnormalities). Newer second-generation antipsychotic agents block serotonin as well as dopamine. The nurse should be familiar with these drugs, their possible side effects, and the interventions required to manage or control side effects.

- Extrapyramidal side effects of antipsychotic drugs may appear early in drug treatment and include acute parkinsonism or pseudoparkinsonism, acute dystonia, and akathisia, but they may also appear later after months or years of treatment. The primary example of late-appearing extrapyramidal side effects is tardive dyskinesia, which is a severe syndrome involving abnormal motor movements of the mouth, tongue, jaw, trunk, fingers, and toes.

- Health promotion and wellness interventions are important for overall well-being. People with schizophrenia spectrum disorders have special challenges because their medications can produce a negative impact on their physical health. Nurses can provide education and guidance for positive activity, exercise, and nutrition strategies that can counteract the effect of the medications and symptoms.

- Because schizophrenia is a lifetime disorder and patients require the continued support and care of mental health professionals and family or friends, one of the primary nursing interventions is ensuring that patients and families are properly educated regarding the course of the disorder, importance of drug maintenance, and need for consistent care and support. Positive interaction between patients and their families is key to the success of long-term treatments and outcomes.

- Other schizophrenia spectrum disorders (e.g., schizoaffective, delusional, and schizotypal disorders, brief psychotic disorder, schizophreniform disorder, and substance/medication induced psychotic disorder) have similar symptom similar to those of schizophrenia. Nursing care should be individualized based on a nursing assessment and current evidence related to care.

CRITICAL THINKING CHALLENGES

1. Describe steps that a nurse should use to make sure an assessment considers the cultural basis of a patient's hallucination and delusions.

2. A patient asks you to explain the difference between "positive" and "negative" symptoms. Develop an answer in "lay" terms for the question.

3. What steps might the nurse take to develop trust in a patient who has hallucinations and delusions and is frightened of other people?

4. Given that a patient with mental illness requires extra efforts at confidentiality and that patients with schizophrenia are often suspicious of their family members, explain ways you can help families and patients develop positive interactions.

5. A patient tells you that she has nothing to live for and everyone would be better off without her. You recognize that she may be having suicidal thoughts. What assessment questions would you ask? How would you help her develop a safety plan?

6. Discuss how therapeutic communication might have to change when working with a person with schizophrenia who is displaying primarily negative symptoms. How will you deal with the person's diminished response to you (both verbally and emotionally) when you are teaching or giving instructions for activities? How will you help the person compensate for some of his or her cognitive deficits?

7. A person with schizophrenia is admitted during a relapse. He said that he did not want to take his haloperidol anymore because it made him shake. The physician prescribes olanzapine. Develop a medication education plan that includes a comparison between olanzapine and haloperidol.

8. Mr. J. has just received a diagnosis of schizophrenia. During a recent outpatient visit, he confides to a nurse that he just has stress and does not think that he really has any psychiatric problems. Identify assessment areas that should be pursued before the patient leaves his appointment. How would you confront the denial?

9. A patient says his medication is not working. He is taking ziprasidone (Geodon) 40 mg twice a day. He tells you that he takes 40 mg before breakfast and 40 mg before bed. What would interventions are needed to increase the effectiveness of the drug?

10. Ms. J. was prescribed olanzapine (Zyprexa) for schizophrenia 1 month ago. Since her last monthly visit, she has gained 15 pounds. She is considering discontinuing her medication regimen because of the weight gain. Develop a plan to address her weight gain and her intention to discontinue her medication regimen.

11. An older adult in a nursing home has a delusion that her husband is having an affair with her sister. Discuss nonpharmacologic nursing interventions that should be implemented with this patient. How would you explain her delusion to her husband? Develop a plan for clinical management, focusing on psychiatric nursing care, for a patient experiencing this condition.

12. Identify health promotion activities for a person with schizophrenia who is gaining weight while taking antipsychotics might pursue.

A Beautiful Mind: (2001). This Academy Award-winning movie starring Russell Crowe is based on the biography by Sylvia Naasar of the mathematician and Nobel Laureate John Nash. It presents the life and experiences of this man as he dealt with schizophrenia. It shows how his life and work were altered and the effects on his relationships with family and colleagues. The movie depicts how this man came to terms with his illness.

Viewing Points: How does the treatment John Nash received in the 1950s differ from treatment today? How would you classify his symptoms according to the *DSM-5*? What is typical or problematic about Mr. Nash's relationship with the medications prescribed for him?

 The Soloist: (2009). Based on a true story, this movie portrays the experience of a reporter/novelist named Steve Lopez (played by Robert Downey, Jr.) when he befriends Nathaniel Anthony Ayers, "the soloist" (played by Jamie Fox), who has severe, persistent, and untreated schizophrenia—and more importantly, exceptional musical talent. Formerly a student at the prestigious Julliard School of Music in New York City, Ayers now lives on the streets of Los Angeles playing his two-string violin. See also the book by the same title.

Viewing Points: What are the risks and rewards of taking on such a personal relationship? How best can nurses advocate for individuals with severe mental illness (and their family and friends) when community resources are inadequate?

M VIE viewing **GUIDES** related to this chapter are available at http://thepoint.lww.com/BoydEssentials.

 A related Psychiatric-Mental Health Nursing video on the topic of Schizophrenia is available at http://thepoint.lww.com/BoydEssentials.

 A Psychiatric-Mental Health Nursing Practice and Learn Activity related to the video on the topic of Schizophrenia is available at http://thepoint.lww.com/BoydEssentials.

REFERENCES

Acosta, F. J., Hernández, J. L., Pereira, J., Herrera, J., & Rodríguez, C. J. (2012) Medication adherence in schizophrenia. *World Journal of Psychiatry, 2*(5), 74–82.

Altamura, A. C., Aguglia, E., Bassi, M., Bogetto, F., Cappellari, L., De Giorgi, S., Gafiolini, et al. (2012). Rethinking the role of long-acting atypical antipsychotics in the community setting (Review). *International Clinical Psychopharmacology, 27*(6), 336–349.

American Psychiatric Association. (2013). *Diagnostic and Statistical Manual of Mental Disorders: Fifth edition.* Arlington, VA: Author.

Auquier, P., Tinland, A., Fortanier, C., Loundou, A., Baumstarck, K. Lanson, C., et al. (2013). Toward meeting the needs of homeless people with schizophrenia: the validity of quality of life measurement. *PLOS One, 8*(10), 1–9.

Austad, F., Joa, I., Johannessen, J. O., & Larsen, T. K. (2015). Gender differences in suicidal behavior in patients with first-episode psychosis. *Early Intervention Psychiatry, 9*(4):300-7. DOI: 10.1111/eip.12113.

Baker, J. T., Holmes, A. J., Masters, G. A, Yeo, B. T., Krienen, F., Buckner, R. L., et al. (2014). Disruption of cortical association networks in schizophrenia and psychotic bipolar disorder. *JAMA Psychiatry, 71*(2), 109–118.

Barajas, A., Usall, J., Baños, I., Dolz, M., Villalta-Gil, V., Vilaplana, et al. (2013). Three-factor model of premorbid adjustment in a sample with chronic schizophrenia and first-episode psychosis. *Schizophrenia Research, 151*(1–3), 252–258.

Birnbaum, R., & Weinberger, D. R. (2013). Functional neuroimaging and schizophrenia: A view towards effective connectivity modeling and polygenic risk. *Dialogues in Clinical Neuroscience, 15*(3), 279–289.

Bolton, J. M., & Robinson, J. (2010). Population-attributable fractions of Axis I and Axis II mental disorders for suicide attempts: Findings from a representative sample of the adult, noninstitutionalized US population. *American Journal of Public Health, 100*(12) 2473–2480.

Bonsch, D., Wunschel, M., Lenz, B., Janssen, G., Weisbrod, M., & Sauer, H. (2012). Methylation matters? Decreased methylation status of genomic DNA in the blood of schizophrenic twins. *Psychiatry Research, 19*(3), 533–537.

Bora, E., Yucel, M., & Pantelis, C. (2009). Cognitive functioning in schizophrenia, schizoaffective disorder and affective psychoses: Meta-analytic study. *British Journal of Psychiatry, 195*(6), 475–482.

Boshes, R. A., Manschreck, T. C., & Konigsberg, W. (2012). Genetics of the schizophrenias: a model accounting for their persistence and myriad phenotypes. *Harvard Review of Psychiatry, 20*(3), 119–129.

Brown, A. S. (2011). The environment and susceptibility to schizophrenia. *Progress in Neurobiology, 93*(1), 23–58. Doi:10.1016/j.pneurobio.2010.09.003

Buchsbaum, M. (1990). The frontal lobes, basal ganglia, and temporal lobes as a site for schizophrenia. *Schizophrenia Bulletin, 16*, 377–387.

Carliner, H., Collins, P. Y., Cabassa, L. J., McNallen, A., Joestl, S. S., & Lewis-Fernández, R. (2014). Prevalence of cardiovascular risk factors among racial and ethnic minorities with schizophrenia spectrum and bipolar disorders: A critical literature review. *Comprehensive Psychiatry, 55*(2), 233–247. Doi: 10.1016/j.comppsych.2013.09.009.

Challis, S., Nielssen, O., Harris, A., & Large, M. (2013). Systematic meta-analysis of the risk factors for deliberate self-harm before and after treatment for first-episode psychosis. *Acta Psychiatrica Scandinavica, 127*(6), 442–454.

Chu, C. M., Thomas, S. D., Ogloff, J., & Daffern, M. (2013). The short-to medium-term predictive accuracy of static and dynamic risk assessment measures in a secure forensic hospital. *Assessment, (20)*2, 230–241.

Cohen, C. I., & Marino, L. (2013). Racial and ethnic differences in the prevalence of psychotic symptoms in the general population. *Psychiatric Services, 64*(11), 1103–1109.

Department of Health Statistics and Information Systems. (2013). *WHO methods and data sources for global burden of disease estimates 2000–2011.* Geneva: World Health Organization.

Fanning, J. R., Bell, M. D., & Fiszdon, J. M. (2012). Is it possible to have impaired neurocognition but good social cognition in schizophrenia? *Schizophrenia Research, 135*(1–3), 68–71.

Fraguas, D., Del Rey-Mejias, A., Moreno, C., Castro-Fornieles, J., Graell, M., Otero, S., et al. (2014). Duration of untreated psychosis predicts functional and clinical outcome of children and adolescents with first-episode psychosis: A 2-year longitudinal study. *Schizophrenia Research, 152*(1), 130–138. Doi: 10.1016/j.schres.2013.11.018.

Franzen, G. (1970). Plasma free fatty acids before and after an intravenous insulin injection in acute schizophrenic men. *British Journal of Psychiatry, 116* (531), 173–177.

Gimblett, D. (2015). Monitoring physical health in patients with serious mental illness. *Mental Health Practice, 18*(5), 20–23.

Goff, D. C. (2013). Future perspectives on the treatment of cognitive deficits and negative symptoms ins schizophrenia. *World Psychiatry, 12*, 99–107.

Goldstein, J. M, Cherkerzian, S., Tsuang, M. T., & Petryshen, T. L. (2013). Sex differences in the genetic risk for schizophrenia: history of the evidence for sex-specific and sex-dependent effects. *American Journal of Medical Genetics, Part B, Neuropsychiatric Genetics. 162B*(7):698–710.

Gray, R., White, J., Schulz, M., & Aberhalden, C. (2010). Enhancing medication adherence in people with schizophrenia: An international programme of research. *International Journal of Mental Health Nursing, 19*(1), 36–44.

Guo, X., Fang, M., Zhai, J., Wang, B., Wang, C., Hu, B., et al. (2011). Effectiveness of maintenance treatments with atypical and typical antipsychotics in stable schizophrenia with early stage: 1-year naturalistic study. *Psychopharmacology, 216*(4), 475–484.

Guo, X., Zhai, J., Fang, M., Liu, Z., Fang, M., Wang, B., Wang, C., et al. (2010). Effect of antipsychotic medication alone vs. combined with psychosocial intervention on outcomes of early-stage schizophrenia: A randomized, 1-year study. *Archives of General Psychiatry, 67*(9), 895–904.

Harding, C., Zubin, J., & Strauss, J. (1987). Chronicity in schizophrenia: Fact, partial fact or artifact? *Hospital and Community Psychiatry, 38*(5), 477–486.

Hawken, E. R., Crookall, J. M., Reddick, D., Millson, R. C., Milev, R., & Delva, M. (2009). Mortality over a 20-year period in patients with primary polydipsia associated with schizophrenia: A retrospective study. *Schizophrenia Research, 107*(2–3), 128–133.

Jaeger, S., Seißhaupt, S., Flammer, E., & Steinert, T. (2014). Control beliefs, therapeutic relationship, and adherence in schizophrenia outpatients: A cross-sectional study. *American Journal of Health Behavior, 38*(6), 914–923.

Johnson, S. L. M., Wang, L., Alpert, K. I., Greenstein, D., Clasen, L., Lalonde, F., et al. (2013). Hippocampal shape abnormalities of patients with childhood-onset schizophrenia and their unaffected siblings. *Journal of the American Academy of Child & Adolescent Psychiatry, 52*(5), 527–536.

Kaplan, G., Casoy, J., & Zummo, J. (2013). Impact of long-acting injectable antipsychotics on medication adherence and clinical, functional, and economic outcomes of schizophrenia. *Patient Preference and Adherence, 7,* 1171–1180.

Kay, S. R., Fiszbein, A., & Opler, L. A. (1987). The Positive and Negative Syndrome Scale (PANSS) for schizophrenia. *Schizophrenia Bulletin, 13,* 261–276.

Kristensen, D., Brandt-Christensen, M., Ockelmann, H. M., & Jørgensen, M. S. (2012). The use of electroconvulsive therapy in a cohort of forensic psychiatric patients with schizophrenia. *Criminal Behavior and Mental Health, 22*(2), 148–156.

Koch, D. A., & Scott, A. J. (2012). Weight gain and lipid-glucose profiles among patients taking antipsychotic medications: comparisons for prescriptions administered using algorithms versus usual care. *Journal of Psychiatric & Mental Health Nursing, 19*(5), 389–394.

Lau, C. I., Wang, H. C., Hsu, J. L., & Liu, M. E. (2013). Does the dopamine hypothesis explain schizophrenia? *Reviews in the Neurosciences, 24*(4), 389–400.

Laursen, T. M., Nordentoft, M., & Mortensen, P. B. (2013). Excess early mortality in schizophrenia. *Annual Review of Clinical Psychology, 10,* 425–48.

Lepage, M., Bodmar, M., & Bowie, C. R. (2014). Neurocognition: clinical and functional outcomes in schizophrenia. *Canadian Journal of Psychiatry, 59*(1), 5–12.

Leshner, A. F., Tom, S. R., & Kern, R. S. (2013). Errorless learning and social problem solving ability in schizophrenia: an examination of the compensatory effects of training. *Psychiatry Research, 206*(1), 1–7.

Lincoln, J., Stewart, M. E., & Preskorn, S. H. (2010). How sequential studies inform drug development: evaluating the effect of food intake on optimal bioavailability of ziprasidone. *Journal of Psychiatric Practice, 16*(2), 103–104.

Loewenstein, D. A., Czaja, S. J., Bowie, C. R., & Harvey, P. D. (2012). Age-associated differences in cognitive performance in older patients with schizophrenia: a comparison with health older adults. *American Journal of Geriatric Psychiatry, 20*(1), 29–40.

MacKinnon, K., Newman-Taylor, K., & Stopa, L. (2011). Persecutory delusions and the self: An investigation of implicit and explicit self-esteem. *Journal of Behavior Therapy and Experimental Psychiatry, 42* (1), 54–64.

Margetić, B., & Aukst-Margetić, B. (2010). Neuroleptic malignant syndrome and its controversies. *Pharmacopepidemiology and Drug Safety, 19*(5), 429–435.

McAuliffe, R., O'Connor, L., & Meagher, D. (2014). Parents' experience of living with and caring for an adult son or daughter with schizophrenia at home in Ireland: a qualitative study. *Journal of Psychiatric & Mental Health Nursing, 21*(2), 145–53.

McDaid, T. M., & Smyth, S. (2015). Metabolic abnormalities among people diagnosed with schizophrenia: a literature review and implications for mental health nurses. *Journal of Psychiatric & Mental Health Nursing, 22*(3), 157–170.

McDonnell, M. G., Strebnik, D., Angelo, F., McPherson, S., Lowe, J. M., Sugar, A., et al. (2013). Randomized controlled trial of contingency management of stimulant use in community mental health patients with serious mental illness. *American Journal of Psychiatry, 170*(1), 94–101.

Meier, M. H., Caspi, A., Reichenberg, A., Keefe, R. S. E., Fisher, H. L., Harrington, H. L., et al. (2013). Neuropsychological Decline in Schizophrenia From the Premorbid to the Post onset Period: Evidence From a Population-Representative Longitudinal Study, *American Journal of Psychiatry, 171*(1):91–101.

Möller, H. J., Jäger, M., Riedel, M., Obermeier, M., Strauss, A., & Bottlender, R. (2010). The Munich 15-year follow-up study (MUFUSSAD) on first-hospitalized patients with schizophrenic or affective disorders: Comparison of psychopathological and psychosocial course and outcome and prediction of chronicity. *European Archives of Psychiatry & Clinical Neuroscience, 260*(5), 367–384.

Mueser, K. T., Deavers, F., Penn, D. L., & Cassisi, J. E. (2013). Psychosocial treatment for schizophrenia. (Review). *Annual Review of clinical Psychology, 9,* 465–497.

National Alliance on Mental Illness (NAMI). (2013). *Trends, themes and best practices in state mental health legislation.* Arlington, VA: Author.

Neugeboren, J. (2006). Meds alone couldn't bring Robert back. *Newsweek.* Retrieved January 31, 2006, from http://www.power2u.org/articles/recovery/meds.html. Retrieved August 3, 2015.

Nilsen, L., Grich, J. C., Friis, S., & Røssberg, J. I. (2014). Patients' and family members' experiences of a psychoeducational family intervention after a first episode psychosis: A qualitative study.*Issues in Mental Health Nursing, 35*(1), 58–68.

Pandya, A., & Myrick, K. (2013). Wellness and recovery programs: a model of self-advocacy for people living with mental illness. (Review). *Journal of Psychiatric Practice, 19*(3), 242–6.

Pfizer. (2014). *GEODON U.S. Physician Prescribing Information including Patient Summary of Information.* Retrieved from http://www.pfizer.com/products/product-detail/geodon.

Pratt, R., MacGregor, A., Reid, S., & Given, L. (2012). Wellness Recovery Action Planning (WRAP) in self-help and mutual support groups. *Psychiatric Rehabilitation Journal, 15*(5), 403–405.

Reutfors, J., Bahmanyar, S., Jönsson, E. G., Ekbom, A., Nordström, P., Brandt, L., et al. (2010). Diagnostic profile and suicide risk in schizophrenia spectrum disorder. *Schizophrenia Research, 123*(2–3), 251–256.

Schimmelbusch, W. H., Mueller, P. S., & Sheps, J. (1971). The positive correlation between insulin resistance and duration of hospitalization in untreated schizophrenia. *British Journal of Psychiatry, 118*(545), 429–436.

Simpson, G. M., & Angus, J. W. S. L. (1970). A rating scale for extrapyramidal side effects. *Acta Psychiatrica Scandinavica, 212*(suppl), 11–19.

Shea, J. M. (2010). Coming back normal: The process of self-recovery in those with schizophrenia. *Journal of the American Psychiatric Nurses Association, 16*(1), 43–51.

Smieskova, R., Marmy, J., Schmidt, A., Bendfeldt, K., Riecher-Rossler, A., Walter, M., et al. (2013). Do subjects a clinical high risk for psychosis differ from those with a genetic high risk?—A systematic review of structural and functional brain abnormalities. *Current Medicinal Chemistry, 20*(3), 467–481.

Sunovion. (2013). *Latuda Prescribing Information* (revised 7/30/2013). Retrieved fromwww.latuda.com/LatudaPrescribingInformation.pdf.

Sprague, R. L., & Kalachnik, J. E. (1991). Reliability, validity, and a total score cutoff for the Dyskinesia Identification Scale System: Condensed User Scale (DISCUS) with mentally ill and mentally retarded populations. *Psychopharmacology Bulletin, 27,* 51–58.

Soundy, A., Muhamed, A., Stubbs, B., Probst, M., & Vancampfort, D. (2014). The benefits of walking for individuals with schizophrenia spectrum disorders: A systematic review. *International Journal of Therapy & Rehabilitation, 21*(9), 410–420.

Soundy, A., Stubbs, B., Roskell, C., Williams, S.E., Fox, A., & Vancampfort, D. (2015). Identifying the facilitators and processes which influence recovery in individuals with schizophrenia: a systematic review and thematic synthesis. *Journal of Mental Health, 24*(2), 103–110.

Stahl, S. (2013). *Stahl's Essential Psychopharmacology: Neuroscientific Basis and Practical Application* (4th ed). Cambridge, United Kingdom: Cambridge University Press.

Tarbox, S. I., Addington, J., Cadenhead, K. S., Cannon, T. D., Cornblatt, B. A., Perkins, D. O., et al. (2013). Premorbid functional development and conversion to psychosis in clinical high-risk youths. *Development and Psychopathology. 25*(4 Pt 1), 1171–1186.

U.S. Food and Drug Administration. (12/11/2014). FDA drug safety communication: FDA reporting mental health drug ziprasidone (Geodon) associated with rare but potentially fatal skin reactions. www.fda.gov/Drugs/DrugSafety/ucm426391.htm?source = govdelivery&utm_medium = email&utm_source = govdelivery. Retrieved January 18, 2015.

Valente, S., & Fisher, D. (2010). Recognizing and managing psychogenic polydipsia in mental health. *The Journal for Nurse Practitioners, 6*(7), 546–552.

Van Os, J., Kenis, G., & Rutten, P. F. (2010). The environment and schizophrenia. *Nature, 468*(7321), 203–212.

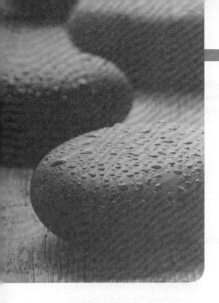

22
Personality and Impulse-Control Disorders

Nursing Care of Persons with Personality and Impulse-Control Disorders

Mary Ann Boyd and Kimberlee Hansen

KEY CONCEPTS

- antisocial personality disorder (ASPD)
- borderline personality disorder (BPD)
- difficult temperament
- emotional dysregulation
- impulse-control disorders
- impulsivity
- personality
- personality disorder
- self-harm
- temperament

LEARNING OBJECTIVES

After studying this chapter, you will be able to:

1. Describe the prevalence and incidence of personality disorders.

2. Delineate the clinical symptoms of borderline personality disorder and antisocial personality disorder with emphasis on emotional dysregulation, self-harm, temperament, and impulsivity.

3. Discuss the theories explaining personality disorders.

4. Identify evidence-based nursing interventions for persons with personality disorders.

5. Discuss communication strategies with persons with personality disorders.

6. Develop recovery-oriented strategies that address the needs of persons with personality disorders.

7. Compare and contrast disruptive impulse-control disorders.

KEY TERMS

- affective instability • avoidant personality disorder • cognitive schemata • conduct disorder • dependent personality disorder • dialectical behavior therapy (DBT) • dichotomous thinking • dissociation • emotional dysregulation • histrionic personality disorder • identity diffusion • impulse control disorders • impulsivity • inhibited grieving • intermittent explosive disorder • invalidating environment • kleptomania • narcissistic personality • obsessive-compulsive personality disorder • oppositional defiant disorder • paranoid personality disorder • parasuicidal behavior • personality disorder • personality traits • projective identification • pyromania • schizoid personality disorder • self-harm • schizotypy • schizotypal personality disorder • separation-individuation • splitting

Case Study: Rebecca

Rebecca is a 23-year-old single female who lives alone. She has few friends, but does attend regular psychotherapy sessions that help her understand her emotions and behaviors. She becomes very upset when her therapist leaves town for a planned vacation. Her family wants to help but are frustrated with Rebecca's inability to deal with every day stresses.

INTRODUCTION

The concept of personality seems deceptively simple but instead is very complex. Historically, the term *personality* was derived from the Greek word *persona*, the theatrical mask used by dramatic players that had the connotation of a projected pretense or allusion. With time, the connotation changed from being an external surface representation to the internal traits of the individual.

| KEYCONCEPT **Personality** is a complex pattern of characteristics, largely outside of the person's awareness, which comprise the individual's distinctive pattern of perceiving, feeling, thinking, coping, and behaving.

Personality traits are prominent aspects of personality that are exhibited in a wide range of social and personal contexts. Intrinsic and pervasive, personality traits emerge from a complicated interaction of biologic dispositions, psychological experiences, and environmental situations that ultimately comprise a distinctive personality (Millon, 2011).

No sharp division exists between normal and abnormal personality functioning. Instead, personalities are viewed on a continuum from normal at one end to abnormal at the other. Many of the same processes involved in the development of a "normal" personality are responsible for the development of a personality disorder.

This chapter provides an overview of personality disorders with borderline personality disorder (BPD) explained in detail and antisocial personality disorder (ASPD) emphasized. Disruptive impulse-control and conduct disorders, a closely related group of disorders, are also discussed.

OVERVIEW OF PERSONALITY DISORDERS

A personality disorder is "an enduring pattern of inner experience and behavior that deviates markedly from the expectations of the individual's culture, is pervasive and inflexible, has an onset in adolescence or early adulthood, is stable over time, and leads to distress or impairment" (American Psychiatric Association [APA], 2013), p. 646).

| KEYCONCEPT A **personality disorder** diagnosis is based on abnormally inflexible behavior patterns of long duration, traced to adolescence or early adulthood that deviate from acceptable cultural norms.

Estimates of the prevalence of personality disorders vary from 4.4% to 13.4% with a median of 9.6% (Samuels, 2011). This rate is of public health significance because of the extreme social dysfunction and high health care use of persons with personality disorders. Many others do not seek treatment for the distress or impairment related to their personality disorder because they do not perceive themselves as having a problem. However, they frequently seek help for concurrent medical or mental health disorders.

At present, 10 personality disorders are recognized in the *DSM-5* within three clusters. Cluster A disorders are characterized by odd or eccentric behavior; Cluster B disorders are characterized by dramatic, emotional, or erratic behavior; in Cluster C disorders, individuals appear anxious or fearful (see Table 22.1) (APA, 2013).

TABLE 22.1   DESCRIPTIONS OF PERSONALITY DISORDERS

Cluster A : Odd and Eccentric

Paranoid	Distrustful and suspicious of others
Schizoid	Detached from social relationships; restricted range of emotional expression
Schizotypal	Discomfort in close relations, cognitive or perceptual distortions, eccentricities

Cluster B: Dramatic, Emotional, or Erratic behavior

Antisocial	Disregard for others and violation of others' rights
Borderline	Instability in interpersonal relationships, self-image. and emotions; impulsive
Histrionic	Excessive emotionality and attention-seeking
Narcissistic	Grandiosity, need for admiration, lack of empathy

Cluster C: Anxious or Fearful

Avoidant	Social inhibition, feelings of inadequacy, hypersensitive to criticism
Dependent	Submissive and clinging behavior; excessive need to be taken care of
Obsessive-Compulsive	Preoccupation with orderliness, perfectionism, and control

Source: APA, 2013.

CLUSTER A: PARANOID, SCHIZOID, AND SCHIZOTYPAL PERSONALITY DISORDERS

Paranoid Personality Disorder

Clinical Course and Diagnostic Criteria

Paranoid personality disorder is characterized by a long-standing suspiciousness and mistrust of people in general. Individuals with these traits refuse to assume personal responsibility for their own feelings, assign responsibility to others, and avoid relationships in which they are not in control or power. These individuals are suspicious, guarded, and hostile. They are consistently mistrustful of others' motives, even those of relatives and close friends. Actions of others are often misinterpreted as deception, deprecation, and betrayal, especially regarding loyalty or trustworthiness of friends and associates (APA, 2013).

People with paranoid personality disorder are unforgiving and hold grudges; their typical emotional responses are anger and hostility. They distance themselves from others and are outwardly argumentative and abrasive; internally, they feel powerless, fearful, and vulnerable. Other hallmark features of paranoid personality disorder are persistent ideas of self-importance and the tendency to be rigid and controlling. Blind to their own unattractive behaviors and characteristics, they often attribute these same traits to others. Their outward demeanor often seems cold, sullen, and humorless. They want to appear controlled and objective, yet often they react emotionally, displaying signs of nervousness, anger, envy, and jealousy. Orderly by nature, they are hypervigilant to any environmental changes that may loosen their control on the world. Occupational problems are common. They do not seek mental health care until they decompensate into psychosis.

Epidemiology and Risk Factors

The prevalence estimate for paranoid personality is 2.3%, whereas the National Epidemiologic Survey on Alcohol and Related Conditions data suggest a prevalence of paranoid personality disorder of 4.4% (APA, 2013).

Etiology

The etiologic factors of paranoid personality remain unclear, but a genetic predisposition for an irregular maturation may be involved. As children, these individuals tend to be active and intrusive, difficult to manage, hyperactive, irritable, and have frequent outbursts of temper.

Nursing Care

Nurses most likely see these patients about other health problems but formulate nursing diagnoses based on the patient's underlying suspiciousness. Assessment of these individuals reveals disturbed or illogical thoughts that demonstrate misinterpretation of environmental stimuli. For example, a man was convinced that his wife was having an affair with the neighbor because his wife and the neighbor left their homes for work at the same time each morning. Although the man's beliefs were illogical, he never once considered that he was wrong. He frequently followed them but never caught them together. He continued to believe they were having an affair. The nursing diagnosis of Disturbed Thought Processes is usually supported by the assessment data.

Because of their inability to develop relationships, these patients are often socially isolated and lack social support systems. However, the nursing diagnosis of Social Isolation is not appropriate for the person with paranoid personality disorder because the person does not meet the defining characteristics of feelings of aloneness, rejection, desire for contact with people, and insecurity in social situations.

Nursing interventions based on the establishment of a therapeutic relationship are difficult to implement because of the patient's mistrust. If a trusting relationship is established, the nurse helps the patient identify problematic areas, such as getting along with others or keeping a job. Through therapeutic techniques such as acceptance, confrontation, and reflection, the nurse and patient examine a problematic area to gain another view of the situation. Changing thought patterns takes time. Patient outcomes are evaluated in terms of small changes in thinking and behavior.

Continuum of Care

Individuals with paranoid personalities are unlikely to participate in treatment or recovery plans. If they have other comorbid disorders and are forced to seek treatment (through loss of their job or being ordered by a court in connection with an offense of a chargeable nature), they may seek help for depression or psychosis.

Schizoid Personality Disorder

Clinical Course and Diagnostic Criteria

People with **schizoid personality disorder** are characterized as being expressively impassive and interpersonally disengaged (Millon, 2011). They tend to be unable to experience the joyful and pleasurable aspects of life. They are introverted, reclusive, and clinically seem distant, aloof, apathetic, and emotionally detached. Typically life-long loners, they have difficulty making friends, seem uninterested in social activities, and appear to gain little satisfaction in personal relationships. In fact, they appear to be incapable of forming social relationships. Their interests are directed at objects, things, and abstractions. They may do well at solitary jobs other people might find difficult to tolerate. Often people with schizoid personality disorders may daydream excessively and become attached to animals, and they frequently do not marry or even form long-lasting romantic relationships. As children, they engage primarily in solitary activities, such as stamp collecting, computer games, electronic equipment, or academic pursuits such as mathematics or engineering. In addition, they seem to have a cognitive deficit characterized by obscure thought processes, particularly about social matters. Communication with others is confused and lacks focus. These individuals reveal minimum introspection and self-awareness, and interpersonal experiences are described in a very mechanical way.

Epidemiology

Schizoid personality disorder is rarely diagnosed in clinical settings. It is estimated that the prevalence is 3.1% (APA, 2013).

Etiology

The etiologic processes are speculative. There may be defects in either the limbic or reticular regions of the brain that may result in the development of the schizoid pattern (Millon, 2011). The defects of this personality may stem from an adrenergic–cholinergic imbalance in which the parasympathetic division of the autonomic nervous system is functionally dominant. Excesses or deficiencies in acetylcholine and norepinephrine may result in the proliferation and scattering of neural impulses that may be responsible for the cognitive "slippage" or affective deficits.

Nursing Care

Impaired Social Interactions and Chronic Low Self-esteem are typical diagnoses of patients with schizoid personality disorder. Major treatment goals are to enhance the experience of pleasure, prevent social isolation, and increase emotional responsiveness to others. Because these individuals often lack customary social skills, social skills training is useful in enhancing their ability to relate in interpersonal situations. The primary focus is to increase the patient's ability to feel pleasure. The nurse balances interventions between encouraging enough social activity to prevent the individual from retreating into a fantasy world and too much social activity that becomes intolerable to the patient.

The nurse may find working with such individuals unrewarding and as a result, the attending nurses may become frustrated, feel helpless, or become bored during the interactions. It is difficult to establish a therapeutic relationship with these individuals because they tend to shy away from interactions and are rarely motivated about treatment. Evaluation of outcomes should be in terms of increasing the patient's feelings of satisfaction with solitary activities.

Continuum of Care

People with schizoid personalities are rarely hospitalized unless they have a comorbid disorder. Family members may seek treatment for them in an outpatient setting.

Schizotypal Personality Disorder
Clinical Course and Diagnostic Criteria

Schizotypal personality disorder is characterized by a pattern of social and interpersonal deficits. The term **schizotypy** refers to traits that are similar to the symptoms of schizophrenia but are less severe. Cognitive perceptual symptoms are a primary characteristic and include magical beliefs (similar to delusions) and perceptual aberrations (similar to hallucinations). Other common symptoms include referential thinking (interpreting insignificant events as personally relevant) and paranoia (suspicion of others).

Schizotypal personality–disordered persons are more dramatically eccentric than those with schizoid personality disorder who are characteristically flat, colorless, and dull (Millon, 2011). These individuals are perceived as strikingly odd or strange in both appearance and behavior, even to laypersons. They may have unusual mannerisms, an unkempt manner of dress that does not quite "fit together," and inattention to usual social conventions (e.g., avoiding eye contact, wearing clothes that are stained or ill fitting, and being unable to join in the give-and-take banter of coworkers). Devoid of any close friends other than first-degree relatives, their mood is constricted or inappropriate, with excessive social anxieties. They usually exhibit an avoidant behavior pattern.

Persons with schizotypal personality disorder may respond to stress with transient psychotic episodes (lasting minutes to hours). Because of their short duration, the symptoms mirror but fall short of features that would justify the diagnosis of schizophrenia. Many individuals (30%– 50%) with schizotypal personality disorder also have a co-occurring major depressive disorder diagnosis when admitted to a hospital (APA, 2013; Cicero & Kerns, 2010). Schizotypal personality disorders may be slightly more common in males (APA, 2013).

Epidemiology and Risk Factors

The lifetime prevalence of schizotypal personality disorder is 3.9% with higher rates among men (4.2%) than women. There is cultural variation with black women and low-income individuals having a greater risk than others (Pulay, Stinson, Dawson, Goldstein, Chou, Huang, et al., 2009).

Etiology

Magnetic resonance imaging (MRI) studies of individuals with schizotypal personality disorder show smaller gray matter volume, which are correlated with negative symptoms. This pattern of gray matter loss is similar to schizophrenia, although there does not appear to be the progression of volume reduction present in schizophrenia (Asami, Whitford, Bouix, Dickey, Niznikiewicz, Shenton, et al., 2013; Rapp, Mutschler, Wild, Erb, Lengsfeld, Saur, et al., 2010).

Nursing Care

Depending on the amount of decompensation (i.e., deterioration of functioning and exacerbation of symptoms), the assessment of a patient with a schizotypal personality disorder can generate a range of nursing diagnoses. If a person has severe symptoms, such as delusional thinking or perceptual disturbances, the nursing diagnoses are similar to those for a person with schizophrenia (see Chapter 21). If symptoms are mild, the typical nursing diagnoses include Social Isolation, Ineffective Coping, Low Self-esteem, and Impaired Social Interactions.

People with schizotypal personality disorder need help in developing recovery-oriented strategies to increase their sense of self-worth and recognize their positive attributes. They can benefit from social skills training and environmental management that increases their psychosocial functioning. Their eccentric thoughts and behaviors alienate them from others. Reinforcing socially appropriate dress and behavior can improve their overall appearance and ability to relate in the environment. Because they have a hard time generalizing from one situation to another, attention to cognitive skills is important.

Continuum of Care

Quality of life for a patient with schizotypal personality disorder can be improved with supportive psychotherapy, but their suspiciousness, lack of trust, or impaired social interactions make it difficult to establish a therapeutic relationship. These individuals do not usually seek treatment unless more serious symptoms appear, such as depression or anxiety. Medications are not generally used unless the individual has coexisting anxiety or depression.

Nursing care is often provided in a home or clinic setting, with the personality disorder being secondary to the purpose of the care. This means that nurses are focusing on other aspects of patient care and may miss the underlying psychiatric disorder. A psychiatric nursing consult may be needed for these patients to help identify the disorder.

CLUSTER B DISORDERS: BORDERLINE, ANTISOCIAL, HISTRIONIC, AND NARCISSISTIC PERSONALITY DISORDERS

Borderline Personality Disorder

People with **borderline personality disorder** (BPD) have problems regulating their moods, developing a self-identity, maintaining interpersonal relationships, maintaining reality-based thinking, and avoiding impulsive or destructive behavior. The severity and difficulty in treating the disorder leads to enormous public health costs from health care utilization and functional disability (Gunderson, Stout, McGlashan, Shea, Morey, Gril, et al., 2011).

> **KEYCONCEPT Borderline personality disorder** (BPD) is characterized by a disruptive pattern of instability related to self-identity, interpersonal relationships, and affect, combined with marked impulsivity and destructive behavior.

Clinical Course

Individuals with BPD appear more competent than they actually are and often set unrealistically high expectations for themselves. When these expectations are not met, they experience intense shame, self-hate, and self-directed anger. Their lives are like soap operas—one crisis after another. Some of the crises are caused by the individual's dysfunctional lifestyle or inadequate social milieu, but many are caused by fate—the death of a spouse or a diagnosis of an illness. They react emotionally with minimal coping skills. The intensity of their emotions often frightens them and others. Friends, family members, and coworkers limit their contact with the person, which furthers the sense of aloneness, abandonment, and self-hatred. It also diminishes opportunities for learning self-corrective measures.

Remissions from the acute symptoms (e.g., self-injurious behaviors, suicide attempts or threats about suicide) are fairly common and the relapse rate is relatively low compared to other disorders. However, psychosocial functioning does not necessarily improve as symptoms decrease. Younger age and higher education levels predict higher functioning (Gunderson, et al., 2011).

Diagnostic Criteria

BPD is a "pervasive pattern of instability of interpersonal relationships, self-image, and affects, and marked impulsivity beginning by early adulthood and present in a variety of contexts" (APA, 2013, p. 663). See Key Diagnostic Characteristics 22.1. Individuals with BPD also exhibit related cognitive and behavioral dysfunctions.

Unstable Interpersonal Relationships

People with BPD have an extreme fear of abandonment as well as a history of unstable or insecure attachments (Miano, Fertuck, Arntz, & Stanley, 2013). Most have never experienced a consistently secure, nurturing relationship and are constantly seeking reassurance and validation. In an attempt to meet their interpersonal needs, they idealize others and establish intense relationships that violate others' interpersonal boundaries, which leads to rejection. When these relationships do not live up to their expectations, they devalue the person. Continually disappointed in relationships, these individuals, who are already intensely emotional and have a poor sense of self, feel estranged from others and inadequate in the face of perceived social standards. Intense shame and self-hate

---

KEY DIAGNOSTIC CHARACTERISTICS 22.1 • BORDERLINE PERSONALITY DISORDER 301.83

Diagnostic Criteria

A pervasive pattern of instability of interpersonal relationships, self-image, and diminished affect, and marked impulsivity, beginning by early adulthood and present in a variety of contexts, as indicated by five (or more) of the following:

1. Frantic efforts to avoid real or imagined abandonment. (Note: Do not include suicidal or self-mutilating behavior covered in Criterion 5.)
2. A pattern of unstable and intense interpersonal relationships characterized by alternating between extremes of idealization and devaluation.
3. Identity disturbance: markedly and persistently unstable self-image or sense of self.
4. Impulsivity in at least two areas that are potentially self-damaging (e.g., spending, sex, substance abuse, reckless driving, binge eating). (Note: Do not include suicidal or self-mutilating behavior covered in Criterion 5.)
5. Recurrent suicidal behavior, gestures, or threats, or self-mutilating behavior.

6. Affective instability due to a marked reactivity of mood (e.g., intense episodic dysphoria, irritability, or anxiety usually lasting a few hours and only rarely more than a few days).
7. Chronic feelings of emptiness.
8. Inappropriate intense anger or difficulty controlling anger (e.g., frequent displays of temper, constant anger, recurrent physical fights).
9. Transient stress-related paranoid ideation or severe dissociative symptoms.

Associated Behavioral Findings

- Pattern of undermining self at the moment a goal is to be realized
- Possible psychotic-like symptoms during times of stress
- Recurrent job losses, interrupted education, and broken marriages
- History of physical and sexual abuse, neglect, hostile conflict, and early parental loss or separation

Reprinted with permission from the *Diagnostic and Statistical Manual of Mental Disorders*, (5th ed.) (Copyright ©2013). American Psychiatric Association. All Rights Reserved.

---

follow. These feelings often result in self-injurious behaviors, such as wrist cutting, self-burning, or head banging.

> **Consider Rebecca:**
> Rebecca hates being alone, but her behaviors drive others away. When she feels rejected, anxious, or angry, she cuts her wrists, which decreases her anxiety.

Unstable Self-Image

These patients appear to have no sense of their own identity and direction; this becomes a source of great distress to them and is often manifested by chronic feelings of emptiness and boredom. It is not unusual for people with BPD to direct their actions in accord with the wishes of other people. For example, one woman with BPD describes herself: "I am a singer because my mother wanted me to be. I live in the city because my manager thought that I should. I become whatever anyone tells me to be. Whenever someone recommends a song, I wonder why I didn't think of that. My boyfriend tells me what to wear."

Unstable Affects

Affective instability (i.e., rapid and extreme shift in mood) is a core characteristic of BPD and is evidenced by erratic emotional responses to situations and intense sensitivity to criticism or perceived slights. For example, a person may greet a casual acquaintance with intense affection yet later be aloof with the same acquaintance.

Friends describe individuals with BPD as moody, irresponsible, or intense. These individuals often fail to recognize their own emotional responses, thoughts, beliefs, and behaviors and have difficulty interpreting the facial affects of others. In this disorder recognizing emotions in others is altered (Mitchell, Dickens, & Picchioni, 2014). See Fame and Fortune.

Cognitive Dysfunctions

People with BPD often have **dichotomous thinking**. That is, they evaluate experiences, people, and objects in terms of mutually exclusive categories (e.g., good or bad, success or failure, trustworthy or deceitful). Their interpretation of normally occurring events is usually extremely positive or extremely negative. Sometimes their thinking becomes disorganized with irrelevant, bizarre notions and vague or scattered thought connections as well as delusions and hallucinations.

Another cognitive dysfunction common in BPD is **dissociation**, or times when thinking, feeling, or behaviors occur outside a person's awareness (van Dijke, van der Hart, Ford, van Son, van der Heijden, & Bühring, 2010). It is a coping strategy for avoiding disturbing events. In dissociating, the person does not have to be aware of or remember traumatic events.

Impaired Problem Solving

In BPD, affected people often fail to engage in active problem-solving. Instead, problem-solving is attempted

FAME & FORTUNE

Lady Diana Frances Spencer
Princess Diana (1961–1997)

PUBLIC PERSONA

Lady Diana was reared in the British upper class and lived her short life in privilege and wealth. She came onto the world stage as the fairy tale princess, when at 21 years of age, she married Prince Charles, age 33 years, in a royal wedding in front of 3,500 guests and an international television audience. Her startling beauty and charm enchanted the world. Publicly, Princess Diana projected grace, kindness, charisma, and vulnerability. Her charitable works related to land mines and AIDS issues brought world attention and understanding to these poignant social problems, creating a legacy. She was frequently photographed around the world as she greeted the public and engaged in charitable works, often including her two young sons in these activities.

PERSONAL REALITIES

Parental divorce resulted in the departure of her mother and emotional withdrawal of her father early in her life. Friends described her low self-esteem and identity confusion. Diana's brother referred to her deep feelings of unworthiness. She looked to the press, the public, and those around her to define her identity. "Diana brought a ferocious intensity to her relationships, pleading for attention and time, and demanding intense loyalty" (Smith, 1999, p. 446). She fluctuated between total intensity to withdrawal with intimate relationships and frequently experienced mercurial moods. Privately, she had episodes of self-mutilation by cutting, but she talked openly of her bouts with bulimia and feelings of emptiness. She admitted to adultery and multiple affairs (Smith, 1999). In tapes broadcast by NBC that were released after her death, Princess Diana talked about her relationship with Prince Charles and her suicide attempts.

Source: Smith, S. B. (1999). Diana in search of herself: Portrait of a troubled princess. New York: Times Books/Crown Publishing.

by soliciting help from others in a helplessly hopeless manner. Suggestions offered are rarely taken up.

Impulsivity

These individuals often have difficulty delaying gratification or thinking through the consequences before acting on their feelings; their actions are often unpredictable. Essentially, they act in the moment and clean up the mess afterward. Gambling, spending money irresponsibly, binge eating, engaging in unsafe sex, and abusing substances are typical of these individuals. They can also be physically or verbally aggressive. Job losses, interrupted education, and unsuccessful relationships are common.

Self-Harm Behaviors

The turmoil and unsuccessful interpersonal relationships and social experiences associated with BPD may lead the

person to undermine him- or herself when a goal is about to be reached. The most serious consequences are a suicide attempt or **parasuicidal behavior** (i.e., deliberate self-injury with intent to harm oneself).

KEYCONCEPT   **Self-harm** is deliberate self-injurious behavior.

Self-harm behavior can be compulsive (e.g., hair pulling), episodic, or repetitive (e.g., cutting wrists, arms, other body parts) and is more likely to occur when the individual with BPD is depressed; has highly unstable interpersonal relationships, especially problems with intimacy and sociability; and is paranoid, hypervigilant (i.e., alert, watchful), and resentful. It is not unusual for persons with this disorder to self-harm in unusual ways such as swallowing pens, staples, and even razor blades, or banging one's head against a brick wall. All self-harm behaviors should be considered potentially life threatening and taken seriously.

Borderline Personality Disorder Across the Life-Span

Many children and adolescents show symptoms similar to those of BPD, such as moodiness, self-destruction, impulsiveness, lack of temper control, and rejection sensitivity. If a family member has BPD, the adolescent should be carefully assessed for this disorder. Because symptoms of BPD begin in adolescence, it makes sense that some children and adolescents would meet the criteria for BPD even though it is not diagnosed before young adulthood. More likely, some personality traits, such as impulsivity and mood instability, in many adolescents should be recognized and treated whether or not BPD eventually develops.

Epidemiology and Risk Factors

The estimated prevalence of BPD in the general population ranges from 0.5% to 2.7%, with a median rate of 1.6%. In clinical populations, BPD is one of the most frequently diagnosed personality disorders with a higher proportion of women (Sansone & Sansone, 2011). One possible explanation for more women being diagnosed more often is that it is more socially acceptable for women than men to seek help from the health care system. Another reason is that childhood sexual abuse, which more commonly affects girls, is one of the strongest risk factors for BPD. Another explanation is that eating disorders are more common in women with BPD and so they have a greater likelihood of also having a mood, anxiety, or posttraumatic stress disorder. Men with BPD are more likely to have a substance use problem and intermittent explosive disorder. Women are more likely to seek treatment than men (Sansone & Sansone, 2011).

Other studies cite parental loss and separation (Steele & Siever, 2010). Clearly, more studies are needed to identify risk factors for the development of BPD.

Comorbidity

Ample clinical reports show the coexistence of personality disorders with other mental disorders such as mood, substance abuse, eating, dissociative, and anxiety disorders and other personality disorders (Gunderson, et al., 2011). The coexistence of BPD with other disorders presents clinicians with the difficult choice of which disorder receives treatment priority. Symptoms associated with this disorder often provoke negative reactions on the part of clinicians, which interfere with clinicians' ability to provide effective care (Fielding, 2013).

Etiology

Evidence supports a biopsychosocial etiology. Recent studies demonstrate differences in brain functioning between those with and without BPD but also provide evidence that psychological and social factors contribute to the development of the disorder (Stone, 2013). The following discussion highlights the leading explanations for BPD.

Biologic Theories

Evidence of central nervous system dysfunction in BPD is now clear, including possible structural changes (Koenigsberg, Denny, Fan, Liu, Guerreri, Mayson, et al., 2014). Biologic abnormalities are associated with three BPD characteristics: affective instability; transient psychotic episodes; and impulsive, aggressive, and suicidal behavior. Associated brain dysfunction occurs in the limbic system and frontal lobe and increases the behaviors of impulsiveness, parasuicide, and mood disturbance (Stone, 2013).

Psychosocial Theories

Psychoanalytic Theories

Using psychoanalytic methodology suggests persons with BPD have not achieved the normal and healthy developmental stage of **separation-individuation**, during which a child develops a sense of self, a permanent sense of significant others (object constancy), and integration of seeing both bad and good components of oneself (Clarkin & De Panfilis, 2013). Those with BPD lack the ability to separate from the primary caregiver and develop a separate and distinct personality or self-identity. **Projective identification** is believed to play an important role in the development of BPD and is a defense mechanism by which people with BPD protect their fragile self-image. For example, when overwhelmed by anxiety or anger at being disregarded by another, they defend against the intensity of these feelings by unconsciously blaming others for what happens to them. They project their feelings onto a significant other with the unconscious hope that that person knows how to deal with it. Projective identification becomes a defensive way of interacting with the world, which leads to more rejection.

Maladaptive Cognitive Processes

Cognitive schemata are patterns of thought that determine how a person interprets events. Each person's cognitive schemata screen, code, and evaluate incoming stimuli. In personality disorders, maladaptive cognitive schemata cause misinterpretation of other people's actions or reactions and of events that result in dysfunctional ways of responding. Cognitive schemata are important in understanding BPD (and antisocial personality disorder as well).

Individuals with BPD develop dysfunctional beliefs and maladaptive schemata early in life, leading them to misinterpret environmental stimuli continuously, which in turn leads to rigid and inflexible behavior patterns in response to new situations and people (Lawrence, Allen, & Chanen, 2011). Because those with BPD have been conditioned to anticipate rejection and disappointment in the past, they become entrenched in a pattern of fear and anxiety regarding encountering new people or situations. They have fears that disaster is going to strike at any minute. The work of cognitive therapists is to challenge distortions in thinking patterns and replace them with realistic ones.

> **Remember Rebecca?**
> Rebecca does not see herself as contributing to her problem but believes her misfortunes are caused by others. For example, when she encounters new people, she shares too much personal information and is disappointed when they do not respond with the same intensity. She interprets their response as rejection.

Social Theories: Biosocial Theories

The biosocial viewpoint proposed by Marsha Linehan and colleagues sees BPD as a multifaceted problem, a combination of innate emotional vulnerability (sensitivity and reactivity to environmental stress), emotional dysregulation (inability to control emotions in social interactions), and the environment (Linehan, 1993) (Box 22.1).

BOX 22.1

Behavioral Patterns in Borderline Personality Disorder

1. *Emotional vulnerability.* Person experiences a pattern of pervasive difficulties in regulating negative emotions, including high sensitivity to negative emotional stimuli, high emotional intensity, and slow return to emotional baseline.
2. *Self-invalidation.* Person fails to recognize one's own emotional responses, thoughts, beliefs, and behaviors and sets unrealistically high standards and expectations for self. May include intense shame, self-hate, and self-directed anger. Person has no personal awareness and tends to blame social environment for unrealistic expectations and demands.
3. *Unrelenting crises.* Person experiences pattern of frequent, stressful, negative environmental events, disruptions, and roadblocks—some caused by the individual's dysfunctional

lifestyle, others by an inadequate social milieu, and many by fate or chance.
4. *Inhibited grieving.* Person tries to inhibit and overcontrol negative emotional responses, especially those associated with grief and loss, including sadness, anger, guilt, shame, anxiety, and panic.
5. *Active passivity.* Person fails to engage actively in solving of own life problems but will actively seek problem solving from others in the environment; learned helplessness, hopelessness.
6. *Apparent competence.* Tendency for the individual to appear deceptively more competent than he or she actually is; usually because of failure of competencies to generalize across expected moods, situations, and time. Person fails to display adequate nonverbal cues of emotional distress.

Adapted from Linehan, M. (1993). Cognitive-behavioral treatment of borderline personality disorder (p. 10). New York: Guilford Press.

> **KEYCONCEPT   Emotional dysregulation** is the inability to control emotions in social interactions and includes an instability of mood, marked shifts to or from depression, stress-related and transient mood crashes, rejection sensitivity, and inappropriate and intense outbursts of anger.

The emotional dysregulation and aggressive impulsivity entail both social learning and biologic regulation. Much of the neurobiologic research is directed at corticolimbic function and other cerebral function (Stone, 2013). In fact, restoring balance in these systems permits more consistent neural firing between the limbic system and the frontal and prefrontal cortices. When these circuits are functional, the person has a greater capacity to think about his or her emotions and modulate behavior more responsibly.

The ability to control emotion is partly learned from private experiences and encounters with the social environment. BPD is believed to develop when emotionally vulnerable individuals interact with an **invalidating environment**, a social situation that negates private emotional responses and communication. When core emotional responses and communications are continuously dismissed, trivialized, devalued, punished, and discredited (invalidated) by respected or valued persons, the vulnerable individual becomes unsure about his or her feelings. A minor example of an invalidating environment or response follows: The parents of Emily, a 4-year-old girl, tell her that the family is going to grandmother's house for a family meal. The child responds, "I am not going to Gramma's. I hate Stevie (her cousin)." The parents reply, "You don't hate Stevie. He is a wonderful child. He is your cousin, and only a spoiled and selfish little girl would say such a thing." The parents have devalued Emily's feelings and discredited her comments, thereby invalidating her feelings and sense of personal worth.

The most severe form of invalidation occurs in situations of child sexual abuse. Often, the abusing adult

has told the child that this is a "special secret" between them. The child experiences feelings of fear, pain, and sadness, yet this trusted adult continuously dismisses the child's true feelings and tells the child what he or she should feel.

Family Response to Borderline Personality Disorder

Individuals with BPD are typically part of a chaotic family system, but their behavior adds to the chaos. Family members often feel captive to these patients. Family members are afraid to disagree with them or refuse to meet their multiple needs, fearing that self-destructive behavior will follow. During the course of the disorder, family members often get "burned out" and withdraw from the patient, only adding to the patient's fear of abandonment (Miano, et al., 2013).

Teamwork and Collaboration: Working Toward Recovery

BPD is a very complex disorder that requires collaboration of treatment by the entire mental health care team. Because BPD patients view the world in absolutes, nurses and other treatment team members are alternately categorized as all good or all bad. This defense is called **splitting** and presents clinicians with a challenge to work openly with each other as well as the patient until the issue can be resolved through team meetings and clinical supervision.

People with BPD are inadvertently highly stigmatized by many clinicians. Staff often accuse these individuals of "manipulation" to get attention and say so in a very derogatory manner. In reality, all of us want attention from significant people in our lives. Most of us have the necessary skills to successfully meet our need for closeness and attention without alienating the very people who are important to us.

People with BPD are unsuccessful in developing long-term meaningful relationships or getting what they want because their approach alienates others. Their need for attention and closeness to others is very normal: it is how they seek attention that is problematic.

Psychotherapy is needed to help the individual with BPD manage the dysfunctional moods, impulsive behavior, and self-injurious behaviors. Specially trained therapists who are comfortable with the many demands of these patients are needed. These therapists represent a variety of mental health disciplines, including psychology, social work, and advanced practice nursing. This is a lifelong disorder requiring ongoing treatment as the individual copes with multiple interpersonal crises. Several types of medications are usually needed, including mood stabilizers, antidepressants, and anxiolytics; careful medication monitoring is necessary.

Dialectical behavior therapy (DBT) combines cognitive and behavior therapy strategies; it was developed for persons with **borderline personality disorder.** Core interventions include problem-solving, exposure techniques (i.e., gradual exposure to cues that set off aversive emotions), skills training, contingency management (i.e., reinforcement of positive behavior), and cognitive modification. Skills groups are an integral part of DBT and are taught in group settings in which patients practice emotional regulation, interpersonal effectiveness, distress tolerance, core mindfulness, and self-management skills (Dimeff, Woodcock, Harned, & Beadnell, 2011; Linehan, 1993).

Safety Issues

Persons with BPD can be extremely volatile emotionally. Because they experience emotions so intensely, they are at high risk for self-harm and suicide. Self-harm threats should be taken very seriously.

Evidence-Based Nursing Care for Persons with Borderline Personality Disorder

Persons with BPD may enter the mental health system early (during young adulthood or even before) because of their chaotic lifestyles. Behavior includes unstable moods, problems with interpersonal relationships, low self-esteem, and self-identity issues. Thinking and behavior are dysregulated (Box 22.2). They have problems in daily living, including maintaining intimate relationships, keeping a job, and living within the law (Box 22.3). (see Nursing Care Plan 22.1, available at http://thepoint.lww.com/BoydEssentials.)

Mental Health Nursing Assessment

Physical Health Assessment

People with BPD are usually able to maintain personal hygiene and physical functioning. Because of the

---

> **BOX 22.2**
>
> ### Response Patterns of Persons with Borderline Personality Disorder
>
> Affective (mood) Dysregulation
> Mood lability
> Problems with anger
> Interpersonal dysregulation
> Chaotic relationships
> Fears of abandonment
> Self-dysregulation
> Difficulties with sense of self
> Sense of emptiness
> Behavioral dysregulation
> Parasuicidal behavior or threats
> Impulsive behavior
> Cognitive dysregulation
> Dissociative responses
> Paranoid ideation
>
> ---
>
> Courtesy of M. Linehan, Department of Psychology, Box 351525, University of Washington, Seattle, WA 98195-1525, 1993.

---

comorbidity of BPD and eating disorders and substance abuse, however, a nutritional assessment may be needed. The assessment should also include the use of caffeinated beverages (e.g., coffee, tea, cola, energy drinks) and alcohol. In patients who engage in binging or purging, assessment should include examining the teeth for pitting and discoloration, as well as the hands and fingers for redness and calluses caused by inducing vomiting. The patient should be queried about physiologic responses of emotion. Sleep patterns also should be assessed because sleep alterations may suggest coexisting depression or mania.

Physical Indicators of Self-Injurious Behaviors

Patients with BPD should be assessed for self-injurious behavior or suicide attempts. It is important to ask the patient about specific self-abusive behaviors, such as cutting, scratching, or swallowing foreign objects. The patient may wear long sleeves to hide injury to the arms. Specifically, asking about thoughts of hurting oneself when experiencing a major upset provides an opportunity for prevention and for coaching the patient toward alternative self-soothing measures.

Medication Assessment

Patients with BPD may be taking several medications. For example, one patient may be taking a small dose of an antipsychotic and a mood stabilizer. Another may be taking a selective serotonin reuptake inhibitor (SSRI). Initially, patients may be reluctant to disclose all the medications they are taking because, for many of them, trial and error has led to repeated represcription. They are fearful of having medication taken away from them.

BOX 22.3 CLINICAL VIGNETTE

Borderline Personality Disorder

Joanne is a 22-year-old single woman who was recently fired from her job as a data entry clerk. She is living with her mother and stepfather, who brought her to the emergency department after finding her crouched in a fetal position in the bathroom, her wrists bleeding. She seemed to be in a daze. This is her first psychiatric admission although her mother and stepfather have suspected that she has "needed help" for a long time. In high school, she received brief treatment for a potential eating disorder. She remains very thin but is able to eat at least one meal per day. During periods of stress, she will go for days without eating. Joanne is the second of three children. Her parents divorced when she was 3 years old. She has not seen her father since he left. Although she has pleasant memories of her father, her mother has told her that he beat Joanne and her sisters when he was drinking. When Joanne was 6 years old, her older sister died as a result of an automobile accident. Joanne was in the car but was uninjured. As a child, Joanne was seen as a potential singing star. Her natural musical talent attracted her teachers' support, which encouraged her to develop her talent. She took singing lessons and entered statewide competitions in high school. Although she enjoyed the attention, she was never really comfortable in the limelight and felt "guilty" about having a talent that she sometimes resented. She was able to make friends but found that she was unable to keep them. They described her as "too intense" and emotional. She had one boyfriend in high school, but she was very uncomfortable with any physical closeness. After ending the relationship with the boyfriend, she concentrated on dieting to have a "perfect body." When her dieting attracted her parents' attention, she vowed to eat just enough to keep them "off her back about it." She spent much of her leisure time with her grandmother. She attended college briefly but was unable to concentrate. It was during college and after her grandmother's death that Joanne began cutting her wrists during periods of stress. It seemed to calm her.

After leaving college, Joanne returned home. She had several jobs and short-lived friendships. She was usually fired from her job because of "moodiness," and it took her several months before she would again find another. She spent days in her room listening to music. Her recent episode occurred after she was fired from work and spent 3 days in her bedroom.

What Do You Think?

- How would you describe Joanne's mood?
- Are Joanne's losses of her father and sister really severe enough to affect her ability to relate to others now? Do the losses seem to relate to the self-injury?
- What behaviors indicate problems with self-esteem and self-identity are present?

Development of rapport with special attention to a nonjudgmental approach is especially important when eliciting current medication practices. The effectiveness of the medication in relieving the target symptom needs to be determined. Use of alcohol, OTC medications, and street drugs should be carefully assessed to determine drug interactions.

Psychosocial Assessment

People with BPD have usually experienced significant losses in their lives that shape their view of the world. They experience **inhibited grieving**, "a pattern of repetitive, significant trauma and loss, together with an inability to fully experience and personally integrate or resolve these events" (Linehan, 1993). They have unresolved grief that can last for years and will avoid situations that evoke those feelings of separation and loss. During the assessment, the nurse can identify the losses (real or perceived) and explore the patient's experience during these losses, paying particular attention to whether the patient has reached resolution. A history of physical or sexual abuse and early separation from significant caregivers may provide important clues to the severity of the disturbances (Box 22.4).

Mood fluctuations are common and can be assessed by any number of the depression and anxiety screening scales or by asking the following questions:

- What things or events bother you and make you feel sad or angry?
- Do these things or events trouble you more than they trouble other people?
- Do friends and family tell you that you are moody?
- Do you get angry easily?
- Do you have trouble with your temper?
- Do you think you were born with these feelings or did something happen to make you feel this way?

BOX 22.4

Research for Best Practice: BPD and Patients' Childhood Experiences

Holm, A. L., Bégat, I., & Severinsson, E. (2009). Emotional pain: Surviving mental health problems related to childhood experiences. Journal of Psychiatric and Mental Health Nursing, 16, 636–645.

THE QUESTION: How do women with borderline personality disorder (BPD) experience emotional pain related to childhood?

METHODS: An exploratory design was used to collect data from 13 women suffering from BDP. An interpretative content analysis was used to analyze the text.

FINDINGS: Women survived their painful childhood experiences of being forced to be silent and hide their feelings. Most escaped emotional despair by running away to their friends or family members with whom they felt safe. Some who had been sexually abused managed to forget the abuse but still felt guilty. As a result of being criticized, rejected, humiliated, beaten, and not respected, most perceived they were not loved and tried anything to get their parents' love and attention. Surviving in an environment where one remains unnoticed leads to an endless need to be empowered, confirmed, and loved.

IMPLICATIONS FOR NURSING: Only when the emotional pain and trauma are understood can the overall situation of these women be understood.

Appearance and activity level generally reflect the person's mood and psychomotor activity. Many of those with BPD have been physically or sexually abused and thus should be assessed for depression. A disheveled appearance can reflect depression or an agitated state. When feeling good, these patients can be very engaging; they tend to be dramatic in their style of dress and attract attention, such as by wearing an unusual hairstyle or heavy makeup. Because physical appearance reflects identity, patients may experiment with their appearance and seek affirmation and acceptance from others. Body piercing, tattoos, and other perceived adornments provide a mechanism to define self.

Rebecca's Assessment

Rebecca loves to project a dramatic appearance when she is feeling good. When she is in a good mood, she projects as an overly confident, engaging person. She has several body piercings. She refuses to discuss any childhood trauma or sexual abuse.

Impulsivity

Impulsivity can be identified by asking the patient whether he or she does things impulsively or spur of the moment. For example: "Have there been times when you were hurt by your actions or were sorry later that you acted in the way you did?" Direct questions about gambling, choices in sexual partners, sexual activities, fights, arguments, arrests, and habits related to consumption of alcohol can also help in identifying areas of impulsive behavior.

From a neurophysiologic perspective, impulsively acting before thinking seems to be mediated by rapid nerve firing in the mesolimbic area. This activates psychomotor responses before pathways reach the prefrontal cortex (Wolf, Sambataro, Vasic, Schmid, Thomann, Bienentreu, et al., 2011). Teaching the patient strategies to slow down automatic responses (e.g., deep breathing, counting to 10) buys time to think before acting.

Cognitive Disturbances

The mental status examination of those with BPD usually reveals normal thought processes that are not disorganized or confused except during periods of stress. Those with BPD usually exhibit dichotomous thinking, or a tendency to view things as absolute, either black or white, good or bad, with no perception of compromise. Dichotomous thinking can be assessed by asking patients how they view other people. Evidence of dichotomous thinking is indicated with responses of "good" or "bad," "wonderful" or "terrible."

Identity Disturbance

Unstable self-image is often manifested as an identity disturbance or **identity diffusion**, a loss of the capacity for self-definition and commitment to values, goals, or relationships. The nurse can recognize identity diffusion if the patient reports an ongoing "emptiness" or contradictory behavior. "I know I should not have gone out with him, but he wanted to see me." The person's thoughts and behavior will seem fragmented and superficial (Goth, Foelsch, Schlüter-Müller, Birkhölzer, Jung, Pick, et al., 2012).

Dissociation and Transient Psychotic Episodes

With BPD, periods of dissociation and transient psychotic episodes may occur. Dissociation can be assessed by asking if there is ever a time when the patient does not remember events or has the feeling of being separate from his or her body. Some patients refer to this as "spacing out." By asking specific information about how often, how long, and when dissociation first was used, the nurse can get an idea of how important dissociation is as a coping skill. It is important to ask the person what is happening in the environment when dissociation occurs. Frequent dissociation indicates a highly habitual coping mechanism that is difficult to change. Because transient psychotic states occur, it is also important to elicit data regarding the presence of hallucinations or delusions and their frequency and circumstances.

Interpersonal Skills

Assessment of the person's ability to relate to others is important because interpersonal problems are linked to dissociation and self-injurious behavior. Information about friendships, frequency of contact, and intimate relationships provide data about the person's ability to relate to others. Patients with BPD often are sexually active and may have numerous sexual partners. Their need for closeness clouds their judgment about sexual partners, so it is not unusual to find these patients in abusive, destructive relationships with people with antisocial personality disorder.

Self-Esteem and Coping Skills

Coping with stressful situations is one of the major problems of people with BPD. Assessment of their coping skills and their ability to deal with stressful situations is important. Self-esteem is closely related to identifying with health care workers. Patients with BPD perceive their families and friends as being weary of their numerous crises and their seeming unwillingness to break the vicious self-destructive cycle. Feeling rejected by their natural support system, these individuals create one within the health system. During periods of crisis, especially during the late evening, early morning, or on weekends, they may call or visit various psychiatric units asking to speak to specific personnel who formerly cared for them. They even know different nurses' scheduled days off and make the rounds to several hospitals and clinics. Sometimes they bring gifts to nurses or call them at home. Because their newly created social support system cannot provide the support that is needed, the patient continues to feel rejected. One of the treatment goals is to help the individual establish a more natural support network.

Functional Assessment

Some individuals with BPD can function very well except during periods when symptoms erupt. They hold jobs, are active in communities, and can perform well. During periods of stress, symptoms often appear. Conversely, some individuals with severe BPD function poorly; they seem to be always in a crisis, which often they have created.

Social Support Systems

Identification of social supports (e.g., family, friends, religious organizations) is the purpose in assessing resources. Knowing how the patient obtains social support is important in understanding the quality of interpersonal relationships. For example, some patients consider as their "best friends" nurses, physicians, and other health care personnel. Because these are false friendships (i.e., not reciprocated), they inevitably lead to frustration and disappointment. However, helping the patient find ways to meet other people and encouraging the patient's efforts are more realistic.

Risk Assessment: Suicide or Self-Injury

It is critical that patients with BPD be assessed for suicidal and self-damaging behavior, including alcohol and drug abuse (see Chapter 15). The assessment should include direct questions, such as asking whether the patient thinks about or engages in self-injurious behaviors. If so, the nurse should continue to explore the behaviors: what is done, how is it done, how frequently is it done, and what are the circumstances surrounding the self-injurious behavior. It is helpful to explain briefly to the patient that sometimes people cut, scratch, or pick at themselves as a way of bringing some relief and comfort. Although the behavior brings temporary relief, it also places the person at risk for infection. Approaching the assessment in this way conveys a sense of understanding and is more likely to invite the patient to disclose honestly.

Strength Assessment

The strength assessment is important because these positive thoughts, skills, and behaviors can be supported as the individuals replace self-defeating behaviors with positive ones. Many of these individuals are extremely resilient despite the trauma that they have often experienced. The person's strength will emerge in the assessment and

increase as the nurse gets to know the patient better. Some key questions include the following:

- How do you make yourself feel better?
- How do you resist the urge to hurt yourself?
- How do you make friends?
- What is the most positive thought, skill, or behavior that you have?

Nursing Diagnoses

One of the first diagnoses to consider is Risk for Self-mutilation because protection of the patient from self-injury is always a priority. If cognitive changes are present (dissociation and transient psychosis), two other diagnoses may be appropriate: Disturbed Thought Process and Ineffective Coping. The Disturbed Thought Process diagnosis is used if dissociative and psychotic episodes actually interfere with daily living. If the individual copes with stressful situations by dissociating or hallucinating, the diagnosis Ineffective Coping is used. Other nursing diagnoses data include Insomnia, Imbalanced Nutrition, Personal Identity Disturbance, Anxiety, Grieving, Chronic Low Self-esteem, Powerlessness, Post-trauma Response, Defensive Coping, and Spiritual Distress.

The strength assessment may generate Readiness for Enhanced Hope, Readiness for Enhanced Coping or Readiness for Enhanced Self-Concept.

Therapeutic Relationship

Psychiatric-mental health registered nurses do not function as the patient's primary therapists, but they do need to establish a therapeutic relationship that strengthens the patient's coping skills and self-esteem and also supports individual psychotherapy. The therapeutic relationship helps the patient to experience a model of healthy interaction with consistency, limit setting, caring, and respect (both self-respect and respect for the patient). Patients who have low self-esteem need help in recognizing genuine respect from others and reciprocating with respect for others. In the therapeutic relationship, the nurse models self-respect by observing personal limits, being assertive, and clearly communicating expectations (Box 22.5). The nurse should always avoid using stigmatizing language, such as describing the person's behavior as manipulating instead of reporting or documenting specific behaviors.

Nurses should use their own self-awareness skills to examine their personal response to the patient. How the nurse responds to the patient can often be a clue to how others perceive and respond to the person. For example, if the nurse feels irritated or impatient during the interview that is a sign that others respond to this person in the same way; conversely, if the nurse feels empathy or closeness, chances are this patient can evoke these same feelings in others. (Norrie, Davidson, Tata, & Gumley, 2013; Wright & Jones, 2012).

BOX 22.5 • THERAPEUTIC DIALOGUE • Borderline Personality Disorder

INEFFECTIVE APPROACH

Rebecca: Hey, you know what? You are my favorite nurse. That night nurse sure doesn't understand me the way you do.

Nurse: Oh, I'm glad you are comfortable with me. Which night nurse?

Rebecca: You know, Sue.

Nurse: Did you have problems with her?

Rebecca: She is terrible. She sleeps all night or she is on the telephone.

Nurse: Oh, that doesn't sound very professional to me. Anything else?

Rebecca: Yeah, she said that you didn't know what you were doing. She said that you couldn't nurse your way out of a paper bag (smiling).

Nurse: She did, did she? (Getting angry.) She should talk.

Rebecca: Well, I gotta go to group. Where will you be? I feel so much better if I know where you are. I don't know how I can possibly be discharged tomorrow.

EFFECTIVE APPROACH

Rebecca: Hey, you know what? You are my favorite nurse. That night nurse sure doesn't understand me the way you do.

Nurse: I really like you, Rebecca. Tomorrow you will be discharged, and I'm glad that you will be able to return home. (Nurse avoided responding to "favorite nurse" statement. Redirected interaction to impending discharge.)

Rebecca: That night nurse slept all night.

Nurse: What was your night like? (Redirecting the interaction to Sara's experience.)

Rebecca: It was terrible. Couldn't sleep all night. I'm not sure that I'm ready to go home.

Nurse: Oh, so you are not quite sure about discharge? (reflection)

Rebecca: I get so, so lonely. Then, I want to hurt myself.

Nurse: Lonely feelings have started that chain of events that led to cutting, haven't they? (validation)

Rebecca: Yes, I'm very scared. I haven't cut myself for 1 week now.

Nurse: Do you have a plan for dealing with your lonely feelings when they occur?

Rebecca: I'm supposed to start thinking about something that is pleasant—like spring flowers in the meadow.

Nurse: Does that work for you?

Rebecca: Yes, sometimes.

CRITICAL THINKING CHALLENGE

• How did the nurse in the first scenario get sidetracked?

• How was the nurse in the second scenario able to keep the patient focused on herself and her impending discharge?

Mental Nursing Interventions

Physical Care

Usually, the person can manage hydration and self-care fairly well. This section focuses on those areas that are more likely to be problematic.

Sleep Hygiene

Disturbed sleep patterns are common in association with BPD. The nurse can intervene by helping the person establish a regular bedtime routine by teaching sleep hygiene strategies such avoiding foods and drinks that could interfere with

sleep. If relaxation exercises are used, they should be adapted to the tolerance of the individual. Special consideration must be made for persons who have been physically and sexually abused and who may be unable to put themselves in a vulnerable position (e.g., lying down in a room with other people or closing their eyes). These patients may need additional safeguards to help them sleep, such as a night light or repositioning the furniture in the room to allow a quick exit.

Teaching Nutritional Balance

The nutritional status of the person with BPD can quickly become a priority, particularly if the patient has coexisting eating disorders, mood disorders, schizophrenia, or substance abuse. Eating is often a response to stress, so patients can quickly become overweight. This is especially a problem when the patient has also been taking medications that promote weight gain, such as antipsychotics, antidepressants, or mood stabilizers. Helping the patient learn the basics of nutrition, make reasonable choices, and develop other coping strategies are useful interventions. If patients are engaging in purging or severe dieting practices, teaching the patient about the dangers of both of these practices is important (see Chapter 24). Referral to an eating disorders specialist may be needed. (Ripoll, 2012; Stoffers, Völlm, Rücker, Timmer, Huband, & Lieb, 2010).

Preventing and Treating Self-Harm

Patients with BPD are usually admitted to the inpatient setting because of threats of self-harm. Observing for antecedents of self-injurious behavior and intervening before an episode are important safety interventions. Patients can learn to identify situations leading to self-destructive behavior and develop preventive strategies.

> **EMERGENCY CARE ALERT** ! Because patients with BPD are impulsive and may respond to stress by harming themselves, observation of the patient's interactions and assessment of mood, level of distress, and agitation are important indicators of impending self-injury.

Remembering that self-harm is an effort to self-soothe by activating endogenous endorphins, the nurse can assist the patient to find more productive and enduring ways to find comfort. Linehan (1993) suggests using the Five Senses Exercise:

- Vision (e.g., go outside and look at the stars or flowers or autumn leaves)
- Hearing (e.g., listen to beautiful or invigorating music or the sounds of nature)
- Smell (e.g., light a scented candle, boil a cinnamon stick in water)
- Taste (e.g., drink a soothing, warm, nonalcoholic beverage)
- Touch (e.g., take a hot bubble bath, pet your dog or cat, get a massage)

Pharmacologic Interventions

Limiting medication is better for people with BPD. Patients should take medications only for target symptoms for a short time (e.g., an antidepressant for a bout with depression) because they may be taking many medications, particularly if they have a comorbid disorder, such as a mood disorder or substance abuse. Medications are used to control emotional dysregulation, impulsive aggression, cognitive disturbances, and anxiety as an adjunct to psychotherapy, but limited studies support the treatment of BPD with medication. Available evidence shows some benefit from atypical antipsychotics and mood stabilizers but little support for the use of antidepressants (Ripoll, 2012; Stoffers, et al., 2010).

Administering and Monitoring Medications

In inpatient settings, it is relatively easy to control medications; in other settings, however, patients must be aware that it is their responsibility to take their medication and monitor the number and type of drugs being taken. Patients who rely on medication to help them deal with stress and those who are periodically suicidal are at high risk for abuse of medications. Patients who experience unusual side effects are also at high risk for noncompliance. The nurse determines whether the patient is actually taking medication, whether the medication is being taken as prescribed, its effect on target symptoms, and the use of any OTC drugs (e.g., antihistamines, sleeping pills or herbal supplements with similar pharmacologic activity).

Managing Side Effects

Patients with BPD appear to be sensitive to many medications, so the dosage may need to be adjusted based on the side effects they experience. Listen carefully to the patient's description of the side effects. Any unusual side effects should be accurately documented and reported to the prescriber.

Teaching Points

Patients should be educated about the precribed medications and their interactions with other drugs and substances, but they should be encouraged to avoid relying on medication alone. Interventions include teaching patients about the medication and how and where it acts in the brain and body, helping establish a routine for taking prescribed medication, reporting side effects, and facilitating the development of positive coping strategies to deal with daily stresses rather than relying on medications. Eliciting the patient's partnership in care improves adherence and thereby outcomes.

Psychosocial Interventions

Addressing Abandonment and Intimacy Fears

One key to helping patients with BPD is recognizing their fears of both abandonment and intimacy. Informing the patient of the length of the therapeutic relationship as much as possible allows the patient to engage in and prepare for termination with the least pain of abandonment. If the patient's hospitalization is time limited, it is important to acknowledge the limit overtly and remind the patient with each contact how many sessions remain.

In day treatment and outpatient settings, the duration of treatment may be indeterminate, but the nurse may not be available that entire time. The termination process cannot be casual; this would stimulate abandonment fears. However, some patients end prematurely when the nurse informs them of the impending end as a way to leave before being rejected. The best approach is to explore these anticipated feelings with the patient. After careful planning, the nurse and patient discuss how to cope with anticipated feelings, including the wish to run away, review the progress the patient has made, and summarize what the patient has learned from the relationship that can be generalized to future encounters.

Establishing Personal Boundaries and Limitations

Personal boundaries are highly context specific; for example, stroking the hair of a stranger on the bus would be inappropriate, but stroking the hair and face of one's intimate partner while sitting together would be appropriate. Clarifying limits requires making explicit what is usually implicit. This may mean having a standing time during each shift that the nurse will talk with the patient. The nurse should refrain from offering personal information, which is frequently confusing to the person with BPD. At times, the person may present in a somewhat arrogant and seemingly entitled way. It is important for the nurse to recognize such a presentation as reflective of internal confusion and dissonance. Responding in a very neutral manner avoids confrontation and a power struggle, which might also unwittingly reinforce the patient's internal sense of inferiority.

Some additional strategies for establishing the boundaries of the relationship include the following:

- Documenting in the patient's chart the agreed-on appointment expectations
- Sharing the treatment plan with the patient
- Confronting violations of the agreement in a nonpunitive way
- Discussing the purpose of limits in the therapeutic relationship and applicability to other relationships

When patients violate boundaries, it is important to respond right away but without taking the behavior personally. For example, if a patient is flirtatious, simply say something like, "X, I feel uncomfortable with your overly friendly behavior. It seems out of place because we have a professional relationship. That would be more fitting for an intimate relationship that we will never have."

Using Behavioral Interventions

The goal of behavioral interventions is to replace dysfunctional behaviors with positive ones. The nurse has an important role in helping patients control emotions and behaviors by acknowledging and validating desired behaviors and ignoring or confronting undesired behaviors. Patients often test the nurse for a response, so nurses must decide how to respond to particular behaviors. This can be tricky because even negative responses can be viewed as positive reinforcement by the patient. In some instances, if the behavior is irritating but not harmful or demeaning, it is best to ignore, rather than focus, on it. However, grossly inappropriate and disrespectful behaviors require confrontation. If a patient throws a glass of water on an assistant because she is angry at the treatment team for refusing to increase her hospital privileges, an appropriate intervention would include confronting the patient with her behavior and issuing the consequences, such as losing her privileges and apologizing to the assistant.

However, such an incident can be used to help the patient understand why such behavior is inappropriate and how it can be changed. The nurse should explore with the patient what happened, what events led up to the behavior, what the consequences were, and what feelings were aroused. Advanced practice nurses or other therapists explore the origins of the patient's behaviors and responses, but the generalist nurse needs to help the patient explore ways to change behaviors involved in the current situation. The laboriousness of this analytic process may be a sufficient incentive for the patient to abandon the dysfunctional behavior.

Challenging Dysfunctional Thinking

The nurse can often challenge the patient's dysfunctional ways of thinking and encourage the person to think about the event in a different way. When a patient engages in catastrophic thinking, the nurse can challenge by asking, "What is the worst that could happen?" and "How likely would that be to occur?" Or in dichotomous thinking, when the patient fixates on one extreme perception or alternates only between the extremes, the nurse should ask the patient to think about any examples of exceptions to the extreme. The point of the challenge is not to debate or argue with the patient but to provide different perspectives to consider. Encouraging patients to keep journals of real interactions to process with the nurse or therapist is another effective way of testing the reality of their thinking and anticipations, affording more choices and flexibility (Box 22.6).

In problem-solving, the nurse might encourage the patient to debate both sides of the problem and then search for common ground. Practicing communication and negotiation skills through role-playing helps the patient make mistakes and correct them without harm to her or his self-esteem. The nurse also encourages patients to use these skills in their everyday lives and report back on the results, asking patients how they feel applying the skills and how doing so affects their self-perceptions.

BOX 22.6
Challenging Dysfunctional Thinking

Ms. S had worked for the same company for 20 years with a good job record. After an accident, she made some minor mistakes in her work that she quickly corrected. She informed her company nurse that her work was "really slipping" and that she was fearful of her coworkers' disapproval and of getting fired from her job. The nurse asked her to keep a journal of coworkers' comments for the next week. At the next visit, the following dialogue occurred:

Nurse: I noticed that you received several compliments on your work. Even a close friend of your boss expressed appreciation for your work.

Ms. S: It was a light week at work. I really don't believe they meant what they said.

Nurse: I can see how you can believe that one or two comments are not genuine, but how do you account for four and five good reports on your work?

Ms. S: Well, I don't know.

Nurse: It looks like your beliefs are not supported by your journal entries. Now, what makes you think that your boss wants to fire you after 20 years of service?

BOX 22.7

Psychoeducation Checklist: Borderline Personality Disorder

When caring for the patient with borderline personality disorder, be sure to include the following topic areas in the teaching plan:

- Management of medication, if used, including drug action, dosage, frequency, and possible adverse effects
- Regular sleep routines
- Nutrition
- Safety measures
- Functional versus dysfunctional behaviors
- Cognitive strategies (e.g., distraction, communication skills, thought stopping)
- Structure and limit setting
- Social relationships
- Recovery strategies
- Community resources

Success, even partial success, builds a sense of competence and self-esteem (Table 22.2).

Psychoeducation

Patient education within the context of a therapeutic relationship is one of the most important, empowering interventions for the generalist psychiatric–mental health nurse to use. Teaching patients skills to resist parasuicidal urges, improve emotional regulation, enhance interpersonal relationships, tolerate stress, and enhance overall quality of life provide the foundation for long-term behavioral changes. These skills can be taught in any treatment setting as a part of the overall facility program (Box 22.7). If nurses are practicing in a facility where DBT is the treatment model, they can be trained in DBT and can serve as group skills leaders.

Teaching Emotional Regulation

A major goal of cognitive therapeutic interventions is emotional regulation—recognizing and controlling the expression of feelings. Patients often fail even to recognize their feelings; instead, they respond quickly without thinking about the consequences. Remember, the time needed for taking action is shorter than the time needed for thinking before acting. Pausing makes up for the momentary lag between the limbic and autonomic response and the prefrontal response. Many of the cognitive interventions discussed in Chapters 16 and 17 can be used with persons with BPD.

TABLE 22.2	THOUGHT DISTORTIONS AND CORRECTIVE STATEMENTS
Thought Distortion	**Corrective Statement**
Catastrophizing	
"This is the most awful thing that has ever happened to me"	*"This is a sad thing but not the most awful."*
"If I fail this course, my life is over."	*"If you fail the course, you can take the course again. You can change your major."*
Dichotomizing	
"No one ever listens to me."	*"Your husband listened to you last night when you told him …"*
"I never get what I want."	*"You didn't get the promotion this year, but you did get a merit raise."*
"I can't understand why everyone is so kind at first and then always dumps me when I need them the most."	*"It is hard to remember those kind things and times when your friends have stayed with you when you needed them."*
Self-Attribution Errors	
"If I had just found the right thing to say, she wouldn't have left me."	*"There is not a single right thing to say, and she left you because she chose to."*
"If I had not made him mad, he wouldn't have hit me."	*"He has a lot of choices in how to respond, and he chose hitting. You are responsible for your feelings and actions."*

Another element of emotional regulation is learning to delay gratification. When the patient wants something that is not immediately available, the nurse can teach patients to distract themselves, find alternate ways of meeting the need, and think about what would happen if they have to wait to meet the need.

Teaching Effective Ways to Communicate

Another important area of patient education is teaching communication skills. Patients lack interpersonal skill in relating because they often had inadequate modeling and few opportunities to practice. The goals of relationship skill development are to identify problematic behavior that interferes with relationships and to use appropriate behaviors in improving relationships. The starting point is with communication. The nurse teaches the patient basic communication approaches, such as making "I" statements, paraphrasing what the other party says before responding, checking the accuracy of perceptions with others, compromising and seeking common ground, listening actively, and offering and accepting reactions. Besides modeling the behaviors, the nurse guides patients in practicing a variety of communication approaches for common situations. When role-playing, the nurse needs to discuss not only what the skills are and how to perform them but also the feelings patients have before, during, and after the role-play.

In day treatment and outpatient settings, the nurse can give the patient homework, such as keeping a journal, applying role-playing skills to actual situations, and observing behaviors in others. In the hospital, the patient can experience the same process, where the nurse is available to offer immediate feedback. Whatever the setting or whatever the specific problems addressed, the nurse must keep in mind and remind the patient that change occurs slowly. Thus, working on the problems occurs gradually, with severity of symptoms as the guide to deciding how fast and how much change to expect.

Building Social Skills and Self-Esteem

In the hospital, the nurse can use group therapy to discuss feelings and ways to cope with them. Women with BPD benefit from assertiveness classes and women's health issues classes. Many of the women are involved in abusive relationships and lack the ability to resolve these relationships because of their extreme anxiety regarding separating from those they love and their extreme need to feel connected. These women verbalize desires to do it, but they do not have the strength and self-confidence needed to leave. Exposing them to a different style of interaction as well as validation from other people increases their self-esteem and ability to get away from negative influences.

Evaluation and Treatment Outcomes

Evaluation and treatment outcomes vary depending on the severity of the disorder, the presence of comorbid disorders, and the availability of resources. For a patient with severe symptoms or continual self-injury, keeping the patient safe and alive may be a realistic outcome. Helping the patient resist parasuicidal urges may take years. In contrast, individuals who rarely need hospitalization and have adequate resources can expect to recover from the self-destructive impulses and learn positive interaction skills that promote a high-quality lifestyle. Most patients fall somewhere in between, with periods of symptom exacerbation and remission. In these patients, increasing the symptom-free time may be the best indicator of outcomes.

Continuum of Care

Treatment and recovery involve long-term therapy. Hospitalization is sometimes necessary during acute episodes involving parasuicidal behavior, but after this behavior is controlled, patients are discharged. It is important for these individuals to continue with treatment in the outpatient or day treatment setting. Because these individuals often appear more competent and in control than they are, nurses must not be deceived by these outward appearances. These individuals need continued follow-up and long-term therapy, including individual therapy, psychoeducation, and positive role models.

ANTISOCIAL PERSONALITY DISORDER

Antisocial personality disorder (ASPD) is defined as "a pervasive pattern of disregard for, and violation of, the rights of others occurring since age 15 years" (APA, 2013), p. 659). This diagnosis is given to individuals 18 years of age or older who fail to follow society's rules—that is, they do not believe that society's rules are made for them and so are consistently irresponsible. For many, evidence suggests a conduct disorder (introduced later in the chapter) before the age of 15 years. The term *psychopath*, or *sociopath*, a person with a tendency toward antisocial and criminal behavior with little regard for others, is often used in describing the behaviors of people with ASPD.

> **KEYCONCEPT** **Antisocial personality disorder** is characterized by a pervasive pattern of disregard for and violation of the rights of others.

Clinical Course and Diagnostic Criteria

ASPD has a chronic course, but the antisocial behaviors tend to diminish later in life, particularly after the age of

40 years (APA, 2013). Individuals with ASPD are arrogant and self-centered and feel privileged and entitled. They are self-serving, and they exploit and seek power over others. They can be interpersonally engaging and charming, which is often mistaken for a genuine sense of concern for other people. In reality, they lack empathy; are unable to express human compassion; and tend to be insensitive, callous, and contemptuous of others. Deceit and manipulation for personal profit or pleasure are central features associated with this disorder. They are behaviorally impulsive and interpersonally irresponsible. Many with this disorder repeatedly perform acts that are grounds for arrest (whether they are arrested or not), such as destroying property, harassing others, stealing,

---

FAME & FORTUNE

David Hampton (1964–2003)

Socialite Imposter

PUBLIC PERSONA

Although his name might not be familiar, his story is. David Hampton was the teenager who gained infamy in the 1980s after conning New York's wealthy elite out of thousands of dollars by convincing them he was the son of actor Sidney Poitier. His now famous elaborate ruse began in 1983, when he and a friend were trying to get into Studio 54. Unable to gain entry, Hampton's friend decided to pose as Gregory Peck's son, while Hampton assumed the persona of "David Poitier" and identified himself as Sidney Poitier's son.

PERSONAL REALITIES

The cost of his deceit and swindling of some of New York's more affluent people ultimately ended in a formal charge of attempted burglary, for which he received 21 months in prison. His story became the inspiration for the play and later the movie titled *Six Degrees of Separation*. Attempting to turn the play's success to his own advantage, David Hampton gave interviews to the press; gate crashed producers' parties; and began a campaign of harassment against the playwright John Guare, which included calls and death threats, prompting Guare to apply for a restraining order against Hampton. Believing others were profiting from his hoax, Hampton filed a $100 million lawsuit, claiming that the play had stolen the copyright on his persona and his story. The lawsuit was eventually dismissed.

Continuing to dupe others for money, attention, and entrée into New York society, Hampton met men in bars, dazzled them with his good looks and intellect, dropped celebrity tidbits, and then fleeced them, often using other aliases. Hampton's name appeared more often in crime reports than society pages for such crimes as fare beating, credit card theft, and threats of violence.

David Hampton's pursuit of a fabulous Manhattan life ended in July 2003 when he died alone of AIDS-related complications in a Manhattan hospital.

Source: Barry, D. (2003, July 19). About New York: He conned the society crowd but died alone. *The New York Times*. Retrieved from http://www.nytimes.com/2003/07/19/nyregion/about-new-york-he-conned-the-society-crowd-but-died-alone.html. Retrieved August 4, 2015.

---

or pursuing other illegal occupations. They act hastily and spontaneously, are temperamentally aggressive and shortsighted, and fail to plan ahead or consider alternatives. They fail to adapt to the ethical and social standards of the community. They lack a sense of personal obligation to fulfill social and financial responsibilities, including those involved with being a spouse, parent, employee, friend, or member of the community. They lack remorse for their transgressions (APA, 2013).

Some of these individuals openly and flagrantly violate laws and end up in jail (see Fame & Fortune). But most people with ASPD never come in conflict with the law and instead find a niche in society, such as in business, the military, or politics that rewards their competitively tough behavior. Although ASPD is characterized by continual antisocial acts, the disorder is not synonymous with criminality. See Key Diagnostic Characteristics 22.2.

Epidemiology and Risk Factors

Twelve-month prevalence rates of ASPD are estimated between 0.2% and 3.3% (APA, 2013). Males with alcohol use disorder and those released from substance abuse clinics, prisons, or other forensic settings have the highest rates. Adverse socioeconomic (i.e., poverty) or sociocultural (i.e., migration) factors also are associated with higher prevalence (APA, 2013). Gender differences also exist in how symptoms are manifest (Box 22.8).

Age of Onset

To be diagnosed with ASPD, the individual must be at least 18 years old and must have exhibited one or more childhood behavioral characteristics of conduct disorder before the age of 15 years, such as aggression to people or animals, destruction of property, deceitfulness or theft, or serious violation of rules. The likelihood of developing adult ASPD is increased if onset of conduct disorder is seen before age 10 years as well as an accompanying childhood attention deficit hyperactivity disorder (ADHD) diagnosis (APA, 2013).

Comorbidity

ASPD is associated with several other psychiatric disorders, including mood, anxiety, and other personality disorders. ASPD is strongly associated with alcohol and drug abuse (Black, Gunter, Loveless, Allen, & Sieleni, 2010). However, a diagnosis of ASPD is not warranted if the antisocial behavior occurs only in the context of substance abuse. For example, some people who misuse substances sometimes engage in criminal behavior, such as stealing or prostitution, only when in pursuit of drugs. Therefore, it is crucial to assess whether the person with possible ASPD has engaged

Diagnostic Criteria

A. A pervasive pattern of disregard for and violation of the rights of others, occurring since age 15 years, as indicated by three (or more) of the following:

1. Failure to conform to social norms with respect to lawful behaviors, as indicated by repeatedly performing acts that are grounds for arrest.
2. Deceitfulness, as indicated by repeated lying, use of aliases, or conning others for personal profit or pleasure.
3. Impulsivity or failure to plan ahead.
4. Irritability and aggressiveness, as indicated by repeated physical fights or assaults.
5. Reckless disregard for safety of self or others.
6. Consistent irresponsibility, as indicated by repeated failure to sustain consistent work behavior or honor financial obligations.
7. Lack of remorse, as indicated by being indifferent to or rationalizing having hurt, mistreated, or stolen from another.

B. The individual is at least age 18 years.
C. There is evidence of conduct disorder with onset before age 15 years.
D. The occurrence of antisocial behavior is not exclusively during the course of schizophrenia or bipolar disorder.

Associated Findings
- Lacking empathy
- Callous, cynical, and contemptuous of the feelings, rights, and suffering of others
- Inflated and arrogant self-appraisal
- Excessively opinionated, self-assured, or cocky
- Glib, superficial charm; impressive verbal ability
- Irresponsible and exploitative in sexual relationships; history of multiple sexual partners and lack of a sustained monogamous relationship
- Possible dysphoria, including complaints of tension, inability to tolerate boredom, and depressed mood

Reprinted with permission from the *Diagnostic and Statistical Manual of Mental Disorders, Fifth Edition* (Copyright ©2013). American Psychiatric Association. All Rights Reserved.

BOX 22.8 CLINICAL VIGNETTE

Antisocial Personality Disorder: Male Versus Female

Stasia (female) and Jackson (male) are fraternal twins, 22 years old, who received diagnoses of antisocial personality disorder. The following are their clinical profiles.

Jackson

Jackson is currently in the county jail for the third time. Although his juvenile records begin at age 9 years and include misdemeanors and class B felonies, his burglary conviction is his first adult crime. His school teachers thought Jackson was very bright but that he had significant difficulty with peers and authority figures. He fought regularly, was described as a bully, and seemed always to be scamming. At age 16 years, Jackson dropped out of school and joined a gang.

Jackson's juvenile probation officer explained that Jackson came from a very violent family and neighborhood and described the situation by saying, "If gangs hadn't gotten him, his father would have." His lawyer described him as "a likeable guy, but I wouldn't turn my back on him."

The jail nurse described Jackson as "a real charmer, but nothing is ever his fault." Oddly, he is the only person in the jail with an adequate supply of cigarettes and music downloads. "We get along fine," the nurse says. "I don't understand why guards have such difficulty with him." Sometimes the guards send Jackson to the dispensary for injuries, and Jackson plaintively explains to the nurse, "Those guards beat me up again; I don't know why."

Stasia

Stasia was recently hospitalized for the sixth time when one of her male friends beat her. She has been working as a prostitute for 5 years. Her physical examination noted not only multiple bruises but also tattoos that cover 50% of her body. In addition, she has piercings of her tongue, ears, eyebrow, lips, and nipples. She is emotionally volatile, manipulative, and angry. Stasia has many acquaintances and sexual partners, but none are truly intimate. She has times when she uses drugs regularly.

Stasia and Jackson's mother was jailed when the twins were 18 months old and did not return until they were 6 years old. They were raised mostly by their paternal grandmother, who hated their mother and reminded Stasia frequently of how much she looked like her mother. Their father, when present, was violent toward Jackson and sexually abused Stasia.

What Do You Think?
- How might gender influence the development of symptoms?
- How might culture influence early recognition of problems and provision of early intervention to prevent future serious mental disorders?
- What are some possible outcomes in this situation?
- How does this case demonstrate the interaction between socialization, biology, and culture?

in illegal activities at times other than when pursuing or using substances.

Etiology

Biologic Theories

Perhaps more than any other personality disorder, an extensive number of biologically oriented studies explore the genetic bases, neuropsychological factors, and arousal levels among this group of pathologies (Millon, 2011). Many of these studies show changes associated with personality disorders or characteristics, but we do not have evidence that these changes caused the disorder. These studies often overlap with studies of aggression, temperament, and substance use (Alcorn, Gowin, Green, Swann, Moeller, & Lane, 2013; Jovev, Whittle, Yücel, Simmons, Allen, & Chanen, 2014).

Early MRI studies showed that persons with ASPD failed to activate the limbic-prefrontal circuit (comprising amygdala, orbitofrontal cortex, insula, and anterior cingulate cortex) during fearful situations (Birbaumer, Veit, Lotze, Erb, Hermann, Grodd, et al., 2005). These findings support the neural basis of fearlessness in these individuals. Impairment in moral judgment is associated with dysfunction of the prefrontal cortex (Taber-Thomas, Asp, Koenigs, Sutterer, Anderson, & Tranel, 2014). Emotional distance, aggression, and impulsivity are consistently associated with neural dysfunction (Millon, 2011).

Psychosocial Theories

Temperament

Scientists believe temperament is neurobiologically determined, and many believe that it is central to understanding personality disorders. A temperament, the natural predisposition to express feelings and actions, is evident during the first few months of life and remains stable through development. For example, whereas some infants are more relaxed or calm and sleep a lot, others are extremely alert, startled by the slightest noise, cry more, and sleep less.

Difficult temperaments are common in ASPD and are often at the basis of their aggression and impulsivity.

> **KEYCONCEPT** **Temperament** comprises a person's characteristic intensity, rhythmicity, adaptability, energy expenditure, and mood. A **difficult temperament** is characterized by withdrawal from stimuli, low adaptability, and intense emotional reactions. Four key behaviors are present in a difficult temperament: aggression, inattention, hyperactivity, and impulsivity.

Temperaments consist of two behavioral dimensions that interact with each other. The activity spectrum varies from intense to passive. The adaptability spectrum varies from having a positive attitude about new stimuli with high flexibility to withdrawal from new stimuli and minimal flexibility in response to change. A strong relationship is found between difficult temperament and ASPD behaviors (Lennox & Dolan, 2014).

Attachment

One of the leading explanations of ASPD is that unsatisfactory attachments in early relationships lead to antisocial behavior in later life. Attachment, attaining and retaining interpersonal connection to a significant person, begins at birth. In a secure attachment, a child feels safe, loved, and valued and develops the self-confidence to interact with the rest of the world. Experiences within the context of secure relationships enable the child to develop trust in others. Strong attachments between parents and child may lower the risk of delinquency, assault, and other offenses that are characteristic of those who develop antisocial behavior (Sousa, Herrenkohl, Moylan, Tajima, Klika, Herrenkohl, et al., 2011).

In individuals with ASPD, a failure to make or sustain stable attachments in early childhood can lead to avoidance of future attachments. Risk factors for developing dysfunctional attachments include parental abandonment or neglect, loss of a parent or primary caregiver, and physical or sexual abuse. Parents who lacked secure attachment relationships in their own childhoods may be unable to form secure attachment relationships with their own children.

Family Issues

In many cases, individuals with ASPD come from chaotic families in which alcoholism and violence are the norm. Individuals who have been victims of abuse or neglect, live in a foster home, or had several primary caregivers are more likely to be victimized by antisocial behaviors, especially aggression (Gao, Raine, Chan, Veneables, & Mednick, 2010). Child abuse and growing up in a home with domestic violence increase risk of antisocial behavior (Sousa, et al., 2011). However, it is difficult to separate the influence of social factors on the development of the disorder because the symptoms of ASPD are expressed as social manifestations, including unemployment, multiple divorces and separations, and violence.

Family Response to Antisocial Personality Disorder

If family members are present in a patient's life, they have probably been abused, mistreated, or intimidated by these patients. For example, one patient sold his mother's possessions while she was at work. Another abused his wife after drinking. However, family members may be fiercely loyal to the patient and blame themselves for his or her shortcomings.

Teamwork and Collaboration: Working toward Recovery

People rarely seek mental health care for ASPD but rather for treatment of depression, substance abuse, uncontrolled anger, or forensic-related problems. Patients with psychiatric disorders who are admitted through the courts often have a comorbid diagnosis of ASPD. Antisocial personality disordered patients usually present for treatment as a result of an ultimatum. Treatment is often a choice between losing a job, being expelled from school, ending a marriage or relationship with children, or giving up on a chance at probation and psychological treatment. Under these circumstances treatment is usually forced on them; most prisons and other correctional facilities require inmates to attend psychotherapy sessions. In either case working with people with ASPD is likely to be a frustrating and exasperating experience for the nurse due to the patient's clear lack of insight and/or motivation to change. Treatment is difficult and involves helping the patient alter his or her cognitive schemata. The overall treatment goals are to develop a nurturing sense of attachment and empathy for other people and situations and to live within the norms of society.

Safety Issues

Although they can be interpersonally charming, these patients can become verbally and physically abusive if their expectations are not met. Protection of other patients and staff is a priority.

Evidence-Based Nursing Care of Persons with Antisocial Personality Disorder

Mental Health Nursing Assessment

ASPD does not significantly impair physical functioning except in the presence of coexisting substance use disorder or another psychiatric diagnosis involved. Because substance abuse is a major problem with this population, the physical effects of chronic use of addictive substances must be considered. Conversely, someone who has health problems secondary to chronic substance misuse should also be assessed for concurrent personality disorders. Many patients with ASPD are committed to mental health care by the court system.

Eliciting psychosocial data from persons with ASPD may be difficult because of their basic mistrust about authority figures. They may not give an accurate history or may embellish aspects to project themselves in a more positive light. They often deny any criminal activity even if they are admitted in police custody.

Key areas of assessment are determining the quality of relationships, impulsivity, and the extent of aggression. These individuals do not assume responsibility for their own actions and often blame others for their misfortune. Their disregard for others is manifested in their interactions. For example, one patient with human immunodeficiency virus was engaging in unprotected sex with several different women because he wanted to "have fun as long as I can." He was completely unconcerned about the possibility of transmitting the virus. These individuals often make good first impressions. Self-awareness is especially important for the nurse because of the initial charming quality of many of these individuals. When these patients realize that the nurse cannot be used or manipulated, they lose interest in the nurse and revert to their normal, egocentric behaviors. Nursing Care Plan 22.1 is available at http://thepoint.lww.com/BoydEssentials.

Nursing Diagnoses

A common nursing diagnosis for persons with ASPD is Risk for Other Directed Violence, Dysfunctional Family Processes. Other typical diagnoses are Ineffective Role Performance, Ineffective Individual Coping, Impaired Communication, Impaired Social Interactions, Low Self-esteem, and Risk for Violence.

Outcomes should be short-term and relevant to a specific problem. For example, if a patient has been chronically unemployed, a reasonable short-term outcome is to set up job interviews rather than obtain a job.

Therapeutic Relationship

Therapeutic relationships are difficult to establish because these individuals do not attach themselves to others and are often unable to use a relationship to change behavior. The goal of the therapeutic relationship is to identify dysfunctional thinking patterns and develop new problem-solving behaviors. After the first few meetings with these patients, the nurse may believe that the relationship has a good start, but in reality, a superficial alliance is usually formed. Additional sessions reveal the lack of patient commitment to the relationship. These patients begin to revisit topics discussed in previous sessions or lose interest in trying to work on problems. By using self-awareness skills and accessing supervision regularly, the nurse can identify blocks in the development of a therapeutic relationship (or lack of) and his or her response to the relationship. See Box 22.9.

Mental Health Nursing Interventions

In instances in which there are concurrent disorders, the patient with ASPD may actually interfere with interventions aimed at improving physical functioning.

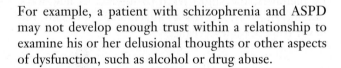

BOX 22.9 • THERAPEUTIC DIALOGUE • Antisocial Personality Disorder

INEFFECTIVE APPROACH

Danny: Hey, I need a light for my cigarette.

Nurse: Really? You know the rules – no smoking on the unit.

Danny: I'm not going to smoke here. I just need a light so that I can have a cigarette when I leave here.

Nurse: I also need your cigarettes. Cigarettes are contraband.

Danny: You are terrible – just like the bitch who kicked me out. Who do you think you are anyway?

Nurse: You need to quiet down.

Danny: Yeah, says who?

Nurse: I will call security if you don't quiet down.

Danny: Call them, I don't care.

EFFECTIVE APPROACH

Danny: Hey, I need a light for my cigarette.

Nurse: A light? I don't have a light.

Danny: I need a light so that I can smoke later.

Nurse: Oh, I see. Did you have a lighter when you were admitted?

Danny: Yea, they took everything away including my belt and shoe laces.

Nurse: The reason for storing everything is for the safety of everyone. When you are discharged you can retrieve everything. I also need to store any cigarettes you have.

Danny: What makes you think I have any cigarettes?

Nurse: Well, you asked for a light. Many patients manage to bring cigarettes into the unit. I need to put them with your things. You can retrieve them when you are discharged.

Danny: This place is something.

Nurse: I will put your cigarettes in a bag with your name on them.

Danny: This sucks. But here they are.

CRITICAL THINKING CHALLENGE

- How did the nurse in the first scenario get sidetracked?
- How was the nurse in the second scenario able to convince Danny to give up his cigarettes without escalating his anger?

For example, a patient with schizophrenia and ASPD may not develop enough trust within a relationship to examine his or her delusional thoughts or other aspects of dysfunction, such as alcohol or drug abuse.

Facilitating Self-Responsibility

Facilitating self-responsibility (i.e., encouraging a patient to assume more responsibility for personal behavior) is an important intervention. The nursing activities that are particularly helpful include holding the patient responsible for his or her behavior, monitoring the extent that self-responsibility is assumed, and discussing the consequences of not dealing with responsibilities. The nurse needs to refrain from arguing or bargaining about the unit rules, such as time for meals, use of the television room, and smoking. Instead, positive feedback is given to the patient for accepting additional responsibility or changing behavior.

Enhancing Self-Awareness

Enhancing self-awareness (i.e., exploring and understanding personal thoughts, feelings, motivation, and behaviors) is another nursing intervention that is helpful in developing an understanding about relating peacefully to the rest of the world. Encouraging patients to recognize and discuss their thoughts and feelings helps the nurse understand how the patient views the world. Some evidence indicates that substance misuse can be improved through cognitive behavioral treatment, but there is little evidence that the core problems of this disorder (aggression, reconviction, global functioning, and social functioning) are improved with psychological interventions (Gibbon, Duggan, Stoffers, Huband, Völlm, Ferriter, et al., 2010).

Teaching Points

Patient education efforts have to be creative and thought provoking. In teaching a person with ASPD, a direct

BOX 22.10

Psychoeducation Checklist: Antisocial Personality Disorder

When caring for the patient with antisocial personality disorder, be sure to include the following topic areas in the teaching plan:

- Positive health care practices, including substance abuse control
- Effective communication and interaction skills
- Impulse control
- Anger management
- Group experience to help develop self-awareness and impact of behavior on others
- Analyzing an issue from the other person's viewpoint
- Maintenance of employment
- Interpersonal relationships and social interactions

approach is best, but the nurse must avoid "lecturing," which the patient will resent. In teaching the patient about positive health care practices, impulse control, and anger management, the best approach is to engage the patient in a discussion about the issue and then direct the topic to the major teaching points. These patients often take great delight in arguing or showing how the rules of life do not apply to them. A sense of humor is important, as are clear teaching goals and avoiding being sidetracked (see Box 22.10).

Group Interventions

Group interventions are more effective than individual modalities because other patients and staff can validate or challenge the patient's view of a situation. Problem-solving groups that focus on identifying a problem and developing a variety of alternative solutions are particularly helpful because patient self-responsibility is reinforced when patients remind each other of better alternatives. Patients are likely to confront each other with dysfunctional schemata or thinking patterns. Teaching patients with ASPD the same communication techniques as those with BPD will also encourage self-responsibility. These patients often attend groups that focus on the development of empathy.

Milieu Interventions

Milieu interventions, such as providing a structured environment with rules that are consistently applied to patients who are responsible for their own behavior, are important. While living in close proximity to others, the individual with ASPD will demonstrate dysfunctional social patterns that can be identified and targeted for correction. For example, these patients often violate ward rules, such as no smoking or limitations on the number of visitors, and may bring contraband, such as illegal drugs, into the unit.

In an inpatient unit, interventions can be more intense and focus on helping the patient develop positive interaction skills and experience a consistent environment. For example, the focus of nursing interventions may be the patient's continual disregard of the rights of others. On one unit, a patient continually placed orders for pizzas in the name of another patient who had limited intelligence and was genuinely afraid of the person with ASPD. The victimized patient always paid for the pizza. When the nursing staff realized what was happening, they confronted the patient with ASPD about the behavior and revoked his unit privileges.

Anger Management

Aggressive behavior is often a problem for these individuals and their family members. Similar to patients with borderline personality disorder (BPD), people with ASPD tend to be impulsive. Instead of self-injury, these individuals are more likely to strike out at those who are perceived to be interfering with their immediate gratification. Anger control assistance (helping to express anger in an adaptive, nonviolent manner) becomes a priority intervention. Because the expression of anger and aggression develops during a lifetime, these individuals can benefit from anger management techniques.

Social Support

Social support for these individuals is often minimal, just as it is for individuals with BPD, but the reasons are different. These individuals have often taken advantage of friends and relatives who, in turn, no longer trust them. Helping the patient build a new support system after new skills are learned is usually the only option. For these individuals to develop friends and re-engage family members, they must learn to interact in new ways, develop empathy, and risk an attachment. For many, this never truly becomes a reality.

Interventions for Family Members

Family members of patients with ASPD usually need help in establishing boundaries. Because there is a long-term pattern of interaction in which family members feel responsible for the patient's antisocial behavior, these patterns need to be stopped. Families need help in recognizing the patient's responsibility for his or her actions.

Evaluation and Treatment Outcomes

The outcomes of interventions for patients with ASPD need to be evaluated in terms of management of specific problems, such as maintaining employment or developing a meaningful interpersonal relationship. The nurse will most likely see these patients for other health care problems, so adherence to treatment recommendations and development of health care practices (e.g., reducing smoking and alcohol consumption) can also be factored into the evaluation of outcomes.

Continuum of Care

People with ASPD rarely seek mental health care (Millon, 2011). Nurses are most likely to see these patients in medical–surgical settings for comorbid conditions. Consistency in interventions is necessary in treating the patient throughout the continuum of care.

OTHER PERSONALITY DISORDERS
Histrionic Personality Disorder
Clinical Course and Diagnostic Criteria

"Attention seeking," "excitable," and "emotional" are terms used to describe people with **histrionic personality disorder.** Histrionic personality disorder is more likely in women. Affected individuals are lively and dramatic and draw attention to themselves by their enthusiasm, dress, and apparent openness. They are the "life of the party" and, on the surface, seem interested in others. Their insatiable need for attention and approval quickly becomes obvious. Their need to be "center stage" arises in two ways: (1) their interests and topics of conversation focus on their own desires and activities, and (2) their behavior, including their speech pattern, continually calls attention to themselves. These needs are inflexible and persistent even after others attempt to meet them. Persons with histrionic personality disorders are quick to form new friendships and just as quick to become demanding. Because they are trusting and easily influenced by other opinions, their behavior often appears inconsistent. Their strong dependency need makes them overly trusting and gullible. They are moody and often experience a sense of helplessness when others are uninterested in them. They are sexually seductive in their attempts to gain attention and often are uncomfortable within a single relationship. Their appearance is provocative and their speech dramatic. They express strong opinions without supporting facts. Loyalty and fidelity are lacking (APA, 2013).

Gender influences the manifestations of this disorder. Women dress seductively, may express dependency on selected men, and may "play" a submissive role. Men may dress in a very masculine manner and seek attention by bragging about athletic skills or successes in their jobs. Individuals with this disorder have difficulty achieving any true intimacy in interpersonal relationships. They seem to possess an innate sensitivity to the moods and thoughts of those they wish to please. This hyperalertness enables them to maneuver quickly to gain their attention. They

then attempt to control relationships by their seductiveness at one level but become extremely dependent on their friends at another level. Their demand for constant attention quickly alienates their friends. They become depressed when they are not the center of attention.

Epidemiology and Risk Factors

The prevalence of histrionic personality disorder is estimated at 1.8% of the general population of the United States (Grant, Hasin, Stinson, Dawson, Chou, Ruan et al., 2004). No gender differences arise in the occurrence of this disorder; however, this diagnosis is seen more frequently in women than men clinically. Risk of occurrence of this disorder is greater among African Americans than whites. Low-income groups and less educated persons are also at higher risk for occurrence of histrionic personality disorder. Widowed, separated, divorced, or people who never married are at greater risk than married ones. This disorder occurs concurrently with other mental disorders; anxiety disorder, obsessive-compulsive syndromes, somatoform syndromes, substance use disorder, and mood disorders in which they overplay their feelings of dysthymia by expressing them through dramatic and eye-catching gestures (Millon, 2011).

Etiology

Research related to this personality disorder is minimal. Some speculate that there is a biologic component and that heredity may play a role but that the biologic influence is less than in some of the previously discussed personality problems. In infancy and early childhood, these individuals are extremely alert and emotionally responsive. The tendencies for sensory alertness may be traced to responses of the limbic and reticular systems. They demonstrate a high degree of dependence on others and a type of dissociation in which they have reduced awareness of their behavior in relation to others (Millon, 2011).

It is believed that these highly alert and responsive infants seek more gratification from external stimulation during their first few months of life. Depending on the responsiveness of caregivers to them, they develop behavior patterns in response to their caregivers. It is believed that these children experience brief, highly charged, and irregular reinforcement from multiple caregivers (parents, siblings, grandparents, foster parents) who are unable to provide consistent experiences.

Parental behavior and role modeling are also believed to contribute to the development of histrionic personality disorder. Many of the women with this disorder reported that they are just like their mother, who is emotionally labile, bored with the routines of home life, flirtatious with men, and clever in dealing with people. It is believed that through role modeling, these children learn and mimic the behaviors observed in caregivers or adults (Millon, 2011).

Nursing Care

The ultimate treatment goal for patients with histrionic personality disorder is to correct the tendency to expect others to fulfill all of their needs. When these individuals seek mental health care, they have usually experienced a period of social disapproval or deprivation. Their hope is that the mental health providers will help fulfill their needs. Specific goals are needed to protect the person from becoming dependent on a mental health system. In the nursing assessment, the nurse focuses on the quality of the individual's interpersonal relationships. It is common that the person is dissatisfied with his or her partner, and sexual relations may be nonexistent.

During the assessment, the patient will make statements that indicate low self-esteem. Because these individuals believe that they are incapable of handling life's demands and have been waiting for a truly competent person to take care of them, they have not developed a positive self-concept or adequate problem-solving abilities.

Nursing diagnoses that are usually generated include Chronic Low Self-esteem, Ineffective Individual Coping, and Ineffective Sexual Patterns. Outcomes focus on helping the patient develop autonomy, a positive self-concept, and mature problem-solving skills.

A variety of interventions support the outcomes. A nurse–patient relationship that allows the patient to explore positive personality characteristics and develop independent decision-making skills forms the basis of the interventions. Reinforcing personal strengths, conveying confidence in the patient's ability to handle situations, and examining the patient's negative perceptions of him- or herself can be done within the therapeutic relationship. Encouraging the patient to act autonomously can also improve the individual's sense of self-worth. Attending assertiveness groups can help increase the individual's self-confidence and improve self-esteem.

Continuum of Care

Patients with histrionic personality disorder do not seek mental health care unless they have a coexisting medical or mental disorder. They are likely to be treated within the community for most of their lives, with the exception of short hospitalizations for nonpsychiatric problems.

Narcissistic Personality Disorder

Clinical Course and Diagnostic Criteria

People with **narcissistic personality disorder** are grandiose, have an inexhaustible need for admiration, and lack empathy. Beginning in childhood, these individuals believe that they are superior, special, or unique and that others should recognize them in this way (APA, 2013). They are often preoccupied with fantasies of unlimited success, power, beauty, or ideal love. They overvalue their personal worth, direct their affections toward themselves, and expect others to hold them in high esteem. They define the world through their own self-centered view. Their sense of entitlement is striking. People with narcissistic personality disorder are benignly arrogant and feel themselves above the conventions of their cultural group. They handle criticism poorly and may become enraged if someone dares to criticize them or else they may appear totally indifferent to criticism. They believe they are entitled to be served and that it is their inalienable right to receive special considerations. People with this disorder want to have their own way and are frequently ambitious for fame and fortune. These individuals are often successful in their jobs but may alienate their significant others, who grow tired of their narcissism. They cannot show empathy, and they feign sympathy only for their own benefit to achieve their selfish ends. Clinically, those with narcissistic personality disorder show overlapping characteristics of BPD and ASPD.

Epidemiology

The prevalence of narcissistic personality disorder is 6.2% of the U.S. general population with rates greater for men (7.7%) than for women (4.8%) according to a recent national epidemiologic survey (Stinson, Dawson, Goldstein, Chou, Huang, Smith, et al., 2008). Narcissistic personality disorder can be found in professionals who are highly respected such as those in law, medicine, and science and those associated with celebrity status. Persons with this disorder may impart an unrealistic sense of omnipotence, grandiosity, beauty, and talent to their children; therefore, children of parents with a narcissistic personality disorder have a higher than usual risk of developing the disorder themselves. It also commonly occurs in only children and among first-born boys in cultural groups in which males have special privileges (Millon, 2011).

Etiology

Limited evidence suggests biologic factors contribute to the development of this disorder. One notion about its development is that it is the result of parents' overvaluation and overindulgence of a child. These children are overly pampered and indulged, with every whim catered to. They learn to view themselves as special beings and to expect special treatment and subservience from others. They do not learn how to cooperate, share, or consider others' desires and interests. An alternate explanation is that the child never truly separated emotionally from his or her primary caregiver and therefore cannot envision functioning independently. According to another set of theories, these individuals try to avoid or reduce intense feelings of shame and engage in diverse strategies to gain attention for themselves (Roepke & Vater, 2014).

Nursing Care

The nurse usually encounters persons with narcissism in medical settings and in psychiatric settings with a coexisting psychiatric disorder. They are difficult patients who often appear snobbish, condescending, and patronizing in their attitudes. It is unlikely that these individuals are motivated to develop sensitivity to others and socially cooperative attitudes and behaviors. Building a therapeutic relationship is a slow process because these patients avoid self-reflection and often reject the clinician's approaches. Nurses need to use their self-awareness skills in interacting with these patients. The nursing process focuses on the coexisting responses to other health care problems (Ronningstam & Weinberg, 2013).

Continuum of Care

Similar to patients with histrionic disorder, those with narcissistic personality disorder do not seek mental health care unless they have a coexisting medical or mental disorder. They are likely to be treated within the community for most of their lives, with the exception of short hospitalizations for nonpsychiatric problems.

AVOIDANT, DEPENDENT, AND OBSESSIVE-COMPULSIVE PERSONALITY DISORDERS

Avoidant Personality Disorder

Clinical Course and Diagnostic Criteria

Avoidant personality disorder is characterized by staying out of social situations in which interpersonal contact with others may be expected. Individuals appear timid, shy, and hesitant; they also fear criticism and feel inadequate. These individuals are extremely sensitive to negative comments and disapproval and appraise situations more negatively than others do. This behavior becomes problematic when it restricts their social activities and work opportunities because of their extreme fear of rejection.

In childhood, they are shy, but instead of growing out of the shyness, it becomes worse in adulthood. They perceive themselves as socially inept, inadequate, and inferior, which in turn justifies their isolation and rejection by others. Vocationally, people with avoidant personality

disorder often take jobs on the sidelines, rarely obtaining personal advancement or exercising much authority, but to employers, they seem shy and eager to please. They are reluctant to enter relationships unless they are given strong assurance of uncritical acceptances, so they consequently often have no close friends or confidants (Millon, 2011).

Epidemiology and Risk Factors

The prevalence of avoidant personality disorder is 2.4% in the general population (APA, 2013), but it has been reported in 10% of outpatients in mental health clinics (Grant, Hasin, Stinson, Dawson, Chou, Ruan, et al., 2004). The problem with examining the epidemiology of avoidant personality disorder is its potential overlap with generalized social phobia. Several studies found that a significant portion of the patients with diagnoses of social phobia also met criteria for avoidant personality disorder (Carter & Wu, 2010; Cox, Pagura, Stein, & Sareen, 2009). More research is needed to clarify the relationship between avoidant personality and anxiety disorders.

Etiology

Experts speculate that individuals with avoidant personality disorder experience aversive stimuli more intensely and more frequently than others do because they may possess an overabundance of neurons in the aversive center of the limbic system (Millon, 2011).

Nursing Care

Assessment of these individuals reveals a lack of social contacts, a fear of being criticized, and evidence of chronic low self-esteem. The nursing diagnoses Chronic Low Self-esteem, Social Isolation, and Ineffective Coping can be used. The establishment of a therapeutic relationship is necessary to be able to help these individuals meet their treatment outcomes. The development of the nurse–patient relationship is a slow process and requires an extreme amount of patience on the part of the nurse. These individuals may not have had positive interpersonal relationships and need time to be able to be sure that the nurse will not criticize and demean them. Interventions should focus on refraining from any negative criticism, assisting the patient to identify positive responses from others, exploring previous achievements of success, and exploring reasons for self-criticism. The patient's social dimension should be examined for activities that increase self-esteem and interventions focused on increasing these self-esteem–enhancing activities. Social skills training may help reduce symptoms.

Continuum of Care

Long-term therapy is ideal for patients with avoidant personality disorder because it takes time to make changes in one's behavior. Mental health nurses may initially see these individuals for other health problems. Encouraging the patient to continue with therapy and contacting the therapist when necessary are important in maintaining continuity of care. These patients are hospitalized only for a coexisting disorder.

Dependent Personality Disorder

Clinical Course and Diagnostic Criteria

People with **dependent personality disorder** cling to others in a desperate attempt to keep them close. Their need to be taken care of is so great that it leads to doing anything to maintain the closeness, including total submission and disregard for themselves.

Decision making is difficult or nonexistent. They adapt their behavior to please those to whom they are attached. They lean on others to guide their lives. They ingratiate themselves with others and denigrate themselves and their accomplishments. Their self-esteem is determined by others. Behaviorally, they withdraw from adult responsibilities by acting helpless and seeking nurturance from others. In interpersonal relationships, they need excessive advice and reassurance. They are compliant, conciliatory, and placating. They rarely disagree with others and are easily persuaded. Friends describe them as gullible. They are warm, tender, and noncompetitive. They timidly avoid social tension and interpersonal conflicts (APA, 2013). However, these individuals are at risk for suicide and parasuicide, perpetration of child abuse, perpetration of domestic violence (in men), and victimization by a partner (in women) (Bornstein, 2012).

Epidemiology and Risk Factors

A recent study estimates the prevalence at 0.49% (APA, 2013). The diagnosis is made more frequently in women than in men. This gender difference may represent a sex bias by clinicians because when standardized instruments are used, men and women receive diagnoses at equal rates. The risk of dependent personality disorder is greater for the least educated and for widowed, divorced, separated, and never married women (Disney, 2013).

Etiology

It is likely that a biologic predisposition exists to develop the dependency attachments of this disorder. However, no research studies support a biologic hypothesis. Dependent personality disorder is most often explained as a result of parents' genuine affection, extreme attachment, and overprotection. Children then learn to rely on others to meet their basic needs and do not learn the necessary skills for autonomous behavior. Persons with chronic physical illnesses in childhood may be prone to developing this disorder.

Nursing Care

Nurses can determine the extent of dependency by assessment of self-worth, interpersonal relationships, and social behavior. They should determine whether there is currently someone on whom the person relies (parent, spouse) or whether there has been a separation from a significant relationship by death or divorce.

Nursing diagnoses that are usually generated from the assessment data are Ineffective Individual Coping, Low Self-esteem, Impaired Social Interaction, and Impaired Home Maintenance Management. Home management skills may be a problem if the patient does not have the useful skills and now has to make decisions related to finances, shopping, cooking, and cleaning. The challenge of caring for these patients is to help them recognize their dependent patterns; motivate them to want to change; and teach them adult skills that have not been developed, such as balancing a checkbook, planning a weekly menu, and paying bills when they are due. Occasionally, if a patient is extremely fatigued, lethargic, or anxious; the disorder interferes with efforts at developing greater independence, antidepressants or antianxiety agents may be used in therapy.

These patients readily engage in a nurse–patient relationship and initially look to the nurse to make all decisions. The nurse can support patients to make their own decisions by resisting the urge to tell them what to do. Ideally, these patients are in individual psychotherapy and working toward long-term personality changes. The nurse can encourage patients to stay in therapy and to practice the new skills that are being learned. Assertiveness training is helpful.

Continuum of Care

Individuals with dependent personality disorder readily seek out therapy and are likely to spend years seeking therapy. Hospitalization occurs for comorbid conditions such as depression.

Obsessive-Compulsive Personality Disorder

Clinical Course and Diagnostic Criteria

Obsessive-compulsive personality disorder (OCPD) stands out because it bears close resemblance to obsessive-compulsive disorder (OCD), and is closely related to anxiety disorder. Although these disorders have similar names, the clinical manifestations are quite different. A distinguishing difference is that those with the OCD tend to use obsessive thoughts and compulsions when anxious but less so when anxiety decreases. Persons with OCPD do not demonstrate obsessions and compulsions but rather a pervasive pattern of preoccupation with orderliness, perfectionism, and control. They also have the capacity to delay rewards; whereas those with OCD do not (Pinto, Steinglass, Greene, Weber, & Simpson, 2013). Individuals with this disorder attempt to maintain control by careful attention to rules, trivial details, procedures, and lists (APA, 2013). They may be completely devoted to work, which typically has a rigid character, such as maintaining financial records or tracking inventory. They are uncomfortable with unstructured leisure time, especially vacations. Their leisure activities are likely to be formalized (e.g., season tickets to sports, organized tour groups). Hobbies are approached seriously.

Behaviorally, individuals with OCPD are perfectionists, maintaining a regulated, highly structured, strictly organized life. A need to control others and situations is common in their personal and work lives. They are prone to repetition and have difficulty making decisions and completing tasks because they become so involved in the details. They can be overly conscientious about morality and ethics and value polite, formal, and correct interpersonal relationships. They also tend to be rigid, stubborn, and indecisive and are unable to accept new ideas and customs. Their mood is tense and joyless. Warm feelings are restrained, and they tightly control the expression of emotions (APA, 2013).

Epidemiology and Risk Factors

OCPD is one of the most prevalent personality disorders in the general population, with estimated prevalence ranging from 2.1% to 7.9% (APA, 2013). This disorder is associated with higher education, employment, and marriage. Subjects with the disorder had a higher income than did those without the disorder.

Etiology

As with some other personality disorders, evidence for a biologic formulation is scant. The basis of the compulsive patterns that characterize OCPD is parental overcontrol and overprotection that is consistently restrictive and sets distinct limits on the child's behavior. Parents teach these children a deep sense of responsibility to others and to feel guilty when these responsibilities are not met. Play is viewed as shameful, sinful, and irresponsible, leading to dire consequences. They are encouraged to resist the natural inclinations toward play and impulse gratification, and parents try to impose guilt on the child to control behavior.

Nursing Care

These individuals seek mental health care when they have attacks of anxiety, spells of immobilization, sexual impotence, and excessive fatigue. The nursing assessment focuses on the patient's physical symptoms (sleep, eating, sexual), interpersonal relationships, and social problems. Typical nursing diagnoses include Anxiety, Risk for Loneliness, Decisional Conflict, Sexual Dysfunction, Insomnia, and Impaired Social Interactions. People with OCPD realize that they can improve their quality of life, but they find it extremely anxiety provoking to make the necessary changes. To change the compulsive pattern, psychotherapy is needed. There may be short-term pharmacologic intervention with an antidepressant or anxiolytic as an adjunct may take place. A supportive nurse–patient relationship based on acceptance of the patient's need for order and rigidity will help the person have enough confidence to try new behaviors. Examining the patient's belief that underlies the dysfunctional behaviors can set the stage for challenging the childhood thinking. Because the compulsive pattern was established in childhood, it will take a long time to modify the behavior.

Continuum of Care

People with OCPD are treated primarily in the community. If there is a coexisting disorder or the person experiences periods of depression is present, hospitalization may be useful for a short period of time.

DISRUPTIVE, IMPULSE-CONTROL, AND CONDUCT DISORDERS

Disruptive, impulse-control, and **conduct disorders** are a group of mental conditions that have the essential feature of irresistible impulsivity. Behaviors associated with these disorders violate the rights of others and/or are in conflict with societal norms (APA, 2013). Disorders discussed include oppositional defiant disorder, conduct disorder, intermittent explosive disorder, kleptomania, and pyromania. ASPD was discussed earlier in this chapter.

> **KEYCONCEPT** **Impulsivity**, acting without considering consequences or alternative actions, results when neurobiologic overactivity is stimulated by psychological, personality, or social factors related to personal needs of the individual (Tansey, 2010).

> **KEYCONCEPT** **Impulse-control disorders** often coexist with other disorders and are characterized by an inability to resist an impulse or temptation to complete an activity that is considered harmful to oneself or others.

Tension increases before the individual commits the act and derives excitement or gratification when the act is committed. The release of tension is perceived as pleasurable, but remorse and regret usually follow the act. The disruptive behavior disorders, which include oppositional defiant disorder and conduct disorder, are a group of conditions marked by significant problems of conduct.

Oppositional defiant disorder is characterized by a persistent pattern of disobedience, argumentativeness, angry outbursts, low tolerance for frustration, and tendency to blame others for misfortunes, large and small. Children with oppositional defiant disorder have trouble making friends and often find themselves in conflict with adults.

Conduct disorder is characterized by more serious violations of social norms, including aggressive behavior, destruction of property, and cruelty to animals. Children and adolescents with conduct disorder often lie to achieve short-term ends, may be truant from school, may run away from home, and may engage in petty larceny or even mugging (Box 22.11).

BOX 22.11 CLINICAL VIGNETTE

Leon (Conduct Disorder)

Leon, a 14-year-old Hispanic boy, was admitted to the child psychiatric inpatient service from the emergency department (ED) after a fight with his mother. His mother reported that she and Leon had argued earlier in the evening and that he stormed out of the house screaming and vowing he would never return. Several hours later, Leon came back, yelling and demanding entry into the apartment. Leon's father was working. While his mother was getting up to open the door, Leon continued to yell and scream, waking the neighbors. This led to further arguing between Leon and his mother. Before long, the police were called, and Leon was taken to the ED.

The admission interview revealed that Leon had run away on several occasions and had even stayed away overnight. Although he strongly denied drug use, he had gotten drunk on several occasions. He had also been in several fights, the latest of which resulted in an expulsion from school. Three months before admission, he was caught trying to steal a CD from a music store. More recently, he boasted that he and his friends had snatched a purse at an outdoor concert and had broken into a car to steal its contents. Leon's school performance has been declining; he was truant on several occasions and will probably have to repeat ninth grade.

Leon was born in Puerto Rico and is the oldest of three children. His family moved to the mainland shortly after his birth, and the primary language at home is Spanish. His father is employed as a janitor and speaks very little English. His mother works as a secretary and has achieved fairly good command of English. He has received no treatment except for consultation with the school social worker.

What Do You Think?

- When conducting a nursing assessment, what would you want to learn about Leon's school performance?
- What information could you provide Leon's parents about pharmacotherapy? About behavior management?

Epidemiology

Disruptive behavior disorders are more common in boys and are associated with lower socioeconomic status and urban living (Rowe, Costello, Angold, Copeland, & Maughan, 2010). These disorders are relatively common in school-aged children and are frequently presenting complaints in child psychiatric treatment settings.

The prevalence of conduct disorder estimates range from 2% up to 10% with a median of 4%. The disorder appears to be fairly consistent across various countries that differ in race and ethnicity. Prevalence rates rise from childhood to adolescence and are higher among males than among females. Males with conduct disorder frequently are involved in fighting, stealing, vandalism, and school disciplinary problems. Females with the diagnosis are more likely to practice lying, truancy, running away, substance use, and prostitution. Whereas males tend to exhibit both physical aggression and relational aggression (i.e., behaviors that harm social relations of others), females tend to exhibit relatively more relational aggression (APA, 2013). Conduct disorder is one of the most frequently diagnosed disorders in children in mental health facilities. Individuals with conduct disorder are at greater risk for experiencing mood or anxiety disorders and substance-related disorders (APA, 2013).

Etiology

The etiologies of oppositional defiant disorder and conduct disorder are complex. More attention has been paid to conduct disorder, probably because it is the more serious of the two. Models used to understand aggressiveness (see Chapter 13) are useful in examining these childhood disorders, which appear to have both genetic and environmental components.

Mental Health Nursing Assessment

The nurse gathers data from multiple sources. Adolescents with these disorders are at high risk for physical injury as a result of fighting and impulsive behavior. Sexual promiscuity is common, resulting in an increased frequency of pregnancy and sexually transmitted diseases.

An important aspect of assessment is to rule out comorbid conditions that may partially explain or complicate the person's lack of behavioral control. These conditions include ADHD, learning disabilities, chemical dependency, depression, bipolar illness, or generalized anxiety disorder. Young people who are chronically depressed may be irritable and easily frustrated. Given the tendency of adolescents to act out their frustration, chronic depression may exacerbate their behavior. Conduct problems can also elevate the risk for depression because young people who regularly elicit negative attention from parents and teachers and are constantly at odds with their environment may become despondent.

Adolescents with conduct problems are usually brought or forced into the mental health system by family, school, or the court system because of fighting, truancy, speeding tickets, car accidents, petty crimes, substance abuse, or suicide attempts. These young people may be hostile, sarcastic, defensive, and provocative. At the same time, they may appear calm, outgoing, and engaging. Inconsistencies, distortions, and misrepresentations of the truth are common when interviewing these children, so obtaining a clear history may be difficult. Therefore, instead of asking whether an event or behavior occurred, it may be better to ask when it occurred. These adolescents are adept at changing the subject and diverting discussions from sensitive issues. They often use denial, projection, and externalization of anger as defense mechanisms when asked for self-disclosure. The assessment, which may take several sessions, should be conducted in a nonjudgmental fashion. High levels of marital conflict, parental substance abuse, and parental antisocial behavior often mark family history.

Nursing Diagnoses

Typical nursing diagnoses are Risk for Other Directed Violence, Risk for Self-directed Violence, and Impaired Verbal Communication, Ineffective Coping, Compromised Family Coping and Impaired Social Interaction

Outcomes are individualized for each patient but can include increased personal responsibility for behavior, increased use of problem-solving skills, decreased rule violations and conflicts with authority figures.

Mental Health Nursing Interventions for the Biologic Domain

Children with oppositional defiant disorder or conduct disorder who also have specific neurodevelopmental disorders should be placed in appropriate programs for remediation. If a diagnosis of ADHD or depression emerges from the evaluation, appropriate pharmacotherapy should be considered (see previous discussion of ADHD and after the discussion regarding depression).

Psychosocial Interventions

In planning interventions for patients with oppositional defiant disorder or conduct disorder, the focus is on problem behaviors. Therapeutic progress may be slow, at least partly because these patients often lack trust in authority figures.

Social Skills Training

The nurse should communicate behavioral expectations clearly and enforce them consistently. Consequences of appropriate and inappropriate actions also should be clear. Specific approaches for improving social and problem-solving skills are fundamental features for school-aged children and adolescents. Insofar as children and adolescents with conduct problems fail to recognize the adverse effects of their verbal and nonverbal behavior, their deficit can be formulated as an interpersonal problem. Social skills training teaches adolescents with these behavior disorders to recognize the ways in which their actions affect others. Training involves techniques such as role-playing, modeling by the therapist, and giving positive reinforcement to improve interpersonal relationships and enhance social outcomes.

Problem-Solving Therapy

In contrast to social skills training, which proposes that problems of conduct are the result of poor interpersonal skills, problem-solving therapy conceptualizes conduct problems as the result of deficiencies in cognitive processes. These processes include assessment of situations, interpretation of events, and expectations of others that are congruent with behavior. These children often misinterpret the intentions of others and may perceive hostility with little or no cause. Problem-solving skills training teaches these children to generate alternative solutions to social situations, sharpen thinking concerning the consequences of those choices, and evaluate responses after interpersonal conflicts.

Parent Management Training and Education

Parent training begins with educating parents about disruptive behavior disorders, focusing particularly on impulsiveness, impaired judgment, and self-control. Children with long-standing problems in these areas often elicit punitive responses and negative attributions about their behavior from their parents. Ironically, because these parental responses focus on the child's failure, they may contribute to the child's behavior problems. An important second step is to clarify parental expectations and interpretation of the child's behavior. Parent management training may be offered to a group of parents or to individuals.

The aims of education are to provide parents with new ways of understanding their child's behavior and to promote improved interactions between parent and child. The most commonly presented techniques include the importance of positive reinforcement (praise and tangible rewards) for adaptive behavior, clear limits for unacceptable behavior, and use of mild punishment (e.g., a time out) (Box 22.12).

Referral to Family Therapy

Family therapy is directed at assisting the family with altering maladaptive patterns of interaction or improving

BOX 22.12

Time-Out Procedure

- *Labeling behavior:* Identify the behavior that the child is expected to perform or cease. The aim of this statement is to make clear what is required of the child. It typically takes the form of a simple declarative sentence: "Threatening is not acceptable."
- *Warning:* In this step, the child is informed that if he or she does not perform the expected behavior or stop the unacceptable behavior, he or she will be given a "time out." "This is a warning: if you continue threatening to hit people, you'll have a time out."
- *Time out:* If the child does not heed the warning, he or she is told to take a time out in simple straightforward terms: "Take a time out."
- *Duration:* The usual duration for a time out is 5 minutes for children 5 years of age or older.
- *Location:* The child sits in a designated time-out chair without toys and without talking. The chair should be located away from general activity but within view. A kitchen timer can be used to mark the time, but the clock does not start until the child sits quietly in the designated spot.
- *Follow-up:* The child is asked to recount why he or she was given the time out. The explanation need not be detailed, and no further discussion of the matter is required. Indeed, long discourse about the child's behavior is not helpful and should be avoided.

adjustment to stressors, such as changes or loss in family membership. Multisystem family therapy, which considers the child in the context of multiple family and community systems, has shown promise in the treatment of adolescents with conduct disorder.

Evaluation and Treatment Outcomes

The nurse can review treatment goals and objectives to assess the child's progress with respect to verbal and physical aggression, socially appropriate resolution of conflicts, compliance with rules and expectations, and better management of frustration. As is true for the initial assessment, evaluation of treatment outcomes relies on input from parents, teachers, and other health care team members.

Continuum of Care

Children and adolescents with conduct disorders may be involved with many different agencies in the community, such as child welfare services, school authorities, and the legal system. Mental health services are requested when a child or adolescent's behavior is out of control or a when comorbid disorder is suspected. Helping the patient and family negotiate their way through this maze of services may be an essential part of the treatment plan.

Intermittent Explosive Disorder

Episodes of aggressiveness that result in assault or destruction of property characterize people with **intermittent explosive disorder.** The severity of aggressiveness is out of proportion to the provocation. The episodes can have serious psychosocial consequences, including job loss, interpersonal relationship problems, school expulsion, divorce, automobile accidents, or jail. This diagnosis is given only after all other disorders with aggressive components (e.g., delirium, dementia, head injury, borderline personality disorder, ASPD, substance abuse) have been excluded. Little is known about this disorder, but it is a more common condition than previously thought. The prevalence of intermittent explosive disorder in the United States is about 2.7%. The onset is most common in childhood or adolescence and rarely begins for the first time after the age 40 years. The mean age at onset is 14 years. It is more prevalent in individuals with a high school education or less (APA, 2013). The anger experience and expression of anger contribute to suicidality (Hawkins & Cougle, 2013).

The treatment of this disorder is multifaceted. Psychopharmacologic agents are sometimes used as an adjunct to psychotherapeutic, behavioral, and social interventions. Serotonergic antidepressants and gamma-aminobutyric acid (GABA)-ergic mood stabilizers have been used. Anxiolytics are used to treat obsessive patients who experience tension states and explosive outbursts. Medication alone is insufficient, and anger management should be included in the treatment plan.

Kleptomania

In **kleptomania,** individuals cannot resist the urge to steal, so they independently steal items that they could easily afford. These items are not particularly useful or wanted. The underlying issue is the act of stealing. The term **kleptomania** was first used in 1838 to describe the behavior of several kings who stole worthless objects (Aboujoude & Koran, 2010). These individuals experience an increase in tension and then pleasure and relief at the time of the theft. Kleptomania occurs in about 4% to 24% of individuals arrested for shoplifting. Its prevalence in the general population however is very rare, at approximately 0.3% to 0.6%. Females outnumber males at a ratio of 3:1 (APA, 2013). Because it is considered a "secret" disorder, little is known about it, but it is believed to last for years despite numerous convictions for shoplifting. It appears that kleptomania often has its onset during adolescence (Grant & Kim, 2005).

Some shoplifting appears to be related to anxiety and stress in that it serves to relieve symptoms. In a few instances, brain damage has been associated with kleptomania (Kozian, 2001). Depression is the most common symptom identified in a compulsive shoplifter.

Kleptomania is difficult to detect and treat and means of treatment are little known. It appears that behavior therapy is frequently used. Antidepressant medication that helps relieve the depression has been successful in some cases. More investigation is needed (Ravindran, Da Siva, Ravindran, Richter, & Rector, 2009).

Pyromania

Irresistible impulses to start fires characterize **pyromania**, repeated fire setting with tension or arousal before setting fires; fascination or attraction to the fires; and gratification when setting, witnessing, or participating in the aftermath of fire. These individuals often are regular "fire watchers" or even firefighters. They are not motivated by aggression, anger, suicidal ideation, or political ideology. Little is known about this disorder because only a small number of deliberate fire starters are apprehended, and of those individuals, only a few undergo a psychiatric evaluation. The prevalence of fire setting in the general population is about 1%, but most fire setting is not done by people with pyromania, which occurs infrequently, mostly in men. However, those with a history of fire setting are most likely male, young, and never married and are more likely to have other psychiatric issues such as ASPD, substance use, and impulsivity (Blanco, Alergria, Petry, Grant, Simpson, Liu, et al., 2010). Prevalence rates are lower among African Americans and Hispanics (Vaughn, Fu, Delisi, Wright, Beaver, Perron, et al., 2010).

Early research demonstrated low serotonin and norepinephrine levels associated with arson. Little is known about treatment, and as with the other impulse-control disorders, no approach is uniformly effective. Historically, fire starters generally possess poor interpersonal skills, exhibit low self-esteem, battle depression, and have difficulty managing anger. Education, parenting training, behavior contracting with token reinforcement, problem-solving skills training, and relaxation exercises may all be used in the management of the patient's responses (Blanco, et al., 2010).

Continuum of Care for Disruptive, Impulse-Control Disorders

Impulse-control disorders require long-term treatment, usually in an outpatient setting. Group therapy is often a facet of treatment because patients can talk in a community where people share common experiences. Hospitalization is rare except when patients have comorbid psychiatric or medical disorders.

SUMMARY OF KEY POINTS

- A personality is a complex pattern of characteristics, largely outside of the person's awareness, that comprise the individual's distinctive pattern of perceiving, feeling, thinking, coping, and behaving.

- A personality disorder is an enduring pattern of inner experience and behavior that deviates markedly from the expectations of the individual's culture, is pervasive and inflexible, has an onset in adolescence or early adulthood, is stable over time, and leads to distress or impairment.

- For many patients with personality disorders, maintaining a therapeutic nurse–patient relationship can be one of the most helpful interventions. Through this therapeutic relationship, the patient experiences a model of healthy interaction, establishing trust, consistency, caring, boundaries, and limitations that help to build the patient's self-esteem and respect for self and others. In some personality disorders, nurses will find it more difficult to engage the patient in a true therapeutic relationship because of the patient's avoidance of interpersonal and emotional attachment (i.e., antisocial personality disorder or paranoid personality disorder).

- Patients with personality disorders are rarely treated in an inpatient facility except during periods of destructive behavior or self-injury. Treatment is delivered in the community and over time. Continuity of care is important in helping the individual change lifelong personality patterns.

- People with borderline personality disorder have difficulties regulating emotion and have extreme fears of abandonment, leading to dysfunctional relationships; they often engage in self-injury.

- Medications, including mood stabilizers, antidepressants, and antipsychotics, are useful in regulating the symptoms. They should, however, only be taken for target symptoms for a short time because patients may already be taking other medications, particularly for a comorbid disorder.

- During hospitalizations, keeping the patients safe by preventing self-harm is priority. Open communication and use of dialectical behavior therapy techniques are important interventions.

- Recovery-oriented approaches are grounded in cognitive behavioral therapy. The interdisciplinary treatment or recovery team needs to maintain open communication to work effectively with a person with BPD.

- Antisocial personality disorder, often synonymous with psychopathy, includes people who have no regard for and refuse to conform to social rules.

- The primary characteristic of disruptive, impulse-control disorders is impulsivity, which leads to inappropriate social behaviors that are considered harmful to oneself or others and that give the patient excitement or gratification at the time the act is committed.

CRITICAL THINKING CHALLENGES

1. Define the concepts *personality* and *personality disorder*. When does a normal personality become a personality disorder?

2. Karen, a 36-year-old woman receiving inpatient care, was admitted for depression; she also has a diagnosis of borderline personality disorder. After a telephone argument with her husband, she approaches the nurse's station with her wrist dripping with blood from cutting. What nursing diagnosis best fits this behavior? What interventions should the nurse use with the patient after the self-injury is treated?

3. A 22-year-old man with borderline personality disorder is being discharged from the mental health unit after a severe suicide attempt. As his primary psychiatric nurse, you have been able to establish a therapeutic relationship with him but are now terminating the relationship. He asks you to meet with him "for just a few sessions" after his discharge because his therapist will be on vacation. What are the issues underlying this request? What should you do? Explain and justify.

4. Compare the biologic theory with the psychoanalytic and Linehan's biosocial theory. What are the primary differences between these theories?

5. Compare the characteristics, epidemiology, and etiologic theories of antisocial and borderline personality disorders.

6. Discuss the differences between histrionic and obsessive-compulsive personality disorder.

7. Compare and contrast antisocial personality disorder with narcissistic personality trait.

8. Define and summarize personality disorders. Compare the following among the Cluster A, B, & C disorders:
   a. Defining characteristics
   b. Epidemiology
   c. Biologic, psychological, and social theories
   d. Key nursing assessment data
   e. Nursing diagnoses and outcomes
   f. Specific issues related to a therapeutic relationship
   g. Interventions

9. Define and summarize the impulse-control disorders. Compare the following among kleptomania, pyromania and conduct disorders:
   a. Defining characteristics
   b. Epidemiology
   c. Biologic, psychological, and social theories
   d. Key nursing assessment data
   e. Nursing diagnoses and outcomes
   f. Interventions

Fatal Attraction: (1987) This award-winning film portrays the relationship between a married attorney, Dan Gallagher (played by Michael Douglas), and Alex Forest, a single woman (played by Glenn Close). Their one-night affair turns into a nightmare for the attorney and his family as Alex becomes increasingly possessive and aggressive, demonstrating behaviors characteristic of borderline personality disorder, including anger, impulsivity, emotional lability, fear of rejection and abandonment, vacillation between adoration and disgust, and self-mutilation.

Viewing Points: Identify the behaviors of Alex that are characteristics of borderline personality disorder. Identify the feelings that are generated by the movie. With which characters do you identify? For which characters do you feel sympathy? If Alex had lived and been admitted to your hospital, what would be your first priority?

Grey Gardens: (1975) This documentary by Albert and David Maysles is the unbelievable true story of Mrs. Edith Bouvier Beale and her daughter Edie, who are the aunt and first cousin of Jacqueline Kennedy Onassis. The film depicts mother and daughter, known as "Big Edie" and "Little Edie," who have descended into a strange life of dependence and eccentricity.

Living in a world of their own in a decaying 28-room East Hampton mansion, their living conditions—infested by fleas, inhabited by numerous cats and raccoons, deprived of running water, and filled with garbage—give viewers a glimpse into schizotypal personality disorder.

Viewing Points: Identify the behaviors of Big Edie and Little Edie that are characteristic of schizotypal personality disorder. Do "Big Edie" and "Little Edie" exhibit a folie à deux (a shared psychotic disorder)? Why or why not?

 M·VIE viewing **GUIDES** related to this chapter are available at http://thepoint.lww.com/BoydEssentials.

 Related Psychiatric-Mental Health Nursing videos on the topics of Antisocial Personality Disorder and Borderline Personality Disorder are available at http://thepoint.lww.com/BoydEssentials.

Related Psychiatric-Mental Health Nursing Practice and Learn Activities related to the videos on the topics of Antisocial Personality Disorder and Borderline Personality Disorder are available at http://thepoint.lww.com/BoydEssentials.

REFERENCES

Aboujaoude, E., & Koran, L.M. (2010). *Impulse control disorders*. New York: Cambridge University Press.

Alcorn, J. L., Gowin, J. L., Green, C. E., Swann, A. C., Moeller, F. G., & Lane, S. D. (2013). Aggression, impulsivity, and psychopathic traits in combined antisocial personality disorder and substance use disorder. *Journal of Neuropsychiatry and Clinical Neurosciences, 25*(3), 229–232.

American Psychiatric Association. (2013). *Diagnostic and statistical manual of mental disorders* (5th ed.). Washington, DC: Author.

Asami, T., Whitford, T. J., Bouix, S., Dickey, C. C., Niznikiewicz, M., Shenton, M. E., et al. (2013). Globally and locally reduced MRI gray matter volumes in neuroleptic-naïve men with schizotypal personality disorder: Association with negative symptoms. *Journal of the American Medical Association Psychiatry, 70*(4), 361–372.

Birbaumer, N., Veit, R., Lotze, M., Erb, M., Hermann, C., Grodd, W., et al. (2005). Deficient fear conditioning in psychopathy: A functional magnetic resonance imaging study. *Archives of General Psychiatry, 62*(7), 799–805.

Black, D. W., Gunter, T., Loveless, P., Allen, J., & Sieleni, B. (2010). Antisocial personality disorder in incarcerated offenders: Psychiatric comorbidity and quality of life. *Annals of Clinical Psychiatry, 22*(2), 113–120.

Blanco, C., Alergria, A. A., Petry, N. M., Grant, J. E., Simpson, B., Liu, S., et al. (2010). Prevalence and correlates of fire-setting in the United States: Results from the National Epidemiologic Surveys on Alcohol and Related Conditions (NESARC). *Journal of Clinical Psychiatry, 71*(9), 1218–1225.

Bornstein, R. F. (2012). Illuminating a neglected clinical issue: Societal costs of interpersonal dependency and dependent personality disorder. *Journal of Clinical Psychology, 68*(7), 766–781.

Carter, S. A., & Wu, K. D. (2010). Relations among symptoms of social phobia subtypes, avoidant personality disorder, panic, and depression. *Behavior Therapy, 41*(1), 2–13.

Cicero, D. C., & Kerns, J. G. (2010). Multidimensional factor structure of positive schizotypy. *Journal of Personality Disorders, 24*(3), 327–343.

Clarkin, J. F., & De Panfilis, C. (2013). Developing conceptualization of borderline personality disorder. *The Journal of Nervous and Mental Disease, 201*(2), 88–93.

Cox, B. J., Pagura, J., Stein, M. B., & Sareen, J. (2009). The relationship between generalized social phobia and avoidant personality disorder in a national mental health survey. *Depression and Anxiety, 26*(4), 354–362.

Dimeff, L. A., Woodcock, F. A., Harned, M. S., & Beadnell, B. (2011). Can dialectical behavior therapy be learned in highly structured learning environments? Results from a randomized controlled dissemination trial. *Behavior Therapy, 42*(2), 263–275.

Disney, K. L. (2013). Dependent personality disorder: A critical review. *Clinical Psychology Review, 33*, 1184–1196.

Fielding, P. (2013). The stigma of diagnosis. *Mental Health Practice, 17*(3), 11.

Gao, Y., Raine, A., Chan, F., Veneables, P. H., & Mednick, S. A. (2010). Early maternal and paternal bonding, childhood physical abuse and adult psychopathic personality. *Psychological Medicine, 40*(6), 1007–1016.

Gibbon, S., Duggan, C., Stoffers, J., Huband, N., Völlm, B. A., Ferriter, M., et al. (2010). Psychological interventions for antisocial personality disorders. *Cochrane Database of Systematic Reviews*, (6):CD007668.

Grant, B. F., Hasin, D. S., Stinson, F. D., Dawson, D. A., Chou, S. P., Ruan, W. J., et al. (2004). Prevalence, correlates, and disability of personality disorders in the United States: Results from the National epidemiologic survey on alcohol and related conditions. *Journal of Clinical Psychiatry, 65*(7), 948–995.

Grant, J. E., & Kim, S. W. (2005). Quality of life in kleptomania and pathological gambling. *Comprehensive Psychiatry, 46*(1), 34–37.

Goth, K., Foelsch, P., Schlüter-Müller, S., Birkhölzer, M., Jung, E., Pick, O., et al. (2012). Assessment of identity development and identity diffusion in adolescence – Theoretical basis and psychometric properties of the self-report questionnaire AIDA. *Child and Adolescent Psychiatry and Mental Health 6*(1):27. doi: 10.1186/1753-2000-6-27.

Gunderson, J. G., Stout, R. L., McGlashan, T. H., Shea, M. T., Morey, L. C., Gril, C. M., et al. (2011). Ten-year course of borderline personality disorder: Psychopathology and function from the collaborative longitudinal personality disorders study. *Archives of General Psychiatry, 68*(8), 827–837.

Hawkins, K. A., & Cougle, J. R. (2013). A test of the unique and interactive roles of anger experience and expression in suicidality. *The Journal of Nervous and Mental Disease. 201*(11), 959–963.

Jovev, M., Whittle, S., Yücel, M., Simmons, J. G., Allen, N. B., & Chanen, A. M. (2014). The relationship between hippocampal asymmetry and temperament in adolescent borderline and antisocial personality pathology. *Development and Psychopathology, 26*(1), 275–285.

Koenigsberg, H. W., Denny, B. T., Fan, J., Liu, X., Guerreri, S., Mayson, S. J., et al. (2014). The neural correlates of anomalous habituation to negative emotional pictures in borderline and avoidant personality disorder patients. *American Journal of Psychiatry, 17*(1), 82–90.

Kozian, R. (2001). Kleptomania in frontal lobe lesion. *Psychiatrische Praxis, 28*(2), 98–99.

Lawrence, K., Allen, J., & Chanen, A. (2011). A study of maladaptive schemas and borderline personality disorder in young people. *Cognitive Therapy and Research, 35*(1), 30–39.

Lennox, C., & Dolan, M. (2014). Temperament and character and psychopathy in male conduct disordered offenders. *Psychiatry Research, 215*(3), 706–710.

Linehan, M. (1993). *Cognitive-behavioral treatment of borderline personality disorder*. New York: Guilford Press.

Miano, A., Fertuck, E. A., Arntz, A., & Stanley, B. (2013). Rejection sensitivity is a mediator between borderline personality disorder features and facial trust appraisal. *Journal of Personality Disorders, 27*(4), 442–446.

Millon, T. (2011). *Disorders of personality: Introducing a DSM/ICD spectrum from normal to abnormal* (3rd ed.). Hoboken, NJ: John Wiley & Sons, Inc.

Mitchell, A. E., Dickens, G. L., & Picchioni, M. M. (2014). Facial emotion processing in borderline personality disorder: A systematic review and meta-analysis. *Neuropsychological Review, 24*(2):166–184.

Norrie, J., Davidson, K., Tata, P., & Gumley, A. (2013). Influence of therapist competence and quantity of cognitive behavioural therapy on suicidal behavior and inpatient hospitalisation in a randomized controlled trial in borderline personality disorder: Further analyses of treatment effects in the BOSCOT study. *Psychology and Psychotherapy, 86*(3), 280–293

Pinto, A., Steinglass, J. E., Greene, A. L., Weber, E. U., & Simpson, H. B. (2013). Capacity to delay reward differentiates obsessive-compulsive disorder and obsessive compulsive personality disorder. *Biological Psychiatry, 75*(8):653–659.

Pulay, A. J., Stinson, F. S., Dawson, D. A., Goldstein, R. B., Chou, S. P., Huang, B., et al. (2009). Prevalence, correlates, disability, and comorbidity of DSM-IV schizotypal personality disorder: Results from the Wave 2 National Epidemiologic Survey on Alcohol and Related Conditions. *Journal of Clinical Psychiatry, 11*(2), 53–67.

Rapp, A. M., Mutschler, D. E., Wild, B., Erb, M., Lengsfeld, I., Saur, R., et al. (2010). Neural correlates of irony comprehension: The role of schizotypal personality traits. *Brain and Language, 113*, 1–12.

Ravindran, A. V., Da Siva, T. L., Ravindran, L. H., Richter, N. A., & Rector, N. A. (2009). Obsessive-compulsive spectrum disorders: A review of the evidence-based treatments. *Canadian Journal of Psychiatry, 54*(5), 331–342.

Ripoll, L. H. (2012). Clinical psychopharmacology of borderline personality disorder: an update on the available evidence in light of the Diagnostic and Statistical Manual of Mental Disorders-5. *Current Opinion in Psychiatry, 25*(1), 52–58.

Roepke, S., & Vater, A. (2014). Narcissistic personality disorder: An integrative review of recent empirical data and current definitions. *Current Psychiatry Reports, 16*(5), 445–453.

Ronningstam, E., & Weinberg, I. (2013). Narcissistic personality disorder: Progress in recognition and treatment. *Focus, 11*(2), 167–177.

Rowe, R., Costello, E. J., Angold, A., Copeland, W. E., & Maughan, B. (2010). Developmental pathways in oppositional defiant disorder and conduct disorder. *Journal of Abnormal Psychology, 119*(4), 728–736.

Samuels, J. (2011). Personality disorders: Epidemiology and public health issues. *International Review of Psychiatry, 23*(3), 223–233.

Sansone, R. A., & Sansone, L. A. (2011). Gender patterns in borderline personality disorder. *Innovations in Clinical Neuroscience, 8*(5), 16–20.

Sousa, C., Herrenkohl, T. I., Moylan, C. A., Tajima, E. A., Klika, J. B., Herrenkohl, R. C., et al. (2011). Longitudinal study on the effects of child abuse and children's exposure to domestic violence, parent-child attachments, and antisocial behavior in adolescence. *Journal of Interpersonal Violence, 26*(1), 111–136.

Steele, H., & Siever, L. (2010). An attachment perspective on borderline personality disorder: in gene-environment considerations. *Current Psychiatry Reports, 12*(1), 61–67.

Stinson, F. S., Dawson, D. A., Goldstein, R. B., Chou, S. P., Huang, B., Smith, S. M., et al. (2008). Prevalence, correlates, disability, and comorbidity of DSM-IV narcissistic personality disorder: Results from the Wave 2 National Epidemiologic Survey on Alcohol and Related Conditions. *Journal of Clinical Psychiatry, 69*(7), 1033–1045.

Stoffers, J., Völlm, B. A., Rücker, G., Timmer, A., Huband, N., & Lieb, K. (2010). Pharmacological interventions for people with borderline personality disorder. *Cochrane Database of Systematic Reviews*, (1), CD005653.

Stone, M. H. (2013). The brain in overdrive: A new look at borderline and related disorders. (2013) *Current Psychiatry Reports, 15*(10), 1–8.

Taber-Thomas, B. C., Asp, E. W., Koenigs, M., Sutterer, M., Anderson, S. W., & Tranel, D. (2014). Arrested development: Early prefrontal lesions impair the maturation of moral judgement. *Brain, 137*(pt 4), 1254–1261.

Tansey, T. N. (2010). Impulsivity: An overview of a biopsychosocial model. *Journal of Rehabilitation, 76*(3), 3–9.

Vaughn, M. G., Fu, Q., Delisi, M., Wright, J. P., Beaver, K. M., Perron, B. E., et al. (2010). Prevalence and correlates of fire-setting in the United States: Results from the national epidemiological survey on alcohol and related conditions. *Comprehensive Psychiatry, 51*(3), 217–223.

van Dijke, A., van der Hart, O., Ford, J. D., van Son, M., van der Heijden, P., & Bühring, M. (2010). Affect dysregulation and dissociation in borderline personality disorder and somatoform disorder: Differentiating inhibitory and excitatory experiencing states. *Journal of Trauma & Dissociation, 11*(4), 424–443.

Wolf, R. C., Sambataro, F., Vasic, N., Schmid, M., Thomann, P. A., Bienentreu, S. D., et al. (2011). Aberrant connectivity of resting-state networks in borderline personality disorder. *Journal of Psychiatry & Neuroscience, 36*(2), 402–411. doi:10.1503/jpn.100150

Wright, K., & Jones, F. (2012). Therapeutic alliances in people with borderline personality disorder. *Mental Health Practice, 16*(2), 31–35.

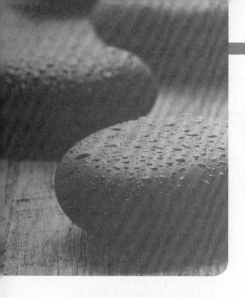

23
Somatic Symptom and Dissociative Disorders

Nursing Care of Persons with Somatization

Mary Ann Boyd and Victoria Soltis-Jarrett

KEY CONCEPT

- somatization

LEARNING OBJECTIVES

After studying this chapter, you will be able to:

1. Explain the concept of somatization and the occurrence of somatic symptom and related disorders in people with mental health problems.

2. Discuss the prevailing theories related to somatic symptom and related disorders.

3. Identify evidence-based nursing assessment and outcomes for persons with somatization and cognitive distortions.

4. Formulate nursing diagnoses based on a mental health nursing assessment of people with somatic symptom and related disorders.

5. Develop recovery-oriented nursing interventions for patients with somatic symptom and related disorders.

6. Discuss special concerns within the therapeutic relationship common for those with somatic symptom and related disorders.

KEY TERMS

- alexithymia • somatic symptom disorder (SSD) • conversion disorder • factitious disorder imposed on another • illness anxiety disorder • pseudologia fantastica • psychosomatic

---

Case Study: Carol

Carol is a 48-year-old woman with obesity who is very angry at being forced to see a mental health care provider. She has had multiple surgeries including hysterectomy, gastric bypass, carpal tunnel release. She suffers from shoulder and neck pain and from vertigo. She takes multiple medications.

INTRODUCTION

The connection between the "mind" and "body" has been hypothesized and described for centuries. The term **psychosomatic** has been traditionally used to describe, explain, and predict the psychological origins of illness and disease. Unfortunately, this notion perpetuates the stigma that certain disorders are purely "psychological" in nature and thus that they are not real or valid. For example, it was formerly believed that people with asthma were behaviorally "acting out" their anger, fear, or emotional pain and were seeking attention rather than experiencing an alteration in their respiratory status.

In contrast, the concept of *somatization* acknowledges and respects that bodily sensations and functional changes are expressions of health and illness, and, even though they may be unexplained, they are not imaginary or "all in the head" (Boutros & Peters, 2012).

> **KEYCONCEPT** **Somatization** (from *soma*, meaning body) is the manifestation of psychological distress as physical symptoms that may result in functional changes, somatic descriptions, or both.

Whereas some evidence suggests that somatization is a result of abnormally high levels of physiologic response (Boutros & Peters, 2012), other evidence supports the idea that somatization is the physical expression of personal problems or the internalization and expression of stress through physical symptoms (Fava, et al., 2012). For example, a woman quits her job complaining of chronic fatigue syndrome rather than recognizing that she is emotionally stressed from the constant harassment of a coworker.

Historically, the concept of somatization was linked to women and was related to a woman's body, mind, or even her soul. For example, the term *hysteria*, frequently associated with somatization, actually comes from ancient times when it was believed that a woman's unfounded physical symptoms were related to her "wandering or discontented uterus." Because *hystera* is the Greek word for uterus, the terms *hysteria* and *hysterical* were used to describe a woman whose physical or emotional symptoms could not be substantiated by physicians at that time.

Today, we understand that somatization is not linked to the uterus nor is it just a problem for women. Men also are affected by somatization. Much research is still needed in this area to be able to make any valid and reliable conclusions about gender and somatization. Somatization also crosses all cultures and is recognized in almost every society (Woolfolk, Allen, & Tiu, 2007). In many cultures, the expression of physical discomfort is more acceptable than acknowledging psychological distress. The disruption of routine body cycles, such as digestion, menstruation, or sleep, is more socially acceptable than having emotional responses related to interpersonal relationships, economic crises, adjustment to marriage, infertility, or the death of a spouse.

This chapter explores the holistic evidenced-based nursing care for people experiencing the DSM-5 group of disorders with the prominent symptom of somatization (American Psychiatric Association [APA], 2013). Somatic symptom disorder (SSD) is highlighted and illness anxiety disorder, conversion disorder, and factitious disorders are discussed.

SOMATIC SYMPTOM DISORDER

Nurses in primary care and medical–surgical settings are more likely than mental health nurses to encounter persons with these problems. Note: the term *somatoform* is no longer used in the DSM-5 to describe these disorders (APA, 2013).

Clinical Course

Somatic symptom disorder (SSD) is one of the most difficult disorders to manage because its symptoms tend to change, are diffuse and complex, and vary and move from one body system to another. For example, initially gastrointestinal (e.g., nausea, vomiting, diarrhea) and neurologic (e.g., headache, backache) symptoms may be presentthat change to musculoskeletal (e.g., aching legs) and sexual issues (e.g., pain in the abdomen, pain during intercourse). Physical symptoms may last for 6 to 9 months.

Individuals with SSD perceive themselves as being "sicker than the sick" and report all aspects of their health as poor. Many eventually become disabled and unable to work. They typically visit health care providers many times each month and quickly become frustrated because their primary health care providers do not appreciate their level of suffering and are unable to validate that a particular problem accounts for their extreme discomfort. Consequently, individuals with SSD tend to "provider shop," moving from one to another until they find one who will give them new medication, hospitalize them, or perform surgery. Because the source of worrisome physical symptoms cannot be determined through medical or laboratory tests, medical or psychiatric interviews, or medical imaging, they repeatedly seek a medical reason for their discomfort and ask for relief from suffering. Depending on the severity, these individuals undergo multiple surgeries and even develop iatrogenic illnesses. People with SSD often evoke negative subjective responses in health care providers, who usually wish that the patient would go to someone else.

The most common characteristics are:

- Reporting the same symptoms repeatedly
- Receiving support from the environment that otherwise might not be forthcoming (e.g., gaining a spouse's attention because of severe back pain)
- Expressing concern about the physical problems inconsistent with the severity of the illness (being "sicker than the sick")

NCLEXNOTE Patients with SSD seek health care from multiple providers but avoid mental health specialists.

Diagnostic Criteria

The diagnostic criteria of SSD include one or more symptoms that cause persistent distress or significant disruption in daily lives for at least 6 months and excessive thoughts about the seriousness of the symptoms, feelings (such as anxiety about the symptoms or overall health), or behaviors related to the symptoms or health concerns (e.g., spending excessive time and energy focusing on these symptoms or health) (APA, 2013). These symptoms may or may not be explained by medical evidence. The expression of the symptoms varies from population to population.

Somatic Symptom Disorder Across the Life-Span

SSD is found in most populations and cultures even though its expression may vary from population to population. In cultures that highly stigmatize mental illness, somatic symptoms are more likely to appear (Dere, Sun, Zhao, Persson, Zhu, Yao, et al., 2013; Zaroff, Davis, Chio, & Madhaven, 2012).

Children and Adolescents

Although many children have somatic symptoms, SSD is not usually diagnosed until adolescence. However, when children have medical symptoms, further evaluation is needed so they are often referred to specialists to rule out physical, sexual, or emotional abuse or a comorbid psychiatric illness, such as depression or anxiety. In children, the most common symptoms are frequent abdominal pain, headache, fatigue, and nausea. Expression of somatic symptom in children tends to be overlooked or minimized when it needs to be identified as a risk factor for follow-up (Schulte & Peterman, 2011). In adolescents, initial symptoms are typically menstrual difficulties, and pelvic or abdominal pain. Risk factors for both children and adolescents need to be taken seriously. Research has shown a link between childhood sexual abuse and somatization, substance use, and depression in adults (Zink, Klesges, Stevens, & Decker, 2009).

Older Adults

SSD can involve a lifelong pattern of symptoms that persists into old age. The symptoms of SSD, however, are often unrecognized by health care providers who tend to accept and minimize them as a part of the natural aging process after no medical cause is found.

Epidemiology

The estimated prevalence of SSD ranges from 5% to 7% (APA, 2013). Millions of dollars of lost revenue and the increased use of short- and long-term disability have prompted employers to study this unique population of employees. In reality, about 20% of persons seeking primary care fall in this group (Fabião, Silva, Fleming, & Barbosa, 2010).

Age of Onset

SSD usually begins before the age of 30 years with the first symptom often appearing during adolescence. Rarely diagnosed until several years later, seeking help can last for many years with the individual frequently going from one health care provider to another to no avail. Most studies report that somatization is more common in middle-aged and older adults (Woolfolk, et al., 2007).

Gender, Ethnic, and Cultural Differences

Epidemiologic studies have reported that SSD occurs primarily in nonwhite, less educated women, particularly those with a lower socioeconomic status and high emotional distress (Woolfolk, et al., 2007). Men are less likely to be diagnosed with SSD, partly because of stereotypic male traits, such as a disinclination to admit discomfort or seek help for their symptoms (APA, 2013).

Risk Factors

SSD tends to run in families, and children of mothers with multiple unexplained somatic complaints are more likely to have somatic problems. Individuals with a tendency toward heightened physiologic arousal and a tendency to amplify somatosensory information have a greater risk of developing this disorder. Adults are also at higher risk for unexplained medical symptoms if they experienced them as children or if their parents were in poor health when the patient was about 15 years old. Data have also confirmed a strong association between sexual trauma exposure and somatic symptoms, illness attitudes, and healthcare utilization in women (Woolfolk, et al., 2007).

Comorbidity

SSD frequently coexists with other psychiatric disorders, most commonly depression and anxiety. Others include panic disorder, mania, social phobia, obsessive-compulsive disorder (OCD), psychotic disorders, and personality disorders (van Dijke, Ford, van der Hart, van Son, van der Heijden, & Bühring, 2010). Older adults are at particularly high risk for comorbid depression (Spangenberg, Forkmann, Brahler, & Glaesmer, 2011).

Ultimately, numerous unexplained medical problems also coexist with this disorder because many patients have received medical and surgical treatments, often unnecessarily, and are plagued with side effects. A disproportionately high number of women who eventually receive diagnoses of SSD have been treated for irritable bowel syndrome, polycystic ovary disease, and chronic pain.

Etiology

Biologic Theories

The cause of SSD is unknown. General agreement exists that somatization has a biopsychosocial basis with the possibility of biologic dysfunction common in depression and chronic fatigue syndrome (Anderson, Maes, & Berk, 2012).

Although SSD has been shown to run in families, the exact transmission mechanism is unclear. Strong evidence suggests an increased risk for SSD in first-degree relatives, indicating a familial or genetic effect. Because many individuals with SSD live in chaotic families, the high prevalence in first-degree relatives could be explained by environmental influence. Some boys and men in these families show a high risk for antisocial personality disorder and substance abuse (Rief & Broadbent, 2007).

Psychological Theories

Somatization has been explained as a form of social or emotional communication, meaning that the bodily symptoms express an emotion that cannot be verbalized by the individual. An adolescent who experiences severe abdominal pain after her parents' argue or a wife who receives nurturing from her husband only when she has back pain are two examples. From this perspective, somatization may be a way of communicating and maintaining relationships. Following this line of reasoning, an individual's physical problems may also become a way of controlling relationships, so somatization becomes a learned behavior pattern. With time, physical symptoms develop automatically in response to perceived threats. Finally, SSD develops when somatizing becomes a way of life.

Consistent with a communication explanation, cognitive behaviorists explain somatization symptoms as an interaction of negative views of the world with physical factors (e.g., pain, discomfort). In this model, individuals have a heightened response based on their experiences with a stressor, especially if the stressor is uncontrollable and unpredictable. Over time, their exaggerated responses become an automatic pattern, resulting in "sick role" behavior, which in turn provokes either a negative or positive response in others (Dumont & Olson, 2012; Mik-Meyer & Obling, 2012).

Another theoretical explanation for somatization is the personality trait **alexithymia**, which is associated with somatic symptom disorder. Individuals with alexithymia have difficulty identifying and expressing their emotions. They have a preoccupation with external events and are described as concrete externally oriented thinkers (Deng, Ma, & Tang, 2013; Pedrosa, Ridout, Kessler, Neuffer, Schoechlin, Traue, et al., 2009).

Social Theories

SSD has been reported globally even though its conceptualization is primarily Western. The symptoms may vary from culture to culture. For example, studies in China have identified and discussed the notion of somatization as a moral issue rather than a medical problem. Somatization is a more socially acceptable way to express behavior in lieu of being diagnosed as depressed because in China, where mental illness is perceived as a character flaw. In many non-Western societies, where the mind–body distinction is not made and symptoms have different meanings and explanations, these physical manifestations are not labeled as a psychiatric

---

BOX 23.1

Somatization in Chinese Culture

In Chinese tradition, the health of the individual reflects a balance between positive and negative forces within the body. Five elements at work in nature and in the body control health conditions (e.g., fire, water, wood, earth, metal), five viscera (e.g., liver, heart, spleen, kidneys, lungs), five emotions (anger, joy, worry, sorrow, fear), and five climatic conditions (e.g., wind, heat, humidity, dryness, cold). All illness is explained by imbalances among these elements. Because emotion is related to the circulation of vital air within the body, anger is believed to result from an adverse current of vital air to the liver. Emotional outbursts are seen as results of imbalances among the natural elements rather than the results of behavior of the person.

The stigma of mental illness in the Chinese culture is so great that it can have an adverse effect on a family for many generations. If problems can be attributed to natural causes, the individual and family are less responsible, so that stigma is minimized. The Chinese have a culturally acceptable term for symptoms of mental distress—the closest translation of which would be *neurasthenia*—which comprises somatic complaints of headaches, insomnia, dizziness, aches and pains, poor memory, anxiety, weakness, and loss of energy.

---

disorder (Box 23.1). In Latin American countries, depression is more likely described in somatic symptoms, such as headaches, gastrointestinal disturbances, or complaints of "nerves," rather than sadness or guilt (Yusim, Anbarasan, Hall, Goetz, Neugebauer, Stewart, et al., 2010).

Family Response to Disorder

Family dynamics are shaped by all members, including the person with SSD. When one member has several ongoing chronic healthissues, family members' activities and interactions are affected. The physical symptoms of the individual become the focus of family life, so activities are planned around that person. Because so much time and so many resources are used trying to discover an underlying illness, resources to other family member are reduced. Because the person is always sick, expressing anger about the situation is difficult. The family members need support as they learn to understand the seriousness and difficulty of experiencing an SSD (Krishnan, Sood, & Chadda, 2013).

Teamwork and Collaboration: Working Toward Recovery

The care of patients with SSD involves three approaches:

- Providing long-term general management of the chronic condition
- Treating symptoms of comorbid psychiatric and physical problems conservatively
- Providing care in special settings, including individual and group treatment and the use of complementary and alternative medicine (Moreno, Gili, Magallón, Bauzá, Rocal, Hoyo, et al., 2013; Woolfolk, et al., 2007).

The cornerstones of management are trust and believing. Ideally, the patient should see only one health care provider at regularly scheduled visits. During each primary care visit, the provider should conduct a partial physical examination of the organ system about which which the patient has complaints. Physical symptoms are treated conservatively using the least intrusive approach. In the mental health setting, the use of cognitive behavior therapy (CBT) is effective (Moreno, et al., 2013).

Evidence-Based Mental Health Nursing Care

Mental Health Nursing Assessment

During the assessment interview, the nurse should allow enough time for the patient to explain all medical problems; a hurried assessment interview blocks communication. Nursing Care Plan 23.1 is available at http://thepoint.lww.com/BoydEssentials.

NCLEXNOTE Encourage and allow patients with SSD to discuss their physical problems before focusing on psychosocial issues.

Physical Health Assessment

Psychiatric–mental health nurses typically see these patients for problems related to a coexisting psychiatric disorder, such as depression, not because of the SSD. While taking the patient's history, the nurse may discover that the individual has had multiple surgeries or medical problems, making SSD a strong possibility. If the patient has not already received a diagnosis of SSD, the nurse should screen for it by determining the presence of the most commonly reported problems associated with this disorder, which include dysmenorrhea, a lump in the throat, vomiting, shortness of breath, burning sensation in the sex organs, painful limbs, and amnesia. If the patient has these symptoms, he or she should be seen by a mental health provider qualified to make the diagnosis. Box 23.2 presents the Health Attitude Survey, which can be used as a screening test for somatization.

Review of Systems

Although these patients' symptoms have usually received considerable attention from the medical community, a careful review of systems is important because the appearance of physical problems is usually related to psychosocial problems. Even as the patient continues to be seen for mental health problems, an ongoing awareness of biologic symptoms is important, particularly because these symptoms are de-emphasized in the overall case management.

Pain is the most common finding in people with this disorder. Because the pain is usually related to symptoms of all the major body systems, it is unlikely that a somatic intervention such as an analgesic will be effective on a

---

BOX 23.2

Health Attitude Survey

On a scale of 1 to 5, please indicate the extent to which you agree (5) or disagree (1).

DISSATISFACTION WITH CARE
1. I have been satisfied with the medical care I have received. (R)
2. Doctors have done the best they could to diagnose and treat my health problems. (R)
3. Doctors have taken my health problems seriously.
4. My health problems have been thoroughly evaluated. (R)
5. Doctors do not seem to know much about the health problems I have had.
6. My health problems have been completely explained. (R)
7. Doctors seem to think I am exaggerating my health problems.
8. My response to treatment has not been satisfactory.
9. My response to treatment is usually excellent. (R)

FRUSTRATION WITH ILL HEALTH
10. I am tired of feeling sick and would like to get to the bottom of my health problems.
11. I have felt ill for quite a while now.
12. I am going to keep searching for an answer to my health problems.
13. I do not think there is anything seriously wrong with my body. (R)

HIGH UTILIZATION OF CARE
14. I have seen many different doctors over the years.
15. I have taken a lot of medicine recently.
16. I do not go to the doctor often. (R)
17. I have had relatively good health over the years.

EXCESSIVE HEALTH WORRY
18. I sometimes worry too much about my health.
19. I often fear the worst when I develop symptoms.
20. I have trouble getting my mind off my health.

PSYCHOLOGICAL DISTRESS
21. Sometimes I feel depressed and cannot seem to shake it off.
22. I have sought help for emotional or stress-related problems.
23. It is easy to relax and stay calm. (R)
24. I believe the stress I am under may be affecting my health.

DISCORDANT COMMUNICATION OF DISTRESS
25. Some people think that I am capable of more work than I feel able to do.
26. Some people think that I have been sick just to gain attention.
27. It is difficult for me to find the right words for my feelings.

(R) indicates items reversed for scoring purposes. Scoring—The higher the score, the more likely somatization is a problem.

From Noyes, R. Jr., Langbehn, D., Happel, R., Sieren, L., & Muller, B. (1999). Health Attitude Survey: A scale for assessing somatizing patients. *Psychosomatics, 40*(6), 470–478.

---

long-term basis. Remember that although no medical explanation exists for the pain, the patient's pain is real and has serious psychosocial implications. A careful assessment should include the following questions:

- What is the pain like?
- What is the extent of the pain?
- What helps the pain get better?
- When is the pain at its worst?
- What has worked in the past to relieve the pain?

Physical Functioning

The actual physical functioning of these individuals is often marginal. They usually have problems with sleep, fatigue, activity, and sexual functioning. Assessment of these areas generates data to be used in establishing a nursing diagnosis. The amount and quality of sleep are important, as are the hours when the individual sleeps. For example, an individual may sleep a total of 6 hours each diurnal cycle but only from 2:00 to 6:00 AM plus an afternoon nap.

Fatigue is a constant problem for many people with SSD, and because various physical problems interfere with normal activity. These patients report an overwhelming lack of energy, which makes maintaining usual routines or accomplishing daily tasks impossible. Fatigue is accompanied by the inability to concentrate on simple functions, leading to decreased performance and disinterest in surroundings. Patients tend to be lethargic and listless and often have little energy (Box 23.3).

Female patients with this disorder usually have had multiple gynecologic problems, so that the physical manifestations of SSD often lead to altered sexual behavior. The reason is not known, but symptoms of dysmenorrhea, painful intercourse, and pain in the "sex organs" suggest involvement of the hypothalamic–pituitary–gonadal axis. Physiologic indicators, such as those produced by laboratory tests, are not available. However, a careful assessment of the patient's menstrual history, gynecologic problems, and sexual functioning is important. It is also important to assess whether abuse occurred in the past or continues in the present, and whether such abuse is sexual, physical, or emotional.

Medication Assessment

A medication assessment of these patients is challenging. Patients with SSD frequently provider shop, perhaps seeing seven or eight different health care providers within a year. Because they often receive medications from each provider, they are usually taking a large number of drugs. They tend to protect their sources and may not be truthful in identifying the actual number of medications they are taking. A medication assessment is needed not only because of the number of medications but also because these individuals frequently have unusual side effects or they report that they are "sensitive" to medications. Because of their somatic sensitivity, they often overreact to medication.

These patients spend much of their lives trying to find out what is wrong with them. When one health care provider after another can find little if any explanation for their symptoms, many become anxious. To alleviate their anxiety, they either self-medicate with over-the-counter (OTC) medications and substances of abuse (e.g., alcohol, marijuana) or find a health care provider who prescribes an anxiolytic. Because the anxiety of their disorder cannot be treated within a few weeks with an anxiolytic,

they become dependent on medication that should not have been prescribed in the first place.

Although anxiolytics have a place in therapeutics, they are not recommended for long-term use and only complicate the treatment of individuals with SSD. These medications should also be avoided because of their addictive qualities. Unfortunately, by the time these individuals see a mental health provider, they have already begun taking an anxiolytic for anxiety, usually a benzodiazepine. Many times, they only agree to see a mental health provider because the last provider would no longer prescribe an anxiolytic without a psychiatric evaluation.

BOX 23.3 CLINICAL VIGNETTE

Somatic Symptom Disorder and Stress

Ms. J, age 42 years, has been coming to the mental health clinic for 2 years for her nerves. She has seen only the physician for medication but now has been referred to the nurse's new stress management group because she is experiencing side effects to all the medications that have been tried. The psychiatrist has diagnosed SSD and wants her to learn to manage her "nerves" without medication.

At the first meeting with the nurse, Ms. J was preoccupied with chest pain and bloating that had lasted for the past 6 months. Her chest pain is constant and sharp at times. The pain does not prevent her from going to her job as a waitress but does interfere with meal preparation at night for her family and her ability to have sexual intercourse. She has numerous other physical problems, including allergies to certain perfumes, dysmenorrhea, ovarian polycystic disease (ovarian cysts), chronic urinary tract infections, and rashes. She is constantly fatigued and has frequent leg cramps. She states that she is too tired to fix dinner for her family. On days off from work, she takes a nap in the afternoon, sleeping until evening. She is unable to fall asleep at night.

She believes that she will soon have to have her gallbladder removed because of occasional referred pain to her back and nausea that occurs a couple hours after eating. She is not enthusiastic about a stress management group and does not believe it will help her problems. However, she has agreed to consider it for as long as the psychiatrist will continue prescribing diazepam (Valium).

What Do You Think?

- How would you prioritize Ms. J's physical symptoms?
- What are some possible explanations for Ms. J's fatigue?

Remember Carol?

Carol has been taking alprazolam for stress for years. Her primary health care provider is refusing to prescribe it again until she has a complete mental health examination. No other health care providers will prescribe alprazolam for her.

Psychosocial Assessment

The mental status of individuals with SSD can be within normal limits, although most patients report frustration, depression, and hopelessness about their situation. What is most noticeable is their intense focus on their bodies and the physical symptoms that are causing them distress and disability.

Generally, cognition is not impaired in people with SSD, but it may be distorted, such as believing the pain means a life-threatening condition. These individuals seem preoccupied with the signs and symptoms of their illnesses and may even keep a record of their experiences. Living with illness, diseases, and suffering truly becomes a way of life.

Some individuals with SSD have intense emotional reactions to life stressors and have led or are leading traumatic or chaotic lives. These patients usually have had a series of personal crises beginning at an early age. Examples include severe sexual and physical abuse and psychological trauma. Typically, a new symptom or medical problem develops during times of emotional stress as well as during anniversaries of losses or traumas that have occurred in the patient's lifetime. It is critical that the link between the physical assessment data and the patient's psychological and social history are considered. A thorough history of major psychological events should be compared with the chronology of physical problems. Special attention should be paid to any history of sexual abuse or trauma in the patient's younger years. Early sexual abuse also may prevent the individual from being able to perform sexually or to have to endure chronic abdominal pain or discomfort during sexual relations.

The individual's mood is usually labile, often shifting from extremely excited or anxious to being depressed and hopeless. Response to physical symptoms is usually magnified, such as interpreting a simple cold as pneumonia or a brief chest pain as a heart attack. Family members may not believe the physical symptoms are real and may view them as attention-getting behavior because symptoms often improve when the patient receives attention. For example, a woman who has been in bed for 3 weeks with severe back pain may suddenly feel much better when her children visit her.

Social Network

People with this disorder spend excessive time seeking medical care and treating their multiple illnesses. Because they believe themselves to be very sick, they also believe that they are disabled and cannot work. Many are unemployed, so frequently these individuals have changed jobs, had multiple positions over their lifetimes or careers, or have had absences or gaps in employment (Sharma & Manjula, 2013).

Because their symptoms are often inconsistent with any identifiable medical diagnosis, these individuals are rarely satisfied with their health care providers who can find nothing wrong. However, their social network often consists of a series of health care providers, rather than peers or family members, who can also become weary of the individual's constant complaints of physical problems. Identifying a support network requires sorting out the health care providers from family and friends.

> **Consider Carol's limited social network**
> Carol has no friends and spends her time going from provider to provider.

Family Issues

Individuals with SSD sometimes live in chaotic families with multiple problems. In assessing the family structure, other members with psychiatric disorders must be identified. Women may be married to abusive men who have antisocial personality disorders; alcoholism is common. Identifying the positive and negative relationships within the family is important.

SSD is particularly problematic because it disrupts the family's social life. Changes in routine or major life events often precipitate the appearance of a symptom. For example, a person may be planning a vacation with the family but at the last minute decides she cannot go because her back pain has returned and she will not be able to sit in the car. These family disruptions are common. In addition, as already noted, employment history for the person with SSD may be erratic.

Strengths Assessment

A person with SSD may have difficulty identifying *any* personal strengths. The nurse should help the person focus on daily activities and suggest strengths that emerge. For example, some strengths might be that the person has a place to live, has a caring family, or some educational attainment. The nurse also elicits motivation to feel better.

Nursing Diagnoses

Because SSD is a chronic illness, patients could have almost any of the nursing diagnoses at some time in their lives. At least one nursing diagnosis likely will be related to the individual's physical state. Fatigue, Pain, and Insomnia are usually supported by the assessment data. Other diagnoses include Anxiety, Ineffective Sexuality Patterns, Impaired Social Interactions, Ineffective Coping, and Ineffective Therapeutic Regimen Management, Ineffective Community Coping, Disabled Family Coping, Social Isolation, Readiness for Hope, and Readiness for Enhanced Comfort. The challenge in devising outcomes for these problems is to avoid focusing on the biologic aspects and instead help the person overcome the fatigue, pain, or sleep problem through biopsychosocial approaches.

Development of a Therapeutic Relationship

The most difficult aspect of nursing care is developing a sound, positive, nurse–patient relationship, yet this relationship is crucial. Without it, the nurse is just one more provider who fails to meet the patient's expectations. Developing this relationship requires time and patience. Therapeutic communication techniques should be used to refocus the patient on psychosocial problems related to the physical manifestations (Box 23.4).

During periods when symptoms of other psychiatric disorders surface, additional interventions are needed.

BOX 23.4 • THERAPEUTIC DIALOGUE • Establishing a Relationship

INEFFECTIVE APPROACH

Nurse: Good morning, Carol.

Carol: I'm in so much pain. Take that breakfast away.

Nurse: You don't want your breakfast?

Carol: Can't you see? I hurt! When I hurt, I can't eat!

Nurse: If you don't eat now, you probably won't be able to have anything until lunch.

Carol: Who cares? I have no intention of being here at lunchtime. I don't belong here.

Nurse: Carol, I don't think that your doctor would have admitted you unless there were a problem. I would like to talk to you about why you are here.

Carol: Nurse, I'm just here. It's none of your business.

Nurse: Oh.

Carol: Please leave me alone.

Nurse: Sure, I will see you later.

EFFECTIVE APPROACH

Nurse: Good morning, Carol.

Carol: I'm in so much pain. Take that breakfast away.

Nurse: (Silently removes tray. Pulls up chair and sits down.)

Carol: My back hurts.

Nurse: Oh, when did the back pain start?

Carol: Last night. It's this bed. I couldn't get comfortable.

Nurse: These beds can be pretty uncomfortable.

Carol: My back pain is shooting down my leg.

Nurse: Does anything help it?

Carol: Sometimes if I straighten out my leg it helps.

Nurse: Can I help you straighten out your leg?

Carol: Oh, it's OK. The pain is going away. What did you say your name is?

Nurse: I'm Susan Miller, your nurse while you are here.

Carol: I won't be here long. I don't belong in a psychiatric unit.

Nurse: While you are here, I would like to spend time with you.

Carol: OK, but you understand, I do not have any psychiatric problems.

Nurse: We can talk about whatever you want. But because you want to get out of here, we might want to focus on what it will take to get you ready for discharge.

CRITICAL THINKING CHALLENGE

- What communication mistakes did the nurse in the first scenario make?
- What communication strategies helped the patient feel comfortable with the nurse in the second scenario?
- How is the first scenario different from the second?

For example, if depression occurs, additional supportive or cognitive approaches may be needed.

> ### Carol's behavior on the mental health unit
> Carol felt she was tricked into agreeing to be admitted to a mental health unit for medication evaluation. She believes she should be on a medical unit for her constant pain.

Mental Health Nursing Interventions

Physical Health Interventions

Nursing interventions that focus on physical health become especially important because medical treatment must be conservative;aggressive pharmacologic treatment must be avoided. Each time a nurse sees the patient, a limited time should be spent respectfully discussing physical complaints. During the discussion, to the nurse must project the belief that the patient is truly experiencing these problems. Several physically focused interventions, including pain management, activity enhancement, nutrition regulation, relaxation, and pharmacologic interventions, may be useful in caring for patients with SSD.

Pain Management

In pain management, a single approach rarely works. Pain is a primary issue and was previously considered a separate disorder. Nursing care focuses on helping patients identify strategies to relieve pain and to examine stressors in their lives. After a careful assessment of the pain, nonpharmacologic strategies should be developed to reduce it. If gastrointestinal pain is frequent, eating and bowel habits should be explored and modified as needed. For back pain, exercises and consultation from a physical therapist may be useful. Headaches are a challenge. Self-monitoring and tracking them engages the patient in the therapeutic process and helps to identify psychosocial triggers. In addition, suggesting or referring the individual for complementary and alternative treatments has been shown to be very useful (Woolfolk, et al., 2007). Relaxation techniques, identifying thoughts and feelings about pain or discomfort, and including family members in the intervention have also been shown to be useful.

Activity Enhancement

Helping the patient establish a daily routine may alleviate some of the difficulty with sleeping, but doing so may be difficult because most of these patients do not work. Encouraging the patient to get up in the morning and go to bed at night at specific times can help the patient to establish a routine. These patients should engage in regular exercise to improve their overall physical state, although they often have numerous reasons why they cannot. This is where the nurse's patience is tested; the nurse ultimately needs to remember that the patient's symptoms are an expression of suffering. Agreeing that daily exercise is difficult but continuing to emphasize the importance of exercise can counter some of the reluctance to exercise.

Nutrition Regulation

Patients with SSD often have gastrointestinal problems and may have special nutritional needs. The nurse should discuss the nutritional value of foods with the patient. Because these individuals often take medications that promote weight gain, weight control strategies may be discussed. For overweight individuals, suggest healthy low-calorie food choices. Teach patients about balancing dietary intake with activity levels to increase their awareness of food choices.

Relaxation

Patients taking anxiety-relieving medication can be taught relaxation techniques to alleviate stress. It is a challenge to help these patients really use these strategies. The nurse should consider various techniques, including simple relaxation techniques, distraction, and guided imagery (see Chapter 9).

Medications Interventions

No medication is specifically recommended for patients with SSD; however, psychiatric symptoms of comorbid disorders, such as depression and anxiety, should be treated pharmacologically as appropriate. Usually, the patients who are depressed or anxious are taking an antidepressant to treat their symptoms (see Chapter 19).

Phenelzine (Nardil) is one of the monoamine oxidase inhibitors (MAOIs) that are effective in treating not just depression but also the chronic pain and headaches common in people with SSD. Food–drug interactions are the most serious side effects of MAOIs (Box 23.5). While taking these agents, patients should avoid foods high in tyramine (e.g., aged cheese, sausage, smoked fish, beer) and some OTC cough and cold medications. Additionally, these medications should not be given with selective serotonin reuptake inhibitors SSRIs (see Chapter 10).

Patients with anxiety are treated pharmacologically, similar to those with depression. The first line of treatment for all anxiety disorders is with an SSRI. Doses for SSD are usually higher than those prescribed for depression to relieve and manage the symptoms of the anxiety disorders, including panic, social phobia, generalized anxiety, OCD, and posttraumatic stress disorder.

Nonpharmacologic approaches such as biofeedback and relaxation are also quite useful in conjunction with

BOX 23.5

Drug Profile: Phenelzine (Nardil)

DRUG CLASS: Monoamine oxidase inhibitor (MAOI)

RECEPTOR AFFINITY: Inhibits MAO, an enzyme responsible for breaking down biogenic amines, such as epinephrine, norepinephrine, and serotonin, allowing them to accumulate in neuronal storage sites throughout the central and peripheral nervous systems

INDICATIONS: Treatment of depression characterized as "atypical," "nonendogenous," or "neurotic" or nonresponsive to other antidepressant therapy or in situations in which other antidepressant therapy is contraindicated

ROUTE AND DOSAGE: Available as 15-mg tablets

Adults: Initially, 15 mg PO tid, increasing to at least 60 mg/d at a fairly rapid pace consistent with patient tolerance. Therapy at 60 mg/d may be necessary for at least 4 weeks before response occurs. After maximum benefit has been achieved, the dosage is reduced gradually over several weeks. The maintenance dose may be 15 mg/d or every other day.

Geriatric: Adjust dosage accordingly because patients older than 60 years of age are more prone to develop side effects.

Pediatric: Not recommended for children younger than 16 years of age

HALF-LIFE (PEAK EFEECTS): Unknown (48–96 h)

SELECTED SIDE EFFECTS: Dizziness, vertigo, headache, overactivity, hyperreflexia, tremors, muscle twitching, mania, hypomania, jitteriness, confusion, memory impairment, insomnia, weakness, fatigue, overstimulation, restlessness, increased anxiety, agitation, blurred vision, sweating, constipation, diarrhea, nausea, abdominal pain, edema, dry mouth, anorexia, weight changes, hypertensive crisis, orthostatic hypotension, and disturbed cardiac rate and rhythm

BOXED WARNING: Suicidality in children and adolescents

WARNINGS: Contraindicated in patients with pheochromocytoma, congestive heart failure, hepatic dysfunction, severe renal impairment, cardiovascular disease, history of headache, and myelography within previous 24 h or scheduled within next 48 h. Use cautiously in patients with seizure disorders, hyperthyroidism, pregnancy, lactation, and those scheduled for elective surgery. Possible hypertensive crisis, coma, and severe convulsions may occur if administered with tricyclic antidepressants; possible hypertensive crisis when taken with foods containing tyramine. Increased risk for adverse interaction is possible when given with meperidine. Additive hypoglycemic effect can occur when taken with insulin and oral sulfonylureas.

SPECIFIC PATIENT/FAMILY EDUCATION

- Take drug exactly as prescribed; do not stop taking it abruptly or without consulting your health care provider.
- Families and caregivers of patients should be advised to observe for the emergence of anxiety, agitation, panic attacks, insomnia, irritability, hostility, aggressiveness, impulsivity, akathisia (psychomotor restlessness), hypomania, mania, other unusual changes in behavior, worsening of depression, and suicidal ideation. Such symptoms should be reported to the patient's prescriber or health professional, especially if side effects are severe, abrupt in onset, or were not part of the patient's presenting symptoms.
- Avoid consuming any foods containing tyramine while taking this drug and for 2 weeks afterward.
- Avoid alcohol, sleep-inducing drugs, over-the-counter drugs such as cold and hay fever remedies, and appetite suppressants, all of which may cause serious or life-threatening problems.
- Report any signs and symptoms of side effects.
- Maintain appointments for follow-up blood tests.
- Report any complaints of unusual or severe headache or yellowing of your eyes or skin.
- Avoid driving a car or performing any activities that require alertness.
- Change position slowly when going from a lying to sitting or standing position to minimize dizziness or weakness.

---

pharmacologic treatment. Benzodiazepines may be used initially in the treatment of those with anxiety but should be slowly decreased and discontinued because of the psychological and physiologic dependence associated with these medications. Buspirone (BuSpar), a nonbenzodiazepine, does not lead to tolerance or withdrawal and may be useful for relief of anxiety. If panic disorder is present, it should be treated aggressively.

Pain medication should be prescribed conservatively. If mood disorders are also present, mood stabilizers not only treat the depression but also may treat the pain (Leiknes, Finset, & Moum, 2010).

Administering and Monitoring Medications

In SSD, patients are usually treated in the community, where they commonly self-medicate. Carefully question patients about self-administered medicine and determine which medicines they are currently taking (including OTC and herbal supplements). Also listen carefully to determine any side effects the patient attributes to the medication. This information should be documented and reported to the rest of the team. The patient should be encouraged to continue taking only prescribed medication and to seek approval before taking any additional OTC or other prescribed medications.

Managing Side Effects

These individuals often have atypical reactions to their medications. Side effects should be assessed, but the patient should be encouraged to compare the benefits of the medication with any problems related to side effects. Patients should also be encouraged to give the medications enough time to be effective because many medications require up to 6 weeks before the patient has a response or experiences a relief of symptoms.

Monitoring for Drug Interactions

In working with patients with SSD, always be on the lookout for drug–drug interactions. Medications these patients take for physical problems could interact with psychiatric medications. Patients may be taking alternative medicines, such as herbal supplements, but they usually willingly disclose doing so. The patient should be encouraged to use the same pharmacy for filling all prescriptions so possible interactions can be checked and monitored.

Psychosocial Interventions

The choice of psychosocial intervention depends on the specific problem the patient is experiencing. The most important and ongoing intervention is the maintenance of a therapeutic relationship.

Reduction of Patient Anxiety About Illness

Several interventions are effective in reducing patients' fears of experiencing serious illnesses. cognitive behavioral therapy (CBT), stress management, and group interventions may lead to a decrease in intensity and increase in control of symptoms (Allen & Woolfolk, 2010). Whether the positive outcomes result from the intervention itself or from the symptom validation and increased attention given to the patient remains unknown. Other interventions include the use of antidepressants in reducing depressive and anxiety-related symptoms. Nursing care should include listening to the patient's report of symptoms and fears, validating it by acknowledging that the fears may be real, asking the patient to monitor symptoms in a journal, and encouraging the patient to bring the journal to the next visit. By reviewing the symptom pattern, it is possible to continue to educate the patient and assess for significant symptoms. The outcome of this approach should be a decrease in fears and better control of the symptoms.

Counseling

Counseling with a focus on problem-solving is needed from time to time. These patients often have chaotic lives and need support through the multitude of crises. Although they may appear fascinating and at times self-assured, they can easily irritate others because of their constant complaints. The consequences of their impaired social interaction with others must be examined within a counseling framework. It will become evident that the patient's problem-solving and decision-making skills could be improved. Identifying stresses and strengthening positive coping responses helps the patient deal with a chaotic lifestyle.

Psychoeducation

Health teaching is useful throughout the nurse–patient relationship. These patients have many questions about illnesses, symptoms, and treatments. Emphasize positive health care practices and minimize the effects of serious illness. Because of problems in managing medications and treatment, the therapeutic regimen needs constant monitoring, resulting in ample opportunities for teaching. Patients with SSD should focus on "staying healthy" instead of focusing on their illnesses. For these individuals, approaching the topic of health promotion usually has to be within the context of preventing further problems. Setting aside time for themselves and identifying activities that meet their psychological and spiritual needs, such as going to church or synagogue, are important in maintaining a healthy balance (Box 23.6).

Social Relationships

Patients with SSD are usually isolated from their families and communities. Strengthening social relationships and activities often becomes the focus of the nursing care. The nurse should help the patient identify individuals with whom contact is desired, ask for a commitment to contact them, and encourage them to reinitiate the relationship. The nurse should counsel patients about talking too much about their symptoms with these individuals and emphasize that medical information should be shared with the nurse instead. The nurse must also ensure that patients know when their next appointments are scheduled.

Group Interventions

Although these patients may not be candidates for insight group psychotherapy, they do benefit from cognitive behavioral groups that focus on developing coping skills for everyday life (Allen & Woolfolk, 2010). Because most are women, participation in groups that address feminist issues should be encouraged to strengthen their assertiveness skills and improve their generally low self-esteem.

When leading a group that has members with this disorder, redirection can keep the group from giving too

---

BOX 23.6

Psychoeducation Checklist: Somatic Symptom Disorder

When caring for a patient with SSD, be sure to include the following topic areas in the teaching plan:

- Psychopharmacologic agents (anxiolytics) if ordered, including drug, action, dosage, frequency, and possible side effects
- Nonpharmacologic pain relief measures
- Exercise
- Nutrition
- Social interaction
- Appropriate health care practices
- Problem-solving
- Relaxation and anxiety-reduction techniques
- Sexual functioning

much attention to a person's illness. However, these individuals need reassurance and support while in a group. They may say that they do not fit in or belong in the group. In reality, they are feeling insecure and threatened by the situation. The group leader needs to show patience and understanding to engage the individual effectively in meaningful group interaction.

Family Interventions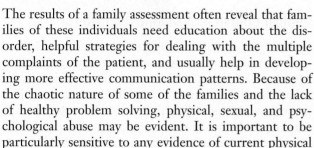

The results of a family assessment often reveal that families of these individuals need education about the disorder, helpful strategies for dealing with the multiple complaints of the patient, and usually help in developing more effective communication patterns. Because of the chaotic nature of some of the families and the lack of healthy problem solving, physical, sexual, and psychological abuse may be evident. It is important to be particularly sensitive to any evidence of current physical or sexual abuse because this may lead to a need for additional interventions.

Evaluation and Treatment Outcomes

Recovery outcomes for patients with SSD should be realistic. Because this is a lifelong disorder, small successes should be expected. Specific outcomes should be identified, such as gradually increasing social contact. Over time, a gradual reduction in the number of health care providers the individual contacts should occur and a slight improvement in the ability to cope with stresses should follow.

Continuum of Care

Inpatient Care

Ideally, individuals with SSD spend minimal time in the hospital for treatment of their medical or comorbid mental disorders. While an inpatient, the patient should have consistency in providers who care or oversee all nursing care. Therapeutic interactions and relationships are very important and can help move the individual toward recovery.

Emergency Care

The emergencies these individuals experience may be physical (e.g., chest pain, back pain, gastrointestinal symptoms) or stress responses related to a psychosocial crisis. Occasionally, these individuals become suicidal and require an intensive level of care. Generally speaking, nonpharmacologic interventions should be tried first, with very conservative use of antianxiety medications. All attempts should be made to retrieve records from other facilities.

Community Treatment

These patients can spend a lifetime in the health care system and still have little continuity of care. Switching from one health care provider to others is detrimental to their long-term care. Most are outpatients. When they are hospitalized, it is usually for evaluation of medical problems or to receive care for comorbid disorders.

ILLNESS ANXIETY DISORDER

Illness anxiety disorder is a new classification in the DSM-5. Previously, the term *hypochondriasis* (or hypochondria) was used to designate this disorder. Most of the persons with hypochondriasis were also diagnosed with somatic symptom disorder. However, there are some individuals who either do not have somatic symptoms or have only very mild symptoms, but who remain preoccupied with having or developing a medical illness (APA, 2013). These individuals would receive the diagnosis of illness anxiety disorder and would be encouraged to seek mental health treatment for their anxiety and preoccupation.

Individuals with illness anxiety disorder are fearful about developing a serious illness based on their misinterpretation of body sensations. The fear of having an illness continues despite medical reassurance and interferes with psychosocial functioning. They spend time and money on repeated examinations looking for feared illnesses. For example, an occasional cough or the appearance of a small sore results in the person's making an appointment with an oncologist. An illness anxiety disorder sometimes appears if the person had had a serious childhood illness or if a family member has a serious illness. See Fame & Fortune.

CONVERSION DISORDER (FUNCTIONAL NEUROLOGIC SYMPTOM DISORDER)

Conversion disorder is a psychiatric condition in which severe emotional distress or unconscious conflict is expressed through physical symptoms (APA, 2013). Patients with conversion disorder have neurologic symptoms that include impaired coordination or balance, paralysis, aphonia (i.e., inability to produce sound), difficulty swallowing or a sensation of a lump in the throat, and urinary retention. They also may have loss of touch, vision problems, blindness, deafness, and hallucinations. In some instances, they may have seizures (Nielsen, Stone, & Edwards, 2013). However, laboratory, electroencephalographic, and neurologic test results are typically negative. The symptoms, different from those with an organic basis, do not follow a neurologic course but rather follow the person's own perceived conceptualization of the problem. For example, if the arm is paralyzed and will not move, reflexes and muscle tone may still be present.

Some evidence suggests that that there are neurobiologic changes in the brains of people with this disorder that may be responsible for the loss of sensation or control of movement. Stress may also be a contributing factor. Published reports state that childhood trauma (e.g., sexual abuse) is associated with the later development of conversion disorder (Kaplan, Dwivedi, Privitera, Isaacs, Hughes, & Bowman, 2013).

It is important to understand that the lack of physical sensation and movement is real for the patient. In approaching this patient, the nurse treats conversion symptoms as real symptoms that may have distressing psychological aspects. Acknowledging the symptoms helps the patient deal with them. As trust develops within the nurse–patient relationship, the nurse can help the patient develop problem-solving approaches to everyday problems.

FACTITIOUS DISORDERS

Persons with **factitious disorders** intentionally cause an illness or injury to receive the attention of health care workers. These individuals are motivated solely by the desire to become a patient and develop a dependent relationship with a health care provider. There are two types of factitious disorders: factitious disorder and factitious disorder imposed on another.

Factitious Disorder

Although feigned illnesses have been described for centuries, it was not until 1951 that the term *Münchausen's*

[sic] *syndrome* was used to describe the most severe form of this disorder, which was characterized by fabricating a physical illness, having recurrent hospitalizations, and going from one health care provider to another (Asher, 1951). Today, this disorder is called *factitious disorder* and is differentiated from malingering, in which the individual who intentionally produces symptoms of illness and is is motivated by another specific self-serving goal, such as being classified as disabled or avoiding work.

Clinical Course and Diagnostic Criteria

Unlike people with borderline personality disorder, who typically injure themselves overtly and readily admit to self-harm, patients with factitious disorder injure themselves covertly. The illnesses are produced in such a manner that the health care provider is tricked into believing that a true physical or psychiatric disorder is present (McDermott, Leamon, Feldman, & Scott, 2010).

The self-produced physical symptoms appear as medical illnesses and involve all body systems. They include seizure disorders, wound-healing disorders, the abscess processes (i.e., introduction of infectious material below the skin surface), and feigned fever (rubbing the thermometer). These patients are extremely creative in simulating illnesses. They tell fascinating but false stories of personal triumph. These tales are referred to as pseudologia fantastica and are a core symptom of the disorder. **Pseudologia fantastica** are stories that are not entirely improbable and often contain a mixture of truth and falsehood. These patients falsify blood, urine, and other samples by contaminating them with protein or fecal matter. They self-inject anticoagulants to receive diagnoses of "bleeding of undetermined origin" or ingest thyroid hormones to produce thyrotoxicosis. They also inflict injury on themselves by inserting objects or feces into body orifices, such as the urinary tract, open wounds, or even intravenous tubing. They produce their own surgical scars, especially abdominal, and when treated surgically, they delay wound healing through scratching, rubbing, or manipulating the wound and introducing bacteria into the wound. These patients put themselves in life-threatening situations through actions such as ingesting allergens known to produce an anaphylactic reaction.

Patients who manifest primarily psychological symptoms produce psychotic symptoms such as hallucinations and delusions, cognitive deficits such as memory loss, dissociative symptoms such as amnesia, and conversion symptoms such as pseudoblindness or pseudoparalysis. These individuals often become psychotic, depressed, or suicidal after an unconfirmed tragedy. When questioned about details, they become defensive and uncooperative.

Sometimes these individuals have a combination of both physical and psychiatric symptoms.

Epidemiology and Risk Factors

The prevalence of factitious disorder is unknown because diagnosing it and obtaining reliable data are difficult. The prevalence was reported to be high when researchers were actually looking for the disorder in specific populations. Within large general hospitals, factitious disorders are diagnosed in about 1% of patients with whom mental health professionals consult. The age range of patients with the disorder is between 19 and 64 years. The median age of onset is the early 20s. formerly thought to occur predominantly in men, this disorder is now reported predominantly in women. No genetic pattern has been identified, but it does seem to run in families. The presence of comorbid psychiatric disorders, such as mood disorders, personality disorders, and substance-related disorders, is common (McDermott, et al., 2010).

Etiology

Many people with factitious disorder have experienced severe sexual or marital distress before the development of the disorder. The psychodynamic explanation is that these individuals, who were often abused as children, received nurturance only during times of illness; thus, they try to recreate illness or injury in a desperate attempt to receive love and attention. During the actual self-injury, the individual is reported to be in a trance-like, dissociative state. Many patients report having an intimate relationship with a health care provider, either as a child or as an adult, and then experiencing rejection when the relationship ended. The self-injury and subsequent attention is an attempt by the individual to re-enact those experiences and gain control over the situation and the other person. Often, the patients exhibit aggression after being discovered, allowing them to express revenge on their perceived tormenter (Feldman, Eisendrath, & Tyerman, 2008).

These patients are usually discovered in medical–surgical settings. They are hostile and distance themselves from others. Their network is void of friends and family and usually consists only of health care providers, who change at regular intervals. In factitious disorder, the patient fabricates a detailed and exaggerated medical history. When the interventions do not work and the fabrication is discovered, the health care team feels manipulated and angry. When the patient is confronted with the evidence, he or she becomes enraged and often leaves that health care system, only to enter another. Eventually, the person is referred for mental health treatment. The course of the disorder usually consists of intermittent episodes (McDermott, et al., 2010).

Evidence-based Nursing Care for Persons with Factitious Disorder

The overall goal of treatment for a patient with factitious disorder is to replace the dysfunctional attention-seeking behaviors with positive behaviors. To begin treatment, the patient must acknowledge the deception. Because the pattern of self-injury is well established and meets overwhelming psychological needs, giving up the behaviors is difficult. The treatment is long-term psychotherapy. The psychiatric–mental health nurse will most likely care for the patient during or after periods of feigned illnesses.

Mental Health Nursing Assessment

A nursing assessment should focus on obtaining a history of medical and psychological illnesses. Physical disabilities should be identified. Early childhood experiences, particularly instances of abuse, neglect, or abandonment, should be identified to understand the underlying psychological dynamics of the individual and the role of self-injury. Family assessment is important because family relationships become strained as the members become aware of the self-inflicted nature of this disorder.

Nursing Diagnoses

The nursing diagnoses could include almost any diagnosis, including Risk for Trauma, Risk for Self-Mutilation, Ineffective Individual Coping, or Low Self-Esteem.

Desired outcomes include decreased self-injurious behavior and increased positive coping behaviors. Any nursing intervention must be implemented within the context of a strong nurse–patient relationship.

Nursing Interventions

The fabrications and deceits of patients with factitious disorder provoke anger and a sense of betrayal in many nurses. To be effective with these patients, it is important to be aware of these feelings and resolve them by developing a better understanding of the underlying psychodynamic issues. Confronting the patient has been reported to be effective if the patient feels supported and accepted and if there is clear communication among the patient, the mental health care team, and family members. All care should be centralized within one facility. The patient should see health care providers regularly even when not in active crisis. Offering the patient a face-saving way of giving up the behaviors is often crucial. Behavioral techniques that shape new behaviors help the patient move forward toward a new life.

The health care team that knows the patient, agrees on a treatment approach, and follows through is crucial to the patient's eventual recovery. For this to happen, the medical, psychiatric, inpatient, and outpatient teams need to communicate with each other on a regular basis. Family members must also be aware of the need for consistent treatment.

Factitious Disorder Imposed on Another

A rare but dramatic disorder, **factitious disorder imposed on another** (previously *factitious disorder by proxy* or *Münchausen's* [sic] *by proxy*), involves a person who inflicts injury on another person. It is commonly a mother, who inflicts injuries on her child to gain the attention of the health care provider through her child's injuries. These actions include inducing seizures, poisoning, or smothering. This most severe form of child abuse is usually identified in the emergency department. The mother rarely admits injuring the child and thus is not amenable to treatment; the child is frequentlyremoved from the mother's care. This form of child abuse is distinguished from other forms by the routine unwitting involvement of health care workers, who subject the child to physical harm and emotional distress through tests, procedures, and medication trials. Some researchers suspect that children who are abused in this way may later experience factitious disorder themselves (McDermott, et al., 2010).

SUMMARY OF KEY POINTS

- Somatization is affected by sociocultural and gender factors. It occurs more frequently in women than men and in those who are less educated. It also has been strongly associated with individuals who have been sexually abused as children.

- SSD is a chronic relapsing condition characterized by multiple physical symptoms of unknown origin that develop during times of emotional distress.

- Conversion disorder is a condition of neurologic symptoms (e.g., impaired voluntary muscles or sensory stimulation) that is associated with severe emotional distress.

- Factitious disorders include two types, factitious disorder and factitious disorder imposed on another. In factitious disorder, physical or psychological symptoms (or both) are fabricated to assume the sick role. In factitious disorder imposed on another, the intentional production of symptoms is in others, usually children.

- Identifying somatic symptom disorders is very complex because patients with these disorders refuse to accept any psychiatric basis to their health problems and often go for years moving from one health care provider to another to receive medical attention and avoid psychiatric assessment.

- These patients are often seen on the medical–surgical units of hospitals and go years without receiving a correct diagnosis. In most cases, they finally receive mental health treatment for comorbid conditions, such as depression, anxiety, and panic disorder.

- The development of the nurse–patient relationship is crucial to assessing these patients and identifying appropriate nursing diagnoses and interventions. Because these patients deny any psychiatric basis to their problem and continue to focus on their symptoms as being medically based, the nurse must take a flexible, relaxed, and nonjudgmental approach that acknowledges the symptoms but focuses on new ways of coping with stress and avoiding recurrence of symptoms.

- Health teaching is important to help the individual develop positive lifestyle changes in place of somatization responses. Identifying personal strengths and supporting the development of positive skills improve self-esteem and personal confidence. Teaching the use of stress management provides the patient with positive coping skills.

CRITICAL THINKING CHALLENGES

1. A depressed young woman is admitted to a psychiatric unit in a state of agitation. She reports extreme abdominal pain. Her admitting provider tells you that she has a classic case of somatization disorder and to de-emphasize her physical symptoms. Under no circumstances can she have any more pain medication. Conceptualize the assessment process and how you would approach this patient.

2. Develop a continuum of "self-injury" for patients with borderline personality disorder, SSD, factitious disorder, and factitious disorder imposed on another.

3. Develop a teaching plan for an individual who has a long history of somatization but who recently received a diagnosis of breast cancer. How will the patient be able to differentiate the physical symptoms of somatization from those associated with the treatment of her breast cancer?

4. A Chinese American patient was admitted for panic attacks and numerous somatic problems, ranging from dysmenorrhea to painful joints. The results of all medical examinations have been negative. She truly believes that her panic attacks are caused by a weak heart. What approaches should the nurse use in providing culturally sensitive nursing care?

5. A person with depression is started on a regimen of phenelzine, 15 mg three times a day. She believes that she is allergic to most foods but insists on having wine in the evenings because it helps digest her food. Develop a teaching plan that provides the knowledge that she needs to prevent a hypertensive crisis caused by excessive tyramine but that is sensitive to the patient's food preferences.

 Safe: 1995. This is a story of Carol White (Julianne Moore), a married stay-at-home mother who appears to have everything. She begins having headaches that lead to a grand mal seizure. As the movie unfolds, she becomes sicker and sicker as she reports she is allergic to environmental toxins. She seeks help from an allergist and psychiatrists. She eventually leaves her husband for a retreat that is actually a scam.

Significance: The film depicts the pain and suffering that is characteristic of somatization and its impact on the family. It also shows how desperate a person can be to seek out relief of symptoms.

Viewing Points: Identify the mistakes in recognizing and treating the somatic disorder.

REFERENCES

Allen, L. A., & Woolfolk, R. L. (2010). Cognitive behavioral therapy for somatoform disorders. *Psychiatric Clinics of North America, 33*(3), 579–593.

American Psychiatric Association (APA). (2013). *Diagnostic and Statistical Manual of Mental Disorders* (5th ed). Arlington, VA: American Psychiatric Association.

Anderson, G., Maes, M., & Berk, M. (2012). Biological underpinnings of the commonalties in depression, somatization, and Chronic Fatigue Syndrome. *Medical Hypotheses, 78*(6), 752–756.

Asher, R. (1951). Münchausen's syndrome. *Lancet, 1,* 339–341.

Boutros, N. N., & Peters, R. (2012). Internal gating and somatization disorders: Proposing a yet un-described neural system. *Medical Hypotheses. 78*(1), 174–178.

Deng, Y., Ma, X., & Tang, Q. (2013). Brain response during visual emotional processing: An fMRI study of alexithymia. *Psychiatry Research, 213*(3), 225–229.

Dere, J., Sun, J., Zhao, Y., Persson, T., Zhu, X., Yao, S., et al. (2013). Beyond "somatization" and "psychologization": Symptom-level variation in depressed Han Chinese and Euro-Canadian outpatients. *Frontiers in Psychology, 4,* 377, doi:10.3389/fpsyg.2013.00377.

Dumont, I. P., & Olson, A. L. (2012). Primary care, expression, and anxiety: Exploring somatic and emotional predictors of mental health status in adolescents. *Journal of the American Board of Family Medicine, 25*(3), 291–299.

Fabião, C., Silva, M. C., Fleming, M., & Barbosa, A. (2010). Somatoform disorders: A revision of the epidemiology in primary health care. *Acta Medica Portuguesa, 23*(5), 865–872.

Fava, G.A., Guidi, J., Porcelli, P., Rafanelli, C., Bellomo, A., Grandi, S., Grassi, L., ...Sonino, M. (2012). A cluster analysis-derived classification of psychological distress and illness behavior in the medically ill. *Psychological Medicine, 42*(2), 401–407.

Feldman, M. D., Eisendrath, S. J., & Tyerman, M. (2008). Psychiatric and behavioral correlates of factitious blindness. *Comprehensive Psychiatry, 49*(2), 159–162.

Leiknes, K. A., Finset, A., & Moum, T. (2010). Commonalities and differences between the diagnostic groups: Current somatoform disorders, anxiety and/or depression, and musculoskeletal disorders. *Journal of Psychosomatic Research, 68*(5), 439–446.

Kaplan, M. M., Dwivedi, A. K., Privitera, M. D., Isaacs, K., Hughes, C., & Bowman, M. (2013). Comparisons of childhood trauma, alexithymia, and defensive styles in patients with psychogenic non-epileptic seizures vs. epilepsy: Implications for the etiology of conversion disorder. *Journal of Psychosomatic Research, 75*(2), 142–146.

Krishnan, V., Sood, M., & Chadda, R. K. (2013). Caregiver burden and disability in somatization disorder. *Journal of Psychosomatic Research, 75*(4), 376–380.

McDermott, B. E., Leamon, M. H., Feldman, M. D., & Scott, C. L. (2010). Factitious disorder and malingering. In R. E. Hales, S. C. Yudofsky, & G. O. Gabbard (Eds.). *The American Psychiatric Publishing Textbook of Clinical Psychiatry* (5th ed.). Arlington, VA: American Psychiatric Publishing.

Mik-Meyer, N., & Obling, A. R. (2012). The negotiation of the sick role: General practitioners; classification of patients with medically unexplained symptoms. *Sociology of Health & Illness, 34*(7), 1025–1038.

Moreno, S., Gili, M., Magallón, R., Bauzá, N., Rocal, M., Hoyo, Y. L., et al. (2013). Effectiveness of group versus individual cognitive-behavioral therapy in patients with abridged somatization disorder: A randomized controlled trial. *Psychosomatic Medicine, 75*(6), 600–608.

Nielsen, G., Stone, J., & Edwards, J. J. (2013). Physiotherapy for functional (psychogenic) motor symptoms: A systematic review. *Journal of Psychosomatic Research, 75*(2), 93–102.

Noyes, R. Jr., Langbehn, D., Happel, R., Sieren, L., & Muller, B. (1999). Health Attitude Survey: A scale for assessing somatizing patients. *Psychosomatics, 40*(6), 470–478.

Pedrosa, G. F., Ridout, N., Kessler, H., Neuffer, M., Schoechlin, C., Traue, H. C., et al. (2009). Facial emotion recognition and alexithymia in adults with somatoform disorders. *Depression and Anxiety, 26*(1), e26–e33.

Rief, W., & Broadbent, E. (2007). Explaining medically unexplained symptoms-models and mechanisms. *Clinical Psychology Review, 27*(7), 821–841.

Schulte, I. E., & Petermann, F. (2011). Somatoform disorders: 30 years of debate about criteria? What about children and adolescents? *Journal of Psychosomatic Research, 70*(3), 218–228.

Sharma, M. P., & Manjula, M. (2013). Behavioural and psychological management of somatic symptom disorders: An overview. *International Review of Psychiatry, 25*(1), 116–124

Spangenberg, L., Forkmann, T., Brahler, E., & Glaesmer, H. (2011). The association of depression and multimorbidity in the elderly: Implications for the assessment of depression. *Psychogeriatrics, 11*(4), 227–234.

van Dijke, A., Ford, J. D., van der Hart, O., van Son, M., van der Heijden, P., & Bühring, M. (2010). Affect dysregulation in borderline personality disorder and somatoform disorder: Differentiating under- and over-regulation. *Journal of Personality Disorders, 24*(3), 296–311.

Woolfolk, R. L., Allen, L. A., & Tiu, J. E. (2007). New directions in the treatment of somatization. *Psychiatric Clinics of North America, 30*(4), 21–44.

Yusim, A., Anbarasan, D., Hall, B., Goetz, R., Neugebauer, R., Stewart, T., et al. (2010). Sociocultural domains of depression among indigenous populations in Latin America. *International Review of Psychiatry, 22*(4), 370–377.

Zaroff, C. M., Davis, J. M., Chio, P. H., & Madhavan, D. (2012). Somatic presentations of distress in China. *Australian and New Zealand Journal of Psychiatry, 46*(11), 1053–1057.

Zink, T., Klesges, L., Stevens, S., & Decker, P. (2009). The development of a sexual abuse severity score: Characteristics of childhood sexual abuse associated with trauma symptomatology, somatization, and alcohol abuse. *Journal of Interpersonal Violence, 24*(3), 395–405.

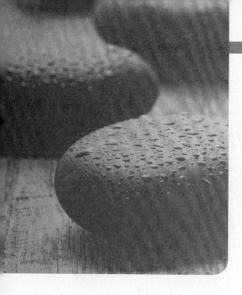

24
Eating Disorders

Nursing Care of Persons with Eating and Weight-Related Disorders

Jane H. White

KEY CONCEPTS

- body dissatisfaction
- body image distortion
- dietary restraint

- drive for thinness
- interoceptive awareness
- perfectionism

LEARNING OBJECTIVES

After studying this chapter, you will be able to:

1. Distinguish the signs and symptoms of anorexia nervosa from those of bulimia nervosa.

2. Describe theories explaining anorexia nervosa and bulimia nervosa.

3. Differentiate binge-eating disorder from anorexia nervosa and bulimia nervosa.

4. Describe the risk factors and protective factors associated with the development of eating disorders.

5. Explain the importance of body image, body dissatisfaction, and gender identity in developmental theories that explain etiology of eating disorders.

6. Explain the impact of sociocultural norms on the development of eating disorders.

7. Formulate the nursing diagnoses for individuals with eating disorders.

8. Analyze special concerns within the therapeutic relationship for the nursing care of individuals with eating disorders.

9. Develop recovery-oriented nursing interventions for individuals with anorexia nervosa and bulimia nervosa.

10. Identify strategies for prevention and early detection of eating disorders.

KEY TERMS

• anorexia nervosa • binge-eating • binge-eating disorder (BED) • bulimia nervosa (BN) • cue elimination • enmeshment • night eating syndrome • self-monitoring • purge • purging disorder

Case Study: Ellen

Ellen is a 20-year old-college sophomore admitted to an inpatient mental health unit after treatment on a medical unit where she was admitted for electrolyte imbalance and dehydration. Ellen has been binging and purging while in college to maintain a normal body weight.

INTRODUCTION

Only since the 1970s have eating disorders received national attention, primarily because several high-profile personalities and athletes with these disorders have received front-page news coverage. Since the 1960s, the increased incidence of anorexia nervosa and bulimia nervosa has prompted mental health professionals to address their causes and to devise effective treatments.

This chapter focuses on anorexia nervosa and bulimia nervosa and more briefly discusses binge-eating-disorder (BED). Eating disorders differ in definition, clinical course, causes, and interventions and are presented separately in this chapter. However, symptoms of these disorders, such as dieting, binge-eating, and preoccupation with weight and shape overlap significantly. Viewing the symptoms along a continuum from less- to more-severe eating behaviors helps with this conceptualization, as shown in Figure 24.1 (Dennard & Richards, 2013). People with eating disorders share common psychological characteristics (Box 24.1). Subclinical cases, also called partial syndromes, are usually diagnosed as Eating Disorder Not Otherwise Specified (EDNOS). These individuals still need treatment despite not meeting criteria for anorexia nervosa or bulimia nervosa.

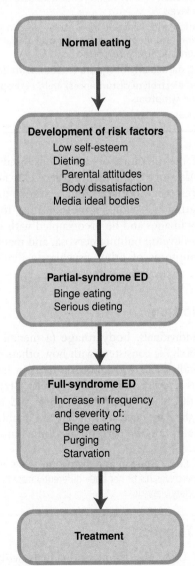

FIGURE 24.1 Progression of symptoms leading to an eating disorder.

BOX 24.1

Psychological Characteristics Related to Eating Disorders

ANOREXIA NERVOSA
Decreased interoceptive awareness
Sexuality conflict or fears
Maturity fears
Ritualistic behaviors

BULIMIA NERVOSA
Impulsivity
Boundary problems
Limit-setting difficulties

ANOREXIA NERVOSA AND BULIMIA NERVOSA
Difficulty expressing anger
Low self-esteem
Body dissatisfaction
Powerlessness
Ineffectiveness
Perfectionism
Dietary restraint
Obsessiveness
Compulsiveness
Nonassertiveness
Cognitive distortions

ANOREXIA NERVOSA

Anorexia nervosa is a mixture of symptoms that include significantly low body weight, intense fear of gaining weight or becoming fat, and a disturbance in experiencing body weight or shape (undue influence or distorted self-evaluation of body weight or shape or lack of recognition of the seriousness of low body weight).

Anorexia nervosa is further categorized into two major types: *restricting* (dieting and exercising with no binge-eating or misuse of laxatives, diuretics, or enemas) and *binge-eating and purging* (binge-eating and misuse of laxatives, diuretics, or enemas). Malnutrition and semistarvation result in a preoccupation with food, binge-eating, depression, obsession, and apathy, as well as compromising several body systems, leading to medical complications and, in some instances, death (American Psychiatric Association [APA], 2013). See Table 24.1 for a list of complications from eating disorders.

Clinical Course

The onset of anorexia nervosa usually occurs in early adolescence. The onset may be slow with serious dieting occurring before an emaciated body—the result of starvation—is noticed. This discovery often prompts diagnosis. Because the incidence of subclinical or partial-syndrome cases, in which the symptoms are not severe enough to diagnose anorexia nervosa, is higher than that of anorexia nervosa, many young women may not receive early treatment for their symptoms, or in some cases, they may

TABLE 24.1	COMPLICATIONS OF EATING DISORDERS
Body System	Symptoms
Relating to Starvation and Weight Loss	
Musculoskeletal	Loss of muscle mass, loss of fat (emaciation), osteoporosis
Metabolic	Hypothyroidism (its symptoms include lack of energy, weakness, intolerance to cold, and bradycardia), hypoglycemia, decreased insulin sensitivity
Cardiac	Bradycardia; hypotension; loss of cardiac muscle; diminished cardiac muscle; cardiac arrhythmias, including atrial and ventricular premature contractions, prolonged QT interval, ventricular tachycardia, sudden death syndrome
Gastrointestinal	Delayed gastric emptying, bloating, constipation, abdominal pain, gas, diarrhea
Reproductive	Amenorrhea, low levels of luteinizing hormone and follicle-stimulating hormone, irregular menses
Dermatologic	Dry cracking skin and brittle nails caused by dehydration, lanugo (fine, baby-like hair over the body), edema, acrocyanosis (bluish hands and feet), thinning hair
Hematologic	Leukopenia, anemia, thrombocytopenia, hypercholesterolemia, hypercarotenemia
Neuropsychiatric	Abnormal taste sensation (related to possible zinc deficiency) Apathetic depression, mild organic mental symptoms, sleep disturbances, fatigue
Related to Purging (Vomiting and Laxative Abuse)	
Metabolic	Electrolyte abnormalities, particularly hypokalemia, hypochloremic alkalosis; hypomagnesemia; increased blood urea nitrogen levels
Gastrointestinal	Salivary gland and pancreatic inflammation and enlargement with increase in serum amylase, esophageal and gastric erosion (esophagitis) rupture, dysfunctional bowel syndrome with dilation, superior mesenteric artery syndrome
Dental	Erosion of dental enamel (perimylolysis), particularly of the front teeth, with decay
Neuropsychiatric	Seizures (related to large fluid shifts and electrolyte disturbances), mild neuropathies, fatigue, weakness, mild organic mental symptoms
Cardiac	Ipecac-related cardiomyopathy arrhythmias

never receive treatment. The individual's refusal to maintain a normal weight because of a distorted body image and an intense fear of becoming fat make individuals with this disorder difficult to identify and treat.

It can be a chronic condition with relapses that are usually characterized by significant weight loss. Reporting conclusive outcomes for anorexia nervosa is difficult because of the plethora of definitions used to signify recovery. Although patients considered to have recovered have restored normal weight, resumed menses, and changed eating behaviors, some continue to have distorted body images and be preoccupied with weight and food; many develop bulimia nervosa; and many continue to have symptoms of other psychiatric illnesses, especially of the anxiety disorders.

Body Distortion

For most individuals, **body image** (a mental picture of one's own body) is consistent with how others view them. However, individuals with anorexia nervosa have a body image that is severely distorted from reality. Because of this distortion, they see themselves as obese and undesirable even when they are emaciated. They are unable to accept objective reality and the perceptions of the outside world.

> **KEYCONCEPT** **Body image distortion** occurs when the individual perceives his or her body differently from how the world or society views it.

Drive for Thinness

Because of body distortion, individuals with anorexia nervosa have an intense drive for thinness. They see

---

FAME & FORTUNE

Karen Carpenter (1950–1983)
An American Musician

PUBLIC PERSONA

Karen Carpenter and her brother were the top best-selling American recording artists and performing musicians of the 1970s. In the United States alone, the Carpenters had eight gold albums, five platinum albums, and 10 gold single recordings—all proof of significant professional success.

PERSONAL REALITIES

In everyday life, however, Karen Carpenter battled with anorexia nervosa for 7 years—starving herself, using laxatives, drinking water, taking dozens of thyroid pills, and purging. Just as she was beginning to overcome the disorder, she died of complications at 32 years of age.

themselves as fat, fear becoming fatter, and are "driven" to work toward "undoing" this fear.

> **KEYCONCEPT** **Drive for thinness** is an intense physical and emotional process that overrides all physiologic body cues.

The individual with anorexia nervosa ignores body cues, such as hunger and weakness, and concentrates all efforts on controlling food intake. The entire mental focus of the young patient with anorexia nervosa narrows to only one goal: weight loss. Typical thought patterns are: "If I gain a pound, I'll keep gaining." This all-or-nothing thinking keeps these patients on rigid regimens for weight loss.

The behavior of patients with anorexia nervosa becomes organized around food-related activities, such as preparing food, counting calories, and reading cookbooks. Much behavior concerning what, when, and how they eat is ritualistic. Food combinations and the order in which foods may be eaten, and under which circumstances, can seem bizarre. One patient, for example, would eat only cantaloupe, carrying it with her to all meals outside of her home and consuming it only if it were cut in smaller than bite-sized pieces and only if she could use chopsticks, which she also carried with her.

Interoceptive Awareness

Feelings of inadequacy and a fear of maturity are also characteristic of individuals with anorexia nervosa. Weight loss becomes a way for these individuals to experience some sense of control and combat feelings of inadequacy and ineffectiveness. Every lost pound is viewed as a success; weight loss often confers a feeling of virtuousness. Because these individuals feel inadequate, they fear emotional maturation and the unknown challenges the next developmental stages will bring. For some, remaining physically small is believed to symbolize remaining childlike. Patients with anorexia nervosa also have difficulty defining their feelings because they are confused about or unsure about emotions and visceral cues, such as hunger. This uncertainty is called a lack of interoceptive awareness.

> **KEYCONCEPT** **Interoceptive awareness** is a term used to describe the sensory response to emotional and visceral cues, such as hunger.

Patients with anorexia nervosa are confused about sensations; therefore, their responses to cues are inaccurate and inappropriate. Often they cannot name the feelings they are experiencing, such as anxiety. This profound lack of interoceptive awareness is thought to be partially responsible for developing and maintaining this disorder and some types of bulimia nervosa.

Perfectionism

Perfectionistic behavior, such as making sure that everything is symmetric or that objects are placed the same distance from each other, is a typically significant symptom of both anorexia nervosa and bulimia nervosa. It is hypothesized to develop long before eating symptoms occur. Perfectionism has been highlighted as a significant personality symptom risk factor in eating disorders (Kaye, Wierenga, Bailer, Simmons, & Bischoff-Greffe, 2013a).

> **KEYCONCEPT** **Perfectionism** consists of personal standards (the extent to which the individual sets and tries to achieve high standards for oneself) and concern over mistakes and their consequences for their self-worth and others' opinions.

It is now accepted that perfectionism precedes the development of weight and shape concerns. The more severe the disorder, the more perfectionistic (Kaye, Weirenga, Bailer, Simmons, Wagner, & Bischoff-Grethe, 2013b). As symptoms are resolved, perfectionism decreases (Bardone-Cone, Strum, Lawson, Robinson, & Smith, 2010).

Guilt and Anger

Patients with anorexia nervosa tend to avoid conflict and have difficulty expressing negative emotions, especially anger (Manuel & Wade, 2013). They have an overwhelming sense of guilt and anger, which leads to conflict avoidance, commonly seen in these families. Because of the ritualistic behaviors, an all-encompassing focus on food and weight, and feelings of inadequacy, social contacts are gradually reduced, so that the patient becomes isolated. With more severe weight loss comes other symptoms, such as apathy, depression, and even mistrust of others.

Outcomes

Short-term outcomes for individuals with anorexia nervosa after hospitalization are poor. About 30% usually have a good outcome, 9% a more intermediate outcome, and 55% a poor outcome (Salbach-Andrae, Schneider, Seifert, Pfeiffer, Lenz, Lehmkuhl, et al., 2009). Poor outcomes are related to a low body mass index (BMI) at the beginning of treatment, premorbid depression, comorbidity, and purging (vomiting and laxative use) (Berner, Shaw, Witt, & Lowe, 2013; Keski-Rahkonen, Raevuori, Bulik, Hoek, Rissanen, & Kaprio, 2014). Readiness to change and the rate of weight restoration are associated with a positive outcome for inpatient treatment (Lund, Hernandez, Yates, Mitchell, & McKee, 2009).

Long-term outcomes are more positive than short-term outcomes, probably because of increased awareness of the disorder, early detection, and outpatient treatment after hospitalization. Approximately 70% of individuals with anorexia nervosa are said to have recovered 5 years after diagnosis (Keski-Rahkonen, Hoek, Susser, Linna, Sihvola, Raevuori, et al., 2007).

Diagnostic Criteria

Anorexia nervosa is diagnosed when a restriction of intake has led to significantly low body weight. The BMI is used as a measure of severity. Other criteria include an intense fear of gaining weight or becoming fat, as well as body image issues including an undue influence of body weight on self-concept and lack of recognition of seriousness of low body weight

(APA, 2103). See Key Diagnostic Characteristics 24.1 for an overview of diagnostic criteria and associated findings.

Epidemiology

In the United States, the lifetime prevalence of anorexia nervosa is reported to be from 0.5% to 1%. Despite prevention and early intervention efforts, the incidence (new cases) for anorexia nervosa has remained the same during the past decade at about 270 per 100,000 (Keski-Rahkonen, et al., 2007). These findings lend support to the hypothesis that a biologic or genetic predisposition for the development of anorexia nervosa exists.

KEY DIAGNOSTIC CHARACTERISTICS 24.1 • ANOREXIA NERVOSA

Diagnostic Criteria

A. Restriction of energy intake relative to requirements, leading to a significantly low body weight in the context of age, sex, developmental trajectory, and physical health. *Significantly low weight* is defined as a weight that is less than minimally normal or, for children and adolescents, less than that is minimally expected.

B. Intense fear of gaining weight or of becoming fat, or persistent behavior that interferes with weight gain, even though at a significantly low weight.

C. Disturbance in the way in which one's body weight or shape is experienced, undue influence of body weight or shape on self-evaluation, or persistent lack of recognition of the seriousness of the current low body weight. *Specify* whether:

- **Restricting type:** During the last 3 months, the individual has not engaged in recurrent episodes of binge-eating or purging behavior (i.e., self-induced vomiting or the misuse of laxatives, diuretics, or enemas). This subtype describes presentations in which weight loss is accomplished primarily through dieting, fasting, and/or excessive exercise.
- **Binge-eating/purging type:** During the last 3 months, the individual has engaged in recurrent episodes of binge-eating or purging behavior (i.e., self-induced vomiting or the misuse of laxatives, diuretics, or enemas).

Specify if:
- **In partial remission:** After full criteria for anorexia nervosa were previously met, Criterion A (low body weight) has not been met for a sustained period, but either Criterion B (intense fear of gaining weight or becoming fat or behavior that interferes with weight gain) or Criterion C (disturbances in self-perception of weight and shape) is still met.
- **In full remission:** After full criteria for anorexia nervosa were previously met, none of the criteria have been met for a sustained period of time.
- *Specify* current severity:
The minimum level of severity is based, for adults, on current body mass index (BMI) (see below) or, for children and adolescents, on BMI percentile. The ranges below are derived from World Health Organization categories for thinness in adults; for children and adolescents, corresponding BMI percentiles should be used. The level of severity may be

increased to reflect clinical symptoms, the degree of functional disability, and the need for supervision.
- **Mild:** BMI $\geq$ 17 kg/m^2
- **Moderate:** BMI 16–16.99 kg/m^2
- **Severe:** BMI 15–15.99 kg/m^2
- **Extreme:** BMI < 15 kg/m^2

Target Symptoms and Associated Findings
- Depressive symptoms such as depressed mood, social withdrawal, irritability, insomnia, and diminished interest in sex
- Obsessive-compulsive features related and unrelated to food
- Preoccupation with thought of food
- Concerns about eating in public
- Feelings of ineffectiveness
- Strong need to control one's environment
- Inflexible thinking
- Limited social spontaneity and overly restrained initiative and emotional expression

Associated Physical Examination Findings
- Complaints of constipation, abdominal pain
- Cold intolerance
- Lethargy and excess energy
- Emaciation
- Significant hypotension, hypothermia, and skin dryness
- Bradycardia and possible peripheral edema
- Hypertrophy of salivary glands, particularly the parotid gland
- Dental enamel erosion related to induced vomiting
- Scars or calluses on dorsum of hand from contact with teeth for inducing vomiting

Associated Laboratory Findings
- Leukopenia and mild anemia
- Elevated blood urea nitrogen
- Hypercholesterolemia
- Elevated liver function studies
- Electrolyte imbalances, metabolic alkalosis, or metabolic acidosis
- Low normal serum thyroxine levels; decreased serum-triiodothyronine levels
- Sinus bradycardia
- Metabolic encephalopathy
- Significantly reduced resting energy expenditure
- Increased ventricular/brain ratio secondary to starvation

Age of Onset

The age of onset is typically between 14 and 16 years but can occur much earlier. Adolescents are vulnerable because of stressors associated with their development, especially concerns about body image, autonomy, and peer pressure, and their susceptibility to such influences as the media, which extols an ideal body type. An important predictor of anorexia nervosa is early-onset menses, as early as 10 or 11 years of age (Favaro, Caregaro, Tenconi, Bosello, & Santonastaso, 2009).

Gender

Females are 10 times more likely than males to develop anorexia nervosa. This disparity has been attributed to society's influence on females to achieve an ideal body type (Zhao & Encinosa, 2011). Box 24.2 highlights some of the findings about eating disorders in males.

Ethnicity and Culture

In the United States, eating disorders occur in all ethnic and racial groups, but they are slightly more common among Hispanic and white populations and less common among African Americans and Asians (Rhea & Thatcher, 2013). Since the 1990s, incidence among various ethnic groups, especially ethnic minority groups, has increased. Contextual variables that may influence eating disorders in women of color are level of acculturation, socioeconomic status, level of education, peer socialization,

family structure, and immigration status (Gordon, Castro, Sitnikov, & Holm-Denoma, 2010).

Comorbidity

Depression is common in individuals with anorexia nervosa, and these individuals are at risk to attempt suicide (Preti, Rocchi, Sisti, Camboni, & Miotto, 2011). However, anxiety disorders such as obsessive-compulsive disorder (OCD), phobias, and panic disorder are even more strongly associated with anorexia nervosa. In many individuals with anorexia nervosa, OCD symptoms predate the diagnosis of anorexia nervosa by about 5 years, leading many researchers to consider OCD a causative or risk factor for anorexia nervosa (Brady, 2014). In fact, perfectionism is an aspect of both OCD and anorexia nervosa and is considered a risk factor for anorexia nervosa (Kaye, et al., 2013a). These comorbid conditions often resolve when anorexia nervosa has been treated successfully.

Etiology

The causes of anorexia nervosa are multidimensional. Some risk factors (discussed later) and etiologic factors overlap. For example, dieting is a risk factor for the development of anorexia nervosa, but it is also a etiologic factor, and in its most serious form—starving—it is also a symptom.

Biologic Theories

Brain structure in the medial orbitofrontal cortex and striatum is altered in eating disorders, suggesting brain circuitry has been altered. Pleasantness in taste and sensitivity to reward in individuals with anorexia nervosa are also associated with alterations in cerebral structures (Frank, Shott, Hagman, & Mittal, 2013).

Genetic Theories

First-degree relatives of people with anorexia nervosa have higher rates of this disorder. Rates of partial-syndrome or subthreshold cases among female family members of individuals with anorexia nervosa are even higher (Kaye, et al., 2013a). Female relatives also have high rates of depression, leading researchers to hypothesize that a shared genetic factor may influence development of both disorders.

Genetic research shows that there is a genetic vulnerability to anorexia nervosa, especially in females (Baker, Maes, Lissner, Aggen, Lichtenstein, & Kendler, 2009; Kaye, et al., 2013a). Genetic heritability accounts for an estimated 50% to 80% of the risk of developing an eating disorder (Kaye, et al., 2013a). Separating genetic influences from environmental influences is difficult when twins share a similar family environment.

BOX 24.2

Boys and Men with Eating Disorders

Eating disorders in boys and men are becoming more prevalent. Men are more likely to have a later onset than women, at around age 20.5 years. Boys and men are also more likely to be involved in an occupation or sport in which weight control influences performance, such as wrestling, or sports in which low body fat is advantageous (Sabel, Rosen, & Mehler, 2014).

Men with anorexia nervosa of the restricting type were found to have lower testosterone levels. In addition to having a drive for thinness, men with disordered eating can also be characterized by a drive to gain weight and put on muscle. Childhood risk factors in men for the development of an eating disorder are similar to those in women in that body-focused and social behaviors were prevalent. In addition, familial taboo about nudity and less caressing from family members are also found in childhood experiences of men who develop eating disorders. Men and women do not differ with regard to comorbid conditions, such as depression and substance abuse, but men have less reported sexual abuse than do women with eating disorders. In community samples, boys and men have higher rates of eating disorders than in clinical samples, leading researchers to the hypothesis that eating disorders may go undiagnosed in boys and men and that rates are higher than commonly reported (Mangweth-Matzek, Rupp, Hausman, Gusmerotti, Kemmler, & Biebl, 2010).

Neuroendocrine and Neurotransmitter Changes

Several neurobiologic changes occur in patients with an eating disorder. An increase in endogenous opioids (through exercise) contributes to denial of hunger. Malnutrition leads to a decrease in thyroid function. Serotonergic functioning is also blunted in low-weight patients (Frank, 2011).

Psychological Theories

Historically, the most widely accepted explanation of anorexia nervosa was the psychoanalytic paradigm that focused on conflicts of separation–individuation and autonomy. Usually diagnosed between 14 and 18 years of age, anorexia nervosa was thought to result from a developmental arrest of normal adolescent struggles around identity and role, body image formation, and sexuality (Bruch, 1973). Dieting and weight control were viewed as a means to defend against these feelings of inadequacy and growing into adulthood.

The psychoanalytic paradigm explained the disparity in the prevalence of eating disorders between boys and girls as being related to the development of self-esteem in adolescent girls. It was believed that the normal adolescent increase in self-doubt was linked to naturally occurring pubertal weight gain, which in turn resulted in confusion about one's identity. Unfortunately, this psychoanalytic perspective tended to blame parents, especially mothers, for the development of their child's illness. Today, the psychoanalytic theory is used in some psychotherapies, but it is no longer a compelling theory of causation.

Internalization of Peer Pressure

Some adolescents have reported that dieting, binge-eating, and purging were learned behaviors, resulting from peer pressure and a need to conform. Peers and friends, as well as peers in the larger school system, influence unhealthy weight-control behaviors among preadolescent and adolescent girls (Cave, 2009; Wilkosz, Chen, Kenndey, & Rankin, 2011).

Body Dissatisfaction

When the body is considered all important, the individual begins to compare her body with others, such as those of celebrities. Images from television and fashion magazines are particularly powerful for young girls and adolescents struggling with the tasks of identity and body image formation. Body dissatisfaction resulting from this comparison, in which one's own body is perceived to fall short of an ideal, may include dissatisfaction about one's weight, shape, size, or even a certain body part. Even in the absence of overweight, most adolescents surveyed in numerous studies were dissatisfied with their bodies (van den Berg, Mond, Eisenberg, Ackard, & Neumark-Sztainer, 2010).

KEYCONCEPT **Body dissatisfaction** occurs when the body becomes overvalued as a way of determining one's worth. Body dissatisfaction is strongly related to low self-esteem (van den Berg, et al., 2010).

Many adolescents attempt to overcome this dissatisfaction through dieting and overexercising. Recently, a study on body dissatisfaction demonstrated that high body mass indices (BMIs) and body dissatisfaction were more likely to occur in adolescents who later developed eating disorder symptoms (Napolitano & Himes, 2011).

Social Theories

More than in any other psychiatric condition, society plays a significant role in the development of eating disorders with conflicting messages that young women receive from society about their roles in life. Young girls may interpret expectations about how they should look, what roles they should perform, and what they should achieve in society as pressures to achieve "all."

The media, the fashion industry, and peer pressure are significant social influences. Magazines, television, videos, and the Internet depict young girls and adolescents, with thin and often emaciated bodies, as glamorous, successful, popular, and powerful. Girls diet because they want to be similar to these models both in character and appearance. Two of the most common adolescent dieting methods—restricting calories and taking diet pills—have been shown to be influenced by women's beauty and fashion magazines (Luff & Gray, 2009).

Preoccupation with body image and weight is also influenced by public awareness of the obesity epidemic (Cave, 2009). Pre-adolescent children are extremely susceptible to the message to reduce intake and increase exercise as a way to lose weight and maintain health. Coupled with Internet videos that sanction self-starvation, emerging adolescents are already dissatisfied with their bodies and have the tools to lose additional weight through dieting and exercise.

Feminists have focused on the role of this pressure as one part of an explanation for the significant increase in eating disorders and for its greater prevalence in females. Box 24.3 outlines some feminist assumptions regarding role, feminism, and the development of eating disorders.

Risk Factors

Several risk factors influence eating disorders. Puberty is a risk period for the development of anorexia nervosa, especially in girls (Klump, 2013). Girls often begin to

BOX 24.3

Feminist Ideology and Eating Disorders

Since the 1970s, proponents of the feminist cultural model of eating disorders have advanced a position to explain the higher prevalence of these disorders in women. Feminists believe there is a struggle women have today similar to ones they believe women have had in history. They believe that during the Victorian era, "hysteria," a then well-known emotional illness, developed as a result of oppression when women were not allowed to express their feelings and opinions and were "silenced" by a male-dominated society. Feminist scholars today have advanced the feminist relational model to understand the development of eating disorders. They view a major issue in development that causes conflict for young girls as the need to be connected versus society's view of the importance of separation. This confusion can be a stress that may be converted into disordered eating. Often at the base of symptoms such as severe food restriction is the gaining of power lost possibly because of this confusion in one's development (Kinsaul, Curtin, Bazzini, & Martz, 2014).

Feminists have taken issue with what they call the bio-medical model of explanation for the development of eating disorders, seeing it as limiting and patriarchal. The recovery of society must take place to decrease the prevalence of eating disorders. Feminists believe that this will occur only when women are emancipated, given a voice, and socialized differently. They call for more research in which women are co-researchers as well as "subjects," helping to provide the investigators with their own stories and perspectives. Feminists underscore the need for research, especially on prevention, and the need to consider society and culture as well as individual risk factors such as internalization of thinness and a negative body image (Piran, 2010).

BOX 24.4

Research for Best Practice: Eating Disorders and Women Athletes

Holm-Denoma, J. M., Scaringi, V., Gordon K. H., Van Orden, K. A., & Joiner, T. E. (2009). Eating disorder symptoms among undergraduate varsity athletes, club athletes, independent exercisers, and nonexercisers. International Journal of Eating Disorders, 42(1), 47–53.

THE QUESTION: Are there differences in eating disorder symptoms among undergraduate varsity athletes, club athletes, independent exercisers, and nonexercisers?

METHODS: A total of 274 female undergraduates completed the eating disorders inventory and the physical activity and sport anxiety scale and reported their exercise habits.

FINDINGS: Women who participated in sports tended to have higher levels of eating disorder symptomatology than those who did not. Higher levels of sports anxiety were predictive of higher levels of bulimic symptoms and drive for thinness. Athletes who had a high level of athletic participation and experienced sports anxiety (emotional response to the demands of the sport) were more likely to have symptoms of an eating disorder.

IMPLICATIONS FOR NURSING: Nurses should be aware that athletes have higher rates of disordered eating and so should be assessed for eating disorders. Nurses can teach parents and adolescents about the value of healthy athletic competition and the need to maintain healthy eating habits. An accurate assessment of each young woman is important.

diet at an early age because of body dissatisfaction, a need for control, and a prepubertal weight gain. Restricting food may lead to starvation, binge-eating, and purging.

Low self-esteem, body dissatisfaction, and feelings of ineffectiveness also put individuals at risk for an eating disorder. Much recent research on these factors has demonstrated that resilience or protective factors, such as healthy eating attitudes; an accepting attitude toward body size; and positive self-evaluation, especially toward physical and psychological characteristics, can mediate these risk factors and prevent development of an eating disorder (Gustafsson, Edlund, Kjellin, & Norring, 2009).

Athletes are at greater risk for developing eating disorders. For athletes, self-esteem, attractiveness, and improving appearance are related to disordered eating. Elite ("leanness" sports such as running and gymnastics) and non-elite athletes ("non-leanness" sports such as soccer) experience a triad of symptoms (disordered eating, menstrual dysfunction, and osteoporosis). See Box 24.4. Athletes involved in "leanness sports" are at the greatest risk (Javed, Tebben, Fischer, & Lteif, 2013).

Family Response to Disorder

Historically, the family of the patient with anorexia nervosa was labeled as being overprotective, enmeshed, being unable to resolve conflicts, and being rigid about boundaries. Although an uninformed family can delay and complicate treatment, no evidence confirms that family interactions are the primary cause of eating disorders (le Grange, Lock, Loeb, & Nicholls, 2010). Some family interactions can be problematic for the adolescent with an eating disorder. For example, when conflict erupts between two family members and direct communication becomes blocked, interaction patterns are changed that may result in a dysfunctional relay of messages through other family members.

Enmeshment refers to an extreme form of intensity in family interactions and represents low individual autonomy in a family. In an enmeshed family, the individual gets lost in the system. The boundaries that define individual autonomy are weak. This excessive togetherness intrudes on privacy (Minuchin, Rossman, & Baker, 1978).

Overprotectiveness is defined as a high degree of concern for one another and can be detrimental to children at high risk for anorexia nervosa. The parents' overprotectiveness retards the child's development of autonomy and competence (Minuchin, Rossman, & Baker, 1978). *Rigidity* refers to families that are heavily committed to maintaining the status quo and so find change difficult. Conflict is avoided, where a strong ethical code or religious orientation is usually the rationale.

BOX 24.5

Research for Best Practice: Family Influence on Disordered Eating

Kluck, A. S. (2010). Family influence on disordered eating: The role of body image dissatisfaction. Body Image, 7(1), 8–14.

THE QUESTION: Does family culture that emphasizes appearance and thinness increase disordered eating and body image dissatisfaction? Do parent comments related to daughter's weight relate to the development of disorder eating?

METHODS: A sample of 268 never-married college women, ranging in age from 16–24 years were recruited to participate in a study. Participants' mean weight was 136.57 pounds; height (65.32 in). Sample included 82.8% white; 6.3% Hispanic; 4.9% African American; 2.6% Asian American; and 3% other racial background. Subjects completed the Body Shape questionnaire and Family Influence Scale.

FINDINGS: The findings support that family focus on appearance and specific types of comments (criticism from mother and teasing from father) that parents make about weight and size were associated with increased difficulties with behaviors associated with disordered eating.

IMPLICATIONS FOR NURSING: Families should be cautioned about the negative impact of emphasizing appearance and made aware that specific comments can lead to their daughter's body dissatisfaction.

BOX 24.6

Criteria for Hospitalization of Patients with Eating Disorders

MEDICAL
- Acute weight loss, <85% below ideal
- Heart rate near 40 beats/min
- Temperature, <36.1°C
- Blood pressure, <80/50 mm/Hg
- Hypokalemia
- Hypophosphatemia
- Hypomagnesemia
- Poor motivation to recover

PSYCHIATRIC
- Risk for suicide
- Severe depression
- Failure to comply with treatment
- Inadequate response to treatment at another level of care (outpatient)

Source: American Psychiatric Association (2006). Treatment of patients with eating disorders, third edition. *American Journal of Psychiatry, 163*(7 suppl), 4–54.

The family, often unwittingly, can transmit unrealistic attitudes about weight, shape, and size. Adolescents are particularly sensitive to comments about their bodies because this is the stage for body image formation. Parental attitudes about weight have been found to influence body dissatisfaction and dieting; parental comments about weight or shape, or even parents' worrying about their own weight can influence adolescents in much the same way the media does (Box 24.5). Children of mothers with eating disorders are at risk for developing such disorders, but the degree of risk depends on environmental factors and specific difficulties, such as the child's temperament. Maladaptive paternal behavior, such as low affection, communication, and time spent with a child, has been associated with the development of eating disorders (McElwen & Flouri, 2009).

Teamwork and Collaboration: Working Toward Recovery

Treatment for the patient with anorexia nervosa focuses on initiating nutritional rehabilitation to restore the individual to a healthy weight, resolving psychological conflicts around body image disturbance, increasing effective coping, addressing the underlying conflicts related to maturity fears and role conflict, and assisting the family with healthy functioning and communication. Several methods are used to accomplish these goals during the stages of illness and recovery.

The medical complications presented in Table 24.1 influence the decision to hospitalize an individual with an eating disorder. Suicidality is another reason for hospitalization. The criteria for hospital admission varies, and evidence-based studies are lacking to determine when adolescents with anorexia nervosa should be hospitalized. The APA criteria are outlined in Box 24.6.

After an acceptable weight (at least 85% of ideal) is established, the patient is discharged to a partial hospitalization program or an intensive outpatient program. The intensive therapies needed to help patients with their underlying issues (e.g., body distortion, maturity fears) and to help families with communication and enmeshment usually begin after refeeding because concentration is usually impaired in severely undernourished patients with anorexia nervosa.

Family therapy typically begins while the patient is still hospitalized. Studies demonstrate that family therapy does not have as significant an effect as individual therapy on the psychopathology and psychological symptoms for adolescents with anorexia nervosa. It does, however, improve overall communication within the family and helps members understand the disorder (Lask & Roberts, 2015).

Interpersonal therapy (IPT) is a treatment that focuses on uncovering and resolving the developmental and psychological issues underlying the disorder. Role transitions and negative social evaluations typically are the focus (Rieger, Van Buren, Bishop, Tanofsky-Kraff, Welch, & Wilfley, 2010).

Safety Issues

Mortality is high among patients with anorexia nervosa; the crude rate has been determined to be between 7% and 10%, and therefore higher than for females without anorexia nervosa in the general population (Franko et al., 2013). Suicide is the leading cause of death for individuals with anorexia nervosa (Suokas, Suvisaari, Grainger, Raevuori, Gissler, & Haukka, 2014). These individuals tend to commit suicide using highly lethal means in which rescue is unlikely. Nurses need to pay special attention to the risk of suicide with such individuals (see Chapter 15).

Evidence-based Nursing Care for Persons with Anorexia Nervosa Disorder

Mental Health Nursing Assessment

Physical Health Assessment

A thorough evaluation of body systems is important because many systems are compromised by starvation. A careful history from both the patient with anorexia nervosa and the family, including the length and duration of symptoms, such as fasting, avoiding meals, and overexercising, is necessary to assess altered nutrition. Nursing management involves various biopsychosocial assessment and interventions. See Nursing Care Plan 24.1, available at http://thepoint.lww.com/BoydEssentials.

Patients with longer durations of these maladaptive behaviors typically have more difficult and prolonged recovery periods.

> **NCLEXNOTE**   Eating disorders are serious, life-threatening psychiatric disorders. Careful assessment and referral for treatment are important nursing interventions.

The patient's weight is determined using the BMI and a scale to measure weight. Currently, criteria for discharge require patients to be at least 85% of ideal weight according to height and weight tables. BMI, thought to reflect weight most accurately because exact height is used, is calculated by dividing weight in kilograms by height in meters squared. An acceptable BMI is between about 19 and 25.

Menses history also must be explored. Most patients with anorexia nervosa have reached menarche but have experienced amenorrhea for some months because of starvation. A return to regular menses after treatment signifies substantial body fat restoration.

Psychosocial Assessment

The psychological symptoms that patients with anorexia experience are listed in Box 24.1. The classic symptoms of body distortion—fear of weight gain, unrealistic expectations and thinking, and ritualistic behaviors—are easily noted during a clinical interview. Often, people with anorexia nervosa avoid conflict and have difficulty expressing negative emotions, such as anger. Other conflicts, such as sexuality fears and feelings of ineffectiveness,

may underlie this disorder. These symptoms may not be apparent during a clinical interview; however, a variety of instruments is available to clinicians and researchers for determining their presence and severity. The Eating Attitudes Test is frequently used in community and clinical samples (Box 24.7). There is also a pediatric version of this test, the CHEAT. The results of these paper-and-pencil tests can help identify the most significant symptoms for an individual patient and indicate a focus for interventions, especially types of therapy.

Assessment should also focus on the family interaction, influence, and peer relationships. The role of the patient in the family and community should be considered, as well as the person's ability to cope in social situations. For adolescents who are attending school, a conference with the teacher or counselor provides information regarding the amount and frequency of social contacts.

Strengths Assessment

Strengths such as motivation to eat differently and have a more normal life may emerge during the interview. The following questions that could be asked to elicit personal strengths:

- Do you remember a time when you did not have to worry about what you ate? If so, how old were you and what did you like to do?
- Have you found any strategy that prevented you from worrying about what you hate about your appearance?
- Are you ready to change your eating patterns? What do you think will help you change your eating patterns?
- When you are successful in other areas (e.g., school, athletics), how do you reward yourself?

Nursing Diagnoses

Nursing diagnoses for persons with anorexia nervosa are Imbalanced Nutrition: Less Than Body Requirements, Anxiety, Disturbed Body Image, and Ineffective coping

Establishing Therapeutic Relationships

Establishing a therapeutic relationship with individuals with anorexia nervosa may be difficult initially because they tend to be suspicious and mistrustful. They often express fear of adults, especially health care professionals, whom they believe want to "make them fat." By the time they are hospitalized, mistrust can almost reach a state of paranoia. Because of their low body weight and starvation, they are often impatient and irritable. A firm, accepting, and patient approach is important in working with these individuals. Providing a rationale for all interventions helps build trust, as does a consistent nonreactive

BOX 24.7

Eating Attitudes Test

Please place an (x) in the column that applies best to each of the numbered statements. All the results will be strictly confidential. Most of the questions relate to food or eating, although other types of questions have been included. Please answer each question carefully. Thank you.

	ALWAYS	VERY OFTEN	OFTEN	SOMETIMES	RARELY	NEVER
1. Like eating with other people	—	—	—	—	—	x
2. Prepare foods for others but do not eat what I cook	x	—	—	—	—	—
3. Become anxious before eating	x	—	—	—	—	—
4. Am terrified about being overweight	x	—	—	—	—	—
5. Avoid eating when I am hungry	x	—	—	—	—	—
6. Find myself preoccupied with food	x	—	—	—	—	—
7. Have gone on eating binges in which I feel that I may not be able to stop	x	—	—	—	—	—
8. Cut my food into small pieces	x	—	—	—	—	—
9. Am aware of the calorie content of foods that I eat	x	—	—	—	—	—
10. Particularly avoid foods with a high carbohydrate content (e.g., bread, potatoes, rice)	x	—	—	—	—	—
11. Feel bloated after meals	x	—	—	—	—	—
12. Feel that others would prefer I ate more	x	—	—	—	—	—
13. Vomit after I have eaten	x	—	—	—	—	—
14. Feel extremely guilty after eating	x	—	—	—	—	—
15. Am preoccupied with a desire to be thinner	x	—	—	—	—	—
16. Exercise strenuously to burn off calories	x	—	—	—	—	—
17. Weigh myself several times a day	x	—	—	—	—	—
18. Like my clothes to fit tightly	—	—	—	—	—	x
19. Enjoy eating meat	—	—	—	—	—	x
20. Wake up early in the morning	x	—	—	—	—	—
21. Eat the same foods day after day	x	—	—	—	—	—
22. Think about burning up calories when I exercise	x	—	—	—	—	—
23. Have regular menstrual periods	—	—	—	—	—	x
24. Am aware that other people think I am too thin	x	—	—	—	—	—
25. Am preoccupied with the thought of having fat on my body	x	—	—	—	—	—
26. Take longer than others to eat	x	—	—	—	—	—
27. Enjoy eating at restaurants	—	—	—	—	—	x
28. Take laxatives	x	—	—	—	—	—
29. Avoid foods with sugar in them	x	—	—	—	—	—
30. Eat diet foods	x	—	—	—	—	—
31. Feel that food controls my life	x	—	—	—	—	—
32. Display self-control around food	x	—	—	—	—	—
33. Feel that others pressure me to eat	x	—	—	—	—	—
34. Give too much time and thought to food	x	—	—	—	—	—
35. Suffer from constipation	—	x	—	—	—	—
36. Feel uncomfortable after eating sweets	x	—	—	—	—	—
37. Engage in dieting behavior	x	—	—	—	—	—
38. Like my stomach to be empty	x	—	—	—	—	—
39. Enjoy trying new rich foods	—	—	—	—	—	x
40. Have the impulse to vomit after meals	x	—	—	—	—	—

Scoring: The patient is given the questionnaire without the Xs, just blank. Three points are assigned to endorsements that coincide with the Xs; the adjacent alternatives are weighted as two points and one point, respectively. A total score of more than 30 indicates significant concerns with eating behavior.

The EAT-40 has been reproduced with permission. Garner & Garfinkel. (1982). The Eating Attitudes Test: Psychometric features and clinical correlates. *Psychological Medicine*, 12, 871–878.

approach. Power struggles overeating are common, and remaining nonreactive is a challenge. During such power struggles, the nurse should always think about his or her own feelings of frustration and need for control.

Physical Health Interventions

Refeeding

Refeeding, the most important intervention during the hospital or initial stage of treatment, is also the most challenging. The nurse will encounter resistance to weight gain and refusal to eat and so must monitor and record all intake carefully as part of the weight gain protocol.

The refeeding protocol typically starts with 1,500 calories a day and is increased slowly until the patient is consuming about 3,500 calories a day in several meals. The usual plan for patients with very low weights is a weight gain of between 1 to 2 pounds a week.

Weight-increasing protocols usually take the form of a behavioral plan using positive reinforcements (i.e., excursion passes) and negative reinforcements (i.e., returning to bed rest) to encourage weight gain. The nurse should help patients to understand that these actions are not punitive. When all staff members agree on a clear protocol for behaviors related to eating and weight gain, reactivity of the staff to the patient is greatly reduced. These protocols provide ready-made consistent responses to food-refusal behaviors and should be carried out in a caring and supportive context. On rare occasions, when the patient is unable to recognize or accept her illness (i.e., denial), nasogastric tube feedings may be necessary.

Electrolytes may be completely depleted in anorexia nervosa, so nursing care involves stabilizing electrolyte balance. Potassium depletion usually results from use of diuretics, diarrhea, and vomiting. Calcium depletion is related to large intake of dietary fiber, which decreases calcium absorption. During hospitalization, these electrolytes are replaced through oral or intravenous therapy.

Promotion of Sleep

Sleep disturbance is also common, because these individuals are viewed as hyperkinetic. They sleep little, but they usually awaken in an energized state. A structured healthy sleep routine must be established immediately to conserve energy and reduce calorie expenditure because of low weight. To further conserve energy, patients are often relegated to bed rest until a certain amount of weight is regained. Exercise is generally not permitted during refeeding and only with caution after this phase. Inpatients must be closely supervised because they are often found exercising in their rooms, running in place and doing calisthenics.

Medication Interventions

The selective serotonin reuptake inhibitor (SSRI) fluoxetine (Prozac) is approved by the Food and Drug Administration for the treatment of anorexia nervosa. Of course, comorbid conditions such as depression or OCD should be treated with appropriate medication. The nurse may be responsible for administering medications or providing patient and family teaching. See Box 24.8.

BOX 24.8

Drug Profile: Fluoxetine Hydrochloride (Prozac)

DRUG CLASS: Selective serotonin reuptake inhibitor

RECEPTOR AFFINITY: Inhibits central nervous system neuronal uptake of serotonin with little effect on norepinephrine; thought to antagonize muscarinic, histaminergic, and α-adrenergic receptors

INDICATIONS: Treatment of depressive disorders, obsessive-compulsive disorder, bulimia nervosa, and panic disorder

ROUTES AND DOSAGE: Available in 10- and 20-mg capsules and 20-mg/5-mL oral solution

Adults: 20 mg/d in the morning, not to exceed 80 mg/d. Full antidepressant effect may not be seen for up to 4 weeks. If no improvement, dosage is increased after several weeks. Dosages greater than 20 mg/d are administered twice daily. For eating disorders: typically 40 mg to 60 mg/d is recommended

Geriatric: Administer at lower or less frequent doses; monitor responses to guide dosage

Children: Safety and efficacy have not been established

HALF-LIFE (PEAK EFFECT): 2 to 3 d (6–8 h)

SELECTED ADVERSE REACTIONS: Headache, nervousness, insomnia, drowsiness, anxiety, tremors, dizziness, lightheadedness, nausea, vomiting, diarrhea, dry mouth, anorexia, dyspepsia, constipation, taste changes, upper respiratory infections, pharyngitis, painful menstruation, sexual dysfunction, urinary frequency, sweating, rash, pruritus, weight loss, asthenia, and fever

BOXED WARNING: Increased risk of suicidal thoughts and behaviors in children, adolescents, and young adults.

WARNINGS: Avoid use in pregnancy and while breastfeeding. Use with caution in patients with impaired hepatic or renal function and diabetes mellitus. Possible risk for toxicity if taken with tricyclic antidepressants.

SPECIAL PATIENT AND FAMILY EDUCATION:
- Be aware that the drug may take up to 4 weeks to get a full antidepressant effect.
- Take the drug in the morning or in divided doses, if necessary.
- Families and caregivers of pediatric patients being treated with antidepressants should monitor patient for agitation, irritation, and unusual changes in behavior.
- Report any adverse reactions.
- Avoid driving a car or performing hazardous activities because the drug may cause drowsiness or dizziness.
- Eat small frequent meals to help with complaints of nausea and vomiting.

TABLE 24.2 **COGNITIVE DISTORTIONS TYPICAL OF PATIENTS WITH EATING DISORDERS, WITH RESTRUCTURING STATEMENTS**	
Distortion	Clarification or Restructuring
Dichotomous or all-or-nothing thinking "I've gained 2 pounds, so I'll be up by 100 pounds soon."	"You have never gained 100 pounds, but I understand that gaining 2 pounds is scary."
Magnification "I binged last night, so I can't go out with anyone."	"Feeling bad and guilty about a binge are difficult feelings, but you are in treatment, and you have been monitoring and changing your eating."
Selective Abstraction "I can only be happy 10 pounds lighter."	"When you were 10 pounds lighter, you were hospitalized. You can choose to be happy about many things in your life."
Overgeneralization "I didn't eat anything yesterday and did okay, so I don't think not eating for a week or two will harm me."	"Any starvation harms the body, whether or not outward signs were apparent to you. The more you starve, the more problems your body will encounter."
Catastrophizing "I purged last night for the first time in 4 months—I'll never recover."	"Recovery includes up and downs. It is to be expected you will still have some mild but infrequent symptoms."

Psychosocial Interventions

Addressing Interoceptive Awareness

For interoceptive awareness problems (inability to experience visceral cues and emotions), the nurse can encourage patients to keep a journal. Most patients use a somatic complaint such as, "I feel bloated" or "I'm fat" to replace a negative emotion such as guilt or anger. Although refeeding following a state of starvation may cause bloating in some cases, such bloating is often imagined and part of body image distortion. Help patients to identify these feelings by having them write a description of the "fat feeling" and list possible underlying emotions and troublesome situations next to this description.

Helping Patients Understand Feelings

Identifying feelings, such as anxiety and fear, and especially negative emotions, such as anger, is the first step in helping patients to decrease conflict avoidance and develop effective strategies for coping with these feelings.

Do not attempt to change distorted body image by merely pointing out that the patient is actually too thin. This symptom is often the last to resolve itself; some individuals may take years to see their bodies realistically. However, although this symptom is difficult to abate, patients can continue to fear becoming fat but not be driven to act on the distortion by starving. The fear of becoming fat eventually lessens with time.

The nurse can help individuals with cognitive distortions and unrealistic assumptions to restructure the way they view the world, especially in terms of food, eating, weight, and body shape. Faulty ways of viewing these situations result in ineffective coping. Table 24.2 lists some distortions commonly experienced by individuals with eating disorders and some typical restructuring responses or statements that challenge the distortion, which the nurse can present as more realistic ways of perceiving situations. Imagery and relaxation are often used to overcome distortions and to decrease anxiety stemming from a distorted body image.

Psychoeducation

When weight is restored and concentration is improved, patients with anorexia nervosa can benefit from psychoeducation. Although these individuals have a wealth of knowledge about food and calories, they also have misinformation that needs clarifying. For example, they are often unclear about the role of "fats" in a healthy diet and try to be as "fat free" as possible. A thorough assessment of their knowledge is important because they seem to be "walking calorie books" with little information on the role of all the nutrients and the importance of including them in a healthy diet.

> **NCLEXNOTE** Setting realistic eating goals is one of the most helpful interventions for patients with eating disorders. Because individuals with anorexia nervosa are often perfectionists, they often set unrealistic goals.

One of the most helpful skills the nurse can teach is to set realistic goals concerning food and other activities or tasks. Because of perfectionism, patients with anorexia nervosa often set unrealistic goals and end up frustrated. The nurse can help them establish smaller, more realistic, attainable goals (Box 24.9).

Evaluation and Treatment Outcomes

Several factors influence the outcome of treatment for individuals with anorexia nervosa. Particularly long duration of symptoms and low weight when treatment begins predict poor outcomes, but family support and involvement generally improve outcomes. Comorbid conditions and their severity also influence recovery. Although patients are discharged from the hospital when their weight has reached 85% of what is considered ideal, restoration of healthy eating and changes in maladaptive thinking may not have occurred yet. Individuals often continue to restrict foods. Therefore, without intensive outpatient treatment, including nutritional counseling and support, they are unlikely to recover fully. Distorted thinking and eating patterns can set the stage for a relapse and later for the possible development of bulimia nervosa.

Continuum of Care

Inpatient

Hospitalization is required based on criteria noted in Box 24.6. Because of its life-threatening nature, anorexia nervosa in its very acute stage is unlikely to be manageable in outpatient settings.

The patient's systems are monitored closely because at the time of admission, most patients are severely malnourished (see Table 24.1). Patients usually are placed on a privilege-earning program in which privileges, such as having visitors and receiving passes to go outside the hospital, are earned based on weight gain. See Chapter 9.

Emergency Care

Emergency care is not usually needed for individuals with anorexia nervosa. Family members and peers usually notice the weight loss and emaciation before patients' systems are compromised to the degree that they require emergency treatment. If systems are compromised enough to warrant emergency treatment, patients usually are admitted immediately for inpatient care.

Outpatient Treatment

After refeeding, treatment of anorexia nervosa takes place on an outpatient basis and involves individual and family therapy, nutrition counseling to reinforce healthy eating patterns and attitudes, and physician visits to monitor weight and evaluate somatic recovery. Support groups, which are often suggested, should not be substituted for therapy. In fact, some self-directed support groups that lack professional leadership can actually delay or prevent needed professional treatment. However, after full recovery is attained, support groups are useful in maintaining it.

Family Interventions

Denial, guilt, and subsequent greater overprotectiveness are common reactions of the family, especially when hospitalization has been necessary. In addition to family therapy with a skilled therapist, the nurse can help family members express their feelings, increase effective communication, decrease protectiveness, and resolve guilt. Often, siblings become resentful of the patient with an eating disorder because of the significant amount of attention they get from their parents. Having siblings discuss these feelings and the effect the illness has had on them is helpful. Families and friends are eager to help the patient with anorexia nervosa but often need direction. Box 24.10 provides a list of strategies that may assist them.

BOX 24.11

Eating Disorder Prevention Strategies for Parents and Children

EDUCATION FOR PARENTS
- Real vs. ideal weight
- Influence of attitudes, behaviors, teasing
- Ways to increase self-esteem
- Role of media: TV, magazines
- Signs and symptoms
- Interventions for obesity
- Boys at risk also
- Observe for rituals
- Supervision of eating and exercise

STRATEGIES FOR CHILDREN
Education
- Peer pressure regarding eating, weight
- Menses, puberty, normal weight gain
- Strategies for obesity
- Ways to develop or improve self-esteem
- Body image traps: media, retail clothing
- Adapting and coping with problems
- Reporting friends with signs of eating disorders

Screening: Screen for risk factors
Assessment: Assess for treatment
Follow-up: Monitor for relapse

School Interventions

Younger patients with anorexia nervosa may have lost some school time because of hospitalization. Integrating back into a school and classroom setting is difficult for most patients. Shame and guilt about having an eating disorder and being hospitalized must be addressed. Because these patients typically have isolated themselves before hospitalization and treatment, renewing friendships and relationships with peers may provoke anxiety. Involving school nurses and teachers in the reentry process may help.

Prevention and early detection strategies for parents and schoolteachers are often the focus of school nurses and mental health nurses who work in the community. Some of these strategies appear in Box 24.11 and are based on the research on risk factors and protective factors.

National eating disorder awareness and advocacy groups work toward educating the general public; those at risk; and those who work with groups at risk, such as teachers and coaches. They also monitor the media and work to remove unhealthy advertisements and articles that appear in magazines appealing to young girls.

BULIMIA NERVOSA

Bulimia nervosa (BN) is a relatively newly identified disorder: Until about 25 years ago, it was thought to be a type of anorexia nervosa. However, findings from extensive investigations have identified its characteristics as a separate entity. It is more prevalent than anorexia nervosa. Individuals with bulimia nervosa are usually older at onset than are those with anorexia nervosa. The disorder generally is not as life threatening as anorexia nervosa. The usual treatment is outpatient therapy. Outcomes are better for bulimia nervosa than for anorexia nervosa and mortality rates are lower.

Clinical Course

Few outward signs are associated with bulimia nervosa. Individuals binge (i.e., eating an excessive amount, usually at one sitting) and **purge** (i.e., purposeful initiation of stomach or bowel evacuation through artificial means such as vomiting or laxatives) in secret and are typically of normal weight; therefore, it does not come to the attention of parents and peers as readily as anorexia nervosa does. Treatment consequently can be delayed for years as individuals attempt on their own to get their eating under control. Patients usually initiate their own treatment when control of their eating becomes impossible. When treatment is undertaken and completed, patients typically recover completely, except in cases in which personality disorders and comorbid serious depression are also present.

Patients with bulimia nervosa present as overwhelmed and overly committed individuals, "social butterflies" who have difficulty with setting limits and establishing appropriate boundaries. They have an enormous number of rules regarding food and food restriction. They feel shame, guilt, and disgust about their binge-eating and purging. They may also be impulsive in other areas of their lives, such as spending.

Diagnostic Criteria

Bulimia nervosa involves eating a large amount of food within a discrete period of time (e.g., 2 hours) and engaging in recurrent episodes of binge-eating and compensatory purging in various forms such as vomiting or using laxatives, diuretics, or emetics or in nonpurging compensatory behaviors, such as fasting or overexercising to avoid weight gain. These episodes must occur at least once a week for a period of at least 3 months to meet the *DSM-5* criteria. Self-evaluation is excessively and inappropriately influenced by body weight and shape. Unlike anorexia nervosa, little or no weight loss occurs. See Box 24.1 for characteristics related to bulimia nervosa.

Remember Ellen?

She is of normal weight but has been vomiting once to twice a week for several months after binging. She has callouses on her hands from from her teeth when she gagged herself. She sees herself as very overweight.

Binge-eating is defined as rapid, episodic, impulsive, and uncontrollable ingestion of a large amount of food during a short period of time, usually 1 to 2 hours. Eating is followed by feelings of guilt, remorse, and often self-contempt, leading to purging. To assuage the out-of-control feeling, severe dieting is instituted, and these restrictions, referred to as *dietary restraint*, precipitate the next binge. The restrictions are viewed as "rules," such as no sweets, no fats, and so forth. Each binge seems to require stricter and stricter rules about what cannot be consumed, leading to more frequent binge-eating. This cycle has prompted clinicians to focus treatment primarily on interventions related to dietary restraint. When the question of dietary restraint is resolved, binge-eating is decreased, as is the purging that follows binge-eating.

| KEYCONCEPT **Dietary restraint** has been described by researchers in the field of eating disorders as a way to explain the relationship between dieting and binge-eating.

Dieters' deprivation, or restraint, whether real or imagined, contributes to overeating and binging. Genetic predisposition for binge-eating and deprivation may make dieters more prone to feel distress over their dietary "failures," especially if dieting has become a way to overcome body dissatisfaction and to compensate for distress through dietary restraint that leads to overeating (Racine, Burt, Iacono, McGue, & Klump, 2011). Whether the eating is influenced by the attraction of forbidden foods or by internal needs to assuage failure, significant evidence suggests that restraining one's intake is a precondition for bouts of overeating.

Bulimia Nervosa Across the Life-span

Bulimia nervosa occurs in all age groups. It is not as common in children as in adolescents and adults; children appear more likely to have binge-eating disorder (BED), discussed later. This finding has only recently been reported and more data are needed to substantiate this theory.

Epidemiology

The lifetime prevalence of bulimia nervosa is reported to be from 1% to 2.3%, depending on whether clinical or community populations are sampled, but it is estimated that less than one third of the cases are detected (Smink, van Hocken, & Hoek, 2012). Stricter criteria are used when clinical groups are studied, lowering the prevalence rate. The occurrence is more common than that of anorexia nervosa. The incidence of bulimia nervosa has been decreasing over the past decade; this decrease is not attributable to changes in service use, thereby suggesting that a change in sociocultural factors is involved in its development (Smink, et al., 2012).

Age of Onset

Typically, the age of onset is between 15 and 24 years. Some women older than the typical age of onset have developed bulimia nervosa and symptomatic cases have been identified as subsequent to life stressors such as a loss of a loved one (Smink, et al., 2012).

Gender

As with anorexia nervosa, females are 10 times more likely than males to experience bulimia nervosa. Box 24.2 highlights differences in males with eating disorders.

Ethnicity and Culture

Bulimia nervosa is related to culture in the same way as anorexia nervosa. In Western cultures and those becoming westernized in their norms, the focus on achieving a thin body ideal underlies the dieting and dietary restraint that sets up the trajectory toward a diagnosable eating disorder. Hispanic and white women have higher rates than Asian and African American women. The difference as noted earlier in the chapter has much to do with how women from specific cultural backgrounds internalize the thin ideal (Murphy, Straebler, Cooper, & Fairburn, 2010).

Comorbidity

The most common comorbid conditions are substance abuse, depression, and OCD. In one study, women continued having OCD after remission of their bulimic symptoms, underlining the notion that some comorbid conditions may occur before the eating disorder, are trait-related features, and may have a role in precipitating the disorder (APA, 2013). Borderline personality disorder and avoidant personality disorder combined with child sexual abuse are also found frequently in these individuals. Many women with bulimia nervosa earlier had anorexia nervosa (Vrabel, Hofart, Ro, Martinson, & Rosenvinge, 2010).

Etiology

As with anorexia nervosa, theories do not individually explain the development of bulimia nervosa. Rather, the convergence of many of these factors at a vulnerable stage of individual development best explains causality.

Some predisposing or risk factors for anorexia nervosa and bulimia nervosa overlap with theories of causality. For example, dieting puts an individual at risk for the development of bulimia nervosa. Dieting can turn into dietary restraint, a symptom that leads to binge-eating and purging. However, not all individuals who diet experience bulimia nervosa. The interplay of other risk factors (e.g., body dissatisfaction, separation individuation issues) most likely explains the development of this disorder.

Biologic Theories

Some progress has been made in understanding the biologic changes in bulimia nervosa. Dieting and binging can affect brain function. Dieting is believed to affect serotonergic regulation and binging affects the dopamine (DA), acetylcholine (ACh), and opioid reward-related systems. The changes are the result of eating dysregulation rather than the cause. As with anorexia nervosa, these changes often disappear when symptoms such as dietary restraint, binge-eating, and purging remit (Avena & Bocarsly, 2012).

Genetic and Familial Predispositions

A specific gene responsible for bulimia nervosa has not been conclusively identified (Boraska, Franklin, Floyd, Thornton, Huckins, Southam, et al., 2014). Published studies of twins have been reviewed to determine the role genetics might play in the development of bulimia nervosa. Whereas it has been widely recognized that environment also plays a role, in several twin studies, genetic influences outweighed environmental ones (Thornton, Mazzeo, & Bulik, 2011).

Biochemical Factors

The most frequently studied biochemical theory in bulimia nervosa relates to lowered brain serotonin neurotransmission. People with bulimia nervosa are believed to have altered modulation of central serotonin neuronal systems (Poisinelli, Levitan, & DeLuca, 2012). Other studies also target the dopamine system in women with bulimia nervosa who experienced childhood abuse (Groleau, Steiger, Joober, Bruce, Israel, Badawi, et al., 2012).

Chronic depletion of plasma tryptophan is thought to be one of the major mechanisms whereby persistent dieting can lead to the development of eating disorders in vulnerable individuals. Studies show that depletion of tryptophan, an amino acid and serotonin precursor, leads to a depressed mood, a desire to binge, and an increase in weight and shape concerns in those who were in the acute state of their illness (Bruce, Steiger, Young, Kin, Israël, & Lévesque, 2009).

Psychosocial Theories

Symptoms of bulimia nervosa develop when psychological, sociocultural, or environmental events occur. Because the age of onset for bulimia nervosa is late adolescence—

going away to college, for example—may represent the first physical separation for some adolescents, who are unprepared for the emotional separation. In addition, an inability to set limits and develop healthy boundaries leads to a sense of being overwhelmed and "drained." Overwhelming feelings often lead to binge-eating, either to avoid or to distract oneself from feelings such as resentment, or binge-eating can serve to assuage emptiness or to fill up a "drained" self with food.

Cognitive Theory

Many experts view bulimia nervosa as a disorder of thinking in that distortions are the basis of behaviors such as binge-eating and purging. Psychological triggering mechanism models explain that cues such as stress, negative emotions, and even environmental cues (e.g., the presence of attractive food) play a role in etiology. However, these cognitive and triggering theories are now viewed as an explanation for maintaining the binge-eating *after* it has been established rather than an explanation of causality.

The same sociocultural factors that underlie anorexia nervosa play a significant role in the development of bulimia nervosa.

> **Consider Ellen:**
> Some of Ellen's triggers are anxiety, boredom, alcohol use, exhaustion, anger, and social situations where food is readily available.

Family Factors

The families of individuals who experience bulimia nervosa are reported to be chaotic, with few rules and unclear boundaries. Often, an overly close or enmeshed relationship exists between the daughter and mother. Daughters may relate that their mother is their "best friend." The boundaries are blurred in that the mother may interact with the daughter as a confidante. This unhealthy relation further impedes the separation–individuation process. The daughters often feel guilty about separation and responsible for their mother's happiness and emotional well-being (Kluck, 2008).

Risk Factors

The risk or predisposing factors for bulimia nervosa are similar to those for anorexia nervosa. Society's influences, such as the media and peer pressure, underlie the desire to achieve an ideal thin body type. Comparing oneself with these ideal body types leads to body dissatisfaction. These factors influence behaviors such as dietary restraint and overexercising. Dietary restraint leads to binge-eating. Purging follows because of a fear of becoming fat.

Sexual Abuse

Conflicting findings from studies of the relationship between eating disorders and sexual abuse are present. Childhood sexual abuse has often been suggested as a risk factor for eating disorders. It is thought that sexual abuse leads body dissatisfaction that in turn, leads to body shape and weight concerns. However, it has been noted that although childhood sexual abuse has occurred in a larger percentage of women with bulimia nervosa than in the general population, this percentage may not be larger than the percentage of women with other psychiatric disorders who have experienced such abuse. It is unclear how other symptomatology or environmental conditions interact with eating disorder symptoms after abuse (Badura, Huefner, & Handwerk, 2012).

Teamwork and Collaboration: Working Toward Recovery

Individuals with bulimia nervosa benefit from a comprehensive multifaceted treatment approach. The goals for treatment for individuals with bulimia nervosa focus on stabilizing and then normalizing eating, which means stopping the binge–purge cycles; restructuring dysfunctional thought patterns and attitudes, (especially about eating, weight, and body shape); teaching healthy boundary setting; and resolving conflicts about separation–individuation. Treatment usually takes place in an outpatient setting, except when the patient is suicidal or when past outpatient treatment has failed (see Box 24.6).

In addition to intensive psychotherapy, usually cognitive behavioral therapy (CBT) or interpersonal psychotherapy (IPT) and pharmacologic interventions are also necessary. Antidepressants demonstrate effectiveness in treating binge-eating and purging even without comorbid depression. Nutrition counseling is an important part of outpatient treatment to stabilize and normalize eating. Some mental health professionals, psychologists, advanced practice psychiatric nurses, and social workers specialize in treating eating disorders, often working with nutritionists who also have expertise in working with this population. Group psychotherapy and support groups are also used. Family therapy is not usually a part of the treatment because many people with bulimia nervosa live on college campuses away from home or are older and on their own. Usually, treatment becomes less intensive as symptoms resolve. Therapy focuses on psychological issues, such as boundary setting and separation–individuation conflicts and on changing problematic behaviors and dysfunctional thinking using CBT.

Both CBT and IPT have been used for individuals with bulimia nervosa. The combination of CBT and pharmacologic interventions is best for producing an initial decrease in symptoms (Murphy, et al., 2010).

Behavioral therapy alone has not been as effective as CBT. IPT has had positive outcomes but may take longer to eliminate binge-eating and purging. Although binge-eating may persist, little work can be done on underlying interpersonal issues, such as boundary setting, because the patient is intent on feeling out of control with eating. Therefore, cognitive therapy is begun first to address the distorted thinking processes influencing dietary restraint, binge-eating, and purging. Decreasing these symptoms will eliminate the out-of-control feelings.

Safety Issues

Bulimia nervosa is associated with a high risk of suicide independent of other comorbid disorders (Bodell, Joiner, & Keel, 2013). They are also often at risk for self-mutilation. Because they display high levels of impulsivity, (including shoplifting and overspending), financial and legal difficulties have been associated with bulimia nervosa.

Evidence-based Nursing Care for Persons with Bulimia Nervosa Disorder

Mental Health Nursing Assessment

Physical Health Assessment

Even though most individuals with bulimia nervosa maintain normal weights, the physical ramifications of this disorder may be similar to those of anorexia nervosa. Hypokalemia can contribute to muscle weakness and fatigability, as well as to the development of cardiac arrhythmias, palpitations, and cardiac conduction defects. Patients who purge risk fluid and electrolyte abnormalities that can further compromise cardiac status. Neuropsychiatric disturbances, (e.g., poor concentration, lack of attention), and sleep disturbances are common.

The nurse should assess current eating patterns, determine the number of times a day the individual binges and purges, and note dietary restraint practices. Sleep patterns and exercise habits are also important.

Psychosocial Assessment

For an individual with bulimia nervosa, psychological assessment focuses on cognitive distortions—cues or stimuli that lead to dysfunctional behavior affecting symptom development—and knowledge deficits. The psychological characteristics typical of patients with bulimia nervosa are presented in Box 24.1.

Individuals with bulimia nervosa display a significant number of cognitive distortions, examples of which are found in Table 24.2. These thought patterns form the basis for "rules" and lead the way to destructive eating patterns. During routine history taking, patients will relate many of these erroneous assumptions. Situations that produce feelings of being overwhelmed and powerless need to be explored, as does the patient's ability to set boundaries, control impulsivity, and maintain quality relationships. These underlying issues precipitate binge-eating. Body dissatisfaction should be openly explored. Mood is an important area for evaluation because many people with bulimia nervosa are also depressed. Symptoms of depression should be thoroughly explored (see Chapter 19).

Strengths Assessment

Persons with bulimia nervosa can usually identify periods of time when they were able to resist binging and purging. They are usually motivated to reduce or eliminate binging and purging. The following questions can be used if the strengths do not emerge during the assessment interview.

- How have you curtailed the binging and purging behavior in the past?
- What do you do to reduce your anxiety (instead of binging and purging)?
- Is there anyone in your life that you feel understands your situation?
- How motivated are you to change your eating behaviors and work on body image issues?

Nursing Diagnoses

Typical diagnoses for the person with bulimia nervosa include Imbalanced Disturbed Body Image, Disturbed Sleep Pattern, Deficient Knowledge, Risk for Dysfunctional Gastrointestinal Motility, Disturbed Thought Processes, and Powerlessness. Other possible nursing diagnoses that are based on an individual's strengths are Readiness for Enhanced Coping, and Readiness for Enhanced Self-Care Management.

Establishing a Therapeutic Relationship

Individuals with bulimia nervosa experience a great deal of shame and guilt. They also often have an intense need to please and be liked and may approach the nurse–patient relationship in a superficial manner. They are too ashamed to discuss their symptoms but do not want to disappoint others, so they may discuss more social or unrelated issues in an attempt to engage the nurse (Box 24.12). A nonjudgmental accepting approach, stressing the importance of the relationship and outlining its purpose, is important at the outset of therapy. Explaining the nature of the relationship and the goals of therapy will help clarify the boundaries.

> ### Ellen's Feelings
> Ellen feels shame and guilt over her binging and purging. She does not like to talk about it and is very reluctant to talk to the nurse about the behavior.

Mental Health Nursing Interventions

Physical Health Interventions

If the patient is admitted to the hospital, meals and all food intake are strictly monitored to normalize eating. Bathroom visits may also be supervised to prevent purging. Outpatients are asked to record their intake, binges, and purges. Because individuals with bulimia nervosa often have chaotic lifestyles and are often overcommitted, sleep may be a low priority. Sleep-deprived individuals may assume that food would be helpful, so they begin to eat, triggering a binge. To encourage regular sleep patterns, sleep hygiene strategies are implemented.

Medication Interventions

Whereas medications are effective for symptom remission in bulimia nervosa, experts continue to agree that the combination of CBT and medication has had the best results (Murphy, et al., 2010). Fluoxetine has been the most studied drug for bulimia nervosa in clinical trials. Effective doses are usually 60 mg per day, a higher dosage than that used to treat individuals with depression. Other SSRIs are also used. The most important concern in using these medications is decreased appetite and weight loss during the first few weeks of administration. Weight should be monitored, especially during this period.

The intake of medication must be monitored for possible purging after drug administration. The effect of the medication depends on whether it has had time to be absorbed.

Teaching Points

Patients should be instructed to take medication as prescribed. SSRIs must be taken in the morning because they can cause insomnia. Patients should be informed that any weight loss they initially experience is temporary and is usually regained after a few weeks when the medication dosage has stabilized.

Psychosocial Interventions

Behavioral Strategies

Behavioral techniques, such as **cue elimination** and response prevention, require self-monitoring to

BOX 24.12 • THERAPEUTIC DIALOGUE • The Patient with an Eating Disorder

INEFFECTIVE APPROACH

Nurse: Ellen, I am glad to see that you ate your lunch.

Ellen: Thanks, I feel so fat after I eat.

Nurse: I will lock the bathroom so you are not tempted to purge.

Ellen: What, don't you trust me?

Nurse: It is not about trust, but I don't feel comfortable leaving you alone with bathroom access.

Ellen: Really? You have your nerve.

Nurse: We are just trying to help.

Ellen: Some help you are. I know you don't trust me.

Nurse: Now, Ellen, that is not what I said.

Ellen: No, but that is what you meant.

EFFECTIVE APPROACH

Nurse: Ellen, how was your lunch?

Ellen: It was okay. I always feel so fat after I eat.

Nurse: That is understandable. How long does that feeling last?

Ellen: Well, it depends on how much I have eaten. Since I didn't eat much, it will last for about an hour.

Nurse: Oh, I see. For many people with bulimia nervosa, the urges to purge are strongest after a meal. Is this a hard time for you?

Ellen: Sometimes it is.

Nurse: How can I help you resist the urges? Would you like me to stay with you until group time?

Ellen: That would be great.

CRITICAL THINKING CHALLENGE

- What effect did the first interaction have on Ellen's behavior? Why?
- In the second interaction, what theories and interventions regarding eating disorders did the nurse use in her approach to Ellen?

individualize the therapy. **Self-monitoring** is accomplished using a diary in which the patient records binges and purges, as well as precipitating emotions and environmental cues. After emotional and environmental cues have been identified, alternative responses are suggested, tried, and reinforced. When a cue or stimulus leads to a dysfunctional or unhealthy response, the response can be eliminated or an alternate healthier response to the cue can be substituted, tried, and then reinforced. Figure 24.2 gives two examples of behavioral interventions. In example 1, for the patient with anorexia nervosa, the response is modified or altered to a healthier one; in example 2, for the patient with bulimia nervosa, the cue is changed to produce a healthier response. Other techniques, such as postponing binges and purges through distraction, a technique to interrupt the cycle, are also effective.

NCLEXNOTE Cognitive interventions within the context of a therapeutic relationship are a priority in the nursing care of patients with eating disorders.

Group Interventions

Group interventions are cost effective and increase learning more effectively than does individual treatment because patients learn from each other as well as from the nurse, therapist, or team leader. Some experts have recommended 12-step programs for treating bulimia nervosa. (Eating Disorders Anonymous, 2015). However, many clinicians who work in this specialty have noted that these programs, with their strict rules, can be counterproductive for patients with bulimia nervosa, who already have rigid rules and are "abstinent" in many ways that lead to binge-eating. Broad parameters regarding food choices (e.g., all foods allowed in moderation) in combination with knowledge about healthy eating should be encouraged instead.

After symptoms subside, patients can concentrate on interpersonal issues in therapy, such as a fused relationship with their mothers or feelings of inadequacy and low self-esteem, which often underlie their lack of assertiveness.

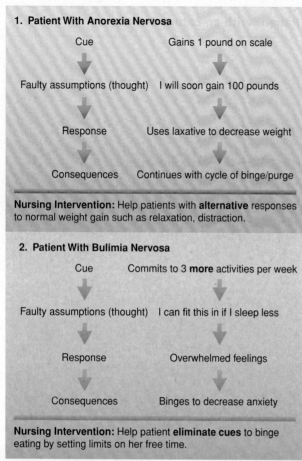

1. Patient With Anorexia Nervosa

Cue	Gains 1 pound on scale
↓	↓
Faulty assumptions (thought)	I will soon gain 100 pounds
↓	↓
Response	Uses laxative to decrease weight
↓	↓
Consequences	Continues with cycle of binge/purge

Nursing Intervention: Help patients with **alternative** responses to normal weight gain such as relaxation, distraction.

2. Patient With Bulimia Nervosa

Cue	Commits to 3 **more** activities per week
↓	↓
Faulty assumptions (thought)	I can fit this in if I sleep less
↓	↓
Response	Overwhelmed feelings
↓	↓
Consequences	Binges to decrease anxiety

Nursing Intervention: Help patient **eliminate cues** to binge eating by setting limits on her free time.

FIGURE 24.2 Examples of the relationship of cues, thoughts, responses, and behavioral interventions.

Psychoeducation

In addition to cognitive and behavioral techniques, educational strategies are also incorporated into treatment. For individuals with bulimia nervosa, psychoeducation focuses on setting boundaries and healthy limits, developing assertiveness, learning nutritional concepts related to healthy eating, and clarifying misconceptions about food. Rules that result from dichotomous thinking also must be addressed because of their role in dietary restraint and resulting binge-eating.

The nurse can assist patients to understand the binge–purge cycle and the role of rigid rules in contributing to this cycle. The value of eating meals regularly to ward off hunger and reduce the possibility of a binge is also important. Patients who abuse laxatives must be taught that although these drugs produce water-weight loss, they are ineffective for true lasting weight loss. Patients also need information about potassium depletion, electrolyte imbalances, dehydration, and the medical consequences of binge-eating and purging. Other topics for psychoeducation are included in Box 24.13.

BOX 24.13

Bulimia Nervosa

When caring for the patient with bulimia nervosa, be sure to include the following topic areas in the teaching plan:

- Psychopharmacologic agents, if used, including drug, action, dosage, frequency, and possible side effects
- Binge–purge cycle and effects on the body
- Nutrition and eating patterns
- Hydration
- Avoidance of cues
- Cognitive distortions
- Limit setting
- Appropriate boundary setting
- Assertiveness
- Resources
- Self-monitoring and behavioral interventions
- Realistic goal setting

Evaluation and Treatment Outcomes

Patients with bulimia nervosa have better recovery outcomes than do patients with anorexia nervosa. Outcomes have improved since the early 1990s, partially because of earlier detection, research on what treatments are most effective, and neuropharmacologic research and advances such as CBT. Experts in the field of eating disorders report a 55% recovery at 5 years (Keski-Rahkonen, Hoek, Susser, Linna, Sihvola, Raevuori, et al., 2009), and in another study, 83% of women recovered with CBT that included exposure and response prevention techniques (McIntosh, Carter, Bulik, Framptom, & Joyce, 2011). Because CBT requires a specialist's care, current treatment research is exploring the use of self-help models, including manuals that can be combined with psychopharmacology (Murphy, et al., 2010).

Continuum of Care

Although patients with bulimia nervosa are less likely than those with anorexia nervosa to require hospitalization, patients with extreme dehydration and electrolyte imbalance, depression and suicidality, or symptoms that have not remitted with outpatient treatment need hospitalization.

However, most treatment takes place in outpatient settings. After treatment, referrals to recovery groups and support groups are important to prevent relapse. As already noted patients with bulimia nervosa rarely require emergency care.

Community Interventions

As with anorexia nervosa, preventing bulimia nervosa requires effort on the part of teachers, school nurses, parents, and society as a whole. Because many of the risk factors are seen early in children attending elementary school, educating school nurses and teachers is an important focus for psychiatric–mental health nurses working in the community. Protective factors that mediate between risk factors and the development of an eating disorder must be emphasized and developed. Box 24.11 covers important prevention strategies for parents and their children or adolescents.

Society has begun to engage in an effort to help young girls. The federal government has developed a website called *girlshealth* (http://girlshealth.gov/) that is devoted to areas such as body changes, body image, relationships, and self-confidence.

BINGE-EATING DISORDER

Another type of disordered eating, **binge-eating disorder** (BED), is now treated as a separate eating disorder in the *DSM-5* (APA, 2013). This disorder is seen in several studies that have uncovered a group of individuals who binge in the same way as those with bulimia nervosa but who do not purge or compensate for binges through other behaviors. Individuals with BED also differ from those with other eating disorders in that most are obese. In addition, investigators have shown that individuals with BED have lower dietary restraint and are heavier than those with bulimia nervosa. It has been estimated that 10% to 30% of obese individuals have BED. Some patients have reported that they binged without purging for several years beginning as young as fifth grade (Combs, Pearson, & Smith, 2011).

The diagnostic criteria for BED consist of binge-eating, which includes both the ingestion of a large amount of food in a short period of time and a sense of loss of control during the binge, distress regarding the binge; eating until uncomfortably full, and feelings of guilt or depression after the binge. As mentioned, purging or other compensatory behavior does *not* follow the binge. The prevalence of BED is estimated to be 1.6% for females and 0.8% for males in the United States (APA, 2013).

Because this is a newly recognized disorder, additional research is needed to clarify its symptoms, etiology, and treatment. Its etiology, however is believed to be similar to that of bulimia nervosa. The treatment of individuals with BED is still in the investigative stages, so most experts use interventions similar to those used for bulimia nervosa.

OTHER EATING DISORDERS

In **purging disorder** frequent purging is frequent, but not binging. Individuals with this disorder purge at least once a week and have an intense fear of gaining weight or becoming fat (APA, 2013). They restrict their dietary intake and purge after eating normal amounts of food due to the fear of eating, gaining weight, and/or appearing "fat." Affected individuals have increased levels of body image disturbance, higher levels of general psychopathology, distress, eating pathology, and personality disorders when compared to a comparable group of persons without purging disorder. Although individuals with this disorder do not overeat as do those with bulimia nervosa, they do report more dietary restraint, greater fear of losing control, and greater guild over eating than control groups. On a continuum of bulimic symptomatology, purging disorder may be the midpoint with BN the more severe (Smith & Crowther, 2013).

In **night eating syndrome,** the individual eats after awakening from sleep or consumes an excessive amount of food after the evening meal (APA, 2013). The person is aware of the overeating that causes significant distress or impairment to the individual. A feeling of loss of control over consumption, sleep fragmentation, and morning anorexia is felt by the patient. Night eating syndrome is conceptualized as a disorder of circadian modulation of food intake and sleep. It is mainly attributed to a endocrinal, metabolic, or psychologic trigger. These individuals typically experience insomnia and nighttime awakenings. A significant association is found between restless legs syndrome and night eating syndrome (Antelmi, Vinai, Pizza, Marcatelli, Speciale, & Provini, 2014).

SUMMARY OF KEY POINTS

- Anorexia nervosa and bulimia nervosa share some common symptoms but are nonetheless classified as discrete disorders.

- Eating disorders are best viewed along a continuum that includes subclinical or partial-syndrome disorders; because these disorders occur more frequently than full syndromes, they are often overlooked but, after they have been identified, they can be prevented from worsening.

- Similar factors predispose individuals to the development of anorexia nervosa and bulimia nervosa; these factors represent a biopsychosocial model of risk. These disorders are preventable; identifying risk factors will assist with prevention strategies.

- Etiologic factors contribute in combination to the development of eating disorders; no single factor provides an explanation.

- Treatment of anorexia nervosa frequently includes hospitalization for refeeding; bulimia nervosa is primarily treated on an outpatient basis.

- CBT and medication improve the symptoms. Both individual and group interpersonal psychotherapy are also effective in self-evaluation and communication.

■ The outcomes for bulimia nervosa are better than those for anorexia nervosa. The type and severity of comorbid conditions and the length of the illness influence outcomes.

■ Binge-eating disorder is characterized by periods of binge-eating not followed by purging or any other compensating behaviors.

CRITICAL THINKING CHALLENGES

1. Discuss the potential difficulties and risks in attempting to treat a patient with anorexia nervosa in an outpatient setting.

2. Parents are often in need of support and suggestions for how to help prevent eating disorders. Develop a teaching program and include the topics and rationale for suggestions chosen.

3. Identify the important nursing management components of a refeeding program for a hospitalized patient with anorexia nervosa.

4. Bulimia nervosa is often described as a closet disorder with secretive binge-eating and purging. Identify the signs and symptoms of each system involved for someone with this disorder.

5. Positive outcomes for the recovery of bulimia nervosa and anorexia nervosa depend on many factors. Identify the factors that promote positive outcomes and those related to poorer outcomes and prognosis.

 M VIE viewing **GUIDES** related to this chapter are available at http://thepoint.lww.com/BoydEssentials.

A related Psychiatric-Mental Health Nursing video on the topic of Eating Disorders is available at http://thepoint.lww.com/Boyd Essentials.

A Psychiatric-Mental Health Nursing Practice and Learn Activity related to the video on the topic of Eating Disorders is available at http://thepoint.lww.com/BoydEssentials.

REFERENCES

American Psychiatric Association. (2013). *Diagnostic and Statistical Manual of Mental Disorders* (5th ed.). Arlington, VA: American Psychiatric Association.

Antelmi, E., Vinai, P., Pizza, F., Marcatelli, M., Speciale, M., & Provini, F. (2014). Nocturnal eating is part of the clinical spectrum of restless legs syndrome and an underestimated risk factor for increased body mass index. *Sleep Medicine, 15*(2), 168–172.

Avena, N. M., & Bocarsly, M. E. (2012). Dysregulation of brain reward systems in eating disorders: Neurochemical information from animal models of binge eating, bulimia nervosa, and anorexia nervosa. *Neuropharmacology, 63*(7), 87–96.

Badura, B. A., Huefner, J. C., & Handwerk, M. L. (2012). The impact of abuse and gender on psychopathology, behavioral disturbance, and psychotropic medication count for youth in residential treatment. *American Journal of Orthopsychiatry, 82*(4), 562–572.

Baker, J. H., Maes, H. H., Lissner, L., Aggen, S. H., Lichtenstein, P., & Kendler, K. S. (2009). Genetic risk factors for disordered eating in adolescent males and females. *Journal of Abnormal Psychology, 118*(3), 576–586.

Bardone-Cone, A. M., Strum, K., Lawson, M. A., Robinson, D. P., & Smith R. (2010). Perfectionism across stages of recovery from eating disorders. *International Journal of Eating Disorders, 43*(2), 139–148.

Berner, L. A., Shaw, J. A., Witt, A. A., & Lowe, M. R. (2013). The relation of weight suppression and body mass index to symptomatology and treatment response in anorexia nervosa. *Journal of Abnormal Psychology, 122*(3), 694–708.

Bodell, L. P., Joiner, T. E., & Keel, P. K. (2013). Comorbidity-independent risk for suicidality increases with bulimia nervosa but not with anorexia nervosa. *Journal of Psychiatric Research, 47*(5), 617–621.

Boraska, V., Franklin, C. S., Floyd, J. A., Thornton, L. M., Huckins, L. M., Southam, L., et al. (2014). A genome-wide association study of anorexia nervosa. *Molecular Psychiatry. 19*(10):1085–94 doi: 10.1038/mp.2013.187

Brady, C. F. (2014). Obsessive-compulsive disorder and common comorbidities. *Journal of Clinical Psychiatry, 75*(1), e02. doi:10.4088/JCP.13023tx1c

Bruce, K. R., Steiger, H., Young, S. N., Kin, N. M., Israël, M., & Lévesque, M. (2009). Impact of acute tryptophan depletion on mood and eating-related urges in bulimic and nonbulimic women. *Journal of Psychiatry and Neuroscience, 34*(5), 376–382.

Bruch, H. (1973). *Eating disorders: Obesity, anorexia nervosa and the person within.* New York: Basic Books.

Cave, K. E. (2009). Influences of disordered eating in prepubescent children. *Journal of Psychosocial Nursing, 47*(2), 21–24.

Combs, J. L., Pearson, C. M., & Smith, G. T. (2011). A risk model for preadolescent disordered eating. *International Journal of Eating Disorders, 44*(7), 599–604.

Dennard, E. E., & Richards, C. S. (2013). Depression and coping in subthreshold eating disorders. *Eating Behaviors, 14*(3), 325–329.

Eating disorders Anonymous. (2015). http://www.eatingdisordersanonymous.org/index.htm Retrieved August 5, 2015.

Favaro, A., Caregaro, L., Tenconi, E., Bosello, R., & Santonastaso, P. (2009). Time trends in age at onset of anorexia nervosa and bulimia nervosa. *Journal of Clinical Psychiatry, 70*(12), 1715–1721.

Frank, G. K. (2011). Reward and neurocomputational processes. *Current Topics in Behavioral Neuroscience, 6*, 95–110.

Frank, G. K., Shott, M. E., Hagman, J. O., & Mittal, V. A. (2013). Alterations in brain structures related to taste reward circuitry in ill and recovered anorexia nervosa and in bulimia nervosa. *American Journal of Psychiatry, 170*(10), 1152–1160.

Franko, D. L., Keshaviah, A., Eddy, K. T., Krishna, M., Davis, M. C., Keel, P. K., et al. (2013). A longitudinal investigation of mortality in anorexia nervosa and bulimia nervosa. *American Journal of Psychiatry, 170*(8), 917–925.

Gordon, K. H., Castro, Y., Sitnikov, L., & Holm-Denoma, J. M. (2010). Cultural body shape ideals and eating disorder symptoms among white, Latina, and Black college women. *Cultural diversity and Ethnic Minority Psychology, 16*(2), 135–143.

Groleau, P., Steiger, H., Joober, R., Bruce, K. R., Israel, M., Badawi, G., et al. (2012). Dopamine-system genes, childhood abuse, and clinical manifestations in women with Bulimia-spectrum Disorders. *Journal of Psychiatric Research, 46*(9), 1139–1146.

Gustafsson, A., Edlund, S., Kjellin, B., & Norring, C. (2009). Risk and protective factors for disturbed eating in adolescent girls—Aspects of perfectionism and attitudes to eating and weight. *European Eating Disorders Review, 17*(5), 380–389.

Javed, A., Tebben, P. J., Fischer, P. R., & Lteif, A. N. (2013). Female athlete triad and its components: Toward improved screening and management. *Mayo Clinic Proceedings, 88*(9), 996–1009.

Kaye, W. H., Wierenga, C. E., Bailer, U. R., Simmons, A. N., & Bischoff-Grethe, A. (2013a). Nothing tastes as good as skinny feels: The neurobiology of anorexia nervosa. *Trends in Neurosciences, 36*(2), 110–120.

Kaye, W. H., Weirenga, C. E., Bailer, U. F., Simmons, A. N., Wagner, A., & Bischoff-Grethe, A. (2013b). Does a shared neurobiology for foods and drugs of abuse contribute to extremes of food ingestion in anorexia and bulimia nervosa? *Biological Psychiatry, 73*(9), 836–842.

Keski-Rahkonen, A., Hoek, H. W., Susser, E. S., Linna, M. S., Sihvola, E., Raevuori, A., et al. (2007). Epidemiology and course of anorexia nervosa in the community. *American Journal of Psychiatry, 164*(8), 1259–1265.

Keski-Rahkonen, A., Hoek, H. W., Susser, E. S., Linna, M. S., Shivola, E., Raevuori, A., et al. (2009). Epidemiology and course of anorexia nervosa in the community. *American Journal of Psychiatry, 164*(8), 1259–1265.

Keski-Rahkonen, A., Raevuori, A., Bulik, C. M., Hoek, H. W., Rissanen, A., & Kaprio, J. (2014). Factors associated with recovery from anorexia nervosa: A population-based study. *International Journal of Eating Disorders, 47*(2), 117–123.

Kinsaul, J. A., Curtin, L., Bazzini, D., & Martz, D. (2014). Empowerment, feminism, and self-efficacy: Relationships to body image and disordered eating. *Body Image, 11*(1), 63–67.

Kluck, A.S. (2008). Family factors in the development of disordered eating: integrating dynamic and behavioral explanation. *Eating Behaviors, 9*(4), 471–483.

Kluck, A. S. (2010). Family influence on disordered eating: The role of body image dissatisfaction. *Body Image, 7*(1), 8–14.

Klump, K. L. (2013). Puberty as a critical risk period for eating disorders: A review of human and animal studies. *Hormones and Behavior, 64*(2), 399–410.

Lask, B., & Roberts, A. (2015). Family cognitive remediation therapy for anorexia nervosa. *Clinical Child Psychology and Psychiatry. 20*, 207–217.

le Grange, D., Lock, J., Loeb, K., & Nicholls, D. (2010). Academy for Eating Disorders Position Paper: The role of the family in eating disorders. *International Journal of Eating Disorders, 43*(1), 1–5.

Luff, G. M., & Gray, J. J. (2009). Complex messages regarding a thin ideal appearing in teenage girls' magazines from 1956 to 2005. *Body Image, 6*(2), 133–136.

Lund, B. C., Hernandez, E. R., Yates, W. R., Mitchell, J. R., & McKee, P. A. (2009). Rate of inpatient weight restoration predicts outcome in anorexia nervosa. *International Journal of Eating Disorders, 42*(4), 301–305.

Mangweth-Matzek, C. I., Rupp, A., Hausman, S., Gusmerotti, G., Kemmler, G., & Biebl, W. (2010). Eating disorders in men: Current features and childhood factors. *Eating and Weight Disorders, 15*(1–2), 15–22.

Manuel, A., & Wade, T. D. (2013). Emotion regulation in broadly defined anorexia nervosa: Association with negative affective memory bias. *Behavior Research and Therapy, 51*(8), 417–424.

McElwen, C., & Flouri, E. (2009). Fathers, parenting, adverse life events and adolescents' emotional and eating disorder symptoms: The role of emotion regulation. *European Child and Adolescent Psychiatry, 18*(4), 206–216.

McIntosh, W., Carter, F. A., Bulik, C. M., Framptom, C. M., & Joyce, P. R. (2011). Five year outcome of cognitive behavioral therapy and exposure with response prevention for bulimia nervosa. *Psychological Medicine, 41*(5), 1061–1071.

Minuchin, S., Rossman, B. L., & Baker, L. (1978). *Psychosomatic families.* Cambridge, MA: Harvard University Press.

Murphy, R., Straebler, S., Cooper, Z., & Fairburn, C. G. (2010). Cognitive behavioral therapy for eating disorders. *Psychiatric Clinics of North America, 33*(3), 611–627.

Napolitano, M. A., & Himes, S. (2011). Race, weight, and correlates of binge eating in female students. *Eating Behaviors, 12*(1), 29–36.

Piran, N. (2010). A feminist perspective on risk factor research and on the prevention of eating disorders. *Eating Disorders, 18*(3), 183–198.

Preti, A., Rocchi, M. B., Sisti, D., Camboni, M. V., & Miotto, P. (2011). A comprehensive meta-analysis of the risk of suicide in eating disorders. *Acta Psychiatrica Scandinavica, 124*(1), 6–17.

Poisinelli, G. N., Levitan, R. N., & DeLuca, V. (2012). 5-HTTLPR polymorphism in bulimia nervosa: A multiple-model meta-analysis. *Psychiatric Genetics, 22*(5), 219–225.

Racine, S. E., Burt, S. A., Iacono, W. G., McGue, M., & Klump, K. L. (2011). Dietary restraint moderates genetic risk for binge eating. *Journal of Abnormal Psychology, 120*(1), 119–128.

Rieger, E., Van Buren, D. J., Bishop, M., Tanofsky-Kraff, M., Welch, R., & Wilfley, E. D. (2010). An eating disorder-specific model of interpersonal psychotherapy (IPT-ED): Causal pathways and treatment implications. *Clinical Psychology Review, 30*, 400–410.

Rhea, D. J., & Thatcher, W. G. (2013). Ethnicity, ethnic identity, self-esteem and at-risk eating disorders behavior differences of urban adolescent females. *Eating Disorders, 21*(3), 223–237.

Sabel, A. L., Rosen, E., & Mehler, P. S. (2014). Severe anorexia nervosa in males: Clinical presentations and medical treatment. *Eating disorders, 22*(3), 209–220.

Salbach-Andrae, H., Schneider, N., Seifert, K., Pfeiffer, E., Lenz, K., Lehmkuhl, U., et al. (2009). Short term outcome of anorexia nervosa in adolescents after inpatient treatment: A prospective study. *European Child and Adolescent Psychiatry, 18*(11), 701–704.

Smink, F. R., van Hocken, D., & Hoek, H. W. (2012). Epidemiology of eating disorders: Incidence, prevalence, and mortality rates. *Current Psychiatry Reports, 14*(4), 404–414.

Smith, K. E., & Crowther, J. H. (2013). An exploratory investigation of purging disorder. *Eating Behaviors. 14*(1), 26–34.

Suokas, J. R., Suvisaari, J. M., Grainger, M., Raevuori, A., Gissler, M., & Haukka, J. (2014). Suicide attempts and mortality in eating disorders: A follow-up study of eating disorder patients. *General Hospital Psychiatry, 36*(3), 355–357.

Thornton, L. M., Mazzeo, S. E., & Bulik, C. M. (2011). The heritability of eating disorders: Methods and current findings. *Current Topics in Behavioral Neurosciences, 6*, 141–156.

van den Berg, P. A., Mond, J., Eisenberg, M., Ackard, D., & Neumark-Sztainer, D. (2010). The link between body dissatisfaction and self-esteem in adolescents: Similarities across gender, age, weight status, race/ethnicity, and socioeconomic status. *Journal of Adolescent Health, 47*(3), 290–296.

Vrabel, K. R., Hofart, A., Ro, Y., Martinson, E. W., & Rosenvinge, J. H. (2010). Co-occurrence of avoidant personality disorder and child sexual abuse predicts poor outcome in long standing eating disorders. *Journal of Abnormal Psychology, 119*(3), 623–629.

Wilkosz, M. E., Chen, J., Kenndey, C., & Rankin, S. (2011). Body dissatisfaction in California adolescents. *Journal of the American Academy of Nurse Practitioners, 23*(2), 101–109.

Zhao, Y., & Encinosa, W. (2011). An Update on Hospitalizations for Eating Disorders, 1999 to 2009 *HCUP statistical brief #120.* Rockville, MD: Agency for Healthcare Research and Quality, Retrieved from https://www.hcup-us.ahrq.gov/reports/statbriefs/sb120.jsp. Retrieved on August 5, 2015.

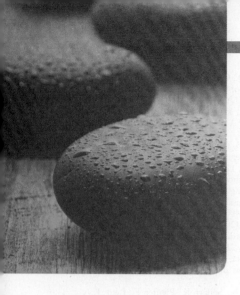

25
Addiction and Substance-Related Disorders

Nursing Care of Persons with Alcohol and Drug Use

Mary Ann Boyd

KEY CONCEPTS
- addiction
- denial
- motivation

LEARNING OBJECTIVES

After studying this chapter, you will be able to:

1. Describe the actions, effects, and withdrawal symptoms of alcohol, marijuana, stimulants, tobacco, hallucinogens, opioids, inhalants, and also gambling disorder.

2. Discuss the evidence that serves as a basis of care and treatment of persons with substance-related and non–substance-related disorders.

3. Formulate nursing diagnoses based on an assessment of people with substance-related disorders.

4. Compare intervention approaches of substance-related and non–substance-related disorders.

5. Implement treatment interventions for patients with substance-related and non–substance-related disorders.

KEY TERMS

- alcohol withdrawal syndrome • Alcoholics Anonymous • brief interventions • codependence • confabulation • confrontation • craving • delirium tremens • denial • detoxification • gambling disorder • hallucinogen • harm reduction • inhalants • intoxication • Korsakoff's amnestic syndrome • methadone maintenance • motivation • motivational interviewing • opioids • relapse • substance induced disorder • substance use disoder • sudden sniffing death • tolerance • Wernicke-Korsakoff syndrome • Wernicke's encephalopathy • withdrawal

Case Study: Gladys

Gladys, a 68-year-old widow, lives by herself in a comfortable apartment. She spends her days with friends and visiting her grandchildren. At night she frequently has an alcoholic drink to relax her and help her sleep. She denies that she has a drinking problem.

INTRODUCTION

The human use and abuse of alcohol and other drugs has been around since the beginning of history; so too have the subsequent social and emotional problems that accompany substance use. This chapter reviews the concept of addiction, types of substance use, biologic and psychological effects, current theories of substance-related disorders, and interventions. Gambling disorder is a non–substance-related disorder that s also discussed in this chapter. Gambling behaviors and their consequences have similar characteristics to the behaviors associated with substance disorders. The nurse's role in helping persons with these disorders recover is discussed within the biopsychosocial nursing model. Professional issues related to chemical dependency within the nursing profession are also examined.

OVERVIEW OF SUBSTANCE USE AND ABUSE

Alcohol, tobacco, marijuana, and illegal prescription drug use have reached epidemic proportions in the United States, with the incidence rising in younger age groups, particularly among adolescents and young adults. One of the goals of *Healthy People 2020* is "to reduce substance abuse to protect the health, safety, and quality of life for all, especially children" (U.S. Department of Health and Human Services, 2010). The overriding concern about using mind-altering substances is that these substances compromise health and continued use will lead to addiction.

> **KEYCONCEPT** **Addiction** is a condition of continued use of substances (or reward-seeking behaviors) despite adverse consequences.

Many mind-altering substances are physiologically addicting and easily can lead to severe health and legal problems. Use by ingestion, smoking, sniffing, or injection of some mind-altering substances such as alcohol, pain medication, tobacco, or caffeine is legal for adults. Other substances such as cocaine and heroin are illegal in the United States. Abuse occurs when a person uses alcohol or drugs for the purpose of intoxication or, in the case of prescription drugs, for purposes other than their intended use. Substance-related disorders involve substances that are commonly abused.

Physiologic dependence can develop with many different types of medications such as beta-blockers, antidepressants, opioids, anti-anxiety agents, and others. As long as medications are used for their intended purposes and under the supervision of qualified health care providers, physiological dependence is a part of treatment. That is, dependence can be a normal response to some medications (American Psychiatric Association [APA], 2013).

Diagnostic Criteria

Substance-related disorders are categorized into two categories: substance use disorders and substance-induced disorders. **Substance-induced disorders** occur when medications used for other health problems or medical/mental health disorders causes **intoxication**, **withdrawal**, or other health-related problems. A **substance use disorder** occurs when an individual continues using substances despite cognitive, behavioral, and physiological symptoms. The *DSM-5* identifies 10 diagnostic categories of substances including alcohol, caffeine, cannabis (marijuana), hallucinogens, inhalants, opioids, sedative–hypnotics, stimulants, tobacco, and others (APA, 2013). Gambling disorder is included within the substance use disorder category because gambling behaviors can activate the brain's reward system similar to the substance use disorders.

A substance use disorder occurs when there is an underlying change in brain circuitry that may persist after **detoxification**, the process of safely and effectively withdrawing a person from an addictive substance, usually under medical supervision. These brain changes lead to pathologic behaviors that occur with repeated relapses and intense drug cravings when exposed to the drug-related cues (e.g., a party, emotional experiences) (APA, 2013).

Epidemiology

Age of Onset

In the United States, alcohol is the most abused substance followed by marijuana. Alcohol use is at historically low levels for adolescents. In 2013, 3.5% of 8th graders, 12.8% of 10th graders, and 26% of 12th graders reported getting drunk in the past month. In 2013, 22.1% of high school seniors reported binge drinking – a drop of almost one third since the late 1990s – but illicit drug use among adolescents is on the rise. In 2013, 7% of 8th graders, 18% of 10th graders, and 22.7% of 12th graders used marijuana within the last 12 months. The rising level of marijuana use reflects a change in attitude and perception that marijuana is a safe drug, especially in light of recent legalization of marijuana in some states (National Institute of Drug Abuse [NIDA], 2014a).

The nonmedical use of prescription and over-the-counter (OTC) medicines continues to represent a significant part of the adolescent drug problems. In 2013, 15% of high school seniors used a prescription drug nonmedically in the past year. Adderall, a stimulant composed of amphetamine and dextroamphetamine used to treat attention deficit hyperactivity disorder (see Chapter 28) was used by 7.4% of high schoolseniors for nonmedical reasons. Fewer teens smoke cigarettes (9.6%) than smoke marijuana (15.6%). The use of other forms of tobacco are increasing with 21.4% of 12th graders smoking hookah water pipes at some point during the past year—an increase from 18.3% in 2012 (NIDA, 2014a).

Ethnicity and Culture

Use of illicit and legal substances among Asians is consistently lower than in the other ethnic groups. In 2012, current illicit drug use was 3.7% among Asians, 7.8% among Native Hawaiians or Other Pacific Islanders, 8.3% among Hispanics, 9.2% among whites, 11.3% among blacks or African Americans, 12.7% among American Indians or Alaska Natives, and 14.8% among persons of two or more races. These statistics have been relatively stable since 2002 except for whites (from 8.5% to 9.2%) and African Americans (from 9.7% to 11.3%) (Substance Abuse and Mental Health Services Administration [SAMHSA], 2013).

The highest use of alcohol was among whites (57.4%) and persons reporting two or more races (51.9%) followed by African Americans (43.2%), Hispanics (41.8%), American Indians or Alaska Natives (41.7%), and Asians (36.9%). The highest tobacco use was reported among the American Indians or Alaska Natives (48.4%) followed by persons reporting two or more races (37.3%), whites (29.2%), African Americans (27.2%), Hispanics (19.2%), and Asians (10.8%) (SAMHSA, 2013).

Comorbidity

Many people who abuse substances have other mental disorders. Some disorders are in part a byproduct of long-term substance use; others predispose the individual to alcohol or drug abuse. Whatever the reason, nurses should be aware that patients who abuse substances often have psychotic, anxiety, or mood disorders (Pope, Joober, & Malla, 2013). Other coexisting mental disorders include attention deficit hyperactivity disorder (ADHD) (Nogueira, Bosch, Valeron, Gómez-Barros, Palomar, Richarte, et al., 2014) and personality disorders (Gonzalez, 2014).

> ### Consider Gladys
> She is also depressed and spends many days in bed. During the last few months her alcohol consumption has increased significantly.

Individuals who abuse substances are at high risk for death from drug overdoses and are at increased risk for death from other causes, including homicide, suicide, and opportunistic infections (such as HIV) secondary to drug injection. Earlier studies have documented the connection between alcohol abuse and increased risk for diabetes mellitus (DM), gastrointestinal problems, hypertension, liver disease, and stroke (Kottke & Pronk, 2010).

Etiology

Substance abuse encompasses the body, the mind, and society's influences (Bowen, Witkiewitz, Clifasefi, Grow, Chawla, Hsu, et al., 2014; Cadet, Bisagno, & Milroy, 2014). Human and animal studies confirm a genetic predisposition for drinking behaviors and self-administering mind-altering drugs, but as yet no precise genetic marker has been established. Temperament, self-concept, age, motivation for change, social consequences for problematic behaviors, parental and family relationships and peer pressure all contribute to expression of substance abuse—a chronic and progressive disorder.

Family Responses to Substance Use and Abuse

Abuse of substances by one or more members has devastating effects on families, their functioning, and the community. Fetal alcohol syndrome (FAS) results from drinking alcohol during pregnancy. Addictions lead to loss of jobs and family relationships. Use of illegal substances can lead to arrest and prison.

Many families try to help their family member learn to abstain or reduce the use of substances. Support groups provide education and help in understanding the addiction. Conversely, some persons who recover from substance abuse find that they must distance themselves from families that are actively using and abusing alcohol and drugs.

Treatment and Recovery

The goal for persons abusing substances is to recover from the abuse. Recovery involves a partnership between health care providers and the individual and family. For many of the individuals, a period of intense treatment is necessary to safely manage the physical and psychological withdrawal symptoms that occur when a substance is no longer used. Specific withdrawal symptoms depend on the addictive substance and are explained below as the substances are discussed. The withdrawal process usually involves detoxification. After a person has safely withdrawn from the substance of abuse, the real work toward recovery can begin. A primary concern is relapse, the recurrence of alcohol- or drug-dependent behavior in an individual who has previously achieved and maintained abstinence for a significant time beyond the period of detoxification.

TYPES OF SUBSTANCES AND RELATED DISORDERS

Table 25.1 provides a summary of the effects of abused substances.

Alcohol

Alcohol (or ethanol) found in various proportions in liquor, wine, and beer relaxes inhibitions and heightens emotions. Mood swings can range from bouts of gaiety to angry outbursts. Cognitive impairments can vary from reduced concentration or attention span to impaired judgment and memory. Alcohol ultimately produces a sedative effect by depressing the central nervous system (CNS). Depending on the amount of alcohol ingested, the effects can range from feelings of mild sedation and relaxation to confusion and serious impairment of motor functions and speech to severe intoxication that can result in coma, respiratory failure, and death.

All patients should be screened not only for alcohol use disorders but also for drinking patterns or behaviors that may place them at increased risk for experiencing adverse

TABLE 25.1	SUMMARY OF EFFECTS OF ABUSED SUBSTANCES, OVERDOSE, WITHDRAWAL SYNDROMES, AND PROLONGED USE			
Substance	**Route**	**Effects (E) and Overdose (O)**	**Withdrawal Syndrome**	**Prolonged Use**
Alcohol	PO	E: Sedation, decreased inhibitions, relaxation, decreased coordination, slurred speech, nausea O: Respiratory depression, cardiac arrest	Tremors; seizures, elevated temperature, pulse, and blood pressure; delirium tremens	Affects all systems of the body. Can lead to other dependencies
Stimulants (e.g., amphetamines, cocaine)	PO, IV, inhalation, smoking	E: Euphoria, initial CNS stimulation and then depression, wakefulness, decreased appetite, insomnia, paranoia, aggressiveness, dilated pupils, tremors O: Cardiac arrhythmias or arrest, increased or lowered blood pressure, respiratory depression, chest pain, vomiting, seizures, psychosis, confusion, seizures, dyskinesias, dystonias, coma	Depression: psychomotor retardation at first and then agitation; fatigue and then insomnia; severe dysphoria and anxiety; cravings, vivid, unpleasant dreams; increased appetite. Amphetamine withdrawal is not as pronounced as cocaine withdrawal.	Often alternates with use of depressants. Weight loss and resulting malnutrition and increased susceptibility to infectious diseases. May produce schizophrenia-like syndrome with paranoid ideation, thought disturbance, hallucinations, and stereotyped movements
Cannabis (marijuana, hashish, THC)	Smoking, PO	E: Euphoria or dysphoria, relaxation and drowsiness, heightened perception of color and sound, poor physical coordination, spatial perception and time distortion, unusual body sensations (e.g., weightlessness, tingling), dry mouth, dysarthria, and cravings for particular foods O: Increased heart rate, reddened eyes, dysphoria, lability, disorientation		Can decrease motivation and cause cognitive deficits (e.g., inability to concentrate, impaired memory)
Hallucinogens (LSD, MDMA)	PO	E: Euphoria or dysphoria, altered body image, distorted or sharpened visual and auditory perceptions, depersonalization, bizarre behavior, confusion, incoordination, impaired judgment and memory, signs of sympathetic and parasympathetic stimulation, palpitations (blurred vision, dilated pupils, sweating) O: Paranoia, ideas of reference, fear of losing one's mind, depersonalization, derealization, illusions, hallucinations, synesthesia, self-destructive or aggressive behaviors, tremors	"Flashbacks" or HPPD may occur after termination of use.	
PCP	PO, inhalation, smoking	E: Feeling superhuman, decreased awareness of and detachment from the environment, stimulation of the respiratory and cardiovascular systems, ataxia, dysarthria, decreased pain perception O: Hallucinations, paranoia, psychosis, aggression, adrenergic crisis (cardiac failure, cerebrovascular accident, malignant hyperthermia, status epilepticus, severe muscle contractions)		"Flashbacks," HPPD, organic brain syndromes with recurrent psychotic behavior, which can last up to 6 months after not using the drug, numerous psychiatric hospitalizations and police arrests
Opioids (heroin, codeine)	PO, injection, smoking	E: Euphoria, sedation, reduced libido, memory and concentration difficulties, analgesia, constipation, constricted pupils O: Respiratory depression, stupor, coma	Abdominal cramps, rhinorrhea, watery eyes, dilated pupils, yawning, "goose flesh," diaphoresis, nausea, diarrhea, anorexia, insomnia, fever (see Table 25.4)	Can lead to criminal behavior to get money for drugs, risk for infection-related to needle use (e.g., HIV, endocarditis, hepatitis).

(Continued)

TABLE 25.1	SUMMARY OF EFFECTS OF ABUSED SUBSTANCES, OVERDOSE, WITHDRAWAL SYNDROMES, AND PROLONGED USE (Continued)			
Substance	**Route**	**Effects (E) and Overdose (O)**	**Withdrawal Syndrome**	**Prolonged Use**
Sedatives, hypnotics, anxiolytics	PO, injection	E: Euphoria, sedation, reduced libido, emotional lability, impaired judgment O: Respiratory depression, cardiac arrest	Anxiety rebound and agitation, hypertension, tachycardia, sweating, hyperpyrexia, sensory excitement, motor excitation, insomnia, possible tonic-clonic convulsions, nightmares, delirium, depersonalization, hallucinations	Often alternated with stimulants, use with alcohol enhances chance of overdose, risk for infection related to needle use
Inhalants (e.g., glue, lighter fluid)	Inhalation	E: Euphoria, giddiness, excitation O: CNS depression: ataxia, nystagmus, dysarthria, coma, and convulsions	Similar to findings with alcohol but milder, with anxiety, tremors, hallucinations, and sleep disturbance as the primary symptoms	Long-term use can lead to hepatic and renal failure, blood dyscrasias, damage to the lungs; CNS damage (e.g., OBS, peripheral neuropathies, cerebral and optic atrophy, parkinsonism)
Nicotine	Smoking	E: Stimulation, enhanced performance and alertness, and appetite suppression O: Anxiety	Mood changes (e.g., craving, anxiety) and physiologic changes (e.g., poor concentration, sleep disturbances, headaches, gastric distress, and increased appetite)	Increased chance for cardiac disease and lung disease
Caffeine	PO	E: Stimulation, increased mental acuity, inexhaustibility O: Restlessness, nervousness, excitement, insomnia, flushing, diuresis, gastrointestinal distress, muscle twitching, rambling flow of thought and speech, tachycardia or cardiac arrhythmia, agitation	Headache, drowsiness, fatigue, craving, impaired psychomotor performance, difficulty concentrating, yawning, nausea	Physical consequences are under investigation

CNS, central nervous system; CVA, cerebrovascular accident; HIV, human immunodeficiency virus; HPPD, hallucinogen persisting perceptual disorder; LSD, D-lysergic acid diethylamide; MDMA, (3-4 methylenedioxymethamphetamine); OBS, organic brain syndrome; PO, oral; PCP, phencyclidine; THC, D-9-tetrahydrocannabinol.

health effects or alcoholism. A frequently used screening tool is the CAGE Questionnaire. This tool consists of four self-report responses to questions about respondents' beliefs of cutting down on their drinking, their experience of others criticizing their drinking, the presence of guilt about drinking, and early morning drinking (Ewing, 1984). People who abuse alcohol exhibit various patterns of use. Some engage in heavy drinking on a regular or daily basis, others may abstain from drinking during the week and engage in heavy drinking on the weekends, and still others experience longer periods of sobriety interspersed with bouts of binge drinking (several days of intoxication). Risky (binge) drinkers who have not yet become addicted to alcohol often can be screened and

receive initial counseling within a primary care setting, but scant evidence suggests that permanent behavior change will occur within the primary care setting (Moyer, LeFevre, Siu, Peters, Baumann, Bibbins-Domingo, et al., 2013; Butler, Simpson, Hood, Cohen, Pickles, Spanou, et al., 2013).

The level of CNS impairment while under the influence of alcohol depends on how much has been consumed in a given period of time and how rapidly the body metabolizes it. Intoxication is determined by the level of alcohol in the blood, called blood alcohol level (BAL). The body can metabolize 1 oz of liquor, a 5-oz glass of wine, or a 12-oz can of beer per hour without intoxication. Table 25.2 lists behavioral responses at various BALs.

TABLE 25.2	BLOOD ALCOHOL LEVELS AND BEHAVIOR	
Number of Drinks	Blood Alcohol Levels (mg%)	Behavior
1–2	0.05	Impaired judgment, giddiness, mood changes
5–6	0.10	Difficulty driving and coordinating movements
10–12	0.20	Motor functions severely impaired, resulting in ataxia; emotional lability
15–20	0.30	Stupor, disorientation, and confusion
20–24	0.40	Coma
25	0.50	Respiratory failure, death

Effects of Long-Term Abuse

People who use alcohol regularly usually develop alcohol **tolerance**, the ability to ingest an increasing amount of alcohol before they experience a "high" and show cognitive and motor effects. The locus ceruleus, which normally inhibits the action of ethanol, is believed to be instrumental in the development of alcohol tolerance. Even though these individuals do not appear intoxicated, their BALs reflect the increased amount of alcohol and are affecting their bodies as described in Table 25.1. Excessive or long-term abuse of alcohol can adversely affect all body systems; the effects can be serious and permanent. Box 25.1 lists the major physical complications of alcohol abuse for the major organ systems.

Alcohol-Induced Amnestic Disorders

Although certain alcohol-related cognitive impairments are reversible with abstinence, long-term alcohol abuse can cause specific neurologic complications that lead to organic brain disorders, known as alcohol-induced amnestic disorders. Alcohol is directly toxic to the brain, causing atrophy of the frontal cortex and eventually chronic brain syndrome. Patients with alcohol-induced amnestic disorders usually have a history of many years of heavy alcohol use and are generally older than 40 years.

Wernicke encephalopathy, a degenerative brain disorder caused by thiamine deficiency, is characterized by vision impairment, ataxia, hypotension, confusion, and coma. **Korsakoff amnestic syndrome**, associated with alcoholism, involves the heart and the vascular and nervous systems, but the primary problem is acquiring new information and retrieving memories. Symptoms include amnesia, **confabulation**, (i.e., telling a plausible but imagined scenario to compensate for memory loss), attention deficit, disorientation, and vision impairment. Although Wernicke encephalopathy and Korsakoff amnestic syndrome can appear as two different disorders, they are generally considered to be different stages of the same

BOX 25.1
Medical Complications of Alcohol Abuse

- **Cardiovascular system:** Cardiomyopathy, congestive heart failure, hypertension
- **Respiratory system:** Increased rate of pneumonia and other respiratory infections
- **Hematologic system:** Anemias, leukemia, hematomas
- **Nervous system:** Withdrawal symptoms, irritability, depression, anxiety disorders, sleep disorders, phobias, paranoid feelings, diminished brain size and functioning, organic brain disorders, blackouts, cerebellar degeneration, neuropathies, palsies, gait disturbances, visual problems
- **Digestive system and nutritional deficiencies:** Liver diseases (fatty liver, alcoholic hepatitis, cirrhosis), pancreatitis, ulcers, other inflammations of the gastrointestinal (GI) tract, ulcers and GI bleeds, esophageal varices, cancers of the upper GI tract, pellagra, alcohol amnestic disorder, dermatitis, stomatitis, cheilosis, scurvy
- **Endocrine and metabolic systems:** Increased incidence of diabetes mellitus, hyperlipidemia, hyperuricemia, and gout
- **Immune system:** Impaired immune functioning, higher incidence of infectious diseases, including tuberculosis and other bacterial infections
- **Integumentary system:** Skin lesions, increased incidence of infection, burns, and other traumatic injury
- **Musculoskeletal system:** Increased incidence of traumatic injury, myopathy
- **Genitourinary system:** Hypogonadism, increased secondary female sexual characteristics in men (hypoandrogenization and hyperestrogenization), erectile dysfunction in men, electrolyte imbalances due to excess urinary secretion of potassium and magnesium

disorder called **Wernicke-Korsakoff syndrome**, with Wernicke's encephalopathy representing the acute phase and Korsakoff amnestic syndrome the chronic phase. Early symptoms can be reversed, but without long-term treatment, the prognosis is poor (Day, Bentham, Callaghan, Kuruvilla, & George, 2013).

Detoxification

When a patient enters treatment for alcohol addiction, alcohol ingestion is immediately stopped, and detoxification begins. Because of physiologic addiction, **alcohol withdrawal syndrome** occurs, with symptoms of increased heart rate and blood pressure, diaphoresis, mild anxiety, restlessness, and hand tremors (Table 25.3). The severity of withdrawal symptoms ranges from mild to severe, depending on the length and amount of alcohol use. In patients with alcoholism and in chronic drinkers, the alcohol withdrawal syndrome usually begins within 12 hours after abrupt discontinuation or attempt to decrease consumption. The most severe symptoms are **delirium tremens** (acute withdrawal syndrome characterized by autonomic hyperarousal, disorientation, hallucinations, and tremors) and grand mal (tonic-clonic) seizures. These symptoms can be life threatening. If seizures occur, they usually do so within the first 48 hours of withdrawal.

TABLE 25.3	ALCOHOL WITHDRAWAL SYNDROME		
	Stage I: Mild	**Stage II: Moderate**	**Stage III: Severe**
Vital signs	Heart rate elevated, temperature elevated, normal or slightly elevated systolic blood pressure	Heart rate, 100–120 bpm; elevated systolic blood pressure and temperature	Heart rate, 120–140 bpm; elevated systolic and diastolic blood pressures; elevated temperature
Diaphoresis	Slight	Usually obvious	Marked
Central nervous system	Oriented; no confusion; no hallucinations; mild anxiety and restlessness; restless sleep; hand tremors; "shakes"; no convulsions	Intermittent confusion; transient visual and auditory hallucinations and illusions (mostly at night) Painful anxiety and motor restlessness; insomnia and nightmares; visible tremulousness, rare convulsions	Marked disorientation, confusion, disturbing visual and auditory hallucinations, misidentification of objects, delusions related to the hallucinations, delirium tremens, disturbances in consciousness Agitation, extreme restlessness, and panic states Unable to sleep Gross uncontrollable tremors, convulsions common
Gastrointestinal system	Impaired appetite, nausea	Anorexia, nausea and vomiting	Rejecting all fluid and food

NCLEXNOTE Alcohol abuse continues to require nursing assessment and interventions in all settings. Patients who abuse alcohol for long periods of time are at high risk for alcohol withdrawal syndrome. Observing for signs of seizure activity is a priority nursing intervention.

Uncomplicated alcohol withdrawal is usually completed within 48 to 96 hours. Assessing for vital sign changes, nausea, vomiting, tremors, perspiration, agitation, headache, and change in mental status are important nursing interventions. The Clinical Institute Withdrawal Assessment for Alcohol Scale (CIWA-Ar) is frequently used for assessment (Box 25.2). Close monitoring of withdrawal symptoms continues until BAL is reduced.

Remember Gladys?

Gladys abruptly stopped her alcohol intake when she was admitted to the hospital for depression and suicidal thoughts. She did not tell her primary care provider that her intake of alcohol was significant. She began to go through withdrawal.

Several medications are used to prevent physiological complications and provide a gradual withdraw from alcohol. Antianxiety and sedating drugs, such as benzodiazepines, are titrated downwardly over several days as a substitution for the alcohol. Chlordiazepoxide (Librium) and diazepam have longer half-lives and smoother tapers. Lorazepam (Ativan) is better for the older adult and people with liver impairment. Antidepressants are usually initiated to treat mood states, and sleep medication is used to promote a regular sleep pattern. Antipsychotic medications are also used if needed.

Prevention of Relapse

Relapse prevention is important in the recovery of people with substance-related disorders, and alcohol addiction is no exception. Psychosocial interventions such as self-help groups, psychoeducation, and cognitive behavioral therapy (CBT) are designed specifically for those with alcohol addictions. These interventions are discussed later in this chapter.

Other medications are used for those who are recovering. Disulfiram (Antabuse) is neither a treatment nor a cure for alcoholism, but it can be used as adjunct therapy to help deter some individuals from drinking while using other treatment modalities to teach new coping skills to alter abuse behaviors (Box 25.3). Disulfiram plus even small amounts of alcohol produces side effects. Severe reactions may include respiratory depression, cardiovascular collapse, arrhythmias, myocardial infarction, acute congestive heart failure, unconsciousness, convulsions, and death.

Naltrexone was originally used as a treatment for heroin abuse, but it is now approved for treatment of alcohol dependence (Box 25.4). Naltrexone is formulated in a once-daily dose in pill form and a monthly injection. The precise mechanism of action for naltrexone's effect is unknown; however, reports from successfully treated patients suggest three kinds of effects: (1) it can reduce craving (the urge or desire to drink despite negative consequences), (2) it can help maintain abstinence, and (3) it can interfere with the tendency to want to drink more if a recovering patient slips and has a drink. Naltrexone may be particularly useful in patients who continue to drink heavily (Franck & Jayaram-Lindström, 2013).

BOX 25.2

Clinical Institute Withdrawal Assessment of Alcohol Scale, Revised (CIWA-Ar)

Patient: _____ Date: _____ Time: _____ (24 hour clock, midnight = 00:00)

Pulse or heart rate, taken for one minute: _____ Blood pressure: _____

NAUSEA AND VOMITING – Ask "Do you feel sick to your stomach? Have you vomited?" Observation.
0 no nausea and no vomiting
1 mild nausea with no vomiting
2
3
4 intermittent nausea with dry heaves
5
6
7 constant nausea, frequent dry heaves and vomiting

TACTILE DISTURBANCES – Ask "Have you any itching, pins and needles sensations, any burning, any numbness, or do you feel bugs crawling on or under your skin?" Observation.
0 none
1 very mild itching, pins and needles, burning or numbness
2 mild itching, pins and needles, burning or numbness
3 moderate itching, pins and needles, burning or numbness
4 moderately severe hallucinations
5 severe hallucinations
6 extremely severe hallucinations
7 continuous hallucinations

TREMOR – Arms extended and fingers spread apart. Observation.
0 no tremor
1 not visible but can be felt fingertip to fingertip
2
3
4 moderate, with patient's arms extended
5
6
7 severe, even with arms not extended

AUDITORY DISTURBANCES – Ask "Are you more aware of sounds around you? Are they harsh? Do they frighten you? Are you hearing anything that is disturbing to you? Are you hearing things you know are not there?" Observation.
0 not present
1 very mild harshness or ability to frighten
2 mild harshness or ability to frighten
3 moderate harshness or ability to frighten
4 moderately severe hallucinations
5 severe hallucinations
6 extremely severe hallucinations
7 continuous hallucinations

PAROXYSMAL SWEATS – Observation.
0 no sweat visible
1 barely perceptible sweating, palms moist
2
3
4 beads of sweat obvious on forehead
5
6
7 drenching sweats

VISUAL DISTURBANCES – Ask "Does the light appear to be too bright? Is its color different? Does it hurt your eyes? Are you seeing anything that is disturbing to you? Are you seeing things you know are not there?" Observation.
0 not present
1 very mild sensitivity
2 mild sensitivity
3 moderate sensitivity
4 moderately severe hallucinations
5 severe hallucinations
6 extremely severe hallucinations
7 continuous hallucinations

ANXIETY – Ask "Do you feel nervous?" Observation.
0 no anxiety, at ease
1 mild anxious
2
3
4 moderately anxious, or guarded, so anxiety is inferred
5
6
7 equivalent to acute panic states as seen in severe delirium or acute schizophrenic reactions

HEADACHE, FULLNESS IN HEAD – Ask "Does your head feel different? Does it feel like there is a band around your head?" Do not rate for dizziness or lightheadedness. Otherwise, rate severity.
0 not present
1 very mild
2 mild
3 moderate
4 moderately severe
5 severe
6 very severe
7 extremely severe

AGITATION – Observation.
0 normal activity
1 somewhat more than normal activity
2
3
4 moderately fidgety and restless
5
6
7 paces back and forth during most of the interview, or constantly thrashes about

ORIENTATION AND CLOUDING OF SENSORIUM – Ask "What day is this? Where are you? Who am I?"
0 oriented and can do serial additions
1 cannot do serial additions or is uncertain about date
2 disoriented for date by no more than 2 calendar days
3 disoriented for date by more than 2 calendar days
4 disoriented for place/or person

Total **CIWA-Ar** Score _____
Rater's Initials _____
Maximum Possible Score 67

The **CIWA-Ar** is not copyrighted and may be reproduced freely. This assessment for monitoring withdrawal symptoms requires approximately 5 minutes to administer. The maximum score is 67 (see instrument). Patients scoring less than 10 do not usually need additional medication for withdrawal.

Sullivan, J. T., Sykora, K., Schneiderman, J., Naranjo, C. A., & Sellers, E. M. (1989) Assessment of alcohol withdrawal: The revised Clinical Institute Withdrawal Assessment for Alcohol scale (**CIWA-Ar**). British Journal of Addiction, 84:1353–1357.

BOX 25.3

Drug Profile: Disulfiram (Antabuse)

DRUG CLASS: Antialcoholic agent, enzyme inhibitor

RECEPTOR AFFINITY: Inhibits the enzyme aldehyde dehydrogenase, blocking oxidation of alcohol and allowing acetaldehyde to accumulate to concentrations 5 to 10 times higher than normal in the blood during alcohol metabolism. Believed to inhibit norepinephrine synthesis.

INDICATIONS: Management of selected patients with chronic alcohol use who want to remain in a state of enforced sobriety

ROUTE AND DOSAGE: Available in 250- and 500-mg tablets

Adults: Initially, a maximum dose of 500 mg/d PO in a single dose for 1–2 weeks. Maintenance dosage of 125 to 500 mg/d PO not to exceed 500 mg/d, continued until patient is fully recovered socially and a basis for permanent self-control is established.

HALF-LIFE (PEAK EFFECT): Unclear (12 h)

SELECTED SIDE EFFECTS: Drowsiness, fatigue, headache, metallic or garlic-like aftertaste. If taken with alcohol: flushing, throbbing in head and neck, throbbing headaches, respiratory difficulty, nausea, copious vomiting, sweating, thirst, chest pain, palpitations, dyspnea, hyperventilation, tachycardia, hypotension, syncope, weakness, vertigo, blurred vision, confusion; severe reactions may include arrhythmias, cardiovascular collapse, acute congestive heart failure, and unconsciousness.

WARNINGS: Never administer to an intoxicated patient or without the patient's knowledge. Do not administer until patient has abstained from alcohol for at least 12 hours.

Contraindicated in patients with severe myocardial disease, coronary occlusion, or psychoses and in patients receiving current or recent treatment with metronidazole, paraldehyde, alcohol, or alcohol-containing preparations. Use cautiously in patients with DM, hypothyroidism, epilepsy, cerebral damage, chronic and acute nephritis, cirrhosis or dysfunction.

POSSIBLE DRUG INTERACTIONS: Concomitant administration of phenytoin, diazepam, or chlordiazepoxide may increase serum levels and risk for drug toxicity. Increased prothrombin time caused by disulfiram may lead to a need to adjust dosage of oral anticoagulants.

SPECIFIC PATIENT AND FAMILY EDUCATION

- Take the drug daily; take it at bedtime if it makes you dizzy or tired. Crush or mix tablets with liquid if necessary.
- Do not take *any* form of alcohol (e.g. beer, wine, liquor, vinegar, cough mixtures, sauces containing alcohol, aftershave lotions, liniments, or cologne); doing so may cause a severely unpleasant reaction.
- Wear or carry medical identification with you at all times to alert any medical emergency personnel that you are taking this drug.
- Keep appointments for follow-up blood tests.
- Avoid driving or performing tasks that require alertness if drowsiness, fatigue, or blurred vision occur.
- Know that the metallic aftertaste is transient and will disappear after use of the drug is discontinued.

PO, oral.

BOX 25.4

Drug Profile: Naltrexone (Trexan)

DRUG CLASS: Narcotic antagonist

RECEPTOR AFFINITY: Binds to opioid receptors in the CNS and competitively inhibits the action of opioid drugs, including those with mixed narcotic agonist–antagonist properties

INDICATIONS: Adjunctive treatment of alcohol or narcotic dependence as part of a comprehensive treatment program

ROUTE AND DOSAGE: Available in 50-mg tablets

Adults: For alcoholism: 50 mg/d PO; for narcotic dependence: initial dose of 25 mg PO; if no signs or symptoms seen, complete dose with 25 mg. Usual maintenance dose is 50 mg/d PO.

Children: Safety has not been established for use in children younger than 18 y.

HALF-LIFE (PEAK EFFECT): 3.9–12.9 h (60 min)

SELECTED SIDE EFFECTS: Difficulty sleeping, anxiety, nervousness, headache, low energy, abdominal pain or cramps, nausea, vomiting, delayed ejaculations, decreased potency, rash, chills, increased thirst, joint and muscle pain

WARNINGS: Contraindicated in pregnancy and patients allergic to narcotic antagonists. Use cautiously in narcotic addiction because may produce withdrawal symptoms. Do not administer unless patient has been opioid free for 7 to 10 d. Also, use cautiously in patients with acute hepatitis, liver failure, depression, or suicidal tendencies and in those who are breast-feeding. Must make certain patient is opioid free before administering naltrexone. Always give naloxone challenge test before using, except in patients showing clinical signs of opioid withdrawal.

SPECIFIC PATIENT AND FAMILY EDUCATION

- Understand that this drug will help facilitate abstinence from alcohol and block the effects of narcotics.
- Wear a medical identification tag to alert emergency personnel that you are taking this drug.
- Avoid use of heroin or other opioid drugs; small doses may have no effect, but large doses can cause death, serious injury, or coma.
- Report any signs and symptoms of adverse effects.
- Notify other health care providers that you are taking this drug.
- Keep appointments for follow-up blood tests and treatment program.

CNS, central nervous system; PO, oral.

Promotion of Health: Adequate Nutrition and Supplemental Vitamins

Multivitamins and adequate nutrition are essential for patients who are withdrawing from alcohol. Because malnutrition is common, other vitamin replacement may be necessary for certain individuals. Thiamine (vitamin B₁) is initiated during detoxification, given to decrease ataxia and other symptoms of deficiency. It is usually given orally, 100 mg three to four times daily, but can be given intramuscularly or by intravenous infusion with glucose. Folic acid deficiency is corrected with administration of 1.0 mg orally four times daily. Magnesium deficiency also is found in those with long-term alcohol dependence. Magnesium sulfate, which enhances the body's response to thiamine and reduces seizures, is given prophylactically for patients with histories of withdrawal seizures. The usual dose is 1.0 g intramuscularly, four times daily for 2 days.

Stimulants

Cocaine

Cocaine (also known as coke, snow, nose candy, flake, blow, big c, lady, white, or snowbirds) is made from the leaves of the *Erythroxylon coca* plant into a coca paste that is refined into cocaine hydrochloride, a crystalline form (thus the white powder appearance), which is commonly inhaled or "snorted" in the nose, injected intravenously (with water), or smoked. The smokeable form of cocaine, often called *free-base cocaine*, can be made by mixing the crystalline cocaine with ether or sodium hydroxide. Crack cocaine, often simply called "crack," is a form of free-base cocaine produced by mixing the crystal with water and baking soda or sodium bicarbonate and boiling it until a rock precipitant remains. The hardened crystal is then broken into pieces ("cracked") and smoked in cigarettes or water pipes. This extremely potent form produces a rapid high with intense euphoria and a dramatic crash. It is extremely addictive because of the intense and rapid onset of euphoric effects, which leave users craving more.

After cocaine is inhaled or injected, the user experiences a sudden burst of mental alertness and energy ("cocaine rush") and feelings of self-confidence, being in control, and sociability, which last 10 to 20 minutes. This high is followed by an intense let-down effect ("cocaine crash") in which the person feels irritable, depressed, tired, and craves more of the drug. Users experience a serious psychological addiction and pattern of abuse. Although cocaine users typically report that the drug enhances their feelings of well-being and reduces anxiety, cocaine also is known to bring on panic attacks in some individuals. Long-term cocaine use leads to increased anxiety. Increased use of cocaine is associated with stress and drug craving (NIDA, 2013a).

Biologic Responses to Cocaine

Cocaine is absorbed rapidly through the blood–brain barrier and is also readily absorbed through skin and mucous membranes. Rapid intoxication occurs when cocaine is injected intravenously or inhaled. Cocaine increases dopaminergic and serotonergic activity by attaching to transport proteins and in turn by blocking neurotransmitter reuptake. Increased dopamine causes euphoria and psychotic symptoms. Cocaine increases norepinephrine levels in the blood, causing tachycardia, hypertension, dilated pupils, and rising body temperatures. Serotonin excess contributes to sleep disturbances and anorexia. With prolonged cocaine use, these neurotransmitters are eventually depleted.

Cocaine Intoxication

Intoxication causes CNS stimulation, the length of which depends on the dosage and route of administration. With steadily increasing doses, restlessness proceeds to tremors and agitation followed by convulsions and CNS depression. In lethal overdose, death generally results from respiratory failure. Toxic psychosis is also possible; it may be accompanied by physical signs of CNS stimulation (e.g., tachycardia, hypertension, cardiac arrhythmias, sweating, hyperpyrexia, convulsions).

Cocaine and alcohol taken together could cause a potentially dangerous reaction. Taken in combination, the two drugs are converted by the body to cocaethylene, which has a longer duration of action in the brain and is more toxic than either drug individually. Notably, this mixture of cocaine and alcohol is a common two-drug combination that frequently results in drug-related death (Pilgrim, Woodford, & Drummer, 2013; Snipes & Benotsch, 2013).

Cocaine Withdrawal

Severe anxiety, along with restlessness and agitation, is among the major symptoms of cocaine withdrawal. Users quickly seek more cocaine or other drugs, such as alcohol, marijuana, or sleeping pills, to rid themselves of the terrible effects of crashing. Withdrawal causes intense depression, craving (i.e., a strong desire to use cocaine despite negative consequences), and drug-seeking behavior that may last for weeks. Individuals who discontinue cocaine use often relapse.

Long-term cocaine use depletes norepinephrine, resulting in a "crash" when use of the drug is discontinued that causes the user to sleep 12 to 18 hours. On awakening, withdrawal symptoms may occur, characterized by sleep disturbances with rebound rapid eye movement (REM) sleep, anergia (i.e., lack of energy), and decreased libido, depression with possible suicidality, anhedonia, poor concentration, and cocaine craving.

Treating individuals with cocaine addiction is complex, because it involves assessing the psychobiologic, social, and pharmacologic aspects of abuse.

> **NCLEXNOTE** In cocaine withdrawal, patients are excessively sleepy because of norepinephrine depletion. Recovery is difficult because of the intense cravings. Nursing interventions should focus on helping patients solve problems related to managing these cravings.

Amphetamines

Amphetamines, known on the street as speed, uppers, ups, black beauties, pep pills, or copilots, were first synthesized for medical use in the 1880s. Amphetamines (Biphetamine, Delcobese, dextroamphetamine,) and other stimulants, such as phenmetrazine (Preludin) and methylphenidate (Ritalin), act on the CNS and peripheral nervous system. They are used to treat attention deficit hyperactivity disorder (ADHD) in children, narcolepsy, depression, and obesity (on a short-term basis). Some people abuse these drugs to achieve the effects of alertness, increased concentration, a sense of increased energy, euphoria, and appetite suppression. Amphetamines are indirect catecholamine agonists and cause the release of newly synthesized norepinephrine. Similar to cocaine, they block the reuptake of norepinephrine and dopamine, but they do not affect the serotonergic system as strongly. They also affect the peripheral nervous system and are powerful sympathomimetics, stimulating both α- and β-receptors. This stimulation results in tachycardia, arrhythmias, increased systolic and diastolic blood pressures, and peripheral hyperthermia. The effects of amphetamine use and the clinical course of an overdose are similar to those of cocaine.

Methamphetamine

Methamphetamine, also known as meth, speed, ice, chalk, crank, fire, glass, and crystal, is an illegal potent CNS stimulant that releases excess dopamine responsible for the drug's toxic effects, including damage to nerve terminals. Highly addictive, it comes in many forms and can be smoked, snorted, orally ingested, or injected. A brief intense sensation, or rush, is reported by those who smoke or inject methamphetamine. Oral ingestion or snorting produces a long-lasting high instead of a rush, which can continue for as long as half a day. This illegal substance is cheap, easy to make, and has devastating consequences.

High doses can elevate body temperature and stimulate seizures. Methamphetamine has a longer duration of action than cocaine and leads to prolonged stimulant effects. Long-term effects include dependence and addiction psychosis (e.g., paranoia, hallucinations), mood disturbances, repetitive motor activity, stroke, weight loss,

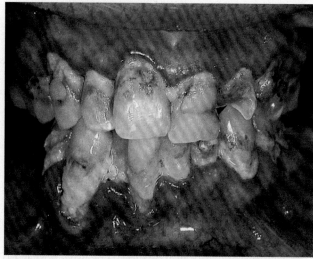

FIGURE 25.1 Severe tooth decay caused by abuse of methamphetamine.

and extensive tooth decay (NIDA, 2013b) (Figure 25.1). Methamphetamine is often used in a "binge and crash" pattern. Tolerance occurs within minutes, and the pleasurable effect disappears even before the drug concentration in the blood falls significantly. After being assessed, referral of the patient to a drug treatment program is necessary.

MDMA and Other Club Drugs

The drug 3-4 methylenedioxymethamphetamine (MDMA), also known as Ecstasy or Molly, is known as a "club drug" because it is used by teens and young adults as part of the nightclub, bar, and rave scenes. MDMA, similar in structure to methamphetamine, causes serotonin to be released from neurons in greater amounts than normal. After being released, this serotonin can excessively activate serotonin receptors. Scientists have also shown that MDMA causes excess dopamine to be released from dopamine-containing neurons. Alarmingly, research in animals has demonstrated that MDMA can damage and destroy serotonin-containing neurons. MDMA can also cause hallucinations, confusion, depression, sleep problems, drug craving, severe anxiety, and paranoia. In higher doses, MDMA can sharply increase body temperature (i.e., malignant hyperthermia), leading to muscle breakdown, kidney and cardiovascular failure, and death (NIDA, 2013c).

Rohypnol gamma-hydroxybutyrate (GHB), and ketamine are predominantly CNS depressants but are also considered "club drugs." Often colorless, tasteless, and odorless, the drugs can be ingested unknowingly. Known also as "date rape" drugs when mixed with alcohol, they can be incapacitating, causing a euphoric, sedative-like effect and producing an "anterograde amnesia," which means that individuals may not remember events they experience while under the influence of these drugs. Ketamine is associated with an increased heart rate and blood pressure, impaired motor function, memory loss, numbness, and vomiting. At high doses, delirium, depression, respiratory depression, and cardiac arrest can occur (NIDA, 2014c).

Nicotine

Nicotine, the addictive chemical mainly responsible for the high prevalence of tobacco use, is the primary reason tobacco is named a public health menace. Smoking is more prevalent among people with alcoholism, polysubstance users, and persons with mental disorders than among the general population. Smoking prevalence among persons with any mental disorders is 36.1% compared to 19.9% adults without mental disorders (Centers for Disease Control and Prevention [CDC], 2013).

Biologic Response to Nicotine

Nicotine stimulates the central, peripheral, and autonomic nervous systems, causing increased alertness, concentration, attention, and appetite suppression. Readily absorbed, it is carried in the bloodstream to the liver where it is partially metabolized. It is also metabolized by the kidneys and excreted in urine (NIDA, 2012a).

Nicotine acts as an agonist of the nicotinic cholinergic receptor sites and stimulates autonomic ganglia in both the parasympathetic and sympathetic nervous systems, resulting in increased release of norepinephrine or acetylcholine. The release of epinephrine by nicotine from the adrenal medulla increases fatty acids, glycerol, and lactate levels in the blood, thereby increasing the risk for atherosclerosis and cardiac muscle pathology.

Other medical complications of nicotine use are numerous. Smoking cigarettes and cigars causes respiratory problems, lung cancer, emphysema, heart problems, and peripheral vascular disease. In fact, smoking is the largest preventable cause of premature death and disability. Cigarette smoking kills at least 440,000 people in the United States each year and makes countless others ill. The use of smokeless tobacco is also associated with serious health problems (CDC, 2013).

Repeated use of nicotine produces both tolerance and addiction. Recent research has shown that nicotine addiction is extremely powerful and is at least as strong as addictions to other drugs, such as heroin and cocaine; most of those who quit relapse within 1 year (NIDA, 2013d).

Nicotine Withdrawal and Smoking Cessation

Nicotine withdrawal is marked by mood changes (e.g., craving, anxiety, irritability, depression) and physiologic changes (difficulty in concentrating, sleep disturbances, headaches, gastric distress, increased appetite). Nicotine replacements such as transdermal patches, nicotine gum, nasal spray, and inhalers have been used successfully to assist in withdrawal by reducing the craving for tobacco. Patches are rotated on skin sites and help maintain a steady blood level of nicotine. Products such as Habitrol, NicoDerm, and ProStep are used daily, with the decrease in strength of nicotine occurring during a period of 6 to 12 weeks.

Successful smoking cessation usually requires more than one type of intervention, including social support and education. However, studies do show that even giving a brief instruction to patients about quitting smoking can be effective. (See Box 25.5). Medications are often used as a smoking cessation strategy. The antidepressant bupropion (Wellbutrin) is marketed as Zyban to help people quit smoking. Another medication, varenicline tartrate (Chantix) reduces the craving and rewarding effects of nicotine by preventing nicotine from accessing one of the acetylcholine receptor sites involved with nicotine dependence, but it can cause depression and related psychiatric symptoms in some people. This side effect limits its usefulness for people with psychiatric disorders (Faessel, Obach, Rollema, Ravva, Williams, & Burstein, 2010; Tranel, McNutt, & Bechara, 2012).

Auricular therapy, or ear acupressure, is being studied as a potential adjunctive treatment for nicotine addiction. Acupressure is based on the principles of an ancient Chinese system of medicine with a goal of returning the

---

BOX 25.5

Research for Best Practices: Nursing Interventions for Smoking Cessation

Rice, V. H., Hartmann-Boyce, J., & Stead, L. F. (2013). Nursing interventions for smoking cessation (Review). The Cochrane Database of Systematic Reviews, 8. Art. No.: CD001188. doi:10.1002/14651848. CD001188.pub4

QUESTION: Which nursing-delivered smoking cessation interventions are effective?

METHODS: Review of 49 studies that were randomized trials of smoking cessation interventions delivered by nurses or health visitors with follow-up of at least 6 months. The main outcome measure was abstinence from smoking. Participants were adult smokers, 18 years and older, of both genders. Primary intervention was advice defined as verbal instruction to stop smoking. This intervention was further categorized into low intensity advice (verbal instruction only) and high intensity (verbal instruction for more than 10 minutes usually with additional materials such as pamphlets).

FINDINGS: Comparing the nursing intervention groups with control groups or to usual care, the studies showed the intervention increased the likelihood of the participants' quitting. Limited indirect evidence showed that interventions were more effective for hospital inpatients with cardiovascular disease than for inpatients with other health conditions. Interventions in nonhospitalized adults also showed evidence of benefit.

IMPLICATIONS FOR NURSING: Even brief instructions to patients regarding the importance of quitting can have a positive effect in changing their smoking behavior.

body to a harmonic balanced state. Through stimulating acupoints on the ear, endogenous endorphin levels and regulation of the sympathetic nervous system changes the taste for tobacco, suppressing nicotine addiction, decreasing nicotine withdrawal symptoms, reducing the desire to smoke, and promoting cessation for a short period of time. Research into this therapy, however, has not yet shown significant effectiveness in smoking cessation (Leung, Neufel, & Marin, 2012; White, Rampes, Liu, Stead, & Campbell, 2014).

Electronic cigarettes (e-cigarettes) were introduced as smoking cessation aids. They are smokeless, battery-operated devices designed to deliver nicotine with flavorings or other chemicals to the lungs without burning tobacco to do so. They resemble regular tobacco cigarettes, cigars, or pipes. More than 250 e-cigarette brands are on the market. E-cigarettes are designed to simulate the act of tobacco smoking without the toxic chemicals produced by burning tobacco leaves. Their safety and effectiveness in smoking cessation are being questioned because e-cigarettes deliver highly addictive nicotine into the lungs and the vapor of some of them contain known carcinogens and toxic chemicals. Additionally, adolescents are increasingly using e-cigarettes believing they are safe, but instead, they may instead serve as a gateway to try other tobacco products (NIDA, 2013e).

Caffeine

Caffeine is a stimulant found in many drinks (coffee, tea, cocoa, soft drinks); chocolate; and OTC medications, including analgesics, stimulants, appetite suppressants, and cold relief preparations. Metabolism of caffeine is very complicated, involving more than 25 metabolites, and varies among different populations (Weldy, 2010). Recently, high energy drinks, consisting of alcohol and caffeine are being marketed to reduce the impairment caused by ingestion of alcohol. The reality is that these energy drinks give a false sense of physical and mental competence and decrease the awareness of impairment. Deaths have been associated with these drinks (Wolk, Ganetsky, & Babu, 2012).

Symptoms of caffeine intoxication can include five or more of the following: restlessness, nervousness, excitement, insomnia, flushed face, diuresis, gastrointestinal disturbance, muscle twitching, rambling flow of thought and speech, tachycardia or cardiac arrhythmia, periods of inexhaustibility, and psychomotor agitation (Echeverri, Montes, Cabrera, Galán, & Prieto, 2010).

Caffeine withdrawal syndrome involves headache, drowsiness, and fatigue, sometimes with impaired psychomotor performance; difficulty concentrating; craving; and psychophysiologic complaints, such as yawning or nausea. Patients with caffeine dependence can be supported in their efforts at withdrawal by learning about the caffeine content of beverages and medication, using decaffeinated beverages, and managing individual withdrawal symptoms.

Cannabis

Marijuana is the common name for the plant *Cannabis sativa*, also known as hemp and many other names. Marijuana's active ingredient is D-9-tetrahydrocannabinol (THC). Hashish, a resin found in flowers of the mature *C. sativa* plant, is its strongest form, containing 10% to 30% THC.

Marijuana is fat soluble and is absorbed rapidly after being smoked or taken orally. After ingestion, THC binds with an opioid receptor in the brain—the μ receptor. This action engages endogenous brain opioid receptors, which are associated with enhanced dopamine activity because THC blocks dopamine reuptake. THC can be stored for weeks in fat tissue and in the brain and is released extremely slowly. Long-term use leads to the accumulation of cannabinoids in the body, primarily the frontal cortex, the limbic areas, and the brain's auditory and visual perception centers. In other areas of the brain, it exerts cardiovascular effects, results in ataxia, and causes increased psychotropic effects. Marijuana use impairs the ability to form memories, recall events, and shift attention from one thing to another. It disrupts coordination of movement, balance, and reaction time. Contrary to popular belief, marijuana is addictive, is an irritant to the lungs and can produce the same respiratory problems experienced by tobacco users (i.e., daily cough, phlegm). People who smoke marijuana miss work more often than those who do not smoke it, but it is not yet known whether marijuana smoke contributes to the risk of lung cancer (NIDA, 2014b).

Marijuana is usually smoked and causes relaxation, euphoria, at times dyscoria (i.e., abnormal pupillary reaction or shape), spatial misperception, time distortion, and food cravings. It also causes relaxation and drowsiness, unlike other hallucinogens, and is often associated with decreased motivation after long-term use. Effects begin immediately after the drug enters the brain and last from 1 to 3 hours.

Two Food and Drug Administration (FDA)-approved drugs, dronabinol and nabilone, contain THC and are used to treat nausea caused by chemotherapy. The known safety issues related to marijuana include impairment of short-term memory, altered judgment and decision making, anxiety, paranoia or psychosis especially in high dose (NIDA, 2014b). Marijuana is legal as a recreational drug in some states in the United States.

"Spice" a term used for synthetic cannabinoid compounds found in various herbal mixtures that produces an experience similar to that of marijuana. Spice mixtures of this type are illegal to sell in the United States because of their addictive properties. Some of these compounds bind more strongly to the same receptors as THC and could produce a more powerful and unpredictable effect. Spice products are popular among young people and are second only to marijuana among illegal drugs used mostly by high school seniors (NIDA, 2012b).

Hallucinogens

The term **hallucinogen** refers to drugs that produce euphoria or dysphoria, altered body image, distorted or sharpened visual and auditory perception, confusion, lack of coordination, and impaired judgment and memory. Severe reactions may cause paranoia, fear of losing one's mind, depersonalization, illusions, delusions, and hallucinations. Hallucinogens typically affect the autonomic and regulatory nervous systems first, increasing heart rate and body temperature and slightly elevating blood pressure. The individual may experience a dry mouth, dizziness, and subjective feelings of being hot or cold. Gradually, these physiologic changes fade, but then perceptual distortions and hallucinations may become prominent. Intense mood and sexual behavior changes may occur; the user may feel unusually close to others or distant and isolated. The true content of hallucinogenic drugs purchased on the street is always in doubt; they are often misidentified or adulterated with other drugs. There are more than 100 different hallucinogens with substantially different molecular structures. Psilocybin (mushroom), D-lysergic acid diethylamide (LSD), phencyclidine (PCP), mescaline, and numerous amphetamine derivatives are examples from a list of many other hallucinogens (NIDA, 2014c).

Patients in acute states of intoxication or in dissociated states may become combative. During the acute state, the primary intervention goals are to reduce stimuli, maintain a safe environment for the patient and others, manage behavior, and observe the patient carefully for medical and psychiatric complications. Instructions to the patient should be clear, short, and simple and delivered in a firm but nonthreatening tone.

Prescription and Over-the-Counter Drugs

Use of prescription drugs for nonmedical purposes has escalated since 2002 with more than 15.2 million Americans taking a pain reliever, tranquilizer, stimulants, or sedative for nonmedical purposes. Abuse of prescription and OTC drugs occurs when one of the following criteria are met:

- Taking a medication that has been prescribed for someone else
- Taking a drug in higher quantity or in another manner than prescribed
- Taking a drug for another purpose than prescribed (NIDA, 2013f)

The **opioids** (e.g., oxycodone, hydrocodone, morphine, fentanyl, codeine) prescribed for pain are some of the more commonly abused prescription medications. The most commonly abused CNS depressants are the barbiturates (e.g., pentobarbital [Nembutal] and benzodiazepines [diazepam, alprazolam, clonazepam, lorazepam), which are prescribed for anxiety and sleep. The *DSM-5* diagnosis, *sedative, hypnotic, or anxiolytic use disorder* would be given when these drugs are abused. Amphetamines (Adderall, Dexedrine) and methylphenidate (Concerta, Ritalin) are stimulants prescribed for ADHD that are also frequently abused. Often, patients combine these drugs with alcohol, which is extremely dangerous and can put patients at risk for overdose, causing coma or death (NIDA, 2013f).

OTC cough medicine containing dextromethorphan (DXM) can produce the same effects as those of ketamine or PCP, such as impaired motor function, numbness, nausea or vomiting, and increased heart rate and blood pressure. In some cases, severe respiratory depression and hypoxia have occurred (NIDA, 2014f).

Opioids and Morphine Derivatives

The term **opioid** refers to any substance that binds to an opioid receptor in the brain to produce an agonist action. Derived from poppies, opioids are powerful drugs that have been used for centuries to relieve pain. They include opium, heroin, morphine, and codeine. Even centuries after their discovery, opioids are still the most effective pain relievers. They also cause CNS depression, sleep, or stupor. Although heroin has no medicinal use, other opioids, such as morphine and codeine, are used to treat pain related to illnesses (e.g., cancer) and during medical and dental procedures. When used as directed by a clinician, opioids are safe and generally do not produce addiction. However, opioids also possess very strong reinforcing properties and can quickly trigger addiction when used improperly.

Two important effects produced by opioids are pleasure (or reward) and pain relief. The brain itself also produces substances known as endorphins that activate the opioid receptors. Opioids cause tolerance and physical dependence that appear to be specific for each receptor subtype. Tolerance develops, particularly to the analgesic, respiratory depression, and sedative actions of opioids. Often, a 100% increase in dose is used to achieve the same physical effects when tolerance exists. Physical dependence can develop rapidly. When use of the drug is discontinued, after a period of continuous use, a rebound hyperexcitability withdrawal syndrome usually occurs. Table 25.4 describes the onset, duration, and symptoms of mild, moderate, and severe withdrawal symptoms.

Heroin is an illegal highly addictive drug that is the most abused and the most rapidly acting of the opioids. Typically sold as a white or brownish powder or as the black sticky substance known as "black tar heroin" on the streets, it is

TABLE 25.4	SEVERITY OF OPIOID WITHDRAWAL SYNDROME		
Initial Onset and Duration	Mild Withdrawal	Moderate Withdrawal	Severe Withdrawal
Onset: 8–12 h after last use of short-acting opioids. 1–3 d after last use for longer acting opioids, such as methadone	Physical: yawning, rhinorrhea, perspiration, restlessness, lacrimation, sleep disturbance	Physical: dilated pupils, bone and muscle aches, sensation of "goose flesh," hot and cold flashes	Nausea; vomiting; stomach cramps; diarrhea; weight loss; insomnia; twitching of muscles and kicking movements of legs; increased blood pressure, pulse, and respirations
Duration: Severe symptoms peak between 48 and 72 h. Symptoms abate in 7–10 d for short-acting opioids. Methadone withdrawal symptoms can last several weeks.	Emotional: increased craving, anxiety, dysphoria	Emotional: irritability, increased anxiety, and craving	Emotional: depression, increased anxiety, dysphoria, subjective sense of feeling "wretched"

frequently "cut" with other substances, such as sugar, starch, powdered milk, quinine, and strychnine or other poisons. It can be sniffed, snorted, and smoked but is most frequently injected, which poses risks for transmission of human immunodeficiency devices (HIV) and other diseases resulting from the sharing of needles or other injection equipment.

Naturally occurring neurotransmitters normally bind to the mu-opioid receptors which are involved in pain, hormonal release, and feelings of well being. When heroin enters the brain, it is converted to morphine and immediately binds to the mu-opioid receptors stimulating the release of dopamine, which causes an intense pleasurable rush. Usually, the individual also experiences a warm flushing of the skin, dry mouth, and a heavy feeling in the limbs. Side effects include nausea, vomiting, and severe itching. Following these initial side effects, drowsiness, clouded mental function, slowing of the heart, and extreme slowing of breathing can occur (NIDA 2014d).

One of the most detrimental long-term side effects of heroin is addiction itself, which causes neurochemical and molecular changes and profoundly alters brain structure and composition. Enlarged ventricular spaces and loss of frontal volume are reported (Cadet, et al., 2014). Heroin also produces profound degrees of tolerance and physical dependence, which are powerful motivating factors for compulsive use and abuse. After becoming addicted, heroin users gradually spend more and more time and energy obtaining and using the drug until these activities become their primary purpose in life (NIDA, 2014d).

Opioid Intoxication or Overdose

Emergency treatment of individuals with opioid intoxication is initiated with an assessment of CNS functioning, specifically arousal and respiratory functioning. Naloxone (Narcan), an opioid antagonist, is given to reverse the side effects of respiratory depression, sedation, and hyperten-

sion. In the presence of physical dependence on opioids, naloxone produces withdrawal symptoms that are related to the dosage and the degree and type of opioid dependence. When administered intravenously, the pharmacologic effect is generally apparent within 2 minutes. When administered intramuscularly, the effect is more prolonged.

Initial Opioid Detoxification

Ideally, opioid detoxification is achieved by gradually reducing an opioid dose over several days or weeks. Many treatment programs include administering low doses of a substitute drug, such as methadone, which can help satisfy the drug craving without providing the same subjective high. If opioids are abruptly withdrawn ("cold turkey") from someone who is physically dependent on them, severe physical symptoms occur, including body aches, diarrhea, tachycardia, fever, runny nose, sneezing, sweating, yawning, nausea or vomiting, nervousness, restlessness or irritability, shivering or trembling, abdominal cramps, weakness, and elevated blood pressure.

Maintenance Treatment

Methadone maintenance is the treatment of people with opioid addiction with a daily stabilized dose of methadone. Methadone is used because of its long half-life of 15 to 30 hours. It is a potent opioid and is physiologically addicting, but it satisfies the opioid craving without producing the subjective high of heroin (Box 25.6).

Detoxification is accomplished by setting the beginning methadone dose and then slowly reducing it during the next 21 days. Treatment programs determine the dose of methadone that will block subjective feelings of craving and will not cause somnolence or intoxication in patients. The initial dose of methadone is determined by the severity of withdrawal symptoms and is usually 20

BOX 25.6

Drug Profile: Methadone (Dolophine)

DRUG CLASS: Narcotic agonist, analgesic

RECEPTOR AFFINITY: Binds to opioid receptors in the CNS to produce analgesia, euphoria, sedation; the receptors mediating the effects of endogenous opioids, which are thought to be enkephalins, endorphins

INDICATIONS: Detoxification and temporary maintenance treatment of narcotic addiction; relief of severe pain

ROUTE AND DOSAGE: Available in 5-, 10-, and 40-mg tablets; oral concentrate

Adults: Detoxification: Initially 15 to 30 mg. Increase dosage to suppress withdrawal signs. 40 mg/d in single or divided dose is usually an adequate stabilizing dose; continue stabilizing dose for 2 to 3 days; then gradually decrease dosage. Usual maintenance dose is 20 to 120 mg/d in single dosing.

HALF-LIFE (PEAK EFFECT):
PO 90–120 min
IM 1–2 h
SC 1–2 h

SELECTED SIDE EFFECTS: Light-headedness, dizziness, sedation, nausea, vomiting, facial flushing, peripheral circulatory collapse, arrhythmia, palpitations, urethral spasm, urinary retention, respiratory depression, circulatory depression, respiratory arrest, shock, cardiac arrest

WARNINGS: Never administer in the presence of hypersensitivity to narcotics, diarrhea caused by poisoning (before toxins are eliminated), bronchial asthma, or chronic obstructive pulmonary disease. Use caution in the presence of acute abdominal conditions and cardiovascular disease. Increased effects and toxicity of methadone if taken concurrently with cimetidine and/or ranitidine. Methadone hydrochloride tablets are for PO administration only and *must not* used for injection. It is recommended that methadone hydrochloride tablets, if dispensed, be packaged in child-resistant containers and kept out of the reach of children to prevent accidental injection.

SPECIFIC PATIENT AND FAMILY EDUCATION
- Take drug exactly as prescribed.
- Avoid use of alcohol.
- Take the drug with food while lying quietly; this should minimize nausea.
- Eat small, frequent meals to treat nausea and loss of appetite.
- If experiencing dizziness and drowsiness, avoid driving a car or performing other tasks that require alertness.
- Administer mild laxative for constipation.
- Report severe nausea, vomiting, constipation, shortness of breath, or difficulty breathing. Methadone products, when used for treatment of narcotic addiction, shall be dispensed only by approved hospital and community pharmacies and maintenance programs approved by the FDA and designated state authority.

CNS, central nervous system; COPD, chronic obstructive pulmonary disease; IM, intramuscular; FDA, Food and Drug Administration; PO, oral; SC, subcutaneous.

---

to 30 mg orally. If symptoms persist after 1 to 2 hours, the dosage can be raised. Dosage should should then be reevaluated daily during the first few days of treatment. Initial doses of exceeding 40 mg can cause severe discomfort as the detoxification proceeds.

Patients receive this dose daily in conjunction with regular drug abuse counseling focused on the elimination of illicit drug use; lifestyle changes, such as finding friends who do not use drugs or achieving stability in one's living situation; strengthening social supports; and structuring time into pursuits that do not involve drug use. After illicit drug use ceases for a period of time, major lifestyle changes have been made, and social supports are in place, patients may gradually detoxify from methadone with continuing support through community support groups, such as Narcotics Anonymous.

The length of methadone treatment varies for each patient. The protocol for starting detoxification from methadone varies widely, depending on the patient's commitment to abstinence, lifestyle changes that have occurred, and strong peer group support, all of which are needed to sustain the patient during methadone detoxification when increased cravings often occur. Methadone treatment combined with behavioral therapy and counseling has been used effectively and safely to treat opioid addiction for more than 40 years. Combined with behavioral therapy and counseling, methadone enables patients to stop using heroin.

Naltrexone has also been used successfully to treat opioid addiction. It binds to opioid receptors in the CNS and competitively inhibits the action of opioid drugs, including those with mixed narcotic agonist–antagonist properties, thereby blocking the intoxicating effects. If an opioid-addicted individual takes naltrexone before he or she is fully detoxified from opioids, withdrawal symptoms may result (see Table 25.4).

Buprenorphine is a long-acting partial agonist that acts on the same receptors as heroin and morphine, relieving drug cravings without producing the same intense "high" or dangerous side effects. At low doses, buprenorphine produces sufficient agonist effect to enable opioid-addicted individuals to discontinue the misuse of opioids without experiencing withdrawal symptoms. Buprenorphine carries a lower risk of abuse, addiction, and side effects compared with full opioid agonists. Buprenorphine is highly bound to plasma proteins and metabolized by the liver. The half-life of buprenorphine is 24 to 60 hours. Buprenorphine has poor oral bioavailability and moderate sublingual bioavailability. Formulations for opioid addiction treatment are given as sublingual tablets.

Buprenorphine and naloxone were recently combined into one formulation with a brand name of *Bunavail, Suboxone, or Zubsolv* and is indicated for maintenance treatment of opioid addiction. The medication is administered sublingually as a single dose.

Inhalants

Inhalants are organic solvents, also known as *volatile substances* that are CNS depressants. When inhaled, they cause euphoria, sedation, emotional lability, and impaired judgment. Intoxication can result in respiratory depression, stupor, and coma. Inhalants are typically abused by young children with adolescents using less than younger children. Different inhalants tend to be used by various age groups. New users (ages 12 to 15) are more likely to abuse glue, shoe polish, spray paints, gasoline, and lighter fluids. The 16- to 17-year olds most commonly abuse nitrous oxide or "whippets" and adults a class of nitrites such as amyl nitrites or "poppers" (NIDA 2012c). Addiction is rare, but inhalants can be intermediate between legal and illegal drugs (Sanchez, Ribeiro, Moura, Noto, & Martins, 2013).

Most inhalants are common household or industrial products that give off mind-altering chemical fumes when sniffed. They include the following:

- *Volatile Solvents:* liquids that vaporize at room temperature such as paint thinners or removers, degreasers, dry-cleaning fluids, gasoline, and lighter fluid. Office supply solvents include correction fluids, felt-tip marker fluid, electronic contact cleaners, and glue.
- *Aerosols:* sprays that contain propellant and solvents such as spray paint, hair spray, fabric protector spray, aerosol computer cleaning products, vegetable oil spray, analgesics, asthma sprays, deodorants, and air fresheners
- *Gases:* household or commercial products such as butane lighters and propane tanks, whipped cream aerosols or dispensers, and refrigerant gases; medical anesthetics such as ether, chloroform, halothane, and nitrous oxide ("laughing gas").
- *Nitrites:* organic nitrites include cyclohexyl, butyl, and amyl nitrites. When marketed for illicit uses, organic nitrates are sold in small brown bottles labeled "video head cleaner," "room odorizer," "leather cleaner," or "room deodorizer" (NIDA, 2012c).

Most inhalants other than nitrites depress the CNS in a manner similar to alcohol (e.g., slurred speech, lack of coordination, euphoria, dizziness). They may cause light-headedness, hallucinations and delusions. The nitrites enhance sexual pleasure by dilating and relaxing blood vessels. They are thought to be antagonistic at the NMDA receptor and may cause neuronal damage in the mesolimbic system (Cousaert, Heylens, & Audenaert, 2013).

Inhalant Intoxication

Inhalants are easily absorbed through the lungs and are widely distributed in the body, reaching the highest concentrations in fat tissue and the nervous system where the most profound effects are exhibited. Mild intoxication occurs within minutes and can last as long as 30 minutes. Often, the drugs are inhaled repeatedly to maintain an intoxicated state for hours. Initially, the person experiences a sense of euphoria, but as the dose increases, confusion, perceptual distortions, and severe CNS depression occurs. Inhalant users are also at risk for **sudden sniffing death**, which can occur when the inhaled fumes replace oxygen in the lungs and CNS, causing the user to suffocate. Inhalants can also cause death by disrupting the normal heart rhythm, which can lead to cardiac arrest (NIDA, 2012b).

Long-Term Complications

Chronic neurologic syndromes can result from long-term use, which is linked to widespread brain damage and cognitive abnormalities that can range from mild impairment to severe dementia. In recent studies, considerably more inhalant users than cocaine users had brain abnormalities and their damage was more extensive. Inhalant users also performed significantly worse on tests of working memory with diminished ability to focus attention, plan, and solve problems. However, inhalants can change brain chemistry and may permanently damage the brain and CNS. Magnetic resonance imaging scans of users demonstrate severe changes in cerebral white matter (Cairney, O'Connor, Dingwall, Maruff, Shafiq-Antonacci, Currie, et al., 2013).

Steroids

Anabolic steroids is the name for synthetic substances related to the male sex hormones (androgens). Developed in the late 1930s to treat hypogonadism, they are also used to treat delayed puberty, some types of impotence, and wasting of the body caused by HIV infection or other diseases. They promote growth of skeletal muscle and the development of male sexual characteristics. More than 100 different types exist; to be used legally, all require a prescription. Some dietary supplements, such as dehydroepiandrosterone (DHEA) and androstenedione (Andro), can be purchased in commercial health stores. They are often used in the belief that large doses can convert into testosterone or a similar compound in the body that promote muscle growth. They can be taken orally or intramuscularly. Some are applied to the skin as a cream or gel. When abused, these preparations are taken at 10 to 100 times higher doses than are used for medical disorders. Although use among men is higher than among women, use among women is growing (NIDA, 2012d).

Case reports and small studies indicate that in high doses, anabolic steroids increase irritability and aggression

(Hallberg, 2011). Some steroid users report that they have committed aggressive acts, such as physical fighting, armed robbery, using force to obtain something, committing property damage, stealing from stores, or breaking into a house or building. Users engage in these behaviors more often when they take steroids than when they are drug free. Other behavioral effects include euphoria, increased energy, sexual arousal, mood swings, distractibility, forgetfulness, and confusion.

Anabolic steroids do not trigger a rapid increase in dopamine or cause the "high" associated with other drugs of abuse. However, long-term use can affect neurotransmitter pathways that regulate mood and behavior. With time, anabolic steroid use is associated with an increased risk for heart attacks and strokes, blood clotting, cholesterol changes, hypertension, depressed mood, fatigue, restlessness, loss of appetite, insomnia, reduced libido, muscle and joint pain, and severe liver problems (including hepatic cancer). Males can have reduced sperm production, shrinking of the testes, and difficulty or pain in urinating. Other undesirable body changes include breast enlargement in men and masculinization of women's bodies. Both sexes may experience hair loss and acne. Intravenous or intramuscular use of the drug and needle sharing puts users at risk for HIV, hepatitis B and C, and infective endocarditis, as well as bacterial infections at injection sites (NIDA, 2012e).

EMERGING DRUGS AND TRENDS

New drugs and drug use trends rapidly enter our communities. The National Institute of Drug Abuse continuously report on these drugs. Some of the newer drugs include synthetic cathinones (bath salts), Krokodil, (toxic homemade opioid), and synthetic hallucinogens (N-bomb).

Bath salts contain cathinone, an amphetamine-like stimulant naturally found in the Khat plant (*Catha edulis*). Severe intoxication and dangerous health effects are associated with these drugs. These drugs, which are chemically similar to methamphetamines and MDMA, produce euphoria, increased sociability, and increased sex drive, as well as paranoia, agitation, and hallucinatory delirium. Indication is that they are strongly linked to abuse (NIDA, 2012e).

Krokodil, a synthetic form of a heroin-like drug called desomorphine, is made by combining codeine tablets with toxic chemicals such as lighter fluid and industrial cleaners. It is used as a cheap substitute for heroin in poor rural areas of Russia but is now making its appearance in the United States. The drug is named Krokodil because a scaly, gray–green dead skin forms at the site of injection (NIDA, 2014e).

Synthetic hallucinogens, (e.g., the N-bomb), are being sold as substitutes for LSD or mescaline. These chemicals, considered more powerful than LSD, act on serotonin receptors and can cause seizures, heart attack, or respiratory arrest and death (NIDA, 2014e).

GAMBLING: A NON–SUBSTANCE–RELATED DISORDER

Social gambling becomes a **gambling disorder** (also referred to as pathologic gambling) when it is persistent and recurrent leading to clinically significant impairment or distress. In the DSM-5, this disorder is classified as an addiction and a non–substance-related disorder (APA, 2013). Individuals with this disorder are preoccupied with gambling and experience an aroused, euphoric state during the actual betting. The action of seeking an aroused state is often more important to the pathologic gambler than the desire for money itself. They are drawn to the games and begin making bigger and bigger bets. Characteristically, they relentlessly chase their losses in an attempt to win them back. They are unable to control their gaming and may lie to family, friends, and employers to hide their gambling habit. They have an intense need to gamble and often turn to gambling when feeling distressed. These individuals are highly competitive, energetic, restless, and easily bored. Some evidence shows that changes in the serotonin system are associated with addiction behavior, similar to results reported for nicotine and alcohol dependence (Wilson, da Silva Lobo, Tavares, Gentil, & Vallada, 2013).

One study found a 1% to 3% lifetime prevalence (Grant, Schreiber, Odlaug, & Kim, 2010). According to the DSM-5, the lifetime prevalence rate is about 0.4% to 1% (APA, 2013). Individuals with gambling problems are more likely to commit suicide than those who do not have a gambling problem and are less likely to seek mental health treatment (Séquin, Boyd, Lesage, McGirr, Suissa, & Tousignant, 2010).

This disorder is conceptualized as similar to alcohol and other substances of dependence. When substances are used in conjunction with gambling, they cause a deterioration in play and accelerate the progression of the gambling disorder. Other comorbid disorders include depression, ADHD, Tourette's syndrome, and personality disorders (Park, Cho, Jeon, Lee, Bae, Park, et al., 2010). The disorder has four phases: winning, losing, desperation, and hopelessness. Pathologic gambling can be treated by psychotherapists experienced in this disorder; for many of these addicts, Gamblers Anonymous is sufficient to curb the disorder.

Compulsive gamblers feel omnipotent in their ability to win back what was lost. This omnipotence serves as self-deception that leads to denial. Care of these patients involves confronting such omnipotent beliefs. These individuals quickly irritate staff with their self-assurance and overbearing attitude. Staff education about the disorder is important. Family involvement is also crucial. Families often have been dealing with the patient in a dysfunctional manner. Relapse prevention involves learning about specific cues that trigger the gambling behavior.

EVIDENCE-BASED NURSING CARE FOR PERSONS WITH SUBSTANCE-RELATED DISORDERS

The assessment process is, in part, a treatment intervention. Patients are often in denial about the severity of the problem and about its emotional, social, legal, vocational, or other consequences (see Nursing Care Plan 25.1, available at http://thepoint.lww.com/BoydEssentials).

Nursing Assessment

Assessment is crucial to understanding level of use, abuse, or dependence and to determining the patient's denial or acceptance of treatment. Assessment is often detailed and may involve family members and other loved ones. Along with the psychiatric nursing interview (see Chapter 9), specific areas should be assessed. Box 25.7 gives examples of typical behaviors exhibited by individuals that are associated with each level of use, abuse, and addiction. The nurse can use the Substance Abuse Assessment as a guide in eliciting a substance use history in the assessment process (Box 25.8).

Usually, nurses encounter individuals during crisis when they are seeking professional help. These situations offer an opportunity to explore the denial that keeps their addiction thriving. The nurse's approach should be caring, matter-of-fact, gentle, and direct. Approaches that are punitive or attempt to elicit feelings of guilt or shame are destructive to the therapeutic relationship.

Denial of a Problem

Denial can be expressed in diverse behaviors and attitudes and may not be expressed as an overt denial of the problem. For example, patients may admit to a problem and even thank you for helping them to realize they have a problem but insist they can overcome the problem on their own and do not need outside help.

> **KEYCONCEPT** **Denial** is the patient's inability to accept his or her loss of control over substance use or the severity of the consequences associated with the substance abuse or addiction.

The following characteristics are typical of a person who has alcoholism and who is in denial:

- Confusion about severity of drinking history: "I went out drinking with friends last week and didn't have any problems; I don't get drunk all the time."
- Difficulty reconciling early positive experiences of alcohol use with current problems: "I used to drink with my buddies after work to unwind. We had a great time. Those were some good times...."
- Confusion regarding the definition of *alcoholic:* "Well, I don't have withdrawal symptoms, so I can't be an alcoholic."
- Relief when they compare themselves with others and find the others in worse condition: "They are the alcoholics, not me!"

BOX 25.7

Behaviors in Substance Use, Abuse, and Addiction

SUBSTANCE USE
- Does not have possible danger or potential legal problems
- Engages in use to enhance social situations and interaction
- Is not intended to result in intoxication
- Has control of the amount and frequency of use
- Exhibits socially acceptable behavior while using

PRESCRIPTION MEDICATION USE
- Use is for the dose, frequency, and indications prescribed.
- Use is for the particular episode of the condition for which it was prescribed.
- Use is coordinated among prescribing physicians.

SUBSTANCE ABUSE
- Use for intoxication or feeling of being "high"
- Use that interferes with normal life functions (e.g., producing sleep when inappropriate, excitability or irritability interfering with social interaction)
- Potential harm to self or others (e.g., driving while intoxicated, use of injection drug equipment)
- Use that has legal consequences (e.g., all use of illicit drugs)
- Use resulting in socially unacceptable behavior (e.g., public drunkenness, verbal or physical abuse)
- Use to alter normal feeling states such as sadness or anxiety

PRESCRIPTION MEDICATION ABUSE
- Use is at a higher dose and greater frequency than prescribed.
- Use is for indications other than prescribed or for self-diagnosed condition.
- Use results in feeling tired, having a clouded mental state, or feeling "hyperactive" or nervous.
- Supplementing medication with alcohol or drugs
- Soliciting more than one physician for the same medication
- Inability to control the amount and frequency of use
- Tolerance to larger amounts of the substance
- Withdrawal symptoms when stopping use
- Severe consequences from alcohol or drug use

SUBSTANCE ADDICTION
- Drug craving
- Compulsive use
- Presence of aberrant drug-related behaviors
- Repeated relapse into drug use after withdrawal

BOX 25.8

Substance Abuse Assessment

DRUG/LAST USE	PATTERN OF USE (AMOUNT, ROUTE, FIRST USE, FREQUENCY, AND LENGTH OF USE)
Alcohol/	
Stimulants/	
Opioids/	
Sedative–hypnotics and anxiolytic agents/	
Hallucinogens/	
Marijuana/	
Inhalants/	
Nicotine/	
Caffeine/	

ABUSE INDICATORS
1. Tolerance (increasing use of drug or alcohol with the same level of intoxication): _____
2. Withdrawal symptoms: a. Shakes? _____ b. Tremors? _____ c. Cramps, diarrhea, or rapid pulse? _____ d. Feeling paranoid, fearful? _____ e. Difficulty sleeping? _____
3. Consequences of use (e.g., presenting problems, persistent or recurrent emotional, social, legal, or other problems): _____
4. Loss of control of amount, frequency, or duration of use: _____
5. Desire or efforts to decrease use or control use: _____
6. Preoccupation (increasing focus or time spent on use and obtaining substances): _____
7. Social, vocational, recreational activities affected by use: _____
8. Previous alcohol or drug abuse treatment: _____

Nursing Diagnoses: _____

- A delusion that drinking can be self-controlled: "If I search hard enough or long enough, I will find a way to control and enjoy drinking."
- Confusion or trouble accepting that behavior is different when intoxicated: "I couldn't have done that; that's just not like me."

This quandary about the nature of the problem has often been met with confrontation by nurses and other professionals in the past. But argumentation, presenting evidence of addiction, and lecturing often fail to elicit admission of a problem or induce behavior change.

> ### Gladys and Denial
> Gladys continues to deny that she has a drinking problem. She is angry with her son for suggesting that she has a problem and refuses to sign a release of information for him.

Motivation for Change

Motivation is a key predictor of whether individuals will change their substance use behavior (Collins, Malone, & Larimer, 2012).

> **KEYCONCEPT**   **Motivation** is a goal-oriented attitude that propels action for change and can help sustain the development of new activities and behaviors.

Ambivalence about substance use is normal and can be dealt with by working with the patients' own concerns about their use of alcohol and other drugs. Motivation is fluid and can be modified. Experiences such as increased distress levels, critical life events, a period of evaluation or appraisal of one's life, recognizing negative consequences of use, and positive and negative external incentives for change can all influence a patient's commitment to change.

Techniques that enhance motivation are associated with increased success in treatment, higher rates of abstinence, and successful follow-up treatment (Lozano, LaRowe, Smith, Tuerk, & Roitzsch, 2013). **Motivational interviewing** is a method of therapeutic intervention that seeks to elicit self-motivational statements from patients, supports behavioral change, and creates a disconnect between the patient's goals and their continued alcohol and other drug use. The acronym FRAMES (which is short form for feedback, responsibility, advice, menu of strategies, empathy, and self-efficacy) summarizes elements of brief interventions with patients using motivational interviewing (Box 25.9).

> **NCLEXNOTE**   Motivational approaches are priority interventions for patients with substance-related disorders. They help patients recognize a problem and develop change strategies.

Countertransference

Countertransference is the total emotional reaction of the treatment provider to the patient (see Chapter 5).

BOX 25.9

FRAMES—Effective Elements of Brief Intervention

FEEDBACK
Provide patients with personal feedback regarding their individual status, such as personal alcohol and other drug consumption relative to norms, information about elevated liver enzyme values, and other factors.

RESPONSIBILITY
Emphasize the individual's freedom of choice and personal responsibility for change. General themes are as follows:
1. It's up to you; you're free to decide to change or not.
2. No one else can decide for you or force you to change.
3. You're the one who has to do it if it's going to happen.

ADVICE
Include a clear recommendation or advice on the need for change, typically in a supportive and concerned, rather than in a judgmental, manner.

MENU
Provide a menu of treatment options from which patients may pick those that seem more suitable or appealing.

EMPATHIC COUNSELING
Show warmth, support, respect, and understanding in communication with patients.

SELF-EFFICACY
Reinforce self-efficacy or an optimistic feeling that he or she can change.

Patients with substance-related disorders can generate strong feelings and reactions in nurses and other health care providers (Table 25.5). These feelings can be generated by overtly unpleasant behaviors of the substance-dependent persons, such as lying, deceit, manipulation, or hostility, or these feelings may be more subconscious and stem from past experiences with people with alcoholism or addicts or even from dealing with situations in the health care provider's own family.

Codependence

The concept of **codependence** emerged out of studies of women's relationships with husbands who abused alcohol. Today, the scope of codependency includes both men and women who grew up in any type of dysfunctional family system in which substance abuse may or may not have been a problem. Codependence has also been described as "enabling," in which an individual in a relationship with a person who abuses alcohol inadvertently reinforces the drinking behavior of the other person. The codependency label remains controversial and is viewed by some as an oversimplification of complex emotions and behaviors of family members. Mental health professionals should be careful not to use it as a catch-all diagnosis and to take special care to assess and plan interventions that address each person's particular situation, problems, and needs (Mental Health America, 2014).

Nursing Diagnoses

Several nursing diagnoses could be generated for persons using and abusing substances. The particular substance and the patient's addiction to it must be considered in forming the nursing diagnoses. For example, a person who is newly diagnosed with alcoholism will be assessed differently than one who has multiple attempts at treatment for cocaine addiction. One common nursing diagnosis is Ineffective Denial.

Therapeutic Relationship

It is critical that the nurse establish a therapeutic relationship with these patients (Box 25.10). Several

TABLE 25.5	PATIENT BEHAVIORS AND COUNTERTRANSFERENCE REACTIONS
Patient Behavior	**Common Nursing Reaction**
Behaves as a victim	Feels a sense of helplessness, increased need to give advice and "fix" the situation and the patient; shows anger toward the patient for not being able to take care of the situation him- or herself
Is intrusive, hostile, belittling	Can be frightened, withdraw from patient, express anger overtly, or be passive-aggressive (i.e., suggesting discharge to the team or ignoring legitimate requests from patient)
Does everything right, is insightful, pleasant, and so forth	Congratulates self on therapeutic interventions; can become bored or complacent
Relapses into drug or alcohol use	Feels angry, personally betrayed; withdraws from other patients; doubts own abilities
Asks personal questions about staff qualifications or prior drug or alcohol abuse	Reveals personal information, resents the intrusion, and may regret divulging information
Is silent or divulges minimal information	Tries harder, doubts own therapeutic ability, is angered by patient's resistance
Tries to "bend" or ignore rules of milieu and group rules	May permit program rule infractions; may feel pressured, angry, or passive-aggressive
Insists that no one can help him or her	Feels pressure to be the one who can help; may feel angry and inept or helpless

Imhof, J. E. (1991). Countertransference issues in alcoholism and drug addiction. *Psychiatric Annals*, 21(5), 292–306.

BOX 25.10 • THERAPEUTIC DIALOGUE • The Patient with Alcoholism

INEFFECTIVE APPROACH

Nurse: I would like to talk with you about your problem with alcoholism.

Gladys: Alcoholism! It's not that bad. Everyone gets loaded!

Nurse: You tell me why you were drinking. Your wife left you. You drink a quart of vodka a day. Your blood alcohol level was 0.15% when you were admitted.

Gladys: So what! I do have some problems or I wouldn't be here. But, I'm not an alcoholic. (Denial)

Nurse: Do you know what an alcoholic is?

Gladys: Sure I do. My father was one. He was a useless bum. I'm not anything like him.

Nurse: It sounds like you are a lot like him.

Gladys: I think I need to rest now. My back is killing me (avoidance).

EFFECTIVE APPROACH

Nurse: I would like to talk with you about what happens when you drink.

Gladys: It's not that bad. Everyone gets loaded!

Nurse: What concerns do you have about your drinking?

Gladys: I'm not really concerned. My son is. He thinks I drink too much.

Nurse: What does he tell you about that?

Gladys: Well, complains about it, but I just have a glass of wine at night.

Nurse: It sounds as if he is concerned about this, but you have your doubts about how serious it is. Your son is invited to our family education group, so he can learn about alcohol abuse.

Gladys: I have a lot of problems besides alcohol. I never use drugs. I only drink because it relaxes me and makes it easier to deal with stress.

Nurse: Many people drink to help them cope with stress. Sometimes the drinking itself can cause stress. While you are here, do you think it would be useful to look at the stress in your life and how it relates to your drinking?

Gladys: Yes. But I only drink when things get too out of hand. My health is pretty good.

Nurse: We can provide information about your health and alcohol use. To evaluate what information may be helpful, I would like to get a little more information about your drinking.

CRITICAL THINKING CHALLENGE

- What effect did the nurse have on the patient in using the word alcoholism in the first interaction?

- Discuss what communication approaches the nurse used in the second scenario to engage the patient in disclosing problems with alcohol and her relationship with her son. How does this nurse's approach vary from the one in the first interaction?

general guidelines are available for establishing therapeutic interactions with patients in substance abuse treatment programs:

- Encourage honest expression of feelings.
- Listen to what the individual is really saying.
- Express caring for the individual.
- Hold the individual responsible for his or her behavior.
- Provide fair and consistent consequences for negative behavior.
- Talk about specific objectionable actions.
- Do not compromise your own values or nursing practice.
- Communicate the treatment plan to the patient and to others on the treatment team.
- Monitor your own reactions to the patient.

Confrontation, or pointing out the inconsistencies in thoughts, feelings, and actions, can promote the person's experience of the natural consequences of one's behavior. Learning from previous behavior and its consequences is how change occurs. Confrontation can be very threatening to patients and should only occur within the context of a trusting relationship.

Mental Health Nursing Interventions

Several treatment modalities are used in most addiction treatment (pharmacologic modalities were discussed earlier in this chapter), including 12-step–program-focused, cognitive or psychoeducation, behavioral, group psychotherapy, and individual and family therapy.

BOX 25.11

Principles of Effective Treatment for Addiction

1. Addiction is a complex but treatable disease that affects brain function and behavior.
2. No single treatment is appropriate for everyone.
3. Treatment needs to be readily available.
4. Effective treatment attends to multiple needs of the individual, not just his or her drug use.
5. Remaining in treatment for an adequate period of time is critical.
6. Behavioral therapies—including individual, family, or group counseling—are the most commonly used forms of drug abuse treatment.
7. Medications are an important element of treatment for many patients, especially when combined with counseling and other behavioral therapies.

8. An individual's treatment and service plan must be assessed continually and modified as necessary to ensure that it meets his or her changing needs.
9. Many drug-addicted individuals also have concurrent mental disorders.
10. Medically assisted detoxification is only the first stage of addiction treatment and by itself does little to change long-term drug abuse.
11. Treatment does not need to be voluntary to be effective.
12. Drug use during treatment must be monitored continuously because lapses during treatment do occur.
13. Treatment programs should provide assessment for HIV/AIDS, hepatitis B and C, tuberculosis, and other infectious diseases, as well as provide targeted risk-reduction counseling, linking patients to treatment as necessary.

National Institute on Drug Abuse. (2012f). *Principles of drug addiction treatment: A research-based guide* (NIH Publication No. 12-4180) (3rd ed., pp. 3–4). Bethesda: MD: Author.

Discharge planning and relapse prevention are also essential components of successful treatment and so are incorporated into most programs. See Table 25.6 for different treatment approaches to chemical addiction and Box 25.11 Principles of Effective Treatment for Addiction.

Because patients with substance-related disorders differ greatly, no single type of treatment program will work for every individual. Often, several approaches can work together, but others may be inappropriate. Treatment programs usually combine many different interventions to provide a comprehensive approach based on the individual's needs. Nursing interventions vary depending on the nature of the current problems and their severity. For a patient who is being detoxified, physical interventions (e.g., monitoring vital signs and neurologic functioning) are necessary. When the substance use disorder is secondary to other physical or psychiatric problems, education of patient and family may be a priority.

Assessment and interventions should include culturally relevant data such as unique physiological responses to substances, behavioral responses to dependence, and social expectations and sanctions. Staff who are knowledgeable about cultural differences and issues are integral to successful treatment.

Brief Intervention

Within the alcohol and other drugs field, brief intervention is a highly developed, researched, and widely accepted approach. A growing body of evidence indicates **brief interventions** are more effective than no treatment and indications suggest that they are as effective as more intensive interventions (Cole, Clark, Seale, Shellenberger, Lyme, Johnson et al., 2012).

Screening and brief intervention are two separate skills that can be used together to reduce risky substance use.

Screening involves asking questions about alcohol or drug use. A **brief intervention** is a negotiated conversation between the professional and patient designed to reduce or eliminate alcohol and drug use.

Not everyone who is screened will need a brief intervention and not everyone who needs a brief intervention will require treatment. In fact, the goals of screening and brief intervention are to reduce risky substance use before people become dependent or addicted.

Brief intervention is effective for several reasons. Research indicates that brief interventions are an appropriate response to patients presenting in a general health or community setting and who are unlikely to need, seek, or attend specialist treatment. Brief intervention—to be given clear concise information by a professional—may be all the patient may want. It is also an important part of the overall approach of harm reduction (discussed later in this chapter).

Brief intervention is most successful when working with people who:

- Are experiencing few problems with their drug use
- Have low levels of dependence
- Have a short history of drug use
- Have stable backgrounds
- Are unsure or ambivalent about changing or ending their drug use

It is recommended that brief intervention at a minimum include:

- Advising how to reduce patient's drug use
- Providing harm reduction information or self-help manuals relevant to the patient
- Giving the patient relevant information about
  - The consequences of a drug conviction in terms of international travel and employment
  - Consequences of further or heavier drug charges

TABLE 25.6 TREATMENT APPROACHES TO CHEMICAL DEPENDENCE

Approach	Conception of Etiology	Conception of Patient	Conception of Treatment Outcome	Conception of Treatment Process	Advantages of Approach	Disadvantages of Approach
Psychiatric	Symptom of underlying emotional problem	Emotionally disturbed	Emotional conflicts are resolved; emotional health improves	Psychotherapy, medication to treat cause of substance abuse	Not punitive, treats comorbidity	Focus is only on treatment of mental disorder
Social	Society and environment cause dependence	Victim of circumstance	Improved social functioning or improved environment	Removal of environmental influences and increasing coping responses to it	Stresses social supports and coping skills	Blames "ills of society"—the person not responsible for addiction
Moral	Person is morally weak—can't say "no"	"Hustler," morally deficient	Moral recovery, increased willpower, self-control, and responsible behavior	"Street addict" behavior and manipulation confronted	Holds person responsible for actions and making amends	Punitive, increases low self-esteem and sense of failure
Learning	Abuse is a learned, reinforced behavior	Has distorted thinking, poor coping skills	Patient learns new ways of thinking and new coping skills	Cognitive therapy techniques and coping skills taught	Not punitive; teaches new coping skills	Places emphasis on control of use
Disease	Probably caused by genetic or biologic factors	Has a chronically progressive disease	Abstinence, arresting disease progression, and beginning of recovery process	Is treated as a primary disease, reinforces patient is an addict and is sick	Not punitive, stresses support and education	Minimizes mental health disorders; discounts return to social use
12-Step	Combination of disease concept and "spiritual bankruptcy"	Has an addiction and is powerless over substances	Abstinence, ongoing spiritual recovery	Use 12 steps, seeking spiritual support, making amends, serving others in need	Widespread success, emphasis is on quality of life and spiritual growth	Self-help group, not a treatment program
Dual diagnosis	Both a primary substance dependency and a mental health disorder	Has both mental and substance abuse disorder	Improvement in both mental health and substance abuse disorders	Concurrent treatment of both disorders	Treats both mental health disorder and dependency, minimizing relapse potential	Not inclusive enough; does not include social or other issues
Biopsychosocial	Biologic basis, with social and psychological influences	Has deficiencies in all three interacting areas	Improvement in mental and physical health, utilization of social supports	Concurrent treatment of all issues	Uses different modalities; is more inclusive	Does not match patient and specific interventions
Multivariant	Many different causes; may be different for each individual	Has multiple issues to be assessed and addressed	Particular issues for individual addressed, so improvement occurs	Treatment strategies are matched with individual patient needs	Treatment matched to individual's needs	Logistical problems can occur during its implementation

Discussing harm reduction strategies, especially those relating to

- Overdose
- Violence
- Driving under the influence
- Safe practices (e.g., safe injecting, safe sex)
- Offering and arranging a follow-up visit

Cognitive and Cognitive Behavioral Interventions and Psychoeducation

Cognitive approaches to addiction hypothesize that if a patient can change the way he or she thinks about a situation, both the emotional reaction to it and the behavioral response will change. Psychoeducational materials, groups, and one-on-one interactions with nurses also impart information to reduce knowledge deficits related to alcohol and drug dependence (Box 25.12). Cognitive behavioral therapy (CBT) is a brief structured treatment that focuses on immediate problems. It enables patients to examine the thinking process that leads to decisions to use substances, analyze distortions in thinking, and develop rational responses to these distortions.

Enhancing Coping Skills

Improving coping skills is thought to be one component of preventing relapse into alcohol and drug use. Coping skills include the ability to use thought, emotion, and action effectively to solve interpersonal and intrapersonal problems and to achieve personal goals. Groups in addiction treatment programs that also have a relapse prevention component look at coping. The skills listed in Box 25.13 are often taught as coping strategies for dealing with alcohol and drug cravings. Patients role-play new behaviors and learn from the feedback they receive from

---

BOX 25.13

Skills Training Group Topics

INTERPERSONAL
Starting conversations
Giving and receiving compliments
Nonverbal communication
Receiving criticism
Receiving criticism about drinking
Drink and drug refusal skills
Refusing requests
Close and intimate relationships
Enhancing social support networks

INTRAPERSONAL
Managing thoughts about alcohol
Problem-solving
Increasing pleasant activities
Relaxation training
Awareness and management of anger
Awareness and management of negative thinking
Planning for emergencies
Coping with persistent problems

---

other group members. They also increase their sense of competency to use these skills in real-life situations.

Group Interventions and Early Recovery

Isolation and alienation from friends and family are common themes in patients with substance-related disorders. In addition, thinking that has become distorted is left unchallenged without contact with others; thus, change is difficult. When a patient enters a group that is working with the goals of continuing recovery, numerous healing advantages can occur.

Groups in treatment settings focus on immediate goals of maintaining sobriety and not on childhood issues. The emphasis is on using problem solving and other skills to deal with stressful events that threaten abstinence. This type of support group is also extremely effective in outpatient treatment settings. After a period of successful abstinence, group therapy can focus more on traditional psychotherapy work.

Individual Therapy

Often, individual therapy is helpful, particularly in conjunction with group therapy or family therapy. In addiction treatment settings, counselors meet with individuals to maintain focus on the goals and objectives of their treatment, to review the fears and anxieties that often arise in early recovery, and to devise new and healthy responses and solutions to stressful and difficult situations.

Family Interventions

Family therapy, a vital part of addiction treatment, can be used in several beneficial ways to initiate change and

---

BOX 25.12

Substance Abuse

When caring for the patient and family with substance abuse, be sure to include the following topic areas in the family's teaching plan:

- Psychopharmacologic agents, if used, including drug action, dosage, frequency, and possible side effects
- Manifestations of intoxication, overdose, and withdrawal
- Emergency medical system activation
- Nutrition
- Coping strategies
- Structured planning
- Safety measures
- Available treatment programs
- Family therapy referral
- Self-help groups and other community resources
- Follow-up laboratory testing, if indicated

help the family when the substance-abusing person is unwilling to seek treatment. Behavioral couples therapy for people with alcoholism can improve family functioning, reduce stressors, smooth marital adjustment, and lessen domestic violence and verbal conflict. When the substance-abusing person seeks help, family therapy can help stabilize abstinence and relationships. Often, inpatient substance abuse treatment programs have family education and group therapy components that help meet these goals. Family therapy can also help to maintain long-term recovery and prevent relapse. Goals of family therapy should be realistic and obtainable. Action plans must be specific and organized into manageable increments. Target dates should be realistic, so pressure is minimal, yet there is motivation to act in a timely manner. Planning for the future is very difficult as long as alcohol or drug abuse continues.

Harm-Reduction Strategies

Harm reduction, a community health intervention designed to reduce the harm of substance use to the individual, the family, and society, has replaced a moral or criminal approach to drug use and addiction. It recognizes that the ideal is abstinence but works with the individual regardless of his or her commitment to reduce use. The goal is to reduce the potential harm of the associated behavior. Harm reduction initiatives range from widely accepted designated driver campaigns to controversial initiatives such as provision of condoms in schools, safe injection rooms, needle exchange programs, and heroin maintenance programs.

Twelve-Step Programs

Alcoholics Anonymous (AA) was the first 12-step, self-help program (see Box 25.14 for a list of these steps). AA is a worldwide fellowship of people with alcoholism who provide support, individually and at meetings, to others who seek help. The program steps include spiritual, cognitive, and behavioral components. Many treatment programs discuss concepts from AA, hold meetings at the treatment facilities, and encourage patients to attend community meetings when appropriate. They also encourage continuing use of AA and other self-help groups as part of an ongoing plan for continued abstinence.

Twelve-step programs do not solicit members, engage in political or religious activities; make medical or psychiatric diagnoses; engage in education about addiction to the general population; or provide mental health, vocational, or legal counseling (Alcoholics Anonymous, 2014). Alternative peer support groups differ from these programs in their approach. Four such groups in the United States are Women for Sobriety, Moderation Management, Men for Sobriety, and SMART Recovery.

BOX 25.14

The Twelve Steps of Alcoholics Anonymous

1. We admitted we were powerless over alcohol—that our lives had become unmanageable.
2. Came to believe that a Power greater than ourselves could restore us to sanity.
3. Made a decision to turn our will and our lives over to the care of God *as we understood Him.*
4. Made a searching and fearless moral inventory of ourselves.
5. Admitted to God, to ourselves, and to another human being the exact nature of our wrongs.
6. Were entirely ready to have God remove all these defects of character.
7. Humbly asked Him to remove our shortcomings.
8. Made a list of all persons we had harmed, and became willing to make amends to them all.
9. Made direct amends to such people wherever possible, except when to do so would injure them or others.
10. Continued to take personal inventory and, when we were wrong, promptly admitted it.
11. Sought through prayer and meditation to improve our conscious contact with God, as we understood Him, praying only for knowledge of His will for us and the power to carry that out.
12. Having had a spiritual awakening as a result of these steps, we tried to carry this message to alcoholics and to practice these principles in all our affairs.

Reprinted with permission from Alcoholics Anonymous World Services (2002). *Alcoholics Anonymous.* New York: Author.

Evaluation and Treatment Outcomes

Recovery from alcoholism is a journey, often lasting a lifetime. Recovery involves a change in lifestyle and, often, new relationships. Short-term outcomes can be evaluated within the treatment setting. Long-term outcomes are established and evaluated by the patient who often continues to use professional and nonprofessional support as needed.

CHEMICAL DEPENDENCY AND PROFESSIONAL NURSES

Although accurate epidemiologic data specific to nursing are scarce, extrapolations from national data reveal an estimated prevalence that 6% to 8% of nurses use alcohol or drugs to the extent to impair professional practice (National Council of State Boards of Nursing [NCSBN], 2011). A nurse is just as susceptible to addiction as any other individual but additional risk factors exist such as access and availability of drugs, training in the administration and injection of drugs, and a familiarity with and a frequency of administering drugs. Difficult working conditions, staffing shortages, acutely ill patients, inadequate patient to nurse ratios, shift rotation, shifts lasting longer than 8 hours and increased overtime all add additional stress to the nurse which increases the risk of substance abuse. Because of the risk of losing a license to practice, nurses are very reluctant to seek help. To protect patients' safety and maintain the standards of the profession, many states have mandatory reporting laws. According to the nurse practice acts, any nurse who knows of any health care provider's incompetent, unethical, or illegal practice must report that information through proper channels.

In 1982, the American Nurses Association House of Delegates adopted a national resolution to provide assistance to impaired nurses. The peer assistance programs strive to intervene early, reduce hazards to patients, and increase prospects for the nurse's recovery. The program offers consultation, referral, and monitoring for nurses whose practice is impaired, or potentially impaired, because of the use of illicit drugs or alcohol or a psychological or physiologic condition.

A referral can be made confidentially by the employer, Employee Assistance Program, coworker, family member, friend, or the nurse her- or himself. If the nurse is willing to undergo a thorough evaluation to determine the extent of the problem and any treatment needed, all information is kept confidential from the Board of Nursing, so that the nurse does not face disciplinary action against his or her nursing license.

Some signs of substance abuse in nurses include mood swings; inappropriate behavior at work; frequent days off for implausible reasons; noncompliance with acceptable policies and procedures; deteriorating appearance; deteriorating job performance; sloppy illegible charting; errors in charting; alcohol on the breath; forgetfulness; poor judgment and concentration; lying; and volunteering to act as the medications nurse.

Other characteristics of nurses with substance abuse include high achievement, both as a student and a nurse; volunteering for overtime and extra duties; no drug use unless prescribed after surgery or for a chronic illness; and family history of alcoholism or addiction.

SUMMARY OF KEY POINTS

- Substance use disorders are categorized according to the following substances: alcohol, caffeine, cannabis (marijuana), hallucinogens, inhalants, opioids, sedative–hypnotics, stimulants, tobacco, and others.

- Addiction is a condition of continued use of substances despite adverse consequences. Abuse occurs when a person uses alcohol or drugs for the purpose of intoxication or, in the case of prescription drugs, for purposes beyond their use.

- Accurate and comprehensive assessment is crucial in planning addiction treatment interventions. This assessment should consider all substances for pattern of use, including factors of tolerance; withdrawal symptoms; consequences of use; loss of control over amount,

frequency, or duration of use; desire or efforts to cease or control use; and social, vocational, and recreational activities affected by use, history of previous addiction treatment, and family and social support systems.

- Denial of a substance use disorder is the individual's attempt to avoid accepting its diagnosis; it can be manifest in attempts to rationalize the substance use, minimize the harmful results, deflect attention from one's own problem to society's or someone else's, or blame childhood trauma.

- Nurses should use a nonconfrontational approach when dealing with patients in denial of their problem. Motivational interviewing approaches are most effective, using empathy and a nonjudgmental approach and to help the patient to realize the discrepancy between life goals and engaging in substance use, thus, motivating patients to change their self-destructive behaviors and make personal choices regarding treatment goals.

- Several effective modalities are used in addiction treatment, and many programs combine them, which may include 12-step programs, social skills groups, psychoeducational groups, group therapy, and individual and family therapies. No one best treatment method exists for all people.

- Substance use disorders have many social and political ramifications. Even the profession of nursing is not immune to substance use disorders among its members.

CRITICAL THINKING CHALLENGES

1. Jeff H, a 35-year-old patient who abuses cocaine, has entered a rehabilitation program. What goals do you believe would be realistic to achieve by the end of his projected 30-day inpatient stay?

2. You are working in an orthopedic unit, and Mary L has been admitted for treatment for a fractured femur. She has been drinking recently and has a blood alcohol level of 0.08%. What further information in the following areas would you need to plan her care?
   a. Medical
   b. Alcohol and drug use related
   c. Other psychosocial issues

3. Normal adolescent behavior is often similar to that associated with substance abuse. How would you differentiate this normal behavior from possible substance abuse or addiction?

4. John M has sought treatment for depression and job stress. He came to your psychiatric assessment unit

smelling of alcohol. He believes that he does not have a drinking problem but a job problem. What interventions would you use for possible alcohol abuse or addiction?

5. Sylvia G has been abusing heroin intravenously heavily for 2 years. She has come into the hospital with an abscess on her leg. What symptoms would you expect to observe as she experiences withdrawal? What medications would likely be used to ease these symptoms?

6. After Sylvia G is free from withdrawal symptoms, she expresses interest in obtaining drug treatment. What are her options? How would you describe them to her?

7. Raymond L has been treated for hypertension at your clinic. You notice that he complains of peripheral neuropathy and has an unsteady gait. What other medical signs would corroborate alcoholism?

8. What laboratory test results would help confirm a diagnosis of alcoholism?

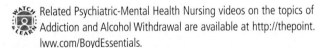 *Ray:* 2004. This award-winning film is based on the life of Ray Charles (played by Jamie Foxx), the musical genius of rhythm and blues. His early childhood experiences included racial discrimination, extreme poverty, an absent father, the traumatic drowning of his younger brother, and the loss of his sight. The film depicts Ray Charles' struggle with his heroin addiction.

Viewing Points: Identify the role of heroin in the development of Ray Charles as a performer, adult, husband, and father. How did denial shape his use of heroin? What was his primary reason for entering treatment? What motivated him to stay clean for the rest of his life?

M◐VIE viewing **GUIDES** related to this chapter are available at http://thepoint.lww.com/BoydEssentials.

Related Psychiatric-Mental Health Nursing videos on the topics of Addiction and Alcohol Withdrawal are available at http://thepoint.lww.com/BoydEssentials.

Psychiatric-Mental Health Nursing Practice and Learn Activities related to the videos on the topics of Addiction and Alcohol Withdrawal are available at http://thepoint.lww.com/BoydEssentials.

REFERENCES

Alcoholics Anonymous. (2014). Alcoholics Anonymous Information on AA. Retrieved April 12, 2014, from http://www.aa.org.

American Psychiatric Association. (2013). *Diagnostic and Statistical Manual of Mental disorders* (5th Ed.), Arlington, VA: American Psychiatric Association.

Bethesda, MD: National Institute on Drug Abuse. (2013a). Cocaine. *Drug Facts*. www.drugabuse.gov. Retrieved 7/15/2105

Bowen, S., Witkiewitz, K., Clifasefi, S. L., Grow, J., Chawla, N., Hsu, S. H., et al. (2014). Relative efficacy of mindfulness-based relapse preventions, standard relapse preventions, and treatment as usual for substance use disorders. *JAMA Psychiatry, 71*(5), 547–556.

Butler, C. C., Simpson, S. A., Hood, K., Cohen, D., Pickles, T., Spanou, C., et al. (2013). Training practitioners to deliver opportunistic multiple behavior changes counselling in primary care: A cluster randomized trial. *British Medical Journal, 346*, f1191. doi:10.1136/bmj.f1191

Cadet, J. L., Bisagno, V., & Milroy, C. M. (2014). Neuropathology of substance use disorders. Review. *Acta Neuropathology, 127*(1), 91–107.

Cairney, S., O'Connor, N., Dingwall, K. M., Maruff, P., Shafiq-Antonacci, R., Currie, J., et al. (2013). A prospective study of neurocognitive changes 15 years after chronic inhalant abuse. *Addiction, 108*(6), 1107–1114.

Centers for Disease Control. (2013). Vital signs: current cigarette smoking among adults aged ≥ 18 years with mental illness-United States, 2009–2011. *Morbidity and Mortality Weekly Report, 62*(5), 81–87.

Cole, B., Clark, D. C., Seale, J. P., Shellenberger, S., Lyme, A., Johnson, J. A., et al. (2012). Reinventing the reel: An innovative approach to resident skill-building in motivational interviewing for brief intervention. *Substance Abuse, 33*(3), 278–281.

Collins, S. E., Malone, D. K., & Larimer, M. E. (2012). Motivation to change and treatment attendance as predictors of alcohol-use outcomes among project-based Housing First residents. *Addictive Behaviors, 37*(9), 931–939.

Cousaert, C., Heylens, G., & Audenaert, K. (2013). Laughing gas abuse is no joke. An overview of the implications for psychiatric practice. *Clinical Neurology and Neurosurgery, 115*(7), 859–862.

Day, E., Bentham, P. W., Callaghan, R., Kuruvilla, T., & George, S. (2013). Thiamine for prevention and treatment of Wernicke-Korsakoff syndrome in people who abuse alcohol (Review). *The Cochran Collaboration, 7*, CD004033. doi:10.1002/14651858.CD004033.pub3

Echeverri, D., Montes, F. R., Cabrera, M., Galán, A., & Prieto, A. (2010). Caffeine's vascular mechanisms of action. *International Journal of Vascular Medicine, 2010*, 834060.

Ewing, J. A. (1984). Detecting alcoholism. *Journal of the American Medical Association, 252*(14), 1905–1907.

Faessel, H. M., Obach, R. S., Rollema, H., Ravva, P., Williams, K. E., & Burstein, A. H. (2010). A review of the clinical pharmacokinetics and pharmacodynamics of varenicline for smoking cessation. *Clinical Pharmacokinetics, 49*(12), 799–816.

Franck, J., & Jayaram-Lindström, N. (2013). Pharmacotherapy for alcohol dependence: Status of current treatments. *Current Opinion in Neurobiology, 23*(4), 692–699.

Gonzalez, D. (2014). Screening for personality disorder in drug and alcohol dependence. *Psychiatry Research, 217*(1–2):121–123.

Grant, J. E., Schreiber, L., Odlaug, B. L., & Kim, S. W. (2010). Pathologic gambling and bankruptcy. *Comprehensive Psychiatry, 51*, 115–120.

Hallberg, M. (2011). Impact of anabolic androgenic steroids on neuropeptide systems. (Review). *Mini-Reviews in Medicinal Chemistry, 11*(5), 399-408.

Kottke, T., & Pronk, N. (2010). Optimal lifestyle adherence and 2-year incidence of chronic conditions. *Clinical Medicine & Research, 8*(3–4), 181–182.

Leung, L., Neufeld, T., & Marin, S. (2012). Effect of self-administered auricular acupressure on smoking cessation-a pilot study. *BMC Complementary and Alternative Medicine, 12*, 11.

Lozano, B. E., LaRowe, S. D., Smith, J. P., Tuerk, P., & Roitzsch, J. (2013). Brief motivational feedback may enhance treatment entry in veterans with comorbid substance use and psychiatric disorders. *American Journal on Addictions, 22*(2), 132–135.

Mental Health America. (2014). Co-dependency. Retrieved April 12, 2014, from http://www.mentalhealthamerica.net/go/codependency.

Moyer, V. A., LeFevre, J. L., Siu, A. L., Peters, J. J., Baumann, L. C., Bibbins-Domingo, K., et al. (2013). Screening and behavioral counseling interventions in primary care to reduce alcohol misuse: U.S. preventive services task force recommendation statement. *Annals of Internal Medicine, 159*(3), 210–218.

National Council of State Boards of Nursing. [NCSBN]. (2011). *Substance use disorders in nursing: A resource manual and guidelines for alternative and disciplinary monitoring programs*. Chicago: National Council of State Boards of Nursing.

National Institute on Drug Abuse. (2012a). Cigarettes and other tobacco products. *Drug Facts*. www.drugabuse.gov. Retrieved 7/15/2105

National Institute on Drug Abuse. (2012b). Spice (Synthetic Marijuana). *Drug Facts*. www.drugabuse.gov. Retrieved 7/15/2105

National Institute on Drug Abuse. (2012c). Inhalants. *Drug Facts*. www.drugabuse.gov. Retrieved 7/15/2105

National Institute on Drug Abuse. (2012d). Anabolic steroids. *Drug Facts*. www.drugabuse.gov. Retrieved 7/15/2105

National Institute on Drug Abuse. (2012e). Synthetic Cathinones ("Bath Salts"). *Drug Facts*. www.drugabuse.gov. Retrieved 7/15/2105

National Institute on Drug Abuse. (2012f). Principles of drug addiction treatment: A research-based guide (NIH Publication No. 12-4180) (3rd ed., pp. 3–4).

National Institute on Drug Abuse. (2013b). *Methamphetamine. Research Report Series.* NIH Publication Number 13-4210.

National Institute on Drug Abuse. (2013c), MDMA ("ecstasy" or "Molly"). *Drug Facts.* www.drugabuse.gov. Retrieved 7/15/2105

National Institute on Drug Abuse. (2013d). Tobacco addiction: A research update from the National Institute on Drug Abuse. *Topics in Brief.* www.drugabuse.gov. Retrieved 7/15/2105

National Institute on Drug Abuse. (2013e). Electronic cigarettes (e-Cigarettes). *Drug Facts.* www.drugabuse.gov. Retrieved 7/15/2105

National Institute on Drug Abuse. (2013f). Prescription and over-the-counter medication. *Drug Facts.* www.drugabuse.gov. Retrieved 7/15/2105

National Institute on Drug Abuse. [NIDA]. (2014a). High school and youth trends. *Drug Facts,* www.drugabuse.gov. Retrieved 7/15/2105

National Institute on Drug Abuse. (2014b). Is marijuana medicine? *Drug Facts.* www.durgabuse.gov. Retrieved 7/15/2105

National Institute on Drug Abuse. (2014c). Hallucinogens and dissociative drugs. *Research Report Series.* NIH Publication Number 14-4209. www.drugabuse.gov. Retrieved 7/15/2105

National Institute on Drug Abuse. (2014d). *Heroin. Research Report Series.* NIH Publication Number 14-0165. www.drugabuse.gov. Retrieved 7/15/2105

National Institute of Drug Abuse. (2014e). *Emerging Trends. Drugs of Abuse.* www.drugabuse.gov/drugs-abuse/emerging-trends. Retrieved 7/15/2105

Nogueira, M., Bosch, R., Valeron, S., Gómez-Barros, N., Palomar, G., Richarte, V., et al. (2014). Early-age clinical and developmental features associated to substance use disorders in attention-deficit/hyperactivity disorder in adults. *Comprehensive Psychiatry, 55*(3), 639–649.

Park, S., Cho, M. J., Jeon, H. J., Lee, H. W., Bae, J. N., Park, J. I., et al. (2010). Prevalence, clinical correlations, comorbidities, and suicidal tendencies in pathological Korean gamblers: Results from the Korean Epidemiologic Catchment Area Study. *Social Psychiatry & Psychiatric Epidemiology, 45*(6), 621–629.

Pilgrim, J. L., Woodford, N., & Drummer, O. H. (2013). Cocaine in sudden and unexpected death: A review of 49 post-mortem cases. *Forensic Science International, 227*(1–3), 52–39.

Pope, M. A., Joober, R., & Malla, A. K. (2013). Diagnostic stability of first-episode psychotic disorders and persistence of comorbid psychiatric disorders over 1 year. *Canadian Journal of Psychiatry, 58*(10), 588–594.

Rice, V. H., Hartmann-Boyce, J., & Stead, L. F. (2013). Nursing interventions for smoking cessation (Review). *The Cochrane Database of Systematic Reviews, 8,* CD001188.

Sanchez, Z. M., Ribeiro, L. A., Moura, Y. G., Noto, A. R., & Martins, S. S. (2013). Inhalants as intermediate drugs between legal and illegal drugs among middle and high school students. *Journal of Addictive Diseases, 32*(2), 217–226.

Séquin, M., Boyd, R., Lesage, A., McGirr, A., Suissa, A., & Tousignant, M. (2010). Suicide and gambling: Psychopathology and treatment-seeking. *Psychology of Addictive Behaviors, 24*(3), 541–547.

Snipes, D. J., & Benotsch, E. G. (2013). High-risk cocktails and high-risk sex: Examining the relations between alcohol mixed with energy drink consumption, sexual behavior, and drug use in college students. *Addictive Behaviors, 38*(1), 1418–1423.

Strang, J., Metrebian, M., Lintzeris, N., Potts, L., Carnwath, T., & Mayet, S., et al. (2010). Supervised injectable heroin or injectable methadone versus optimised oral methadone as treatment for chronic heroin addicts in England after persistent failure in orthodox treatment (RIOTT): A randomised trial. *The Lancet, 375*(9729), 1885–1895.

Substance Abuse and Mental Health Services Administration. (2013). Results from the 2012 *National Survey on Drug Use and Health: Summary of National Findings.* NSDUH Series H-46, HHS Publication NO. (SMA) 13-4795. Rockville, MD: Substance Abuse and Mental Health Services Administration.

Tranel, D., McNutt, A., & Bechara, A. (2012). Smoking cessation after brain damage does not lead to increased depression: Implications for understanding the psychiatric complications of varenicline. *Cognitive & Behavioral Neurology, 25*(1), 16–24.

U.S. Department of Health and Human Services. (2010). *Healthy people 2020.* Washington, DC: U.S. Government Printing Office. Retrieved from http://www.healthypeople.gov. Retrieved 6/15/2105

Weldy, D. L. (2010). Risks of alcoholic energy drink for youth. *The Journal of the American Board of Family Medicine, 23*(4), 555–558.

White, A. R., Rampes, H., Liu, J. P., Stead, L. F., & Campbell, J. (2014). Acupuncture and related interventions for smoking cessation. *Cochrane Database System Review, 1,* CD000009

Wilson, D., da Silva Lobo, D. S., Tavares, H., Gentil, V., & Vallada, H. (2013). Family-based association analysis of serotonin genes in pathological gambling disorder: Evidence of vulnerability risk in the 5HT-2A receptor gene. *Journal of Molecular Neuroscience, 49*(3), 550–553.

Wolk, B. J., Ganetsky, M., & Babu, K. M. (2012), Toxicity of energy drinks. *Current Opinion in Pediatrics, 24*(2), 243–251.

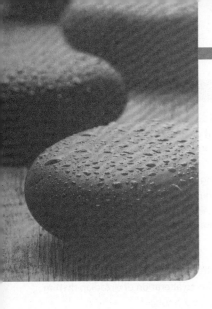

26
Sleep–Wake Disorders

Nursing Care of Persons with Insomnia and Sleep Problems

Sheri Compton-McBride

KEY CONCEPTS

- Insomnia

LEARNING OBJECTIVES

After studying this chapter, you will be able to:

1. Identify common sleep–wake disorders that co-occur with other mental disorders.

2. Discuss the impact of changes in sleep associated with psychiatric disorders.

3. Perform a sleep history during a patient's assessment.

4. Formulate a model nursing care plan for patients with sleep–wake disorders.

KEY TERMS

- circadian rhythm • insomnia disorder • non–rapid eye movement (NREM) • rapid eye movement (REM) sleep
- sleep diary • sleep–wake disorders • sleep latency • somnambulism

Case Study: Michael

Michael is a 20-year-old student who is majoring in nursing. He presents himself at Student Health Services with a complaint of insomnia. In assessing his problem, the nurse ascertains that he falls asleep 2 to 3 hours after turning lights out.

INTRODUCTION

Many Americans are severely sleep deprived. Implications for public safety, increased use of health care services, and morbidity are associated with sleep disturbances (Centers for Disease Control and Prevention [CDC], 2012). The average sleep duration of adults in the United States has plateaued to between 6 and 6.5 hours from a high of 8.5 hours in 1960 (Adenekan, Pandey, McKenzie, Zizi, Casimir, & Jean-Louis, 2013).

Sleep–Wake Disorders

The *DSM-5* identifies ten **sleep–wake disorders**. Sleep–wake disorders include insomnia, hypersomnolence, and narcolepsy. See Table 26.1. This chapter presents an overview of sleep–wake disorders. Insomnia disorder is covered in greater detail.

INSOMNIA DISORDER

> KEYCONCEPT **Insomnia,** which is Latin for "no sleep," refers to difficulty falling asleep or maintaining sleep when opportunity and circumstances are adequate for sleep. Dissatisfaction with sleep quantity or quality may also be present (Matthews, Arnedt, McCarthy, Cuddihy, & Aloia, 2013).

Clinical Course

Few studies describe the course of insomnia disorder which can last for short periods in some patients and for

TABLE 26.1	SLEEP–WAKE DISORDERS
Sleep–Wake Disorders	Description
Insomnia	Dissatisfaction with sleep quality, quantity, and difficulty initiating or maintaining sleep with waking up and unable to return to sleep
Hypersomnolence	Excessive sleepiness lasting at least 7 hours
Narcolepsy	Irrepressible need to sleep; napping and lapsing into sleep, involuntarily
Breathing-Related Disorders	Includes 3 disorders related to difficulty breathing while sleeping: obstructive sleep apnea hypopnea, central sleep apnea, sleep related hypoventilation
Obstructive Sleep Apnea	Nocturnal breathing disturbances including snoring, snorting/gasping, or pauses in breathing while sleeping
Central Sleep Apnea	Five or more periods of apnea within 1 hour
Sleep-Related Hypoventilation	Periods of decreased respiration associated with elevated CO_2 levels
Circadian Rhythm Sleep–Wake Disorder	Recurrent pattern of sleep disruption primarily due to alteration of circadian rhythm
Delayed Sleep Phase Type	Delay in the timing of major sleep period (usually 2 hours)
Advanced Sleep Phase Type	Sleep-wake times several hours earlier than desired or conventional times
Irregular Sleep-Wake Type	Insomnia at night, excessive sleepiness during the day
Non-24-hour Sleep-Wake Type	Insomnia or excessive sleep related to abnormal synchronization between 24 hour light-dark cycle & endogenous circadian rhythm
Shift Work Type	Impaired sleep due to shift work or traveling across time zones
Parasomnias	Abnormal behavioral, experiential or physiologic events associated with sleep.
Non-Rapid Eye Movement Sleep Arousal Disorders	Sleep walking, sleep terrors, nightmare disorder, restless legs syndrome
Nightmare Disorder	Extremely upsetting dreams, well-remembered that usually involve threats to survival, security, or physical integrity
Rapid Eye Movement Sleep Behavior Disorder	Repeated episodes of arousal during sleep associated with vocalization and/or complex motor behaviors.
Restless Legs Syndrome	Urge to move the legs; usually uncomfortable with unpleasant sensation in legs
Substance/Medication-Induced Sleep Disorder	Symptoms develop after use of a specific substance or medication

Source: APA 2013.

decades in others. Limited data show that symptoms are usually of long duration (Mysliwiec, Matsangas, Baxter, McGraw, Bothwell, & Roth, 2014).

Diagnostic Criteria

Insomnia disorder is characterized by dissatisfaction with sleep quantity or quality and difficulty initiating or maintaining sleep, or in waking early in the morning, and being unable to return to sleep at least 3 nights per week for at least 3 months (American Psychiatric Association [APA], 2013).

During insomnia therapy, patients may deny fighting sleep or falling asleep unintentionally during the day.

Epidemiology and Risk Factors

Of all sleep-related problems, insomnia is the most prevalent, with an estimated 23.6% of noninstitutionalized adults; the prevalence of chronic or severe insomnia is estimated to range from 10% to 15% (Kessler, Berglund, Coulouvrat, Fitzgerald, Hajak, Roth, et al., 2012; Kraus & Rabin, 2012). Insomnia is one of the most prevalent complaints in primary health care (Morin & Benca, 2012).

Insomnia has a greater prevalence among older people and among divorced, separated, and widowed adults. Increasing age, female sex, and comorbid disorders (e.g., medical, mental disorders, and substance use) are all risks for developing insomnia disorder.

Comorbidity

Sleep–wake disorders occur independently of the diagnosis of other mental disorders, but they are also seen in people with mental disorders. For example, a core feature of posttraumatic stress disorder (PTSD) is sleep disturbance (Lauterbach, Behnke, & McSweeney, 2011). Insomnia often increases the risk for relapse of the mental disorder. Documented comorbid conditions include cardiovascular disorders, diabetes, musculoskeletal disorders (e.g., arthritis, chronic back/neck pain), respiratory disorders (e.g., chronic obstructive pulmonary disease [COPD], seasonal allergies, chronic bronchitis, emphysema), digestive disorders (e.g., gastroesophageal reflux disease, irritable bowel syndrome), pain conditions, and mental disorders including depression, PTSD, and other sleep disorders such as sleep apnea, and restless legs syndrome (RLS) (Kessler, et al., 2012).

Etiology

Many factors affect sleep, but one of the major reasons for insomnia is depression, which accounts for most cases. However, most people with insomnia do not have a psychiatric diagnosis (Kraus & Rabin, 2012).

Family Response to Disorder

Living with a family member with insomnia disorder is challenging. Irritability, complaints of sleeplessness, and chronic fatigue interfere with quality interpersonal relationships. Family members become "exhausted" by living with someone who never sleeps.

Teamwork and Collaboration: Working Toward Recovery

Sleep disorders are best treated by clinicians specializing in this area, but primary and mental health care professionals should be able to identify sleep disturbances and provide education and interventions for normalizing sleep. However, because sleep disorders are common in individuals with mental health problems, psychiatric–mental health nurses should be prepared provide care for those with sleep disorders.

Priority Care Issues

Safety is a priority for people with insomnia disorder. Sleep deprivation can lead to accidents, falls, and injuries, especially in older patients. Sedating medication could potentially increase falls (Kessler, et al., 2012).

Evidence-Based Nursing Care for Persons with Insomnia

Nursing Assessment

Assessment of a patient's sleep pattern is a part of every psychiatric nursing assessment (see Chapter 9). If a patient has a sleep disorder, a detailed sleep history should be included in the assessment process. During the patient interview, the description, duration (when problem began), stability (every night?), and intensity (how bad is it?) should be determined (Box 26.1). A sleep history includes current sleeping patterns, medical problems, current medications (including over-the-counter [OTC] and dietary supplements), current life events, use of alcohol and caffeine, and emotional and mental status that might be affecting sleep (see Box 26.2 and Box 26.3). A **sleep diary**, a person's written account of the sleep experience, is useful in determining the extent of the sleep problem (Arora, Broglia, Pushpakumar, Lodhi, & Taheri, 2013). The diary may cover a few days to several weeks. A simple diary is typically a daily record of

the patient's bedtimes, rising times, estimated time to fall asleep, number and length of awakenings, and naps. More complicated sleep diaries involve recording the amount and time of alcohol ingestion, ratings of fatigue, medication, and stressful events.

> ### Consider Michael
>
> His problem falling asleep occurs 3 nights a week—on Mondays, Wednesdays, and Fridays. He exercises vigorously during his physical education class (7–9 PM) on these three evenings. He denies any sleep problems during a spring break trip.

The assessment also includes evaluating the behavioral and social factors related to sleep problems. Recent changes in relationships, particularly a divorce or death of a loved one, can interfere with sleep significantly. A recent move, travel, and addition of a new family member can impact sleep. Fatigue and stress increase when individuals assume the role of caregiver in their personal lives and in those with occupations as professional health care providers. Shift work compromises the **circadian rhythm** (a daily cycle of biologic activity based on a 24-hour period influenced by regular variation including alteration of night and day) and contributes to insomnia.

Nursing Diagnoses

The nursing diagnosis usually applied to the patient with a sleep disorder is Sleep Pattern Disturbance, Insomnia or Sleep Deprivation (see Nursing Care Plan 26.1, available at http://thepoint.lww.com/BoydEssentials).

Interventions

Physical Health Interventions

Nonpharmacologic health-promoting interventions are the first choice before administering pharmacologic agents (Morin & Benca, 2012). Sleep hygiene strategies can be effective and should be encouraged (Box 26.4). The goal is to normalize sleep patterns to improve well-being.

Activity, Exercise, Nutrition, and Thermoregulation Interventions

Exercise promotes sleep, but regular exercise should be planned to end 3 hours before bedtime. Routines are important, especially when preparing your body to sleep. Engaging in a quiet relaxing activity, such as listening to soft music or reading nonstimulating material, is often suggested. Additional interventions include avoiding eating a heavy meal, and avoiding drinking alcohol or caffeinated beverages. Patients should be encouraged to evaluate the temperature of the room. Generally, a cooler environment enhances sleep.

BOX 26.1 • THERAPEUTIC DIALOGUE • Sleep Assessment

INEFFECTIVE APPROACH

Nurse: What time do you go to bed at night?

Michael: Oh, my bedtime varies between 10 PM and 2 AM.

Nurse: What time do you get up?

Michael: I get up anywhere between 6 AM and noon.

Nurse: How do you sleep during the night?

Michael: OK.

Nurse: OK?

Michael: Yeah, no problems sleeping.

EFFECTIVE APPROACH

Nurse: What time do you go to bed at night and what time do you get up?

Michael: Oh, my bedtime varies between 10 PM and 2 AM. I get up anywhere between 6 AM and noon.

Nurse: Let's be more specific. During a week's time, what time do you go to bed each night?

Michael: Well, this semester I have a morning clinical rotation Monday through Thursday. I'm usually up till 11 or midnight preparing for the next day. On Friday and Saturday nights, I typically go out with my friends and get to bed around 2 AM. On Sunday night, I get in to bed around 10 PM.

Nurse: What time do you get up each day of the week?

Michael: On the mornings that I have clinicals, I have to get up around 6 AM to be at the hospital by 6:45 AM. On Friday, I get up at 8 AM for a 9 o'clock class. Saturday morning, I get up around 8 AM so I can go to my part-time job. On Sunday, I get up by noon.

Nurse: How long do you take to fall asleep?

Michael: That's gotten much better. I fall asleep in 15 minutes or so.

Nurse: Do you take any naps?

Michael: Outside of class, I don't have time to nap. I'm just too busy with my classes, clinical, homework, job, and social life.

Nurse: Before this semester, how much sleep did you get?

Michael: That was last summer; I had a job that started at 1:30 PM, so I could sleep as late as I wanted. I bet I got 8 or even 9 hours of sleep every night. I don't remember being sleepy then.

CRITICAL THINKING CHALLENGE

- Compare the quality and quantity of elicited data in the two scenarios.
- What conclusions could be drawn from the first scenario?

- Are the conclusions different for the second scenario? Explain.

BOX 26.2

Sleep History

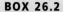

Perception of sleep problem
Sleep schedule (bedtime and rise time)
Difficulty falling asleep or maintaining sleep
Quality of sleep
Daytime sleepiness and impact of the sleep disorder on daytime functioning
General emotional and physical problems (e.g., stress)
Sleep hygiene (e.g., consuming caffeine immediately before bed)
Sleep environment (e.g., room temperature, noise, light)

Adapted from Kessler, T. A. & Kurtz, C. P. (2014). Sleep and sleep disorders. In Porth, C. M. (Ed.), *Pathophysiology: Concepts of altered health states* (pp. 525–543). Philadelphia: Wolters Kluwer Health | Lippincott Williams & Wilkins.

Pharmacologic Interventions

Types of drugs used to treat symptoms of insomnia include benzodiazepine receptor agonists, melatonin receptor agonists, sedating antidepressants, and OTC medications and dietary supplements.

Remember Michael?

Michael has tried over-the-counter sleep medication but does not remember the name of it. When he took these pills, he was able to fall asleep better, but found the pills to be costly. He wants a medication that will be covered by his student health insurance.

BOX 26.3
Medications and Other Substances and Their Effects on Sleep

ALCOHOL
- Increases TST during the first half of the night
- Decreases TST during the second half
- Decreases REM sleep during the first half of the night
- Withdrawal from long-term use of alcohol decreases TST, increased wakefulness after sleep onset, and REM rebound.

AMPHETAMINES
- Disrupt sleep–wake cycle during acute use
- Decrease TST
- Decrease REM sleep
- Withdrawal may cause REM rebound.

ANTIDEPRESSANTS (TRICYCLICS AND MAOIS)
- Sleep effects vary with sedative potential
- Increase slow-wave sleep (i.e., a recurrent period of very deep sleep, typically totaling 5 or 6 hours a night.)
- Decrease REM sleep

BARBITURATES
- Increase TST
- Decrease WASO
- Decrease REM sleep
- Withdrawal may cause a decrease in TST and REM rebound.

BENZODIAZEPINES
- Drugs vary in onset and duration of action.
- Decrease SL
- Increase TST
- Decrease WASO

- Decrease REM sleep
- Daytime sedation may occur with long-acting drugs.

β-ADRENERGIC BLOCKERS
- Decrease REM sleep
- Increase WASO, nightmares
- Daytime sedation may occur

CAFFEINE
- Increases SL
- Decreases TST
- Decreases REM sleep

L-DOPA
- Vivid dreams and nightmares

LITHIUM
- Increases slow-wave sleep
- Decreases REM sleep

OPIOIDS
- Effects vary with specific agents
- Increase WASO
- Decrease REM sleep
- Decrease slow-wave sleep

PHENOTHIAZINES
- Increase TST
- Increase slow-wave sleep

STEROIDS
- Increase WASO

MAOI, monoamine oxidase inhibitor; REM, rapid eye movement; SL, sleep latency; TST, total sleep time; WASO, wake after sleep onset.

BOX 26.4
Sleep Hygiene Tips

Nurses are often involved in helping patients develop and maintain good sleep habits. Teaching tips include the following:

1. The most important healthy sleep habit is to *establish and maintain a regular bedtime and rising time.* Even if you awaken feeling unrefreshed, get up and out of bed at a regular, consistent time. "Sleeping in" can disturb sleep on the subsequent night. For most, time in bed should be limited to 8 hours.
2. Avoid naps.
3. Abstain from alcohol. Although alcohol may assist with sleep onset, there is an alerting effect when it wears off.
4. Refrain from caffeine after midafternoon. Avoid nicotine before bedtime and during the night. Caffeine and nicotine are strong stimulants and fragment sleep.
5. Exercise regularly, avoiding the 3 hours before bedtime. Exercising 6 hours before bedtime tends to strengthen the circadian rhythms of body temperature and sleepiness.
6. Use the bedroom only for sleep and sex. Promote the bedroom as a stimulus for sleep, not for studying, watching television, or socializing on the telephone.
7. Set a relaxing routine to prepare for sleep. Avoid frustrating or provoking activities before bedtime.
8. Provide for a comfortable environment. A cool room temperature, minimal light, and limiting noise are suggested.

Benzodiazepine Receptor Agonists (BzRAs)

The BzRA hypnotics have U.S. Food and Drug Administration (FDA) approval for insomnia. They include the benzodiazepines (e.g., triazolam, temazepam, estazolam, quazepam, and flurazepam) and the nonbenzodiazepines (e.g., zolpidem, zolpidem extended release, zaleplon, and eszopiclone) (Table 26.2). All these medications bind to benzodiazepine receptors and exert their effects by facilitating gamma-aminobutyric acid (GABA) effects. GABA, the most common inhibitory neurotransmitter, must be

TABLE 26.2	HYPNOTICS: BENZODIAZEPINE RECEPTOR AGONISTS	
	Dosage (mg)	Half-life (h)
Estazolam	1–2	10–24
Flurazepam	15–30	48–120
Temazepam (Restoril)	15–30	8–20
Triazolam (Halcion)	0.125–0.25	2.4
Quazepam (Doral)	7.5–15	48–120
Zolpidem (Ambien)	5–10	1.4–3.8
Zolpidem ER (Ambien)	6.25–12.5	2.8
Zaleplon (Sonata)	5–20	1
Eszopiclone (Lunesta)	1–3	6

present at the benzodiazepine receptor for the BzRA to exert its effect. These medications are all absorbed rapidly and reduce **sleep latency** (the amount of time it takes to fall asleep after the lights have been turned off) with medication at recommended doses (Riemann & Perlis, 2009). Nonbenzodiazepine hypnotics, which provide immediate relief, are often used for short-term treatment of insomnia. The most common side effects are headache, dizziness, and residual sleepiness (Box 26.5).

The BzRAs are Schedule IV controlled substances by federal regulation, have abuse and dependence potential, and produce withdrawal signs and symptoms after abrupt discontinuation. The risk for residual sedation on the day after using hypnotic medication is determined by the dose and rate of elimination (Riemann & Perlis, 2009). The recommended dose for women using zolpidem (immediate release) was lowered from 10 to 5 mg and zolpidem CR be lowered from 12.5 to 6.25 mg.

Melatonin Receptor Agonist

Melatonin, a hormone released from the pineal gland, aids in the regulation of the sleep–wake cycle through activation of MT_1 and MT_2 receptors. Melatonin has been shown to shift circadian rhythm, decrease body temperature, alter reproductive rhythm, enhance immune function, and decrease alertness. Normally, levels of melatonin increase with decreasing exposure to light. Ramelteon (Rozerem), indicated for insomnia, is a melatonin receptor agonist

---

BOX 26.6

Psychoeducation Checklist: Sleep Disorders

When teaching patients with sleep disorders, be sure to include the following topics:

- Maintenance of a sleep log
- Foods to avoid before going to bed
- Importance of developing a bedtime ritual and good sleep habits
- Use of sleep medications as prescribed
- Avoidance of caffeine and rigorous exercise within the 6 hours before bedtime
- Avoidance of cigarette smoking 1 hour before bedtime and during nighttime awakenings
- Allowing for 8 hours of sleep per night
- Maintenance of a regular sleep schedule, specifically a routine rise time
- An occasional "bad night" happens to nearly everyone
- Avoidance of alcohol because it disrupts sleep and is a poor hypnotic
- Daytime sleepiness as a symptom of sleep disorders
- How to do relaxation exercises
- Bedroom rituals
- Appropriate family support

---

with high affinity for melatonin receptors MT_1 and MT_2. This pharmacologic activity is believed to be related to its sleep-promoting properties (Box 26.6). Ramelteon has a low abuse potential and is not a controlled substance (Feren, Schweitzer, & Walsh, 2011).

Orexin Receptor Antagonist

Orexins (also known as hypocretins) are neurotransmitter produced in the hypothalamus that trigger wakefulness, while low levels result in sleep. A deficiency is associated with narcolepsy. Suvorexant (Belsomra) is an orexin receptor antagonist approved for the treatment of insomnia. Blocking the binding of orexins to receptors is thought to suppress the wake drive. This antagonism may also trigger signs of narcolepsy/cataplexy. The relatively new medication should be given in the lowest dose possible because of its long half-life (Kishi, Matsunaga, & Iwata, 2015).

Over-the-Counter Medications and Dietary Supplements

OTC sleeping pills are usually antihistamines. The most common agents are doxylamine and diphenhydramine. These histamine-1 antagonists have a central nervous system (CNS) effect that includes sedation, diminished alertness, and slowing of reaction time. These drugs also produce anticholinergic side effects, such as dry mouth, accelerated heart rate, urinary retention, and dilated pupils. Drowsiness lasts from 3 to 6 hours after a single dose. Next-morning hangover can be a problem. Diphenhydramine decreases sleep latency and improves quality of sleep for those with occasional sleep problems but is not as effective as benzodiazepines for chronic sleep disturbances (Feren, et al., 2011).

BOX 26.5

Drug Profile: Zaleplon (Sonata)

DRUG CLASS: Sedative–hypnotic (pyrazolopyrimidine nonbenzodiazepine hypnotic). It is readily absorbed and metabolized with only about 1% of zaleplon eliminated in urine.

RECEPTOR AFFINITY: Zaleplon acts at the gamma-aminobutyric acid–benzodiazepine receptor complex.

INDICATION: Treatment of onset or maintenance insomnia

ROUTES AND DOSING: Zaleplon is available in 5- and 10-mg capsules. It should be taken at bedtime or after a nocturnal awakening with difficulty falling back to sleep (but at least 4 hours before the desired rise time).

Adults: The recommended starting dose is 10 mg with a maximum of 20 mg. An initial dose of 5 mg should be considered in adults with low body weight. Doses of over 20 mg have not been sufficiently studied.

Geriatric: Initially, 5 mg is recommended as a starting dose. Older adults should not exceed a 10-mg dose.

HALF-LIFE (PEAK PLASMA CONCENTRATION): 1 hour

SELECTED SIDE EFFECTS: Abdominal pain, headache, dizziness, depression, nervousness, difficulty concentrating, back pain, chest pain, migraine, conjunctivitis, bronchitis, pruritus, rash, arthritis, constipation, and dry mouth

WARNINGS: Zaleplon should not be administered to patients with severe hepatic impairment. Zaleplon potentiates the psychomotor impairments of ethanol consumption.

Exogenous melatonin has long been available OTC and has been shown to have mild sleep-promoting properties when given outside the period of usual secretion. That is, melatonin can advance the sleep–wake cycle by making it easier to fall asleep earlier than usual. Some evidence suggests that in young and older individuals with insomnia, melatonin can be beneficial in ameliorating the symptoms (Cortesi, Giannotti, Sebastiani, Panunzi, & Valente, 2012).

Valerian, a dietary supplement, is used as a medicinal herb in many cultures. The mechanism of action is not fully understood and is believed to inhibit GABA reuptake. Valerian may be useful for sleeplessness, but not enough evidence from double-blind studies exists to confirm this. Mild side effects include headaches, dizziness, upset stomach, and tiredness the morning after its use (National Center for Complementary and Alternative Medicine, 2012).

Administering and Monitoring Medication

Sleeping medications are commonly used in all settings. They are usually given nightly for a short period of time to establish a wake–sleep pattern. Rebound insomnia can occur if a drug is abruptly discontinued. This side effect can be minimized or prevented by giving the lowest effective dose and tapering before discontinuing. Nurses should assess for confusion, memory problems, excessive sedation, and risk of falls.

Monitoring for Drug-to-Drug Interactions

Sleep medications generally have increased depressive effects when given with other CNS depressants. Sleep medications can interact with oral contraceptives, isoniazid (an antibiotic), fluvoxamine (a serotonin reuptake inhibitor [SSRI]), and verapamil (a calcium channel blocker) (see Chapter 10). Grapefruit juice should be avoided when taking these drugs. Ramelteon should not be given with fluvoxamine.

Teaching Points

Pharmacologic agents should complement sleep hygiene practices. These medications can be useful on a short-term basis. Alcohol use should be avoided when taking sleeping medications. Patients should use these medications when time for sleeping is adequate (at least 8 hours). Most sleep-related medications should be taken at bedtime. Patients should be instructed about the safe use of these medications and possible side effects.

Sleep Hygiene

The nurse can help the patient develop bedtime rituals and good sleep hygiene. Bedtime should be at a regular hour and the bedroom environment should be conducive to sleep. Preferably, the bedroom should not be where the individual watches television or does work-related activities. The bedroom should be viewed as a room for either resting or sleep (see Box 26.4).

Behavioral Interventions

Stimulus control is a technique used when the bedroom environment no longer provides cues for sleep but has become the cue for wakefulness. Patients are instructed to avoid behaviors in the bedroom incompatible with sleep, including watching television, doing homework, and eating. This allows the bedroom to be reestablished as a stimulus for sleep.

Another behavioral intervention is sleep *restriction*. Patients often increase their time in bed to provide more opportunity for sleep, resulting in fragmented sleep and irregular sleep schedules. Patients are instructed to spend less time in bed and avoid napping.

Relaxation training is used when patients complain of difficulty relaxing, especially if these patients are physically tense or emotionally distressed. Various procedures to reduce somatic arousal can be used, including progressive muscle relaxation, autogenic training, and biofeedback. Imagery training, meditation, and thought stopping are attention-focusing techniques that center on cognitive arousal (see Chapter 9).

Cognitive Behavioral Therapy

Cognitive behavioral (CBT) therapy is useful in changing negative learned responses that perpetuate insomnia. This approach is especially helpful for those who also have comorbid depression or anxiety. The objective of CBT is to change the belief system that results in improvement of the self-efficacy of the individual (Morin & Benca, 2012). See Chapter 19.

Psychoeducation

Education regarding interventions is crucial for patients with sleep disorders. An explanation of the sleep cycle and the factors that influence sleep are important for these patients. For those with insomnia, teaching about avoiding foods and beverages that might interfere with sleep should be highlighted (Box 26.6).

Family Education

Family and friends should be encouraged to support the new habits the patient is trying to establish. Patients, spouses, and friends must understand that activities engaged in just before sleep can greatly affect sleep patterns and sleep difficulties, such as socializing, alcohol consumption, use of caffeine, and engaging in stimulating activities. Relaxing activities before bedtime are vital contributors to establishing a routine conducive to sleep. Family and friends can help create a positive environment with an emphasis on sleep as a priority.

Evaluation and Treatment Outcomes

The primary treatment outcome is establishing a normal sleep cycle. Changes in diet and behavior (e.g., initiation of an exercise program) should be evaluated for their impact on the individual's sleep. Environmental modifications, such as a change in the level of lighting in the bedroom, decreased stimulation (e.g., turning off cell phone or moving the television out of the bedroom), or modification in room temperature, can be monitored for any changes affecting the sleep cycle.

HYPERSOMNOLENCE DISORDER

The essential characteristic of hypersomnolence disorder is excessive sleepiness at least three times a week for at least 3 months (APA, 2013). Sleepiness occurs on an almost daily basis and causes significant impairment in social and occupational functioning. Affected patients have an excessive quantity of sleep (typically 8–12 hours per night), deteriorated quality of wakefulness, and sleep inertia (a period of impaired performance occurring during the sleep–wake transition characterized by confusion, ataxia, or combativeness) (APA, 2013). This diagnosis is reserved for individuals who have no other causes of daytime sleepiness (e.g., narcolepsy, OSA syndrome).

NARCOLEPSY

The overwhelming urge to sleep is the primary symptom of narcolepsy. This irresistible urge to sleep occurs at any time of the day, regardless of the amount of sleep the patient has had. Falling asleep often occurs in inappropriate situations, such as while driving a car or reading a newspaper. These sleep episodes are usually short, lasting 5 to 20 minutes, but may last up to an hour if sleep is not interrupted. Individuals with narcolepsy may experience sleep attacks and report frequent dreaming. They usually feel alert after a sleep attack, only to fall asleep unintentionally again several hours later.

BREATHING-RELATED DISORDERS

The DSM-5 identifies three breathing disorders including obstructive sleep apnea–hypopnea, central sleep apnea, and sleep-related hypoventilation. This section discusses obstructive sleep apnea–hypopnea disorder (obstructive sleep apnea syndrome) (APA, 2013). The term obstructive sleep apnea (OSA) syndrome is more commonly used in nonpsychiatric areas and will be used in this section instead of the term obstructive apnea–hypopnea disorder. Central sleep apnea and sleep-related hypoventilation will not be discussed.

OBSTRUCTIVE SLEEP APNEA SYNDROME

Obstructive sleep apnea syndrome, the most commonly diagnosed breathing-related sleep disorder, may affect up to 20% of the U.S. adults (Santarnecchi, Sicilia, Richiardi, Vatti, Polizzotto, Marina, et al., 2013). OSA is characterized by snoring during sleep and episodes of sleep apnea (i.e., cessation of breathing) that disrupt sleep and contribute to daytime sleepiness. The hallmark symptoms are snoring and daytime sleepiness. Often, snoring is so loud and disturbing that partners choose separate bedrooms for sleeping. Approximately 50% of the U.S. population snores (Ram, Seirawan, Kuma, & Clark, 2009).

CIRCADIAN RHYTHM SLEEP DISORDER

The chief feature of a circadian rhythm sleep disorder is the mismatch between the individual's internal sleep–wake circadian rhythm and the timing and duration of sleep (Dodson & Zee, 2010). People with these disorders complain of insomnia at particular times during the day and excessive sleepiness at others. This diagnosis is reserved for those individuals who present with marked sleep disturbance or significant social or occupational impairment.

The DSM-5 identifies a broad group of subtypes, including the following (APA, 2013).

- *Delayed sleep phase type:* Individuals with delayed sleep phase type, or "night owls," tend to be unable to fall asleep before 2 to 6 AM; hence, their whole sleep patterns shift, and they have difficulty rising in the morning.
- *Advanced sleep phase type:* Opposite of the night owls, these individuals are "larks" or earlier risers. They are unable to stay awake in the evening and consistently wake up early.
- *Irregular sleep–wake type:* People with this type have a temporarily disorganized sleep pattern that varies in a 24-hour period.
- *Non-24-hour sleep–wake type:* Individuals with this type have an abnormal synchronization between the 24-hour light–dark cycle and their endogenous circadian rhythm, which leads to periods of insomnia, excessive sleepiness, or both. This type is most common among blind or visually impaired individuals.

Chan, M. F. (2009). Factors associated with perceived sleep quality of nurses working on rotating shifts. Journal of Clinical Nursing, 18(2) 285–293.

THE QUESTION: Do nurses perceive that rotating shifts contribute to insufficient sleep quality?

METHODS: A cross-sectional study was conducted in two hospitals in Hong Kong. Nurses (*n* = 163) completed a self-reported questionnaire that included information on health status, strain and symptom levels, and perceived sleep quality.

FINDINGS: More than 70% of the nurses reported having insufficient sleep; more advanced age, perceived poor sleep status, gastrointestinal symptoms, and higher strain and symptom levels were risk factors that contributed to insufficient sleep.

IMPLICATIONS FOR NURSING: Nurses, especially older nurses, who rotate shifts are at risk for sleep disorders and other health problems.

• *Shift work type:* The endogenous sleep–wake cycle is normal but is mismatched to the imposed hours of shift work. Rotating shift schedules are disruptive because any consistent adjustment is prevented. Compared with day and evening shift workers, night and rotating shift workers have a shorter sleep duration and poorer quality of sleep. They may also be sleepier while performing their jobs. This disorder is further exacerbated by insufficient daytime sleep resulting from social and family demands and environmental disturbances (i.e., traffic noise, telephone). Because of the job requirements of the profession, nurses often experience this disorder. Furthermore, 20% of the U.S. work force is engaged in shift work and thereby at risk for circadian rhythm disorders. See Box 26.7.

One of the circadian rhythm sleep–wake disorders not included in the DSM-5 is the jet lag type that occurs after travel across time zones, particularly in coast-to-coast and international travel. The normal endogenous circadian sleep–wake cycle does not match the desired hours of sleep and wakefulness in a new time zone. Individuals traveling eastward are more prone to jet lag because it involves resetting one's circadian clock to an earlier time—it is easier to delay the endogenous clock to a later time period than adjust it to an earlier one.

PARASOMNIAS

Parasomnias are sleep–wake disorders that occur in association with sleep, specific sleep stages, or sleep–wake transitions. They are characterized by abnormal behavioral,

experiential, or physiologic events (APA, 2013). **Non–rapid eye movement** (NREM) sleep arousal disorders including sleepwalking and sleep terror types, usually occur during the first third of the major sleep episode. Nightmare disorder is a **rapid eye movement** (REM) disorder that generally occurs during the second half of the major sleep episode (APA, 2013). RLS is considered a sleep disorder and is classified as a parasomnia.

SLEEP TERRORS AND SLEEPWALKING

In sleep terrors (also called night terrors or pavor nocturnus), episodes of screaming, fear, and panic occur, causing clinical distress or impairing social, occupational, or other areas of functioning. Sleep terrors usually last 1 to 10 minutes, are frightening to the person and to anyone witnessing them. Often, individuals abruptly sit up in bed screaming; others have been known to jump out of bed and run across the room. Other symptoms include a rapid heart rate and breathing, dilated pupils, and flushed skin. Usually, the person having a sleep terror is inconsolable and difficult to awaken completely. Efforts to awaken the individual may prolong the episode. Once they are awake, most are unable to recall the dream or event that precipitated such a response. A few report a fragmentary image. Often, the individual does not fully awaken and cannot recall the episode the next morning (Carter, Hathaway, & Lettieri, 2014).

In sleepwalking or **somnambulism**, repeated episodes of complex motor behavior during sleep may involve getting out of bed and walking around. While sleepwalking, people typically have a blank stare and are difficult to awaken. Often, they awaken to find themselves in a different place from where they went to sleep. If awakened during the episode, a brief period of confusion follows. See Box 26.8.

• Ensure adequate sleep. The occurrence of sleepwalking dramatically increases after sleep loss.
• Anticipate sleepwalking sleep loss is significant. Family members should be aware of the likelihood of sleepwalking for the first 2 to 3 hours after the sleepwalker goes to bed.
• Keep a sleep log to assist in identifying how much sleep is needed to prevent a sleepwalking event.
• Consider use of a noise devices on the door of the sleepwalker's room to alert others that the sleepwalker is up.
• Deadbolt locks should be installed on doors leading outside. Windows should be secured to limit their opening.
• When the sleepwalker is spending the night away from home, alert appropriate individuals to the possibility that sleepwalking may occur. Ensure adequate sleep on the preceding nights.

NIGHTMARE DISORDER

The repeated occurrence of frightening dreams that fully awaken an individual is the essential characteristic of nightmare disorder. Typically, the individual can recall detailed dream content that involves physical danger (e.g., attack or pursuit) or perceived danger (e.g., embarrassment or failure). On awakening, the individual is fully alert and experiences a persisting sense of anxiety or fear. Many people have difficulty returning to sleep. Multiple same-night nightmares may be reported. Some people avoid sleep because of their fear of nightmares. Consequently, people may report that excessive sleepiness, poor concentration, and irritability disrupt their daytime activities. The occurrence of nightmares may be more serious than previously suspected. Nightmares are commonly experienced by military combat personnel who have PTSD (see Chapter 17).

RESTLESS LEGS SYNDROME

RLS is a sleep–wake disorder characterized by an urge to move the legs that begins or worsens at rest or periods of inactivity, typically in the evening or at night. The urge to move legs is reduced or relieved by movement (APA, 2013).

SUMMARY OF KEY POINTS

■ Assessment is key. Information should focus on a comprehensive sleep history, including specific details of the sleep complaint, current sleep patterns, and sleep patterns before sleep difficulties, medical problems, current medications, current life events, and emotional and mental status.

■ Nursing interventions for sleep disorders focus on nonpharmacologic approaches (e.g., exercise, nutrition, activity, thermoregulation) and pharmacologic interventions.

■ Psychosocial nursing interventions for sleep disorders include educating patients about good sleep habits, instructing patients in relaxation exercises and sleep-promoting activities, providing patients with nutritional suggestions regarding foods and substances to avoid, and educating family members and friends regarding the importance of supporting the need for making high-quality sleep a priority.

■ Insomnia disorder is characterized by difficulty falling asleep or difficulty maintaining sleep. Insomnia is often precipitated by feelings of stress or tension, with associations and behaviors persisting after the crisis or stressful situation has passed.

■ Obstructive sleep apnea syndrome is a diagnosed breathing-related sleep disorder characterized by excessive snoring and episodes of apnea (i.e., cessation of breathing). These episodes disrupt sleep and may cause daytime sleepiness.

■ In circadian rhythm sleep–wake disorders a mismatch takes place between the individual's internal sleep–wake circadian rhythm and the timing and duration of sleep.

■ Parasomnias occur in association with sleep, specific sleep stages, or sleep–wake transitions and include sleepwalking, sleep terrors, nightmare disorders, and restless legs syndrome. They are characterized by abnormal behavioral, experiential, or physiologic events. The etiology is unknown but appears to be of genetic predisposition. Unrestorative sleep, excessive sleepiness, poor concentration, and irritability are often the result.

CRITICAL THINKING CHALLENGES

1. Describe the sleep hygiene interventions that would be useful for the person with insomnia disorder.

2. Identify the primary problems related to the sleep–wake disorders.

3. A 25-year-old woman reports that she is has not slept for 3 days. What are the primary assessment questions for her?

4. A 55-year-old truck driver presents reporting excessive daytime sleepiness. Develop a list of assessment questions that could be used to investigate his chief complaint.

5. Outline nursing interventions and educational highlights for the parents of a 12-year-old child diagnosed with sleepwalking disorder.

 Insomnia: 1997. This movie is a compelling thriller that occurs in a state of perpetual light. The setting is north of the Arctic Circle in the middle of summer, where it is daylight 24 hours a day. Jonas Engström (Stellan Skarsgård) and Erik Vik (Sverre Anker Ousdal) are cops from Oslo brought into a small town to help with a murder investigation. Things go wrong, and Engström finds himself trapped in a web of deceit. His guilty conscience and the never-ending light keep him awake at night, and the lack of sleep makes him increasingly desperate and error prone. **Viewing Points:** How did the lack of sleep have an impact on Engström's ability to make sound decisions? If the setting of this movie were in an area that had normal nighttime darkness, would the outcome have been different? If you were conducting a sleep assessment, what nursing diagnosis would be generated from the data?

REFERENCES

Adenekan, B., Pandey, A., McKenzie, S., Zizi, F., Casimir, G. H., & Jean-Louis, G. (2013). Sleep in America: role of racial/ethnic differences. *Sleep Medicine Reviews.* 17(4), 255–262.

American Psychiatric Association. (2013). *Diagnostic and Statistical Manual of Mental Disorders* (5th ed.). Arlington, VA: Author.

Arora, T., Broglia, E., Pushpakumar, D., Lodhi, T., & Taheri, S. (2013). An investigation into the strength of the association and agreement levels between subjective and objective sleep duration in adolescents. *PLoS ONE, 8*(8), E72406.

Carter, K. A., Hathaway, N. E., & Lettieri, C. F. (2014). Common sleep disorders in children. *American Family Physician, 89*(5), 368–377.

Centers for Disease Control and Prevention. (2012). Short sleep duration among workers–United States, 2010. *Morbidity and Mortality Weekly Report, 61*(16), 281–285.

Cortesi, F., Giannotti, F., Sebastiani, T., Panunzi, S., & Valente, D. (2012). Controlled-released melatonin, singly and combined with cognitive behavioral therapy, for persistent insomnia in children with autism spectrum disorders: A randomized placebo-controlled trial. *Journal of Sleep Research, 21*(6), 700–709.

Dodson, E. R., & Zee, P. C. (2010). Therapeutics for circadian rhythm sleep disorders. *Sleep Medicine Clinics, 5*(4), 701–715.

Feren, S., Schweitzer, P., & Walsh, J. (2011). Pharmacotherapy for insomnia. In P. J. Vinken, & G. W. Bruyn (Eds.). *Handbook of clinical neurology* (pp. 747–762). Philadelphia: Elsevier.

Kessler, R., Berglund, P. A., Coulouvrat, C., Fitzgerald, T., Hajak, G., Roth, T., et al. (2012). Insomnia, comorbidity and risk of injury among insured Americans: Results from the America Insomnia survey. *Sleep, 35*(6), 825–834.

Kishi, T., Matsunaga, S., & Iwata, N. (2015). Suvorexant for primary insomnia: A systematic review and meta-analysis of randomized placebo-controlled trials. *PLOS ONE.* August 28, 2015. doi: 10.1371/journal.pone.0136910.

Kraus, S. S., & Rabin, L. A. (2012). Sleep America: Managing the crisis of adult chronic insomnia and associated conditions. *Journal of Affective Disorders, 138*(3), 192–212.

Lauterbach, D., Behnke, C., & McSweeney, L. B. (2011). Sleep problems among persons with a lifetime history of posttraumatic stress disorder alone and in combination with a lifetime history of other psychiatric disorders: A replication and extension. *Comprehensive Psychiatry.* 52(6), 580–586.

Matthews, E. E., Arndt, J. R., McCarthy, M. S., Cuddihy, L. J., & Aloia, M. S. (2013). Adherence to cognitive behavioral therapy for insomnia: A systematic review. *Sleep Medicine Reviews, 17*(6), 453–464.

Morin, C. M., & Benca, R. (2012). Chronic insomnia. *The Lancet, 379*(9821), 1129–1141.

Mysliwiec, F., Matsangas, P., Baxter, T., McGraw, L., Bothwell, N. E., & Roth, B. J. (2014). Comorbid insomnia and obstructive sleep apnea in military personnel: correlation with polysomnographic variables. *Military Medicine, 179*(3), 294–300.

National Center for Complementary and Alternative Medicine. (2012). Valerian: Herbs at a glance. Washington, DC: National Institutes of Health, U.S. Department of Health and Human Services. NCCAM Publication No. D272.

Porth, C. M. (Ed.) (2010). Sleep and sleep disorders. *Pathophysiology: Concepts of altered health states* (pp. 1281–1297). Philadelphia, PA: Lippincott Williams & Wilkins.

Ram, S., Seirawan, H., Kuma, S., & Clark, G. (2009). Prevalence and impact of sleep disorders and sleep habits in the United States. *Sleep & Breathing, 14*, 63–70.

Riemann, D., & Perlis, M. L. (2009). The treatments of chronic insomnia: A review of benzodiazepine receptor agonists and psychological and behavioral therapies. *Sleep Medicine Review, 13*(3), 204–214.

Santarnecchi, E., Sicilia, I., Richiardi, J., Vatti, G., Polizzotto, N. R., Marina, D., et al. (2013). Altered cortical and subcortical local coherence in obstructive sleep apnea: a functional magnetic resonance imaging study. *Journal of Sleep Research, 22*(3), 337–347.

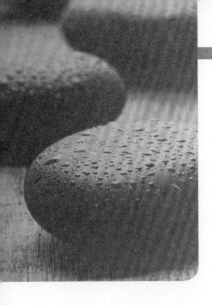

27
Sexual Disorders

Nursing Care of Persons with Sexual Dysfunction

Mary Ann Boyd

This chapter is available at http://thepoint.lww.com/BoydEssentials and in the CoursePoint ebook.

27

Sexual Disorders

Nursing Care of Persons with Sexual Dysfunction

Mary Ann Boyd

This chapter is available at http://thepoint.lww.com/Boyd/Essentials and in the CoursePoint eBook.

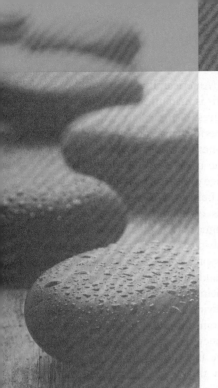

28

Mental Health Disorders of Childhood and Adolescence

Mary Ann Boyd

KEY CONCEPTS

- attention
- neurodevelopmental delay
- hyperactivity
- impulsiveness
- tics

LEARNING OBJECTIVES

After studying this chapter, you will be able to:

1. Describe mental disorders usually diagnosed in childhood or adolescence.

2. Discuss prevailing theories relevant to the mental health disorders in childhood and adolescence.

3. Discuss the nursing care of children with neurodevelopmental disorders.

4. Analyze the nursing assessment, diagnosis, intervention, and evaluation processes in caring for a child or adolescent with attention-deficit hyperactivity disorder.

5. Discuss the epidemiology, etiology, medications, and nursing care of children with tic disorders.

6. Discuss the nursing care of children and adolescents with separation anxiety and obsessive-compulsive disorders.

7. Discuss the significance of behavioral intervention strategies for children who have elimination disorders.

8. Compare the nursing care of children and adolescents with mood disorders and schizophrenia with that for adults with similar disorders.

KEY TERMS

- adaptive behavior • attention-deficit hyperactivity disorder (ADHD) • autism spectrum disorder (ASD) • communication disorders • dyslexia • encopresis • enuresis • intellectual disability • learning disorder • motor tics • phonic tics
- phonologic processing • separation anxiety disorder • Tourette disorder

INTRODUCTION

Psychiatric problems are less easily recognized in children than in adults. Normal growth and development behaviors of one age group may be a symptom of a disorder in another age group. For example, an imaginary friend is age appropriate for a 4-year-old child but not for an adolescent. Despite the difficulty in diagnosis, about 20% of U.S. youth in their lifetimes are affected by a mental disorder that impairs their ability to function (Merikangas, He, Burstein, Swanson, Avenevoli, Cui, et al., 2010). Only a minority of youths with mental disorders receive services for their illnesses (Costello, Jian-ping, Sampson, Kessler, & Merikangas, 2014). Major depressive disorder, schizophrenia, and bipolar disorder are the main causes of disability worldwide among young people ages 10 to 24 years (Gore, Bloem, Patton, Ferguson, Joseph, Coffey, et al., 2011).

This chapter presents an overview of selected childhood disorders and discusses nursing care for children and their families with these problems. Because it is beyond the scope of this text to present all child psychiatric disorders, this chapter discusses selected ones, including intellectual disability, autism spectrum disorder, tic disorders, obsessive-compulsive disorder, and elimination disorders. Oppositional defiant and conduct disorders are discussed in Chapter 22. Attention-deficit hyperactivity disorder is highlighted in this chapter.

> **NCLEXNOTE** All the psychiatric disorders of childhood and adolescence should be viewed within the context of growth and development models. Safety and self-esteem are priority considerations.

NEURODEVELOPMENTAL DISORDERS OF CHILDHOOD

Under the primary influences of genes and environment, neurodevelopment of attention, cognition, language, affect, and social and moral behavior proceeds along several pathways. Developmental pathways and developmental delays are closely interwoven. For example, a language delay can interfere with a child's social development and contribute to behavior problems (Foster-Cohen, Friesen, Champion, & Woodward, 2010). This section discusses neurodevelopmental disorders of childhood that include several conditions that are etiologically unrelated; however, their common feature is a significant delay in one or more lines of development.

> **KEYCONCEPT** **Neurodevelopmental delay** means that the child's development in attention, cognition, language, affect, and social or moral behavior is outside the norm and is manifested by delayed socialization, communication, peculiar mannerisms, and idiosyncratic interests.

INTELLECTUAL DISABILITY

Intellectual disability is defined as a disability characterized by significant limitations in both intellectual function and in adaptive behavior that covers many everyday social and practical skills (American Association on Intellectual and Developmental Disabilities [AAIDD], 2015). The disability begins before the age of 18 years.

Diagnostic Criteria and Clinical Course

The diagnosis of intellectual disability involves an assessment of intellectual function such as reasoning, problem solving, and adaptive function in personal independence and social responsibility (American Psychiatric Association [APA], 2013). A diagnosis is made through clinical assessment of behavioral features; historical accounts from parents and teachers; and performance on standardized tests such as the Stanford-Binet or the Wechsler Intelligence Scales for Children. The usual threshold for intellectual disability is an intelligence quotient (IQ) of 70 or less (i.e., two standard deviations below the population mean).

Adaptive behavior is composed of three skill types: *conceptual skills* (e.g., language and literacy, money, time, number concepts, and self-direction); *social skills* (e.g., interpersonal skills, social responsibility, self-esteem, gullibility, social problem-solving, and the ability to follow rules and obey laws and to avoid being victimized); and *practical skills* (e.g., activities of daily living [ADLs], occupational skills, health care, travel and transportation, schedules and routines, safety, use of money, use of telephone) (AAIDD, 2015). Impaired adaptive functioning is primarily a clinical judgment based on the child's capacity to manage age-appropriate ADLs. However, standardized assessment instruments are available to assist with determination of the child's capabilities (Lecavalier & Butter, 2010).

An intellectual disability is not necessarily lifelong. Some children may be diagnosed at school age as having an intellectual disability, but with guidance and education, they may no longer meet the criteria as adults.

Epidemiology and Etiology

A large meta-analysis estimated the prevalence of intellectual disabilities to be about 1% in the United States and worldwide (Maulik, Mascarenhas, Mathers, Dua, & Saxena, 2011). A considerable variability worldwide exists, with low- and middle-income countries (e.g., Pakistan, Bangladesh) reporting higher rates of disability than high-income countries such as the United States (Maulik, et al., 2011). The rate of co-occurring psychiatric disorders is estimated between 10% and 39%. In children and adolescents with intellectual disabilities, mental health problems are three to seven times higher than in those without an intellectual disability (Toth & King, 2010).

Intellectual disabilities result from a variety of causes with the most common etiology related to genetic syndromes. Chromosomal changes or defects (e.g., Down syndrome) and exposure to toxins during prenatal development (e.g., fetal alcohol syndrome), heredity, pregnancy and perinatal complications, medication conditions, and environmental influences are all associated with intellectual disabilities. The cause is unknown in about 50% of the cases (Toth & King, 2010).

Nursing Care of Children with Intellectual Disability

Assessment of a child with an intellectual disability focuses on current adaptive skills, intellectual status, and social

History and Hallmarks of Childhood and Adolescent Disorders

- Maternal age and health status during pregnancy
- Exposure to medication, alcohol, or other substances during pregnancy
- Course of pregnancy, labor, and delivery
- Infant's health at birth
- Eating, sleeping, and growth in first year
- Health status in first year
- Interest in others in first 2 years
- Motor development
- Mastery of bowel and bladder control
- Speech and language development
- Activity level
- Response to separation (e.g., school entry)
- Regulation of mood and anxiety
- Medical history in early childhood
- Social development
- Interests

functioning. A developmental history is a useful way to gather information about past and current capacities (Box 28.1). The nurse compares these data with normal growth and development. Developmentally delayed children who have not had a psychological evaluation should be considered for referral. These children also require evaluation for other comorbid psychiatric disorders, which may be a challenge because of the child's cognitive limitations. Discussions about feelings and behavior may be too complex for these children. If children or adolescents with intellectual disabilities have a comorbid mental disorder or serious behavioral problems, a carefully constructed interdisciplinary behavioral plan will guide care and treatment.

The nurse also assesses the child's support systems (family, school, rehabilitative, and psychiatric) to ensure that the child's special needs have been identified and are being addressed. For example, occupational therapy may be recommended to improve motor coordination, but the family may not have transportation to these services available, so availability to alternative services should be explored.

The child and family's response to intellectual disability and other comorbid conditions will determine the nursing diagnoses, planning, and implementation of nursing interventions. Associated nursing diagnoses include Ineffective Coping, Delayed Growth and Development, and Interrupted Family Processes. Nursing interventions include promoting coping skills (i.e., interventions directed at building strengths, adapting to change, and maintaining or achieving a higher level of functioning), patient education, and parent education.

The overall goals of treatment and nursing care are an optimal level of functioning for the family and eventual independent functioning within a normal social environment for the child. For many children with intellectual disability, achieving independence in adulthood will be delayed but not impossible.

Continuum of Care

Children and families may require varying levels of interventions at different times throughout the life cycle. When a child is young, the family requires special educational support and, for some, residential services. The need for psychiatric intervention varies according to the severity of disability, family functioning, and the coexistence of other disorders. Feelings of grief and loss in family members (especially parents) related to having a child with a disability may be relieved through family therapy. More specific parent training may be needed to deal with emerging maladaptive behaviors.

AUTISM SPECTRUM DISORDER

Autism spectrum disorder (ASD) is characterized by persistent impairment in social communication and social interaction with others (APA, 2013). Children with ASD may or may not have an intellectual disability, but they commonly show an uneven pattern of intellectual strengths and weaknesses. This condition may be a lifelong pattern of being rigid in manner, intolerant of change, and prone to behavioral outbursts in response to environmental demands or changes in routine. Two conditions, autism disorder and Asperger syndrome, were previously diagnosed as separate disorders. However, because they have many overlapping symptoms and are difficult to differentiate from each other, the DSM-5 no longer considers autism and Asperger syndrome as separate disorders, but considers both as an ASD differentiated by language or intellectual impairment (APA, 2013).

ASD with restricted repetitive patterns of behavior such as stereotypic or repetitive motor movement, use of objects, inflexible adherence to routine or ritualized patterns, and fascination with lights or movement has been a subject of considerable interest and research effort since its original description more than 70 years ago. Leo Kanner (1943) described the profound isolation of these children and their extreme desire for sameness. These children appear aloof and indifferent to others and often seem to prefer inanimate objects.

Impairment in communication is severe and affects both verbal and nonverbal communication. Children with ASD may manifest delayed and deviant language development, as evidenced by echolalia (repetition of words or phrases spoken by others) and a tendency to be extremely literal in interpretation of language. Pronoun reversals and abnormal intonation are also common. Other common features of ASD are stereotypic behavior, self-stimulating, nonfunctional repetitive behaviors, such as repetitive rocking, hand flapping, and an extraordinary insistence on sameness. These children may also engage in self-injurious behavior, such as hitting, head banging, or biting. In some children, their unusual interests may evolve into fascination with specific objects, such as fans or air conditioners, or a particular topic, such as U.S. Civil War generals.

A child with ASD may have age-appropriate language and intelligence but also have severe and sustained impairment in social interaction and restricted, repetitive patterns of behavior, interests, and activities. This type of ASD was previously known as Asperger syndrome and appears to be a milder form of ASD. These children have social deficits marked by inappropriate initiation of social interactions, an inability to respond to normal social cues, and a tendency to be literal in their interpretation of language (APA, 2013). They may also display stereotypic behaviors, such as rocking and hand flapping, and have highly restricted areas of interest, such as train schedules, fans, air conditioners, or dogs. Signs of developmental delay may not be apparent until preschool or school age, when social deficits become evident (Box 28.2).

BOX 28.2 CLINICAL VIGNETTE

Frank (Autism Spectrum Disorder Asperger Syndrome)

A pediatrician refers Frank, age 5 years, 6 months, for an evaluation because of Frank's unusual preoccupation with ceiling fans and lawn sprinklers. According to his mother, Frank became interested in ceiling fans at age 3 years when he began drawing them, tearing pictures of them out of magazines, and engaging others in discussions about them. In the months before the evaluation, Frank also became fascinated by lawn sprinklers. These preoccupations so dominated Frank's interactions with others that he was practically incapable of discussing any other topics. He remained on the periphery of his kindergarten class and had few friends. Although he tried to make friends, his approaches were inept and he had trouble reading others.

Frank was the product of a full-term uncomplicated pregnancy, labor, and delivery to his then 25-year-old mother. It was her first pregnancy, and both parents eagerly anticipated Frank's birth. As an infant, Frank was healthy but seemed to cry a lot and was difficult to comfort, causing his mother to feel inadequate and depleted. His motor development was also delayed, and at age 3 years, nonfamily members had difficulty understanding his speech. His articulation, however, was within normal limits at the time of consultation. Frank received regular pediatric care and had no history of serious illness or injury. There was no family history of intellectual disability or psychiatric illness; results of genetic testing for chromosomal abnormality were negative.

In addition to his unusual preoccupations and social deficits, Frank resisted any change in his routine, was easily frustrated, and was prone to temper tantrums. His parents sharply disagreed about the nature of and appropriate response to his problems.

What Do You Think?

- What effect do you think Frank's preoccupation may have on his family and their relationships?
- What kind of teaching program would you develop if you were the nurse assigned to this family?

Epidemiology and Etiology

ASD is estimated to occur in 2.64% of the general population (Kim, Leventhal, Koh, Fombonne, Laska, Lim, et al., 2011). It occurs in boys more often than girls (Brugha, McManus, Bankart, Scott, Purdon, Bebbington, et al., 2011). About half of children with ASD have an intellectual disability and about 25% have seizure disorders. Published claims that the prevalence of autism is increasing are confounded by improved methods of diagnosis (Pickles, Simonoff, Chandler, Louicas, & Baird, 2011).

Research is accelerating in understanding the etiology of ASD because structural and functional imaging studies provide intriguing leads for future inquiry (Figure 28.1). Multiple etiological hypotheses are related to this disorder. Recent studies support a shared genetic etiology between autism spectrum disorder and schizophrenia (McCarthy, Gillis, Kramer, Lihm, Yoon, Berstein, et al., 2014). Expression of multiple genes related to the regulation of neurogenesis, brain, and differentiation process are implicated in ASD (Vaishnavi, Manikandan, & Munirajan, 2014). One line of research is determining defects in the metabolism of cellular antioxidants (Raymond, Deth, & Ralston, 2014). Studies show that higher levels of lead and mercury and lower levels of antioxidants are found in inpatients with autism spectrum disorder when compared to control groups (Alabdali, Al-Ayadhi, & El-Ansary, 2014). Symptoms of gastrointestinal disturbance has focused other research on the role of the GI microbiota and their fermentation products (Wang, Conlon, Christophersen, Sorich, & Angley, 2014). Other researchers suggest a role for maternal autoantibodies in the fetal brain in some cases (Elamin & Al-Ayadhi, 2014).

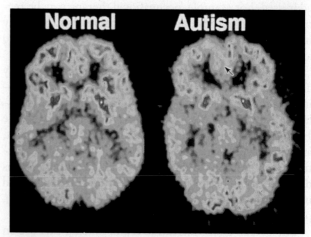

FIGURE 28.1 Patients with autism (*right*) may have decreased metabolic rates in the cingulate gyrus and other associated areas; however, wide heterogeneity in brain metabolic patterns is seen in patients with autism. (Courtesy of Monte S. Buchsbaum, MD, The Mount Sinai Medical Center and School of Medicine, New York.)

Teamwork and Collaboration: Working Toward Recovery

ASDs require long-term care at various levels of intensity. Treatment consists of designing academic, interpersonal, and social experiences that support the child's development. Children with autism, even those who are severely affected, may be able to live at home and attend special schools that use behavioral techniques. Other outpatient services may include family counseling, home care, and medication. As the child moves toward adulthood, living at home may become more difficult given the appropriate need for greater independence. The level of structure required depends primarily on IQ and adaptive functioning.

Planning interventions for children with an ASD considers the child; family; and community supports, such as schools, rehabilitation centers, or group homes. First and foremost, the clinicians involved in the child's treatment should collaborate with the family toward the same general goals. As the number of clinicians and educators involved increases, the chance of fragmentation in treatment planning also increases. The nurse can serve as a case coordinator.

Residential care may be necessary in some cases. After making the decision to place a child into a residential facility, family members may experience guilt, loss, and a sense of failure concerning their inability to care for the child at home.

EVIDENCE-BASED NURSING CARE FOR CHILDREN WITH AUTISM SPECTRUM DISORDER

Mental Health Nursing Assessment

Physical Health Assessment

Physical health assessment should include a review of physical health and neurologic status, giving particular attention to coordination, childhood illnesses, injuries, and hospitalizations. The nurse should assess sleep, appetite, and activity patterns because they may be disturbed in affected children. Lack of adequate sleep can increase irritability. Comorbid seizure disorders are common in those with autism; depression is often seen concurrently even when no intellectual or language impairment is evident. Thus, the nurse should consider these conditions in the assessment.

Children with additional psychiatric disorders or seizures may be receiving multiple medications and require the care of several clinicians. Therefore, assessment should include a careful review of current medications and treating clinicians.

Psychosocial Assessment

Communication, behaviors, and flexibility are critical assessment areas. Direct behavioral observation is important to evaluate the child's ability to relate to others, to verify the selection of age-appropriate activities, and to watch for stereotypic behaviors. Assessment of the child with ASD can be based on the following categories:

- Communication
  - Verbal and nonverbal
  - Use of picture cards, writing, or drawing
  - Comfortable with eye contact
  - Understand emotional cues
  - Presence of pain
  - Preoccupation with restricted interests
- Behaviors
  - Items of fixation (how does family manage?)
  - Triggers for agitation
  - Early signs that indicate beginning of agitation
  - Interventions that work when child is overstimulated or agitated
  - Repetitive behaviors
- Flexibility or adherence to routine
  - Home schedule
  - What aggravates or irritates the person
  - Early warning signs of agitation
  - When overagitated, what interventions work best (Scarpinato, Bradley, Kurbjun, Bateman, Holtzer, & Ely, 2010).

The child's behavior, need for structure, and communication style can affect family functioning. Having a child with ASD is bound to influence family interaction; responding to the child's needs may adversely affect family functioning. For example, sleep disruption in family members who care for these children may increase family stress.

Nursing Diagnoses

Assessment data generate several potential nursing diagnoses, including Self-Care Deficits, Delayed Growth and Development, Disturbed Sleep Pattern, Anxiety, Disturbed Thought Processes, and Social Isolation Treatment outcomes need to be individualized to the child, family, and social environment and may change with time (Herdman & Kamitsuru, 2014).

Nursing Interventions

Physical Health Interventions

In teaching self-care skills, the nurse needs to consider the child's current adaptive skills and language limitations. Developing a list of activities for the child to post in his or her bedroom may be effective for some children. Drawings or symbols may be useful for nonverbal children. Physical safety is an important concern for children who are cognitively delayed and may have impaired judgment.

No medication has proved effective at changing the core social and language deficits of autism. However, some atypical antipsychotics (i.e., risperidone, aripirazole) are approved for the treatment of irritability associated with autism. Weight gain and metabolic syndrome are concerns with these agents. Evidence is minimal that anticonvulsants and traditional mood stabilizers are useful in managing mood lability and aggression. (Politte, Henry, & McDougle, 2014; Baribeau & Anagnostou, 2014).

Psychosocial Interventions

When working with children with neurodevelopmental disorders, building on their strengths and using positive reinforcement are very important. If these children feel that they are constantly criticized or need "fixing," their self-esteem will be eroded and they will be unlikely to cooperate and learn (Scarpinato, et al., 2010).

Promoting Interaction

Structuring interventions for social isolation should fit the child's cognitive, linguistic, and developmental levels. Interventions fostering nonverbal social interactions may be more useful than those based on speech. For higher functioning children, activities such as getting the mail, passing out snacks, or taking turns in the context of simple games can engage them in social activities without requiring the use of their limited language skills. Structuring social interactions so that the child shares a task with another, such as carrying a load of books, may help boost confidence in relating to others.

Caring for children with ASD requires extraordinary patience and determination. With help, these children can learn social and communication skills, such as taking turns in conversation and warning the listener before changing the subject in the context of milieu.

Ensuring Predictability and Safety

When children with autism spectrum disorders are hospitalized, milieu management—a consistent, structured environment with predictable routines for activities, mealtimes, and bedtimes—is necessary for successful treatment. Changes in routine may provoke disorganization in the child, leading to emotional dysequilibrium and explosive behavior. The safety of the inpatient unit offers an opportunity to try behavioral strategies, such as rewards for managing transitions. Health care professionals can pass on successful strategies to parents or primary caretakers (Reaven, 2009).

A structured physical environment will most likely be important to a child with a development disorder. Keeping furniture, dishes, and toys in the same place helps ease anxiety and fosters secure feelings. The nurse should identify the child's individually specific needs for structure.

Behavioral Interventions

Children with ASDs often need specific behavioral interventions to reduce the frequency of inappropriate or aggressive behavior (Scarpinato, et al., 2010). For example, a child may have angry outbursts in response to routine transitions. If the tantrum is dramatic, the consequence may be that the transition does not take place. By structuring the environment and using visual cues to signal the end of one activity and the start of another, it may be possible to reduce the number and intensity of responses to transitions. Safety is always a concern. Self-injury and aggression are sometimes present, so children may need to be protected from hurting themselves and others. If aggressive or assaultive behavior is a problem, a brief "time out" followed by prompt reentry into activities is usually effective.

Managing the repetitive behaviors of these children depends on the specific behavior and its effects on others or the environment. If the behavior, such as rocking, has no negative effects, ignoring it may be the best approach. If the behavior, such as head banging, however, is unacceptable, redirecting the child and using positive reinforcement are recommended. In some cases, especially in severely delayed children, these strategies may not work, and environmental alterations and perhaps protective headgear will be needed.

Supporting Family

Unfortunately, lack of integration of medical, psychiatric, social, and educational services can add to the family's burden. Parents may manifest denial, grief, guilt, and anger at various points as they adjust to their child's disability. The nurse can offer parents the opportunity to express their frustrations and disappointments and can be alert for indications that parents are in need of additional assistance, such as parent support groups or respite care.

Family interventions include support, education, counseling, and referral to self-help groups. Whenever possible, the nurse provides education to help parents determine appropriate expectations for their child and to meet the child's special needs. The following are examples of potentially useful nursing interventions focusing on the family:

- Interpreting the treatment plan for parents and child
- Modeling appropriate behavior modification techniques
- Including the parents as cotherapists for the implementation of the care plan
- Assisting the family in identifying and resolving their sense of loss related to the diagnosis
- Coordinating support systems for parents, siblings, and family members
- Maintaining interdisciplinary collaboration

Evaluation and Treatment Outcomes

Evaluation of patient and family outcomes is an ongoing process. Short-term outcomes might consist of discrete behavioral improvements, such as reducing self-injurious behavior by 50%. The long-term goal is for the patient to achieve the highest level of functioning.

ATTENTION-DEFICIT HYPERACTIVITY DISORDER

Attention-deficit hyperactivity disorder (ADHD) is one of the most commonly diagnosed disorders in school-aged children (Centers for Disease Control and Prevention [CDC], 2013). It is almost certainly a heterogeneous disorder with multiple etiologies. The relatively high frequency of ADHD and associated behavior problems virtually guarantees that nurses will meet affected children in all pediatric treatment settings. ADHD is also diagnosed in adults, but it is less common than in children (Kessler, Green, Adler, Barkley, Chatterji, Faraone, et al., 2010).

Clinical Course and Diagnostic Criteria

A persistent pattern of inattention, hyperactivity, and impulsiveness that interferes with functioning characterizes ADHD (APA, 2013). A diagnosis is made based on school behavior, parents' reports, and direct observation of inattention and hyperactivity-impulsivity that are inconsistent with developmental level. Parents and teachers describe children with ADHD as restless, always on the go, highly distractible, unable to wait their turn, heedless, and frequently disruptive. Indeed, it is often disruptive behavior that brings these children into treatment.

KEYCONCEPT   **Attention** involves concentrating on one activity to the exclusion of others, as well as the ability to sustain focus.

In ADHD, the person finds it difficult to attend to one task at a time and is easily distracted. For some, the lack of attention is related to being unable to filter incoming information, which leads to being unable to screen and select the important information. That is, all incoming stimuli are treated the same (e.g., directions from a teacher elicits the same importance as noise in the hallway). For others, the distractibility may be related to stimuli-seeking behavior. Given the heterogeneity of ADHD, either of these models may explain problems of attention for subgroups of affected children.

Children with ADHD are prone to impulsive, risk-taking behavior and often fail to consider the consequences of

their actions (Shaw, Gilliam, Liverpool, Weddle, Malek, Sharp, et al., 2011). They tend to exercise poor judgment and seem to have more than the usual lumps, bumps, and bruises because of their risk-taking behavior. They often require a high degree of structure and supervision (Davis & Williams, 2011).

KEYCONCEPT   **Impulsiveness** is the tendency to act on urges, notions, or desires without adequately considering the consequences.

Although hyperactivity is a characteristic often associated with ADHD, controversy is long-standing about whether attention-deficit disorder can occur without overactivity. In many cases, the hyperactivity prompts the search for treatment. Parents typically report that a child's hyperactivity was manifested early in life and is evident in most situations (APA, 2013). Hyperactivity and impulsivity in childhood are associated with conduct disorder (Chapter 22) and intimate partner violence perpetration in adults (Fang, Massetti, Ouyan, Srosse, & Mercy, 2010).

KEYCONCEPT   **Hyperactivity** is excessive motor activity, as evidenced by restlessness, an inability to remain seated, and high levels of physical motion and verbal output.

ADHD Across the Life-span

ADHD is usually diagnosed in childhood and was traditionally viewed as a problem of children. We now understand that ADHD persists into adulthood and it is sometimes first diagnosed later than in childhood. In adults, symptoms of hyperactivity and impulsivity tend to decline with age and deficit of attention persist and become more varied (Kessler, et al., 2010). However, the majority of the adults with ADHD are undiagnosed and untreated (Waite & Ramsay, 2010). Many of the adults with ADHD become the parents of children with the same disorder (Mokrova, O'Brien, Calkins, & Keane, 2010).

Epidemiology and Risk Factors

Although prevalence estimates vary depending on the diagnostic criteria used, the sources of data, and the sampling procedure, ADHD in school-aged children is about 6%, with a range of 2% to 14% (Kessler, et al., 2010; Syed, Masaud, Nkire, Iro, & Garland, 2010). Boys are twice as likely as girls to be diagnosed with ADHD (CDC, 2013). A familial history of ADHD, bipolar disorder, or substance use (Kessler, et al., 2010), early exposure to pesticides (Kuehn, 2011), prenatal tobacco exposure, and high blood lead concentrations (Polanska, Jurewicz, & Hanke, 2012) are associated with increasing the risk for ADHD.

Etiology

No single explanation for the occurrence of ADHD exists; instead, this disorder is viewed as having multiple causes. Genetic factors are implicated in the etiology of ADHD. They clearly play a fundamental role in the manifestation of the ADHD behavior (Gagne, Saudino, & Asherson, 2011). In some children, ADHD may have developed because of being hypersensitive to environmental stimuli such as foods. This hypersensitivity to foods may be allergies to specific foods (e.g.,wheat, milk, peanuts, eggs, soy) or to other substances such as artificial dyes and flavors or salicylates (Stevenson, Buitelaar, Cortese, Ferrin, Konofal, Lecendreux, et al., and members of the European ADHD Guidelines Group, (2014).

Biologic Theories

Although the etiology of ADHD is uncertain, evidence about neurobiologic dysfunction is pervasive. Several lines of research have shown that the frontal lobe and functional connections are impacted with specific subcortical structures also dysregulated. One clearly dysfunctional area is the dorsolateral prefrontal cortex, the center of directed attention and the ability to manage emotions or delay emotional reactions (Manos, Tom-Revzon, Bukstein, & Crismon, 2007). Several neurotransmitters (e.g., dopamine, serotonin) are dysregulated (Halmey, Johansson, Winge, McKinney, Knappskog, & Haavik, 2010). Clinically, the hyperactive-impulsive behavior characteristic of ADHD has been shown to be predominantly related to biologic factors, not psychosocial factors (Freitag, Hänig, Schneider, Switz, Palmason, & Meyer, 2012).

Psychosocial Theories

Although genetic endowment is clearly a fundamental element in the etiology of ADHD, psychosocial factors are also important risk factors, particularly those related to inattention (Freitag, et al., 2012). Family stress, marital discord, and parental substance use are also associated with ADHD (Palcic, Jurbergs, & Kelley, 2009). Other implicated psychosocial factors are poverty, overcrowded living conditions, and family dysfunction.

Family Response to ADHD

Living with a child who has ADHD is a challenge for all family members, particularly those members who also have issues similar to those of the affected child. The family will not only be raising a child who needs a structured environment that helps support focus and attention, but the parents have to partner with their children's school system. For some families, the relationship with the school is positive and supportive. For others, the relationship with the school can be strained and lead to additional stress. It is important that the teachers and parents work together and provide consistent directions to the child.

If parents also have problems related to attention, impulse, and hyperactivity, home chaos and ineffective parenting practices can occur (Mokrova, et al., 2010). If the parents also have ADHD, they might not be able to provide a calm structured environment for the child. Effective parenting requires the ability to resist overreacting emotionally, to focus on the child, to keep track of activities, and to provide consistency in discipline.

Teamwork and Collaboration: Working Toward Recovery

Children with ADHD and their families benefit from symptom management, education, and support from various disciplines to have a high-quality life. Successful recovery efforts involve early recognition and treatment. By recognizing the problem early, family members and teachers can structure the child's interactions, develop meaningful discipline strategies, and modify the physical environment so the child can learn coping skills to deal with impulsivity, distractibility, and hyperactivity. Evidence has accumulated over the years that medication is helpful, especially in the early years, but for long-term effects, a combination of medication management and behavioral approaches results in the best outcomes for the children and their families (Moriyama, Polanczyk, Terzi, Faria, & Rhode, 2013).

ADHD is not an easy disorder to treat or manage. Comorbidity complicates successful recovery. Children with ADHD have more conduct problems (e.g., run-ins with police), depression, and psychiatric admissions (McQuade, Vaughn, Hoza, Murray-Close, Molina, Arnold, et al., 2014). Many other problems interfere with recovery efforts, such as family disruptions and economic problems, as well as naturally occurring changes such as maturational issues during their adolescent years. Additionally, children from disadvantaged backgrounds fare worse than those children who have socioeconomic and educational support (Law, Sideridis, Prock, & Sheridan, 2014).

Safety Issues

Children, adolescents, and adults with ADHD are high risk for moodiness that could lead to risk-taking behavior and suicide ideation or attempts (Balazs, Miklósi, Keresztény, Dallos, & Gádoros, 2014). Mood lability, the presence of depression, and potential for self-harm should be carefully assessed in these individuals. These children are also at risk for depression and suicidal ideation, especially in adolescence. Girls and those with mothers who experience depression when the child is

4 to 6 years of age are more likely to attempt suicide 5 to 13 years later (Chronis-Tuscano, Molina, Pelham, Applegate, Dahlke, Overmyer, et al., 2010).

EVIDENCE-BASED NURSING CARE FOR CHILDREN WITH ADHD

The planning of nursing interventions must be done within the context of the family, treatment setting, and school environment. With the parents, clinical team members, and school personnel, the nurse participates in designing a plan of care that fits the child's and family's needs. Persons with ADHD and their families will benefit from nursing care at many different times in the course of the disorder. Unless hospitalized for a comorbid mental health problem, most treatment will occur outside the mental health system. School nurses often provide most of the nursing care and family education.

Mental Health Nursing Assessment

In the school setting, the primary focus of the assessment is the impact of ADHD on classroom behavior and school performance. In the hospital, the nurse tries to determine the contribution of ADHD to the acute psychiatric problem. In both cases, the nurse collects assessment data through direct interview, observation of the child and parent, and teacher ratings. Because children with ADHD may have difficulty sitting through long sessions, interviews are typically brief. Parents and teachers are extremely important sources for assessment data. To this end, the nurse can make use of several standardized instruments (Box 28.3). See Nursing Care Plan 28.1 at http://thepoint.lww.com/BoydEssentials.

Physical Health Assessment

As with other psychiatric disorders with onset in childhood, the nursing assessment of children with ADHD begins with identification and exploration of the presenting problems, usually hyperactivity, impulsivity, and inattention. This typically entails a review of the child's developmental course, the onset and pattern of the current symptoms, factors that have worsened or improved the child's problems, and prior treatment or self-initiated efforts to remedy the situation. Medical history is also essential, consisting of perinatal course, childhood illnesses, hospital admissions, injuries, seizures, tics, physical growth, general health status, and date of the child's last physical examination.

The behavior of these children is characteristically very active and can often be observed in the office. They cannot sit still. They fidget. Even in sleep, they may be more active than normal children. Thus, a careful assessment of eating, sleeping, and activity patterns is essential. Assessing daily food intake, typical diet, and frequency

---

BOX 28.3

Standardized Tools for ADHD Diagnosis*

CONNERS QUESTIONNAIRES
The Conners Parent Questionnaire is a 48-item scale that a parent completes about his or her child. Each item is a statement that the parent rates on a 4-point scale from 0 (not at all) to 3 (very much). The Conners Teacher Questionnaire is a 28-item questionnaire that the child's teacher completes according to the same 4-point scale as the Parent Questionnaire. Both questionnaires have been standardized by age and gender for a mean of 50 and a standard deviation of 10 (Conners, 1989; Goyette, Connors, & Ulrich, 1978).

CHILD BEHAVIOR CHECKLIST
The Child Behavior Checklist (CBCL) is a 118-item questionnaire that a parent completes. In addition to the 118 questions about specific behaviors and psychiatric symptoms, the CBCL also includes questions concerning the child's competence in social and academic spheres as well as age-appropriate activities. Normative data are available, allowing the conversion of raw scores to standard scores for age and gender. A teacher version of this scale is also available.

*Note that the diagnosis of ADHD is not made on the basis of questionnaires alone. Data from these rating scales augment the information gathered through interview and observation. These questionnaires can be especially useful before and after initiating a treatment plan to measure change.

---

of eating will help identify any nutritional problems. Caffeinated products can contribute to hyperactivity in some children. Sleep is often disturbed for children with ADHD and consequently also the family. A detailed sleep assessment can provide points for interventions and help the interpretation of drug effects.

Psychosocial Assessment

Data regarding school performance, behavior at home, and comorbid psychiatric disorders are essential for developing school interventions and behavior plans and establishing the baseline severity for medication. Children with ADHD are more likely to have problems with their cognitive process during changing demands of teachers and parents (Mulder, M. J., Bos, D., Weusten, van Belle, van Dijk, Simen, et al., 2011; Shaw, et al., 2011). Consequently, they may have more difficulty in school with decision-making. These children are often behind in their work at school because of poor organization, off-task behavior, and impulsive responses.

Dysfunctional interactions can develop within the family. Discipline is frequently an issue because parents may have difficulty controlling their child's behavior, which is disruptive and occasionally destructive. They can exhaust their parents, aggravate teachers, and annoy siblings with their intrusive and disruptive actions. Reviewing the problem behaviors and the situations in which they occur is a way to identify negative interaction patterns.

Because ADHD often occurs in the context of psychosocial adversity, it is important to review the family situation, including parenting style, stability of household membership, consistency of rules and routines, and life events (e.g., divorce, moves, deaths, job loss). Identification of these factors can be useful in shaping a care plan that builds on potential strengths and mitigates the effects of environmental factors that may perpetuate the child's disruptive behavior.

Nursing Diagnoses

Depending on the severity of the responses, family situation, and school environment, several nursing diagnoses could be generated from the assessment data, including Self-Care Deficit, Risk for Imbalanced Nutrition, Risk for Injury, Disturbed Sleep Pattern, Anxiety, Defensive Coping Impaired Social Interaction, Ineffective Role Performance, and Compromised Family Coping (Herdman & Kamitsuru, 2014). The outcomes should be individualized to the child. Short-term outcomes, such as decreasing the number of classroom ejections within a 2-week period, may be useful for one child, but reducing the frequency and amplitude of angry outbursts at home may be relevant to another child.

Nursing Interventions

Physical Health Interventions

Modifying Nutrition

A link between adverse reaction to food (e.g., dietary salicylates and artificially added food colors, flavors, preservatives) and ADHD was suggested many years ago when the Feingold diet was introduced (Feingold, 1975). Over the years, interest in the link between food and behavior continues to spark interest in ADHD as a problem related to food. Study outcomes are mixed. Agreement exists that in some children the behaviors associated with ADHD can be decreased with diet changes (Ghuman, 2011; Pelsser, Frankena, Toormam, Savelkoul, Dubois, Pereira, et al., 2011). The Restricted Elimination Diet has been shown to improve behavior in some children and can be used as an instrument to determine whether ADHD behaviors are induced by food. In this diet, all-natural, chemical-free foods are eaten, and most of the foods that are regularly eaten are removed (Lomangino, 2011). Fruits, vegetables, nuts, nut butters, beans, seeds, gluten-free grains such as rice and quinoa, fish, lamb, wild game meats, organic turkey and large amounts of water are consumed. This diet is very restricted and consequently difficult to follow all of the time (Pelsser, et al., 2011).

If patients adhere to this diet, the nurse should support the patient and family in providing the nutritional information needed for this diet. Additionally, the patient and family will need education regarding those foods that are chemical free. A referral to a dietitian will benefit both patient and family.

A subgroup of children with ADHD show inattention, impulsivity, and hyperactivity following ingestion of foods containing artificial food color (Nigg, Lewis, Edinger, & Falk, 2012; Stevens, Kuczek, Burgess, Stochelski, Arnold, & Galland, 2013). The reason some children seem susceptible to artificial food color, however, is unclear so more research is needed in this area.

Supplementation with free fatty acids has been shown to be helpful for children who have deficiencies in free fatty acid such as omega-3 free fatty acid, omega-6 free fatty acid, and linolenic acid. This supplementation is usually achieved with capsule-containing oils or diets rich in fish products (Stevenson, et al., 2014).

Children with ADHD seem to be more susceptible to being overweight and developing obesity (Pauli-Pott, Albayrak, Hebebrand, & Pott, 2010). Because of the impulsivity and inattention characteristic of ADHD, these children may be unable to resist external cues for high-fat foods. The nurse can help the family and patient structure the external environment so the child has healthy choices available.

Promoting Sleep

Sleep can be a problem for children with ADHD for many reasons. The overactivity of the disorder itself and the side effects of the psychostimulants contribute to sleep problems. A sleep history should be taken before medications are prescribed. If problems exist, atomoxetine (Strattera) should be considered before the psychostimulants (see next section). If sleep problems arise while taking medications, sleep diaries should be kept. Sleep hygiene and behavior therapy techniques should be implemented (Graham, Banaschewski, Buitelaar, Coghill, Danckaerts, Dittmann, et al., 2011). See Chapter 26.

Using Pharmacologic Interventions

The first-line recommended medications for ADHD symptoms are the psychostimulants and atomoxetine (Strattera). Alpha$_{2A}$ agonists, guanfacine extended release (Intuniv) is also approved for the treatment of ADHD alone or adjunctive to stimulants (Hirota, Schwartz, & Correll, 2014).

Psychostimulants

Psychostimulants (see Chapter 10) are by far the most commonly used medications for the treatment of ADHD. These medications enhance dopamine and norepinephrine activity and thereby improve attention and focus, increase inhibition of impulsive actions, and quiet the "noise" associated with distractibility and shifting attention (Moriyama, et al., 2013).

Methylphenidate (Ritalin) has a total duration of action of about 4 hours (Box 28.4). Thus, parents or

BOX 28.4
Drug Profile: Methylphenidate (Ritalin)

DRUG CLASS: Central nervous system stimulant

RECEPTOR AFFINITY: The mechanisms of pharmacologic effect are not completely clear. At low doses, it provides mild cortical stimulation similar to that of amphetamines. This stimulation results from methylphenidate's ability to promote release and interfere with the reuptake of dopamine in the synaptic cleft. Main sites appear to be the brain stem arousal system and cortex to produce its stimulant effect.

INDICATIONS: Treatment of narcolepsy, attention-deficit disorders, and hyperkinetic syndrome.

ROUTES AND DOSAGE: Available in 5- to 10-mg immediate-release tablets and 20-mg sustained-release tablets (Ritalin-SR). Newer long-acting preparations such as Concerta and Metadate, in various dose strengths, are also available.

Adult dosage: Must be individualized; range from 10 to 60 mg/d orally in divided doses bid (twice a day) to tid (three times a day), preferably 15 to 30 min before meals. If insomnia is a problem, drug should be administered before 6 PM.

Child dosage: The immediate-release formulation can be started at 5 mg twice or three times daily on a 4-hour schedule with weekly increases depending on response. Starting doses of the long-acting preparations are equivalent to the total tid dose (e.g., 5 tid of short-acting would translate into 18 mg of Concerta). Usually given on a tid schedule, with the last dose being roughly half that of the first and second dose. Daily dosage of more than 60 mg is not recommended. Discontinue after 1 month if no improvement is seen.

PEAK EFFECT: 1 h; half-life: 3–4 h for the immediate-release preparations

SELECT SIDE EFFECTS: Nervousness, insomnia, dizziness, headache, dyskinesias (including tics), toxic psychosis, anorexia, nausea, abdominal pain, increased pulse and blood pressure, palpitations, tolerance, psychological dependence

WARNING: The drug is discontinued periodically to assess the patient's condition. Contraindications include marked anxiety, tension and agitation, glaucoma, severe depression, and obsessive-compulsive symptoms. Use cautiously in patients with a personal or family history of tic disorders, seizure disorders, hypertension, drug dependence, alcoholism, or emotional instability.

SPECIFIC PATIENT AND FAMILY EDUCATION
- Do not chew or crush sustained-release tablets; they must be swallowed whole.
- Take the drug exactly as prescribed; if insomnia is a problem, the time and dose may need adjustment. The drug is rarely taken after 5 PM.
- Avoid alcohol and over-the-counter products, including decongestants, cold remedies, and cough syrups; these could accentuate side effects of the stimulant.
- Keep appointments for follow-up, including evaluations for monitoring the child's growth and use of parent and teacher ratings to monitor benefit.
- Note that the prescriber may discontinue the drug periodically to confirm effectiveness of therapy.

Concerta, Ritalin LA, and Metadate or amphetamine–dextroamphetamine (Adderall), do not require such frequent dosing and may be a better fit with a school day schedule.

One major concern with the psychostimulants is the potential for abuse. With the increase in recognition of ADHD, psychostimulant prescriptions have increased, as well as an increase in teen and preteen abuse of amphetamine products. These abused prescription medications most often belong to the adolescents or a friend. Nurses should caution parents about the potential for abuse and prevent their child's medication from being a source of recreational use.

Atomoxetine

Atomoxetine (Strattera), a noradrenergic reuptake inhibitor, is not classified as a stimulant and is effective in the treatment of ADHD, especially when it is used in combination with the psychostimulants. Because it has little risk of abuse or misuse, it is often used for those who have a comorbid substance abuse issue (Murthy & Chand, 2012). It is also helpful in treating comorbid anxiety and inattention (Wagner & Pliszka, 2011). This medication is generally well tolerated in children and adults. Common side effects include headache, abdominal pain, decreased appetite, vomiting, somnolence, and nausea (Childress & Berry, 2012).

Teaching Points

Medication can help the child's hyperactivity, impulsiveness, and inattention; therefore, teaching the parent, child, and school personnel about the importance of the medication in ADHD and the potential side effects is a place to begin. Explaining to the child that the medication improves concentration and the ability to sit still can help strengthen patient motivation.

Many times parents are reluctant to initiate treatment with psychostimulants because of the fear that their use in childhood will increase the risk of using substances in adulthood. Studies show that treatment of ADHD is not associated with a risk of substance use disorders (Humphreys, Eng, & Lee, 2013). Teaching patients and families about the biologic basis of ADHD helps parents understand that these children are not "bad" kids but that they have problems with impulse control and attention. It may be helpful to review the purposes of the medications and assure parents that evidence shows medications help most affected children.

Psychosocial Interventions

Behavioral programs based on rewards for positive behavior, such as waiting turns and following directions, can foster new social skills. Behavioral parent training, behavioral classroom management, and behavioral peer

teachers often describe a return of overactivity and distractibility as the first dose of medication wears off. This "rebound effect" can often be managed by moving the second dose of the day slightly closer to the first dose. Longer acting preparations of methylphenidate, such as interventions are well-established treatments. Specific cognitive behavioral techniques are helpful in which the child learns to "stop, look, and listen" before doing. These approaches have been refined and several useful treatment manuals are available (Evans, Owens, & Bunford, 2014). In general, interactions with children can be guided by the following:

• Set clear limits with clear consequences. Use few words and simplify instructions.
• Establish and maintain a predictable environment with clear rules and regular routines for eating, sleeping, and playing.
• Promote attention by maintaining a calm environment with few stimuli. These children cannot filter out extraneous stimuli and react to all stimuli equally.
• Establish eye contact before giving directions; ask the child to repeat what was heard.
• Encourage the child to do homework in a quiet place.
• Help the child work on one assignment at a time (reward with a break after each completion).

Family treatment is nearly always a component of cognitive behavioral treatment approaches with the child. This may involve parent training that focuses on principles of behavior management, such as appropriate limit setting and use of reward systems, as well as revising expectations about the child's behavior. School programming often involves increasing structure in the child's school day to offset the child's tendency to act without forethought and to be easily distracted by extraneous stimuli. Specific remediation is required for the child with comorbid deficits in learning or language. Some children may require small self-contained classrooms.

Evaluation and Treatment Outcomes

Children may not notice any effects after taking medication, but people in their environment do. Often, within 1 to 2 weeks of initiating therapy, children with ADHD become more attentive, less impulsive, and less active. Parents and teachers are often the first to notice improvement. With time, academic achievement also may improve (Figure 28.2).

Continuum of Care

Treatment of ADHD typically is conducted in outpatient settings. Optimal treatment is multimodal (i.e., includes several types of interventions), encompassing four main areas: individual treatment for the child, family treatment, school accommodations, and medication. Parent training and social skills training also help diminish disruptive and defiant behavior.

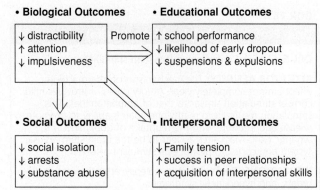

FIGURE 28.2   Long-term outcomes of optimal treatment for patients with attention-deficit hyperactivity disorder.

OTHER NEURODEVELOPMENTAL DISORDERS

Other neurodevelopmental disorders are characterized by a narrower range of deficits. These include specific neurodevelopmental disorders generally classified as learning, communication, and motor skills disorders. This section focuses primarily on learning and **communication disorders.**

Specific Learning Disorders

Generally, a **learning disorder** (also called learning disability) is defined as a discrepancy between actual achievement and expected achievement based on the person's age and intellectual ability. The definition varies depending on the source and state statute. Learning disorders are typically classified as verbal (e.g., reading, spelling) or nonverbal (e.g., mathematics).

Reading disability, also called **dyslexia**, has been recognized for more than 100 years. It is defined as a significantly lower score for mental age on standardized tests in reading that is not the result of low intelligence or inadequate schooling. This relatively common problem affects about 5% of school-aged children, with some studies reporting higher prevalence. In clinical samples, dyslexia affects boys more often than girls; however, a large community-based sample of children with reading disorders found no gender difference. This discrepancy suggests that the observed difference in clinic samples may be related to biases in seeking treatment rather than a true gender difference (Ferrer, Shaywitz, Holahan, Marchione, & Shaywitz, 2010; Stoeckel, Colligan, Barbaresi, Weaver, Killian, & Katusci, 2013).

Although it is clear that no single cause will provide a sufficient explanation for reading disability, the underlying problem appears to be a deficit in **phonologic processing**, which involves the discrimination and interpretation of speech sounds. A disturbance in the development of the left hemisphere is believed to cause this deficit. Both genetic and environmental factors have been implicated in the etiology of reading disability. Data from family studies show that reading disability is familial and that shared environmental factors alone cannot explain the high rate of recurrence in affected families (van der Leij, van Bergen, van Zuijen, de Jong, Maurits, & Maassen, 2013).

Less is known about the prevalence of nonverbal learning disorder (i.e, mathematics disorder), with estimates of occurrence ranging from 0.1% to 1.0% of school-aged children and no apparent difference between boys and girls. Mathematical ability is moderately inheritable and negatively associated with inattentiveness and hyperactivity-impulsivity symptoms of ADHD (Greven, Kovas, Willcutt, Petrill, & Plomin, 2014).

Communication Disorders

Communication disorders involve speech or language impairments. *Speech* refers to the motor aspects of speaking; *language* consists of higher order aspects of formulating and comprehending verbal communication. Communication disorders are fairly common and are yet more common in children with ASDs, ADHD, anxiety, and conduct disorders (Mackie & Law, 2010). As with reading disability, undoubtedly multiple causes of speech or language deficit may be present.

A delay in speech or language development can adversely affect the child's socialization and education. For example, peers may rebuff or tease a child with an articulation defect or stutter, contributing to withdrawal and a negative self-image. The resulting isolation could limit opportunities to negotiate rules, take turns, and learn cooperation. These same tasks could also be difficult for children with language delay. Moreover, language appears to play a role in the regulation of behavior and impulses (Mackie & Law, 2010).

Evidence-Based Nursing Care for Children with Communication Disorders

Nursing assessment of children with a known specific developmental disorder includes (1) evidence of interference in daily life, (2) determination of the child's ability (and limitations) to communicate during the interview, (3) assessment of the child's perception about his or her disability, (4) observation for impaired learning and communication, and (5) past and current interventions for the learning or communication deficit with data gathered through direct interview of the child and significant others such as parents. Several nursing diagnoses can be generated from these data, such as Impaired Verbal Communication and Social Isolation.

For the child with learning disabilities, nurses can focus on building self-confidence and helping the family connect with guidance and educational resources that support the child's development into adulthood. For the child with communication disorders, the interventions focus on fostering social and communication skills and making referrals for specific speech or language therapy. Modeling appropriate communication in spontaneous situations with the child can be a useful intervention for some children. The following is an overview of nursing interventions for the child with specific developmental difficulties:

- Introduce strategies for increasing communication skills (e.g., initiating conversation, taking turns in conversation, facing the listener).
- Identify and develop specific intervention strategies for problems secondary to learning communication disorders, such as low self-esteem.
- Provide parental support for coping with the disorder.
- Maintain interdisciplinary medical, dental, and speech therapy, and also educational collaboration.
- Refer to learning or speech specialist for evaluation and assistance.

Continuum of Care

Children with learning disabilities obviously require careful psychoeducational and cognitive testing to identify their strengths and deficits. School or clinical psychologists usually perform this type of specialized testing. When a learning disability has been identified, the U.S. Education for All Handicapped Children Act (Public Law 94-142) mandates that public school systems provide remedial services in the least restrictive educational setting. Families occasionally need help in advocating for these services.

The same is true for children with communication disorders, although the services requested may be different. Speech pathologists conduct the diagnostic assessment of speech and language disorder. Nurses may be involved with formal screening for communication disorders. Services such as speech therapy (directed at the motor aspects of speaking) or social skills groups (directed at the social and interpersonal aspects of language) are often available in school districts and can be obtained if a speech or language disorder has been identified. For some children with communication disorders, the services offered by the school may be insufficient. In such cases, the nurse can help the family locate a facility that can provide these needed services.

■ TIC DISORDERS AND TOURETTE DISORDER

Tics are a part of several mental health problems. **Motor tics** are usually quick jerky movements of the eyes, face, neck, and shoulders, although they may involve other muscle groups as well. Occasionally, tics involve slower, more purposeful, or dystonic movements. **Phonic tics** typically include repetitive throat clearing, grunting, or other noises but may also include more complex sounds, such as words; parts of words; and in a minority of patients, obscenities. Transient tics by definition do not endure over time and appear to be fairly common in school-aged children. *Tic disorder* is a general term encompassing several syndromes that are chiefly characterized by motor tics, phonic tics, or both.

> **KEYCONCEPT** **Tics** are sudden, rapid, repetitive, stereotyped motor movements or vocalizations.

Tourette disorder, the most severe tic disorder, is defined by multiple motor and phonic tics for at least 1 year. Because no diagnostic tests are used to confirm this disorder, the diagnosis is based on the type and duration of tics present (Jankovic, Gelineau-Kattner, & Davidson, 2010). The typical age of onset for tics is about 7 years; motor tics generally precede phonic tics. Parents often describe the seeming replacement of one tic with another. In addition to this changing repertoire of motor and phonic tics, Tourette disorder exhibits a waxing and waning course. The child can suppress the tics for brief periods. Thus, it is not uncommon to hear from parents that their child has more frequent tics at home than at school. Older children and adults may describe an urge or a physical sensation before having a tic. The general trend is for tic symptoms to decline by early adulthood.

EPIDEMIOLOGY AND ETIOLOGY

The prevalence of Tourette disorder is estimated to be between one and 3 to 6 per 1,000 in school-aged children, with boys being affected three to six times more often than girls (Centers for Disease Control and Prevention [CDC], 2014). Obsessive-compulsive disorder (OCD) frequently occurs in association with Tourette disorder (Matthews & Grados, 2011).

The precise nature of the underlying pathophysiology in this primarily inherited disorder is unclear, but the basal ganglia and functionally related cortical areas are presumed to play a central role. Findings from neuroimaging studies are consistent with the presumption that a dysregulation of the cortico–striatal–thalamic circuitry of the brain underlies Tourette disorder. Additionally, multiple genes on different chromosomes interacting with environmental factors are involved. Several neurochemical systems have been implicated in the etiology of Tourette disorder, including dopamine systems, noradrenaline, endogenous opioids, and serotonin (Scharf, Yu, Mathews, Neale, Stewart, Fagerness, et al., 2013).

FAMILY RESPONSE TO DISORDER

Before evaluation and diagnosis of Tourette disorder, most families struggle with various explanations for the child's tics. Because tics fluctuate in severity with time and may be more prominent in some settings than in others, family members may have difficulty understanding their involuntary nature. Some parents may be convinced that the tics are deliberate and done to secure attention; others may judge that the tics are "nervous habits" indicative of underlying trouble. Such views require reconciliation with the currently accepted view that tics are involuntary. Some parents may conclude that the child is incapable of controlling any behavior because of Tourette disorder. They may subsequently feel uncertain about setting limits. In these families, delineating the boundaries of Tourette disorder can be helpful (Cavanna & Seri, 2014; CDC, 2014).

On learning that this disorder is probably genetic, some parents may harbor guilt for having passed it on to their child. The nurse can assist such families by listening to these concerns and providing information about the natural history of Tourette disorder—it is not a progressive condition, tics often diminish in adulthood, and it need not restrict what the child can achieve in life.

EVIDENCE-BASED NURSING CARE FOR CHILDREN WITH TOURETTE DISORDER

Mental Health Nursing Assessment

Nursing assessment of a child with tics includes a review of the onset, course, and current level of the symptoms. Goals of the assessment are to identify the frequency, intensity, complexity, and interference of the tics and their effects on functioning; determine the child's level of adaptive functioning; identify the child's areas of strength and weakness in general and in school; and identify social supports for the child and family.

Another important aspect of the assessment is to determine the effects of the tic symptoms on the child and family. Some children and families adjust well; however, others are embarrassed or devastated and tend to withdraw socially. Some children with Tourette disorder have ADHD, and a substantial percentage have symptoms of OCD (Matthews & Grados, 2011). Therefore, in addition to inquiring about tics, the nurse should assess the child's overall development, activity level, and capacity to concentrate and persist with a single task, as well as explore repetitive habits and recurring worries.

Nursing Diagnoses

Nursing diagnoses could include Ineffective Coping, Impaired Social Interaction, Anxiety, and Compromised Family Coping (Herdman & Kamitsuru, 2014). Children with Tourette disorder typically have normal intelligence, but their tics can interfere with their ability to relate to others and perform in school.

Nursing Interventions

The approach to planning nursing interventions depends on the primary source of impairment: tics themselves; OCD symptoms; or the triad of hyperactivity, inattention, and poor impulse control. The nurse can provide counseling and education for the patient, education for the parents, and consultation for the school. Most children and their families need some education about Tourette disorder. Individual psychotherapy with a mental health specialist (e.g., a psychologist or an advanced practice nurse) may be indicated for some children and adolescents with Tourette disorder to deal with maladaptive responses to the chronic condition.

Medications

Two classes of drugs are commonly used in the treatment of tics: antipsychotics and α-adrenergic receptor agonists. Aripiprazole is replacing the use of older antipsychotics, such as haloperidol and pimozide (Cavanna & Seri, 2013). These potent dopamine blockers are often effective at low doses. Attempts to eradicate all tics by increasing the dosages of these antipsychotics almost certainly will result in diminishing therapeutic returns and additional side effects. The

most frequently encountered side effects include drowsiness, dulled thinking, muscle stiffness, akathisia, increased appetite and weight gain, and acute dystonic reactions. Long-term use carries a small risk for tardive dyskinesia.

Psychoeducation

Teachers, guidance counselors, and school nurses may need current information about Tourette disorder and its related problems. Discussions with school personnel often include issues such as how to deal with tic behaviors that are disruptive in the classroom, how to manage teasing from other children, and how to handle medication side effects. A careful discussion of the boundaries of Tourette disorder and tic symptomatology usually can resolve these matters. Teachers who understand the involuntary nature of tics can often generate creative solutions, such as excusing the child to do errands. This strategy allows the child to step out of the classroom briefly to release a bout of tics, thereby reducing stress. In some situations, a brief presentation about Tourette disorder to the class will reduce teasing and help both teachers and classmates tolerate the tic symptoms (Box 28.5).

Before initiating these interventions with the school personnel, it is essential to identify the child's needs and

---

BOX 28.5 • THERAPEUTIC DIALOGUE • Tics and Disruptive Behaviors

INEFFECTIVE APPROACH

Teacher: I see the tics. He jerks his head, makes faces, and flicks his hands.

Nurse: What do you do about them?

Teacher: What can I do? If he isn't disrupting the class, I leave him alone. Even when he is throwing spitballs.

Nurse: Spitballs! He shouldn't be allowed to throw spitballs.

Teacher: Oh, I thought that was a part of his problem.

Nurse: Well, throwing spitballs has nothing to do with tics.

EFFECTIVE APPROACH

Teacher: I see the tics. He jerks his head, makes faces, and flicks his hands.

Nurse: He cannot help the tics that you are seeing. Tic disorders can exhibit a wide range of severity, from mild to severe and from simple to complex. Some complex tics may be difficult to distinguish from habits or rituals.

Teacher: What about things like throwing spitballs? When he does things like that, I try to ignore that behavior.

Nurse: Sounds like you give him the benefit of the doubt. (Validation) However, throwing a spitball is not a tic behavior.

Teacher: What should I do?

Nurse: How do you usually handle that type of behavior? (A modification of reflection)

Teacher: I'd ask him to stop and sometimes go into the hall.

Nurse: Disruptive behavior that is voluntary in a student with a tic disorder should be handled as you would handle any other child.

CRITICAL THINKING CHALLENGE

• Compare the responses of the nurse in these scenarios. What made the difference in the teacher's responsiveness to the nurse?

to pursue these strategies in collaboration with the family and other clinical team members. The Education for the Handicapped Act (Public Law 94–142) ensures that children with conditions such as Tourette disorder are eligible for special education services even if they do not meet full criteria for having a learning disability. Thus, if evidence shows that Tourette disorder is hindering academic progress, parents can demand special education services for their child. Nurses can help families negotiate with the school to obtain appropriate services.

EVALUATION AND TREATMENT OUTCOMES

Treatment outcomes will vary over the years and will be influenced by growth and development changes, family interaction and understanding of the disorder, and reduction or elimination of the frequency of the tics. Outcomes should include improvement of the child's quality of life and ability to learn to manage the symptoms of the disorder.

SEPARATION ANXIETY DISORDER

Anxiety disorders are the most common mental disorders in children and adolescents (Beesdo, Knappe, & Pine, 2009). Nearly one in three adolescents (31%) meets the criteria for an anxiety disorder. Although some degree of worry and fearfulness is considered normal during the course of childhood, in children and adolescents with anxiety disorders, the level of anxiety is excessive and hinders daily functioning. This section focuses on separation anxiety, a disorder diagnosed in childhood, and OCD, a disorder that occurs in both adults and children. For a discussion of other anxiety disorders, see Chapter 16.

Separation anxiety is normal for very young children, but typically declines between ages 3 to 5 years of age. When the child's fear and anxiety around separation become developmentally inappropriate, **separation anxiety disorder** is diagnosed. Although many children experience some discomfort on separation from their attachment figures, children with separation anxiety disorder suffer great worry or fear when faced with ordinary separations or being away from home, such as when going to school. When separation is about to occur, children often resist by crying or hiding from their parents (Milrod, Markowitz, Gerber, Cyranowski, Altemus, Shaprio, et al., 2014). When asked, most children with separation anxiety disorder will express worry about harm to or permanent loss of their major attachment figure. Other children may express worry about their own safety.

A common manifestation of anxiety is school phobia, in which the child refuses to attend school, preferring to stay at home with the primary attachment figure. The

term *school phobia* was coined to distinguish it from truancy; whether it is a phobia in the usual sense is a matter of some debate. However, school phobia is common in other disorders such as general anxiety disorder, social phobia, OCD, depression, and conduct disorder. When a comorbid disorder such as depression is identified, it becomes the focus of treatment. In some cases, school phobia may resolve when the primary disorder is successfully treated.

EPIDEMIOLOGY AND ETIOLOGY

The prevalence of separation anxiety disorder is estimated at 2% to 8% of school-aged children, with an onset usually between 7 and 9 years of age; thus, it is relatively common (Merikangas, et al., 2010). Insecure attachment, difficult temperaments, and genetic factors contribute to the development of separation anxiety disorder. Anxiety disorders are often familial, so it appears that both environmental and genetic factors affect the risk for separation anxiety disorder. For example, separation anxiety may emerge after a move, change to a new school, or death of a family member or pet.

No single etiological factor, but instead several risk factors are associated with the onset of the disorder. For example, children of parents with at least one anxiety disorder have an increased risk of also having an anxiety disorder. The risk increases even more when two parents are affected. Parental depression is also associated the anxiety disorders in children (Milrod, et al., 2014).

FAMILY RESPONSE TO DISORDER

There is no single family response to a child who is experiencing separation anxiety. Parenting style, life events, and environmental factors vary from family to family. The family dynamics related to the child's behavior have to be carefully assessed. In some instances, the family may be undergoing a separation of a significant family member through death, divorce, or military deployment. In other situations, the arrival of a new family member may precede the child's separation anxiety. A family assessment is important in determining the relationship of the child's fears and anxiety and the family dynamics.

TEAMWORK AND COLLABORATION: WORKING TOWARD RECOVERY

An interdisciplinary approach is needed for the treatment of separation anxiety disorder. Effective treatment includes child and parent psychoeducation, school consultation, cognitive-behavioral therapy, and selective serotonin reuptake inhibitors (SSRIs) (Rapp, Dodds, Walkup, & Rynn, 2013).

EVIDENCE-BASED NURSING CARE FOR CHILDREN WITH SEPARATION ANXIETY DISORDER

School refusal is often what prompts the family to seek consultation for the child. Because school refusal can be a behavioral manifestation of several different child psychiatric disorders, it requires careful assessment. Issues to consider are whether the parents have been aware that the child is avoiding school (separation anxiety versus truancy); what efforts the family has used to return the child to school; the presence of significant subjective distress in the child with anticipation of going to school; and whether the school refusal occurs in the context of other behavioral, social, or emotional problems. The nurse should also review the purpose and dose of current medications.

The child's developmental history and response to new situations and prior separations provide essential background information for understanding the child's current separation anxiety. The assessment should also include a review of recent life events and the methods the family has used to promote the child's return to school. Finally, the family history with respect to anxiety, panic attacks, or phobias is also informative.

Nursing diagnosis and interventions will depend on the role of the nurse (school nurse, acute care, or community practice) and the relationship with the child and family. In some instances, the nurse will be responsible for education of the child and family. If the child is receiving medication, nursing care related to administration of medications and education should be implemented. Nurses will also be involved in educating teachers and serving as a liaison between treating physicians, family and child, and school.

OBSESSIVE-COMPULSIVE DISORDER

OCD is characterized by intrusive thoughts that are difficult to dislodge (i.e., obsessions) or ritualized behaviors that the child feels driven to perform (i.e., compulsions) (see Chapter 18). Children tend to exhibit both multiple obsessions and compulsions that relate to fear of catastrophic family event, contamination, sexual or somatic obsessions, and overly moralistic thoughts. Washing, checking, repeating and ordering are the most commonly reported compulsions (Geller, 2010).

Epidemiology and Etiology

The prevalence rate of OCD is estimated at 1% to 2% with two peaks of incidence across the life-span, one occurring in pre-adolescent children and later a peak in early adult life (Geller, 2010). More than half of the cases of OCD in youth involve a comorbid disorder such as a tic, mood, or anxiety disorder. The etiology of OCD in children is thought to be similar to that of adults (see Chapter 18). However, there is a subset of children whose OCD behavior that may be related to an immune response to group A beta-hemolytic streptococcal infections that led to inflammation of the basal ganglia (Geller, 2010).

Family Response to Disorder

Parents' responses to their child's obsessions and compulsions depend on their understanding of the thoughts and behaviors. Because OCD is highly familial, if the parents are recovering from their disorder, they may be able to support their child's ability to begin to deal with the symptoms. Conversely, the parents may find their child's thoughts and behaviors tiring so they become easily irritated with the multiple obsessions and compulsions. Parents need education and support to help their child.

Teamwork and Collaboration: Working Toward Recovery

Interdisciplinary treatment including school personnel is important for the child and family with OCD. Cognitive behavior therapy (CBT), including psychoeducation, cognitive training, exposure and response preventions, and relapse prevention is the treatment of choice

Evidence-Based Nursing Care for Children with OCD

Recurrent worries and ritualistic behavior can occur normally in children at particular stages of development. The first step in the assessment of OCD in children is to distinguish between normal childhood rituals and worries and pathologic rituals and obsessional thoughts. Obsessional thoughts are recurrent, nagging, and bothersome. Although children may describe obsessions as occurring "out of the blue," external events may trigger obsessions. For example, a child may fear contamination whenever he or she is in contact with a certain person or object. Likewise, compulsions waste time, cause distress, and interfere with daily life (Box 28.6).

The severity of the child's and family's response to OCD will determine the appropriate nursing diagnoses. When the obsessions and compulsions emerge, these children or adolescents are in distress because of the disturbing and relentless nature of the symptoms. Ineffective Coping, Compromised Family Coping, and Ineffective Role Performance are likely nursing diagnoses (Herdman & Kamitsuru, 2014).

Nursing interventions will be guided by the needs of the family and the developmental needs of the child or adolescent. If medication is prescribed, it is important to emphasize safe management of medications. Because the antidepressants have a "black box" warning regarding

BOX 28.6 CLINICAL VIGNETTE

Kimberly and OCD

Kim, an 11-year-old fifth grader, comes for evaluation because her mother and teacher have become increasingly concerned about her repetitive behaviors. In retrospect, Kim's mother recalls first noticing repetitive rituals about 2 years before, but she did not become alarmed about these behaviors until recently when they began to interfere with daily living. At the time of referral, Kim exhibits complicated jumping rituals that involve a specific number of jumps and a particular manner of jumping. She also turns light switches off and on and performs complex movements, such as blinking in patterns and thrusting her arms back and forth a certain number of times. Her mother also reports Kim's near-constant request for reassurance about her own safety. In recent months, her incessant demands for reassurance have been more frequent and elaborate. For example, Kim's mother has to answer three times that everything is all right and then say, "I swear to it."

At the evaluation, Kim expresses fears that some ill fate, such as catastrophic illness or injury, will befall her. This fear is triggered by contact with any individual who seems sick, chance exposures to foul smells or dirt, and minor scrapes or bumps. When the fear is triggered, she becomes increasingly anxious and consumed with the fear that she will develop an illness and die. Sometimes her fears are specific, such as cancer or AIDS. Other times her fears are more ambiguous, as evidenced by statements such as, "Something bad will happen" if she doesn't complete the ritual. Kim acknowledges that the ritual is probably not related to the feared event, but she is reluctant to take a chance. If the ritual does not reduce her anxiety, she seeks reassurance from her mother.

Kim's medical history was negative for serious illness or injury. She was born after an uncomplicated pregnancy, labor, and delivery and achieved developmental milestones at appropriate times. Indeed, her mother could recall no unusual problems in the first few years of life except that Kim was typically anxious in unfamiliar situations. Kim's mother reports a prior history of panic attacks, but the family history is otherwise negative for anxiety disorders, including OCD.

What Do You Think?

• What assessment information would you want to elicit from Kim?
• What additional information should be considered from Kim's mother about her history of panic attacks?
• What nursing interventions should be considered if Kim were your patient?

suicide risk in adolescents, the nurse must discuss with the parents and child the importance of monitoring moods and keeping regularly scheduled mental health appointments.

ELIMINATION DISORDERS

ENURESIS

Enuresis is the involuntary excretion of urine after the age at which the child should have attained bladder control. It usually involves involuntary bed-wetting at night, but repeated urination on clothing during waking hours can occur (diurnal enuresis). Enuresis is a self-limiting disorder, with most children experiencing a spontaneous remission.

Epidemiology and Etiology

The prevalence of nocturnal enuresis varies with age and gender, being most common in young boys—an estimated 5% to 10% of 5-year-old boys, and 3% to 5% in 10-year old boys have nocturnal enuresis (Mikkelsen, 2014). The frequency in girls is about half that of boys in each age group. The etiology of enuresis is unknown, with probably no single cause. Most children with nocturnal enuresis are urologically normal. Some evidence has shown that at least some children with nocturnal enuresis secrete decreased amounts of antidiuretic hormone during sleep, which may play a role in enuresis (Mikkelsen, 2014).

Nursing Care

Nursing assessment should include the child's developmental history, the onset and course of enuresis, prior treatment, presence of emotional problems, and medical history. The nurse should also explore the family's home environment, family attitudes about the child's enuresis, and the family's medical history. Routine laboratory tests such as urinalysis and a urine culture are used to identify the presence of infection. The nurse should obtain baseline data regarding toileting habits, including daytime incontinence, urinary frequency, and constipation. He or she should refer children with persistent daytime enuresis for consultation with an urologist.

In many cases, limiting fluid intake in the evening and treating constipation (if present) is sufficient to decrease the frequency of bed-wetting. One of the most effective methods is the bell and pad. In this approach, the child sleeps on a pad that has wires on it, and when the child voids, a bell sounds, waking up the child. With use, the child either wakes up to urinate or learns to sleep through the night without voiding. A more temporary solution is the use of desmopressin (DDAVP), a synthetic antidiuretic hormone that actually inhibits production of urine. After medication is withdrawn, the enuresis frequently returns (Mikkelsen, 2014).

ENCOPRESIS

Encopresis involves soiling clothing with feces or depositing feces in inappropriate places. Additional diagnostic criteria include that the child is older than 4 years; that the soiling occurs at least once per month; and that the soiling is not the result of a medical disorder, such as congenital aganglionic megacolon (Hirschsprung disease). The most common form of encopresis is fecal impaction accompanied by leakage around the hardened mass of stool. Because of the loss of muscle tone in the lower bowel, the child loses the usual urge to defecate and may not feel the leakage. Surprisingly, the child may not detect the smell of the stool because the olfactory apparatus becomes accustomed to the odor. If left untreated, this problem generally resolves independently by middle adolescence. Nonetheless, the social consequences may be substantial (Mikkelsen, 2014).

Epidemiology and Etiology

As with enuresis, encopresis is more common in boys, and the frequency of the condition declines with age. The current estimate of prevalence is 1.5% of school-aged children aged 7 to 8 years old, with boys three times more likely to have encopresis than girls (Mikkelsen, 2014).

The reasons for withholding stool and starting the cycle of fecal impaction are unclear but are not usually the result of physical causes. However, as noted, when fecal impaction occurs, there is an accompanying loss of tone in the bowel and subsequent leakage.

Nursing Care

Assessment includes a detailed interview with the child and parent regarding the pattern of the encopresis. A calm matter-of-fact approach can help to reduce the child's embarrassment. Physical examination is also necessary; thus, collaboration with the child's primary care provider or consulting pediatric specialist is essential. The presence of encopresis does not necessarily signal severe emotional or behavioral disturbances, but the nurse should inquire about other psychiatric disorders. Diagnosis of encopresis is presumed given a history of intermittent constipation and soiling. Collaboration with primary care consultants is often helpful to rule out rare medical conditions, such as Hirschsprung disease.

Effective intervention begins with educating the parents and the child about normal bowel function and the self-perpetuating cycle of fecal impaction and leakage of stool around the hardened mass of feces. The short-term goal of this educational effort is to decrease the anger and recrimination that often complicate the picture in these families. Because encopresis often results in a loss of bowel tone, it may help to motivate children by emphasizing the need to strengthen their anal muscles.

In many cases, cleaning out the bowel is necessary before initiating behavioral treatment. The bowel catharsis is usually followed by administration of mineral oil, which is often continued during the bowel retraining program. A high-fiber diet is often recommended.

The behavioral treatment program involves daily sitting on the toilet after each meal for a predetermined period (e.g., 10 minutes). The child and parents can measure the time with an ordinary kitchen timer. The parents can encourage the child to read or look at picture books while sitting. They can give the child rewards in the form of stars, stickers, or points for complying with the retraining program and add bonuses for successful defecation. The family can tally stickers or points on a calendar, and the child can "cash in" collected points for small prizes.

Caring for children with encopresis on an inpatient unit is a challenge, because very little research provides direction for positive outcomes. Staff can become frustrated with the child's seemingly unwillingness to cooperate. Possible interventions include maintaining discretion, assisting children with the development of age-appropriate social skills and empathy, and providing positive peer pressure (Hardy, 2009).

OTHER MENTAL DISORDERS

MOOD DISORDERS

Mood disorders in children and adolescents are a major public health concern. The prevalence of mood disorder in adolescents is estimated to be 14.3%, with depression representing the largest percentage (11.7%) and bipolar I or II disorder comprising 2.9% (Merikangas, et al., 2010). (See Chapters 19 and 20 for a complete discussion of these disorders.) Girls are more likely to meet the diagnostic criteria for these disorders, which cause severe impairment in 11% of the adolescents diagnosed.

Children with mood disorders may not spontaneously express feelings (e.g., sadness, irritability) and are more likely to show their suffering through their behavior. These children may act out their feelings rather than discuss them. Thus, behavior problems may accompany depression. Reports from parents are important sources of information about changes in sleep patterns, appetite, activity level and interests, and emotional stability.

Nursing diagnoses for children or adolescents who are depressed are similar to those for adults, including Ineffective Coping, Risk for Suicide, Chronic Low Self-Esteem, Disturbed Thought Processes, Self-Care Deficit, Imbalanced Nutrition, and Disturbed Sleep Pattern (Herdman & Kamitsuru, 2014).

Treatment goals include improving the mood and restoring sleep, appetite, and self-care. Interventions for responses to mood disorders in children and adolescents are also similar to those for adults. The psychiatric nurse develops a therapeutic relationship with the child and provides parent education and support. Developing sensitivity to the influence of environmental events on the

Mrs. S has just returned with her son Jared to the child psychiatric inpatient services facility after an overnight pass. She reports that the visit did not go well because of Jared's anger and defiance. She remarked that this behavior was distressingly similar to his behavior before the hospitalization. She expressed additional concern because of the upcoming discharge from the hospital. After saying goodbye to Jared, she pulled the nurse aside and stated that she had decided to file for divorce.

Mrs. S indicated that she had not told her husband or the family therapist. When asked whether Jared knew about her decision, Mrs. S suddenly realized that he may have overheard her discussing the matter with her sister on the telephone during this home visit.

How should the nurse approach this situation?

Choice	Possible Outcomes
Discuss her hypothesis about Jared's behavior and his uncertainty.	Mother can see relationship between Jared's behavior and her plan for divorce. Mother ignores the nurse. Mother is interested but does not see the connection.
Ignore the statement	Child and family did not learn about the connection between Jared's behavior and the events at home.
Encourage Jared's mother to sort out her problems.	The focus is then on mother's problems.

ANALYSIS

The best response is focusing on the possible relationship between Jared's recent behavioral deterioration and his uncertainty about his family's future. If the nurse ignores the statement or focuses on the mother's interpretation of Jared's behavior, the mother is less likely to appreciate the connection between her pending divorce and Jared's behavior. The nurse should also emphasize the importance of discussing the matter in family therapy.

child is important for the nurse, parents, and teachers (Box 28.7).

Children and adolescents may be treated with medication. Antidepressants medications are used for depression and mood antipsychotics for bipolar disorder. The controversy surrounding the use of SSRIs in children reminds us that all treatments involve a risk–benefit equation. Given the modest benefit of the SSRIs and the potential for side effects, these medications merit careful monitoring in children and adolescents. Patient monitoring should focus on evidence of benefit and side effects, including sleep problems, hyperactivity, sudden changes in mood or behavior, suicidal ideation, or self-injurious behavior.

CHILDHOOD SCHIZOPHRENIA

Childhood (early-onset) schizophrenia is diagnosed by the same criteria as those used in adults (see Chapter 21).

Difficulty in diagnosing a psychiatric disorder in children has led to years of debate and controversy regarding whether childhood schizophrenia differs from the adult type or is merely an early manifestation of the same disorder. For many years, it was believed that autism represented the childhood form of schizophrenia. However, today autism and childhood schizophrenia are differentiated (Kuniyoshi & McClellan, 2010). As currently defined, childhood schizophrenia (onset before the age of 13 years) is very rare, but prevalence increases sharply during adolescence, especially in young men. There are reports of children diagnosed with schizophrenia younger than the age of 6 years, but the validity of such diagnosis has not been established (Kuniyoshi & McClellan, 2010).

Childhood schizophrenia is usually characterized by poorer premorbid functioning than later onset schizophrenia. Common premorbid difficulties include social, cognitive, linguistic, attentional, motor, and perceptual delays. Taken together, these findings suggest that early-onset schizophrenia is a more severe form of the disorder.

Nursing care for children with schizophrenia follows an approach similar to that for ASD. Antipsychotic medications are not generally approved for use in children, although the newer atypical antipsychotic medications appear to have a lower risk for neurologic effects; other side effects such as weight gain also warrant careful monitoring.

Development of an individualized care plan for children with schizophrenia begins with a nursing assessment to identify functional problems specific to the child. Similarly, the recognition that childhood schizophrenia is a chronic and severe condition should guide the identification of outcomes. Goals should be realistic; the nurse should pay special attention to the child's support systems. Parent education about the disorder, medications, and long-term management (including use of community resources) is an essential part of the treatment plan. Long-term management also requires monitoring of chronic antipsychotic therapy.

SUMMARY OF KEY POINTS

- An estimated 20% of American youths are affected by a mental disorder that impairs their ability to function.

- In addressing intellectual disabilities, the emphasis is on determining adaptive behaviors (e.g., conceptual skills, concepts, self-direction), social skills, and practical skills. With guidance and education, many children will no longer have a disability as adults.

- Children with ASD benefit from structure and specific behavioral interventions.

- ADHD is defined by the presence of inattention; impulsiveness; and in most cases, hyperactivity. As currently defined, ADHD is the most common disorder of childhood. This heterogeneous disorder affects boys more often than girls. Nursing interventions involve family and child education and support. The family must partner with the school system to help the child receive the best educational experience. Effective treatment of ADHD often involves multiple approaches, including medication and parental education and support.

- Tourette disorder is a tic disorder characterized by motor and phonic tics. It is a frustrating disorder that requires patience and understanding. About half of the children with this disorder also have ADHD.

- Separation anxiety is relatively common in school-aged children. OCD becomes more common in adolescents. Treatment of separation anxiety and OCD may include medication, behavioral therapy, or a combination of these treatments.

- Elimination disorders include encopresis and enuresis. Behavioral therapy approaches are the most effective treatment for these disorders. Medication may also be used.

- Major depression in children is believed to be similar to major depression in adults.

- Childhood schizophrenia is a rare disorder, so other diagnoses should be carefully considered. Nursing care is similar to care of children with ASDs.

CRITICAL THINKING CHALLENGES

1. Interview parents of a child with an intellectual disability. Determine their approach to providing support in education and socialization.

2. Examine the differences and similarities between ASD with and without intellectual and language impairment. Determine whether differences exist in the nursing care according to the diagnoses. Develop a teaching plan for parents of children who have ASD and are trying to understand the underlying problems related to the disorder.

3. Compare and contrast nursing approaches for a child with ADHD with those used for a child with ASD. How are they different? How are they similar?

4. Learning disabilities and communication disorders are more common in children with psychiatric disorders than in the general population. How might a learning disability or a communication disorder complicate a psychiatric illness in a school-aged child?

5. How would you answer these questions from a parent: "What causes ADHD? Is it my fault?"

6. A child is threatening to kill himself. What information is needed in order to keep this child safe?

 Rain Man: 1988. This classic film stars Dustin Hoffman as Raymond Babbitt, a man who has autism (savant). Tom Cruise plays his brother Charlie, a self-centered hustler who believes that he has been cheated out of his inheritance. Discovering Raymond in an institution, Charlie abducts Raymond in a last-ditch effort to get his fair share of the family estate. The story revolves around the relationship that develops as the brothers drive across the country.

Dustin Hoffman brilliantly portrays the behaviors and symptoms of high-functioning autism, such as the monotone speech, insistence on sameness, and repetitive behavior.

Viewing Points: Identify and describe Raymond's ritualistic behaviors. Observe Raymond's language patterns and any distinct abnormalities. What happens when Raymond's rituals are interrupted?

REFERENCES

Alabdali, A., Al-Ayadhi, L., & El-Ansary, A. (2014). A key role for an impaired detoxification mechanism in the etiology and severity of autism spectrum disorders. *Behavioral and Brain Functions, 10*(1), 14.

American Association on Intellectual and Developmental Disabilities. (2015). Definition of intellectual disability. Retrieved on June 17, 2015, from http://www.aamr.org.

American Psychiatric Association. (2013). *Diagnostic and Statistical Manual of Mental Disorders*, (5th ed). Arlington, VA: Author.

Balazs, J., Miklósi, M., Keresztény, A., Dallos, G., & Gádoros, J. (2014). Attention-deficit hyperactivity disorder and suicidality in a treatment naïve sample of children and adolescents. *Journal of Affective Disorders, 152–154*, 282–287. http://dx.doi.org/10.1016/j.jad.2013.09.026

Baribeau, D. A., & Anagnostou, E. (2014). An update on medication management of behavioral disorders in autism. *Current Psychiatry Reports, 16*(3), 437.

Beesdo, K., Knappe, S., & Pine, D. S. (2009). Anxiety and anxiety disorders in children and adolescents: Developmental issues and implications for DSM-V. *Psychiatric Clinics of North America, 32*(3), 483–524.

Brugha, T. S., McManus, S., Bankart, J., Scott, F., Purdon, S., Bebbington, P., et al. (2011). Epidemiology of autism spectrum disorders in adults in the community in England. *Archives of General Psychiatry, 68*(5), 459–465.

Cavanna, A. E., & Seri, S. (2013). Tourette's syndrome. *Clinical Review BMJ, 347*, f4964. doi:10.1136/bmj.f4964

Centers for Disease Control and Prevention. (2013). Mental health surveillance among children-United States, 2005–2011. *Morbidity and Mortality Weekly Report [MMWR], 62*(Suppl), 1–35. www.cdc.gov/mmwr/preview/mmwrhtml/su6202a1.htm?s

Centers for Disease Control and Prevention. (2014). *Tourette syndrome, data & statistics. National Center on Birth Defects and Developmental Disabilities.* http://www.cdc.gov/ncbddd/tourette/facts.html

Childress, A. C., & Berry, S. A. (2012). Pharmacotherapy of attention-deficit disorder in adolescents. (Review). *Drugs, 72*(3), 309–325.

Chronis-Tuscano, A., Molina, B. S., Pelham, W. E., Applegate, B., Dahlke, A., Overmyer, M., et al. (2010). Very early predictors of adolescent depression and suicide attempt in children with attention-deficit/hyperactivity disorder. *Archives of General Psychiatry, 67*(10), 1044–1051.

Conners, C. K. (1989). *Conners' Rating Scales Manual.* North Tonawanda, NY: Multi-Health Systems.

Costello, E. J., Jian-ping, H., Sampson, N. A., Kessler, R. C., & Merikangas, K. R. (2014). Services for adolescents with psychiatric disorders: 12-month data from the National Comorbidity Survey Adolescent, *Psychiatric Services, 65*(3), 359–366.

Davis, D. W., & Williams, P. G. (2011). Attention-deficit hyperactivity disorder in preschool-aged children: Issues and concerns. *Clinical Pediatrics, 50*(2), 144–152.

Elamin, N. E., & Al-Ayadhi, L. Y. (2014). Brain autoantibodies in autism spectrum disorders. *Biomarkers in Medicine, 8*(3), 345–352.

Evans, S. W., Owens, J. S., & Bunford, N. (2014). Evidence-based psychosocial treatments for children and adolescents with attention-deficit/hyperactivity disorder. *Journal of Clinical Child and Adolescent Psychology, 43*(4), 527–551.

Fang, X., Massetti, G. M., Ouyan, L., Srosse, S. D., & Mercy, J. A. (2010). Attention-deficit/hyperactivity disorder, conduct disorder and young adult intimate partner violence. *Archives of General Psychiatry, 67*(11), 1179–1186.

Feingold, B. M. (1975). Hyperkinesis and learning disabilities linked to artificial food flavors and colors. *American Journal of Nursing, 75*(5), 797–783.

Ferrer, E., Shaywitz, B. A., Holahan, J. M., Marchione, K., & Shaywitz, S. E. (2010). Uncoupling of reading and IQ over time: Empirical evidence for a definition of dyslexia. *Psychological Science, 21*(1), 93–101.

Foster-Cohen, S. H., Friesen, M. D., Champion, P. R., & Woodward, L. J. (2010). High prevalence/low severity language delay in preschool children born very preterm. *Journal of Developmental and Behavioral Pediatrics, 31*(8), 658–667.

Freitag, C. M., Hänig, S., Schneider, A., Switz, D., Palmason, H., & Meyer, R. W. (2012). Biological and psychosocial environmental risk factors influence symptom severity and psychiatric comorbidity in children with ADHD. *Journal of Neural Transmission, 119*(1), 81–94.

Gagne, J. R., Saudino, K. J., & Asherson, P. (2011). The genetic etiology of inhibitory control and behavior problems at 24 months of age. *Journal of Child Psychology and Psychiatry, 52*(11), 1155–1163.

Geller, D. (2010). Obsessive-compulsive disorder. In M. K. Dulcan (Ed.), *Dulcan's textbook of child and adolescent psychiatry.* Arlington, VA: American Psychiatric Publishing.

Ghuman, J. K. (2011). Restricted elimination diet for ADHD: The INCA study. *The Lancet, 377*(9764), 446–448.

Gore, F. M., Bloem, P. J., Patton, G. C., Ferguson, J., Joseph, V., Coffey, C., et al. (2011). Global burden of disease in young people aged 10–24 years: A systematic analysis. *The Lancet, 377*(9783), 2093–2102.

Goyette, C. H., Connors, C. K., & Ulrich, R. F. (1978). Normative data on the Connors Parent and Teachers Rating Scales. *Journal of Abnormal Child Psychology, 6*(2), 221–236.

Graham, J., Banaschewski, T., Buitelaar, J., Coghill, D., Danckaerts, M., Dittmann, R. W., et al. (2011). European guidelines on managing adverse effects of medications for ADHD. *European Child & Adolescent Psychiatry, 20*(1), 17–37.

Greven, D. U., Kovas, Y., Willcutt, E., Petrill, S. A., & Plomin, R. (2014). Evidence for shared genetic risk between ADHD symptoms and

reduced mathematics ability: A twin study. *Journal of Child Psychology and Psychiatry, 55*(1), 39–48.

Halmey, A., Johansson, S., Winge, I., McKinney, J. A., Knappskog, P. M., & Haavik, J. (2010). Attention-deficit/hyperactivity disorder symptoms in offspring of mothers with impaired serotonin production. *Archives of General Psychiatry, 67*(10), 1033–1043.

Hardy, L. T. (2009). Encopresis: A guide for psychiatric nurses. *Archives of Psychiatric Nursing, 23*(5), 351–358.

Herdman, T. H., & Kamitsuru, S. (Eds.). (2014). *NANDA International Nursing Diagnoses: Definitions and Classification 2015-2017* (11th ed.). Oxford: Wiley-Blackwell.

Hirota, T., Schwartz, S., & Correll, C. U. (2014). Alpha-2 agonists for attention-deficit/hyperactivity disorder in youth: A systematic review and meta-analysis of monotherapy and add-on trials to stimulant therapy. *Journal of the American Academy of Child and Adolescent Psychiatry, 53*(2), 153–173.

Humphreys, K. L., Eng, T., & Lee, S. S. (2013). Stimulant medication and substance use outcomes: A meta-analysis. *JAMA Psychiatry, 70*(7), 740–749.

Jankovic, J., Gelineau-Kattner, R., & Davidson, A. (2010). Tourette's syndrome in adults. *Movement Disorders, 25*(11), 2171–2175.

Kanner, L. (1943). Autistic disturbances of affective contact. *Nervous Child, 2,* 217–250.

Kessler, R. C., Green, J. G., Adler, L. A., Barkley, R. A., Chatterji, S., Faraone, S. V., et al. (2010). Structure and diagnosis of adult attention-deficit/hyperactivity disorder: Analysis of expanded symptom criteria from the Adult ADHD Clinical Diagnostic Scale. *Archives of General Psychiatry, 67*(11), 1168–1178.

Kim, Y. S., Leventhal, B. L., Koh, Y. J., Fombonne, E., Laska, E., Lim, E. C., et al. (2011). Prevalence of autism spectrum disorders in a total population sample. *American Journal of Psychiatry, 168*(9), 904–912.

Kuehn, B. M. (2011). Increased risk of ADHD associated with early exposure to pesticides, PCBs. *Journal of the American Medical Association, 304*(1), 26–28.

Kuniyoshi, J. S., & McClellan, J. M. (2010). Early-onset schizophrenia. In M. K. Dulcan (Ed.), *Dulcan's textbook of child and adolescent psychiatry.* Arlington, VA: American Psychiatric Publishing.

Law, E. C., Sideridis, G. D., Prock, L. A., & Sheridan, M. A. (2014). Attention-deficit/hyperactivity disorder in young children: Predictors of diagnostic stability. *Pediatrics, 133*(4), 659–667.

Lecavalier, L., & Butter, E. M. (2010). Assessment of social skills and intellectual disability. In D. W. Nangle, D. Hansen, D. A. Erdley, & P. F. Norton (Eds.), *Practitioner's guide to empirically based measures of social skills* (pp. 179–192). New York: Springer.

Lomangino, K. (2011). Benefit for elimination diet in ADHD? *Clinical Nutrition Insight, 37*(4), 8–9, 11.

Mackie, L., & Law, J. (2010). Pragmatic language and the child with emotional/behavioural difficulties (EBDP: A pilot study exploring the interaction between behaviour and communication disability. *International Journal of Language & Communication Disorders, 45*(4), 397–410.

Manos, M. J., Tom-Revzon, C., Bukstein, O. G., & Crismon, M. L. (2007). Changes and challenges: Managing ADHD in a fast-paced world. *Journal of Managed Care Pharmacy, 13*(9 suppl), S2–S16.

Matthews, C. A., & Grados, M. A. (2011). Familiarity of Tourette syndrome, obsessive-compulsive disorder, and attention-deficit/hyperactivity disorder: Heritability analysis in a large sib-pair sample. *Journal of the American Academy of Child & Adolescent Psychiatry, 50*(1), 46–54.

Maulik, P. K., Mascarenhas, M. N., Mathers, C. D., Dua, R., & Saxena, S. (2011). Prevalence of intellectual disability: A meta-analysis of population-based studies. *Research in Developmental Disabilities, 32*(2), 419–436.

McCarthy, S. E., Gillis, J., Kramer, M., Lihm, J., Yoon, S., Berstein, Y., et al. (2014). De novo mutations in schizophrenia implicate chromatin remodeling and support a genetic overlap with autism and intellectual disability. *Molecular Psychiatry, 19*(6), 652–658. doi:10.1038/mp.2014.29

McQuade, J. D., Vaughn, A. M., Hoza, B., Murray-Close, D., Molina, B., Arnold, L. E, et al. (2014). Perceived social acceptance and peer status differentially predict adjustment in youth with and without ADHD. *Journal of Attention Disorders, 18*(1), 31–43.

Merikangas, K. R., He, J., Burstein, M., Swanson, S. A., Avenevoli, S., Cui, L., et al. (2010). Lifetime prevalence of mental disorders in U.S. adolescents: Results from the National Comorbidity Survey Replication–Adolescent supplement (NCS-A). *Journal of the American Academy of Child & Adolescent Psychiatry, 49*(10), 980–989.

Mikkelsen, E. J. (2014). Elimination disorders. In R. E. Hales, S. C. Yudofsy, & L. W. Roberts (Eds.). *The American Psychiatric Publishing textbook of psychiatry* (6th ed.). Arlington, VA: American Psychiatric Publishing. www.psychiatryonline.org. http://dx.doi.org/10.1176/appi.books.9781585625031.rh01

Milrod, B., Markowitz, J. C., Gerber, A. J., Cyranowski, J., Altemus, M., Shaprio, T., et al. (2014). Childhood separation anxiety and the pathogenesis and treatment of adult anxiety. *American Journal of Psychiatry, 171*(1), 34–43.

Molina, B. S., Hinshaw, S. P., Swanson, J. M., Arnold, L. E., Vitiello, B., Jensen, P. S., et al. (2009). The MTA at 8 years: Prospective follow-up of children treated for combined-type ADHD in a multisite study. *Journal of the American Academy of Child & Adolescent Psychiatry, 48*(5), 484–500.

Mokrova, I., O'Brien, M., Calkins, S., & Keane, S. (2010). Parental ADHD symptomology and ineffective parenting: The connecting link of home chaos. *Parenting: Science and Practice, 10*, 19–135.

Moriyama, T. S., Polanczyk, F. V., Terzi, F. S., Faria, K. M., & Rohde, L. A. (2013). Psychopharmacology and psychotherapy for the treatment of adults with ADHD—a systematic review of available meta-analysis. *CNS Spectrums, 18*(6), 296–306.

Mulder, M. J., Bos, D., Weusten, J. M., van Belle, J., van Dijk, S. C., Simen, P., et al. (2011). Basic impairments in regulating the speed-accuracy tradeoff predict symptoms of attention-deficit/hyperactivity disorder. *Biological Psychiatry, 68*(12), 1114–1149.

Murthy, P., & Chand, P. (2012). Treatment of dual diagnosis disorders. (Review). *Current Opinion in Psychiatry, 25*(3), 194–200.

Nigg, J. T., Lewis, K., Edinger, T., & Falk, M. (2012). Meta-analysis of attention-deficit/hyperactivity disorder or attention-deficit/hyperactivity disorder symptoms, restriction diet, and synthetic food color additives. *Journal of the American Academy of Child & Adolescent Psychiatry, 51*(1), 86–97.

Palcic, J. L., Jurbergs, M., & Kelley, M. L. (2009). A comparison of teacher and parent delivered consequences: Improving classroom behavior in low-income children and ADHD. *Child & Family Behavior Therapy, 31*(2), 117–133.

Pauli-Pott, U., Albayrak, O., Hebebrand, J., & Pott, W. (2010). Association between inhibitory control capacity and body weight in overweight and obese children and adolescents: Dependence on age and inhibitory control component. *Child Neuropsychology, 16*(6), 592–603.

Pelsser, L. M., Frankena, K., Toorman, J., Savelkoul, H. F., Dubois, A. E., Pereira, R. R., et al. (2011). Effects of a restricted elimination diet on the behavior of children with attention-deficit hyperactivity. *The Lancet, 377*(9764), 494–503.

Pickles, T., Simonoff, E., Chandler, S., Louicas, T., & Baird, G. (2011). IQ in children with autism spectrum disorders: Data from the Special Needs and Autism Project (SNAP). *Psychological Medicine, 41*(3), 619–627.

Polanska, K., Jurewicz, J., & Hanke, W. (2012). Exposure to environmental and lifestyle factors and attention-deficit/hyperactivity disorder in children—a review of epidemiological studies. *International Journal of Occupational Medicine and Environmental Health, 25*(4), 330–355.

Politte, L. C., Henry, C. A., & McDougle, C. J. (2014). Psychopharmacological interventions in autism spectrum disorder. *Harvard Review of Psychiatry, 22*(2), 76–92.

Rapp, A., Dodds, A., Walkup, J. T., & Runn, M. (2013). Treatment of pediatric anxiety disorders. *Annals of the New York Academy of Sciences, 1304*, 52–61.

Raymond, L. J., Deth, R. C., & Ralston, N. V. (2014). Potential role of selenoenzymes and antioxidant metabolism in relation to autism etiology and pathology. *Autism Research and Treatment, 2014*, 164938. doi:10.1155/2014/164938

Reaven, J. A. (2009). Children with high-functioning autism spectrum disorders and co-occurring anxiety symptoms: Implications for assessment and treatment. *Journal of Specialists in Pediatric Nursing, 14*(3), 192–199.

Scarpinato, N., Bradley, J., Kurbjun, K., Bateman, X., Holtzer, B., & Ely, B. (2010). Caring for the child with an autism spectrum disorder in the acute care setting. *Journal of Specialists in Pediatric Nursing, 15*(3), 244–254.

Scharf, J. M., Yu, D., Mathews, C. A., Neale, B. M., Stewart, S. E., Fagerness, J. A., et al. (2013). Genome-wide association study of Tourette's syndrome. *Molecular Psychiatry, 18*(6), 721–728.

Shaw, P., Gilliam, M., Liverpool, M., Weddle, C., Malek, M., Sharp, W., et al. (2011). Cortical development in typically developing children with symptoms of hyperactivity and impulsivity: Support for a dimensional view of attention deficit hyperactivity disorder. *American Journal of Psychiatry, 168*(2), 143–151.

Stevens, L. J., Kuczek, T., Burgess, J. R., Stochelski, M. A., Arnold, L. E., & Galland, L. (2013). Mechanisms of behavioral, atopic and other reactions to artificial food colors in children. *Nutrition Reviews, 71*(5), 268–281.

Stevenson, J., Buitelaar, J., Cortese, S., Ferrin, M., Konofal, E., Lecendreux, M., et al., and members of the European ADHD Guidelines Group. (2014). Research review: The role of diet in the treatment of attention-deficit/hyperactivity disorder—an appraisal of the evidence on efficacy and recommendations on the design of future studies. *Journal of Child Psychology and Psychiatry, 55*(5), 416–427.

Stoeckel, R. E., Colligan, R. C., Barbaresi, W. J., Weaver, A. L., Killian, J. M., & Katusci, S. K. (2013). Early speech-language impairment and risk for written language disorder: A population-based study. *Journal of Developmental and Behavioral Pediatrics, 34*(1), 38–44.

Syed, H., Masaud, T. M., Nkire, N., Iro, C., & Garland, M. R. (2010). Estimating the prevalence of adult ADHD in the psychiatric clinic: A cross-sectional study using the ADHD self-report scale (ASRS). *Journal of Psychological Medicine, 27*(4), 195–197.

The Foundation for Medical Practice Education. (2009). ADHD rating scale. Retrieved from http://www.fmpe.org/en/documents/appendix/Appendix%201%20-%20ADHD%20Rating%20Scale.pdf.

Toth, K., & King, B. H. (2010). Intellectual disability. In M. K. Dulcan (Ed.), *Dulcan's textbook of child and adolescent psychiatry* (pp. 151–172). Arlington, VA: American Psychiatric Publishing.

Vaishnavi, V., Manikandan, M., & Munirajan, A. K. (2014). Mining the 3'UTR of autism-implicated genes for SNPs perturbing microRNA regulation. *Genomics Proteomics Bioinformatics, 12*(2), 92–104. doi:10.1016/j.gpb.2014.01.003

Van der Leij, A., van Bergen, E., van Zuijen, T., de Jong, P., Maurits, N., & Maassen, B. (2013). Precursors of developmental dyslexia: An overview of the longitudinal Dutch Dyslexia Programme study. *Dyslexia, 19*(4), 191–213.

Wagner, K. D., & Pliszka, S. R. (2011). Treatment of child and adolescent disorders. In A. F. Schatzberg & C. B. Nemeroff (Eds.), *The American Psychiatric Publishing Textbook of Psychopharmacology* (4th ed.). Arlington, VA: American Psychiatric Publishing.

Waite, R., & Ramsay, J. R. (2010). Adults with ADHD: Who are we missing? *Issues in Mental Health Nursing, 31*, 670–678.

Wang, L., Conlon, M. A., Christophersen, C. T., Sorich, M. J., & Angley, M. T. (2014). Gastrointestinal microbiota and metabolite biomarkers in children with autism spectrum disorders. *Biomarkers in Medicine, 8*(3), 331–334.

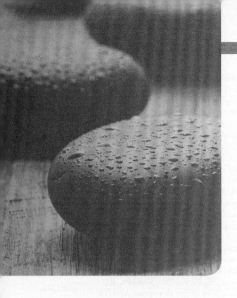

29
Mental Health Disorders of Older Adults

Mary Ann Boyd

KEY CONCEPTS

- cognition
- delirium
- dementia
- memory

LEARNING OBJECTIVES

After studying this chapter, you will be able to:

1. Distinguish the clinical characteristics, onset, and course of delirium and dementia.

2. Integrate biologic, psychological, and social theories related to delirium and dementia.

3. Discuss the nursing care of persons with delirium and dementia.

KEY TERMS

- acetylcholine (ACh) • acetylcholinesterase (AChE) • acetylcholinesterase inhibitors (AChEIs) • agnosia • aphasia • apraxia • beta-amyloid plaques • catastrophic reactions • cortical dementia • disinhibition • disturbance of executive functioning • hypersexuality • hypervocalization • illusions • impaired consciousness • neurocognitive disorders • neurofibrillary tangles • oxidative stress • subcortical dementia

INTRODUCTION

The chapters in Unit V integrate content related to the impact of the disorders on the older adult. Most mental disorders occur throughout the lifespan. This chapter presents new content that focuses on changes in cognitive functioning and neurocognitive disorders that are associated with the older adult.

Cognition is an intellectual process of acquiring, using, or manipulating perceptions and information. It involves the perception of reality and an understanding of its representations. Cognitive functions to be noted include the acquisition and use of language, the orientation of time and space, and the ability to learn and solve problems. Cognition also is the basis of judgment, reasoning, attention, comprehension, concept formation, planning, and the use of symbols (e.g., numbers and letters used in mathematics and writing).

> **KEYCONCEPT** **Cognition** is based on a system of interrelated abilities, such as perception, reasoning, judgment, intuition, and memory that allow one to be aware of oneself and one's surroundings. Impairments in these abilities can result in a failure of the afflicted person to recognize that he or she is ill and in need of treatment.

Memory, a facet of cognition, refers to the ability to recall or reproduce what has been learned or experienced. It is more than simple storage and retrieval; it is a complex cognitive mental function that includes most areas of the brain, especially the hippocampus, which is believed to be essential to the transfer of some memories from short- to long-term storage. Defects of memory are an essential feature of many cognitive disorders, particularly dementia.

> KEYCONCEPT **Memory** is a facet of cognition concerned with retaining and recalling past experiences, whether they occurred in the physical environment or internally as cognitive events.

Neurocognitive disorders are characterized by a decline in cognitive function from a previous level of functioning. These disorders are acquired and have not been present since early life. The diagnosis of a neurocognitive disorder is based on deficits in the following cognitive domains: *attention* (distractibility with multiple stimuli), *executive function* (planning, decision making, working memory), *learning and memory* (recall and recognition), *language* (expressive including naming, work finding, fluency, grammatical syntax, and receptive language), *perceptual-motor* (visual perception, visuoconstructional, perceptual-motor), and *social cognition deficits* (recognition of emotions, ability to consider another's mental state) (American Psychiatric Association [APA], 2013).

The neurocognitive disorders discussed in this chapter include delirium, a disorder of acute cognitive impairment usually caused by a medical condition (e.g., infection), substance abuse, or multiple etiologies and dementia, characterized by chronic cognitive impairments. Dementia is differentiated from delirium by underlying cause, not by symptom patterns, which are often similar.

> KEYCONCEPT **Delirium** is a disorder of acute cognitive impairment that is caused by a medical condition (e.g., infection), substance abuse, or multiple etiologies.

> KEYCONCEPT **Dementia** is characterized by chronic cognitive impairments and is differentiated by underlying cause, not by symptom patterns. Dementia can be further classified as cortical or subcortical to denote the location of the underlying pathology.

Cortical dementia results from a disease process that globally afflicts the cortex. **Subcortical dementia** is caused by dysfunction or deterioration of deep gray- or white-matter structures inside the brain and brain stem. Symptoms of subcortical dementia may be more localized and tend to disrupt arousal, attention, and motivation, but they can produce a variety of clinical behavioral manifestations. In this chapter, one type of cortical dementia, Alzheimer disease (AD), is highlighted because it is the most prevalent form of dementia.

DELIRIUM

Clinical Course

Delirium is a disturbance in consciousness and a change in cognition that develops over a short time. It is usually reversible if the underlying cause is identified and treated quickly. It is a serious disorder and should always be treated as a medical emergency.

> EMERGENCY CARE ALERT **!** Individuals with delirium are in a state of confusion and disorientation that develops during a period of a few hours or days. If delirium is not treated in a timely manner, irreversible neurologic damage can occur. Delirium is a common complication in patients admitted to intensive care units and inpatient psychiatric units (Tang, Patel, Khubchandani, & Grossberg, 2014; Bryczkowski, Lopreiato, Yonclas, Sacca, & Mosenthal, 2014).

Diagnostic Criteria

Impaired consciousness is the key diagnostic criterion for delirium. The patient becomes less aware of his or her environment and loses the ability to focus, sustain, and shift attention. Cognitive changes include problems with memory, orientation, and language. The patient may not know where he or she is, may not recognize familiar objects, or may be unable to carry on a conversation. This problem developed during a short period (compared with dementia, which develops gradually) (APA, 2013). Delirium is different than dementia, although the presenting symptoms are often similar. Impaired alertness, apathy, anxiety, disorientation, and hallucinations commonly occur. Table 29.1 highlights the differences between delirium and dementia.

> NCLEXNOTE Delirium and dementia have similar presentations. Because delirium can be life threatening, identifying the potential underlying cause for the symptoms is a priority.

Although delirium may occur in any age group, it is most common among older adults. In this age group, delirium is often mistaken for dementia, which in turn leads to inappropriate treatment. Patients with delirium have a reduced ability to focus, difficulty in sustaining or shifting attention, changes in cognition, or perceptual disturbances (Mattison, Catic, Davis, Olveczky, Moran, Yang, et al., 2014).

Epidemiology and Risk Factors

Statistics concerning prevalence are based primarily on older adults in acute care settings. Estimated prevalence rates range from 10% to 50% of patients. Delirium is particularly common in older postoperative patients. In some groups, such as those with dementia, the prevalence may be nearer 90% (Flaherty, 2011).

Preexisting cognitive impairment is one of the greatest risk factors for delirium. (Voyer, Richard, Doucet, & Carmichael, 2011). See Boxes 29.1 and 29.2.

Etiology

Delirium in the older adult is associated with medications, infections, fluid and electrolyte imbalances, metabolic

TABLE 29.1	DIFFERENTIATING DELIRIUM FROM DEMENTIA	
Characteristics	Delirium	Dementia
Onset	Sudden	Insidious
24-h course	Fluctuating	Stable
Consciousness	Reduced	Clear
Attention	Globally disoriented	Usually normal
Cognition	Globally disoriented	Globally impaired
Hallucinations	Visual auditory	Possible
Orientation	Usually impaired	Often impaired
Psychomotor activity	Increased, reduced, or shifting	Often normal
Speech	Often incoherent; slow or rapid	Often normal
Involuntary movement	Often asterixis or coarse tremor	Rare
Physical illness or drug toxicity	One or both	Rare

Source: Lee, L., Weston, W. W., Heckman, G., Gagnon, M., Lee, F. J., & Stoke, S. (2013). Structured approach to patients with memory difficulties in family practice. *Canadian Family Physician*, *59*(3), 249–254.

disturbances, hypoxia, or ischemia. The probability of the syndrome developing increases if some predisposing factors, such as advanced age, brain damage, or dementia, are also present. Sensory overload or underload, immobilization, sleep deprivation, and psychosocial stress also contribute to delirium (Flaherty, 2011).

Teamwork and Collaboration: Working Toward Recovery

Although delirium may be recognized and diagnosed in any health care setting, appropriate intervention usually requires that the patient be admitted to an acute care setting for rigorous assessment and rapid treatment. Priority in care is identifying the underlying cause of the delirium. Interdisciplinary management of delirium includes

two primary aspects: (1) elimination or correction of the underlying cause and (2) symptomatic and supportive measures (e.g., adequate rest, comfort, maintenance of fluid and electrolyte balance, and protection from injury).

Safety Issues

If possible, the use of all suspected medications should be stopped and vital signs should be monitored at least every 2 hours. Close observation of the patient with particular regard to changes in vital signs, behavior, and mental

---

BOX 29.1

Risk Factors for Delirium

Advanced age
Preexisting dementia
Functional dependence
Endocrine and metabolic disorders
Bone fracture
Infection (pneumonia, urinary tract)
Medications (anticholinergic side effects)
Changes in vital signs (including hypotension and hyper- or hypothermia)
Electrolyte or metabolic imbalance (dehydration, renal failure, hyponatremia)
Admission to a long-term care institution
Postcardiotomy
AIDS
Pain
Acute or chronic stress
Substance use and alcohol withdrawal

BOX 29.2 CLINICAL VIGNETTE

Delirium

Margaret, a widowed 72-year-old woman living in her own home, has been having trouble sleeping. Her daughter visits her and suggests that she try an over-the-counter (OTC) sleeping medication. Margaret also takes antihistamines for allergies and the antidepressant amitriptyline. Three nights later, a neighbor calls the daughter, concerned because Margaret is wandering the streets, unable to find her home. When the neighbor approached Margaret to help her home, she began to scream and strike out at the neighbor.

The daughter visits immediately and discovers that her mother does not know who she is, does not know what time it is, appears disheveled, and is suspicious that people have been in her home stealing the things she cannot find. Margaret does not recall taking any medication, but when her daughter investigates, she finds that 10 pills of the new sleeping aid have already been used.

What Do You Think?
- Identify risk factors that may have contributed to Margaret's experiencing delirium.
- How could the addition of an OTC sleeping medication interact with the antihistamine and antidepressant to be responsible for Margaret's delirium?

status is required. Patients are monitored until the delirium subsides or until discharge. If the delirium still exists at discharge, it is critical that referrals for postdischarge follow-up assessment and care be implemented.

Evidence-Based Nursing Care for Persons with Delirium

The best management is prevention or early recognition of delirium. Special efforts should be made to include family members in the nursing process.

Mental Health Nursing Assessment

The onset of symptoms is typically signaled by a rapid or acute change in behavior. Assessing the symptoms first requires knowing what is normal for the individual. Caregivers, family members, or significant others should be interviewed because they can often provide valuable information. Family members may be the only resource for accurate information.

Physical Health Assessment

History should include a description of the onset, duration, range, and intensity of associated symptoms. Recent physical illness, dementia, depression, or other psychiatric illnesses should be identified. A physical examination should be conducted. Vital signs are crucial. Changes in activities of daily living (ADLs), use of sensory aids (eyeglasses and hearing aids), pain and sleep should be documented.

Medication Assessment

Many medications are associated with delirium. See Table 29.2. Medications and recent changes in the type and number, including over-the counter (OTC) medications should be documented.. Combinations of medications can interact and cause delirium. Cold medications, taken in sufficient quantities may cause confusion, especially in older adults. A substance use history (including alcohol intake and smoking history) should be taken.

TABLE 29.2	EXAMPLES OF DRUGS THAT CAN CAUSE DELIRIUM		
Class	**Specific Drugs**	**Class**	**Specific Drugs**
Anticholinergic	Antihistamines Chlorpheniramine Antiparkinsonian drugs (e.g., benztropine [Cogentin], biperiden [Akineton], or trihexyphenidyl) Atropine Belladonna alkaloids Diphenhydramine Phenothiazines Scopolamine Tricyclic antidepressants	Cardiac	β-Blockers Propranolol (Inderal) Clonidine (Catapres) Digitalis (Digoxin, Lanoxin) Lidocaine (Xylocaine) Methyldopa (Aldomet) Quinidine Procainamide (Pronestyl)
		Sedative—hypnotic	Barbiturates Benzodiazepines
Anticonvulsant	Phenobarbital Phenytoin (Dilantin) Sodium valproate (Depakene, Depakote)	Sympathomimetic	Amphetamines Phenylephrine Phenylpropanolamine
Antiinflammatory	Corticosteroids Ibuprofen (Motrin, Advil) Indomethacin (Indocin) Naproxen (Naprosyn)	Over-the-counter medications	Compoz Excedrin PM Sleep-Eze Sominex
Antiparkinsonian	Amantadine Carbidopa (Sinemet) Levodopa (Larodopa)	Miscellaneous	Acyclovir (antiviral) Aminophylline Amphotericin (antifungal) Bromides Cephalexin (Keflex) Chlorpropamide (Diabinese) Cimetidine (Tagamet) Disulfiram (Antabuse) Lithium Metronidazole (Flagyl) Theophylline Timolol ophthalmic
Antibiotics	Isoniazid Rifampin		
Analgesic	Opioids Salicylates Synthetic narcotics		

Source: Wynn, G. H., Oesterheid, J. R., Cozza, K. I., Armstrong, S. C. (2009). *Clinical Manual of Drug Interaction: Principles for Medical Practice.* Arlington, VA: American Psychiatric Publishing, Inc.

Psychosocial Assessment

Mental Status

Rapid onset of global cognitive impairment that affects multiple aspects of intellectual functioning is the hallmark of delirium. Mental status evaluation reveals several changes:

- Fluctuations in level of consciousness with reduced awareness of the environment
- Difficulty focusing and sustaining or shifting attention
- Severely impaired memory, especially immediate and recent memory

Patients may be disoriented to time and place but rarely to person. Environmental perceptions are often disturbed. The patient may believe shadows in the room are really people. Thought content is often illogical; speech may be incoherent or inappropriate to the context. Mental status tends to fluctuate over the course of the day.

Behavior

Persons with delirium exhibit a wide range of behaviors, complicating the process of making a diagnosis and planning interventions. At times, the individual may be restless or agitated and at other times lethargic and slow to respond.

Family Environment

An assessment of living arrangements may provide information about sensory stimulation or social isolation. Assessing family interactions, support for the patient, and family members' ability to understand delirium is also important. The behaviors exhibited by the person experiencing delirium may be frightening or at least confusing for family members. Some family members may actually contribute to the patient's increased agitation. At the same time, however, the family's presence may help to calm and reassure the patient.

Nursing Diagnoses

The nursing diagnoses typically generated from assessment data are Acute Confusion, Disturbed Thought Processes, Disturbed Sensory Perception (visual or auditory). Risk for Injury is a high-priority diagnosis because individuals with delirium are more likely to fall or injure themselves during a confused state. However, an astute nurse will also use nursing diagnoses based on other indicators, such as Hyperthermia, Acute Pain, Risk for Infection, and Insomnia.

Nursing Interventions

Important interventions include providing a safe and therapeutic environment; maintaining fluid and electrolyte balance and adequate nutrition and preventing aspiration and decubitus ulcers, which are common complications. Other interventions relate to a particular nursing diagnosis focused on individual symptoms and underlying causes (e.g., for patients with Insomnia, the Sleep Enhancement intervention is appropriate).

Safety Interventions

Behaviors exhibited by the person with delirium, such as hallucinations, delusions, illusions, aggression, or agitation (restlessness or excitability), may pose safety problems. The patient must be protected from physical harm by using low beds, guardrails, and careful supervision. Delirium management and fall prevention may be implemented for any patient at risk for falls.

Medications

As the underlying medical problem is treated, the person may be given medication to treat the symptoms associated with delirium, such as agitation, inattention, combativeness, insomnia, and psychosis. Dosages are usually kept very low, especially with older adults and the medication is selected in light of the potential side effects (particularly anticholinergic effects, hypotension, and respiratory suppression). A limited role for antipsychotics may be present for use among a targeted group of patients who experience hallucinations or delusions associated with delirium (Flaherty, 2011). Benzodiazepines are also used when the delirium is related to alcohol withdrawal. In some patients, benzodiazepines may further impair cognition because of the sedation.

Patients should be monitored for sedation, hypotension, or extrapyramidal symptoms. Although mental status often fluctuates during delirium, it may also be influenced by these medications, so any changes or worsening of mental status after administration of the medication should be reported immediately to the prescriber. Some side effects may also be confused with the symptoms of delirium. For example, akathisia (see Chapter 10), a side effect of antipsychotics, may appear as agitation or restlessness. Medications for treating symptoms related to delirium should be discontinued as soon as possible.

Teaching Points

To prevent future occurrences, provide education to the patient and family about the underlying cause of the delirium. If the delirium is not resolved before discharge, family members need to know how to care for the patient at home.

Psychosocial Interventions

Patients with delirium need frequent interaction and support if they are confused or hallucinating. Patients should be encouraged to express their fears and discomforts that result from frightening or disconcerting psychotic experiences. Adequate lighting, easy-to-read calendars and clocks, a reasonable noise level, and frequent verbal orientation may reduce this frightening experience. If the patient wears eyeglasses or uses a hearing aid, these devices should be used. Including familiar personal possessions in the environment may also help. Interventions that may be useful for these individuals are discussed in detail later in the chapter (see the section on dementia).

A safe environment is important to protect the patient from injury. A predictable, orienting environment will help to reestablish order to the patient's life. That is, a calendar, clocks, and other items may be provided to help orient the patient to time, place, and person. If the patient is agitated, de-escalation techniques should be used (see Chapter 13). Physical restraint should be avoided.

Families can also be encouraged to work with staff to reorient the patient and provide a supportive environment. Families need to understand that important decisions requiring the patient's input should be delayed if at all possible until the patient has recovered. Although patients may be able to participate in decision making, they may not remember the decision later; therefore, it is important to have several witnesses present.

Evaluation and Treatment Outcomes

The primary treatment goal is prevention or resolution of the delirious episode with return to previous cognitive status. Outcome measures include

- Correction of the underlying physiologic alteration
- Resolution of confusion
- Family member verbalization of understanding of confusion
- Prevention of injury

Resolution of confusion is the primary goal; however, the nursing care provided makes important contributions to all four of these outcomes. The end result of delirium may be full recovery, incomplete recovery, incomplete recovery with some residual cognitive impairment, or a downward course leading to death.

Continuum of Care

Patients with delirium may present in a number of treatment settings (e.g., home, nursing home, ambulatory care, day treatment, outpatient setting, hospital). Patients usually are admitted to an acute care setting for rapid evaluation and treatment of the underlying etiology. For more information on caring for patients with delirium, see Box 29.3.

BOX 29.3

Psychoeducation Checklist: Delirium

When caring for the patient with delirium, be sure to include the caregivers, as appropriate, and address the following topic areas in the teaching plan:

- Psychopharmacologic agents, if used, including drug action, dosage, frequency, and possible adverse effects
- Underlying cause of delirium
- Mental status changes
- Safety measures
- Hydration and nutrition
- Avoidance of restraints
- Decision-making guidelines

ALZHEIMER DISEASE

Clinical Course

Alzheimer Disease (AD) is a degenerative, progressive, neuropsychiatric disorder that results in cognitive impairment, emotional and behavioral changes, physical and functional decline, and ultimately death. Gradually, the patient's ability to carry out ADLs declines, although physical status often remains intact until late in the disease. Although primarily a disorder of older adults, AD has been diagnosed in patients as young as age 35 years.

Two subtypes have been identified: early onset AD (age 65 years and younger) and late onset AD (age older than 65 years). Late-onset AD is much more common than early-onset AD, but early-onset AD has a more rapid progression. AD is also routinely conceptualized in terms of three stages: mild, moderate, and severe. Signs and symptoms of AD change as the patient passes from one phase of the illness to another (Figure 29.1).

Diagnostic Criteria

The diagnosis of AD is made on clinical grounds, but verification is only confirmed during autopsy. The essential feature of AD is cognitive decline from a previous level of functioning in one or more cognitive domains (attention, executive function, learning and memory, language, perceptual-motor or social cognition) (APA, 2013). These deficits interfere with independence in ADLs. Typical deficits include **aphasia** (i.e., alterations in language ability), **apraxia** (i.e., impaired ability to execute motor activities despite intact motor functioning), **agnosia** (i.e., failure to recognize or identify objects despite intact sensory function), or a **disturbance of executive functioning** (i.e., ability to think abstractly, plan, initiate, sequence, monitor, and stop complex behavior).

Mild neurocognitive impairment (MCI) is diagnosed if a modest cognitive decline from a previous level of function is found in one or more of the cognitive domains,

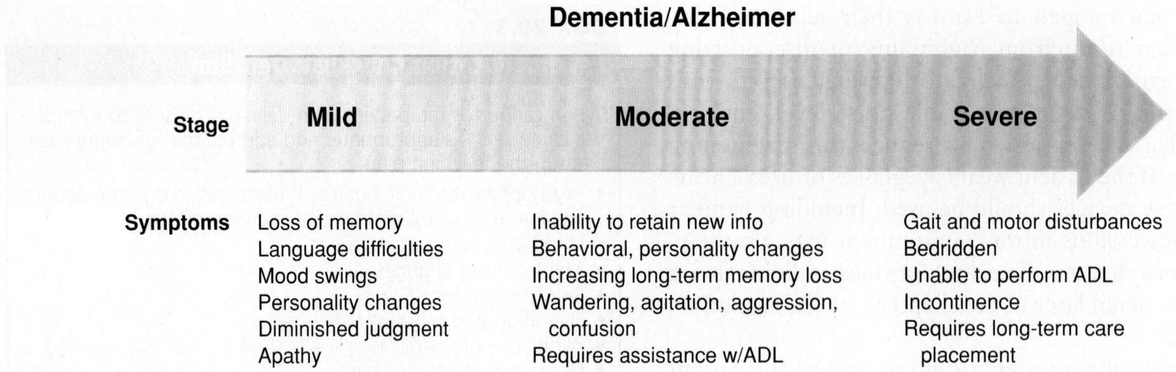

Dementia/Alzheimer

Stage	Mild	Moderate	Severe
Symptoms	Loss of memory Language difficulties Mood swings Personality changes Diminished judgment Apathy	Inability to retain new info Behavioral, personality changes Increasing long-term memory loss Wandering, agitation, aggression, confusion Requires assistance w/ADL	Gait and motor disturbances Bedridden Unable to perform ADL Incontinence Requires long-term care placement

FIGURE 29.1 Alzheimer disease progression.

but the cognitive deficits do not interfere with independence in daily activities (APA, 2013). MCI is thought to be related to multiple causes and some, but not all, progress to AD (Desai & Schwarz, 2011).

Epidemiology and Risk Factors

In 2014, an estimated 5.2 million Americans had AD, 1 in 9 older than 65 years old. Conservative projections estimate that by the year 2025, the number of cases of AD in the United States will be 7.1 million. Almost two thirds of Americans with AD are women. Dementia appears to affect all groups, but studies in the United States reveal a higher incidence in African Americans and Latinos than in whites. Currently, AD is the fifth leading cause of death among older adults in the United States (Alzheimer's Association, 2014a).

AD can run in families. Compared with the general population, first-degree biologic relatives of individuals with early-onset AD are more likely to experience the disorder. Studies show that those with fewer years of education or those who have had a prior head injury are at higher risk of developing Alzheimer's disease (U.S. Department of Health and Human Services [USDHHS], 2015).

Etiology

Researchers have yet to identify a definitive cause of AD, but a combination of genetic, environmental, and lifestyle factors influence a person's risk for developing the disease. In general, the brain appears normal in the early phases of AD, but it undergoes widespread atrophy as the disease progresses (USDHHS, 2015).

Beta-Amyloid Plaques

One piece of the puzzle is partially explained by a leading theory that **beta-amyloid plaques**, made up of proteins, which clump together in the brain and destroy cholinergic neurons. Beta-amyloid is hypothesized to interfere with the process of storing memories through interrupting synaptic connection. Symptoms such as aphasia and visuospatial abnormalities are attributable to plaque formation (USDHHS, 2015).

Neurofibrillary Tangles

Neurofibrillary tangles are made of abnormally twisted protein threads found inside the brain cells. The main component of the tangles is *tau*, a protein that stabilizes the microtubules of transport cells. In AD, tau separates from the microtubules. Loose tau proteins tangle with each other, causing the characteristic neurofibrillary tangles. When microtubules disintegrate, the neuron's transport system collapses, resulting in cell death (USDHHS, 2015) (Figure 29.2).

Cell Death and Neurotransmitters

In patients with AD, neurotransmission is reduced, neurons are lost, and the hippocampal neurons degenerate. Several major neurotransmitters are affected. Cellular loss leads to reduced **acetylcholine** (ACh) important in cognitive functioning and memory (see Chapter 6). See Figure 29.3. Norepinephrine and serotonin are also affected (USDHHS, 2015).

Genetic Factors

Approximately half the cases of early-onset AD appear to be transmitted as a purely genetic, autosomal dominant trait caused by mutations in genes on chromosomes 1 and 14 (USDHHS, 2015). Mutations on chromosome 14 account for most cases of early-onset familial AD. Chromosome 21 is also associated with AD because amyloid plaques and neurofibrillary tangles accumulate consistently in older people with Down syndrome (i.e., trisomy 21) who have AD. Mutations in one of three genes (APP, PSEN1, and PSEN2) have been identified that alter

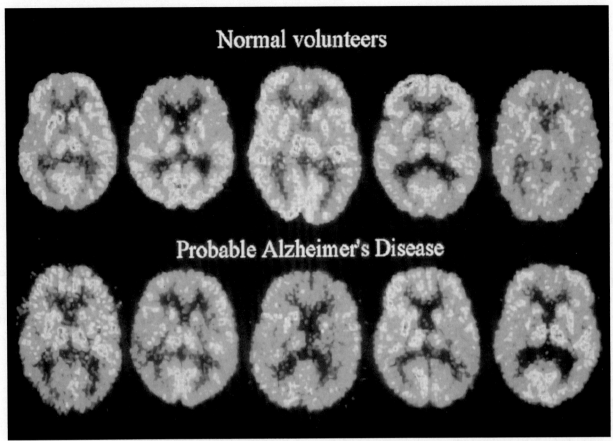

FIGURE 29.2 Series comparison of elderly control subjects (*top row*) and patients with Alzheimer's disease (AD) (*bottom row*). Although some decreases in metabolism are associated with age, in most patients with AD, marked decreases are seen in the temporal lobe, an area important in memory functions. (Courtesy of Monte S. Buchsbaum, MD, The Mount Sinai Medical Center and School of Medicine, New York.)

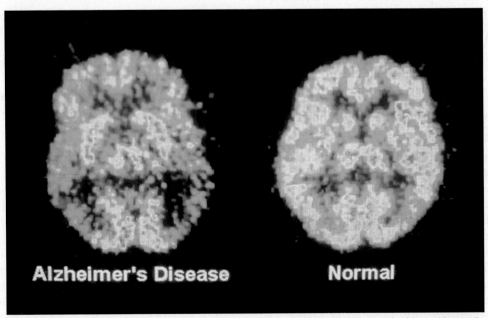

FIGURE 29.3 Metabolic activity in a subject with Alzheimer's disease (*left*) and control subject without AD (*right*). (Courtesy of Monte S. Buchsbaum, MD, The Mount Sinai Medical Center and School of Medicine, New York.)

Aβ processing (Bateman, Xiong, Benzinger, Fagan, Goate, Fox, et al., 2012).

Oxidative Stress, Free Radicals, and Mitochondrial Dysfunction

It is hypothesized that in AD-affected brains, there is a rapid increase in formation of free radicals (i.e., highly reactive molecules) that can lead to **oxidative stress** that damages other cellular molecules such as proteins, lipids, and nucleic acid. Recent studies suggest that oxidative stress may result in changes in chromatin (a complex of DNA and proteins), which may lead to dysfunctional gene expression (Frost, Hemberg, Lewis, & Feany, 2014).

Inflammation

Inflammation is now considered as one of many factors that contribute to the development of Alzheimer' Disease. The hypothesis is that inflammation may damage small blood vessels and brain cells, initiating a cascade of pathologic events related to oxidative damage and dysregulated amyloid metabolism (Marchesi, 2014).

Family Response to Disorder

Families are the first to be aware of the cognitive problem, often before the patient, who can be unaware of the extent of memory impairment. When finally confirmed, the actual diagnosis can be devastating to the family. Unlike delirium, a diagnosis of AD means long-term care responsibilities while the essence of a family member diminishes day by day. Most families keep their relative at home as long as possible to maintain contact and to avoid costly nursing home placement. The two symptoms that often result in nursing home placement are incontinence that cannot be managed and behavioral problems, such as wandering and aggression.

Teamwork and Collaboration: Working Toward Recovery

The nature and range of services needed by patients and families throughout the illness can vary dramatically at different stages. As with any other patient, the person with Alzheimer's Disease should be the center of the decision-making process. The plan should include educational and supportive programs individualized for the person's self-identified needs. Ideally, plans should be designed to support self-awareness, self-esteem, maintenance of abilities, and management of behavioral symptoms and health promotion (Fortinsky & Downs, 2014).

Treatment efforts currently focus on managing cognitive symptoms, delaying cognitive decline (e.g., memory loss; confusion; and problems with learning, speech, reasoning), treating the noncognitive symptoms (e.g., psychosis, mood symptoms, agitation), and supporting the caregivers to improve the quality of life for both patients and their caregivers.

Safety Issues

The priority of care changes throughout the course of AD. Initially, the priority is delaying cognitive decline and supporting family members. Later, the priority is protecting the patient from injury because of lack of judgment. Near the end, the physical needs of the patient are the focus of care.

Evidence-Based Nursing Care for Persons with Alzheimer Disease

Development and implementation of appropriate, effective, and safe nursing services for the care and support of patients with Alzheimer's Disease and their families is a particular challenge because of the complex nature of the illness. See Nursing Care Plan 29.1, available at http://thepoint.lww.com/BoydEssentials.

> **NCLEXNOTE**   Needs and problematic behaviors of patients with Alzheimer's Disease vary throughout the course of the disorder. Early in the disorder, the nurse focuses on support, education, and cognitive interventions for depression. As the Alzheimer's Disease progresses, priority care becomes safety interventions.

Mental Health Nursing Assessment

Physical Health Assessment

A review of body systems must be conducted on each patient suspected of having Alzheimer's Disease. Neurologic function of the patient with AD is usually preserved through the early and middle stages of the disease, although seizures, gait disturbances, and tremors may occur at any time. In the later stages of the disease, neurologic signs, such as flexion contractures and primitive reflexes, are prominent features.

Physical Functions

Assessment of physical functions includes ADLs, recent changes in functional abilities, use of sensory aids (e.g., eyeglasses, hearing aids), activity level, and assessment of pain. Eyeglasses and hearing aids may need to be in place before other assessments can be made.

At first, limitations may primarily involve instrumental activities of daily living (IADLs), (e.g., shopping, preparing meals, performing other household chores). Later in the disease process, basic physical dysfunctions occur, such as incontinence, ataxia, dysphagia, and contractures. Incontinence can be a major source of stress and a considerable burden to family caregivers. Evaluation of the patient's functional abilities includes bathing, dressing, toileting, feeding, nutritional status, physical mobility, sleep patterns, and pain.

Self-Care

Alterations in the central nervous system (CNS) associated with Alzheimer's Disease impair the patient's ability to collect information from the environment, retrieve memories, retain new information, and give meaning to current situations. Therefore, patients with Alzheimer's Disease often neglect self-care activities. Periodically, biologic assessment parameters need to be reevaluated because patients with Alzheimer's Disease may neglect activities such as bathing, eating, or skin care.

Sleep–Wake Disturbances

Patients with Alzheimer's Disease have frequent daytime napping and nighttime periods of wakefulness, with little rapid eye movement (REM) sleep. Lowered levels of REM sleep are associated with restlessness, irritability, and general sleep impairment (Garcia-Alberca, Lara, Cruz, Garrido, Gris, & Barbancho, 2013).

Activity and Exercise

One of the earliest symptoms of AD is withdrawal from normal activities. Motor activity is affected in the mild stages of AD and can lead to early problems in functional performance (Alzheimer's Association, 2014a). As the disease progresses, the patient may just sit staring at a blank wall.

Nutrition

Eating can become a problem for a patient with Alzheimer's Disease and is associated with rapid cognitive decline (Soto, Secher, Gillette-Guyonnet, van Kan, Andrieu, Nourhashemi, et al., 2012; Gomes, Martins, Fonseca, Oliveira, Resende, & Pereira, 2014). As the disease progresses, patients may lose the ability to feed themselves or recognize that what is being offered is food. Some patients with Alzheimer's Disease are bulimic or hyperoral (eating or chewing almost everything possible and sometimes with an insatiable appetite). Other patients with Alzheimer's Disease experience anorexia and have no appetite.

Pain

Although AD is not usually considered a physically painful disorder, patients often have other comorbid physical diseases that may be painful. In the early stages of AD, the patient can usually respond to verbal questions regarding pain. Later, it may be difficult to assess the comfort level objectively, especially if the patient cannot communicate. Some patients in the end stage of Alzheimer's Disease become hypersensitive to touch.

Subtle behavioral changes, such as lethargy, anxiety, or restlessness, or more obvious physical signs, such as pyrexia, tachypnea, or tachycardia, may be the only indications of actual or impending illness. Observing for changes in patterns of nonverbal communication, such as facial expressions, may help in identifying indicators of pain. Hypervocalizations (disturbed vocalizations), restlessness, and agitation are other possible signs of pain.

Psychosocial Assessment

Personality changes almost always accompany Alzheimer's Disease. Researchers have identified two contrasting patterns. One is marked by apathy, lack of spontaneity, and passivity. The other involves growing irritability, sarcasm, self-preoccupation, and intolerance of and lack of concern for others.

Cognitive Status

The mental status assessment can be difficult for the patient with Alzheimer's Disease because cognitive disturbance is the clinical hallmark of AD. However, family members should also be a part of any assessment, especially early in the disease process. The AD8 is a brief, sensitive measure that differentiates between those with and without dementia (Galvin, Roe, Powlishta, Coats, Muich, Grant, et al., 2005; Galvin, Roe, Xiong, & Morris, 2006). The AD8 (Razavi, Tolea, Margrett, Martin, Oakland, Tscholl, et al., 2013) contains eight questions asking the family member to rate any change (yes or no) in memory, problem-solving abilities, orientation, and ADLs. The higher the number of changes, the more likely dementia is present (Figure 29.4). If cognitive deterioration occurs rapidly, delirium should be suspected.

Memory. The most dramatic and consistent cognitive impairment is in memory. Patients with dementia appear mildly forgetful and repetitive in conversation. They misplace objects, miss appointments, and forget what they were just doing. They may lose track of a conversation or television show. Initially, they may complain of memory problems, but rapidly in the course of the illness, insight is lost, and they become unaware of what is lost. Sometimes they may confabulate, making what appears to be an appropriate explanation of why the information or object is missing. Eventually, all aspects of memory are impaired and even long-term memories are affected. During the interview, short-term memory loss is usually readily evident by the patient's inability to recall three or four words given to him or her at the beginning of the assessment. Often, the earliest symptom of AD is the inability to retain new information.

Language. Language is also progressively impaired. Individuals with AD may initially have agnosia (difficulty finding a word in a sentence or in naming an object).

Remember, "Yes, a change" indicates that there has been a change in the last several years caused by cognitive (thinking and memory) problems.	Yes, A change	No, No change	N/A, Don't know
1. Problems with judgment (e.g., problems making decisions, bad financial decisions, problems with thinking)			
2. Less interest in hobbies/activities			
3. Repeats the same things over and over (questions, stories, or statements)			
4. Trouble learning how to use a tool, appliance, or gadget (e.g., VCR, computer, microwave, remote control)			
5. Forgets correct month or year			
6. Trouble handling complicated financial affairs (e.g., balancing checkbook, income taxes, paying bills)			
7. Trouble remembering appointments			
8. Daily problems with thinking and/or memory			

The final score is a sum of the number of items marked "Yes, A change".

Based on clinical research findings from 995 individuals included in the development and validation samples, the following cut points are provided:
• 0-1: Normal cognition
• 2 or greater: Cognitive impairment is likely to be present

Interpretation of the AD8 (Adapted from Galvin, JE et al, The AD8, a brief informal interview to detect dementia, Neurology 2005; 58: 589-364)

Scores in the impaired range indicate a need for further assessment. Scores in the "normal" range suggest that a dementing disorder is unlikely, but a very early disease process cannot be ruled out. More advanced assessment may be warranted in cases where other objective evidence of impairment exists.

FIGURE 29.4 AD8 tool. (Used with permission from James E. Galvin, MD, MSc, Assistant Professor, Director of the Memory Diagnostic Center, Washington University School of Medicine, St. Louis.)

They may be able to talk around it, but the loss is noticeable. Later, fluent aphasia develops; comprehension diminishes; and, finally, they become mute and unresponsive to directions or information.

Visuospatial Impairment. Deficits in visuospatial tasks that require sensory and motor coordination develop early, drawing is abnormal, and the ability to write may change. An inaccurate clock drawing is diagnostic of impairment in this area (Figure 29.5). Sequencing tasks, such as cooking or other self-care skills, become impaired. The individual becomes unable to complete complex tasks that require calculations, such as balancing a checkbook.

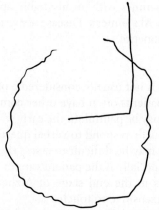

FIGURE 29.5 Clock drawing by a patient with moderate Alzheimer disease. The patient was asked to draw a clock at 3:00 PM.

Executive Functioning. Judgment, reasoning, and the ability to problem solve or make decisions are also impaired later in the disorder, closer to the time of nursing home placement. It is hypothesized that as the disease progresses, the degeneration of neurons is spread diffusely throughout the neocortex.

Psychotic Symptoms. Delusional thought content and hallucinations are common in people with AD. These psychotic symptoms differ from those of schizophrenia.

Suspiciousness, Delusions, and Illusions. **Illusions**, or mistaken perceptions, are also common in patients with AD. For example, a woman with AD mistakes her husband for her father. He resembles her father in that he is roughly her father's age when the father was last alive. If an illusion becomes a false fixed belief, it is a delusion.

As the disease progresses, delusions develop in 34% to 50% of the people with AD. These characteristic delusions are different from those discussed in the psychotic disorders. Common delusional beliefs include the following:

* Belief that his or her partner is engaging in marital infidelity
* Belief that other patients or staff are trying to hurt him or her
* Belief that staff or family members are impersonators
* Belief that people are stealing his or her belongings
* Belief that strangers are living in his or her home
* Belief that people on television are real and not actors

Hallucinations. Visual, rather than auditory, hallucinations are the most common in AD. A frequent complaint is that children, adults, or strange creatures are entering the house or the patient's room. These hallucinations may not seem unusual to the patient. If possible, the content and form of hallucination should be ascertained because this information may suggest a treatable disorder. For example, an auditory hallucination commanding the patient to commit suicide may be caused by a treatable depression, not AD. In some cases, hallucinations may be pleasant, such as children being in the room, or the hallucinations may be frightening and uncomfortable.

Mood Changes

A depressed mood is common, but major depression and AD appear to be separate disorders (Verdelho, Madureira, Moleiro, Ferro, O'Brien, Poggesi, et al., 2013) Many people with AD experience one or more depressive episodes with symptoms such as psychomotor retardation, anxiety, feelings of guilt and worthlessness, sadness, frequent crying, insomnia, loss of appetite, weight loss, and suicidal rumination. Depressive symptoms are most prevalent in the early stages of AD, which may be attributed to the patient's awareness of cognitive changes, memory loss, and functional decline.

Anxiety

Moderate anxiety is a natural reaction to the fear engendered by gradual deterioration of intellectual function and the realization of impending loss of control over one's life. Failure to complete a task formerly regarded as simple creates a source of anxiety in patient with AD. As patients with AD become unsure of their surroundings and the expectations of others, they frequently react with fear and distress. It is thought that anxious behavior occurs when the patient is pressed to perform beyond his or her ability.

Catastrophic Reactions

Catastrophic reactions are overreactions or extreme anxiety reactions to everyday situations. Catastrophic responses occur when environmental stressors are allowed to continue or increase beyond the patient's threshold of stress tolerance. Behaviors indicative of catastrophic reactions typically include verbal or physical aggression, violence, agitated or anxious behavior, emotional outbursts, noisy behavior, compulsive or repetitive behavior, agitated night awakening, and other behaviors in which the patient is cognitively or socially inaccessible. Factors that contribute to catastrophic responses in patients with progressive cognitive decline include fatigue, a change in routine (e.g., faster pace, caregiver), demands beyond the patient's ability, overwhelming sensory stimuli, and physical stressors (e.g., pain, hunger).

Behavioral Responses

Apathy and Withdrawal

Apathy, the inability or unwillingness to become involved with one's environment, is common in AD, especially in the moderate-to-late stages. Apathy leads to withdrawal from the environment and a gradual loss of empathy for others. This lack of empathy is very difficult for families and friends to understand.

Restlessness, Agitation, and Aggression

Restlessness, agitation, and aggression are relatively common in the moderate-to-late stages of AD. Restlessness should be further evaluated to determine its underlying cause. If the restlessness occurs during medication change or adjustment, side effects should be suspected.

Aberrant Motor Behavior

Symptoms such as fidgeting, picking at clothing, wringing hands, loud vocalizations, and wandering may all be signs of such underlying conditions as dehydration, medication reaction, pain, or infection (suggesting delirium). One of the most difficult behaviors for which to determine an underlying cause is **hypervocalization**, a term comprising the screams, curses, moans, groans, and verbal repetitiveness that are common in the later stages of AD in cognitively impaired older adults, often occurring during a hospitalization or nursing home placement. In the assessment of these hypervocalizations, it is important to identify when the behavior is occurring; antecedents of the behavior; and any related events, such as a family member leaving or a change in stimulation.

Disinhibition

One of the most frustrating symptoms of AD is **disinhibition**, acting on thoughts and feelings without exercising appropriate social judgment. In AD, the patient may decide that he or she is more comfortable naked than with clothes. Or the patient may not be able to find his or her clothes and may walk into a room of people without any clothes on. This behavior is extremely disconcerting to family members and can also lead to nursing home placement.

Hypersexuality

A closely related symptom is **hypersexuality**, which is inappropriate and socially unacceptable sexual behavior. The patient begins talking and behaving in ways that are uncharacteristic of premorbid behavior. This behavior is very difficult for family members and nursing home staff.

Stress and Coping Skills

Patients with AD seem extremely sensitive to stressful situations and often do not have the coping abilities to deal with such situations. A careful assessment of the triggers that precede stressful situations will help in understanding a provoking event.

Social Interaction

AD interferes with a person's ability to interact socially as much as it disrupts intellectual functioning. The patient's whole social network is affected by AD and the primary caregiver of a person with AD (usually the partner or offspring in a community setting) is often considered a copatient. It is important to assess the family caregiver's ability to use supportive mechanisms to maintain his or her own integrity throughout the disease process.

If the patient still resides in the community, a home visit will prove useful because it provides information about the patient in the natural environment. From this assessment, the situational and psychosocial stressors that affect the family and patient can be identified, so interventions to strengthen coping strategies, including the ability to seek help from appropriate community resources, can be developed.

Nursing Diagnoses

The unique and changing needs of these patients present a challenge for nurses in all settings. A multitude of potential nursing diagnoses can be generated from the assessment. A sample of common nursing diagnoses include Bathing/Hygiene Self-Care Deficit; Dressing/Grooming Self-Care Deficit; Fatigue; Insomnia; Pain; Impaired Memory; Disturbed Thought Processes; Chronic Confusion; Disturbed Sensory Perception; Risk for Violence: Self-Directed or Directed at Others; Risk for Loneliness; Risk for Caregiver Role Strain; Ineffective Sexuality Patterns; Hopelessness; Powerlessness; and Risk for Social IsolationOutcomes are determined according to nursing diagnoses.

Nursing Interventions

Self-Care Interventions

Patients should be encouraged to maintain as much self-care as possible. If eyeglasses and hearing aids are needed but not used, patients are more likely to have false perceptual experiences (hallucinations). Oral hygiene can be a problem and requires excellent basic nursing care. Aging and many medications reduce salivary flow, which can lead to a painfully dry and cracking oral mucosa. For patients with xerostomia (dry mouth) hard candy or chewing gum may stimulate salivary flow or modification of the drug regimen may be necessary. Glycerol mouthwash can provide as much relief from xerostomia as artificial saliva.

During later stages of AD, bathing can be problematic for the patient and nursing staff. Bath time is a high-risk time for agitation and aggression (Whall, Hyojeong, Colling, Gwi-Ryung, DeCicco, & Antonakos, 2013). The person-centered approach focuses on personalizing care to meet residents' needs, accommodating to residents' preferences, attending to the relationship and interaction with the resident, using effective communication and interpersonal skills, and adapting the physical environment and bathing procedures to decrease stress and discomfort (Fortinsky & Downs, 2014).

Physical Health Interventions

Supporting Bowel and Bladder Function

Urinary or bowel incontinence affects many patients with AD. During the middle phases of the disease, incontinence may be caused by the patient's inability to communicate the need to use the toilet or locate a toilet quickly, undress appropriately to use the toilet, recognize the sensation of fullness signaling the need to urinate or defecate, or apathy with lack of motivation to remain continent.

For the patient who is incontinent because of an inability to locate the toilet, orientation may be helpful. Signs and active training should help to modify disorientation. Displaying pictures or signs on bathroom doors provides visual cues; words should use appropriate terminology.

Sleep Interventions

Sedative–hypnotic agents may be prescribed for a short time for restlessness or insomnia, but they may also cause a paradoxic reaction of agitation and insomnia (especially in older adults). Sleep hygiene interventions are appropriate for patients with AD, although morning and afternoon naps (or rest periods for patients who do not nap) may be the most effective intervention for a patient with altered diurnal rhythms.

Activity and Exercise Interventions

Activity and exercise are important nursing interventions for patients with AD. To promote a feeling of success, any activity or exercise plan must be culturally sensitive and adapted to the patient's functional ability and interests. The activity or exercise must be designed to prevent excess stress (both physical and psychological), which means that it must be individualized for each patient with AD based on his or her relative strengths and deficits.

Nutritional Interventions

Maintenance of nutrition and hydration are essential nursing interventions. The patient's weight, oral intake, and hydration status should be monitored carefully. Patients with AD should eat well-balanced meals appropriate to their activity level and eating abilities, with special attention given to electrolyte balance and fluid intake.

Watch for swallowing difficulties that may put the patient at risk for aspiration and asphyxiation. Swallowing difficulties may result from changes in esophageal motility and decreased secretion of saliva.

Pain and Comfort Management

Nursing care of noncommunicative patients who have AD and who also have pain can be challenging. Because of the difficulty in identifying and monitoring the pain, the patients are often undertreated. However, several measures may be used to assess the efficacy of pharmacologic interventions, such as decreased restlessness and agitation. Small doses of oral morphine solution appear to reduce discomfort during routine nursing procedures. The main side effect of morphine is constipation.

Relaxation

Approaching patients in a calm, confident, unhurried manner; maintaining a soothing, quiet environment; avoiding unnecessary noise or chatter around patients and lowering vocal tone and rate when addressing them; maintaining eye contact; and using touch judiciously are likely to promote a sense of security conducive to patient relaxation and comfort. Simple relaxation exercises can be used to reduce stress and should be performed by the patient.

Medications

Medications have two goals: restoration or maintenance of cognitive function and treatment of related psychiatric and behavioral disturbances that cause discomfort for the patient, interfere with treatment, or worsen the individual's cognitive status. Doses must be kept extremely low, and patients should be monitored closely for any side effects or worsening of cognitive status. "Start low and go slow" is the principle guiding the administration of psychopharmacologic agents in older patients.

Cholinesterase Inhibitors. **Acetylcholinesterase inhibitors** (AChEIs) are the mainstay of pharmacologic treatment of AD because they inhibit **acetylcholinesterase** (AChE), an enzyme necessary for the breakdown of aceytlcholine. Inhibition of AChE results in an increase in cholinergic activity. Because these medications have been shown to delay the decline in cognitive functioning but generally do not improve cognitive function after it has declined, it is important that this medication be started as soon as the diagnosis is made. The primary side effect of these medications is gastrointestinal distress, including nausea, vomiting, and diarrhea.

Cholinesterase inhibitors are indicated for the treatment of AD. These drugs may help to delay or prevent symptoms from becoming worse. See Table 29.3. Cholinesterase inhibitors are oral medications usually taken once or twice a day. The earlier in the disease process these medications are initiated, the more likely they will delay cognitive decline. Although there are no special monitors for the cholinesterase inhibitors, the prolonged concurrent use of nonsteroidal anti-inflammatory drugs (NSAIDs) with them can increase the risk of stomach ulcers. With cholinesterase inhibitors, patients should not take any anticholinergic medication (USDHHS, 2015).

N-Methyl-D-Aspartic Acid Antagonists. In AD, it is hypothesized that the chronic release of glutamate leads to neuronal degeneration. Memantine (Namenda XR) is an *N*-Methyl-D-Aspartic Acid (NMDA)-receptor antagonist that has been shown to improve cognition and ADLs in patients with moderate to severe symptoms of AD (Tucci, et al., 2014) (Box 29.4).

Other Medications. Antipsychotics are not approved for the use dementia-related psychosis and have a boxed warning for this population. The evidence for the use of antidepressants for treating depression is inconclusive (Leong, 2014), but there is limited research support for their use in reducing agitation (Porsteinsson, Drye,

TABLE 29.3   CHOLINESTERASE INHIBITORS

Drug	Dose	Common Side Effects	Drug–Drug Interactions
Galantamine (Razadyne) Prevents breakdown of acetylcholine and modulates nicotinic receptors which releases acetylcholine in the brain	4 mg bid Titrate to 16–24 mg/day over 8 weeks	Nausea, vomiting, diarrhea, weight loss	Some antidepressants, such as paroxetine, amitriptyline, fluoxetine, fluvoxamine, and other drugs with anticholinergic action, may cause retention of excess galantamine in the body. NSAIDs should be used with caution in combination with this medication.
Rivastigmine (Exelon) Prevents the breakdown of acetylcholine and butyrylcholine in the brain	1.5 mg bid Titrate to 24 mg/day by increasing 3 mg/day every 2 weeks	Nausea, vomiting, weight loss, upset stomach, muscle weakness	None observed in laboratory studies; NSAIDs should be used with caution in combination with this medication
Donepezil (Aricept) Prevents the breakdown of acetylcholine in the brain	5 mg once a day Increase after 4–6 weeks to 10 mg/day	Nausea, diarrhea, vomiting	None observed in laboratory studies. NSAIDs should be used with caution in combination with this medication

bid, twice a day; NSAIDs, nonsteroidal antiinflammatory drug

Adapted from USDHHS (2015). Alzheimer's disease medications fact sheet. Washington, DC: Alzheimer's Disease Education & Referral (ADEAR) Center, National Institute on Aging, National Institutes of Health, NIH Publication N. 08–3431. Retrieved on August 12, 2015 from http://www.nia.nih.gov/alheimers/publication/alzheimers-disease-medications-factsheet.

Pollock, Devannand, Grangakis, Ismail, et al., 2014). Benzodiazepines should be used with caution and only on a short-term basis to treat anxiety in older adults. Anticholinergic medications should be avoided in patients with AD if at all possible. See Box 29.5 for examples of medications that are commonly prescribed in older adults that have anticholinergic properties.

Psychosocial Interventions

The therapeutic relationship is the basis for interventions for the patient and family with dementia. Care of the patient entails a long-term relationship needing much support and expert nursing care. Interventions should be delivered within the relationship context.

BOX 29.4

Drug Profile: Memantine (Namenda XR)

DRUG CLASS: N-methyl-D-aspartate (NMDA) receptor antagonist

RECEPTOR AFFINITY: Low to moderate affinity uncompetitive (open-channel) NMDA receptor antagonist, which binds preferentially to the NMDA receptor

INDICATIONS: For treatment of moderate to severe dementia of the Alzheimer type.

ROUTES AND DOSAGE: 7, 14, 21, and 28 mg tablets; oral solution, 2 mL/mg

The recommended starting dose of Namenda XR is 7 mg once daily. The recommended target dose is 28 mg once daily. The dose should be increased in 7 mg increments to 28 mg once daily. The minimum recommended interval between dose increases is 1 week and only if the previous dose has been well tolerated. Maximum dose is 28 mg daily.

HALF LIFE (PEAK EFFECT): Terminal half-life, 60 to 80 hours (peak effect, 3–7 hours)

SELECT ADVERSE REACTIONS: Dizziness, headache, constipation; reduce dosage in patients with severe renal damage

PRECAUTIONS: Avoid use during pregnancy; effect during lactation has not been determined. May cause drowsiness or dizziness; use caution while driving and performing other activities requiring mental alertness

SPECIFIC PATIENT AND FAMILY EDUCATION: Caregivers should be instructed in the recommended administration (twice per day for doses above 5 mg) and dose escalation (minimum interval of 1 week between dose increases).
- This drug does not alter the Alzheimer's disease process, and the efficacy of the medication may decrease over time.
- Continue using other medications for dementia as prescribed by the health care provider.
- Review the Patient Information.
- Teach preparation of oral solution (attach the green cap and plastic tube to new bottles of oral solution, withdraw prescribed dose using dosing syringe, and administer the dose).
- Do not discontinue the drug or change the dose unless advised by the health care provider.
- Do not increase the dose of memantine if Alzheimer's disease symptoms do not appear to be improving or appear to be getting worse; notify the health care provider.
- Memantine may cause drowsiness or dizziness. Use caution while driving and performing other activities requiring mental alertness and coordination until tolerance is determined.
- Do not use any prescription or over-the-counter medications, dietary supplements, or herbal preparations unless advised by the health care provider.
- Follow-up visits may be required to monitor therapy and to keep appointments.

Memory Enhancement

The sooner patients begin taking AChEIs, the slower the cognitive decline will be. However, pharmacologic agents are only a small part of the intervention picture. The nursing goal is to maintain memory function as long as possible. When caring for a patient with AD, a concerted effort should be made to reinforce short- and long-term memory. For example, reminding patients what they had for breakfast, which activity was just completed, or who their visitors were a few hours ago will reinforce short-term memory. Encouraging patients to tell the stories of their earlier years will help bring long-term memories into focus. In the earlier stages of AD, there is considerable frustration when the patient realizes that he or she has short-term memory loss. In a matter-of-fact manner, help "fill in the blanks" and then redirect to another activity. Pictures of familiar people, places, and activities are also important tools in memory retrieval. Using scents (perfume, shaving lotions, spices, different foods) to stimulate memory retrieval and asking patients to relate their memories are also useful. Formalized reminiscence groups also help patients relive their earlier experiences and support maintenance of long-term memories.

Orientation Interventions

To enhance cognitive functioning, attempts should be made to remind patients of the day, time, and location. However, if the patient begins to argue that he or she is really at home or that it is really 1992, the patient need not be confronted by facts. Any confrontation could easily escalate into an argument. Instead, either redirect the patient or focus on the topic at hand (Box 29.6).

Maintaining Language

Losing the ability to name an object (i.e., agnosia) is frustrating. For example, the patient may describe a flower in terms of color, size, and fragrance but never be able to name the flower. When this happens while interacting with a patient, immediately say the name of the item. This reinforces cognitive functioning and prevents disruption in the interaction. Referral to speech therapists may also be useful if the language impairment impedes communication.

Supporting Visuospatial Functioning

The patient with visuospatial impairments loses the ability to sequence automatic behaviors, such as getting dressed or eating with silverware. For example, patients often put their clothes on backward, inside out, or with undergarments over outer garments. After they are dressed, they become confused as to how they arrived at their current state. If this happens, it may help to place clothes for dressing in a sequence for the patient so they patient can move from one article to the next in the correct sequence. This same technique can be used in other situations, such as eating, bathing, and toileting.

Managing Suspicions, Illusions, and Delusions

Delusions often occur when patients are placed in a situation they cannot master cognitively. The principle of nonconfrontation is most important in dealing with formation of suspiciousness and delusion. Efforts should be directed at determining the circumstances that trigger suspicion or delusion formation and creating a means of avoiding these situations.

Frequent causes of suspicion occur when changes in daily routine occur. The common accusations that "Someone has entered my room," or "Someone has changed my room" can be managed by asking, "Do you want to see if anything is missing?" Such accusations usually arise when a patient cannot remember what the room looked like or when the room was rearranged or cleaned.

Patients with AD often have delusions that a spouse, child, or other significant person is an impostor. If this situation occurs, it is important to assert in a matter-of-fact manner, "This is your wife Barbara" or "I am your daughter Jenny." More vigorous assertions, such as offering various types of proof, tend to increase puzzlement as to why a person would go so far to impersonate the spouse or child.

When patients experience illusions, find the source of the illusion and remove it from the environment if possible. For example, if a patient is watching a television program featuring animals and then verbalizes that the animal is in the room, switch the channel and redirect the conversation.

BOX 29.6 • THERAPEUTIC DIALOGUE • The Patient with Dementia of the Alzheimer Type

Lois's daughter has told the home health agency nurse that on several occasions, Lois has been found cowering and fearful under the kitchen table, saying she was hiding from voices. The nurse also knows that Lois denies having any difficulty with her memory or her ability to care for herself.

INEFFECTIVE APPROACH

Nurse: I'm here to see you about your health problems.

Patient: I have no problems. Why are you here?

Nurse: I'm here to help you.

Patient: I do not need any help. I think there is a mistake.

Nurse: Oh, there is no mistake. Your name is Ms. W, isn't it?

Patient: Yes, but I don't know who you are or why you are here. I'm very tired, please excuse me.

Nurse: OK. I will return another day.

EFFECTIVE APPROACH

Nurse: Hello, my name is Susan Miller. I'm the home health nurse, and I will be spending some time with you.

Patient: Oh, alright. Come in. Sit here.

Nurse: Thank you.

Patient: There is nothing wrong with me, you know.

Nurse: Are you wondering why I am here? (Open-ended statement)

Patient: I know why you are here. My children think that I cannot take care of myself.

Nurse: Is that true? Can you take care of yourself? (Restatement)

Patient: Of course I can care for myself. When people get older, they slow down. I'm just a little slower now, and that upsets my children.

Nurse: You are a little slower? (Reflection)

Patient: I sometimes forget things.

Nurse: Such as…(open-ended statement)

Patient: Sometimes I cannot remember a telephone number or a name of a food.

Nurse: Does that cause problems?

Patient: According to my children, it does!

Nurse: What about you? What causes problems for you?

Patient: Sometimes the radio says terrible things to me.

Nurse: That must be frightening. (Acceptance)

Patient: It's terrifying. Then, my daughter looks at me as if I am crazy. Am I?

Nurse: It sounds like your mind is playing tricks on you. Let's see if we can Figure out how to control the radio. (Validation)

Patient: Oh, OK. Will you tell my daughter that I am not crazy?

Nurse: Sure, I would be happy to meet with both you and your daughter if you would like. (Acceptance)

CRITICAL THINKING CHALLENGE

- How did the nurse's underlying assumption that the patient would welcome the nurse in the first scenario lead to the nurse's rejection by the patient?

- What communication techniques did the nurse use in the second scenario to open communication and set the stage for the development of a sense of trust?

Some patients with AD may no longer recognize the reflections in the mirror as themselves and become agitated, thinking that a stranger is staring at them. Potentially misleading or disturbing stimuli, such as mirrors or art work, can be easily covered or removed from the environment.

Managing Hallucinations

Reassurance and distraction may be helpful for the hallucinating patient. For example, an 89-year-old patient with AD in a residential care facility would get up each night, walk to the nursing station, and whisper to the nurses, "There's a man in my bed who won't let me sleep.

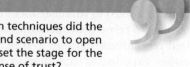

You should patrol this place better!" If the hallucination is not too disturbing for the patient, it can often be dismissed calmly with diversion or distraction. Because this patient did not seem too concerned by the man in her bed, the nurse may gently respond by saying, "I'm sorry you have to put up with so much. Just wait here (or come with me) and I'll make sure your room is ready for you." The nurse should then take the patient back to her room and help her into bed.

Frightening hallucinations and delusions usually require antipsychotic medications to dampen the patient's emotional reactions, but they can also be dealt with by optimizing perceptual cues (e.g., cover mirrors, turn off the television) and by encouraging patients to stay physically close to their caregivers. For example, one patient complained to her visiting nurse that she was being poisoned by deadly bugs that crawled up and down her arms and legs while she tried to sleep at night. Antipsychotic medication may help this patient sleep at night and she would also likely benefit from reassurance and protection.

Interventions for Mood Changes

Managing Depression

Psychotherapeutic nursing interventions for depression that accompanies AD are similar to interventions for any depression. It is important to spend time alone with patients and to personalize their care as a way of communicating the patient's value. Encouraging expression of negative emotions is helpful because patients can talk honestly to a nonjudgmental person about their feelings. Although depressed patients with AD are likely to be too disorganized to commit suicide, it is wise to remove potentially harmful objects from the environment.

Managing Stress and Anxiety

Cognitively impaired patients are particularly vulnerable to anxiety. Patients with AD become unsure of their surroundings or of what is expected of them and then tend to react with fear and distress. They may feel lost, insecure, and left out. Failure to complete a task formerly regarded as simple creates anxiety and agitation. Often, they cannot explain the source of their anxiety. In many cases, lowering the demands, simplifying routines, and reducing the number of choices alleviates the anxiety.

Managing Catastrophic Reactions

If a patient reacts catastrophically, remain calm, minimize environmental distractions (quiet the environment), get the patient's attention, and softly assure the patient that he or she is safe. Give information slowly, clearly, and simply, one step at a time. Let the patient know that you understand the fear or other emotional response, such as anger or anxiety.

As nursing skills are developed in identifying antecedents to the patient's catastrophic reactions, it becomes possible to avoid situations that provoke such reactions. Patients with AD respond well to structure but poorly to change. Attempts to argue or reason with them will only escalate their dysfunctional responses.

Managing Apathy and Withdrawal

As the patient withdraws and becomes more apathetic, it becomes more challenging to engage the patient in meaningful activities and interactions. Providing this level of care requires knowing the premorbid functioning level of the patient. Close contact with family helps provide ideas about meaningful activities.

Managing Restlessness and Wandering

Restlessness and wandering are major concerns for caregivers, especially in the community (home) or long-term care setting. The principal means of dealing with restless patients who wander into other patients' rooms or out the door is to have an adequate number of staff (or caregivers in the home setting) to provide supervision, as well as electronically controlled exits. Wandering behavior may be interrupted in more cognitively intact patients by distracting them verbally or visually. Patients who are beyond verbal distraction can be distracted by physically joining them on their walk and then interrupting their course of action and gently redirecting them back to the house or facility. Many times, wandering is a result of a patient's inability to find his or her own room or may represent other agenda-seeking behaviors such as trying to find a bathroom.

Managing Agitated Behavior

Agitated behavior is likely to occur when patients are pressed to assist in their own care. A calm, unhurried, and undemanding approach is usually most effective. Attempts at reasoning may only aggravate the situation and increase the patient's resistance to care. If unable to determine the source of the patient's anxiety, the patient's restless energy can often be channeled into activities such as walking. Relaxation techniques also can be effective for reducing behavioral problems and anxiety in patients with AD.

Managing Aberrant Behavior

When patients are picking in the air or wringing hands, simple distraction may work. Hypervocalizations are another story. Direct care staff tend to avoid these patients, which only makes the vocalizations worse. In reality, these vocalizations may have meaning to the patient. Instead, develop strategies to try to reduce the frequency of vocalizations (Table 29.4).

Reducing Disinhibition

Anticipation of disinhibiting behavior is the key to nursing interventions for this problem. Disinhibition can

TABLE 29.4	MESSAGES, MEANINGS, AND MANAGEMENT STRATEGIES
Possible Underlying Meanings	**Related Management Strategies**
"I hurt!" (e.g., from arthritis, fractures, pressure ulcers, degenerative joint disease, cancer)	• Observe for pain behaviors (e.g., posture, facial expressions, and gait in conjunction with vocalizations). • Treat suspected pain judiciously with analgesics and nonpharmacologic measures (e.g., repositioning, careful manipulation of patient during transfers and personal care, warm or cold packs, massage, relaxation).
"I'm tired." (e.g., sleep disturbances possibly related to altered sleep–wake cycle with day–night reversal, difficulty falling asleep, frequent night awakenings)	• Increase daytime activity and exercise to minimize daytime napping and promote night-time sleep. • Promote normal sleep patterns and biorhythms by strengthening natural environmental cues (e.g., provide light exposure during the day; avoid bright lights at night), provide large calendars and clocks. • Establish a bedtime routine. • Reduce night awakenings: avoid excess fluids, diuretics, caffeine at bedtime, minimize loud noises, consolidate nighttime care activities (e.g., changing, medications, treatments).
"I'm lonely."	• Encourage social interactions between patients and their family, caregivers, and others. • Increase time the patient spends in group settings to minimize time in isolation. • Provide opportunity to interact with pets.
"I need…" (e.g., food, a drink, a blanket, to use the toilet, to be turned or repositioned)	• Anticipate needs (e.g., assist the patient to toilet soon after breakfast when the gastrocolic reflex is likely). • Keep the patient comfort and safety in mind during care (e.g., minimize body exposure to prevent hypothermia).
"I'm stressed." (e.g., Inability to tolerate sensory overload)	• Promote rest and quiet time. • Minimize "white noise" (e.g., vacuum cleaner) and background noise (e.g., televisions and radios). • Avoid harsh lighting and busy, abstract designs. • Limit patient's contacts with other agitated people. • Reduce behavioral expectations of patient, minimize choices, and promote a stable routine.
"I'm bored." (e.g., lack of sensory stimulation)	• Maximize hearing and visual abilities (e.g., keep external auditory canals free from cerumen plugs, ensure that glasses and hearing aids are worn, provide reading material of large print, soften lighting to reduce glare). • Play soft classical music for auditory stimulation. • Offer structured diversions (e.g., outdoor activities).
"What are you doing to me?" (e.g., personal boundaries are invaded)	• Avoid startling patients by approaching them from the front. • Always speak before touching the patient. • Inform patients what you plan to do and why before you do it. • Allow for flexibility in patient care.
"I don't feel well." (e.g., a urinary or upper respiratory tract infection, metabolic abnormality, fecal impaction)	• Identify the etiology through patient history, examination, possible tests (e.g., urinalysis, blood work, chest radiography, neurologic testing). • Treat underlying causes.
"I'm frustrated—I have no control." (e.g., loss of autonomy)	• When possible, allow patient to make their own decisions. • Maximize patient involvement during personal care (e.g., offer the patient a washcloth to assist with bathing). • Treat patients with dignity and respect (e.g., dress or change patients in private).
"I'm lost." (e.g., memory impairment)	• Maintain familiar routines. • Label the patient's room, bathroom, drawers, and possessions with large name signs. • Promote a sense of belonging through displays of familiar personal items, such as old family pictures.
"I feel strange." (e.g., side effects from medications that may include psychotropics, corticosteroids, beta-blockers, NSAIDs)	• Minimize the overall number of medications; consider nondrug interventions when possible. • Begin new medications one at a time; start with low doses and titrate slowly. Suspect a drug reaction if the patient's behavior (e.g., vocal) changes. • Educate caregivers about the patient's medications.
"I need to be loved!"	• Provide human contact and purposeful touch. • Acknowledge or verify the patient's feelings. • Encourage alternative, nonverbal ways to express feelings, such as through music, painting, or drawing. • Stress a sense of purpose in life, acknowledge achievement, and reaffirm that the patient is still needed.

NSAID, nonsteroidal anti-inflammatory drug.

From Clavel, D. S. (1999). Vocalizations among cognitively impaired elders. *Geriatric Nursing, 20,* 90–93. Reprinted with permission from Elsevier.

take many forms, from undressing in a public setting to touching someone inappropriately to making cruel but factual statements. This behavior can usually be viewed as normal by itself but abnormal within its social context. Keen behavioral assessment of the patient increases the ability to anticipate the likely socially inappropriate behavior and redirect the patient or change the context of the situation. If the patient starts undressing in the dining room, offering a robe and gently escorting him or her to another part of the room might be all that is needed. If a patient is trying to fondle a staff member, having the staff member leave the immediate area or redirecting the patient may alleviate the situation.

Safety Interventions

In the early stages of the illness, safety may not seem to be a prime issue because the individual is cognitively intact. However, early behaviors suggesting AD are often related to safety, such as the patient getting lost while driving or going the wrong way on the highway. Patients may be prevented from driving even though they can continue to live at home. Safety continues to be an issue in the home when patients engage in unsupervised cooking, cleaning, or household tasks. Day care centers provide a structured yet safe environment for these individuals. Family members should be encouraged to assess continually the abilities of members to live at home safely.

During hospitalizations or nursing home care, the safety issues are different. Most geropsychiatric units are kept locked and a dementia unit often has an electronic alarm system to alert staff about patients attempting to leave the secured floor. Staff and visitors need to be vigilant for perilous situations.

Milieu Management

Overstimulating activities (e.g., social outing, family visit) can result in an outburst of delusional accusations or agitation. The nurse should attempt to determine each patient's optimal level of stimulation at various times of the day. It may be that stimulating environments can be tolerated early in the morning but not in the afternoon when the patient is tired.

Socialization Activities

Overlearned social skills are rarely lost in patients with AD. It is not unusual for patients with dementia to respond appropriately to a handshake or smile well into the disease process. Even patients who are no longer able to communicate coherently will carry on long discussions with people who are willing to listen and respond (to language that does not make sense). The risk for social isolation is strong in patients with AD because of communication difficulties. Reinforcing social remarks and gestures, such as eye contact, smiling, greetings, and farewells, can promote a sense of competency and self-esteem. Pet therapy and "stuffed animal" therapy can also enhance social interaction in cognitively impaired individuals. It is important to remember that patients with AD do not lose their ability to laugh and play and the psychosocial benefits of humor are well known.

Activities that elicit pleasant memories from an earlier time in the patient's life (reminiscence) may produce a soothing effect. Eliciting pleasant memories may be enhanced by gentle stimulation of the patient's senses, for example, viewing and discussing photo albums, looking at personal memorabilia, providing a favorite food item, playing a musical instrument, or listening to music the person preferred in younger years. It may be useful to incorporate movement or dance along with a singing exercise.

If the patient with AD resists structured exercise, it may be because of a fear of falling or injury or of demonstrating to others that his or her health is failing. Patients with AD often forget how to move or how to coordinate their movements in relation to objects. Therefore, exercise should be light and enjoyable. Encourage the patient to take rest periods at intervals throughout the activity in an effort to minimize stress.

Home Visits

The goal of in-home and community-based long-term care services is to maintain patients in a self-determining environment that provides the most home-like atmosphere possible, allows maximum personal choice for care recipients and caregiver and encourages optimal family caregiving involvement without overwhelming the resources of the family network. All services for patients with AD and their families must be provided within a context of continuity of care, a concept that mandates access to various health and supportive services over an unpredictable and changing clinical course.

Community Actions

Nurses working with patients with AD are especially knowledgeable about all aspects of the illness and care. These nurses are often involved in local organizations, such as the Alzheimer's Association. Issues of care and safety and reimbursement for services often require professional expertise and influence.

Family Interventions

Especially in AD, the needs of family members should also be considered. Caring for a family member with dementia takes its toll. Eighty percent of the home care

Psychoeducation Checklist: Tips for Caregivers

When caring for the patient with dementia, be sure to include the caregivers, as appropriate, and address the following topic areas in the teaching plan:

- Psychopharmacologic agents, if used, including drug action, dosage, frequency, and possible adverse effects
- Rest and activity
- Consistency in routines
- Nutrition and hydration
- Sleep and comfort measures
- Protective environment
- Communication and social interaction
- Diversional measures
- Community resources

is provided by family caregivers. Most of the caregivers are women (65%), and 21% are over the age of 65 years. Caregivers' health often declines and directly affects their ability to provide care (Alzheimer's Association, 2014a). Caregivers are faced with extreme pressures and often feel isolated, frustrated, and trapped. The potential for patient abuse is significant, especially if agitated and aggressive behaviors are present in the relative.

Caregivers should be encouraged to attend support groups and carve out personal time. Educational and training programs may help in understanding the

BOX 29.8

Research for Best Practice: Easing the Burden of Caregivers

Lewis, M., Hobday, J. V., & Hepburn, K. W. (2011). Internet-based program for dementia caregivers. American Journal of Alzheimer's Disease & Other Dementias, 25(8), 674–679.

THE QUESTION: Will a face-to-face psychoeducation program for caregivers be effective as an internet program to provide caregivers the knowledge, skills, and outlook to undertake and succeed in the caregiving role?

METHODS: The Internet-Based Savvy Caregiver Program merged an effective psychoeducation intervention with the access and interactivity of the Internet to make available this beneficial service. Content from four modules were selected for the program, including (1) the effects of dementia on thinking, (2) taking charge and letting go, (3) providing practical help, and (4) managing daily care and difficult behavior. Each of the storyboard documents were between 30 and 50 pages in length. A total of 47 family caregivers participated in a pilot project that was based on qualitative analysis of open ended questions.

FINDINGS: The participants provided positive ratings for the program and endorsed the program's acceptability and usability.

IMPLICATIONS FOR NURSING: The Internet format is acceptable and another option for caregivers who have a computer access. Nurses should consider encouraging caregivers to participate in high-quality Internet-based psychoeducation programs.

complex nature of the disorder (Boxes 29.7 and 29.8). Community resources, such as day care centers, home health agencies, and other community services, can be an important aspect of nursing care for the patient with dementia.

Evaluation and Treatment Outcomes

The objectives of nursing interventions are to help the patient with AD remain as independent as possible and to function at the highest cognitive, physical, emotional, spiritual, and social levels. The maximum level of functional ability can be promoted when nursing care is related to and based on the remaining abilities of the patient.

Continuum of Care

Community Care

It is estimated that more than 60% to 70% of older adults with AD live at home. Almost 80% of home care is provided by family and friends. Unpaid caregivers provide $202 billion economic worth (Alzheimer's Association, 2014a). Use of community-based services (e.g., home health aides, home-delivered meals, adult day care centers, respite care, caregiver support groups) often extends the amount of time an individual with AD or a related disorder can safely remain in the home.

Inpatient-Focused Care

Comprehensive admission assessment followed by the development of an individualized (and constantly updated) care plan that involves the patient, significant others, and diverse health care professionals is the foundation of an effective and efficient postdischarge plan. Attention to all aspects of this process is necessary to ensure that the goal of continuity of care is achieved. The hospital-based nurse may initiate family education and counseling as part of discharge planning.

Nursing Home Care

As the AD progresses, many patients are placed in a nursing home for care. Nursing care in a nursing home is usually delivered by nurses' aides, who need support and direction. Interestingly, people with AD require complex nursing care, but the skill level of people caring for these individuals often is minimal. Education and support of the direct caregiver is the focus of most nursing homes.

OTHER DEMENTIAS

Dementia symptoms may occur as a result of a number of disorders and underlying etiologies. The subsequent sections provide a brief description of some of the dementias listed in the *DSM-5*. In each case, the classic symptoms of dementia (e.g., memory impairment with a number of other cognitive deficits) must be present. Nursing interventions for all dementias are similar to those described for individuals with AD.

Vascular Neurocognitive Disorder

Vascular neurocognitive disorder (also known as *vascular dementia*) is a decline in thinking skill caused by conditions that block or reduce blood flow to the brain and the second most common type of dementia. Slightly more men than women are affected. Vascular dementia results when a series of small strokes damage or destroy brain tissue. These are commonly referred to as "ministrokes" or transient ischemic attacks (TIAs) and several TIAs may occur before the affected individual becomes aware of the symptoms of vascular dementia. Most often, a blood clot or plaques (fatty deposits) block the vessels that supply blood to the brain, causing a stroke. However, a stroke can also occur when a blood vessel bursts in the brain (Alzheimer's Association, 2014b).

Symptoms of vascular neurocognitive disorder usually begin more suddenly rather than in AD. Often, the neurologic symptoms associated with a TIA are minimal and may last only a few days, including slight weakness in a limb, dizziness, or slurred speech. Thus, the clinical progression is often described as intermittent and fluctuating or of steplike deterioration, with the patient's cognitive and functional status improving or plateauing for a period of time followed by a rapid decline in function after another series of TIAs. Treatment aims to reduce the primary risk factors for vascular dementia, including hypertension, diabetes mellitus, and additional strokes.

Dementia Caused by Parkinson Disease

In individuals with Parkinson disease, 75% will develop neurocognitive dementia (APA, 2013). Although investigators do not know why, pathologic overlap is considerable between Parkinson disease and AD. It is important to know that in patients with dementia caused by Parkinson disease, anticholinergic medications are likely to increase cognitive impairment (Katzenschlager, Sampaio, Costa, & Lees, 2009).

Dementia Caused by Huntington Disease

Huntington's disease is a progressive, genetically transmitted autosomal dominant disorder characterized by choreiform movements and mental abnormalities. The onset is usually between the ages of 30 and 50 years, but onset occurs before 5 years of age in the juvenile form or as late as 85 years of age in the late-onset form. The disease affects men and women equally. A person with Huntington's disease usually lives for approximately 15 years after diagnosis (APA, 2013). The dementia syndrome of Huntington's disease is characterized by insidious changes in behavior and personality. Typically, the dementia is frontal, which means that the person demonstrates prominent behavioral problems and disruption of attention.

FRONTOTEMPORAL NEUROCOGNITIVE DISORDER

Progressive development of behavioral and personality change and/or language impairment characterizes frontotemporal neurocognitive disorder which has distinct patterns of brain atrophy and distinctive neuropathology. Individuals with this disorder have varying degrees of apathy or disinhibition. They may lose interest in socialization, self-care, and personal responsibilities. Family members report socially inappropriate behaviors, but afflicted individuals show little insight. The cognitive deficits are typically in the area of planning, organization, and judgments. They are easily distracted (APA, 2013).

NEUROCOGNITIVE DISORDER WITH LEWY BODIES

Progressive cognitive decline with visual hallucination, rapid eye movement sleep disorder, and spontaneous parkinsonism characterizes dementia with Lewy bodies, a major neurocognitive disorder. Cognitive symptoms occur several months before motor symptoms. These symptoms fluctuate and may resemble delirium. These individuals are at high risk for falls because of periods of syncope and transient episodes of consciousness. Orthostatic hypotension and urinary incontinence may occur. The cause is unknown, but evidence implies a genetic component (Bruni, Conidi, & Bernardi, 2014). The pathology involves Lewy bodies found in the cortical location in the brain which are thought to be responsible for the disorder.

The estimated prevalence of this dementia ranges from 0.1% to 5% of the general elderly population with men slightly more affected (APA, 2013). This onset of disorder is typically in the sixth to ninth decades and is progressive with a 5- to 7-year survival rate. These individuals are more functionally impaired than those with other types of dementia (e.g., AD) and are very sensitive to psychotropic medication, especially antipsychotics.

NEUROCOGNITIVE DISORDER DUE TO PRION DISEASE

Neurocogntive disorder due to prion-related comprises a group of spongiform encephalopathies including Creutzfeldt–Jakob disease, a rare, rapidly fatal, brain disorder, and mad cow disease, which is a bovine disorder. A prion is a small infectious particle composed of abnormally folded protein that causes progressive neurodegeneration. Many of the symptoms seen in Creutzfeldt–Jakob disease are similar to those found in AD and other dementias. However, changes in the brain tissue are different in Creutzfeldt–Jakob disease and are best differentiated with surgical biopsy or during autopsy (APA, 2013). Common symptoms include fluctuating fever, difficulty swallowing, incontinence, tremors, seizures, and sensitivity to touch and environmental noise.

At present, no effective treatment for the disease exists and nothing has been found to slow progression of the illness, although antiviral drug studies are ongoing. Person-to-person transmission of Creutzfeldt-Jakob disease is rare (but possible) and it can be transmitted from people to animals and between animals. Because of the transmissible nature of Creutzfeldt-Jakob disease and because the virus is not easily destroyed, strict criteria for the handling of infected tissues and other contaminated materials have been developed.

NEUROCOGNITIVE DISORDER DUE TO TRAUMATIC BRAIN INJURY

Traumatic brain injury (TBI) affects about 1.4 to 1.7 million people in the United States each year resulting in various symptoms including neurological, cognitive, behavioral, and emotional impairments (APA, 2013); (Lee, Y., Hou, Lee, C. Hsu, Huang, & Su, 2013). Repeated concussions can lead to brain injury with long-term TBI. Evidence suggests that even mild TBI is a significant risk factor of developing dementia (Lee, et al., 2013).

SUBSTANCE/MEDICATION-INDUCED NEUROCOGNITIVE DISORDER

If dementia results from the persisting effects of a substance (e.g., drugs of abuse, a medication, exposure to toxins), substance-induced neurocognitive disorder is diagnosed. Other causes of dementia (e.g., dementia

caused by a general medical condition) must always be considered even in a person with a dependence on or exposure to a substance. For example, head injuries often result from substance use and may be the underlying cause of the neurocognitive changes (APA, 2013). Prescription drugs are the most common toxins in older adults.

SUMMARY OF KEY POINTS

- Neurocognitive disorders are characterized clinically by significant deficits in cognition or memory that represent a clear-cut change from a previous level of functioning. In some disorders, the loss of cognitive function is progressive, such as in AD. It is important to recognize the differences because the interventions and expected outcomes of the two syndromes are different.

- Delirium is characterized by a disturbance in consciousness and a change in cognition that develops over a short period of time. It requires rapid detection and treatment.

- The primary goal of treatment of individuals with delirium is prevention or resolution of the acute confusional episode with return to previous cognitive status and interventions focusing on (1) elimination or correction of the underlying cause and (2) symptomatic and safety and supportive measures.

- Dementia is characterized by the gradual onset of decline in cognitive function, especially memory, usually accompanied by changes in behavior and personality.

- AD is an example of a progressively degenerative dementia. Treatment efforts currently focus on reduction of cognitive symptoms (e.g., memory loss; confusion; and problems with learning, speech, and reasoning) in attempts to improve the quality of life for both patients and their caregivers.

- Research efforts continue to focus on understanding the relationship among the development of the beta-amyloid plaques, neurofibrillary tangles, and cell death.

- Nursing care of a person with dementia depends on the stage of the disease and the availability of family caregivers.

- Educating and supporting families and caregivers through the progressive cognitive decline and behavior changes is essential to ensuring proper care.

■ Several mental health strategies (exercise, education, cognitive stimulation) support and protect a person's cognitive reserve. A healthy cognitive reserve is thought to be protective against neuropathologic insults.

■ Other neurocognitive disorders may be related to specific brain changes (Lewy bodies), infections (prion disease), genetic diseases (Huntington), and substances/medications.

CRITICAL THINKING CHALLENGES

1. What factors should be considered in differentiating AD from vascular dementia?

2. Suggest reasons that older adults are particularly vulnerable to the development of neurocognitive disorders.

3. Compare the nursing care of a person with delirium versus one with dementia. What are the similarities and differences in the care?

4. The physical environment is particularly important to the patient with dementia. Visualize your last experience in a health care setting (e.g., hospital, nursing home, day care program, home care setting). Identify environmental factors that could be misleading or stress producing to a person with impaired cognition (dementia), and identify ways to modify this environment to alleviate some of the stressors or misleading stimuli.

5. Mr. J. has been recently diagnosed with mild AD and is asking for advice about deciding on his care in the future. His wife and daughter believe that he does not have the ability to make these decisions and asks for the nurse's advice. How should the nurse respond? Explain the rationale.

Iris: (2001) This film tells the story of British novelist Iris Murdoch (played by Kate Winslet and then by Judi Dench when Iris is much older) and her relationship with her husband John Bayley (played by Hugh Bonneville and Jim Broadbent) during the last 5 years of her life. Based on Bayley's memoir, *Elegy for Iris*, the film depicts Ms. Murdoch's decline into dementia and the stress associated with caregiving. This wonderful movie shows the suffering of AD but also shows the strength of relationships. The film contrasts the start of their relationship when Iris was an outgoing but dominant individual and John was a timid, shy, scholarly partner with the two older adults who created a loving bond that provided the fabric of the last days of Iris' life. **Viewing Points:** Identify the symptoms of the progressive illness throughout the film. Were there any "breaking points" for the caregiver? Were there aspects of Iris' personality that were sustained throughout the course of her life that were evident at the end? What nursing interventions would have been helpful to support her cognitive functioning?

MOVIE viewing GUIDES related to this chapter are available at http://thepoint.lww.com/BoydEssentials.

REFERENCES

Alzheimer's Association. (2014a). *2014 Alzheimer's disease facts and figures.* Chicago: Alzheimer's Association.

Alzheimer's Association. (2014b) *Vascular dementia.* http://www.alz.org/dementia/vascular-dementia-symptoms.asp. Retrieved May 10, 2014.

American Psychiatric Association. (2013). *Diagnostic and Statistical Manual of Mental Disorders* (5th ed.). Arlington, VA: Author.

Bateman, R. J., Xiong, C., Benzinger, T. L., Fagan, A. M., Goate, A., Fox, N. C., et al. (2012). Clinical and biomarker changes in dominantly inherited Alzheimer' Disease. *The New England Journal of Medicine, 367*(9), 795–804.

Bruni, A. C., Conidi, M. E., & Bernardi, L. (2014). Genetics in degenerative dementia: Current status and applicability. *Journal of Alzheimer Disease & Associated Disorders, 28*(3), 199–205.

Bryczkowski, S. B., Lopreiato, M. C., Yonclas, P. P., Sacca, J. J., & Mosenthal, A. C. (2014). Delirium prevention program in the surgical intensive care unit improved the outcomes of older adults. *Journal of Surgical Research, 190*(1), 280–288. doi:10.1097/TA.0000000000000427.

Clavel, D. S. (1999). Vocalizations among cognitively impaired elders: What is your patient trying to tell you?* *Geriatric Nursing, 20,* 90–93.

Desai, A. K., & Schwarz, L. (2011). Subjective cognitive impairment: When to be concerned about "senior moments." *Current Psychiatry, 10*(4), 31–44.

Garcia-Alberca, J. M., Lara, J. P., Cruz, B., Garrido, V., Gris, E., & Barbancho, M. A. (2013). Sleep disturbances in Alzheimer's disease are associated with neuropsychiatric symptoms and antidementia treatment. *Journal of Nervous & Mental Disease. 201*(3), 251–257.

Flaherty, J. H. (2011). The evaluation and management of delirium among older persons. *Medical Clinics of North America, 95*(3), 555–577.

Fortinsky, R. H., & Downs, M. (2014). Optimizing person-centered transitions in the dementia journey: A comparison of national dementia strategies. *Health Affairs, 33*(4), 566–573.

Frost, B., Hemberg, M., Lewis, J., & Feany, M. B. (2014). Tau promotes neurodegeneration through global chromatin relaxation. *Nature Neuroscience, 17*(3), 357–366.

Galvin, J. E., Roe, C. M., Powlishta, K. K., Coats, M. A., Muich, S. J., Grant, E., et al. (2005). The AD8: A brief informant interview to detect dementia. *Neurology, 65*(4), 559–564.

Galvin, J. E., Roe, C. M., Xiong, C., & Morris, J. C. (2006). Validity and reliability of the AD8 informant interview in dementia. *Neurology, 67*(11), 1942–1948.

Gomes, S., Martins, I., Fonseca, A. C., Oliveira, C. R., Resende, R., & Pereira, C. M., (2014). Protective effect of leptin and ghrelin against toxicity induced by amyloid- oligomers in a hypothalamic cell line. *Journal of Neuroendocrinology, 26*(3), 176–185.

Katzenschlager, R., Sampaio, C., Costa, J., & Lees, A. (2009). Anticholinergics for symptomatic management of Parkinson's disease. *The Cochrane Database of Systematic Reviews,* (2), CD003735.

Lee, Y., Hou, S., Lee, C., Hsu, C., Huang, Y., & Su, Y. (2013). Increased risk of dementia in patients with mild traumatic brain injury: A nationwide cohort study. *PLoS One, 8*(5), e62422.

Leong, D. (2014). Antidepressants for depression in patients with dementia: A review of the literature. *The Consultant Pharmacist, 29*(4), 254–263.

Lewis, M., Hobday, J. V., & Hepburn, K. W. (2011). Internet-based program for dementia caregivers. *American Journal of Alzheimer's Disease & Other Dementias, 25*(8), 674–679.

Marchesi, V. T. (2014). Alzheimer's disease and CADASIL are heritable, adult-onset dementias that both involve damaged small blood vessels. *Cellular and Molecular Life Sciences, 71*(6), 949–955.

Mattison, M. L., Catic, A., Davis, R. B., Olveczky, D., Moran, J., Yang, J., et al. (2014). A standardized, bundled approach to providing geriatric-focused acute care. *Journal of the American Geriatrics Society, 62*(5), 936–942. doi:10.1111/jgs.12780

Porsteinsson, A. P., Drye, L. T., Pollock, B. F., Devannand, D. P., Grangakis, C., Ismail, Z., et al. (2014). Effect of citalopram on agitation in Alzheimer disease: The CitAD randomized clinical trial. *The Journal of the American Medical Association, 311*(7), 682–691.

Razavi, M., Tolea, M., Margrett, J., Martin, P., Oakland, A., Tscholl, D. W., et al. (2013). Comparison of 2 informant questionnaire screening tools for dementia and mild cognitive impairment AD8 and IQCODE. *Alzheimer Disease Association Disorders, 28*(2), 156–161. doi:10.1097/WAD.0000000000000008

Soto, M. E., Secher, M., Gillette-Guyonnet, S., van Kan, G. A., Andrieu, S., Nourhashemi, F., et al. (2012). Weight loss and rapid cognitive decline in community-dwelling patients with Alzheimer's disease. *Journal of Alzheimer's Disease, 28*(3), 647–654.

Tang, S., Patel, P., Khubchandani, J., & Grossberg, G. T. (2014). The psychogeriatric patient in the emergency room: Focus on management and disposition. *ISRN Psychiatry*, doi:10.1155/2014/413572. doi 10.1155/2014/413572.ecollection 2014.

Tucci, P., Mhillaj, E., Morgese, M.G., Colaianna, M., Zotti, M., Schiavone, S., Cicerale, M., Trabace, L., et al. (2014). Memantine prevents memory consolidation failureinduced by soluble beta amyloid in rats. *Frontiers in Behavioral Neuroscience, 8*, 332. doi 10.3389/fnbeh.2014.00332,

U.S. Department of Health and Human Services. (2014). 2012–2013 Progress report on Alzheimer's disease: Translating new knowledge. Washington, DC: Alzheimer Disease Education and Referral (ADEAR) Center, National Institute on Aging, National Institutes of Health. Retrieved April 29, 2014, from http://www.nia.nih.gov/Alzheimers/Publications/ADProgress2009.

Verdelho, A., Madureira, S., Moleiro, C., Ferro, J. M., O'Brien, J. T., Poggesi, A., et al. (2013). Depressive symptoms predict cognitive decline and dementia in older people independently of cerebral white matter changes: The LADIS study. *Journal of Neurology, Neurosurgery, & Psychiatry, 84*(11), 1250–1254.

Voyer, P., Richard, S., Doucet, L., & Carmichael, P. H. (2011). Factors associated with delirium severity among older persons with dementia. *Journal of Neuroscience Nursing, 43*(2), 62–69.

Whall, A. L., Hyojeong, K., Colling, K. B., Gwi-Ryung, H., DeCicco, B., & Antonakos, C. (2013). Measurement of aggressive behaviors in dementia. *Research in Gerontological Nursing, 6*(3), 171–177.

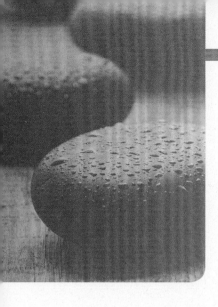

30
Mental Health Care for Survivors of Violence

Beverly Baliko, Mary R. Boyd, and Stephanie Burgess

This chapter is available at http://thepoint.lww.com/BoydEssentials and in the CoursePoint ebook.

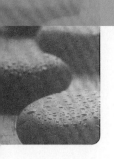

Appendix A, B, C, and the Glossary

Appendix A, Brief Psychiatric Rating Scale; Appendix B, Abnormal Involuntary Movement Scale (AIMS); Appendix C, Simplified Diagnosis for Tardive Dyskinesia (SD-TD); and the Glossary are available at http://thepoint.lww.com/BoydEssentials and in the CoursePoint ebook.

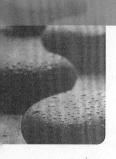

Index

NOTE: Locators followed by 'b', 'f' and 't' refer to boxes, figures and tables respectively. Page numbers preceded by "e-" indicate pages from Chapters 27 and 30, which can be found at http://thepoint.lww.com/BoydEssentials and in the CoursePoint ebook.